Burrows

TEXTBOOK OF MICROBIOLOGY

TWENTY-SECOND EDITION

BOB A. FREEMAN, Ph.D.

Vice Chancellor for Academic Affairs and
Professor of Microbiology,
The University of Tennessee Center for the Health Sciences
Memphis, Tennessee

1985 W.B. SAUNDERS COMPANY
Philadelphia London Toronto Mexico City Rio de Janeiro Sydney Tokyo

W. B. Saunders Company: West Washington Square
Philadelphia, PA   19105

1 St. Anne's Road
Eastbourne, East Sussex BN21 3UN, England

1 Goldthorne Avenue
Toronto, Ontario M8Z 5T9, Canada

Apartado 26370—Cedro 512
Mexico 4, D.F., Mexico

Rua Coronel Cabrita, 8
Sao Cristovao Caixa Postal 21176
Rio de Janeiro, Brazil

9 Waltham Street
Artarmon, N.S.W. 2064, Australia

Ichibancho, Central Bldg., 22-1 Ichibancho
Chiyoda-Ku, Tokyo 102, Japan

Library of Congress Cataloging in Publication Data

Burrows, William, 1908–

Burrows Textbook of microbiology.

1. Medical microbiology.   I. Freeman, Bob A.   II. Title.
   III. Title: Textbook of microbiology.

QR46.B84 1985   616'.01   83–18902

ISBN 0–7216–3868–6

Listed here is the latest translated edition of this book together
with the language of the translation and the publisher.

Spanish (*20th Edition*)—NEISA, Mexico 4, D.F., Mexico

Spanish (*21st Edition*)—Nueva Editorial Interamericana, S.A. de C.V.,
           Mexico City, Mexico

Burrows Textbook of Microbiology   ISBN   0-7216-3868-6

Last digit is the print number: 9   8   7   6   5   4   3   2   1

To the Memory of
WILLIAM BURROWS
and
VERNON T. SCHUHARDT

Contributors

BARON, LOUIS S., Ph.D.

Chief, Department of Bacterial Immunology, Walter Reed Army Institute of Research, Washington, D.C.
Gene Expression and Evolution in Bacteria

DORSETT, PRESTON H., Ph.D.

Associate Professor of Microbiology, The University of Tennessee Center for the Health Sciences, Memphis, Tennessee
Fundamentals of Animal Virology

DUSANIC, DONALD G., Ph.D.

Professor of Life Sciences, Indiana State University; Adjunct Professor of Microbiology, Indiana University School of Medicine, Terre Haute Center for Medical Education, Terre Haute, Indiana
Medical Parasitology

KOPECKO, DENNIS J., Ph.D.

Senior Research Scientist and Head, Molecular Genetics Unit, Department of Bacterial Immunology, Walter Reed Army Institute of Research, Washington, D.C.
Gene Expression and Evolution in Bacteria

MILLER, TERRY L., Ph.D.

New York Department of Health Wadsworth Center for Laboratories and Research, Albany, New York
Bacterial Metabolism; Physical Agents, Disinfectants, and Chemotherapeutic Agents

PEARSON, GARY R., Ph.D.

Professor, Mayo Foundation/Mayo Medical School, Rochester, Minnesota
Introduction to Immunology; Humoral and Cellular Immune Reactions; Immunogenetics and Cellular Regulation of the Immune Response; Transplantation Immunology: Transplantation Immunity and Hypersensitivity; Immunity, Autoimmunity, and Immunopathology

RIPPON, JOHN W., Ph.D.

Associate Professor of Medicine, University of Chicago; Director, Mycology Reference Laboratory, University of Chicago Medical Center, Chicago, Illinois
Medical Mycology

WOLIN, MEYER J., Ph.D.
Chief Research Scientist, Division of Environmental Sciences Center for Laboratories and Research, Albany, New York
Bacterial Metabolism; Physical Agents, Disinfectants, and Chemotherapeutic Agents

Preface

The successive editions of a textbook must reflect the metamorphosis of the science it represents, with changes in emphasis, expansion into new areas of knowledge, and deletion of the outmoded—all dictated by the maturation of the discipline. Yet, it also necessarily reflects the interests, as well as the prejudices, of its author. This textbook began in 1908 as **General Bacteriology,** authored by Edwin O. Jordan. The first edition of 545 pages set forth the essential knowledge of microorganisms of that era. In 1938, William Burrows assumed authorship, and through nine editions, each bearing his unmistakable imprimatur, the textbook has evolved into its present place in the literature of medical microbiology. The present edition seeks to retain the philosophy, established by William Burrows, that it must represent more than a compendium of facts; it must offer to the student an understanding of the science, based on historical evolution and experimental findings.

This edition has been completely revised and rewritten to improve readability, delete outmoded information, incorporate new material, and delineate new directions in medical microbiology; new sections will be found throughout the book. Rigorous attention has been given to the concepts of microbiology that promote an understanding of infectious diseases. Thus, the book is especially suitable for students of medicine and pathogenic microbiology.

This book could not have been completed without the aid and cooperation of many colleagues; the author is especially grateful to those who contributed chapters in their respective specialties. Dr. M. J. Wolin has been joined by his colleague, Dr. T. L. Miller, in his extensive revision of the chapters on microbial metabolism and the effects of physical and chemical agents on microorganisms. Drs. D. J. Kopecko and L. S. Baron have continued their development of the concepts of gene expression and evolution in bacteria in the chapter on microbial genetics. Dr. Preston H. Dorsett has effectively revised the chapter on basic aspects of animal virology, and Dr. J. W. Rippon continues his association with this book by the addition of new material to the chapter on medical mycology. The author is indebted to two new contributors, Drs. Gary R. Pearson and Donald G. Dusanic. Dr. Pearson has reorganized and rewritten the section on immunology, including new developments and perspectives in this exciting discipline; Dr. Dusanic ably succeeds Dr. R. M. Lewert as author of the chapter on medical parasitology. The writer also extends his thanks to Dr. William M. Todd for his critical review of the manuscript and for his many helpful suggestions.

The author is indebted to the many colleagues who contributed illustrative material and to the editors and staff of the W. B. Saunders Company for their invaluable support and cooperation. Finally, special appreciation is expressed to Rosemary Freeman, who has undertaken bibliographic tasks for the book and has aided in countless other ways toward its completion.

BOB A. FREEMAN

Contents

ix

CHAPTER 1

Historical Perspectives in Microbiology

MICROSCOPY
SPONTANEOUS GENERATION
FERMENTATION AND
  BIOCHEMICAL PHYSIOLOGY
INFECTIOUS DISEASE

VIROLOGY
IMMUNITY
CHEMOTHERAPY
MICROBIAL GENETICS
RECONSIDERATION

MI·CRO·BI·OL·O·GY (mī′krō-bī-ŏl′ə-jē) *n.*
The science that deals with microscopic living organisms and, especially, their effects on other forms of life. (From Greek *mikros,* small + *bios,* life.)

The term microbiology is commonly used in a more narrow sense than its etymology suggests. Although it may be used to describe the broader subject of small or minute living organisms, it generally refers to a study of those microscopic life forms that are directly or closely related to human activity and welfare.

In the early history of the science, it was traditional to consider microorganisms as belonging to either the plant or the animal kingdom. In modern concepts of biology, however, the bacteria and blue-green algae are regarded as belonging to a third kingdom, the Procaryotae. The microscopic members of the animal and plant kingdoms—protozoa, fungi, and most algae—share with higher life forms a unit structure, the eucaryotic cell, which is of great organizational complexity. The cellular unit of procaryotes, in contrast, is much more simple in organization and structure (Chapter 2). The viruses represent a special case in that they are noncellular and are distinguished by their obligate parasitic relationship to the cells of their hosts; their evolutionary position is uncertain (Chapter 38).

Although the concept and demonstration of living microorganisms is a relatively recent development in biology, their activities have been familiar to man from prehistoric times. Decomposition of organic matter and especially spoilage of foods, acetic and lactic acid

fermentations and alcoholic fermentation, degradation of proteins with the production of new and desirable flavors in certain foods, and the occurrence of infectious disease are obvious examples of familiar phenomena now known to be of microbial origin.

The existence of these biological entities is inferred from the consequences of their activity; their living nature is evident when the observed effects are reproduced in series, *e.g.,* by transfer of a small portion of a fermenting mixture to a fresh, unfermented substrate. Such inferences may be found in statements made in both ancient and later writings. Thus, Lucretius wrote of "the seeds of disease" in his *De Rerum Natura,* Fracastorius of Verona in 1546 suggested a *contagium vivum* as a cause of disease, and Benjamin Marten in 1720 speculated that minute animals were responsible for consumptive disease.

These suggestions were perhaps too abstract for general acceptance, and the beginning of the science of microbiology awaited a concrete demonstration of the existence of these agents; this was accomplished by optical systems so precise as to permit direct visualization of microscopic, living forms.

MICROSCOPY

The name of Antony van Leeuwenhoek (1632–1723) is inseparably associated with the

1

unquam ſanguinem emittat. Nec tan
ſunt puri, quin, ubi eos per ſpeculc
tuerer, viderim creſcentem inter de
qua
ſitic
len
cer
dig
me
eſſe
plu
ani
ſali
ore
aeri
ſem
exci

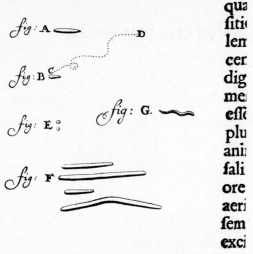

Figure 1–1. The first pictorial representation of bacteria. (Reproduced from *Arcana Naturae Delecta Ab Antonio van Leeuwenhoek.* Delphis Batavorum apud Henricum Crooneveld. 1695.)

early development of microscopy. He held a political sinecure in Delft and devoted the greater part of his time to the hobby of lens grinding. He not only made the best lenses available at that time, but used them to examine a wide variety of materials that interested him. It was characteristic that he first observed bacteria in an attempt to discern in visual terms the nature of the taste of pepper. There is no doubt that he actually observed these microorganisms, for he made recognizable drawings of them that were reproduced in reports of his observations to the Royal Society.[2]

A few of the hundreds of microscopes he constructed are still extant, and it is evident that the maximum magnification he reached was approximately 300 diameters. This is not sufficient to allow observation by transmitted light of objects as small as bacteria. While van Leeuwenhoek was never willing to reveal his method of illumination, it seems probable that he used reflected light as it is used in the modern darkfield microscope.[5]

The direct demonstration of living organisms of such small dimensions was a notable achievement, but any relation of such forms to natural phenomena such as fermentation or infectious disease either escaped van Leeuwenhoek or was of no interest to him. Their possible relation to gross phenomena was ap-

parent to at least some of the scientific men of his day. For instance, in a comment on a report of an epidemic disease of cattle published five years later, his contemporary, Slare, wrote:[11]

I wish Mr. Leeuwenhoek had been present at some of the dissections of these infected Animals, I am perswaded he would have discovered some strange Insect or other in them.

But systematic study was delayed for many years, and it was nearly a century later, in 1786, that a Danish zoologist, O. F. Müller, discovered many of the details of bacterial structure. He left drawings so accurate that the bacteria he showed can be identified today as belonging to one or another of the chief divisions. Somewhat later, in 1838, Ehrenberg published *Infusionstierchen,* in which he put the study of these microorganisms on a systematic basis. He established a number of groups by clearly recognizing fundamental morphological distinctions, such as those differentiating the spirochetes from certain of the protozoa. Some of the names he used, such as "bacterium" and "spirillum," are still current in bacteriological nomenclature though with somewhat changed significance.

The perfection of the modern compound microscope, with achromatic and later apochromatic objective lenses, markedly facilitated the study of the morphology of microorganisms. These permitted observations of certain gross internal structures of the bacterial cell, as well as some of the larger viruses. This made possible accurate differentiation of microorganisms on a morphological basis and provided basic criteria for characterization of the larger forms—fungi, protozoa, and metazoa. Phase microscopy, introduced in the 1940s, further facilitated certain aspects of microscopy, especially the observation of microorganisms in the living state, by accentuation of slight differences in the refractive indices of intracellular elements.

Optical microscopy is nevertheless limited by the resolution that may be obtained with visible light. The lower limit of resolution is about 0.2 μm., with practical magnifications no greater than 1000 to 2000 diameters. It is obvious that these resolution limits are inadequate for details of the intracellular structure and organelles of bacteria. The darkfield microscope, although facilitating the observation of tenuous microorganisms such as spirochetes and structures such as flagella, shows minute objects only as points of light against a dark background without improving resolution.

Table 1–1. **Early Developments in Microscopy**[3]

Date	Name	Contribution
(*ca.*) 1600	Hans and Zaccharias Janssen; Cornelius Drebbel	Developed the earliest compound microscopes. These were crude and imperfect and were little more than magnifying lenses. Bacteria could not be resolved.
1665	Robert Hooke	Designed and built microscopes through which he observed small animals. He published these illustrations in *Micrographia*.
1673	Antony van Leeuwenhoek	First of van Leeuwenhoek's letters to the Royal Society. For a period of 50 years he continued this correspondence, communicating his observations of the microscopic world. In 1683, in his 39th letter, he provided the first unequivocal description of bacteria, found in tooth plaque.
1733	Chester Hall; John Dolland	Credited with independent invention of achromatic lenses, correcting for chromatic aberration.
1830	Joseph J. Lister (Father of Lord Lister)	Contributed major improvements in microscopes, leading to modern microscopy.
1878	Ernst Abbe	Invention of homogeneous immersion lenses.
1911	Oskar Heimstadt	Invention of the fluorescence microscope.
1932	Max Knoll and Ernst Ruska	First description of the electron microscope.
1935	Frits Zernike	First description of the phase-contrast microscope.

Beginning in the 1930s, the electron microscope was developed in practical, usable form. It constituted an important advance in microscopy in that an object or structure casting a "shadow" in the electron beam may be resolved, and working magnifications of 30,000 diameters with excellent resolution were obtained. Thus it became possible to view microorganisms beyond the limits of optical resolution and to visualize structures as small as the individual subunits of the virus coat. The subsequent development of the scanning electron microscope opened new dimensions in the visualization of cell topography; the three-dimensional quality of these high resolution images has yielded new information on cell surfaces and cellular interactions.

SPONTANEOUS GENERATION

For many years it was believed that living organisms could arise *de novo* and fully formed from decomposing organic matter. The development of snakes from horse hairs standing in stagnant water and the appearance of mice in decomposing fodder were, at one time, popular legends. The fallacies in such beliefs were suspected by some, and in the seventeenth century a number of individuals carried out experiments designed to show whether living organisms had their origin only in other living organisms (biogenesis), or appeared spontaneously in decomposing organic matter (abiogenesis).

In the middle of the seventeenth century, the poet-physician Redi performed experiments showing, contrary to popular belief, that maggots were not formed spontaneously in decomposing meat but were fly larvae hatched from eggs deposited in the meat. Spallanzani, an Italian monk, showed further that putrescible meat infusions did not spoil when properly heated and did not contain living organisms. Needham, an Irish priest, took issue with Spallanzani on the basis of similar experiments in which spoilage took place and living organisms appeared in spite of previous heating. A second series of elaborate experiments by Spallanzani corroborated his earlier findings and exposed the fallacies in Needham's experiments. It was evident that microorganisms were carried in air, and this was convincingly demonstrated by many other workers, including Schulze, Schwann, Schröder and von Dusch, and Tyndall.

The whole question seemed settled conclusively in favor of biogenesis when it was raised again in the middle of the nineteenth century by the work of the eminent French chemist

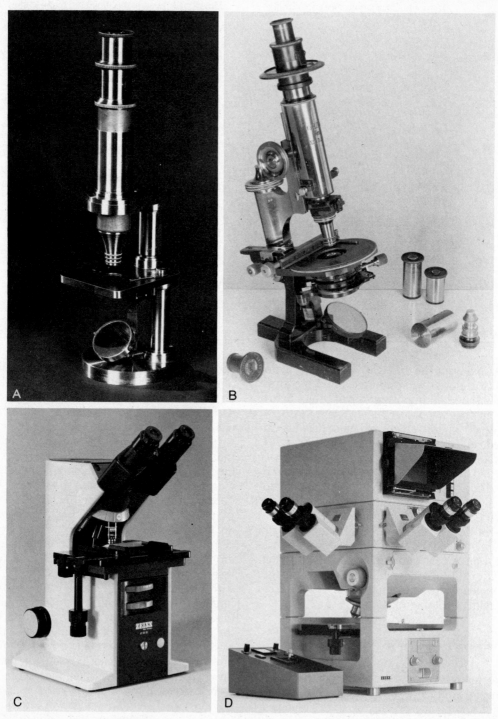

Figure 1–2. Development of light microscopes. *A*, Zeiss microscope, ca. 1860; *B*, Zeiss polarization microscope, ca. 1890; *C*, Zeiss microscope KM; *D*, Zeiss Axiomat NDC microscope. (Courtesy of Carl Zeiss, West Germany.)

Pouchet. He made the same kind of technical errors as some of his predecessors, so that his evidence supported the hypothesis of spontaneous generation of life. It was at this point that Pasteur entered the renewed controversy through his early studies on fermentation. By ingenious and incontrovertible experiments, he demonstrated that microorganisms carried in air were responsible for Pouchet's erroneous results.

The validity of biogenesis has not since been seriously questioned. While biogenesis may seem self-evident today, its establishment was of fundamental importance to the development of modern biological science. Had this not been done, the specific microbic etiology of fermentation, decay, infectious disease, and similar phenomena could not have been established. At the same time, present concepts of evolution, and biochemical evidence in particular, seem to point inevitably toward an original emergence of life from the nonliving.[12]

FERMENTATION AND BIOCHEMICAL PHYSIOLOGY

By the middle of the nineteenth century the general nature of organic material was becoming relatively clear, but the natural decomposition of these substances was not, in that the part played by microorganisms in the processes of putrefaction, decay, and fermentation was not known.

The plant-like nature of yeast had been shown by Schwann in 1837 and Cagniard-Latour in 1838, but the preeminent chemists of the day, Liebig, Berzelius, and Wöhler, regarded the presence of yeast cells in a fermenting mixture as no more than incidental to the decomposition, which was considered by them to have a purely inanimate basis.

Pasteur (1822–1895), originally trained as a chemist, had done his early work on stereoisomerism. The formation of optically active amyl alcohol during the course of the lactic acid fermentation led him to study the processes of fermentation. Having first established the validity of biogenesis, it was not difficult to prove that fermentations resulted from physiological activity of living, growing microorganisms.

Pasteur further established the principle that fermentations are specific, *i.e.,* that different kinds of fermentations, each yielding different end products, result from the activities of specific microorganisms. He applied this principle in work on the "diseases" of beer and wine, showing that these represented secondary fermentations by contaminating microorganisms to produce undesirable end products. It was then logical to control the fermentative process by gently heating the fermentable solution to eliminate undesirable contaminants, followed by inoculation with microorganisms that brought about the desired fermentation. This method of gentle heating, now widely applied to destroy pathogenic microorganisms in milk and other products, is known as pasteurization.

Study of the mechanisms of fermentation was tremendously stimulated by the commercial value of end products such as ethanol, lactic and acetic acids, glycerol, butanol, and acetone. These considerations led to the development of new industries concerned with the large-scale production of organic solvents and subsequently of other microbial products, especially vitamins and antibiotics.

The chemical study of microorganisms grew side by side with the chemical approach to mammalian physiology, eventually fusing into the present-day science of biochemistry. The initial common ground was carbohydrate metabolism and the respiratory processes, astonishingly similar in such widely dissimilar organisms. Thus, the phenomenon of anaerobic respiration, first observed by Pasteur in fermenting mixtures and received with incredulity at the time, is now commonplace in biochemical physiology. More detailed study showed that the catalysis of the processes of respiration is substantially the same also, and characterization of respiratory enzymes, for example, was markedly facilitated by their availability in microorganisms. Many of the vitamins required by mammals, especially those of the B group, are also required by microorganisms, and function in a similar manner.

In other respects, the biochemical potential of microorganisms goes far beyond that of any other living organisms. While some microorganisms simulate mammalian metabolism, others are photosynthetic. These may resemble green plants in the photochemical reduction of carbon dioxide or differ when the photochemical reactions are coupled with the metabolism of inorganic sulfur compounds. Still others are chemoautotrophic, deriving energy for the reduction of carbon dioxide from the oxidation of inorganic substrates such as hydrogen, or inorganic compounds of nitrogen, sulfur, iron, and manganese. The nitrogen-fixing bacteria assimilate atmospheric nitrogen either alone or in symbiosis with leguminous plants. Clearly, the ecological distribution of microorganisms is a function of their physiological properties.[1]

INFECTIOUS DISEASE

Sometimes new vistas are opened prematurely and not appreciated at the time, or too late and are anticlimactic, but occasionally new concepts coincide with an unusually receptive segment of the general stream of thought. Such a monumental coincidence of thought took place with the conceptual transition from the specific microbic etiology of fermentations, advanced by Pasteur, to that of infectious diseases. Inexorably, this transition was to reveal the causes, prevention, control, and possible cure of the rampant infectious diseases, capturing popular imagination as it developed.

The conceptual transition from the specific microbic etiology of fermentations to that of infectious disease was more readily reached than might appear.

The implications of Pasteur's studies on fermentation for infectious disease were almost immediately perceived, notably by the British surgeon Lord Lister. He applied the basic principles to his own work, controlling infection in the operating room by liberal use of phenol. An era of antiseptic surgery, initiated by Lister in 1867, led to a remarkable reduc-

tion in intercurrent infection and mortality. These practices were displaced within the next two decades by those of aseptic surgery, largely by von Bergmann in Berlin, following a growing appreciation of infected persons as the primary source of sepsis.

It remained for the German physician Koch (1843–1910) to develop the experimental methods that proved a causal relation between bacteria and infectious disease. From the first applications of microscopy to the study of microorganisms, it was clear that different morphological types existed and that these usually occurred in nature in mixed populations. It was evident also from the early studies on pyemia that morphological criteria did not suffice to differentiate and characterize the bacteria, since morphologically identical forms differed markedly in pathogenic properties. It was essential to separate such microorganisms from one another and to grow each kind in pure culture.

Initially this had been approximately accomplished by diluting mixed bacterial populations in liquid culture mediums; when replicates of high inoculum dilutions showed irregular occurrence of growth, it was assumed that the

Table 1–2. **Significant Developments in the Germ Theory of Disease**

Date	Name	Contribution
Biblical	Leviticus:13, 14	Refers to contagious nature of disease; contains instructions for sanitation and hygiene to inhibit spread of leprosy.
(ca.) 430 B.C.	Thucydides	Infers contagious nature of certain plagues in Athens.
1546	Hieronymus Fracastorius	In a series of books on contagion, wrote of *seminaria* (seeds or germs) of disease. Whether he recognized "seeds" as living is unlikely. Recognized (1) transmission by "fomites" and direct contact, (2) organ specificity of certain infections, (3) age specificity of disease, and (4) resistance to second attacks of the same disease.
1720	Benjamin Marten	In *A New Theory of Consumptions: More Especially of a Phthisis or Consumption of the Lungs* (London), speculated that minute animalcula were responsible for disease. Marten's theories are remarkably similar to modern ideas of infectious diseases.
1872	C. J. Davaine	Experimentally transmitted septicemia in rabbits by serial injections (passage) of "putrid" blood, with observations of increasing virulence.
1878	Robert Koch	In *Etiology of Traumatic Infectious Disease*, Koch undertook to prove experimentally that infectious diseases were due to specific parasitic microorganisms.
1880 – 1883	Alexander Ogston	Building on Koch's studies, Ogston concluded that inflammation and suppuration of acute abscesses are due to micrococci, based on microscopic observations and bacteriological cultures.
1884	Robert Koch	First complete statement of Koch's postulates.

bacteria growing in these tubes were descendants of a single viable cell and thus constituted a pure culture. Probably one of the greatest single contributions to technical bacteriology was the method for isolation of pure cultures developed by Koch. The inoculum was diluted and cultured on a nutrient medium solidified as a gel by the addition of gelatin. Individual viable cells were separated on the solidified medium and their progeny developed as discrete masses of cells of single ancestry—a "clone" in zoological terminology. Modern microbiology was in large part made possible by, and is based upon, this simple technique.

The specific microbial etiology of infectious disease was first clearly established in studies on anthrax, an epidemic and highly fatal disease of cattle and other domestic animals. The microorganism now known as *Bacillus anthracis* had been observed by Pollender in 1849 in the blood and organs of infected animals and by Davaine and Rayer in 1850. The disease was transmitted by Brauell in 1867 by inoculating normal animals with infected blood. It is generally conceded that modern medical microbiology began with Koch's studies on anthrax in 1878, in which he developed conclusive evidence that the anthrax bacillus is causally related to the disease. In this and succeeding works he advanced the conceptual rules, later to bear his name as Koch's postulates, which outline the proof necessary to establish a specific microorganism as the etiological agent of disease.

These advances, coupled with the development of staining methods by Koch, Ehrlich, Weigert, and others, provided tremendous stimulus to the study of infectious diseases, resulting in an immense accumulation of new knowledge within the ensuing two decades. Indeed, most of the principal bacterial pathogens were described and isolated before the turn of the century.

Characterization of the pathogenic bacteria in morphological, physiological, and pathological terms, and studies of their persistence under adverse conditions and behavior in the infected host were obvious and essential corollaries. Out of this kind of information grew an understanding of the basic elements of the spread of infection, providing a firm foundation to the science of epidemiology. In 1854, Snow deduced the presence of the causative agent of Asiatic cholera in the feces of diseased persons and its transmission to others by way of common contaminated water supply in the famous Broad Street Pump epidemic in London. The nature of waterborne enteric disease was to become clear, however, only after the actual isolation and study of enteric pathogens such as the cholera vibrio and the typhoid and dysentery bacilli.

Effective control was an inevitable consequence of the developing understanding of infectious diseases and their dissemination. The application of indicated control measures, such as chlorination of water and pasteurization of milk, coupled with artificial immunization, has been astonishingly successful. The result has been the virtual disappearance of many of the great killing diseases, such as smallpox, typhoid fever, Asiatic cholera, diphtheria, and plague, and tremendous reduction in others, such as tuberculosis. All of this stems in large part from an understanding of the principle of specific microbial etiology of infectious disease.

VIROLOGY

Early in the study of infectious diseases, it became apparent that there were putative agents of disease which could neither be seen with the light microscope nor be cultivated apart from living host cells. Iwanowski in 1892 and Beijerinck in 1899 observed the first of these agents—that causing mosaic disease of the tobacco plant—which Beijerinck described as a *contagium vivum fluidum,* since it was present in bacteria-free filtrates of infected juice. A similar agent causing foot-and-mouth disease of cattle was described in 1897 by Löffler and Frosch, and the causative agent of yellow fever by the American Army Commission under the direction of Reed in 1900. Other such agents producing a transmissible lysis of bacteria were found by Twort in 1916 and d'Herelle in 1917, to give three groups of agents now known as the plant, animal, and bacterial viruses, respectively.

Prior to 1930, the term virus referred to any living agent of disease, including bacteria. During the period from 1930 to 1940, filterable virus was the name used to describe infective agents that would pass through special filters that retained bacteria. Since about 1940, **virus** has been applied only to extremely small, noncellular particles which infect and replicate only within living host cells.

Physical and morphological evidence has shown that these agents range from a diameter of 200 nm., or just at the limits of resolution of the light microscope, to infectious particles as small as 10 nm., visualized only by electron microscopy. Further, chemical analyses revealed that the larger forms contained protein, polysaccharide, and lipid in biologically reasonable proportions, and thus resembled bacteria, while the smaller forms appeared to possess only nucleoproteins. Some of the latter were, in fact, prepared in crystalline form; the first was tobacco mosaic virus, which was prepared as needle-shaped paracrystals in 1935. Subsequently other plant viruses were prepared in the form of true crystals, *viz.,* tomato bushy stunt virus was isolated as uniform rhombic dodecahedral crystals, and in 1955 a strain of the poliomyelitis virus, one of the smallest animal viruses, was prepared as bipyramidal tetragonal prisms. From such data as these, it was obvious that the viruses do not constitute a homogeneous group of infectious agents.

Other microorganisms, more closely resembling known bacteria, were described as the causative agents of a number of febrile diseases. The etiological agent of spotted fever was discovered by Ricketts in 1909. Subsequently, da Rocha Lima, von Prowazek, and others found similar organisms causing fevers of the typhus group; Q fever was later shown to be of similar etiology. These microorganisms, known as rickettsiae, were in the size range of small bacteria and so were visible by light microscopy, but like the viruses they would proliferate only as intracellular parasites within appropriate host cells.

As a consequence of this apparent dependence of the viruses and rickettsiae on living host cells, a variety of methods for their propagation have been developed since the early part of the twentieth century. Propagation of viruses in the embryonated hen's egg was described in the early 1930s as proliferation on the chorioallantoic membrane, in the allantoic cavity or yolk sac, or in the tissues of the embryo itself, depending on the agent and the route of inoculation. Viruses and rickettsiae may also be grown in animal cell cultures. In virus-infected cell cultures, host cells are often adversely affected, giving rise to cytopathic effects that make it possible to demonstrate their presence. With the advent of antibiotics in the 1940s, it became possible to control the bacterial contamination of cultures of animal cells and tissues, resulting in the development of readily applicable methods of tissue culture for the propagation of viruses. The stimulus to virology was similar to that given to bacteriology by Koch's method of isolating bacteria in pure culture.

This dependence upon the host cell that early was found to characterize the viruses and rickettsiae raised the concept of parasitism to one in which there is a high degree of intimacy. With only a few exceptions, these agents have been found to have no independent metabolism and thus to parasitize the metabolic mechanisms of the host cell. Some of them appear to consist of little more than genetic material which, on entry into the host cell, dominates its normal directive mechanisms to force the synthesis of new virus substance. It then became possible to show that nucleic acids, separated from the virus particle, gave rise to the synthesis of complete virus on introduction into the host cell. The fundamental significance of such observations is obvious, and it becomes more and more difficult to differentiate between the living and the nonliving.

IMMUNITY

It has long been a matter of common knowledge that the individual who had recovered from infectious disease was often specifically refractory to subsequent attacks of that disease, and that this refractory state, or acquired immunity, persisted in some instances for many years. The practice of deliberate exposure to the infectious agent in order to produce the disease and the subsequent immunity persists to this day in a few diseases such as mumps and measles, which are milder and less complicated in children than in adults. It reached a culmination of a sort in the practice of variolation, the deliberate inoculation of a susceptible person with pustular material from an individual with smallpox (variola). The disease so produced was less often fatal than naturally acquired smallpox and provided a more or less permanent protection against it. Variolation had been practiced in the Near East for an unknown time prior to its introduction to Western Europe in 1718 by Lady Mary Wortley Montague, wife of the British ambassador in Constantinople.

Artificial inoculation with an infectious agent of reduced virulence to produce a mild infection and consequent protection against naturally occurring disease began with the work of the Englishman Jenner. Noting the infrequent occurrence of smallpox in milkmaids who had been infected with cowpox (vaccinia), he undertook deliberate inoculation of people with vaccinia, followed by inoculation with variola some weeks later. He reported in 1796 that such prior infection conferred a high degree of protection against smallpox; this method of vaccination was widely practiced thereafter.

With the discovery of pathogenic microorganisms, it became possible to study immunity to infectious disease in a systematic way. Pasteur, working first with chicken cholera and later with anthrax and swine erysipelas, showed that the basic principle uncovered by Jenner could be generalized to include disease other than smallpox. His most striking application of it was the development of a rabies prophylactic in the form of rabies virus that had been reduced in virulence for man by successive passages in the rabbit. Not long afterward, the American workers Salmon and Theobald Smith found that inoculation with killed microorganisms could also stimulate the development of immunity. In 1890 von Behring and Kitasato laid the basis for antitoxic immunity through their discovery of tetanus and diphtheria antitoxins. This rounded out the approach to effective prophylaxis of infectious disease by acquired immunity, which could be produced in response to the artificial inoculation of modified microorganisms, of killed microorganisms, or of relevant products of microorganisms.

It soon became evident that immunized animals characteristically show at least two kinds of immune response—humoral and cellular immunity. Humoral immunity is indicated by the appearance of antibodies, serum globulins that react specifically with microorganisms or their products. Cellular immunity connotes an enhanced capacity of phagocytic cells to ingest and dispose of microorganisms and the production, by certain lymphocytes, of substances that aid and control the immune response.

Humoral immunity was studied intensively by many workers, including Bordet, Ehrlich, and others, with two general approaches being distinguished. One has been concerned with the relation of humoral immunity to effective immunity. In some cases, such as antitoxic immunity, this seemed clear; in others, such as antibacterial and antiviral immunity, the immune state is more complex and presents many problems that are still unresolved.

The other approach has been immunochemical in nature and is concerned with the nature of antigenic specificity, which was elucidated largely through the work of Landsteiner in the 1920s; the nature of antibody; and the nature of the antigen-antibody reaction in physicochemical terms. Serology, the *in vitro* study of reactions between antigens and antibodies, led to the development of highly specific and sensitive tests that have been useful in diagnosis of disease. By application of the methods of antigenic analysis, microorganisms are characterized on the basis of their constituent antigens. Physicochemical methods have been applied to the study of antibodies and have led to the discovery of different classes of these immunoglobulins, elucidation of their functions, and identification of the active portion of antibody molecules.

Cellular immunology, associated with the activity of phagocytic cells, was initially developed by Metchnikoff in the late 1880s and thereafter. Proceeding from studies with *Daphnia,* he expanded the phenomenon of engulfment and destruction of invading microorganisms by polymorphonuclear leucocytes and macrophages into a new system of immunology. On this foundation Aschoff described and defined the free and fixed tissue phagocytes of the reticuloendothelial system and Maximov elucidated the developmental potencies of lymphoid cells. There followed a generalized concept of the inflammatory reaction and cellular response to infection as a process of mobilization of phagocytes and destruction of microorganisms, followed by tissue repair through the development of macrophages into fibroblasts.

While the concepts of cellular and humoral immunity developed somewhat apart, it was early apparent that they are both facets of the host defense mechanism. They are obviously linked by the occurrence of circulating opsonic antibody and by the intimate relation of cells of the lymphoid-macrophage system to antibody formation.

CHEMOTHERAPY[9]

Around the turn of the century, after the microbial etiology of many infectious diseases had been established, Paul Ehrlich, an eminent German medical scientist and younger colleague of Koch, founded the modern science of chemotherapy. He proposed a chemical "magic bullet," a substance nontoxic to the host that would search out and kill invading microorganisms. Ehrlich tested hundreds of arsenicals before discovering salvarsan, a substance effective in the treatment of African sleeping sickness and syphilis. Complemented by a vast chemical industry and guided by the genius of Ehrlich, Germany became the focus of studies on chemotherapy. At about the same time, a laboratory for chemotherapy was established at the Pasteur Institute and headed by Ernest Fourneau. In both France and Germany the screening of possible chemotherapeutic agents led to discovery of compounds that were reasonably effective against animal parasites, but for many years all efforts to prepare similar substances active in bacterial infections were fruitless.

In retrospect it is clear that the fallacy was the unquestioned acceptance of the working hypothesis that a substance must be bactericidal in order to be therapeutically effective. Only in the early 1930s did it become apparent that a bacteriostatic effect, inhibiting reproduction of the invading microorganism, is sufficient to tip the balance in favor of the host, with actual microbial destruction being accomplished largely by host defenses.

Drawing upon the tremendous research efforts in both France and Germany, the chemotherapeutic efficacy of the sulfonamides was discovered in the 1930s. These were the first effective antibacterial drugs, but their fundamental importance was not evident until the early 1940s, following the accumulation of detailed information on bacterial nutrition. Indeed, early studies on the sulfonamides were not considered very promising because their action was primarily bacteriostatic rather than bactericidal.

The first rational basis for chemotherapy was provided by Wood's observation in 1940 that the antibacterial activity of sulfonamides was specifically antagonized by p-aminobenzoic acid, an essential growth factor for many kinds of bacteria. The structural similarity of p-aminobenzoic acid to the active portion of the drug molecule, p-aminobenzene sulfonic acid, suggested that the antibacterial activity of the latter was the result of specific interference with the synthesis of an essential metabolite. Proof of this hypothesis established the general principle of using structural and functional analogues of essential metabolites to exploit small differences, either qualitative or quantitative, between metabolic reactions of the host and parasite cells. Its general significance is illustrated in the modern chemotherapy of neoplastic diseases.

During the latter stages of the development of synthetic chemicals for therapy of infectious diseases, parallel studies on microbial antagonisms would revolutionize, in an even more dramatic way, the treatment of infections.

Since the beginnings of bacteriology, it had been noted that in mixed cultures, one kind of microorganism often exerted an adverse effect on others. Even in folklore, the beneficial effect of moldy bread in preventing wound infection was recognized. In many instances, the antagonistic effect was found to be due to substances formed by one microorganism and toxic to others. An example of such a substance is the pigment pyocanin, produced by *Pseudomonas* and known since the middle of the nineteenth century, which was later used to treat certain bacterial infections.

The great majority of these microbial substances, called antibiotics, were quite toxic to higher animals and thus were of limited use in chemotherapy. Interest in them waned until Fleming discovered penicillin in 1929. Following its development by the Oxford group in the 1940s, penicillin was widely used in a variety of infections as the first antibiotic of low toxicity. In a relatively short time a succession of other antibiotics were discovered, including streptomycin in 1943, chloramphenicol in 1947, and the tetracyclines in 1948, 1950, and 1954.

It would be difficult to overemphasize the profound effects of antibiotics on human health. Most of the major bacterial infections have yielded to treatment and control by these substances. Remaining unconquered, however, are the viral diseases, although some chemotherapeutic agents, such as adenine arabinoside (Ara-A), hold some promise in this regard. It is predictable that the science founded by Ehrlich will ultimately triumph over viral infections as well.

MICROBIAL GENETICS

Variability of microorganisms was obvious from the beginning of their systematic study. Variability is exemplified as alterations in certain bacterial properties produced inadvertently during maintenance on artificial culture mediums or as changes deliberately induced by laboratory manipulation. Alteration in bacterial properties appears with some facility not as a consequence of an unusual plasticity, but rather because of their short generation time and occurrence as populations made up of huge numbers of individuals. Because of the relative structural simplicity of bacteria and viruses, the bacteriologist lacked a system of comparative anatomy such as that available to the botanist and zoologist. He was forced to rely on such seemingly ephemeral characters as fermentation, nutritive requirements, and antigenic constitution, all of which varied, and had no means of knowing whether any of these were biologically trivial or fundamental.

In the 1920s, studies with yeasts showed that the ability to ferment various carbohydrate substrates was genetically determined; a Mendelian segregation of characters occurred in the exchange of nuclear material during spore formation. This work was largely neglected by bacteriologists, and the demonstration of conjugation between physiologically different bacterial cells was not observed until the 1940s.

While the importance of establishing that genes control the characters used for differentiation and identification of bacteria is unquestionable, research in microbial genetics contributed uniquely to and markedly broadened the science of heredity by providing information on phenomena hitherto not demonstrable in other forms.

In 1928 it was shown that immunological types of living pneumococci could be changed by growing them in the presence of killed pneumococci of another type.[8] Further refinement made it clear that the active principle in the dead pneumococci was a highly polymerized deoxyribonucleic acid (DNA) that could be separated from the cells and purified in the test tube before addition to the living culture. This phenomenon (later called transformation) was found to occur also with other kinds of bacteria. Thus, foreign DNA becomes functional in directing the metabolism of the host cell so that it synthesizes a new substance and persists as an integral part of the genetic apparatus of the recipient.

Still another kind of modification of hereditary mechanisms, transduction, was described in the early 1950s. In this process, a bacterial virus infecting a new bacterial cell transmits physiological characters that appear as stable inheritable elements in the recipient host cell. Finally, it has long been known that alteration in the physiological behavior of bacteria may be induced specifically by environmental changes even in the absence of cell multiplication. Studies of induced enzyme synthesis have led to the concepts of genetic control of regulation and to an understanding of induction and repression of physiological reactions in microbial systems.

Out of this seeming disorder of microbial variation there has come, by way of analysis on a molecular basis, an orderly array of widely applicable general principles. This has led to a new era of biology, termed molecular biology, and modern genetics is, in large part, microbial genetics.[4]

RECONSIDERATION

The microbiologist has been something of a renegade, by necessity a master of many trades but a servant of none, and showing a certain lack of respect for the classic and established. Pasteur was not impressed with the opinions of Liebig and Berzelius, nor was it of any concern to Koch that no self-respecting physician would work with a disease of domestic animals. The microbiologist has taken what he needed from zoology, botany, chemistry, physiology, pathology, and medicine to create a new discipline, and it is apparent from even a cursory survey of the more important developments tracing its growth over a century that remarkable results have been achieved.

It is literally true that the majority of the important infectious diseases were conquered, for they were so effectively controlled as to remove them as leading causes of death; this was probably the largest single contribution to increased human life expectancy. New industries have been created, notably the fermentation industry with its ramifications into the production of antibiotics and chemicals. Less obvious, but more important, has been a large number of unique contributions to biology, ranging from the creation of the new science of immunology, through much of biochemical physiology, to a greatly broadened concept of hereditary mechanisms that provide the basis for modern genetics and molecular biology.

Aside from such highly successful practical and theoretical applications, microbiology owes its important position in biological science to its general significance. There is no question that microbiology has produced a change in man's conception of the world around him so sweeping as to deserve the term revolutionary. Up to the middle of the nineteenth century the character of many of the most familiar natural processes was entirely misunderstood. Spontaneous generation of at least the lower forms of life was the generally accepted belief; infectious diseases were not differentiated from one another, and the most fantastic hypotheses were advanced to explain their existence.

Although the great mass of material in other sciences had been brought into apparent orderliness and system, here was a region in which the unscientific imagination rioted in mystery and extravagance. The penetration of this realm of obscurity by the discoveries of microbiologists gave the human race for the first time in its history a rational theory of disease, dispelled the myths of spontaneous generation, and set the process of decay and kindred phenomena in their true relation to the great cycle of living and nonliving matter.

The new conception of the microscopic underworld that microbiology brought into biological science must be reckoned as a conspicuous landmark and, insofar as it has changed the attitude of man toward the universe, may be regarded as one of the most important triumphs of natural science.

REFERENCES

1. Alexander, M. 1971. Biochemical ecology of microorganisms. Ann. Rev. Microbiol. **25**:361–392.
2. Brock, T. D. (Ed.). 1961. Milestones in Microbiology. Prentice-Hall, Englewood Cliffs, N.J.
3. Bulloch, W. 1960. The History of Bacteriology. Heath Clark Lectures, 1936. Reprinted, Oxford University Press, London.
4. Cairns, J., G. S. Stent, and J. D. Watson (Eds.). 1967. Phage and the Origins of Molecular Biology. Cold Spring Harbor Laboratory of Quantitative Biology, Cold Spring Harbor, N.Y.
5. Casida, L. E., Jr. 1976. Leeuwenhoek's observation of bacteria. Science **192**:1348–1349.
6. Dobell, C. 1932. Antony van Leeuwenhoek and His "Little Animals." Harcourt, Brace and Co., New York.
7. Doetsch, R. N. 1978. Benjamin Marten and his "New Theory of Consumptions." Microbiol. Rev. **42**:521–528.
8. Hayes, W. 1966. The discovery of pneumococcal type transformation: an appreciation. J. Hygiene **64**:177–184.
9. Lechevalier, H. A., and M. Solotorovsky. 1965. Three Centuries of Microbiology. Peter Smith, Gloucester, Mass.
10. van Leeuwenhoek, A. 1677. Observations, communicated to the publisher by Mr. Antony van Leeuwenhoek, in a Dutch letter of the 9th of Octob. 1676 here Englished: Concerning little animals observed by him in rain- well- sea- and snow water, as also in water wherein pepper had lain infused. Phil. Trans. Roy. Soc. **11–12**:821.
11. Slare, F. 1682. An abstract of a letter from Dr. Wincler, chief physician of the Prince Palatine, Dat. Dec. 22, 1682 to Dr. Fred Slare, Fellow of the Royal Society, containing an account of a Murren in Switzerland and the method of its cure. A further confirmation of the above mentioned contagion, of its nature and manner of spreading by way of Postscript from the ingenious Fred Slare, M.D. and R.R.S., Dat. March 27, 1683. Phil. Trans. Roy. Soc. **13**:93.
12. Symposium. 1957. Modern ideas on spontaneous generation. Ann. N.Y. Acad. Sci. **69**:255–376.
13. Waterson, A. P., and L. Wilkinson. 1978. An Introduction to the History of Virology. Cambridge University Press, London.

Bacterial Anatomy, Physiology, and Genetics

The Morphology and Structure of Bacteria

For several centuries, long before the beginnings of biology as a science, it was recognized that living forms occurred in two major divisions—plants and animals. As biological science developed, these divisions were perpetuated in the two recognized kingdoms. Even after the discovery of microscopic life forms, the distinctions between bacteria and certain animal and plant cells were not easily resolved by the available techniques of light microscopy. The development of electron microscopy, with its increased resolution and magnification, made it possible to visualize the organizational components and fine structure of all kinds of cells. From these studies came the recognition that a fundamental distinction exists at the level of cellular organization and that two basic cell types occur.[61] On the one hand are the **eucaryotic** cells, the unit structure of higher plants and animals, fungi, protozoa, and most kinds of algae; eucaryotes are characterized by their true nuclei, which are bound by a nuclear membrane, and by chromosomes that undergo mitotic division. Such cells also possess a variety of cellular organelles, such as endocytoplasmic reticulum and Golgi bodies. Less abundant in nature and considerably simpler in organization are the **procaryotic** cells, the cell type of bacteria and blue-green algae. In procaryotes, the nuclear structures are without limiting membranes and do not divide by mitosis. The cell is usually enclosed in a rigid cell wall with muramic acid as a unique constituent.

14

All cells, whether eucaryotic or procaryotic, have certain similarities that indicate a common evolutionary stem. All cells utilize similar genetic codes, with corresponding mechanisms for replication, transcription, and translation of the genetic message, and show homologies in the biosynthesis of major cellular constituents. Although it is not yet possible to establish the precise evolutionary relationships between the two cell types, many favor the view that both arose from a common ancestral form. Stanier[58] provides a thoughtful and provocative discussion of this issue.

MICROSCOPY[2, 24]

A review of the various methods for demonstrating size, shape, and structure of microorganisms is an essential preliminary to a consideration of the morphology of these forms. In general, these methods are of two kinds, *viz.*, those utilizing light and those making use of a focused beam of electrons.

The Compound Microscope

With the ordinary microscope, objects are viewed by transmitted light (brightfield). In order to be seen and delineated (resolved) the object must be sufficiently large to cast a shadow; the critical size, or **limit of resolution**, is approximately half the wavelength of the light used. Thus in the range of blue (500 nm.) or yellow (550 nm.) light, the smallest object that can be resolved is a sphere having a diameter of 250 to 275 nm. Although ultraviolet (250 nm.) light may be used to extend resolution to 125 nm., technical difficulties make its use impractical.

The Darkfield Microscope

In the darkfield microscope, reflected rather than transmitted light is used, taking advantage of the familiar Tyndall effect most commonly seen in the appearance of particles of dust in a shaft of sunlight in a darkened room. The ordinary compound microscope may be employed by substituting a darkfield condenser for the brightfield substage condenser. The object is illuminated by light striking it from an oblique angle, and appears brilliantly lighted against a dark background. There is an illusion of increased resolution, since extremely small objects appear as bright points of light (in contrast with the minute shadows cast in transmitted light) but, in fact, resolution is not increased beyond the critical limits noted above. Thus, the darkfield microscope has not contributed appreciably to bacterial cytology. It has, however, considerable utility in the demonstration of very slender microorganisms, especially spirochetes, as in exudate from a syphilitic chancre or leptospira in the blood (Chapter 32).

The Phase Microscope

Light passing through an object of different thickness or refractive index from that of the surrounding fluid is scattered, with the result that it is out of phase and reduced in amplitude, *i.e.*, the distance from the crest to the trough of the light wave is reduced. Differences in amplitude are visible and allow the observation of the subject as a relatively faint shadow against its background. Bacteria may be so observed in the living unstained state, usually in a wet preparation.

While differences in phase are not ordinarily visible, they may be made so by treating the light scattered by the object and that coming through the surrounding fluid independently, so that they interact, either to interfere with one another to darken the image, or to reinforce one another to brighten it. Microscopes that are modified to accomplish this are phase-contrast microscopes and may be either dark or bright phase.

Phase-contrast microscopy has been particularly useful in the study of structures in the living cell, unmodified by the artifacts inherent in the processes of fixing and staining. The phase microscope is, however, subject to the same limits in ultimate resolving power as the brightfield microscope.

The Electron Microscope[11, 41]

The electron microscope operates on a different principle from that of optical microscopes in that a stream of electrons is used rather than a beam of light. The electron beam is focused by magnetic lenses and the interposed object intercepts the beam to cast a shadow, which is recorded on a photographic plate to give an electron micrograph. Remarkable resolution (0.5 nm.) is possible at magnifications of 10,000 to 50,000 diameters and, because of the small aperture used, the depth of focus is considerably greater than that obtained in high-resolution light microscopy.

Specimen preparation is critical and has been developed into a high art. The conditions of observation, involving high vacuums, requires fixation to minimize distortion and staining to provide proper deflection of the electron beam, particularly when thin sections are employed. External structures are often examined after shadow-casting with heavy metals vaporized under high vacuum and deposited at an angle on the preparation. The metal film is opaque to electrons, and the resulting electron micrograph has a luminous, three-dimensional appearance. The technique of negative staining with reagents such as phosphotungstate is analogous to the negative staining in light microscopy (see following discussion). It has been particularly useful in elucidating the structure of virus particles, since it shows fine structures not apparent in thin sections. When cells are frozen and subsequently fractured, by the techniques of freeze-fracture and freeze-etching, many internal structures are revealed without the distortion inherent in fixation, embedding, and staining.

The recent development of **scanning electron microscopy**[29] has permitted yet another view of cellular morphology by providing a detailed, three-dimensional image of the surface topography of microorganisms.

Application of electron microscopy has made it possible to see details of microbial structures beyond the limits of optical resolution and to determine directly the size and shape of small viruses. The results of electron microscopy must be interpreted with some caution because specimens can be examined only as dead, dry material due to the high vacuum required and are subject to the very considerable distortion of drying.

STAINING OF BACTERIA

In order to be seen clearly by light microscopy, bacterial cells are usually fixed and stained. The intact bacterial cell stains readily with basic dyes such as crystal violet, methylene blue, and basic fuchsin, but relatively poorly with acidic dyes such as eosin. Irregular staining, with differentiation of more deeply staining areas or granules, is often observed in old cells and is characteristic of a few kinds of bacteria, but most bacteria stain uniformly without the differentiation of internal structure often demonstrable in mammalian tissue cells.

The marked affinity for basic dyes is indicative of an acidic protoplasm containing unusually large amounts of nucleic acids more or less uniformly distributed; ribonucleic and deoxyribonucleic acids make up from 5 to 30 per cent of the dry weight of microbial cell substance.

The reactions of intact bacterial cells to these simple stains are remarkably uniform. More fruitful for differentiation are the reaction to the Gram staining procedure and the high resistance to both penetration of dye and decolorization characterizing the acid-fast bacilli.

The Gram Stain

This differential staining procedure was devised in 1884 by the histologist Christian Gram as a method of staining bacteria in tissues. It is an arbitrary procedure consisting of four steps, *viz.*, (1) primary staining with a triphenylmethane dye such as crystal violet and usually containing a mordant such as ammonium oxalate; (2) the application of dilute iodine solution; (3) decolorization, most commonly with 95 per cent ethanol; and (4) counterstaining with a dye of contrasting color, usually safranin. When bacteria are stained by this method, they are separated into two groups. The gram-positive bacteria are those which retain the primary stain and are deep violet in color; the gram-negative bacteria are those which are decolorized and are lightly stained by the counterstain, pink in the case of safranin.

The gram-positive reaction is relatively rare in biology. It occurs only among the bacteria, yeasts, and filamentous fungi. A very few biological structures are gram-positive, including chromosomes of certain species, mitochrondria, centrosomes, and centromeres.

The reaction of bacteria to the Gram stain is correlated with a number of other characteristics; representative differences are shown in Table 2–1. Such differences are only relative and are not completely consistent. For instance, the pathogenic *Neisseria* species, though gram-negative, behave in many respects, such as susceptibility to the antibacterial activity of penicillin, as though they are gram-positive (see Chapter 16).

These differences between gram-positive and gram-negative bacteria reach an impressive total and suggest that the reaction to the Gram stain is a reflection of fundamental differences between the two kinds of bacteria. Consequently, the mechanism of the Gram reaction has been of considerable interest.

Many theories have been proposed to account for the Gram staining reaction; they may be divided into two major categories. Proposals in the first group assume a chemical mechanism with a Gram-staining substrate unique to gram-positive bacteria. In the second group, a permeability difference is proposed to exist between gram-positive and gram-negative bac-

Table 2–1. **Differences Between Gram-Positive and Gram-Negative Bacteria**

Gram-Positive Bacteria	Character	Gram-Negative Bacteria
More susceptible	Antibacterial activity of basic dyes, anionic and cationic detergents, phenol, sulfonamides, penicillin	More resistant
More resistant	Antibacterial activity of azides, tellurites, oxidizing agents, streptomycin	More susceptible
More resistant	Digestion by proteolytic enzymes, lytic action of alkali	More susceptible
Susceptible	Lytic action of lysozyme	Resistant
Resistant	Lytic action of specific antibody and complement	Often susceptible
Higher	Mechanical stability	Lower
Absent	Lipopolysaccharides in cell wall	Usually present
Often present	Teichoic acids in cell wall	Absent (?)
1–4%	Lipids in cell wall	11–22%
Some lacking	Amino acids in cell wall	All present

teria. The predominant evidence now supports the second of these theories and is based upon the structure and composition of the bacterial cell wall. When the bacterial cell is stained with the crystal violet–iodine complex, the complex is trapped within gram-positive organisms and cannot easily be removed by the alcohol solvent because of the physicochemical nature of their cell walls; gram-positive cell walls are known to be less permeable to smaller molecules after treatment with high concentrations of alcohol. The different nature of the cell wall in gram-negative bacteria, however, permits the removal of the dye-iodine complex by alcohol treatment; this removal may be facilitated by the higher lipid content of gram-negative cell walls (see The Cell Envelope, p. 30).

The Acid-Fast Stain

Early in the history of microbiology, it was observed that certain bacteria were stained only with difficulty and, after staining, could not be destained with highly effective agents such as acid-alcohol. Because of this resistance to decolorization they were termed acid-fast. The acid-fast bacteria form a homogeneous group making up the genus *Mycobacterium*, which includes the tubercle and leprosy bacilli (Chapter 31). These bacteria are characterized by a high lipid content, ranging to 40 per cent of the dry weight of the cell. Demonstration of acid-fastness requires the application of a dye, usually basic fuchsin in phenol solution, followed by destaining with a dilute mineral acid in ethanol. The acid-fast bacteria retain the stain as a consequence of the hydrophobic barrier of the cell wall lipids—principally mycoloyl-arabinogalactan—that prevent the penetration of the decolorizer.[22]

The acid-fast property of mycobacteria is of considerable importance in the identification of the tubercle and leprosy bacilli. Aside from the mycobacteria, only a few species of actinomycetes and corynebacteria are acid-fast. Bacterial spores also show this characteristic, but the mechanism of staining is believed to be different.

The Morphology of Bacteria[27, 30, 60]

Bacterial morphology may be considered in two general categories: (1) individual cells (and groups of cells) as observed by microscopy, and (2) bacterial colonies developing on solid mediums, visible to the unaided eye, and consisting of very large numbers of cells. In the first instance, differences in size, shape, and certain structural details are characteristic of at least the main groups of bacteria and provide the primary basis for their systematic study. Similarly, bacterial colonies, composed of masses of individual cells, have character-istics of size, consistency, texture, and color that are of differential value, but do not have the fundamental significance of cellular morphology.

THE SIZE OF BACTERIA

One of the most striking aspects of the morphology of microorganisms is their extremely small size. Their order of size is such that they are most conveniently measured in the units of the micron or micrometer (μm. = 10^{-3} millimeter) and the nanometer (nm. = 10^{-6} millimeter). The bacteria proper, *i.e.,* those capable of independent metabolic existence and which may be grown on lifeless nutrient mediums (axenic cultivation), exhibit remarkable size variation. As shown in Table 2–2, they range in size from the large bacilli, such as *Bacillus anthracis,* to such minute forms as *Francisella tularensis.* The obligately parasitic rickettsiae and viruses form a continuous series of even smaller forms, most below the limits of optical resolution. The rickettsiae, which resemble other small bacteria, and the poxviruses also overlap the smallest bacteria. From this maximum, the viral agents range downward to nearly macromolecular dimensions, *viz.,* 25 nm. for poliomyelitis virus and 22 nm. for foot-and-mouth disease virus. The small viruses are only slightly larger than some protein molecules; the egg albumin molecule, for example, measures 2.5 × 10 nm.

There is some variation in size of bacterial cells within the same species; this variation is not constant, being greatest in the bacillary forms and least in the spherical types. Excluding filamentous and swollen forms that may be produced under certain conditions and usually regarded as aberrant, the maximum difference in size between mature individual cells is about four- to fivefold.

The size continuum of microbial cells and viruses may best be illustrated by comparing them to the familiar lymphocytes, among the smallest of mammalian cells (Table 2–2). They are many times larger than the bacteria, as exemplified by the largest of the medically important bacteria, *B. anthracis,* and the smallest, *F. tularensis.* The last appears to represent the minimum size that permits the degree of

organization necessary for independent metabolism and growth, since the smaller rickettsiae and viruses are obligate intracellular parasites.

The size range of rickettsiae and viruses overlaps that of the true bacteria. The larger rickettsiae, such as *Coxiella burnetii,* and the largest viruses, such as vaccinia virus, are larger than *F. tularensis* and other extremely small bacteria. The smallest viruses, however, represented by the virus of foot-and-mouth disease, can at best contain only relatively few molecules.

THE SHAPES OF BACTERIA

The most obvious difference among bacteria is their shape, and three general morphological types are clearly evident. These are the spherical form or coccus; the rod-shaped form or bacillus; and the spiral forms, with subtypes of vibrio, spirillum, and spirochete.

Coccus

The spherical bacteria are by far the most homogeneous with respect to size and, in general, have a diameter of 0.6 to 1.0 μm., although both smaller and larger varieties have been described. There is some small deviation from the spherical, including lanceolate, coffee bean–like, or coccobacillus shapes, seen in certain species.

Morphological subtypes of cocci are differentiated on the basis of cell groupings. These arise as a consequence of two factors—the plane or planes of cell division and the tendency of daughter cells to remain attached to one another after division is complete.

Those cocci that separate completely after division (regardless of the plane of division)

Table 2–2. **Comparative Sizes of Representative Mammalian and Bacterial Cells and Viruses**

Cells	Dimensions	Minimum Volume (μm³)
Mammalian lymphocytes	10 μm.	524
Bacteria		
Bacillus anthracis	1–1.3 × 3–10 μm.	2.4
Francisella tularensis	0.2 × 0.2–0.7 μm.	0.004
Rickettsiae		
Coxiella burnetii	0.2 × 0.5–1.5 μm.	0.015
Viruses		
Vaccinia virus	200–250 × 250–350 nm.	0.008
Foot-and-mouth disease virus	22–25 nm.	0.000004

appear to occur singly, and this form is called **micrococcus.** When there is a slight tendency of daughter cells to remain attached and cell division occurs in only one plane, the predominant grouping of cocci is in pairs, called **diplococcus.** If the attachment is more marked, longer chains of four or more cocci are seen; this grouping is termed **streptococcus.**

When the cocci divide in a variety of planes, and the tendency to remain attached is marked, the cocci occur in irregular groups, much like a cluster of grapes, called **staphylococcus.**

In a relatively few cocci, cell division takes place in two or three perpendicular planes and the cells remain adherent, resulting in packets of four (tetrads) or in cubical packets of eight cells. Several of the coccal cell groupings are illustrated in Figure 2–1.

The cell groupings of cocci, and some other bacteria discussed below, are most effectively demonstrated in wet mounts observed by phase microscopy, since fixation and staining often result in distortion of the typical groups. Moreover, the separation into morphological subtypes is not completely sharp—diplococci are often seen admixed with single cells, streptococcus chains are interspersed with paired and single cells, and clusters of staphylococcus often appear in the same microscopic field as single, paired, and short chains of cocci. In spite of this, morphological groups are of great practical value in the identification and classification of cocci.

Bacillus

The rod-shaped, or bacillary, form of bacteria collectively embraces a variety of morphological subtypes, since the morphology of individual rod-shaped bacteria differs considerably among genera and even species. Not only is there variation in size, but the shape of individual cells differ, sometimes markedly, as shown in Figure 2–2. Morphological variables, including width, length, and shapes of the ends of the cell, give considerable heterogeneity to

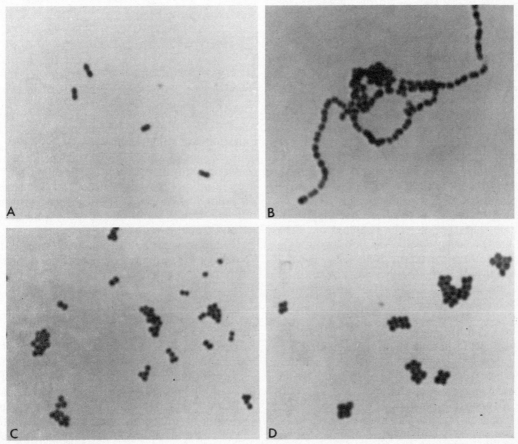

Figure 2–1. Representative cell groupings and relative sizes of spherical bacteria. *A,* Diplococcal grouping of *Streptococcus pneumoniae. B,* Chains of *Streptococcus pyogenes. C,* Grape-like clusters of *Staphylococcus aureus. D,* Packets of *Micrococcus luteus.* All ×2300.

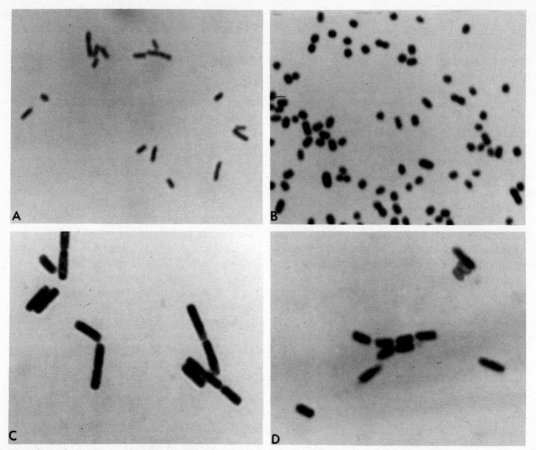

Figure 2–2. Morphology of representative bacilli. *A, Pseudomonas aeruginosa. B, Escherichia coli. C, Bacillus mycoides. D, Bacillus cereus.* All ×2300.

the bacillary form. A given shape is relatively constant, however, within a species, although the length to width ratio may vary, owing in large part to elongation of individual cells prior to cell division.

Like the cocci, some of the bacillary forms assume characteristic cell groupings but these are limited because cell division occurs only in the plane vertical to the long axis. Thus, if daughter cells remain adherent, chains of bacilli may be seen. Other cell groups are a consequence of post-fission movements of the daughter cells.

Post-fission Movements. The post-fission movements of bacilli are of two general kinds. One, known as **slipping,** consists of a sliding movement of the cells against one another with the long axes parallel, resulting in groups of cells with a palisade-like appearance. Slipping appears to be a consequence of space limitations interfering with continued extension of growth in a longitudinal axis. In the other kind of movement, termed **snapping**, the daughter cells bend sharply with respect to one

another after division to give a V-shaped arrangement of cells. When such cells remain adherent through several division cycles, they resemble a split-rail fence.[30] The snapping movement may be due to a localized rupture of the outer layer of the cell wall during growth.[37]

While to a certain extent characteristic, the bacillary cell groupings do not assume the same differential significance as those of cocci.

Spirals

The third principal morphological type of bacteria is the spiral form, which may be regarded as a bacillus twisted into a helix. The curved rods may be regarded as intermediate, on a morphological, but not phylogenetic basis. Although curvature of rods is occasionally observed in many bacillary forms, in the genus *Vibrio* it is sufficiently constant to have differential significance. Vibrios may superficially resemble the spiral form when the cells remain attached end-to-end.

The "true" spiral bacteria are of two general

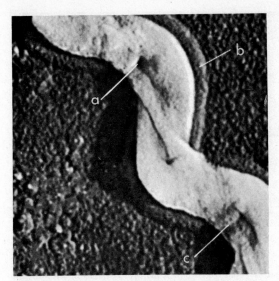

Figure 2–3. Electron micrograph of a chromium-shadow-cast preparation of *Leptospira interrogans*. The axial filament is separated from the protoplasmic spiral by a narrow space at *(a)* and is more closely approximated at *(c)*. The sheath is shown at *(b)*. ×125,000. (C. F. Simpson, and F. H. White, J. Infect. Dis. **109**:243, 1961.)

kinds—one in which the spiral is rigid, exemplified by members of the genus *Spirillum*, and the other in which it is flexible. The latter are separated into several genera, based upon such morphological criteria as tightness of the coiling, hook-like bends at the ends of the cell, the presence of an outer sheath, and the composition of the axial filament. Figure 2–3 illustrates the general nature of such cells and some of the fine structural elements.

Taken together, the flexible spiral forms are casually referred to as **spirochetes**. Classification and differentiation of the pathogenic spirochetes have emphasized morphological criteria, since many have not been grown on laboratory mediums and their physiological activity remains largely unknown (Chapter 32).

Involution Forms

The great majority of bacteria are relatively constant in shape and size in young cultures growing actively under favorable conditions. In older cultures, however, this constancy may disappear; the cell structures are weakened or break down and aberrant forms arise. These include balloon-like cells, Y-shaped forms, and cells with a granular appearance. These are involution forms, which are degenerative in origin, resulting from breakdown of the mechanisms of selective permeability with imbibition of water, autolysis by enzymes, and other causes.

Aberrant bacterial forms may also be produced by cultivation under adverse conditions, such as above optimum temperatures, or in the presence of relatively high concentrations of inorganic salts or sublethal concentrations of antibacterial substances.

COLONIAL MORPHOLOGY OF BACTERIA

When bacteria are grown on the surface of a solid nutrient medium, the proliferating cells remain approximately fixed in position and form masses of many millions of cells that are visible to the naked eye. The colonies so formed range from a minute, barely visible size to masses several millimeters in diameter. They have characteristics of size, shape, texture, and, in some instances, color. While these are often dependent upon the nature of the culture medium and the conditions of incubation, when conditions are carefully controlled they are more constant and often of considerable differential value. Colonial morphology is, then, one of the basic characteristics of bacteria, and one that is indispensable in preliminary identification.

The size of bacterial colonies is, assuming favorable cultural conditions, quite uniform within a species or type. Streptococcus colonies are, for example, relatively small (1 mm. or less in diameter), while those of staphylococcus and enteric bacteria are somewhat larger, and those of *Bacillus* may be several millimeters in diameter.

The shape of the colony is determined by its edge and by its thickness. The edge may be smooth, or it may be irregular and serrated. When the thickness is much greater in the center, diminishing uniformly to the edge, the colony is said to be raised, occasionally so much so as to approach a hemispherical form. Alternatively, it may be relatively uniform so that the colony appears to be little more than a disk on the surface of the medium. Several types of bacterial colonies are illustrated in Figure 2–4.

The consistency and texture of the mass of cells are also distinguishing features of colonial morphology. Bacterial colonies may range in consistency from dry and friable to butyrous, or butter-like, to viscid and sticky. The surface of the colony may be uniformly smooth and glistening, rough and granular, or striated with indentations. On examination with transmitted light, the cell mass may appear to be amor-

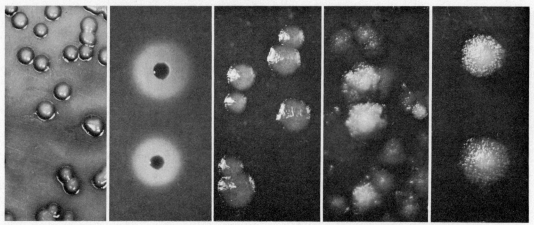

Figure 2–4. Morphological types of bacterial colonies. *From left to right,* the raised, smooth, viscous colonies of the gonococcus on chocolate agar; β-hemolytic streptococcus colonies on blood agar showing the cleared zones of hemolysis and the slightly matte, slightly irregular edge of the typical colony; colonies of the typhoid bacillus on nutrient agar, showing the typical irregular edge (maple leaf appearance) and irregular but smooth surface; colonies of the tubercle bacillus on Löwenstein's medium showing the characteristic roughened appearance; and colonies of the anthrax bacillus on nutrient agar in the typically rough, virulent form.

phous or granular in texture and vary from almost complete translucency, with perhaps a bluish cast, through varying degrees of opalescence to a white or yellowish opacity.

Not all bacterial colonies are pigmented, and pigmentation is more common among the saprophytic bacteria. Since most bacterial pigments are of the carotenoid series, the cell mass may appear red, orange, or yellow. Of the pathogens, one of the more important pigmented forms is *Staphylococcus aureus*, whose colonies are usually golden yellow in color. Pigmentation is not apparent in the individual cells, for the pigment occurs in intracellular granules too small to be resolved with visible light.

Since these characteristics occur in varying degree and combination from one kind of bacterium to another, colonial appearance is often quite characteristic, and kinds of bacteria may be differentiated from others in mixed or contaminated cultures. Differentiation on the basis of colonial morphology has hardly more than tentative status, however, and detailed study of the physiological and immunological characteristics of a bacterium is ordinarily required for identification.

Colonial morphology is analogous to a statistic in that it is derived from the individual cells but is a characteristic of the entire cell mass. Thus, pigmentation is apparent not in the individual cell but in the colony; the viscous consistency of the colony may derive from the capsular substance of heavily encapsulated bacteria; the coiled texture of *Bacillus* colonies is due to the tendency of the cells to form long filaments; and actively motile bacteria, such as *Proteus*, actually move or swarm over the surface of the medium to give a continuous film of growth. In this way colonial morphology may be associated with other significant characteristics of the bacterium; for example, among the pathogenic bacteria virulence may be associated with capsule formation; when this is true, the colony of the virulent form is smooth or mucoid in appearance and texture, and that of the nonencapsulated, avirulent form is rough.

Colonial characteristics may be accentuated or induced by cultivation of the bacterium on so-called **differential** culture mediums which exploit relevant physiological properties. When certain bacteria are grown on an agar medium containing blood, the erythrocytes may be lysed by **hemolysins** produced by the bacteria, resulting in a more or less clear zone surrounding the colony (Chapter 12). The ability of diphtheria bacilli to reduce tellurium salts gives rise to black colonies on tellurite differential mediums. Similarly, a sugar such as lactose may be incorporated in the medium together with an acid-base indicator, so that colonies of bacteria fermenting the sugar and accumulating acidic end products are colored by the indicator. Colonial morphology on such mediums is almost invariably a special case in that the medium is devised for the purpose of inducing or enhancing a colonial appearance that will facilitate identification of a specific bacterium in a mixed culture.

The Ultrastructure of Bacterial Cells[11]

Procaryotic bacterial cells are fundamentally different from the eucaryotic cells of higher plants and animals, although they share some similarities, as noted earlier. Procaryotic cells do not contain the great variety of cellular organelles seen in eucaryotes and are therefore considered to be simpler. Simplicity is, however, only relative, and the organization and structure of bacterial cells is still being elucidated and explained.

Earlier studies on bacterial structure depended largely upon light microscopy to describe gross morphology, with a few aspects of internal structure derived from differential staining and other cytochemical reagents. Knowledge of chemical constitution was limited to information gained by extracting and analyzing large populations or masses of cells. Only after the development of modern electron microscopy, coupled with sophisticated physical and chemical methods, has the orga-

nization, composition, structure, and function of bacterial cells begun to emerge.

In the discussions to follow, bacterial fine structure will be considered at three levels, *viz.*, the structures and components located external to the cell envelope, the cell envelope proper, and those elements enclosed within the cell envelope. The individual components and their spatial relationships are shown diagramatically in Figure 2–5.

EXTERNAL STRUCTURES

Three kinds of structures may be encountered on the external aspects of bacterial cells. These are the flagella, or organelles concerned with locomotion and chemotaxis; the fimbriae, or pili; and the capsule, or slime layer, surrounding the cell. None are essential to the continued existence of the cell; they may be

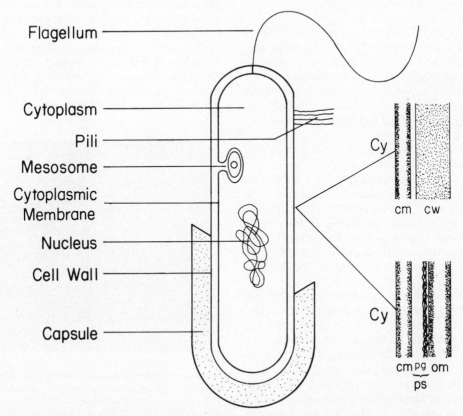

Figure 2–5. Diagrammatic representation of a typical bacterial cell. Not all structures are encountered in all cells. The insert at upper right shows structural details of the cell envelope of gram-positive cells; lower insert shows that of gram-negative cells. *Cy,* cytoplasm; *cm,* cell membrane; *cw,* cell wall of gram-positive bacteria; *om,* outer membrane of gram-negative cell envelope; *pg,* peptidoglycan layer; *ps,* periplasmic space.

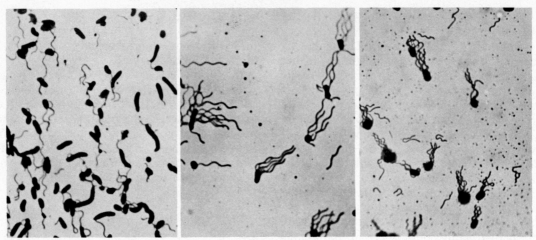

Figure 2–6. Flagella of bacteria in stained smears examined with the optical microscope. *Left,* single polar flagellum of a water vibrio; *center,* peritrichous flagella of *Salmonella typhimurium; right,* peritrichous flagella of *Rhizobium leguminosarum.* ×2000. (Kral.)

removed by mechanical or enzymatic means without inhibition of growth or metabolic function.

FLAGELLA[16, 31, 54]

The bacterial flagellum is a long filamentous appendage that arises in the cell envelope and extends beyond the cell surface. Morphological features of flagella and the relationship to the bacterial cell are shown in Figure 2–6. Flagella are responsible for locomotion of bacterial cells and are involved in chemotaxis and bacterial sensing.

In living cells, the flagellar filament is coiled in the form of a rigid or semirigid helix, but appears in dried preparations as a wavy filament. Because of their slender nature, flagella are rarely seen in the living state by phase-contrast or darkfield microscopy. They may be stained and observed by conventional light microscopy after deposition of a mordant to increase the apparent diameter of the flagellar filament.

Flagella occur most commonly, although not exclusively, among the rod-shaped bacteria. They may be attached either at or near the ends of the cell, or distributed over the cell surface. The location and number are relatively constant within bacterial species. Bacteria with a single polar flagellum are designated **monotrichous**, those with two or more flagella at one end of the cell are **lophotrichous,** those with tufts at both ends are **amphitrichous**, and those with flagella distributed over the cell surface are **peritrichous** (Fig. 2–7).

The complex structure of flagella was suggested when they were separated from the parent cell, purified, and observed by electron microscopy (Fig. 2–8). Morphological, biochemical, and genetic studies have led to the present concepts of their ultrastructure and function. The flagella comprise three morphological components—the filament, the hook, and the basal body—illustrated diagramatically in Figure 2–9 as they occur in gram-negative bacteria. The external filament terminates proximally in the hook structure, which in turn is linked to the basal body. The

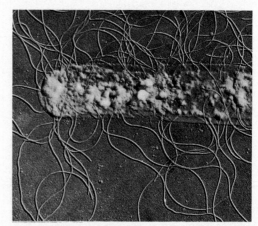

Figure 2–7. Electron micrograph of shadow-cast preparation showing the flagella of *Proteus vulgaris.* The bacteria were grown to the swarming stage on agar, refrigerated at 5° C. for 16 to 20 hours, floated off in 5 per cent formalin, and washed twice before mounting on collodion. The preparation is very transparent and flattens completely so that certain of the internal structures are demonstrable by shadowing. The flagella originate in small, spherical bodies about 100 nm. in diameter, and their remarkably uniform size is clearly shown. (van Iterson.)

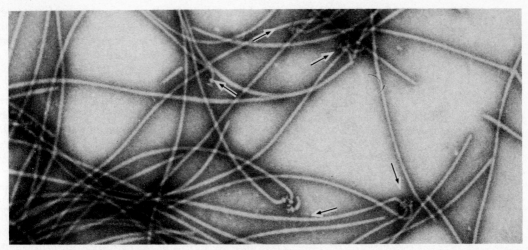

Figure 2–8. Purified intact flagella from *Escherichia coli* stained negatively with uranyl acetate, pH 4.5. A hook-basal body complex is visible at one end of many of the filaments (arrows). ×66,000. (M. L. DePamphilis and J. Adler, J. Bacteriol. **105**:376, 1971.)

latter is associated with the cell envelope and constitutes the flagellar motor.

Filament. The distal filament portion is usually 12 to 15 nm. in diameter, without taper, and of variable length. It may range from 1 to 70 μm., but is ordinarily 15 to 25 μm. in length. The filament is composed of more or less parallel subfibrils of protein, called flagel-

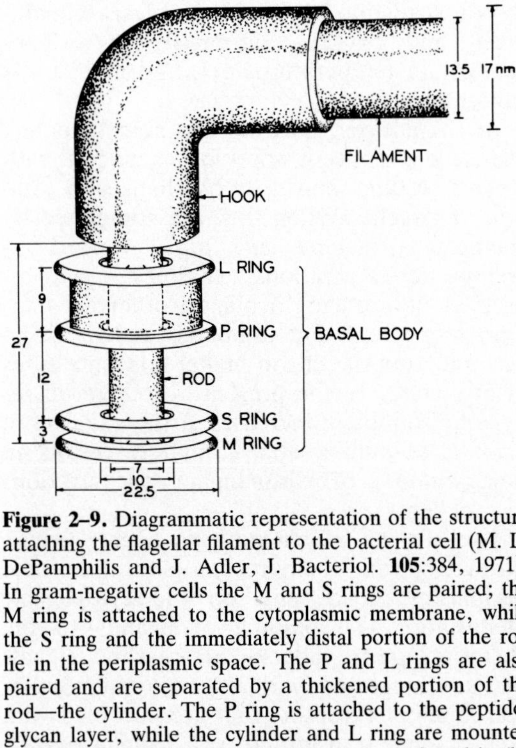

Figure 2–9. Diagrammatic representation of the structure attaching the flagellar filament to the bacterial cell (M. L. DePamphilis and J. Adler, J. Bacteriol. **105**:384, 1971). In gram-negative cells the M and S rings are paired; the M ring is attached to the cytoplasmic membrane, while the S ring and the immediately distal portion of the rod lie in the periplasmic space. The P and L rings are also paired and are separated by a thickened portion of the rod—the cylinder. The P ring is attached to the peptidoglycan layer, while the cylinder and L ring are mounted in the outer membrane. Only two rings are found in the basal body of gram-positive cells and are analogous to the S and M rings.

lin, combined to form a hollow cylinder. The filament is a twisted helix, normally left-handed in most bacteria, and is rigid or semirigid in nature.

The filament protein, **flagellin**, is easily separated from the remainder of the flagellum and has been shown to vary among bacterial species in both antigenic specificity and molecular weight (33,000 to 60,000 daltons). Flagellin is also antigenically distinct from the remainder of the flagellar structural proteins and from those of the cell proper. When motile, flagellated cells are treated with specific antifilament antibody, the organisms become immobilized because of agglutination and entanglement of the flagella.

In some bacteria, the filament may be enclosed in a seemingly amorphous sheath, chemically and antigenically distinct from the filament (Fig. 2–10).

Flagellin is a protein with the critical property of self-assembly. Flagellin monomers bind or polymerize to the end of existing filaments or to the distal end of flagellar hooks, undergo a conformational change, and then serve as the nucleus for further polymerization and growth of the filament.

Hook. The flagellar hook is a single polypeptide unit, slightly larger in diameter than the filament and slightly curved; it is distal to the basal body (Fig. 2–9). The hook is believed to act as a "universal joint," permitting the transmission of rotary motion from the basal body to the helical filament.

Basal Body. The basal structure is the most complex portion of the flagellar organelle. It is situated within the cell envelope and is composed of a central core or rod upon which

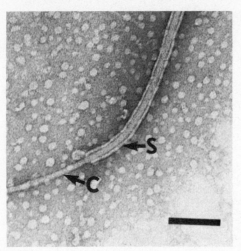

Figure 2–10. Electron micrograph of the polar flagellum of *Vibrio cholerae*. Note the presence of a sheath *(S)* surrounding the flagellar filament *(C)*. Bar represents 0.1 μm. (G. C. Yang, G. D. Schrank, and B. A. Freeman, J. Bacteriol. **129**:1121, 1977.)

are mounted two or four ring-like structures (Fig. 2–9). The rings are attached at their outer edge to one of the layers of the cell envelope (Fig. 2–5). In gram-negative cells, the basal body consists of four rings, whereas in gram-positive cells, only two rings are present, reflecting differences in the cell wall attachment sites in the two kinds of cells.

The component parts of the basal body are constructed of proteins. In basal bodies of gram-negative cells, at least 10 structural proteins have been identified, ranging in molecular weight from 9000 to 60,000 daltons. The genes involved in their synthesis are designated *fla*, and the chromosomal location of many of these has been mapped (Chapter 6).

Motility[40]

The rate of movement of motile bacteria is often surprisingly rapid. For example, peritrichously flagellated gram-negative bacteria have been found to average speeds of 25 to 30 μm. per second and the monotrichous cholera vibrio to move as fast as 55 μm. per second.

With few exceptions, bacterial motility is the consequence of flagellar motion. Bacteria swim by rotation of the rigid or semirigid, helically coiled flagella, with torque provided by the flagellar motor (basal body).

Two types of motility are observed: smooth swimming and tumbling. **Smooth swimming, or translational motion,** occurs when the flagella, which normally is a left-handed helix, is rotated in a counterclockwise direction. If the bacterium is multiflagellated, the filaments

form a bundle during smooth swimming and trail behind the moving cell. When the flagellar motor is reversed, **tumbles,** or **twiddles,** occur; this reversal of torque causes the filament to form a right-handed helix and the bundles of filaments unwind and are dispersed. In a homogeneous environment, a typical bacterial cell will undergo frequent and random changes in flagellar rotation that induce alternating periods of swimming and tumbling. The cell will then move randomly in a three-dimensional walk.

The energy for the flagellar motor is not derived from the hydrolysis of ATP, but instead arises from the electrochemical potential of protons moving across the membrane—proton motive force, or PMF. Both transmembrane potential and transmembrane pH contribute to the total proton motive force (Chapter 4). The manner of coupling of PMF to mechanical rotation is not yet established.

Bacterial Sensing.[35, 36, 45] It has been known for many years that under certain circumstances, bacterial motility is not without purpose or direction; bacteria are capable of avoiding unfavorable environments and are attracted to favorable ones, *e.g.,* the presence of nutrients. They must, then, be able to detect and react to environmental stimuli. It has been established that motile bacteria can react to concentration gradients of certain chemicals **(chemotaxis)** and oxygen **(aerotaxis)**, as well as changes in temperature, pH, and light levels **(phototaxis)**.

In chemotaxis, bacteria are able to detect changes in concentration of chemicals with respect to time, and react by changes in rotation of flagella. When they are stimulated by chemical attractants and move toward increased concentrations, tumbles are suppressed, introducing a bias in otherwise random movement that ultimately results in an accumulation of cells in higher concentrations of attractant. In the presence of chemical repellents, tumbling increases at the expense of smooth swimming and ultimately results in lower numbers of cells in higher concentrations of repellents.

The sensing of chemotactic agents occurs through specific chemoreceptors located in the periplasmic space and on the cytoplasmic membrane. The binding of ligands to the chemoreceptors induces cytoplasmic signals that are integrated (with respect to the number and kinds of receptors that are occupied with ligands) and transmitted to a flagellar switch that controls the rotational direction of the flagellar motor.

Motility of Spirochetes.[3, 10] In spirochetes, the flexible spiral-shaped bacteria (Fig. 2–11), motility is not associated with the rotation of free flagella. Rather, motility is related to one or more structures that are unique to these organisms (Chapter 32).

Several types of motion are encountered in spirochetes, *viz.,* translational motion, rotation about the longitudinal axis, and flexing. The latter may occur as bending, lashing, whipping, or propagation of waves along the cell.

It is generally believed that spirochetal motion is associated with the axial filament, which extends longitudinally beneath the outer sheath from attachments at either end (Fig. 2–3). Each of the fibrils that make up the axial bundle is anchored at only one pole of the cell; individual fibrils may then overlap, near the central region, with those originating from the opposite pole. The fibrils are physically and chemically similar to the flagella encountered in other bacteria and presumably are also capable of rotation. They do not, however, extend into the surrounding menstruum, since they are enclosed in the outer sheath; thus, they cannot propel the cell in the manner described for flagella.

Although the mechanism for locomotion is not certain, one theory supposes that the rotation of the axial fibrils causes the helical cylinder to rotate within the outer sheath, causing the cell to move through the medium in a screw-like fashion. In this theory, a part of the thrust is generated by the resulting roll of the flexible outer sheath. This mechanism of propulsion possibly accounts for the ability of spirochetes to move in environments of high viscosity, conditions that inhibit the movement of flagellated bacteria.

Significance of Bacterial Motility. The capacity of bacteria to sense chemical gradients, as well as changes in temperature and light, with resulting changes in motive behavior undoubtedly provides them with certain ecological advantages. It is not surprising, therefore, that chemotactic responses are observed in the association of certain pathogenic bacteria with mucosal surfaces, where they may subsequently adhere and multiply (Chapter 12). The ability of spirochetes to move effectively in high-viscosity environments may also be important in pathogenesis, since it could theoretically permit them to penetrate the membranes of mammalian cells.

FIMBRIAE (PILI)[44]

Electron microscopy of bacterial flagellation led to the discovery in 1949 of minute filamentous appendages appearing on many kinds of bacteria, which have subsequently been referred to as bristles, filaments, fuzz, pili, or fimbriae. The two latter terms have gained general acceptance.

Fimbriae are not related to locomotion, although there is some superficial resemblance to flagella. Like flagella, they are made up of regularly arranged protein subunits (fimbrilin or pilin), often with a hollow core. Fimbriae are, however, considerably smaller than flagella and tend to be straight. They range in diameter from 3 to 25 nm. and are generally 300 to 1000 nm. in length. They may occur at the ends of the cell or may be distributed over the surface in numbers from one to several hundred per cell (Fig. 2–12). Fimbriae appear to arise in the cytoplasmic membrane and project through the cell wall. The ultrastructure of the insertion apparatus is not well known; hooks have not been observed and structures similar to flagellar basal bodies are only rarely seen.

Not all bacteria possess fimbriae; they are most common in gram-negative bacilli, but are found in some gram-positive bacteria as well. There are several morphological and functional varieties. Some, called **sex pili**, are involved in specific pair formation during bac-

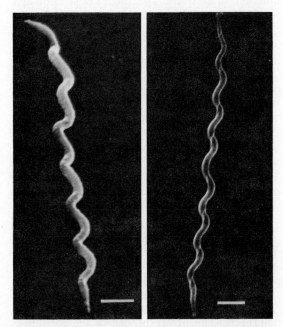

Figure 2–11. Scanning photomicrograph of spirochetes. *Left, Treponema pallidum,* Nichols strain; *Right, Borrelia turicatae.* Bar = 0.5 μm. (D. E. Stephan, and R. C. Johnson, Infect. Immun. **32**:937, 1981.)

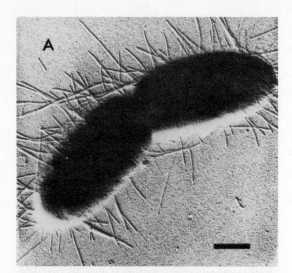

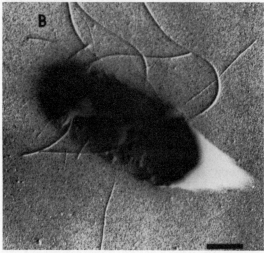

Figure 2–12. Electron micrograph of *Escherichia coli* showing fimbriated cells *(A)* from a 12 hour aerobic static culture and non-fimbriated, but flagellated, cells *(B)* from a 48 hour culture. Gold-palladium shadowed. Bar = 0.5 μm. (D. C. Clegg and S. Old, J. Bacteriol. **137**:1008, 1979.)

terial conjugation and serve to initiate cellular contact, draw the mating cells together, and aid in the transfer of genetic material (Chapter 6). Sex pili are distinguished from other fimbriae by greater diameter (6 to 14 nm.) and length (up to 20 μm.); they are also generally fewer in number, from 1 to 10 per cell. Other fimbriae appear to have **adhesive** properties that facilitate attachment to other kinds of cells, *e.g.,* erythrocytes, leucocytes, and mucosal cells. Thus, fimbriae play a role in certain kinds of hemagglutination reactions. Fimbrial adhesion is also related to the ability of certain bacteria to attach to mucosal and other cell surfaces as a first step in bacterial colonization of host animals (Chapter 12).

CAPSULES[13, 59, 62]

Most bacteria, possibly all wild type cells, are surrounded by a layer of gelatinous, poorly defined, and poorly staining material that has been termed the capsule, slime layer, or glycocalyx. The term **capsule** is generally applied to the material surrounding a single cell, while **slime layer** is often used to describe the matrix that envelops a microcolony or group of cells. Such distinctions are arbitrary, and many prefer **glycocalyx** to describe the extracellular polysaccharides composing this bacterial organelle.

Bacterial capsules are not stained by the usual procedures because they fail to retain dyes. They may be demonstrated in the light microscope by suspending the cells in diluted India ink, called **negative staining.** The capsule displaces the colloidal carbon particles, and the cells appear to lie in lacunae, representing the capsules, in the dark background (Fig. 2–13). Not all capsules, however, are impervious to penetration by the carbon particles and cannot be discerned in this way.

Similarly, capsules are not easily demonstrated by the usual techniques of electron microscopy. Because of their chemical makeup, capsules are not electron-dense and thus show little or no contrast in electron micrographs. Further, since they contain about 99 per cent water, they tend to collapse when vacuum dried during specimen preparation and observation.

Many morphological features can be preserved, however, by stabilizing the structure with specific antibody and staining with polyanion-specific stains, usually ruthenium red. Electron micrographs prepared in this way reveal that capsules are highly ordered, fibrillar matrices surrounding the bacterial cell. Figures 2–14 and 2–15 show the appearance of capsules by electron microscopy, using different preparative procedures.

The apparent size of the capsule varies widely. In heavily encapsulated forms such as the pneumococcus and *Klebsiella,* the thickness of the capsule as seen in India ink preparations is frequently greater than the diameter of the cell proper and is often continuous over adjacent cells. In other bacteria, it may be no more than a thin layer, not visible in the light microscope and demonstrable only by electron microscopy or by chemical or immunological methods. The apparent size of the capsule is dependent upon several factors, including density and solubility in the surrounding fluid. In spite of the difficulties in visualizing capsules,

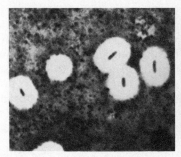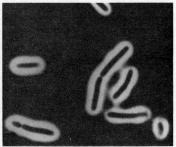

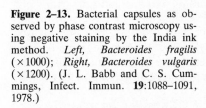

Figure 2–13. Bacterial capsules as observed by phase contrast microscopy using negative staining by the India ink method. *Left, Bacteroides fragilis* (×1000); *Right, Bacteroides vulgaris* (×1200). (J. L. Babb and C. S. Cummings, Infect. Immun. **19**:1088–1091, 1978.)

it is a widely held belief that most, if not all, bacteria possess capsules when growing in their natural environments.

The Nature of Capsular Substance. With rare exceptions, the capsular substance of bacteria is polysaccharide in nature, varying greatly in composition and complexity. The simplest are the homopolysaccharides—polymers of a single monosaccharide—that include the bacterial celluloses, levans, dextrans, and glucans. Most are more complex heteropolysaccharides, often with uronic acid as an additional constituent. The monomeric constituents of these polysaccharides include the neutral hexoses, especially D-glucose, D-galactose, and D-mannose; methyl pentoses, *e.g.*, L-fucose and L-rhamnose; polyols, *e.g.*, ribitol and glycerol; amino sugars; and the uronic acids already mentioned. Phosphorus is also

frequently present, especially in those polysaccharides containing polyols and resembling teichoic acids. The polysaccharide chains may be either linear or branched, which accounts in part for the differences in the physical nature of capsular materials.

The biosynthesis of most capsular polysaccharides appears to occur at the cytoplasmic membrane and involves nucleoside diphosphate sugars and isoprenoid lipid intermediates (Chapter 4); the products are then extruded

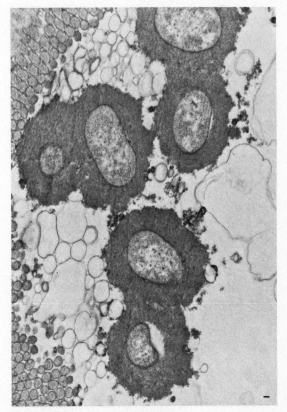

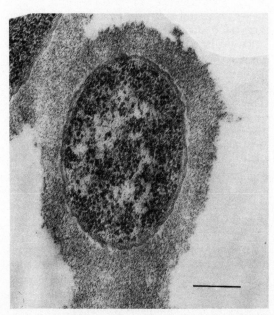

Figure 2–14. Thin section of encapsulated *Escherichia coli.* The capsule has been stabilized by treatment with specific anticapsular antibody before dehydration and embedding. Bar = 250 nm. (M. E. Bayer and H. Thurlow, J. Bacteriol. **130**:911, 1977.)

Figure 2–15. Electron micrograph of a ruthenium red–stained, antibody-stabilized preparation from the ileum of a neonatal calf infected with enterotoxigenic *Escherichia coli.* Note the antibody-stabilized glycocalyx surrounding the bacterial cells. Bar = 0.1 μm. (R. Chan, S. D. Acres and J. W. Costerton, Infect. Immun. **37**:1170–1180, 1982.)

to the extracellular location. In some cases, the synthesis is less complex, and the products, *e.g.*, dextrans and levans, are formed by extracellular processes that do not involve the nucleoside diphosphate sugars or lipid carriers. For example, the cell-free culture fluid of *Leuconostoc mesinteroides*, a bacterium associated with slime formation in sugar refining, polymerizes sucrose to form the dextran capsular substance.

In a few instances, notably in the genus *Bacillus*, the bacterial capsular substance is not polysaccharide but polypeptide in nature. That of the anthrax bacillus is a D-glutamyl polypeptide, while those of nonpathogenic *Bacillus* species contain both D and L isomers of glutamic acid; no polysaccharide appears to be present in these capsular materials.

Role of Bacterial Capsules. For many decades, interest in bacterial capsules centered upon their interference with ingestion of bacteria by the phagocytic cells of the body. It was generally known that the virulence of many encapsulated bacteria was directly associated with this property and that antibody specifically directed against the capsule could promote phagocytosis, with subsequent intracellular destruction of the invading bacterium (Chapter 12). Otherwise, the capsule, regarded simply as a secretory product of cellular metabolism, did not seem to be of great importance to the existence of the bacteria in nature.

This view has recently been challenged, and it now seems clear that capsules play a pivotal role in microbial ecology, not only in the host-parasite relationship, but in survival and growth in natural environments as well. Bacteria found in nature, whether derived from water or soil, from animal mucosal surfaces (*e.g.*, intestine), or from blood and tissues of infected hosts, almost always possess a capsular glycocalyx. Only after continued cultivation in artificial environments and cultures is the glycocalyx lost or diminished. The glycocalyces surrounding individual cells or composing the matrix surrounding microcolonies in these natural environments serve several purposes. Bacteria are protected from toxic heavy metals, from desiccation, and from bacterial viruses (bacteriophages) by their surrounding matrix. The anionic nature and physical structure of the glycocalyx also promotes the concentration of nutrients from the surrounding environment. Of perhaps greatest importance, however, is the adherence of encapsulated bacteria to inert surfaces in natural environments and to cells of an appropriate host in infection and disease, permitting the establishment of microcolonies with increased potential for survival and growth (Chapter 12).

When invading microorganisms gain entry to host tissues, the capsular material not only helps to protect the bacterium from phagocytosis, but in the case of gram-negative bacteria also offers resistance to the bactericidal action of complement and serum components (Chapter 12).

The Specific Capsular Reaction. As just noted, the capsular substance is usually immunogenic and the antibody induced reacts with the capsular substance. Antibody acts as an opsonin, promoting phagocytosis of the encapsulated bacteria, or as a precipitin, penetrating the capsular matrix and reacting with the fibrillar strands of polysaccharide. This microprecipitation alters the refractive index of the capsule so that it appears better defined and even swollen in wet unstained preparations observed microscopically. This **capsular swelling**, or **Quellung** reaction, was applied by Neufeld to the serological identification of pneumococci in 1902 and has subsequently been used in the serological identification and typing of a number of encapsulated bacteria, including *Streptococcus*, *Neisseria*, *Klebsiella*, *Haemophilus*, and *Yersinia*.

THE CELL ENVELOPE[4, 6, 12]

The bacterial cell proper is bounded by an integrated structure, the cell envelope, which is varied in complexity. In most cells the cell envelope consists of the cell wall proper and the underlying cytoplasmic membrane.

The occurrence of bacteria in shapes other than spherical is evidence of a rigidity of structure sufficient to withstand surface tension and the internal turgor of the cell. This rigidity, and the resulting cell shape, are largely attributed to the cell wall component. Both the cell wall and the underlying cytoplasmic membrane are demonstrable in electron micrographs of thin sections or in freeze-fracture preparations, as seen in Figure 2–16.

The bacterial cell may be disrupted by physical means and the resulting cell wall fragments dried from the frozen state. When these fragments are observed by electron microscopy, distortion is minimal and the walls retain their original size and shape (Fig. 2–17).

Mechanical Stability

Because of their cell wall, bacteria are, in general, resistant to mechanical disruption but

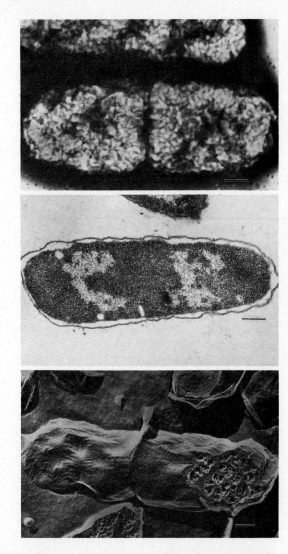

Figure 2–16. Comparative electron micrographs of *Escherichia coli. Top,* surface topography of cells after negative staining in silicotungstate. *Center,* thin-section after fixation with osmium tetroxide shows cell wall and underlying cytoplasmic membrane (evaporated during preparation). *Bottom,* freeze-etched preparation. The intact surface is shown on the left, the cytoplasmic membrane is exposed in the center, and cytoplasm is seen in the right portion. Bar = 250 nm. (M. E. Bayer and C. C. Remsen, J. Bacteriol. **101**:304–313, 1970.

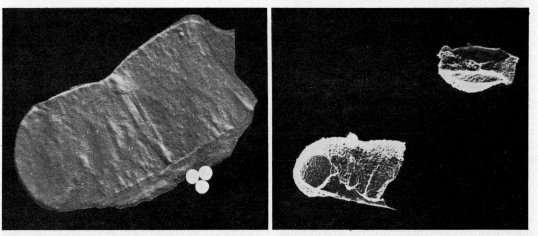

Figure 2–17. Cell walls of *Bacillus megaterium. Left,* an air-dried preparation which superficially exaggerates the size of the cell; the thickened band represents cell wall synthesized during the early stages of cell division, and the spherical particles are latex. ×11,500. *Right,* freeze-dried preparation showing the three-dimensional structure of the cell wall, corresponding more closely to the size of the intact cell. × 12,250. (M. J. R. Salton and R. C. Williams, Biochem. Biophys. Acta **14**:455, 1954.)

with considerable variation among different types. When subjected to shear forces or ultrasonic vibration, fragile organisms such as the cholera vibrio are easily disrupted within a few minutes. Others, such as staphylococci and streptococci, are highly resistant and may require treatment for up to one hour. In general, gram-positive bacteria are more difficult to disrupt by mechanical means than are gram-negative cells. This reflects differences in the architecture of their cell walls, as detailed below.

Nature of the Cell Envelope

Among bacteria, the nature of the cell envelope varies considerably in architectural complexity and degree of differentiation. The simplest in this respect, exemplified by members of the genus *Mycoplasma,* possess only a simple membrane as the outer limiting structure. This membrane, usually about 7.5 nm. in thickness, combines the function of both cell wall and cytoplasmic membrane, which it resembles. Such cells do not contain peptidoglycans (see below), and the limited cellular stability is presumably due to environmental factors.

The envelope structure of gram-positive bacteria is somewhat more complex. In addition to the cytoplasmic membrane enclosing the cytoplasm and appearing as a "double-track" membrane by electron microscopy of thin sections, the cell is surrounded by an amorphous cell wall. In profile, the cell wall does not exhibit the layered appearance of the cytoplasmic membrane and is considerably thicker, usually 15 to 50 nm.

The cell envelope of gram-negative bacteria has been most extensively studied and is considered the most complex. Typically, the envelope is made up of two parallel, multilayered membranes as observed in thin sections by electron microscopy. The inner, or cytoplasmic, membrane is similar to that seen in gram-positive cells. The cell wall is composed of a second or outer membrane, sometimes wrinkled in appearance. Closely apposed to the inner surface of this membrane, and often not visible as a separate layer, is a thin peptidoglycan layer. The gram-negative wall is usually about 10 to 15 nm. in thickness; it is, therefore, thinner than that of gram-positive bacteria. Figure 2–5 shows the relationship of cell envelope structures to other components of a typical bacterial cell. The insets in this figure demonstrate the basic architecture of gram-positive and gram-negative cell envelopes.

THE CYTOPLASMIC MEMBRANE[34, 51]

The cytoplasmic, or plasma, membrane is an indispensable structure of all bacterial cells. It lies on the inner surface of the cell wall and encloses the cytoplasm of the cell.

Bacterial cytoplasmic membranes are similar in composition and structure to other biological membranes and are made up of a phospholipid bilayer with proteins interspersed in the membrane. The membrane contains 50 to 75 per cent protein and 20 to 35 per cent lipid and makes up about 10 per cent of the dry weight of the cell.

The bilayered membrane, with a median hydrophobic zone, is traversed by proteins, many believed to be permeases involved in the active transport of small substrates, such as amino acids and carbohydrates, to the cell interior. Membrane structural proteins may be associated with either the inner or the outer leaflets of the membrane. Other proteins of the membrane are related to enzymatic functions, notably oxidative phosphorylation and macromolecular synthesis, including the synthesis of cell wall components. Within the inner leaflet, or cytoplasmic side of the membrane, are located enzymes associated with cytoplasmic functions.

The cytoplasmic membrane has little mechanical strength and does not contribute significantly to maintenance of cell shape, since rod-shaped cells tend to assume a spherical form after removal of the cell wall. The membrane is forced against the cell wall by internal hydrostatic pressure, as much as 20 atmospheres, corresponding to the osmotic pressure differential across the membrane. While the cytoplasmic membrane is a structure distinct from the cell wall, the two are joined by more than lateral cohesion, and available evidence suggests some sort of bonding or zones of adhesion between the two structures.

Mesosomes[25]

The cytoplasmic membrane may be invaginated to form internal organelles known as mesosomes. These can assume a vesicular, lamellar, or tubular form, and more than one type may be encountered in a single cell. In gross chemical composition mesosomes do not differ from the cytoplasmic membrane. They occur predominantly, and in all morphological forms, in gram-positive bacteria; in gram-negative cells they are typically of the lamellar type. Although many functions have been proposed for mesosomes, none have been firmly established. For example, mesosomes have been linked, largely on morphological grounds, with replication and apportionment of deoxyribonucleic acid to daughter cells during cell division. It has also been proposed, with some substantiating evidence, that mesosomes act as septum initiators during cell division.

PEPTIDOGLYCAN LAYER[52]

The shape and cellular rigidity of bacterial cells are due almost entirely to the presence of a large polymeric supporting structure that lies just external to the cytoplasmic membrane and has been variously called peptidoglycan, murein, mucopeptide, and glycosaminopeptide; current usage tends to favor peptidoglycan as the most descriptive term. Only a few bacterial forms—*Mycoplasma* and some marine halophiles—lack this structure.

The peptidoglycan layer may be envisioned as a single, large, bag-shaped macromolecule entirely surrounding the cytoplasmic elements of the cell. The peptidoglycan is composed of glycan strands cross-linked by short peptides. These glycan strands consist of repeating units of β-1,4-N-acetylglucosamine—β-1,4-N-acetylmuramic acid (see chemical structure, p. 100). Muramic acid, which is the 3-*O*-lactyl ether of D-glycosamine, appears to be peculiar to the peptidoglycans of bacterial cell walls. In individual glycan strands the chain length may vary between 10 and 64 disaccharide units. The detailed structure of peptidoglycan is illustrated on page 101 (Chapter 4).

The glycan strands are cross-linked by short peptide chains. The N-terminus of the peptide subunit is bound through the carboxyl group of muramic acid. The amino acid sequence is usually L-alanine—D-glutamine—L-diamino acid—D-alanine. In most cases, the diamino acid is *meso*-diaminopimelic acid. These peptide subunits of adjacent glycans are then joined directly through the unbound amino group of the diamino acid and the C-terminal of D-alanine, or indirectly through an interpeptide bridge. Although there is a remarkable degree of constancy in the composition of the glycan strands, different groups of bacteria show some variation in the composition of the interpeptide bridges and, to a lesser extent, in the peptide subunits.

The peptidoglycans are susceptible to the hydrolytic activities of a number of enzymes. The best known of these is lysozyme or N-acetylmuramidase. This enzyme hydrolyzes the glycosidic linkages between N-acetylmuramic acid and N-acetylglucosamine in the glycan strand. As would be expected, such enzymes can depolymerize the peptidoglycan and, in gram-positive bacteria particularly, lead to breakdown of the cell wall and subsequent lysis of the cell.

CELL WALL OF GRAM-POSITIVE BACTERIA[48]

Electron micrography of thin sections of gram-positive bacteria usually shows an amorphous, electron dense layer without a notable fine structure surrounding the cell. This cell wall is normally 15 to 50 nm. in thickness and constitutes 20 to 40 per cent of the dry weight of the cell. The cell wall of gram-positive bacteria is composed largely of peptidoglycan, and measurements of its thickness indicate a structure with 15 to 50 peptidoglycan layers, assuming a monolayer thickness of 1 nm.

Intercalated within the cell wall, or occurring as surface layers, are a variety of proteins, polysaccharides, and teichoic acids. Many of these surface components are immunologically specific substances as exemplified by the C polysaccharide and type-specific surface proteins of streptococci.

The teichoic acids of gram-positive cell walls merit special attention.[64] The teichoic acids are a group of cell wall and membrane constituents having several chemical similarities. The basic structure of the teichoic acids is that of a polymer of glycerol or ribitol units joined together by phosphodiester linkages (Chapter 4). D-alanine and carbohydrate substituents may be ether-linked to this linear backbone structure. In a few instances, sugar residues or N-acetylglucosamine are encountered as a part of the backbone structure. These teichoic acids occur in gram-positive bacteria as membrane-associated (glycerol-type) or wall-associated (either glycerol- or ribitol-type).

The membrane-associated teichoic acids are covalently linked to the glycolipids of the cytoplasmic membrane and are generally known as lipoteichoic acids. The glycolipid portion of the molecule is anchored in the outer leaflet of the membrane with hydrophilic polyglycerol phosphate chains extending outward into the cell wall, as illustrated in Figure 2–18. The wall-associated teichoic acids are covalently linked to the glycan chains of the peptidoglycans of the cell wall structure. Since these teichoic acids can participate in serological reactions, they may be partly exposed on the surface, or the wall may constitute an open

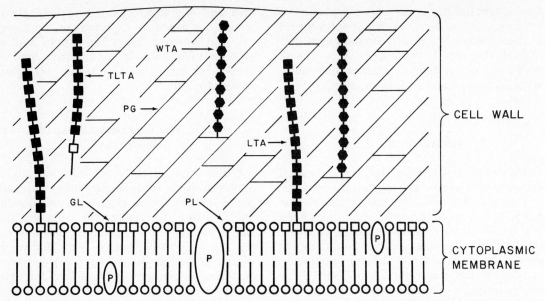

Figure 2–18. Model of the gram-positive cell wall. The cytoplasmic membrane is surrounded by the cell wall peptidoglycan *(PG)*. Lipoteichoic acids *(LTA)* are anchored to the cytoplasmic membrane; when released from the membrane, they are transient *(TLTA)* in the cell wall. The wall-associated teichoic acids *(WTA)* are linked to *PG*. *P,* proteins; *PL,* phospholipid; *GL,* glycolipid.

network that permits penetration by antibodies and other molecules.[18, 33] The teichoic acids probably serve to stabilize the cell wall and maintain its association with the cytoplasmic membrane. They are believed to contribute to magnesium binding and thus maintain proper ionic conditions for cation-dependent enzymes in the cell envelope. Since they behave as cation-binding polymers, they can act as ion-exchangers in a manner similar to that described for polysaccharides of the glycocalyx. Their presence at the cell surface may also permit them to participate in the mucosal attachment and adherence of gram-positive cells in pathogenesis (Chapter 12).

Although not usually immunogenic in the isolated state, teichoic acids induce specific antibody formation when combined with other cell constituents in the whole cell. They are therefore important as surface antigenic components in many gram-positive bacteria.

The topography of the outer surface of bacterial cells is of considerable interest in that it provides insight into the localization of wall components.[57] In this regard, thin-sectioning has not been particularly informative, but negative staining or freeze-etching often reveals regular arrays of macromolecules on the cell surface, designated the S layer. Most of these surface patterns in gram-positive bacteria consist of subunit arrays with tetragonal symmetry, with center-to-center spacing ranging from

about 7 to 16 nm. These seem to be composed of single subunit species, usually protein, and normally cover the entire surface of the cell. Relatively few bacteria have been thoroughly examined for S layers, and their function is largely obscure, although a barrier function seems reasonable.

CELL WALL OF GRAM-NEGATIVE BACTERIA[5]

The cell walls of gram-negative cells have proved to be considerably more complex than those of gram-positive bacteria and have been more extensively studied. Electron micrographs of thin sections usually show an electron-translucent zone immediately external to the cytoplasmic membrane. This zone is, in turn, enclosed by a double-track membrane, the outer membrane. Whether this "space" between the cytoplasmic and outer membranes actually exists in the intact cell is problematical. At any rate, the peptidoglycan layer is found between these two membranes as a part of what has been termed the periplasmic zone.

The cell wall of gram-negative bacteria is somewhat thinner than that of gram-positive cells. The peptidoglycan layer is 3 to 8 nm. thick, while the outer membrane generally ranges between 6 and 10 nm. in thickness and is often wavy or undulating in appearance.

Also in contrast to gram-positive cells, the gram-negative cell wall constitutes only about 20 per cent of the dry weight of the cell and contains significant quantities of lipids, approximately 20 per cent of the dry weight of the cell wall.

Periplasmic Zone

This is regarded as an enzyme-containing compartment located between the outer and cytoplasmic membranes. The outer membrane acts as a molecular sieve to retain enzymes, principally hydrolases, in this zone. Also occupying the zone is the thin peptidoglycan layer, responsible for the morphological control of the cell. The peptidoglycan layer is joined to the outer membrane by lipoproteins.

Outer Membrane[15, 43]

The outer membrane of gram-negative bacteria is similar in morphology and constitution to other biological membranes, including the underlying cytoplasmic membrane. Compared to the cytoplasmic membrane, the outer membrane contains less phospholipid and fewer proteins, but possesses a unique constituent, bacterial lipopolysaccharide. The outer membrane appears in electron micrographs as an electron-translucent middle layer sandwiched between two electron-dense outer layers.

This membrane constitutes the external layer of most gram-negative bacteria and is functionally distinct. It behaves as a hydrophobic diffusion barrier against a variety of substances, it contains receptors for bacteriophages and bacteriocins, it participates in conjugation and in cell division, and it contains a number of systems mediating the uptake of nutrients and passive diffusion of small molecules into the periplasmic space. In concert with the thin peptidoglycan layer, the outer membrane lends structural integrity to the bacterial cell.

Lipopolysaccharide. Occurring as a part of the outer membrane are the lipopolysaccharides, which are unique to gram-negative bacteria and are important structural and functional components of the cell surface. Lipopolysaccharides are the major surface antigenic components, the somatic O antigens, and are responsible for the endotoxic activity of gram-negative cells (Chapter 12). These high molecular weight complexes may be regarded as having three regions: a lipid portion, termed lipid A; a core polysaccharide which may be similar within a genus; and a specific polysaccharide region, the O-specific chains.

Lipopolysaccharides are represented diagrammatically:

O-Specific Side Chains	Core Region	Lipid A

The O-specific chains project from the surface of the outer membrane and thus protect the cell from the action of antibody and complement by preventing their intimate contact with the outer membrane.

The lipid A region is believed to be responsible for the endotoxin activity of bacterial lipopolysaccharide. This lipid portion of the complex is oriented in the hydrophobic zone of the outer membrane.

Outer Membrane Proteins. Many of the properties of the outer membrane described above are attributable to the proteins that occur within the membrane. Those proteins present in greatest amounts are designated major outer membrane proteins, although they comprise only a few different protein species. The major proteins may be divided into three groups: the pore-forming proteins or porins, the nonporin proteins, and the lipoproteins.

The proteins of the gram-negative outer membrane act generally to facilitate the permeation of solutes through the membrane. The simplest, or matrix porins, form transmembrane channels through which flow hydrophilic solutes of low molecular weight; solutes do not interact with the porins in this passive permeation. Other porins have more specific permeation functions and, in some instances, may interact with the substrate as a part of its translocation through the membrane. Porins are thought to have a trimer subunit structure that spans the entire outer membrane.

Nonporin proteins are not as well understood as the porins. Some are known to span the outer membrane and to be associated with the peptidoglycan layer. These proteins may serve as receptors for a variety of ligands, regulate exopolysaccharide biosynthesis, or serve to stabilize the cell envelope.

The lipoproteins are the smallest of the outer membrane proteins, but often occur in the greatest number. Lipoproteins are often covalently bound to the peptidoglycan and are then an essential component for stabilization of the cell envelope. The role of free, or unbound, lipoprotein is not yet established.

The relationships of gram-negative cell envelope components are diagrammed in Figure 2–19.

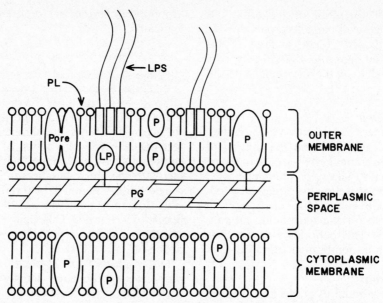

Figure 2–19. Model of the gram-negative cell envelope. In the outer membrane, the lipopolysaccharide *(LPS)* is located in the outer leaflet, with the polysaccharide portion projecting from the membrane surface. The outer leaflet contains relatively smaller amounts of phospholipid *(PL)*. The pore structure traverses the outer membrane and is a protein trimer. The outer membrane is anchored to the peptidoglycan *(PG)* layer through lipoproteins *(LP)* and certain proteins *(P)*.

Topography of the Cell Surface.[4, 57] The topography of the cell surface of gram-negative cells, like that of gram-positive bacteria, has not been completely elucidated. The S, or surface, layers are often present, but are predominantly hexagonal in symmetry; otherwise their morphology and constitution are similar to the gram-positive cell structures. An example of such surface structures is shown in Figure 2–20. The surface of many gram-nega-tive cells is wrinkled or rugose in appearance when negatively stained, as displayed in Figure 2–16.

FUNCTION OF THE CELL ENVELOPE

Osmotic Regulation[49]

While the cell wall and cytoplasmic membrane are distinct and artificially separable

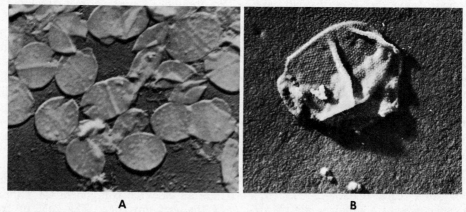

A   B

Figure 2–20. Cell wall preparations. *A,* Unwashed cell walls of *Streptococcus faecalis* prepared in the Mickle apparatus, showing the splitting of the cell wall which allows the contents to escape, the small electron-dense bodies adhering to the cell wall, and the thickened bands occurring in the early stages of cell division. × 12,000. *B,* Freeze-dried preparation of the cell wall of *Rhodospirillum rubrum* showing the surface arrays on the cell wall of this microorganism. × 42,000. *(A,* M. J. R. Salton and R. W. Horne, Biochem. Biophys. Acta 7:177, 1951; *B,* M. J. R. Salton and R. C. Williams, Biochem. Biophys. Acta **14**:455, 1954.)

structures, in the bacterial cell they make up an integrated unit. Together their function is, in part, that of an osmotic barrier and regulatory system separating the cell plasma from the suspending medium and implementing the relatively isolated environment required by free-living organisms.

The contribution of the cell wall to this joint function is largely that of a supporting structure, but in gram-negative bacteria the outer membrane also contributes to the permeability of the intact cell. The outer membrane is only slightly permeable to hydrophobic solutes, presumably attributable to the lipopolysaccharide component. It is also a barrier to hydrophilic solutes with molecular weights of about 1000 daltons or more. While this is not essential to the physiological economy of the cell (see below), it does provide some protection against substances of high molecular weight, including antibodies and lytic enzymes. The cytoplasmic membrane functions as the significant osmotic barrier of the cell and exhibits the usual properties of living semipermeable membranes — selective permeability and the transport of substances across the barrier against concentration gradients.

Membrane Transport[28, 49, 50]

Many low molecular weight solutes equilibrate across bacterial membranes by an energy-dependent mechanism of either passive or facilitated diffusion; the process may or may not involve specific recognition by porin proteins (see above). Most solutes, however, enter the cell by more complex mechanisms. In these cases, the solute accumulates intracellularly against a concentration gradient. If the solute is not modified and energy is required, the

process is known as **active transport**. The process of active solute transport may be considered in three parts: binding of the solute to a receptor or recognition site, translocation of the complex across the membrane, and coupling of these transport systems to metabolic energy sources. Energy sources may be chemical, chemiosmotic, or electrical, interconverted by proton translocating transport systems in the membrane.

Receptor binding or recognition of solutes is associated with the presence of certain binding proteins. In gram-negative bacteria these are located in the periplasmic space. In translocation, the solute-carrier complex probably undergoes a conformational change, which promotes a transfer through the cytoplasmic membrane; energy may or may not be required.

Active transport mechanisms are largely responsible for transport of ions, amino acids, and sugars into bacterial cells. Many of the sugars and amino acids are transported into the cell without metabolic alterations. Some sugars, however, may be phosphorylated and transfer accomplished by a phosphotransferase system, a process known as **group translocation**.

Bacterial Protoplasts[63]

Upon enzymatic degradation of the peptidoglycan layer of the living bacterial cell, *e.g.*, by treatment of gram-positive bacteria with lysozyme, a protoplast is formed. The cell first swells, and the protoplasm becomes partially detached from the disintegrating cell wall; following complete dissolution of the cell wall, the cell content assumes the spherical shape of the protoplast (Fig. 2–21), with the cell pro-

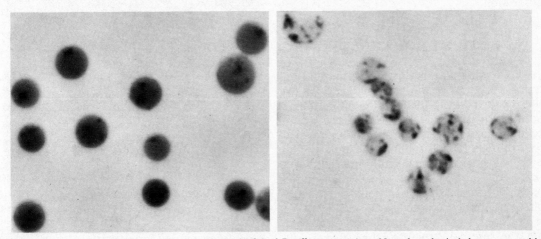

Figure 2–21. Protoplasts *(left)* and protoplast ghosts *(right)* of *Bacillus megaterium*. Note the spherical shape assumed by the bacillary form on dissolution of the cell wall. Phase contrast photomicrographs. × 3000. (C. Weibull, J. Bacteriol. **66**:696, 1953.)

toplasm enclosed in the cytoplasmic membrane.

The protoplast is a fragile structure because the cytoplasmic membrane has little mechanical strength. When the wall of gram-positive cells is removed by enzymatic dissolution in physiological saline, the protoplasts break up almost as soon as they are formed, first to an empty membrane or "ghost," followed by fragmentation of the membrane. Sucrose, polyethylene glycol, sodium chloride, or phosphate buffers can act as stabilizing agents. If the cell wall is removed from cells suspended in solutions of these agents, the protoplast can be stable for a period of several hours. Stabilized protoplasts suspended in sucrose solution with magnesium salts may be lysed by reduction of the sucrose concentration to give stable "ghosts." Gram-negative cells behave in a somewhat different manner. The outer membrane is ordinarily impervious to lytic enzymes such as lysozyme. If the membrane is modified by treatment with ethylenediamine tetraacetic acid, the lysozyme gains access to the peptidoglycan layer. The cell is then transformed to a spherical body, but the residual outer membrane serves in a slightly protective role. Termed **spheroplasts**, these forms are somewhat less osmotically fragile than protoplasts. Spheroplasts may also be induced by agents such as penicillin that interfere with the synthesis of peptidoglycan.

Physiological studies on stabilized protoplasts have shown that the competency of the intact cell persists, to a major extent, in the protoplast. The protoplast is, however, significantly impaired in growth and division and in those functions that require the participation of cell wall receptors, such as bacteriophage adsorption.

INTERNAL STRUCTURES[11]

The dividing line between external and internal structures of the bacterial cell is not a sharp one and is justified on little more than a utilitarian basis. Thus, the protoplast is a subcellular element, yet flagella remain attached to it through their basal bodies. Similarly, the bacterial spore is formed within the cell, but it represents a stage in the life history of the bacterium rather than a subcellular structure in the ordinarily accepted sense.

Enclosed within the cytoplasmic membrane are the internal structures that include the cytoplasm, with a variety of intracytoplasmic inclusions and submicroscopic particulates; the bacterial nucleus or nucleoid; and, in some, the bacterial spore.

THE BACTERIAL NUCLEUS[46]

It has been noted above that most actively growing bacterial cells stain uniformly with basic dyes. This basophilic property is indicative of the relatively large amounts of nucleic acid in the cell. These ordinary simple stains do not, of course, distinguish between ribonucleic acids (RNA) of the cytoplasm and the deoxyribonucleic acids (DNA) of the genetic apparatus. The DNA may be demonstrated if the RNA is selectively removed by mild acid hydrolysis or by treatment with ribonuclease. Subsequent staining with appropriate basic dyes, such as Giemsa, reveals the masses of DNA, or **chromatinic bodies**, illustrated in Figure 2–22.

The persisting identity of a given strain of bacteria is evidence of a hereditary-controlling mechanism, and it is clear that the DNA-containing chromatinic bodies are nuclei with respect to function. There are often two or more such structures in actively growing cells, since cell division usually lags behind nuclear division. These procaryotic nucleoids are simple in structure and are not enclosed within a limiting membrane (Fig. 2–23).

The morphology of the bacterial nucleus or nucleoid has been deduced from genetic and biochemical studies combined with electron microscopy, as detailed in Chapter 6. The

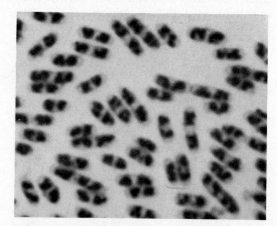

Figure 2–22. Light microscope photomicrograph of a two and one-half hour culture of *Escherichia coli*, fixed with osmium tetroxide vapor and alcoholic mercuric chloride, hydrolyzed at 56° to 60° C. with normal hydrochloric acid, and stained with Giemsa. The deeply staining bodies are chromatinic bodies. (Robinow.)

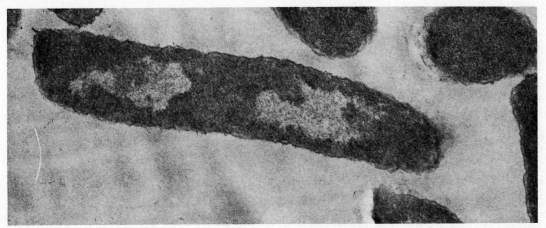

Figure 2–23. The DNA chromatinic bodies in *Escherichia coli* K-12S during the exponential growth phase. Note the apparent lack of a limiting membrane. Section fixed in osmium tetroxide; ×40,000. (Kellenberger.)

entire genome of the cell is contained in a single DNA duplex that, when fully extended, is 100 to 1400 μm. long, with the individual genetic determinants arranged in linear order along its length. Experiments that involve release of the DNA and subsequent spreading and disentanglement of the molecule have revealed that the chromosome is **circular** in structure. In the cell, the circular DNA exists in a supercoiled configuration, a property that results in decreased viscosity as well as decreased sensitivity to shear forces; this configuration is apparently stabilized by association with the cytoplasmic membrane. As seen in electron microscopy of ultrathin sections, bacterial nucleoids appear as fibrillar masses, representing the condensed and folded DNA (Fig. 2–23). When the cell is lysed and the DNA is spread onto supporting film under appropriate conditions, the presence of loops can be discerned.

CYTOPLASM[32]

The cytoplasm of bacterial cells appears to be much less complex than that of eucaryotic cells. The endocytoplasmic reticulum of eucaryotic cells is absent, although gram-positive bacterial cells may possess a fine fibrous network that is not clearly differentiated.

The cytoplasm may be viewed as a gel containing ribosomes, enzymes, and, frequently, granules that may represent storage products.

Cytoplasmic Inclusions[53]

Many procaryotic cells contain a variety of cytoplasmic granules that can be seen by both light and electron microscopy. The most com-

monly observed are those that stain with certain basic dyes and are variously termed **volutin**, **metachromatic**, or **Babès-Ernst granules**. These are readily observed in corynebacteria when stained with alkaline methylene blue or toluidine blue (Fig. 2–24) and as polar granules in other bacteria, such as plague bacilli fixed with methanol before staining (Fig. 2–25).

These granules are primarily composed of polyphosphate, often of high molecular weight. The spherical granules are not membrane bound and are quite variable in size, depending upon the particular organism and the aggregational state of the particles. They are found in greatest number during exponen-

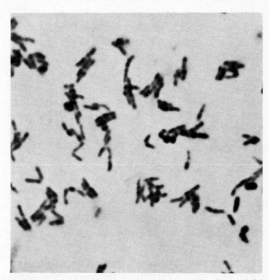

Figure 2–24. Metachromic granules and bipolar staining in the diphtheria bacillus. Note the differences between these organisms and the plague bacillus (Fig. 2–25). Methylene blue; × 1975.

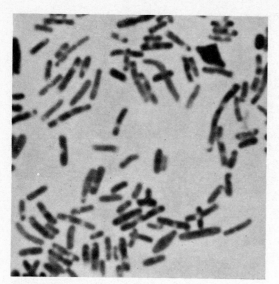

Figure 2–25. Irregular and bipolar staining of the plague bacillus. Note the heavily stained areas and metachromatic granules. Fixed in methyl alcohol and stained with methylene blue; × 2400.

tial growth, diminishing in later growth phases or when phosphates are limited. Functionally, the polymers conserve phosphate, and may also serve for energy storage.

Many bacterial cells store polysaccharide as granular inclusions. Polysaccharide granules are composed of high molecular weight, branched polymers of glucose resembling glycogen or amylopectin. Like volutin granules, they are not usually enclosed by membranes; they range in size from 20 to 100 nm.

Somewhat more complex in nature are the membrane-enclosed granules containing polymers of β-hydroxybutyrate. These granules, somewhat larger than polysaccharide granules, are surrounded by a single-layered, protein membrane. They are regarded as storehouses for energy and reutilizable carbon. These inclusions are morphologically similar to the lipid deposits seen by light microscopy after staining with Sudan black and certain other basic dyes.

Submicroscopic Particles

In addition to the above inclusion granules, bacterial protoplasm contains minute granules or particulates that are separable from the soluble constituents of the cell by ultracentrifugation of lysates. These particles are not seen in electron micrographs of ultrathin sections, but are observed in freeze-etched preparations.

Ultracentrifugal analysis of lysates of disrupted bacterial cells, exclusive of such large fragments as cell wall and inclusion granules, consistently shows several distinct macromolecular components. There is usually a broad, slowly moving band at 5 S, and peaks at 8 S, 20 to 30 S, and 40 S. The 5 S fraction is a heterogeneous mixture of substances making up the ground material of the cytoplasm. The 8 S fraction contains the major portion, 80 to 90 per cent, of the cellular DNA, suggesting that the DNA is quite fragile and is fragmented by these procedures. This fraction also contains the unstructured RNA of the cytoplasm. The majority of the RNA is found in the remaining fractions; ribosomes are present in the 20 to 30 S and the 40 S fractions.

Ribosomes.[8, 26, 38, 42] Of the submicroscopic particulates, the ribosomes have been of special interest, since they are intimately associated with protein synthesis, so much so that they cannot be considered apart from this function.

The cytoplasmic RNA of the bacterial cell is of three kinds with respect to function, *viz.*, **ribosomal RNA** (rRNA); amino acid transfer, or **transfer RNA** (tRNA); and **messenger RNA** (mRNA). Of these, the rRNA makes up about 80 per cent of the total cell RNA. All three kinds of RNA are synthesized on the complementary templates of nuclear DNA.

The rRNA-containing particulates are of four sizes—the 30 S, 50 S, and 70 S particles, and aggregates of the 70 S particles joined by attachment to a common strand of mRNA. In general, the 70 S particle is considered to be the ribosome, the 30 S and 50 S particles to be subunits of the ribosome, and the larger aggregates to be polyribosomes or polysomes. Recent studies have established that the ribosomal subunits are not exactly spherical, but have an irregular shape. Apparent dimensions differ with the techniques of measurement, but electron microscopy suggests approximate dimensions of 80 × 100 × 190 Å for the 30 S subunit and 160 × 200 × 230 Å for the 50 S subunit.

About two-thirds of the mass of the ribosome is rRNA; the remainder is protein. In *Escherichia coli*, 21 distinct proteins are demonstrable in the 30 S particle and at least 31 proteins in the 50 S particle. Certain of these proteins appear to be functional with respect to protein synthesis, and others may be important in ribosomal assembly through protein-protein and protein-RNA interactions.

The subunits, ribosomes, and polysomes act during the cyclic process of protein synthesis. The cycle is initiated by the formation of a complex of the 30 S subunit with mRNA and formyl-methionyl tRNA. With the attachment to mRNA, the complex is joined by a 50 S subunit, and as the ribosomes are formed and attached to a common strand of mRNA, the polysome is formed.

There are many kinds of tRNA in that there are one to four kinds for each of the amino acids. The amino acid is activated by a specific enzyme, and transferred to specific tRNA. The mRNA functions as the template for protein synthesis, *i.e.,* determines the order of amino acids in the peptide chain; there are many different kinds of mRNA, each corresponding to a specific protein. Operatively, the appropriate tRNA-amino acid complexes associate with the predetermined sites on the mRNA template, each amino acid residue being brought into place by its tRNA and inserted into the peptide chain. As additional ribosomes become attached to the mRNA strand, apparently moving from one end to another, there is a continuous synthesis of protein in various stages of development at the points of ribosome attachment. Upon reaching the end of the mRNA strand, the ribosome and the peptide are released. The 70 S particle tends to become dissociated to give rise to a subunit pool from which the 70 S complex and polysomes recur in the cycle of protein synthesis.

THE BACTERIAL SPORE[1, 19, 20, 23]

The bacterial spore, or endospore, is a refractile, oval body formed within the bacterial cell; it represents a dormant and highly resistant stage in the life history of the bacterium. Its high resistance to injury serves to carry the bacterial species through unfavorable circumstances and therefore has survival value. Spore formation is uncommon among bacteria and is confined largely to bacilli. The aerobic spore-forming bacilli make up the genus *Bacillus,* while the obligate anaerobic or microaerophilic bacilli that form spores are members of the genus *Clostridium.* Both are widely distributed in nature. Because it represents a primitive form of differentiation, spore formation is of interest to the cell biologist, but in a practical sense the resistance of spores to physical and chemical agents dictates the sterilization procedures employed by all who are concerned with microorganisms and their activities.

The bacterial spore is a complex structure formed within the parent bacterial cell (sporangium). In the usual stained smear, spores may be seen intracellularly or, after disintegration of the vegetative parent, lying extracellularly (Fig. 2–26). Within the vegetative cell, the spore is an oblate spheroid with its long axis parallel to that of the bacillus. Its breadth may be essentially the same as the width of the parent cell, or it may be greater, bulging the vegetative cell wall. The latter appearance is most commonly seen in the genus *Clostridium* and is the basis for its name (Gr. *klōstēr,* spindle).

The relative size of the spore is constant, and its location reasonably so, within species.

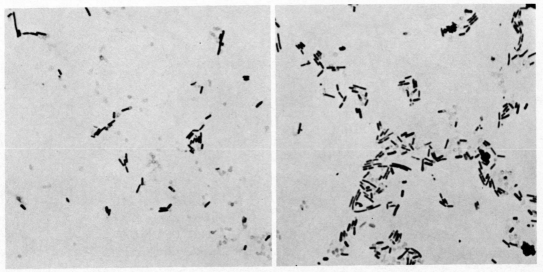

Figure 2–26. Spore formation by bacteria. *Left, Clostridium botulinum* type B, showing the typical endospores separated from disintegrated vegetative cells. *Right, Clostridium sporogenes,* showing a subterminal clostridial spore. These preparations are all stained with a single stain in the usual way; the vegetative cells take up the dye, but the spores remain unstained. Fuchsin; × 1050.

It may be located in the center of the vegetative cell (central), or it may be found part way between the center and end of the cell (subterminal), or it may occur at the end of the cell (terminal). Its size and location result in a characteristic morphology, *e.g.*, the large terminal spore of the tetanus bacillus gives the spore-containing vegetative cell a drumstick appearance.

Spores may be observed in the living state by phase-contrast microscopy. They do not stain, however, by usual methods, requiring heat for stain penetration. Once stained, they are generally difficult to decolorize with reagents such as alcohol, acid-alcohol, or acetone-alcohol. Consequently, differential staining is a simple matter; the smear may be stained with hot carbol-fuchsin, decolorized with alcohol, and counterstained with a contrasting dye, such as methylene blue, to give a red spore in a blue vegetative cell.

In electron micrographs of thin-sectioned or freeze-etched preparations, the spore is seen as a complex organelle (Figs. 2–27, 2–28, and 2–29). The spore protoplast, with a limiting membrane analogous to the cytoplasmic membrane of the vegetative cell, is surrounded by the cortex, a loosely woven, modified peptidoglycan layer of variable thickness. The cortex is enclosed in one or more complex protein layers, which constitute the spore coat; coat proteins are unique to the spore and are not found in vegetative cells. Finally, the mature spore may be surrounded by a thin, often loosely fitting, bag-like exosporium. A diagrammatic section of the spore is illustrated in Figure 2–30.

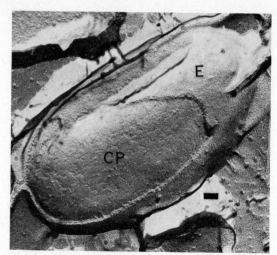

Figure 2–28. Electron micrograph of a freeze-etched spore of *Bacillus cereus*. The exosporium *(E)* is cleaved off the cross-patched *(CP)* coat layer. Bar = 100 nm. (A. I. Aronson and P. Fitz-James, Bact. Rev. **40**:360–402, 1976.)

Dormancy[23]

Bacterial endospores are physiologically dormant, often extremely so. In many cases there is no detectable endogenous metabolism; in others, glucose may be oxidized and a few other enzymatic reactions detected. It is clear that the spore has the necessary metabolic machinery for germination and outgrowth (see below), but these systems may be in an inactive state. It is thought that dormancy may be associated with the presence of a unique spore constituent, dipicolinic acid (pyridine 2,6-dicarboxylic acid), which chelates calcium and results in the high calcium content of spores.

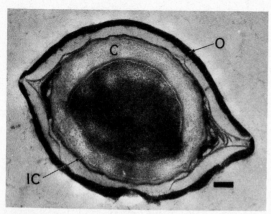

Figure 2–27. Thin-section of a *Bacillus megatherium* spore, showing two spore coats (*IC*, inner coat; *O*, outer coat). The germ cell wall of the spore coat is seen immediately underlying the thick cortex *(C)*. Bar = 100 nm. (A. I. Aronson and P. Fitz-James, Bact. Rev. **40**:360–402, 1976.)

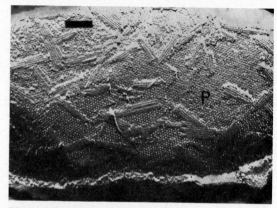

Figure 2–29. *Bacillus cereus* treated with sodium sulfite during coat formation to inhibit formation of the outer CP layer (see Fig. 2–28), revealing the inner coat *(P)* layer. Bar = 100 nm. (A. E. Aronson and P. Fitz-James, Bact. Rev. **40**:360–402, 1976.)

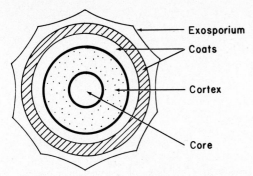

Figure 2–30. Diagrammatic representation of a typical endospore.

Resistance

The spore is an extremely resistant stage in bacterial development. Not only is the spore relatively impermeable to dyes, but it is also much more resistant than vegetative cells to the injurious effects of heat, desiccation, hydrostatic pressure, and many chemical agents.

Sterilization procedures (Chapter 5) are necessarily directed toward the destruction of ubiquitous microbial spores. Some, such as those organisms causing flat sours in canned foods, may be extremely resistant to heat and require autoclaving at 121°C. for as long as 3 hours to insure destruction. Most are not this resistant and are killed by moist heat at 115°C. to 120°C. for 15 to 20 minutes. Still others are destroyed by boiling for a short time, but few if any are killed by treatment at 58°C. to 60°C. for 30 minutes, a procedure that destroys most vegetative cells. They are also quite resistant to desiccation; the classic example is that of the viability, after 60 years, of anthrax spores dried on silk threads in Koch's laboratory.

The ratio of the concentration of bactericidal compounds lethal to the vegetative cell to that lethal for the spore is of the order of 10^3 to 10^4 for many disinfectants such as hypochlorites and phenols. Interesting and significant exceptions are the alkylating agents, including ethylene oxide, for which the ratio ranges from 0.5 to 15.

Heat resistance of bacterial spores is thought to be due to reduced amounts of water in the dense core structure. Whether the lowered water content is due to cortex contraction or expansion is not yet established, but in either case the result is a compression of the core that regulates its state of hydration and thereby its relative resistance to elevated temperatures.

Sporogenesis

Spore formation presents a relatively simple model for cell differentiation and morphoge-

nesis, a fact that has spurred recent research into this phenomenon.

In general, spores are formed most readily under optimal conditions for growth of the vegetative cell, and spore formation begins toward the end of, or just following, the phase of exponential growth (Chapter 3).

The effects of environmental conditions on spore formation vary from one kind of bacterium to another. For example, the anthrax bacillus forms spores only under aerobic conditions; spores are not found in the tissues of infected animals because of insufficient free oxygen. The temperature of incubation may also be a factor; it is common knowledge that aerobic sporulating bacilli fail to form spores when grown at maximum temperatures tolerated for growth. In fact, permanently asporogenous variants can be produced by continued cultivation at maximum growth temperatures.

The initiation of sporogenesis in actively growing cells is usually induced by depletion of nutrients, most often carbon or nitrogen sources, but occasionally by phosphate starvation. Cytological, biochemical, and genetic studies have shown that sporulation follows a multistage succession of events resulting in the release of a mature spore from the sporangium.[17, 47] The stages of sporulation are diagrammed in Figure 2–31.

Only one spore is formed by a single cell, and spore formation cannot be regarded as a method of multiplication. The spore is known to contain antigens, probably coat proteins, that are not present in the vegetative cell; sporulation is, therefore, more than just assembly and concentration of vegetative cell components. Spore antigens are specific in that spores from immunologically distinct vegetative cell species do not share common spore antigens.

Germination

When the spore is placed in an environment favorable to the growth of vegetative cells, it germinates, *i.e.*, dormancy is broken, and the cell begins a new vegetative cycle, or outgrowth. The first step in germination is activation of the spore, which is usually accomplished experimentally by short exposure to sublethal temperatures, by treatment with oxidizing agents, or by treatment at low pH. Germination, a rapid, irreversible, degradative process, may then be induced by a variety of stimulants, including amino acids, nucleosides, or glucose.

The first microscopic evidence of germination is a change in spore refractility, accom-

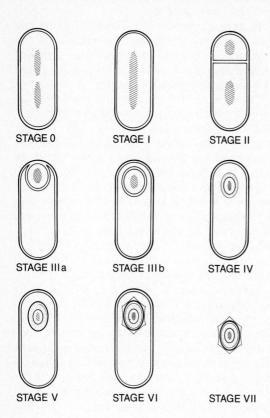

STAGE 0   STAGE I   STAGE II

STAGE IIIa   STAGE IIIb   STAGE IV

STAGE V   STAGE VI   STAGE VII

Figure 2–31. The stages of sporulation in bacteria. At initiation of sporulation the growing vegetative cell contains two chromosomes (Stage 0), which subsequently condense to a single broad filament that characterizes Stage I. As Stage II begins, the chromosomes separate and one moves terminally in the cell. This is followed by the formation of a septum between the two, but without cell wall formation. Near the end of this stage, two daughter protoplasts of unequal size are contained in the cell envelope. In Stage III the larger of the protoplasts engulfs the smaller; the smaller protoplast, or forespore, then lies within the cytoplasm of the larger and is surrounded by two membranes. The outer, or forespore membrane, is "inside-out," since it is derived from the larger protoplast. Stage IV is characterized by the development of the cortex between the two membranes. During this stage the spore becomes refractile to transmitted light. The multiple layers of the spore coat are laid down during Stage V; the spore continues to mature in Stage VI and becomes increasingly resistant to heat. The release of the spore occurs in Stage VII when the mother cell lyses.

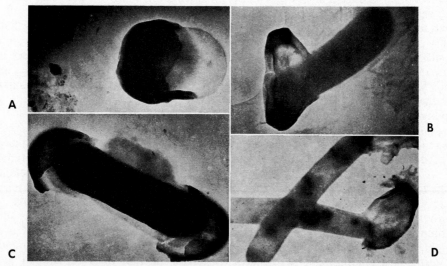

A   B   C   D

Figure 2–32. Electron micrographs illustrating the process of germination of spores of *Bacillus mycoides*. In *A* the vegetative cell is just beginning to emerge from the spore case. In *B* the vegetative cell is growing out of the side of the spore case and in *C* has broken the case into two parts. In *D* germination is complete. The darker areas in the vegetative cells are regarded by some as nucleus-like in nature. (*D*, G. Knaysi and R. F. Baker, J. Bacteriol. **53**:539, 1947; *A, B, C*, G. Knaysi, R. F. Baker, and J. Hillier, J. Bacteriol. **53**:525, 1947.)

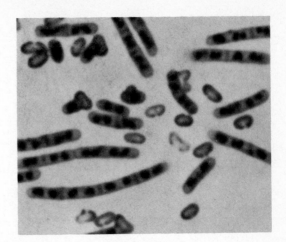

Figure 2–33. Recently germinated vegetative cells of *Bacillus mesentericus*, showing discarded spore cases. Note the cell boundaries in the long filaments made up of cells attached end to end. The deeply staining areas are chromatinic bodies. Osmium tetroxide-hydrochloric acid fixation, Giemsa; × 4000. (Robinow.)

panied by increased permeability to dyes and loss of heat resistance. Depending upon the bacterial species, the spore wall may become thin and stretch to assume the shape of the bacterial cell. In other instances, the vegetative cell emerges from the split spore casing, which is cast off as an empty hull (Figs. 2–32 and 2–33). The anthrax bacillus grows out of one side of the spore integument, whereas the closely related *Bacillus subtilis* grows out of opposite sides of its spore casing simultaneously. Irregularities may occur in germination, even in the same bacterial species.

Physiologically, germination occurs in several steps. The presence of a stimulant triggers the initial reaction, followed by activation of enzymes which degrade the cortex, releasing peptides, calcium, and dipicolinic acid.

As outgrowth begins, ribonucleic acid synthesis is initiated, followed closely by protein synthesis and later by deoxyribonucleic acid synthesis, signaling the start of a new vegetative cycle. Thus, outgrowth represents a successive series of degradative, energy-yielding, and biosynthetic events.

The Taxonomy of Bacteria[7, 21]

From the time of their discovery, the taxonomic position of bacteria has been a matter of controversy. Some microorganisms, such as the fungi, are clearly part of the plant kingdom, while others, commonly referred to as the animal parasites, are unicellular or multicellular forms belonging to the animal kingdom. For a long period, bacteria were considered to represent simple forms of the plant and, in some cases, the animal kingdoms.

When cytochemical and physiological studies led to a clear delineation of the two general patterns of cellular organization—procaryotes and eucaryotes—a conceptual basis was established for bacterial taxonomy. These concepts are formalized in the taxonomic system of *Bergey's Manual of Determinative Bacteriology*,[9] in which bacteria and the blue-green algae are placed in the Kingdom Procaryotae. A summary of the classification of bacteria of medical importance is presented in Table 2–3. The classifications of medically important fungi

and animal parasites are discussed in Chapters 43 and 44, while that of viruses is summarized in Chapter 38.

Although the interrelationships among bacteria present problems that are in many ways new to the taxonomist, certain "natural" groups are apparent. Of these, the most obvious is that based on division into spherical, rod-shaped, and spiral forms, and subdivisions based on size, ultrastructure, and staining reactions. Earlier classifications were constructed on these foundations and exerted a strong influence on modern taxonomy.

Morphology is, however, an inadequate framework for separation of bacterial species, for many morphologically similar bacteria differ markedly in other respects. Physiological differences, generally readily determined in the laboratory, have been widely used.

Beyond such primary subdivisions, classification becomes increasingly difficult, and attempts to provide a sound basis for bacterial

Table 2–3. **Classification of Medically Important Bacteria***

Vernacular Name	Family	Genus	Principal Disease Entity
The Spirochetes	Spirochetaceae	Treponema	Syphilis; yaws; pinta
		Borrelia	Relapsing fever
		Leptospira	Leptospirosis; infectious jaundice
Spiral and Curved Bacteria	Spirillaceae	Spirillum	Rat-bite fever
		Campylobacter	Enteritis and other human infections; animal abortions
Gram-Negative Aerobic Rods	Pseudomonadaceae	Pseudomonas	Opportunistic infections; melioidosis; glanders
	Legionellaceae	Legionella	Acute respiratory illness
	Uncertain Affiliation	Brucella	Undulant fever; contagious abortion
		Bordetella	Pertussis
		Francisella	Tularemia
		Alcaligenes	Opportunistic infections
Gram-Negative Facultatively Anaerobic Rods	Enterobacteriaceae	Escherichia	Gastroenteritis; neonatal meningitis
		Shigella	Bacillary dysentery
		Edwardsiella	Occasional diarrheas
		Salmonella	Typhoid fever; gastroenteritis
		Arizona	Nosocomial infections
		Klebsiella	Bacterial pneumonia
		Enterobacter	Nosocomial infections
		Serratia	Nosocomial infections
		Proteus	Urinary tract infections; nosocomial infections
		Providentia	Nosocomial infections
		Yersinia	Plague; gastroenteritis
	Vibrionaceae	Vibrio	Asiatic cholera; gastroenteritis
		Aeromonas	Opportunistic infections; diarrheas
		Plesiomonas	Diarrheas
	Uncertain Affiliation	Flavobacterium	Nosocomial infections of neonates
		Haemophilus	Meningitis; conjunctivitis; chancroid
		Pasteurella	Hemorrhagic septicemia of animals
		Actinobacillus	Actinobacillosis; endocarditis
		Cardiobacterium	Endocarditis
		Streptobacillus	Rat-bite fever
		Calymmatobacterium	Granuloma inguinale
Gram-Negative Anaerobic Bacteria	Bacteroidaceae	Bacteroides	}Intra-abdominal infections
		Fusobacterium	

Table continued on opposite page

taxonomy have led to a number of approaches. Inevitably, a sound taxonomy must be based on microbial genetics and fertility systems, the latter in the broad sense to include transduction and sexual recombination (Chapter 6). Still other approaches include the occurrence of key cellular constituents identified by biochemical analysis. It has been shown, for example, that biochemical differences in the amino acid constituents of the peptide bridges in the peptidoglycans of gram-negative bacteria can illuminate taxonomic differences.[51] Purine and pyrimidine base ratios in bacterial DNA, as well as DNA homologies, can show similarities between bacteria and thereby aid in their classification into genera and species (see below).

A useful system of bacterial taxonomy is tripartite and must include (1) orderly classifi-cation, in which like is grouped with like; (2) identification, whereby the relevant information on an isolated microorganism is derived and assembled; and (3) nomenclature, or the assignment of codified descriptions and names to species of bacteria.

A variety of formal classification systems have been prepared over the years, including that of Bergey's Manual, mentioned previously. This and other classification systems have attempted to recognize and formalize phylogenetic relationships. Although the Bergey classification is widely used by American workers, universal agreement on a single classification is not yet attained. There are also practical problems of identification, as for medical diagnostic purposes, and general acceptance of a common nomenclature. The identification problem is recognized in the

Table 2–3. **Classification of Medically Important Bacteria*** (*Continued*)

Vernacular Name	Family	Genus	Principal Disease Entity
Gram-Negative Cocci and Coccobacilli	Neisseriaceae	Neisseria	Gonorrhea; meningitis
		Branhamella	Opportunistic infections
		Moraxella	Eye and respiratory tract infections
		Acinetobacter	Opportunistic infections
Gram-Positive Cocci	Micrococcaceae	Staphylococcus	Suppurative infections; food poisoning; toxic shock
	Streptococcaceae	Streptococcus	Pharyngitis; glomerulonephritis; pneumonia; etc.
		Aerococcus	Endocarditis; urinary tract infections
	Peptococcaceae	Peptococcus	Abscesses; septic arthritis
		Peptostreptococcus	
Endospore-Forming Bacteria	Bacillaceae	Bacillus	Anthrax; food poisoning
		Clostridium	Tetanus; gas gangrene; food poisoning; pseudomembranous colitis
Gram-Positive Asporogenous Rods	Uncertain Affiliation	Listeria	Meningitis
		Erysipelothrix	Erysipeloid
Actinomyces and Related Organisms	Coryneform Bacteria	Corynebacterium	Diphtheria
	Propionibacteriaceae	Propionibacterium	Endogenous infections
		Eubacterium	
	Actinomycetaceae	Actinomyces	Actinomycoses
		Arachnia	
		Bifidobacterium	
	Mycobacteriaceae	Mycobacterium	Tuberculosis and similar diseases; leprosy
	Nocardiaceae	Nocardia	Nocardiosis
		Actinomadura	Mycetoma
	Streptomycetaceae	Streptomyces	Mycetoma
The Rickettsias	Rickettsiaceae	Rickettsia	Typhus, spotted fevers; etc.
		Rochalimaea	Trench fever
		Coxiella	Q fever
	Bartonellaceae	Bartonella	Oroya fever
	Chlamydiaceae	Chlamydia	Oculo-urogenital diseases; psittacosis; ornithosis; etc.
The Mycoplasmas	Mycoplasmataceae	Mycoplasma	Primary atypical pneumonia
		Ureaplasma	Urethritis

*Adapted from R. E. Buchanan and N. E. Gibbons (Eds.), Bergey's Manual of Determinative Bacteriology, 8th ed. Williams & Wilkins Co., Baltimore, 1974.

preparation of keys, such as that of Skerman[55] based on the Bergey classification and that of Cowan[14] covering the pathogenic forms.

NUMERICAL TAXONOMY

With the availability of computers and the spreading conviction of the futility of phylogenetic classification of bacteria, considerable interest has developed in numerical taxonomy. In general, the system is based upon a variety of unit characters—morphological, biochemical, physiological, and cultural—to reveal the similarities and dissimilarities of strains (operational taxonomic units; OTU) of microorganisms. A relatively large number of unit characteristics, usually 50 to several hundred, must be used to give reasonable confidence levels to the results. The use of many bacterial strains gives a cross section of the group analyzed. The unit characters may or may not be weighted; weighting obviously presents special problems in assigning relative importance to one or more characteristics.

From these data, coefficients of similarity or percentages of similarity may be calculated between strains. Cluster analysis is carried out by forming taxonomic groups of strains that show greatest similarities. For example, strains that show similarities greater than about 90 per cent might be considered members of the same species, while those with similarities of 70 per cent or greater might be classified in a single genus.

Although such a system is not without difficulties, *e.g.*, the selection and weighting of unit characters, it can provide a practical means of classification and identification for some clinical and applied laboratories.

NUCLEIC ACID HOMOLOGY

Since the morphological, physiological, biochemical, and cultural characteristics of a bacterial strain derive from its genetic potential, the ultimate taxonomy of bacteria should be based upon similarities in their deoxyribonucleic acid (DNA). The measurement of the degree of relatedness of DNA from different bacteria takes several forms, *viz.*, size of the bacterial genome, the guanine plus cytosine (G + C) content, and the determination of common nucleotide sequences by the techniques of DNA hybridization.

Both genome size and guanine plus cytosine content (Table 2–4) vary greatly among bacteria. It is clear that unrelated bacteria may have similar genome size, thereby requiring other criteria for their classification. On the other hand, microorganisms that have phenotypic similarities must be considered unrelated if their genome size is markedly different.

Table 2–4. **The Guanosine plus Cytosine Content of DNA from Representative Bacteria***

Genus	G + C (mole %)	Species	G + C (mole %)
Bacillus	32–62	B. cereus	32–38
		B. subtilis	42–48
Bacteroides	28–58	B. fragilis	40–44
		B. melaninogenicus	41–51
Bordetella	66–70	B. bronchiseptica	65–70
		B. pertussis	66
Brucella	56–58	B. abortus	56
Campylobacter	30–65	C. fetus	32–36
Clostridium	21–58	C. botulinum	22–28
		C. novyi	23–29
		C. perfringens	24–43
		C. tetani	25
Corynebacterium	47–76	C. diphtheriae	52–60
Escherichia	49–52	E. coli	49–52
Haemophilus	38–55	H. influenzae	38–41
Klebsiella	52–60	K. pneumoniae	57–59
Mycobacterium	62–78	M. bovis	66
		M. kansasii	64–68
		M. tuberculosis	64–66
Pseudomonas	43–73	P. aeruginosa	67–68
		P. fluorescens	59–64
Salmonella	50–55	S. typhimurium	52–55
Staphylococcus	30–40	S. aureus	30–39
		S. epidermidis	30–37
Streptococcus	33–87	S. pyogenes	35–39
		S. pneumoniae	39–42
Vibrio	29–52	V. parahemolyticus	44–48
Yersinia	46–49	Y. enterocolitica	47–49

*Data compiled from R. E. Buchanan and N. E. Gibbons (Eds.), Bergey's Manual of Determinative Bacteriology, 8th ed. Williams & Wilkins Co., Baltimore, 1974, and R. Hollander and S. Phol, Zentbl. Bakt. I. Abt. Orig. A **246**:236–275, 1980.

Similar admonitions apply to the use of G + C content.

DNA Hybridization

The genomic DNA of bacterial cells is double-stranded, with the two polynucleotide strands cross-linked by hydrogen bonding between complementary bases, adenine and thymine or cytosine and guanine (Chapter 6). If the DNA from one organism is dissociated into single strands, each is complementary to the other in nucleotide sequence and when they are reassociated they form a double-stranded molecule. If single-stranded DNA from different organisms are appropriately combined, the degree of association between the two strands is directly dependent upon the sequences of complementary nucleotides in the two strands. Thus, DNA from the same organism should show up to 100 per cent relatedness, while that of other members of the same species would be expected to show lesser, but significant relatedness, perhaps 70 to 100 per cent. The methods for DNA homology are sophisticated and complex. They are, therefore, not yet adapted to the routine classification and identification of bacteria, but are of great theoretical significance.

CLASSIFICATION OF BACTERIA

Nomenclature

An official International Code of Nomenclature of Bacteria has been developed by the International Committee on Systematic Bacteriology,[39] and lists of approved bacterial names are published periodically.[56] Bacterial names are binomial, consisting of a generic name (always capitalized) and a species name (not capitalized). The complete name is usually italicized. The generic name may or may not be descriptive, *e.g, Bacillus,* a small rod; or *Pasteurella,* in honor of Pasteur. The species name may be an adjective *(Staphylococcus aureus,* the golden staphylococcus), a noun indicating possession *(Bacillus pasteurii,* the bacillus of Pasteur), or a noun in apposition *(Bacillus ruminicola,* the rumen-dwelling bacillus). Although common names are frequently used, *e.g.,* typhoid bacillus or pneumococcus, these have no taxonomic standing.

Genera

Ideally, bacteria with similar phenotypic and genetic characteristics should be grouped within a genus. There is, however, no uniform and satisfactory agreement as to the meaning of "similar," particularly in the establishment of new genera. Many generic names have wide currency, however, and are acceptable to most bacteriologists because they are applied to distinct groups of microorganisms and have genuine classificatory value.

Species

The differentiation of species is made for the most part on their phenotypic characteristics, including morphology and biochemical reactions, and to a growing extent on DNA-relatedness. A single character, no matter how striking and seemingly important, is insufficient for differentiation. The use of a number of characters has become the rule, particularly with the increasing importance of numerical taxonomy and DNA-relatedness.

Types

Within a species, it is frequently useful to designate subgroups, or types, that may have epidemiological or other special interest. These may be set apart by immunological, biochemical, or pathogenic characters, or by susceptibility to bacteriophages or bacteriocins. They are variously designated as serotypes (or serogroups), biotypes, bioserotypes, pathotypes, or phage types.

REFERENCES

1. Aronson, A. I., and P. Fitz-James. 1976. Structure and morphogenesis of the bacterial spore coat. Bacteriol. Rev. **40**:360–402.
2. Barer, R. 1974. Microscopes, microscopy and microbiology. Ann. Rev. Microbiol. **28**:371–389.
3. Berg, H. C., D. B. Bromley, and N. W. Charon. 1978. Leptospiral motility. Symp. Soc. Gen. Microbiol. **28**:285–294.
4. Beveridge, T. J. 1981. Ultrastructure, chemistry, and function of the bacterial wall. Internat. Rev. Cytol. **72**:229–317.
5. Braun, V. 1978. Structure-function relationships of the gram-negative bacterial cell envelope. Symp. Soc. Gen. Microbiol. **28**:111–138.
6. Braun, V., and K. Hantke. 1974. Biochemistry of bacterial cell envelopes. Ann. Rev. Biochem. **43**:89–121.
7. Brenner, D. J. 1980. Taxonomy, classification, and nomenclature of bacteria. pp. 1–6. *In* E. H. Lennette, *et al.* (Eds.): Manual of Clinical Microbiology. 3rd ed. American Society for Microbiology, Washington, D.C.
8. Brimacombe, R. 1978. The structure of the bacterial ribosome. Symp. Soc. Gen. Microbiol. **28**:1–26.
9. Buchanan, R. E., and N. E. Gibbons (Eds.). 1974. Bergey's Manual of Determinative Bacteriology. 8th ed. Williams & Wilkins Co., Baltimore.
10. Canale-Parola, E. 1978. Motility and chemotaxis of spirochetes. Ann. Rev. Microbiol. **32**:69–99.
11. Costerton, J. W. 1979. The role of electron micros-

copy in the elucidation of bacterial structure and function. Ann. Rev. Microbiol. **33**:459–479.

12. Costerton, J. W., J. M. Ingram, and K.-J. Cheng. 1974. Structure and function of the cell envelope of gram-negative bacteria. Bacteriol. Rev. **38**:87–110.

13. Costerton, J. W., R. T. Irvin, and K.-J. Cheng. 1981. The bacterial glycocalyx in nature and disease. Ann. Rev. Microbiol. **35**:299–324.

14. Cowan, S. T. 1974. Cowan and Steel's Manual for the Identification of Medical Bacteria. 2nd ed. Cambridge University Press, London.

15. DiRienzo, J. M., K. Nakamura, and M. Inouyi. 1978. The outer membrane proteins of gram-negative bacteria: biosynthesis, assembly, and functions. Ann. Rev. Biochem. **47**:481–532.

16. Doetsch, R. N., and R. D. Sjoblad. 1980. Flagellar structure and function in eubacteria. Ann. Rev. Microbiol. **34**:69–108.

17. Doi, R. H. 1977. Genetic control of sporulation. Ann. Rev. Genet. **11**:29–48.

18. Duckworth, M. 1977. Teichoic acids. pp. 177–208. *In* I. Sutherland (Ed.): Surface Carbohydrates of the Prokaryotic Cell. Academic Press, London.

19. Dworkin, M. 1979. Spores, cysts, and stalks. pp. 1–84. *In* J. R. Sokatch and L. N. Ornston (Eds.): The Bacteria. Vol. VII, Mechanisms of Adaptation. Academic Press, New York.

20. Ellar, D. J. 1978. Spore specific structures and their function. Symp. Soc. Gen. Microbiol. **28**:295–325.

21. Goodfellow, M., and R. G. Board (Eds.). 1980. Microbiological Classification and Identification. The Society for Applied Bacteriology Symposium Series No. 8. Academic Press, London.

22. Goren, M. B., M. Cernich, and O. Brokl. 1978. Some observations on mycobacterial acid-fastness. Amer. Rev. Resp. Dis. **118**:151–154.

23. Gould, G. W. 1977. Recent advances in the understanding of resistance and dormancy in bacterial spores. J. Appl. Bacteriol. **42**:297–309.

24. Gray, P. 1973. The Encyclopedia of Microscopy and Microtechnique. Van Nostrand Reinhold Co., New York.

25. Greenawalt, J. W., and T. L. Whiteside. 1975. Mesosomes: membranous bacterial organelles. Bacteriol. Rev. **39**:405–463.

26. Grunberg-Manago, M., *et al.* 1978. Structure and function of the translation machinery. Symp. Soc. Gen. Microbiol. **28**:27–110.

27. Gunsalus, I. C., and R. Y. Stanier (Eds.). 1960. The Bacteria. Vol. I, Structure. Academic Press, New York.

28. Hamilton, W. A. 1977. Energy coupling in substrate and group translocation. Symp. Soc. Gen. Microbiol. **27**:185–216.

29. Heywood, V. H. (Ed.). 1971. Scanning Electron Microscopy. Academic Press, New York.

30. Hoffman, H., and M. E. Frank. 1965. Time-lapse photomicrography of lashing, flexing, and snapping movements in *Escherichia coli* and *Corynebacterium* microcultures. J. Bacteriol. **90**:789–795.

31. Iino, T. 1977. Genetics of structure and function of bacterial flagella. Ann. Rev. Genet. **11**:161–182.

32. van Iterson, W. 1965. Symposium on the fine structure and replication of bacteria and their parts. II. Bacterial cytoplasm. Bacteriol. Rev. **29**:299–325.

33. Knox, K. W., and A. J. Wicken. 1973. Immunological properties of teichoic acids. Bacteriol. Rev. **37**:215–257.

34. Korn, E. D. 1969. Cell membranes: structure and synthesis. Ann. Rev. Biochem. **38**:263–288.

35. Koshland, D. E., Jr. 1980. Bacterial Chemotaxis as a Model Behavioral System. Raven Press, New York.

36. Koshland, D. E., Jr. 1981. Biochemistry of sensing and adaptation in a simple bacterial system. Ann. Rev. Biochem. **50**:765–782.

37. Krulwich, T. A., and J. L. Pate. 1971. Ultrastructural explanation for snapping postfission movements in *Arthrobacter crystallopoietes.* J. Bacteriol. **105**:408–412.

38. Kurland, C. G. 1977. Structure and function of the bacterial ribosome. Ann. Rev. Biochem. **46**:173–200.

39. Lepage, S. P., *et al.* (Eds.). 1975. International code of nomenclature of bacteria and statutes of the International Committee on Systematic Bacteriology and statutes of the bacteriology section of the International Association of Microbiological Societies. Bacteriological Code, 1976 revision. American Society for Microbiology, Washington, D.C.

40. Macnab, R. M. 1978. Bacterial motility and chemotaxis: the molecular biology of a behavioral system. CRC Crit. Rev. Biochem. **5**:291–341.

41. Mercer, E. H., and M. S. C. Birbeck. 1972. Electron Microscopy. A Handbook for Biologists. 3rd ed. Blackwell, Oxford.

42. Nomura, M., A. Tissières, and P. Lengyel. 1974. Ribosomes. Cold Spring Harbor Laboratory, New York.

43. Osborn, M. J., and H. C. P. Wu. 1980. Proteins of the outer membrane of gram-negative bacteria. Ann. Rev. Microbiol. **34**:369–422.

44. Ottow, J. C. G. 1975. Ecology, physiology and genetics of fimbriae and pili. Ann. Rev. Microbiol. **29**:79–108.

45. Parkinson, J. S. 1977. Behaviorial genetics in bacteria. Ann. Rev. Genet. **11**:397–414.

46. Pettijohn, D. E. 1976. Procaryotic DNA in nucleoid structure. CRC Crit. Rev. Biochem. **4**:175–202.

47. Piggot, P. J., and J. G. Coote. 1976. Genetic aspects of bacterial endospore formation. Bacteriol. Rev. **40**:908–962.

48. Rogers, H. J., J. B. Ward, and I. D. J. Burdett. 1978. Structure and grow of the walls of gram-positive bacteria. Symp. Soc. Gen. Microbiol. **28**:139–176.

49. Rosen, B. P. (Ed.). 1978. Bacterial Transport. Marcel Dekker, Inc., New York.

50. Saier, M. H., Jr. 1979. The role of the cell surface in regulating the internal environment. pp. 167–227. *In* J. R. Sokatch and L. N. Ornston (Eds.): The Bacteria. Vol. VII, Mechanisms of Adaptation. Academic Press, New York.

51. Salton, M. R. J. 1967. Structure and function of bacterial cell membranes. Ann. Rev. Microbiol. **21**:417–442.

52. Schleifer, K. H., and O. Kandler, 1972. Peptidoglycan types of bacterial cell walls and their taxonomic implications. Bacteriol. Rev. **36**:407–477.

53. Shively, J. M. 1974. Inclusion bodies of prokaryotes. Ann. Rev. Microbiol. **28**:167–187.

54. Silverman, M., and M. I. Simon. 1977. Bacterial flagella. Ann. Rev. Microbiol. **31**:397–419.

55. Skerman, V. B. D. 1974. A key for the determination of the generic position of organisms listed in the manual. pp. 1098–1146. *In* R. E. Buchanan and N. E. Gibbons (Eds.): Bergey's Manual of Determinative Bacteriology. 8th ed. Williams & Wilkins Co., Baltimore.

56. Skerman, V. B. D., V McGowan, and P. H. A. Sneath. 1980. Approved list of bacterial names. Internat. J. Syst. Bacteriol. **30**:225–420.

57. Sleytr, U. B. 1978. Regular arrays of macromolecules on bacterial cell walls: structure, chemistry, assembly, and function. Internat. Rev. Cytol. **53**:1–64.

58. Stanier, R. Y. 1970. Some aspects of the biology of cells and their possible evolutionary significance. Symp. Soc. Gen. Microbiol. **20**:1–38.

59. Sutherland, I. (Ed.). 1977. Surface Carbohydrates of the Prokaryotic Cell. Academic Press, London.

60. Symposium. 1965. Function and Structure in Microorganisms. Society for General Microbiology, 15th Symposium. Cambridge University Press, London.

61. Symposium. 1970. Organization and Control in Prokaryotic and Eukaryotic Cells. Society for General Microbiology, 20th Symposium. Cambridge University Press, London.

62. Troy, F. A., II. 1979. The chemistry and biosynthesis of selected bacterial capsular polymers. Ann. Rev. Microbiol. **33**:519–560.

63. Ward, J. B. 1978. The reversion of bacterial protoplasts and L-forms. Symp. Soc. Gen. Microbiol. **28**:249–269.

64. Ward, J. B. 1981. Teichoic and teichuronic acids: biosynthesis, assembly, and location. Microbiol. Rev. **45**:211–243.

3

The Growth of Bacteria

The growth of microorganisms is essentially the specific, balanced synthesis of the components of protoplasm from the nutritive substances present in the immediate environment. In addition, the newly synthesized constituents must be assembled and appropriately packaged to yield replicates of the original unit. The specificity of the entire process is dependent upon the operation of directive mechanisms, or genetic controls, which have the unique property of self-replication so that they appear as intrinsic parts of the new units.

This complex process is obviously dependent upon, and affected by, the kinds and concentrations of nutrient substances present in available form and upon a continuous supply of energy required for the endothermic reactions of synthesis.

Studies of microbial growth may be approached in a number of ways. The most obvious are: (1) the cytological approach, *i.e.,* growth and development of individual cells, (2) that of growth of microorganisms as populations, and (3) investigation of the nature of the biochemical processes involved. Such separations are artificial in that they represent no more than relative emphasis on one or another view of the same process, but they are useful for purposes of discussion. The first two will be considered here, and the last elsewhere (Chapter 4).

THE GROWTH AND DIVISION OF BACTERIAL CELLS[2, 4, 5, 10, 11]

Growth of bacteria may be considered from two viewpoints. The first is the enlargement or elongation of an individual cell with the synthesis of new cytoplasmic and cellular constituents. The second is an increase in cell numbers when the mother cell divides to produce two daughter cells.

By far the most common mode of multiplication in bacteria is binary fission. In a complex series of correlated steps, some overlapping and some sequential, the chromosome divides and separates, followed by constriction or septum formation to form two daughter cells. Fission occurs in a single plane at right angles to the long axis of bacillary and spiral forms. It may occur in one or more planes in spherical forms, making possible the characteristic morphological groupings described earlier (Chapter 2). Bacilli and spirochetes show some elongation prior to fission; as a rule, the cocci do not, although there may be some increase in the diameter of the cell while retaining its spherical form. The size that a single cell must reach before fission is remarkably constant, although differences in this maximum are associated with the age of the culture (see below).

More precise definition of bacterial cell fine structure as well as developments in bacterial genetics have clarifed the cytological and biochemical aspects of cell division. Bacterial reproduction begins with the initiation of chromosome synthesis by mechanisms that are essentially unknown, but may include accumulation of initiator proteins. Duplication, followed by separation of the daughter chromosomes, then ensues. The mechanisms responsible for the separation of the two chromosomes are obscure; the chromosomes apparently are attached to the cytoplasmic membrane, and often associated with mesosomes, and many believe that membrane growth may serve to separate the daughter chromosomes. The next step is the formation of a septum, or cell plate, across or slightly oblique to the long axis in the case of bacillary forms, dividing the cell contents into approximately equal portions. In gram-positive bacteria, and probably in many gram-negative bacteria as well,[3] the septum develops by centripetal growth and annular closing of the cytoplasmic membrane, followed closely by synthesis and deposition of new cell wall. The manner in which this occurs is not entirely clear, *viz.*, whether the plasma membrane grows by extension or whether its formation is associated with mesosome activity. At any rate, in gram-positive as well as some gram-negative bacteria, the growth of the cell wall appears to be localized near the site of septum formation. In other gram-negative bacteria, growth of the cell wall appears to be general rather than local, followed by constriction prior to cell division. Finally the daughter cells separate. This separation is likely mediated by amidases, enzymes that hydrolyze linkages in the peptidoglycan layer.

Unlike eucaryotic cells, in which the processes of reproduction begin anew at each cell division, some of the processes in procaryotic cells, such as chromosomal replication, may extend over more than one division cycle. Thus, cell division, although somehow correlated with nuclear division, is a separate process. For example, in rapidly growing cultures, chromosomal replication and division may outpace septum formation and division, so that several pairs of chromosomes may be apparent before the next round of cell division is complete.

The division cycle in bacteria does not always proceed as smoothly as indicated above. Cell division is subject to inhibition by a variety of physical and chemical agents, resulting in the continued growth of the cell, but without production of daughter cells, forming long filaments in the case of bacilli. In many cases, other chemical agents may restore the capacity of these filaments to divide. Such observations, coupled with genetic studies employing mutant strains unable to carry out certain reproductive functions under restrictive conditions, indicate the operation of mechanisms controlling division sites and thus regulating the size and uniformity of cells in the population. Occasionally, failure of some of these controls results in the production of small anucleate cells, called minicells, which do not reproduce further.

While bacterial multiplication usually takes place by transverse fission, other kinds of cell division may occur. Some, such as the diphtheria and tubercle bacilli, show true branching that is characteristic of some of the higher fungi, and budding, similar to the budding of yeast cells, has been described by some workers.

The generation time in binary fission, *i.e.,* the time elapsing between cell divisions, is minimal during the exponential growth phase (see below) of the bacterial culture. Certain forms, such as the cholera vibrio and coliform bacilli, are among the most rapidly proliferating bacteria, with generation times of 20 minutes or less, and one marine *Pseudomonas* species has been found to have a generation time as short as 9.8 minutes. More slowly growing bacteria, such as the tubercle bacilli, have generation times of several hours or even days.

The rapidity of cell division among the bacteria is not unique, as is sometimes supposed, for embryonic cells of higher forms may show equally rapid division. The unique aspect of the rate of bacterial multiplication lies, rather, in the fact that such a short time is required for the bacterial cell to reach full maturity.

THE GROWTH OF BACTERIAL POPULATIONS[6]

For obvious practical reasons bacteria are ordinarily manipulated and studied not as individuals but as aggregates made up of very large numbers of cells. Bacterial growth may be considered as the growth of populations of many millions of cells whose characteristics are essentially statistical ones, and the behavior of individual cells is assayed as a frequency.

Measurement of Growth

Bacterial growth in culture may be measured by following, experimentally, increases in cell substance (protoplasm) or increases in cell numbers. Measurement of cellular material may be accomplished by direct methods such as dry weight or volume of cell mass after centrifugation; indirect measurements usually involve the determination of some relatively constant cellular component, such as protein nitrogen, nucleic acids, or specific enzymes. Numbers of cells may be measured directly by microscopic counting or by quantitative dilution and plate culture. Indirect methods include turbidimetric measurements translated into cell numbers using a previously prepared calibration curve.

Mathematics of Growth

When all, or practically all, of the cells are viable and multiplying by binary fission, the rate of growth is exponential. This potential rate of multiplication may be realized only up to a certain point. As numbers increase in the microcosm of the culture tube, competition between individual organisms for foodstuffs, oxygen, and the like progressively reduces the opportunity for further growth until a saturating population density is reached.

If no increasingly effective retardation were operative, the potential increase would be expressed by the relation:

$$\frac{dY}{dt} = bY$$

where Y is equal to the number of individuals per unit volume, and b to the rate of growth, or generation time, of the microorganism. When there is a maximal possible cell density, K, this geometric rate of increase is only partially realized, the extent of the realization depending on how near the culture is to its maximum density at any given time. Or, mathematically:

$$\frac{dY}{dt} = bY\frac{K-Y}{K}$$

This is the differential equation of the logistic function:

$$Y = \frac{K}{1 + e^{a-bx}}$$

This function, plotting as a symmetrical S-shaped curve, describes the growth of populations of a variety of living organisms. If the numbers of bacteria in a growing culture are measured periodically and plotted against time of incubation, the points fall on a similar S-shaped curve, but one that is asymmetrical in that the point of inflection is not halfway between the upper and lower asymptotes. Such curves are ordinarily plotted on semilog paper, *i.e.*, the logarithms of the numbers of bacteria are plotted against time on an arithmetic scale. This procedure gives a more nearly symmetrical curve and has the advantage not only of minimizing errors in counting, but also, when microorganisms are multiplying at an exponential rate, of the points falling on a straight line, and the generation time being expressed as the slope of the straight-line portion of the curve. Considerably more complex mathematical analysis of bacterial growth may be applied,[9]

but the foregoing simplification suffices for present purposes.

The bacterial growth curve, shown in schematic form in Figure 3–1, is divided into segments, or growth phases. The significant portions are the lag phase during which little or no increase in numbers occurs, the logarithmic or exponential growth rate phase during which the bacteria are multiplying at a maximum rate, and the stationary phase when the maximum total growth has been reached. The positive and negative growth acceleration phases at either end of the period of exponential growth are sometimes differentiated but are of limited utility. Following the stationary phase, death of some portion of the cells present usually occurs, rapidly or slowly and at an exponential rate; microbial death is considered elsewhere (Chapter 5).

It is obvious from even casual consideration of the development of the bacterial culture that descriptions such as "good growth" and "poor growth" have little meaning. Good growth may mean rapid growth and result from a relatively short latent or lag period and/or a short generation time during the exponential growth phase, or it may mean heavy growth in the sense that the maximal population density is high. These are not necessarily synonymous; the cholera vibrio, for example, grows equally rapidly in the logarithmic phase in aerated culture in peptone water, or peptone water enriched by the addition of serum to 10 per cent, but the maximal density is considerably greater in the enriched medium. The meaning of "growth" is, then, variable, and the growth response, however and to what purpose it may be defined, is a function of the environment in the microcosm of the culture vessel. The rate of growth under natural conditions is a function of many factors and is more complex than that studied in pure culture in the laboratory.[1]

The Lag Phase

When bacteria are inoculated into fresh medium, an appreciable time, or latent period, is required for adaptation to an environment new in the sense that it differs from that of the established parent culture. There is convincing evidence that this period is divisible into an apparent and a true lag phase. The first is a consequence of the presence of cells in the inoculum which are not viable in the sense that they will not reproduce, although they may continue to metabolize, and thus reduce the size of the effective inoculum. Within limits, the length of the lag phase is directly

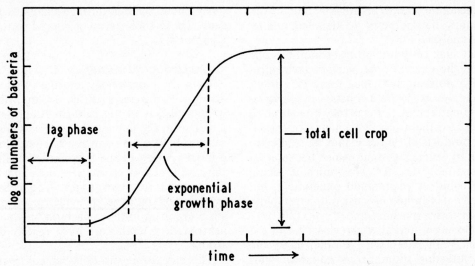

Figure 3–1. Diagrammatic representation of bacterial growth when the logarithms of the numbers of cells are plotted against incubation time.

related to the size of the effective inoculum, and the numbers of cells present during the subsequent exponential growth phase at successive points in time may be predicted from these considerations.

The true lag phase, in contrast, is the period required for the viable cells of the inoculum to accumulate enzymes, diffusible coenzymes, and essential intermediates in the synthesis of cell substance to the balanced concentrations consistent with synthesis at a maximum rate. When the inoculum is taken from a culture in the exponential growth phase, the lag is largely, or entirely, eliminated, since the cells are already in a state of physiological balance, making possible synthesis at a maximal rate.

On the other hand, the lag phase may be prolonged indefinitely by interference with processes of adaptation. Vigorous aeration prevents growth and multiplication by preventing the accumulation of small amounts of carbon dioxide from endogenous respiration that are essential to growth. Similarly, the addition of antibacterial substances whose activity is primarily bacteriostatic, *i.e.*, growth-inhibiting rather than killing, results in an indefinite extension of the lag phase. Such substances include those of practical importance as chemotherapeutic agents, such as the sulfonamides and certain of the antibiotics, as well as other substances, as for example certain dyes. These act by interfering with essential metabolic reactions, such as the synthesis of enzymes (Chapter 5), and when their effect is neutralized, as by *p*-aminobenzoic acid when growth is inhibited by sulfonamides, growth

proceeds. The effect of many chemotherapeutic drugs is, then, in a sense an indefinite prolongation of the lag phase of bacterial growth.

The Exponential Growth Phase

The stage in the development of the bacterial culture during which cells are replicating at a constant and geometric rate represents an approximate, limited, steady state in the relation between the bacteria and their environment. The steady state is approximate because the environment is continuously altered by the microorganisms, and limited in that it persists over only a portion of the life history of the culture.

The rate of growth is obviously determined by limiting factors. These may be intrinsic in the physiological potential of the cell, *e.g.*, the rate of transport of nutrients across the cell membrane. Alternatively, they may be extrinsic in that they may be environmental factors, such as the concentration of an essential nutrient, concentration of oxidizable substrate, and the rate of diffusion of oxygen into the culture.

Continuous Flow Culture. Bacterial cultures may be partially maintained in the exponential growth phase by frequent successive transplant of cells already in this phase, but much more precisely by cultivation of the bacteria in a continuous flow of fresh medium. A considerable number of devices for this purpose have been constructed in which fresh medium is introduced into a growth chamber at a rate that permits bacterial growth at a near maximum rate. The steady state so obtained may be subjected to detailed mathematical analysis.

Under such constant cultural conditions one factor in the environment, such as concentration of a nutrient substance, may be varied, while the others are held constant in excess so that rate-determining effects may be measured precisely. Furthermore, the kinetics of formation of products of synthesis may be studied in relation to generation time, which becomes an experimental parameter. Theoretically, such a culture could be maintained indefinitely, but in practice it is limited because of the instability of the directive mechanisms of synthesis, *i.e.,* mutations occur and alter the character of the microbial population. On the other hand, the factors affecting spontaneous mutation rates may be studied under constant defined environmental conditions.

Synchronous Cell Division. In the usual bacterial culture, cell division is not synchronized, and generation or division time is a statistical average of the entire population. For some purposes, it is desirable to force the majority of cells to divide more or less simultaneously and thus synchronize cell division. This may be approximately achieved by subjecting the culture to alternate chilling and incubation temperatures.

Cessation of Cell Division

Termination of the exponential phase of growth is marked by a relatively rapid decrease in the rate of cell division, which signals the beginning of the stationary phase. Cell division does not stop entirely in the stationary phase, but the cells begin to die and occasional division counteracts deaths so that the number of viable microorganisms remains relatively constant for a time. This period may be relatively short so that within a few hours a decline in numbers of viable cells assumes an exponential rate, or the numbers of viable organisms may fluctuate about some median value that is usually less than the maximum cell density.

The decreasing rate of cell division may be accounted for in a variety of ways. Essential nutrients may be depleted and become a limiting factor for growth. There may be a reduction in oxidizable substrates for energy production or oxygen diffusion may be inadequate at high cell densities. Alternatively, there may be an accumulation of toxic or inhibitory metabolic products, such as organic acids. Some of these end products may also participate in biosynthetic control through feedback regulation. These topics are considered in detail in Chapter 4.

Morphological Variation

Both the morphology and the physiological activity of bacteria differ in the different growth phases of the culture. As growth gets under way, the maximum size that a given cell reaches before fission increases somewhat, and a large portion of the bacteria in a culture at this stage of development are appreciably larger than at other times. The cells stain evenly, and there is no evidence of granular structure even in those bacteria in which metachromatic granules are most readily demonstrable.

The rate of respiration per cell increases, reaching a maximum at the end of the phase of accelerating growth rate, and declining as the culture goes into the logarithmic growth phase. This increased metabolic rate is more apparent than real for it is quantitatively related to cell size.

The cell size decreases also as the culture goes into the logarithmic phase of growth, although the individual cells remain homogeneous and stain uniformly. By the time the stationary phase is reached, the bacterial cells are uniformly smaller, and in cultures of spore-forming bacteria, many are forming spores. When the viable count begins to decrease, the cells no longer stain uniformly, but begin to show granular structure, and involution forms appear.

Temperature and Growth

The temperature restrictions on the growth of any living form generally fall between the freezing point of water and the temperature at which essential cellular constituents are inactivated. Practically, this temperature range is from just under 0°C. to a maximum of about 65° to 75°C. The temperature range permitting growth of complex eucaryotic cells is generally narrower than this, but procaryotic cells are more versatile and the extremes over which bacteria may grow are from −7.5° to +75°C. Bacteria may be ordered on the basis of their optimum temperature, which is generally taken to mean the temperature supporting the greatest rate of growth. Psychrophilic bacteria are those forms with an optimum temperature of 15°C. or below and with growth temperature ranges from about 0° to 20°C.[8] In nature, psychrophiles are often found in colder climates, in frozen soils, and in water; they assume some importance as they grow in refrigerated foods and other products. At the other extreme are the thermophilic bacteria, with optimum temperatures above 45°C. or so, and whose maximum growth temperature may be as high as 75°C. Such microorganisms may be encountered in soils and water, particularly those with higher environmental temperatures. The mesophilic bacteria are those with temperature optima in the middle range, often near 37°C.; the great majority of bacteria are in this group. Most, if not all, of the pathogenic bacteria are mesophilic and frequently their optimum temperature is close to that of their natural hosts.

THE PHYSIOLOGY OF GROWTH

The physiological capabilities of microorganisms are inversely related to their nutritional requirements, since the synthesis of cell substance from inorganic and simple organic compounds is obviously a more complex process than if the starting products are complex organic substances chemically more similar to the final cellular constituents. Taken as a whole, bacteria range in continuous series with respect to their requirements for growth. At one extreme are the autotrophic forms capable of living in an inorganic environment and deriving their energy either from the oxidation of inorganic substrates (the chemolithotrophs) or by using a photosynthetic process to assimilate nitrogen, carbon, and other constituents from inorganic sources (the phototrophs). At the other end of the spectrum are the obligate intracellular bacteria incapable of any but the most rudimentary independent physiological activity. The details of the processes of respiration, synthesis, and assimilation are considered elsewhere (Chapter 4).

Only the autotrophs are completely independent of the activities of other living organisms. Physiological limitations begin to appear in the heterotrophic forms, whose characteristic requirements of organic substrates for growth appear first as a requirement for organic carbon both as a source of energy and as a source of intermediates for the synthesis of cell substance. Among the more nutritionally fastidious kinds of microorganisms, the requirements for growth become more specific in that certain molecular structures, such as those represented in amino acids and fragments of enzymes or enzyme precursors, must be supplied preformed, but the microorganism is still physiologically independent in that it constitutes a complete physiological system, capable of growth and reproduction when supplied with required nutrients.

Finally, the obligate intracellular parasites are set apart in that they are not complete physiological systems but are dependent upon the synthetic mechanisms of living host cells for their replication. It is more than coincidence that lack of independent metabolic activity is associated with the most minute forms, for there is literally not room within the small virus particle for the unknown but relatively large number of enzyme molecules required by a physiologically independent unit (Chapter 38).

Since growth is the replication of the individual unit, and the replication is necessarily a directed process if individuality is to be maintained, microorganisms of diverse physiological capabilities may be equated on this common ground. The directive mechanism, or genetic control of biosynthesis, resides in the deoxyribonucleic acid. The mechanisms of the replication of DNA *in situ* by DNA polymerases and the direction of the processes of protein synthesis through the mediation of the various kinds of RNA and ribosomes have now become clarified.

The growth of microorganisms can be regarded primarily as an expression of DNA replication, complicated to a greater or lesser extent by the side reactions of synthesis of the remainder of the unit. Such a view not only places the multiplication of diverse microorganisms on a common ground, but also provides a basic working hypothesis for an interpretation of the ways in which the hereditary mechanisms of these forms may be altered.[7]

REFERENCES

1. Brock, T. D. 1971. Microbial growth rates in nature. Bacteriol. Rev. **35**:39–58.
2. Donachie, W. D., N. C. Jones, and R. Teather. 1973. The bacterial cell cycle. Symp. Soc. Gen. Microbiol. **23**:9–44.
3. Gilleland, H. E., Jr., and R. G. E. Murray. 1975. Demonstration of cell division by septation in a variety of gram-negative rods. J. Bacteriol. **121**:721–725.
4. Helmstetter, C. E., *et al.* 1979. Control of cell division in *Escherichia coli.* pp. 517–579. *In* J. R. Sokatch and L. N. Ornston (Eds.): The Bacteria. Vol. VII, Mechanisms of Adaptation. Academic Press, New York.

5. Koch, A. L. 1977. Does the initiation of chromosome replication regulate cell division? Adv. Microbial Physiol. **16**:49–98.

6. Mandelstam, J., and K. McQuillen (Eds.). 1968. Biochemistry of Bacterial Growth. John Wiley & Sons, New York.

7. Mendelson, N. H. 1977. Cell growth and division: a genetic viewpoint. pp. 5–24. *In* D. Schlessinger (Ed.): Microbiology—1977. American Society for Microbiology, Washington, D.C.

8. Morita, R. Y. 1975. Psychrophilic bacteria. Bacteriol. Rev. **39**:144–167.

9. Painter, P. R., and A. G. Marr. 1968. Mathematics of microbial populations. Ann. Rev. Microbiol. **22**:519–548.

10. Sargent, M. G. 1978. Surface extension and the cell cycle in prokaryotes. Adv. Microbial Physiol. **18**:105–176.

11. Slater, M., and M. Schaechter. 1974. Control of cell division in bacteria. Bacteriol. Rev. **38**:199–221.

CHAPTER 4

Bacterial Metabolism

M. J. Wolin, Ph.D.
T. L. Miller, Ph.D.

The basic functions of the microbial cell may be illustrated with *Salmonella typhimurium,* a motile, rod-shaped microorganism which will synthesize cell substance, divide, and move about when inoculated into a medium containing glucose, inorganic ammonium, phosphate and sulfate salts, and trace elements (Mg, Mn, Fe, Co, Zn, Cu, Mo).

Glucose is its carbon and energy source. A large array of the two to three thousand enzymes in the cell transforms the glucose into building blocks and then uses these precursors for the construction of the fundamental macromolecules of which all cells are composed: proteins, nucleic acids, carbohydrates, and lipids. Since most of the macromolecules contain nitrogen, phosphorus, and sulfur, these elements are attached to the appropriate carbon building blocks used for the synthesis of particular macromolecules. Synthesis and movement require energy, which is supplied by special enzymatic transformations of glucose.

Bacteria as a group use an almost bewildering array of energy sources. Some make use of light as an energy source, and the others use chemicals, both organic and inorganic. Fortunately, there are some fundamental rules for the process of transforming the energy of the source into a chemical form that can be used for the energy-requiring processes of the cell. Additionally, it is found that almost all pathways of energy generation lead to adenosine triphosphate (ATP) and reduced pyridine nucleotides (PNH), the currency of chemical energy in cells, and all pathways of energy utilization lead from ATP and PNH. ATP participates in biosynthetic reactions by reacting with precursors to give intermediates that form the new carbon–carbon and carbon–nitrogen bonds of the building blocks. PNH, *i.e.,* reduced nicotinamide adenine dinucleotide (NADH) or reduced nicotinamide adenine dinucleotide phosphate (NADPH), is a source of electrons for the many biosynthetic reactions that require a reducing agent.

The pathways for using ATP and PNH in the microbial world are not universal, but they are by no means as diverse as the pathways for ATP and PNH production. ATP and PNH are used in the formation of building blocks, precursors of macromolecules, and significant diversity exists in precursor formation among the bacteria. *Salmonella typhimurium* synthesizes the carbon skeleton of histidine from glucose, but species of *Chromatium* synthesize their carbon compounds from carbon dioxide. Obviously, there are differences in the progression these two organisms follow from their carbon source to histidine. Although there are differences in the pathways organisms use to form ATP and PNH, there is great uniformity in the pathways for using ATP and building blocks for synthesis of cellular macromolecules.

Energy[8, 11, 31]

Sources of Energy

If a bacterium uses light as an energy source, it is called **phototrophic.**[19] If it uses chemicals as an energy source, it is called **chemotrophic,** Chemotrophs fall into two major categories, chemolithotrophs and chemoorganotrophs. **Chemolithotrophs** obtain energy from inorganic compounds,[18] and **chemoorganotrophs** use organic compounds as energy sources. A given organism may or may not fit exclusively into one of these categories. *Steptococcus pyogenes* is completely chemoorganotrophic; it generally uses carbohydrates as energy sources. *Rhodospirillum rubrum* grows as a phototroph, but it can also grow chemoorganotrophically in the dark. Some bacteria can grow chemolithotrophically or chemoorganotrophically (see **4–1** for typical energy-yielding reactions).

The inorganic substrates for chemolithotrophic growth are ferrous compounds, reduced sulfur compounds such as sulfide and thiosulfate, ammonia and nitrite, and hydrogen. Almost all organic compounds can serve as energy sources for microorganisms. A few synthetic organic compounds, *e.g.,* DDT and some detergents, are "recalcitrant molecules," *i.e.,* they are not biodegradable and they persist in nature. Some bacteria are fairly restrictive with respect to the classes of organic compound used for energy.

Streptococcus pyogenes is a member of an entire family of bacteria (the lactic acid bacteria, Lactobacillaceae) which obtains energy mainly by fermenting carbohydrates. The family includes several genera: *Streptococcus, Lactobacillus, Leuconostoc, Pediococcus,* and *Bifidobacterium.* By contrast, a single species of the genus *Pseudomonas, P. multivorans,* can use amino acids, fatty acids, carbohydrates, and aromatic compounds (*e.g.,* benzoic acid) as energy sources. Bacteria are known to grow on hydrocarbons—from the gases methane, ethane, and propane, to the complex hydrocarbons found in petroleum.

This tremendous capacity for using organic energy sources gives microorganisms their important role in nature in cycling the elements of the natural food chain. A simplified outline of this cycling follows:

1. Inorganic carbon, nitrogen, sulfur, and phosphorus are converted to plant organic matter (photosynthesis).
2. Plant organic matter is converted to animal organic matter.
3. Plant and animal organic matter are converted to inorganic carbon, nitrogen, sulfur, and phosphorus by microorganisms. The mineralization process is mainly an energy-yielding process for microorganisms.
4. Repetition of step 1.

High-Energy Phosphate and ATP

Phosphorus is present in all cells in macromolecules (*e.g.,* nucleic acids) and in small molecular weight intermediates of the pathways for energy generation and biosynthesis. The two most important kinds of phosphorus compounds are phosphate esters and phosphate anhydrides. The difference between

4–1.

Typical Energy Sources for Microorganisms

Organism	Energy Source
(*1*) Phototrophs	
Rhodospirillum rubrum	Light
Chromatium okenii	Light
(*2*) Chemotrophs	
(*a*) Chemolithotrophs	
Thiobacillus thiooxidans	$H_2S + 2\ O_2 \rightarrow H_2SO_4$
Nitrosomonas europaea	$NH_3 + 1\frac{1}{2}\ O_2 \rightarrow HNO_2 + H_2O$
Methanobacterium **bryantii**	$4\ H_2 + CO_2 \rightarrow CH_4 + 2\ H_2O$
(*b*) Chemoorganotrophs	
Streptococcus faecalis	glucose $\rightarrow$ 2 lactate
Propionibacterium shermanii	$1\frac{1}{2}$ glucose $\rightarrow$ 2 propionate + acetate + CO_2
Clostridium tetanomorphum	2 glutamate + 2 $H_2O \rightarrow$
	butyrate + 2 acetate + 2 CO_2 + 2 NH_3
Saccharomyces cerevisiae, and	glucose + 6 $O_2 \rightarrow$ 6 CO_2 + 6 H_2O
Escherichia coli (aerobic)	
Methanomonas methanica	$CH_4 + 2\ O_2 \rightarrow CO_2 + 2\ H_2O$

these two phosphate groups (*A* and *B*) is illustrated by the important metabolic intermediate, 1.3-bisphosphoglyceric acid.

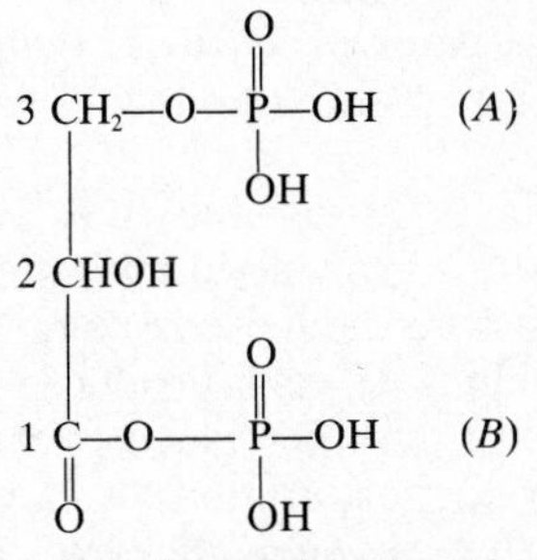

$$3\ CH_2-O-\overset{\overset{\displaystyle O}{\|}}{\underset{\underset{\displaystyle OH}{|}}{P}}-OH \quad (A)$$

$$2\ CHOH$$

$$1\ \underset{\underset{\displaystyle O}{\|}}{C}-O-\overset{\overset{\displaystyle O}{\|}}{\underset{\underset{\displaystyle OH}{|}}{P}}-OH \quad (B)$$

1,3-bisphosphoglyceric acid

Phosphate group A
1. The phosphate group is united with the rest of the molecule through an ester linkage with a primary alcohol group.
2. By analogy with simple and familiar organic compounds, this linkage may be compared with the ester bond joining ethanol and acetic acid in ethyl acetate.

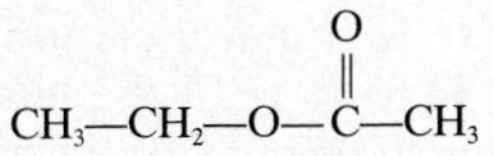

$$CH_3-CH_2-O-\overset{\overset{\displaystyle O}{\|}}{C}-CH_3$$

ethyl acetate

3. Like ethyl acetate, this phosphate ester is not easily hydrolyzed and liberates little heat (energy) on hydrolysis.
4. For these reasons organic phosphate esters, as well as inorganic phosphate salts, are said to contain low-energy phosphate bonds, which are often designated by the shorthand notation R—P.

Phosphate group B
1. The phosphate group is united with the rest of the molecule through an anhydride linkage to a carboxyl group.
2. By analogy, this bond may be compared to the anhydride bond between two molecules of acetic acid in acetic anhydride.

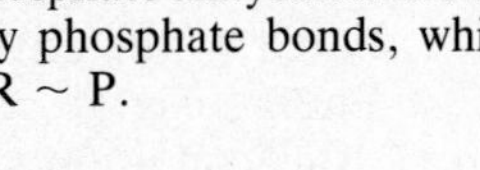

$$CH_3-\overset{\overset{\displaystyle O}{\|}}{C}-O-\overset{\overset{\displaystyle O}{\|}}{C}-CH_3$$

acetic anhydride

3. Like acetic anhydride, this phosphate anhydride is readily hydrolyzed and liberates large amounts of heat (energy) on hydrolysis.
4. Organic phosphate anhydrides are said to contain high-energy phosphate bonds, which are represented as R ~ P.

ATP (see **4–2**) has one ester-linked, low-energy phosphate attached to carbon 5 of the ribose of adenosine. The two terminal phosphates, however, are joined to each other and to the innermost phosphate by high-energy anhydride linkages between the phosphoric acid groups. A strategy of metabolism is the conversion of some of the energy of light and chemical substrates to these phosphoanhydride linkages which then provide chemical energy for energy-requiring cellular processes. The phosphoanhydride bonds are continually being

4–2.

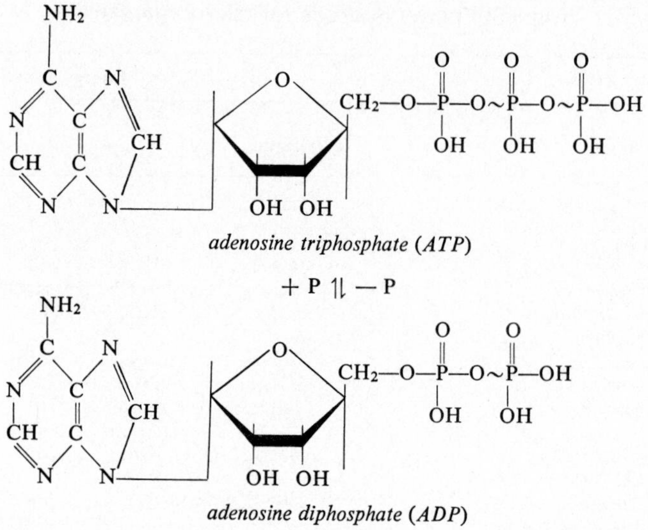

adenosine triphosphate (ATP)

$+ P \updownarrow - P$

adenosine diphosphate (ADP)

made and used as a cell extracts energy from its environment for growth and division.

Immediate products of the use of the high-energy bonds are the lower-energy compounds, adenosine diphosphate (ADP, one ~ P) and adenosine monophosphate (AMP, no ~ P). A cell that is actively using energy for biosynthesis would have a relatively low proportion of its adenine nucleotide pool in the form of ATP and ADP and a high proportion in the form of AMP because of the rapid use of ~ P. When energy use slows relative to production, the pool composition reverses with the ~ P forms (ADP, ATP) increasing in relative concentration. A cell in the former state has a low "energy charge" and in the latter, a high one. Some enzymes involved in energy generation and biosynthesis have been shown to be regulated by the energy charge of the cell.[1] A low-energy charge condition calls for more energy; this condition stimulates energy generation and slows down energy use. The reverse would hold for a high energy charge. Energy charge oscillations operate as a governor that helps to gear the rates of energy production to the rates of utilization.

Growth Yields[16, 17]

Construction of a new cell is a quantitative process. A quantity of ATP has to be generated from a quantity of the energy source for synthesis of the relatively constant amount of macromolecules that make up a cell. It is possible to determine experimentally the amount of energy source that has to be used to produce a certain amount of new cells. The strategy of the experiment is to grow the cells in a medium where all nutrients are in excess except the energy source. Growth then becomes proportional to the amount of energy source supplied.

Streptococcus faecalis uses glucose as an energy source and stops growing in an otherwise complete medium when glucose is completely used. The dry weight of cells produced with varying amounts of limiting glucose can be measured. When the experiment is done, a constant relationship between the dry weight of cells produced and the moles of glucose used is found. The **molar growth yield,** *i.e.,* dry weight per mole glucose used (abbreviated $Y_{glucose}$), is found to be 21.0 gm./mol. Since the molecular weight of glucose is 180, this means that *S. faecalis* needs 180 grams of glucose to obtain sufficient energy to make 21 grams of new cells.

Since many bacteria, *e.g., Salmonella typhimurium,* use glucose not only as an energy source but also as a major carbon source, how do we know that some of the glucose used by *S. faecalis* was used not for energy generation but as a precursor of cell macromolecules? *Streptococcus faecalis* has a very limited ability to synthesize the building block precursors of macromolecules, especially amino acids, purines, and pyrimidines, and these have to be supplied preformed in the medium. When radioactive [14C] glucose is supplied to *S. faecalis* in a growth yield experiment, only a negligible proportion is incorporated into cells, as compared to the amount used for energy generation.

Almost all of the glucose used by *S. faecalis* is converted to lactic acid. The fermentation is identical to that of muscle glycolysis and the energetics are well known. The overall fermentation equation is

$$C_6H_{12}O_6 + 2\text{ ADP} + 2\text{ P}_i \rightarrow$$
$$2\text{ CH}_3\text{CHOHCO}_2\text{H} + 2\text{ ATP}$$

Since 2 ATP are produced per mole of glucose, the 21.0 grams of cells produced per mole of glucose were formed per 2 moles of ATP, or 10.5 grams of cells per mole of ATP ($Y_{ATP} = 10.5$). Similar types of growth yield experiments carried out with other bacteria and yeast give approximately the same value for Y_{ATP}. $Y_{substrate}$ is not a constant because the ATP produced per mole of substrate can vary with substrate and with the pathway of catabolism. For example, *Leuconostoc mesenteroides* uses a pathway for glucose fermentation which leads to the overall equation:

$$C_6H_{12}O_6 + \text{ADP} + \text{P}_i \rightarrow$$
$$\text{CH}_3\text{CHOHCO}_2\text{H} + \text{CH}_3\text{CH}_2\text{OH} + \text{CO}_2 + \text{ATP}$$

Here, $Y_{glucose}$ is 10.5 and Y_{ATP} is 10.5.

The Y_{ATP} value provides a guide to the amount of growth one might expect when energy is limiting and the ATP yield per mole of energy source is known. For example, 1 ml. of normal human blood contains about 1 mg. of glucose, or about 5.6 μmol. per ml. This could support the growth of 21 × 5.6, or 118 μg. of streptococci which ferment glucose like *Streptococcus faecalis*. Since a streptococcal cell weighs about 10^{-6} μg., a final population of 1.2 × 10^8 streptococci per ml. would be attained when blood glucose is exhausted. A good laboratory medium is easily capable of supporting growth to such a level if sufficient glucose is available. If one is studying an organism with an unknown pathway for energy generation from a substrate, the Y_{ATP} value can also be used to obtain a rough approximation of the ATP yield per mole substrate used by growing the organism on limiting substrate and dividing $Y_{substrate}$ by 10.5.

Light and ATP Formation

Energy from a source has to be converted to the phosphoanhydride bonds of ATP and used for the reduction of the pyridine nucleotides, nicotinamide adenine dinucleotide

(NAD), and nicotinamide adenine dinucleotide phosphate (NADP) in order for biosynthesis to occur. Almost all major biological energy generation reactions are built around the theme of oxidation-reduction reactions that release energy from a chemical source or are used to convert the energy of light into chemical energy. There is good reason to believe that systems for converting light into chemical energy were early developments in the evolution of biological energy-generating systems.[14]

As seen in nature today, the photochemical energy systems start with the absorption of light quanta by subcellular structures that contain chlorophyll. In green plants, the chlorophyll is located in the complex membrane system of the subcellular organelle, the chloroplast. In procaryotic bacteria, the chlorophyll is contained in subunits (chromatophores) of the single membrane of phototrophs. Although the details of the activation of chlorophyll by light absorption are complex, the result can be thought of as the ejection of an electron from the chlorophyll molecule. The ejected electron is transferred through a series of cellular electron carriers and finally back to the electron-deficient chlorophyll to restore it to its ground state.

In effect, light-activated chlorophyll is a powerful reducing agent. It has a low oxidation-reduction (O–R) potential. Light energy is thus converted into a form of potential chemical energy, an activated chlorophyll that can reduce more oxidized electron acceptors in the membrane. The electron carriers are a series of compounds of increasing O–R potential such that after one gets reduced, it reduces the next higher O–R potential compound in turn. The carriers include the protein ferredoxin, probably the first carrier reduced by the activated chlorophyll, flavoproteins, quinones, and cytochromes. Once chemical energy is available in the form of activated chlorophyll, all subsequent O–R reactions proceed spontaneously, although most of them require enzyme catalysis.

All spontaneous reactions proceed with the release of energy. The amount of useful chemical energy available from any chemical reaction is designated $\triangle G$. $\triangle G^0$ is the standard free energy change, *i.e.,* the free energy when all reactants and products are at unit activity. $\triangle G^0$ is related to the equilibrium constant (K_{eq}),

$$\triangle G^0 = -RT \ln K_{eq}$$

where R is the gas constant (1.99 cal./mol. deg.) and T is the absolute temperature. To illustrate the significance of this relationship, we will use a hypothetical reaction between a reducing agent (electron donor), AH_2, and an oxidizing agent (electron acceptor), B. We will set their initial concentrations at 10^{-6} M and we will imagine that they react at 37° C. such that only 10^{-9} M AH_2 and B are left at equilibrium, and approximately 10^{-6} M, A and BH_2 are present at equilibrium. Then,

$$\Delta G^0 = -RT \ln \frac{(10^{-6})\,(10^{-6})}{(10^{-9})\,(10^{-9})}$$
$$= -1.99 \times 310$$
$$\times 2.3^* \,[(-12 - (-18)]$$
$$= -8513 \text{ cal./mol.}$$

It should be emphasized that $\triangle G^0$ is not the free energy change at equilibrium. It is the free energy change for a specified set of standard conditions, i.e., unit activity. The free energy change for any condition is given as $\triangle G$ and is related to $\triangle G^0$ and the other parameters of the oxidation-reduction reaction by

$$\Delta G = \Delta G^0 + RT \ln \frac{(A)(BH_2)}{(AH_2)(B)}$$

Thus, at equilibrium, $\triangle G = 0$, which is understandable because no net reaction takes place. When (A), (BH_2), (AH_2), and (B) are 1, i.e., at unit activity, then $\triangle G = \triangle G^0$ (ln 1 = 0).

The oxidation-reduction potential (voltage, measured in volts, V.) difference between an electron donor and an electron acceptor is directly related to the free energy change of the O–R reaction. O–R potential is a measure of the potential of a compound to donate electrons to a proton to form H_2 under the conditions of a standard H_2 half-cell (H^+/H_2) or for a compound to accept electrons from H_2, under the same conditions, to become reduced. The standard H_2 half-cell is H_2 at 1 atm. pressure and H^+ at unit activity and is defined as having an O–R potential of zero.

In biology, the convention is used that the more negative an O–R potential, the greater the tendency to donate electrons. Thus, if the system (A/AH_2) has a potential of -0.100 V., it has the capability of donating electrons to the standard H_2 electrode; if (B/BH_2) has a potential of $+0.085$ V., it has the capability of accepting electrons from the standard H_2 electrode and from the system (A/AH_2).

E_0 is the standard potential for a half-cell and is the potential when the oxidized form is

*ln = 2.3 (log 10)

equal to the reduced form, i.e., A = AH_2. The standard free energy change between two half-cells, e.g., A/AH_2 and B/BH_2, is related to the difference in the standard potentials by

$$\Delta G^0 = -nF \triangle E_0$$

where n equals the number of electrons per gram-equivalent transferred from the electron donor to the electron acceptor and F is the Faraday constant (23,000 calories per absolute volt-equivalent). For the reaction

$$AH_2 + B \rightleftarrows A + BH_2$$

two electrons and two protons are transferred from AH_2 to B and, using the potentials given above for half-cell potentials,

$$\Delta G° = -2(23,000)[0.085 - (-0.100)]$$
$$= -8510 \text{ cal./mol.}$$

This is essentially the same value obtained using the equilibrium constant for the reaction.

The equations and computations show the relationships between free energy changes, equilibrium constants, and O–R potentials. The activation of a chlorophyll molecule by light provides a low O–R potential source of energy. Stepwise movement of electrons from activated chlorophyll through a chain of electron carriers with increasing O–R potential will proceed spontaneously with energy release. Enzyme catalysis of electron transfer of any reaction only accelerates the rate of the reaction and has no effect on the final equilibrium or the free energy change.

Phototrophic organisms have the ingredients for using the energy of light to drive energy-yielding electron transfer reactions. They also have the ingredients for trapping some of the chemical energy in ATP for use in energy-requiring reactions. This can be demonstrated experimentally. Chromatophores can be isolated from disrupted cells of phototrophic bacteria. If the chromatophores are provided with light, ADP, and P_i, ATP is formed as a product:

$$ADP + P_i \xrightarrow{\text{light}} ATP$$

The chromatophore is a self-contained ATP manufacturer. It has chlorophyll and all of the electron transport agents necessary for cycling electrons from activated chlorophyll back to electron-deficient chlorophyll. The machinery is present for coupling the released chemical energy to ATP synthesis in a process called cyclic photophosphorylation (see **4–3**).

Light-activated chlorophyll can serve as a source of electrons to form the reduced pyridine nucleotides necessary for biosynthesis. Extraction of an electron from an excited chlorophyll molecule for formation of PNH, however, robs electrons from the chain which leads from the ejected electron to electron-deficient chlorophyll. An exogenous electron source is necessary to restore the chlorophyll to its initial ground state. In green plants, H_2O provides the exogenous electron source necessary for sustaining phototrophic growth through the reaction

$$H_2O + NADP^+ \xrightarrow{\;hv\;} NADPH + H^+ + \tfrac{1}{2}O_2$$

Photoevolution of oxygen is a complex reaction involving light energy and electron transport components between chlorophyll and NADP. The only procaryotes that carry out this reaction are the blue-green algae. Oxygen evolution is considered to be a highly advanced evolutionary mechanism for providing the reducing power for reductive biosynthesis.[14] The introduction of this mechanism is considered to be the evolutionary origin of atmospheric oxygen, and the prelude for the evolution of organisms that use oxygen in respiratory energy-generating systems and in other aspects of their metabolism.

Earlier phototrophic organisms, the bacteria, used electron donors other than H_2O for providing the electrons needed in reductive biosynthesis. These systems are reflected in those used by contemporary phototrophic bacteria. The purple sulfur and green sulfur phototrophic bacteria are anaerobic and use H_2S as an electron source:

$$H_2S + 4\,H_2O + 4\,NADP^+ \rightarrow$$
$$4\,NADPH + H_2SO_4 + 4\,H^+$$

Some of these bacteria and some of the non-sulfur purple phototrophic bacteria can use H_2 as an electron source:

$$H_2 + NADP^+ \rightarrow NADPH + H^+$$

A few of the purple sulfur and green sulfur and all of the nonsulfur purple bacteria can use organic compounds as electron sources; for example, some can use ethanol:

$$C_2H_5OH + 2\,NADP^+ + H_2O \rightarrow$$
$$CH_3CO_2H + 2\,NADPH + 2\,H^+$$

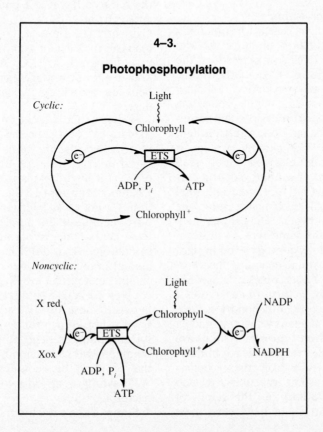

4–3.

Photophosphorylation

All of these processes are anaerobic, requiring light and an exogenous electron donor. Only the nonsulfur purple bacteria can grow in the presence of O_2, but when they do, they do not grow phototrophically. Oxygen represses the formation of chromatophores and the nonsulfur purple bacteria grow chemotrophically by oxidizing organic compounds when grown aerobically.

The use of the electron sources to effect a net reduction of NADP and reductive biosynthesis does not interfere with electron transfer through the electron chain from reduced chlorophyll to oxidized chlorophyll. The exogenous electron donor allows reductive biosynthesis and ATP formation to take place simultaneously, but it is a noncyclic process and is called noncyclic photophosphorylation (see **4–3**).

Light energy from the sun is the primary source of energy for almost all biological reactions. Green plants and many phototrophic bacteria use light-generated ATP and NADPH to synthesize cells from CO_2 and inorganic forms of the other elements of protoplasm. The synthesized organic compounds are then available as food for the many forms of life on this planet that require preformed organic compounds for energy and as building blocks for synthesis of cell macromolecules.

Oxidative Phosphorylation[5]

A general mechanism used for obtaining energy from the oxidation of inorganic and organic compounds is closely related to the phototrophic mechanism. Chemolithotrophic and chemoorganotrophic oxidation-reduction reactions, however, begin with preexisting sources of primary electron donors and terminal electron acceptors and do not rely on light for their generation. The general strategy is the same; low potential electron donors feed electrons into a chain of cellular electron carriers with increasing O–R potential and final transfer to a terminal electron acceptor, the most common being oxygen. The cellular electron carriers are of the same type as those of the electron transport system involved in phototrophic energy generation, including flavoproteins, quinones, and cytochromes organized in a membranous energy factory. In eucaryotes a subcellular organelle, the mitochondrion, contains the membranous energy factory, and in procaryotes the electron transport systems are organized in the single cytoplasmic membrane.

The formation of ATP from these chemotrophic electron transport reactions, termed **oxidative phosphorylation,** and the details of the electron transport chain have been most intensively studied in animal mitochondria. The two key donors that feed electrons into the mitochondrial membrane electron transport system are NADH and succinate. NADH is formed from NAD by enzymatic reduction using electrons from metabolites derived mainly in the breakdown of the important energy sources of animal cells, carbohydrates, and lipids. Succinate is a key electron donor because of the central role of the tricarboxylic acid cycle in oxidizing acetate, a major metabolite produced from carbohydrate and lipid energy sources. In mitochondria, the following reactions take place:

$$NADH + H^+ + \tfrac{1}{2}O_2 + 3\ ADP + 3\ P_i \rightarrow$$
$$NAD^+ + H_2O + 3\ ATP$$

and,

$$HO_2C(CH_2)_2CO_2H + \tfrac{1}{2}O_2 + 2\ ADP + 2\ P_i \rightarrow$$
succinate
$$HO_2CCH{=}CHCO_2H + H_2O + 2\ ATP$$
fumarate

Electrons are transferred from either substrate to a flavin prosthetic group of a specific dehydrogenase located in the membrane and then enzymatically moved sequentially from the reduced flavin to a quinone (coenzyme Q) and cytochromes b, c_1, c, a, and a_3 to O_2. Cytochromes a and a_3 constitute cytochrome oxidase, the enzyme complex directly involved in reducing O_2 to H_2O. ATP is generated at known specific voltage gaps in the chain, *e.g.*, between cytochrome c and cytochrome oxidase.

Bacteria that obtain energy for growth by oxidation of inorganic and organic compounds, in principle, use the same general mechanism as do mitochondria for trapping chemical energy through oxidative phosphorylation. Chemoorganotrophs that oxidize carbohydrates using O_2 as a terminal electron acceptor have membrane-bound electron transport systems containing flavoproteins, quinones, and cytochromes that differ in detail from those of animal mitochondria but essentially carry out similar oxidations of NADH and succinate coupled to ATP synthesis. The stoichiometry between substrate oxidized and ATP synthesized is not known for certain in any bacterial system, but it is believed to be less than that obtained with mitochondria. In other words, the coupling between available energy and ATP synthesis appears to be less efficient in bacterial systems.

Some of the cytochrome-containing bacteria

can substitute nitrate for O_2 as a terminal electron acceptor. For example, some members of the *Bacillus* and *Pseudomonas* genera can oxidize glucose either aerobically, reducing O_2 to H_2O, or anaerobically, reducing nitrate to nitrous oxide and nitrogen gas. Both processes permit ATP synthesis via oxidative phosphorylation.

The specific compounds that serve as electron donors to the membrane electron transport system will vary with different organisms, depending on the nature of the substrates used for growth. Chemoorganotrophs have to metabolize their large variety of organic substrates to obtain a product, *e.g.*, NADH or succinate, that can directly reduce the components of the electron transport chain. Chemolithotrophs, *e.g.*, Fe^{2+} and H_2 oxidizers, depend entirely on the terminal electron transport system and oxidative phosphorylation for energy generation, whereas chemoorganotrophs can obtain energy from organic substrate phosphorylations, as will be discussed later.

ATP generation through oxidative phosphorylation is not restricted to the use of O_2 as a terminal electron acceptor (as was already pointed out with the example of nitrate reduction), nor is it restricted to cytochrome-containing organisms. Some cytochrome-containing bacteria, the sulfate-reducing bacteria, obtain energy for growth by coupling the oxidation of organic compounds like lactate to the reduction of sulfate to sulfide; in these bacteria oxidative phosphorylation is involved in ATP formation. Many methane-forming bacteria do not contain cytochromes, but they obtain energy for growth from the following reaction:

$$4 H_2 + CO_2 \rightarrow CH_4 + 2 H_2O$$

In these bacteria ATP formation must be entirely associated with the transfer of electrons from H_2 to CO_2.

Energy and Chemiosmotic Mechanisms[6]

The electron transport systems that produce significant amounts of useful energy are bound to cell membranes. Enzymes and electron carriers of the systems are fixed in specific sites in the membrane and have specific spatial orientations with respect to one another and to the inside and outside surfaces of membranes. Electrons and protons are removed from internal substrates, *e.g.*, NADH, and the electrons are transferred within the membrane to the terminal electron acceptor, *e.g.*, oxygen. The protons are ejected to the outside of the

membrane with a net accumulation of hydroxyl ions inside. The membrane is impermeable to protons and hydroxyl ions. An electrical force, called the **protonmotive force,** is created that is composed of the membrane potential and the pH gradient. Since the membrane involved in electron transport in bacteria is the cytoplasmic membrane, the inside of bacterial cells is negatively charged. The protonmotive force is used to synthesize ATP from ADP and inorganic phosphate, to transport solutes in and out of the cell against concentration gradients, and to provide the energy required for motility.

ATP is synthesized by a membrane-associated enzyme that catalyzes the reaction:

$$ADP + P_i \rightarrow ATP + H+(inside) + OH-(outside).$$

This synthesis of the terminal high-energy bond of ATP is possible because the enzyme is oriented in the membrane in a way which allows the proton product to enter the inside of the cell where it is neutralized by internal OH-. The OH- product is simultaneously ejected outside where it is neutralized by external H+. Therefore, separation of H+ and OH- caused by electron transport is used to pull the reaction toward ATP synthesis by removing products that would otherwise cause reversal of the reaction. The protonmotive force can also be used to form high affinity, protonated complexes between specific membrane carriers and solutes which then move to the inside of the membrane where the proton is neutralized and the solute is released. External protons can also be used to "energize" proteins of the motility apparatus.

The protonmotive force can be used to couple electron transport to the formation of ATP, and ATP formed by substrate phosphorylation can be used to set up a protonmotive force that can in turn be used to drive active transport and motility. Generation of ATP by the protonmotive force occurs as a result of light-dependent electron transport in photosynthetic bacteria as well as in the membrane electron transport systems of chemotrophs. The concept of protonmotive force is derived from the chemiosmotic hypothesis that was proposed by Mitchell in 1961. A substantial body of experimental evidence has accumulated since then that supports the hypothesis.

Substrate Phosphorylation

ATP can also be formed from organic energy sources by a process called substrate phosphorylation. The energy substrates are enzymatically converted to specific compounds that have part of the potential chemical energy of the parent compound concentrated in high-energy phosphate bonds. This type of energy trapping is illustrated by the fermentation of glucose by muscle. The fermentation pathway, called the Embden-Meyerhof-Parnas (EMP) pathway, is shown in **4–4**.

These chemical reactions, catalyzed by enzymes, shift, split, oxidize, hydrate, dehydrate, and add phosphate to bonds derived from the original glucose molecule. From the point of view of trapping the energy of glucose in the form of ATP, all are aimed at providing two particular substrates for two particular enzyme reactions. One substrate is 3-P-glyceraldehyde and the other is phosphoenolpyruvate.

The 3-P-glyceraldehyde dehydrogenase oxidizes the aldehyde group of the phosphate ester with the simultaneous reduction of NAD. The aldehyde group is oxidized through an intermediate enzyme thioester:

$$R-CHO + E-SH + NAD^+ \rightarrow E-S\sim\overset{\overset{O}{\|}}{C}-R + NADH + H^+$$

E—SH is enzyme (E) with — SH representing the sulfhydryl group of the amino acid cysteine in the protein. The thioester is a high-energy bond in which the energy of the oxidation-reduction reaction is temporarily stored. Inorganic phosphate reacts with the enzyme intermediate to give a phosphoanhydride, 1,3-bisphosphoglyceric acid:

$$E-S\sim\overset{\overset{O}{\|}}{C}-R + H_3PO_4 \rightarrow E-SH + R-\overset{\overset{O}{\|}}{C}\sim OPO_3H_2$$

The phosphoanhydride bond is a high-energy phosphate bond and it can be directly transferred to ADP in a reaction catalyzed by phosphoglyceric acid kinase:

$$R-\overset{\overset{O}{\|}}{C}-O\sim PO_3H_2 + ADP \rightarrow ATP + R-\overset{\overset{O}{\|}}{C}\diagdown_{OH}$$

The second reaction that leads to a high-energy phosphate compound is catalyzed by the enzyme enolase:

$$\begin{array}{ccc} CO_2H & & CO_2H \\ | & & | \\ HC-O-PO_3H_2 & \rightarrow & C-O\sim PO_3H_2 + H_2O \\ | & & \| \\ CH_2OH & & CH_2 \end{array}$$

2-phospho-glyceric acid   *phosphoenolpyruvic acid*

This is a dehydration, and some of the potential energy of the 2-phosphoglyceric acid is concentrated in the enol-phosphate bond. The phosphate is then ready for transfer to ADP in a reaction catalyzed by phosphoenolpyruvate kinase:

$$\begin{array}{ccc} CO_2H & & CO_2H \\ | & & | \\ C-O\sim PO_3H_2 + ADP \rightarrow & C=O + ATP \\ \| & & | \\ CH_2 & & CH_3 \end{array}$$

pyruvic acid

Since 2 moles of 3-P-glyceraldehyde and 2 moles of phosphoenolpyruvate are formed from each mole of glucose fermented, a total of 4 moles of ATP are formed per mole of glucose. It is necessary, however, to use up 2 moles of ATP in the reactions which convert the glucose molecule to the specific high-energy phosphate precursors of ATP (see **4–4**). The net yield of ATP per mole of glucose is 2.

Although one of the reactions which require ATP is written as the hexokinase reaction,

glucose + ATP → glucose-6-phosphate + ADP

it is now known that many bacteria use a different method for forming glucose-6-phosphate:

glucose + phosphoenolpyruvate →
glucose-6-phosphate + pyruvate

This is a complex reaction carried out by enzymes in the cell membrane, and it is used not only to phosphorylate glucose but also to transport glucose from the external medium, through the membrane, and into the cell.[7, 24] No ATP is made from the 1 phosphoenolpyruvate formed from glucose, but since no ATP is used to make glucose-6-phosphate either, the net yield of ATP per mole of glucose is still 2. A similar phosphoenolpyruvate: sugar phosphotransferase is used to transport other sugars into bacterial cells.

There is one oxidative reaction in the EMP scheme, the oxidation of 3-P-glyceraldehyde to 1,3-bisphosphoglyceric acid. NAD is reduced to NADH. Since NAD is only produced in small amounts in the cell, its reduction without reoxidation would stop glucose breakdown. Some NADH can be reoxidized by reductive biosynthetic reactions, but the number of these reactions is small and unable to provide sufficient conversion of glucose to pyruvate to satisfy the ATP need for growth and

4–4.

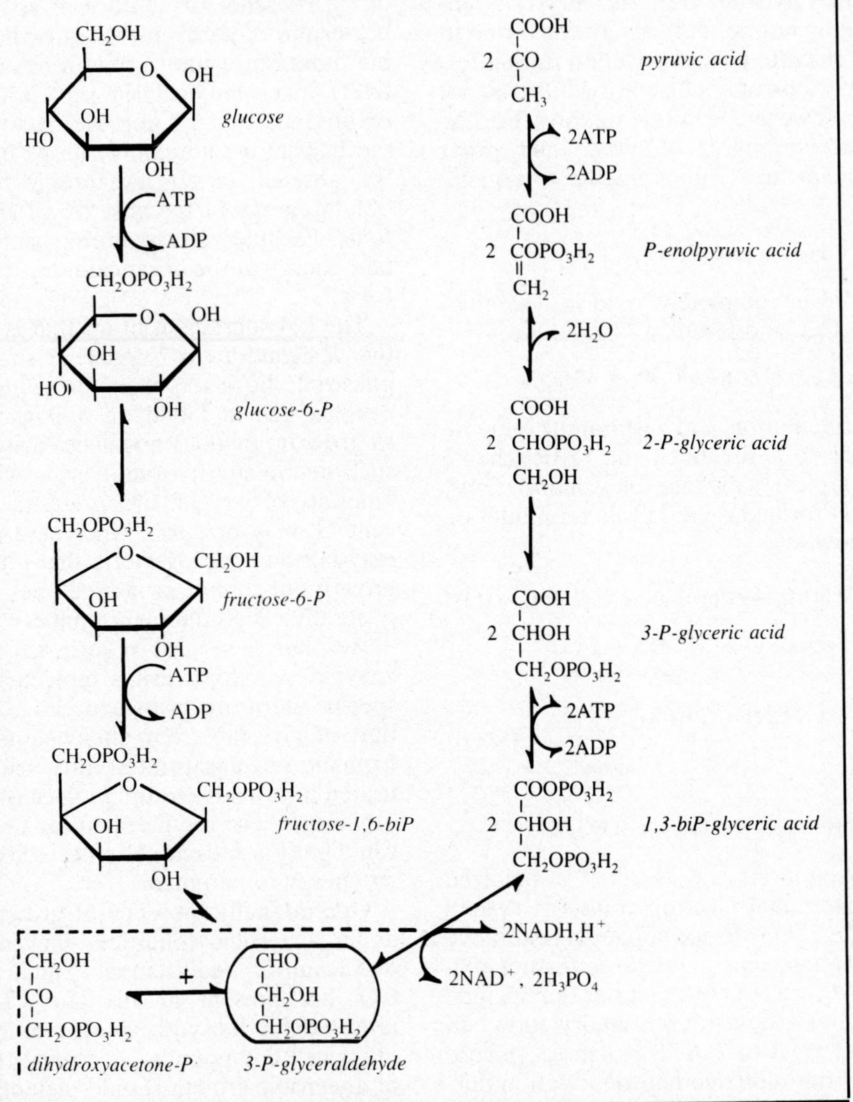

division. Streptococci and muscle have a simple method for rapidly oxidizing NADH back into NAD to sustain the energy-generating system. They use the lactic dehydrogenase reaction,

$$H^+ + NADH + pyruvate \rightarrow NAD^+ + lactate$$

The overall fermentation of glucose to lactic acid does not require the addition of an exogenous electron acceptor, but oxidation-reduction reactions are still essential for driving the system toward ATP synthesis. In effect, an O–R reaction, 3-P-glyceraldehyde dehydrogenase, combined with some nonoxidative re-

actions, leads to the formation of substrates for another O–R reaction, lactic dehydrogenase. The terminal O–R reaction drives the overall sequence by the reoxidation of NADH.

The term "fermentation" is often loosely used to describe a variety of distinctly different metabolic processes. For the purposes of this discussion, the term will be used to signify only oxidation-reduction processes whereby single organic compounds are catabolized to products in the absence of an added electron acceptor substrate. Although carbohydrates are the most familiar substrates for fermentation, the definition does not exclude other common compounds used as energy sources through oxidation-reduction-based pathways. Lactic acid and some amino acids, for example, can be fermented by some bacteria. Substrate energy is mainly but not exclusively converted to ATP via substrate phosphorylation during fermentation. Substrate phosphorylation is not restricted, however, to fermentations. For example, *Saccharomyces cerevisiae* and other yeasts ferment (anaerobic) glucose to ethanol and CO_2,

$$C_6H_{12}O_6 \rightarrow 2\ C_2H_5OH + 2\ CO_2$$

and they also completely oxidize (aerobic) glucose to CO_2 and H_2O:

$$C_6H_{12}O_6 + 6\ O_2 \rightarrow 6\ CO_2 + 6\ H_2O$$

During fermentation and respiration, glucose is converted to pyruvate by the EMP scheme with the typical substrate phosphorylations. The NADH formed is used up in fermentation by the following:

glucose $+\ 2\ NAD^+ \rightarrow 2$ pyruvate $+\ 2\ NADH + 2\ H^+$

2 pyruvate $\rightarrow 2\ CH_3CHO + 2\ CO_2$
acetaldehyde

2 $CH_3CHO + 2\ NADH + 2\ H^+ \rightarrow$
$2\ C_2H_5OH + 2\ NAD^+$
ethanol

Sum:

glucose $\rightarrow 2$ ethanol $+\ 2\ CO_2$

During respiration, the NADH is oxidized through a terminal electron transport system to NAD and H_2O with accompanying oxidative phosphorylation, and pyruvate is further oxidized to CO_2 and H_2O by reactions that include substrate and oxidative phosphorylation. In yeast, a net yield of 2 ATP per mole glucose is derived from substrate phosphorylation during fermentation. A net yield of 36 ATP per mole glucose is derived from the oxidation of glucose: 2 from substrate phosphorylation from glucose to pyruvate and H_2O, 2 from substrate phosphorylation from pyruvate to CO_2 and H_2O, and all the rest from oxidative phosphorylation. In general, oxidation of a substrate with O_2 as an electron acceptor provides a cell with more ATP per mole substrate than does fermentation of the same substrate, and the increase is generally large when the cell is capable of synthesizing ATP by oxidative phosphorylation.

Relationship to Oxygen[13]
Bacteria are commonly designated as **aerobic**, **facultatively anaerobic**, or **anaerobic**.

Strictly speaking, the terms are operational and refer to the ability of an organism to grow in the presence or absence of air. An aerobic bacterium requires air for growth, an anaerobic organism cannot grow in air, and facultatively anaerobic bacteria grow in the presence or absence of air. Aerobic bacteria have no mechanism for obtaining energy for growth in the absence of air. Anaerobic bacteria can obtain energy in the absence of air, but air is toxic. Facultatively anaerobic bacteria can obtain energy in the absence of air, but air is not toxic.

The key ingredient of air that is the basis of the designations is oxygen. It should be emphasized, however, that air contains 20 per cent oxygen and that an organism's inability to grow in air does not necessarily mean that such an organism cannot grow when smaller amounts of oxygen are present; *i.e.*, 20 per cent O_2 may be toxic, whereas 2 per cent O_2 may not be toxic. Bacteria that require O_2 for growth but cannot grow in 20 per cent O_2 are generally called **microaerophilic**.

Aerobes may also require O_2 for specific enzyme reactions using molecular O_2 as a specific substrate in biosynthesis. The formation of tyrosine from phenylalanine and the formation of unsaturated fatty acids from saturated fatty acids require molecular O_2 in some organisms. The requirement for O_2, therefore, can signify a biosynthetic necessity as well as an energy requirement.

Operationally, absence of growth observed under anaerobic conditions may not even be due to an O_2 requirement. Small amounts of CO_2 are present in air, and CO_2 may be required for biosynthesis of amino acids and other cell compounds. A critical test for lack of anaerobic growth should include some CO_2 in the anaerobic atmosphere, *e.g.*, nitrogen, to restrict the designation aerobe to the organism's relationship to O_2.

Facultatively anaerobic bacteria may or may not use oxygen in energy metabolism. *Escherichia coli* and *Saccharomyces cerevisiae* ferment carbohydrates in the absence of O_2 and oxidize carbohydrates to CO_2 and H_2O in the presence of O_2. Many carbohydrate-fermenting bacteria, *e.g.*, most streptococci and other lactic acid bacteria, simply survive in the presence of air. Oxygen can be metabolically inert for these organisms.

The mechanism of O_2 toxicity for anaerobes is not fully understood, and there may be more than one mechanism operating. Oxygen could act through the production of toxic substances, such as hydrogen peroxide or organic peroxides. It is believed that the superoxide radical, O_2^-, formed by the oxidation of reduced flavins, quinones, and other electron carriers, is more toxic than hydrogen peroxide. Many bacteria that tolerate the presence of O_2 (aerotolerant organisms) produce the enzyme superoxide dismutase that destroys the radical as follows:

$$O_2^- + O_2^- + 2H^+ \rightarrow H_2O_2 + O_2$$

Many of the same bacteria contain catalase, an enzyme that produces water and oxygen from hydrogen peroxide, and/or peroxidases that use electron donors such as NADH to reduce hydrogen peroxide to water:

$$2H_2O_2 \rightarrow 2H_2O + O_2 \ (catalase)$$

$$\underset{\substack{\text{(electron} \\ \text{donor)}}}{AH_2} + H_2O_2 \rightarrow \underset{\substack{\text{(oxidized} \\ \text{donor)}}}{A} + 2H_2O \ (peroxidase)$$

Oxygen could also act by causing the oxidation of essential reduced substances in the cell, *e.g.*, sulfhydryl groups, which cannot easily be regenerated by the anaerobic organisms. In this case, O_2 toxicity would involve direct destruction of an essential ingredient rather than production of a toxic agent that, in turn, destroys some key cellular process.

Metabolic Reactions

CARBOHYDRATE BREAKDOWN[37]

Carbohydrates are fermented and oxidized to provide energy for growth and, in many cases, the pathways used for energy generation feed small molecules into biosynthetic pathways. There are a large number of carbohydrates in nature, including polysaccharides, oligosaccharides, and monosaccharides. Hexoses and pentoses are the major monosaccharides existing as free compounds or as oligosaccharide and polysaccharide constituents. Glucose is by far the most common monosaccharide in nature as a free sugar; as the sole sugar component in cellulose, starch, and glycogen; and as a component of other oligo- and polysaccharides.

The general pattern for the use of all carbohydrates is their enzymatic funneling into a few central pathways for catabolism of a few key sugar phosphates. The enzymes of the pathways degrade the sugar phosphates to low-molecular-weight compounds, mainly pyruvate, acetate, and carbon dioxide. Pyruvate rarely accumulates as a product and is further metabolized to fermentation products or oxidized, in respiring organisms, to acetate or to CO_2 and H_2O. Acetate may be a terminal product or it may be oxidized to CO_2 and H_2O.

To understand the catabolism of a specific carbohydrate by a specific bacterium, it is necessary to understand the following:

1. How the carbohydrate enters the central pathway.

2. What central pathway is used.

3. What the products are, and how they are formed.

4. What O–R reactions are involved (related to questions 2 and 3).

5. Where ATP is synthesized (related to questions 2 and 3).

6. How the catabolic pathway provides the ingredients for biosynthesis.

7. How catabolism is regulated.

Polysaccharides and Oligosaccharides[28]

Polysaccharides and oligosaccharides are generally funneled into the major pathways by first being degraded to the constituent monosaccharides. For example, organisms that use cellulose as an energy source contain cellulases that hydrolyze cellulose to glucose. Xylan is hydrolyzed to xylose, starch to glucose, lactose to glucose and galactose, sucrose to glucose and fructose, and so forth. The enzymes are specific for the substrates used and in most cases, hydrolytic:

$$(\text{monosaccharide})_n + (n - 1) \ H_2O \rightarrow n \text{ monosaccharide}$$

When the carbohydrate is large (n is large), as in cellulose or starch, the hydrolytic enzymes are located on the cell surface or excreted into the environment because of the difficulty of transporting the high-molecular-weight compounds through the cell membrane.

There are a few exceptions to the hydrolytic mechanisms for forming monosaccharides from disaccharides. A few organisms have phosphorolytic enzymes that phosphorylyze the disaccharide to a sugar phosphate and a free sugar, *e.g.*,

sucrose (glucose-fructose) + P_i →

glucose-1-phosphate + fructose

In *Staphylococcus aureus,* and probably in many other bacteria, lactose (glucose-galactose) is transported into the cell by the phosphoenol pyruvate phosphotransferase system to give the following sequence[4]:

lactose + phosphoenolpyruvate →
(outside cell)

$$\text{lactose phosphate} + \text{pyruvate}$$
(inside cell)

lactose phosphate → glucose-6-P + galactose

Another method used for disaccharide breakdown is restricted to sucrose breakdown and to a few species of lactic acid bacteria. The method involves polymerization of one portion of the sucrose molecule with the release of the other portion as the free sugar. A fructose polymer (levan) is made if the organism has a transfructosylating enzyme (levansucrase):

$$n \text{ glucose-fructose} \rightarrow n \text{ glucose} + (\text{fructose})_n$$
levan

A glucose polymer (glucan or dextran) is the result of the action of a transglucosylating enzyme,

$$n \text{ glucose-fructose} \rightarrow n \text{ fructose} + (\text{glucose})_n$$
*(glucan
or dextran)*

Bacterial dextrans have been used as blood extenders, and they are used for separation of compounds by molecular weight differences in a separation method known as gel filtration. Glucan production by *Streptococcus mutans* has been strongly implicated in caries formation in man and lower animals.[26] The *S. mutans* glucan produced from sucrose glues the organism to tooth surfaces where it, along with other trapped organisms, can produce acid fermentation products that dissolve the tooth enamel.

In human infections, the breakdown of polysaccharides and oligosaccharides to free sugars is probably not important for organisms that invade normally sterile habitats, such as the blood and specific organ tissues. The major carbohydrate energy source in these environments is glucose. There are some exceptions, *e.g.,* glycogen in the liver and lactose, the sugar in milk. Staphylococci infecting a breast after delivery no doubt get energy for growth from lactose.

However, bacteria normally exist in great numbers in nonsterile parts of the body: in the oral cavity and the lower part of the gastrointestinal tract. These bacteria are sustained by energy sources in human food. Sucrose, starch, and even cellulose, which the human being ingests but does not use as an energy source, can be used by one or another of the bacteria in these habitats. Catabolism of these carbohydrates would then be important in infections of these "open" cavities, such as in caries formation, periodontal disease, throat infections, and intestinal tract infections. Energy from carbohydrates in food would also be important in the harboring of potential pathogens that gain entry into normally sterile environments by entry into the lungs from the oral cavity or into the blood and tissues through lesions in the intestinal tract.

Monosaccharide Conversions

Once monosaccharides are formed, they have to be converted to a sugar phosphate intermediate of the central pathway or pathways used by the organism. The degree of difficulty (amount of enzyme manipulation) necessary to accomplish this depends on the relationship of the monosaccharide to the sugar phosphates of the pathway. A starch-fermenting streptococcus, for example, has only to phosphorylate the derivative glucose to produce a key intermediate of the EMP scheme, glucose-6-phosphate. The conversion of galactose, formed from lactose, to glucose-6-phosphate involves a series of enzyme reactions:

galactose + ATP → galactose-1-P + ADP

uridine diphosphate glucose + galactose-1-P →
uridine diphosphate galactose + glucose-1-P

uridine diphosphate galactose →
uridine diphosphate glucose

glucose-1-P + glucose-6-P

Sum:

galactose + ATP → glucose-6-P + ADP

The purpose of this entire sequence is to epimerize the hydroxyl on carbon 4 of the galactose to make glucose. Galactose and glucose are identical except for the configuration of the hydroxyl group on carbon 4 (see **4–5**). The structure of uridine diphosphate glucose is shown in **4–5**.

The general strategy for converting a "foreign" monosaccharide to a "native" structure of the central pathway is to use epimerization and isomerization reactions to bring the hydroxyl groups and carbonyl groups into line. Sometimes this involves a sugar nucleoside

4–5.

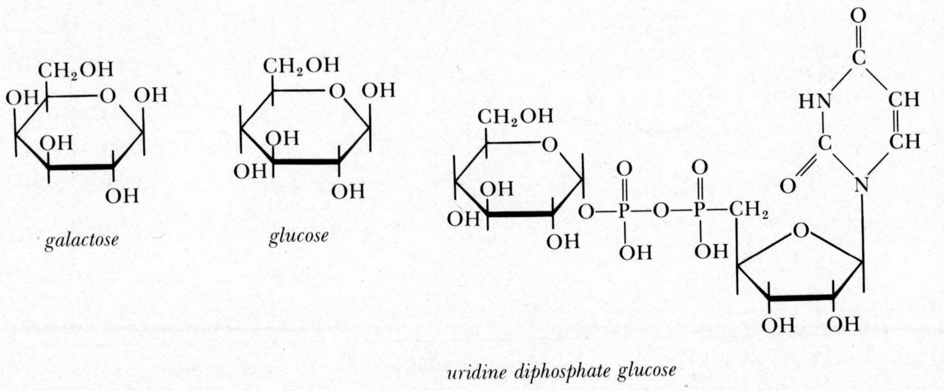

galactose *glucose*

uridine diphosphate glucose

derivative as with galactose and sometimes enzymes manipulate free monosaccharides to achieve the goal. In the fermentation of L-arabinose, an important constituent of plant hemicellulose, by some lactic acid bacteria, it is necessary to form D-xylulose-5-phosphate from L-arabinose. D-Xylulose-5-phosphate is a central compound in the fermentation of pentoses by microorganisms. The conversion is accomplished by reactions which do not involve nucleoside sugar derivatives (see **4–6**).

The D-galactose → D-glucose and L-arabinose → D-xylulose conversions are illustrations of a large number of similar types of conversions of the large variety of monosaccharides encountered by microorganisms in nature. Similar reactions are also used to transform central pathway sugars to special monosaccharides for biosynthesis of specific cell components. Microorganisms encounter a variety of compounds related to the aldo- and keto-sugars, such as amino sugars, polyhydric alcohols (derived from reduction of the sugar car-

bonyl to a hydroxyl group), and compounds in which the sugar aldehyde group has been converted to a carboxyl group (aldonic acids) or the hydroxyl farthest from the carbonyl has been converted to a carboxyl group (uronic acids). Obviously, mechanisms exist for conversion of these energy sources to the phosphate esters of the central pathway, but the details are beyond the scope of this discussion.

CENTRAL HEXOSE PATHWAYS

Several different pathways have evolved for breaking down hexoses into smaller molecular weight compounds. In the EMP pathway (see **4–4**), the hexose molecule is split into two 3-carbon units before any O–R reactions occur. Three different pathways, however, involve prior oxidation of the aldehyde group to a carboxyl group before the carbon chain is cleaved. The pathways all begin with phosphorylating and oxidative reactions leading to the

4–6.

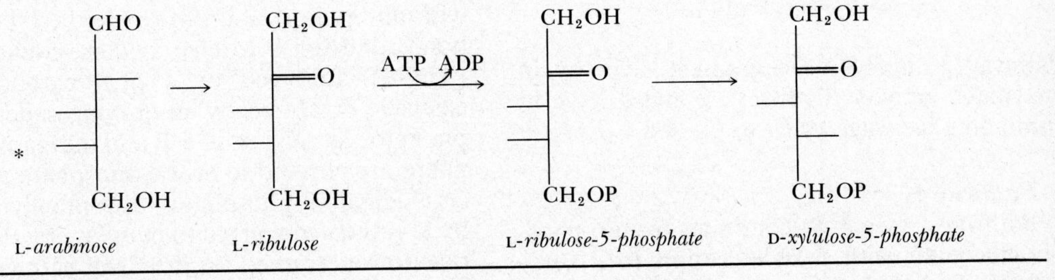

L-arabinose *L-ribulose* *L-ribulose-5-phosphate* *D-xylulose-5-phosphate*

*Single bars represent hydroxyl groups.

4–7.

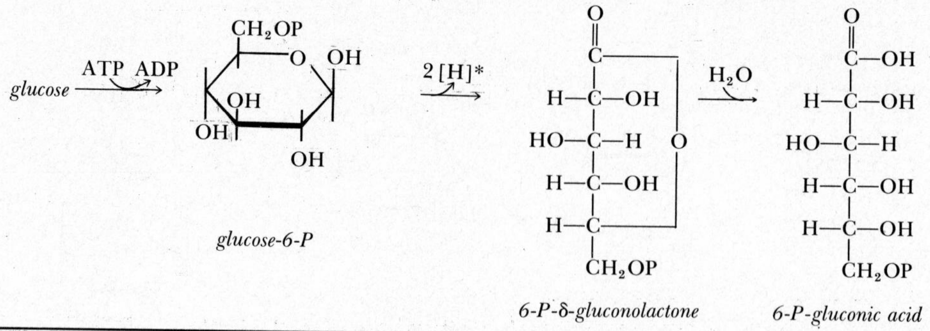

glucose $\xrightarrow{\text{ATP ADP}}$ glucose-6-P $\xrightarrow{2\,[\text{H}]^*}$ 6-P-δ-gluconolactone $\xrightarrow{\text{H}_2\text{O}}$ 6-P-gluconic acid

*[H] is a general way of indicating removal of two protons and two electrons without specifying the electron acceptor.

formation of 6-phosphogluconate from glucose (see **4–7**). Before detailing the important subsequent enzyme reactions in these three pathways, we will look at the respective breaking patterns that lead to the formation of smaller compounds from the 6-carbon compound:

Pathway 1

$$C_6 \rightarrow 2\,C_3$$

Pathway 2

$$C_6 \rightarrow C_5 + C_1$$
$$C_5 \rightarrow C_3 + C_2$$

Sum:

$$C_6 \rightarrow C_3 + C_2 + C_1$$

Pathway 3

$$3\,C_6 \rightarrow 3\,C_5 + 3\,C_1$$
$$2\,C_5 \rightarrow C_7 + C_3$$
$$C_7 + C_3 \rightarrow C_6 + C_4$$
$$C_5 + C_4 \rightarrow C_6 + C_3$$
$$2\,C_6 \rightarrow 4\,C_3$$

Sum:

$$3\,C_6 \rightarrow 5\,C_3 + 3\,C_1$$

Pathway 3 involves the greatest diversity in enzymatic activity. Pathways 2 and 3 have in common a cleavage of C_6 to C_5 and C_1.

Pathway 1

Pathway 1 (see **4–8**) continues from 6-phosphogluconate with a dehydration to 2-keto-3-deoxy-6-phosphogluconic acid (KDPG). KDPG is then cleaved between carbon atoms 3 and 4 to yield 3-P-glyceraldehyde and pyruvate. Then 3-P-glyceraldehyde is converted to pyruvate by exactly the same reactions used in the EMP scheme. This pathway is usually referred to as the Entner-Doudoroff (ED) pathway, after the original discoverers. Although the pathway differs from the EMP pathway, both produce 2 moles of pyruvate per mole of glucose. Since 1 ATP is used to make 1 phosphorylated hexose, and 2 ATP are formed when the hexose is converted to pyruvate, the net yield of ATP per mole glucose is 1 in contrast to the net yield of 2 for the EMP scheme.

Pathways 2 and 3

Pathways 2 and 3 proceed identically from 6-phosphogluconate to a C_5 and C_1 unit. A single enzyme, 6-phosphogluconate dehydrogenase, catalyzes the oxidative decarboxylation of 6-phosphogluconate to ribulose-5-phosphate (Ru-5-P) and CO_2 with a pyridine nucleotide as an electron acceptor (see **4–9**). In both pathways, two oxidative reactions operate to achieve the primary cleavage of the C_6 unit.

Pathway 2. Pathway 2 (see **4–10**) continues with an epimerization of the hydroxyl on carbon 3 of Ru-5-P to give xylulose-5-phosphate (Xu-5-P) followed by a final carbon chain cleavage catalyzed by an enzyme called phosphoketolase. Xylulose-5-P and inorganic phosphate are cleaved to acetyl-phosphate and glyceraldehyde-3-phosphate. Phosphoglyceraldehyde is then converted to pyruvate by the same reactions described for the EMP pathway. The phosphorolytic split of xylulose-5-phosphate leads to the formation of a product with a

4–8.

Pathway 1—Entner-Doudoroff (ED) Scheme

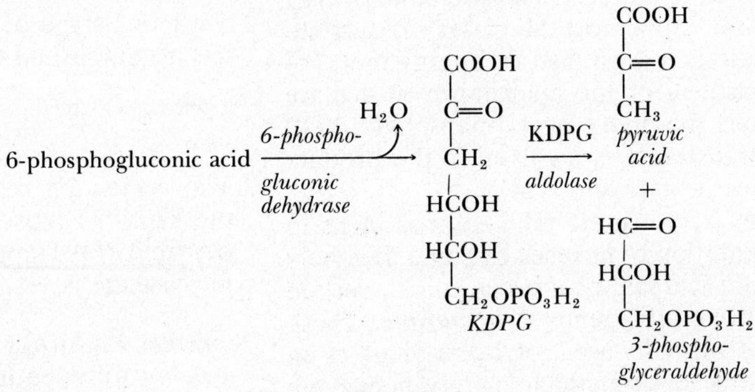

$$6\text{-phosphogluconic acid} \xrightarrow[\substack{\textit{gluconic} \\ \textit{dehydrase}}]{\textit{6-phospho-}} \quad \begin{array}{c} COOH \\ | \\ C{=}O \\ | \\ CH_2 \\ | \\ HCOH \\ | \\ HCOH \\ | \\ CH_2OPO_3H_2 \\ \textit{KDPG} \end{array} \xrightarrow[\textit{aldolase}]{\textit{KDPG}} \quad \begin{array}{c} COOH \\ | \\ C{=}O \\ | \\ CH_3 \\ \textit{pyruvic} \\ \textit{acid} \\ + \end{array} \begin{array}{c} HC{=}O \\ | \\ HCOH \\ | \\ CH_2OPO_3H_2 \\ \textit{3-phospho-} \\ \textit{glyceraldehyde} \end{array}$$

(with H_2O entering at the 6-phosphogluconic dehydrase step)

$$3\text{-P-glyceraldehyde} \xrightarrow{2\ ADP + 2\ P_i + 2\ NAD^+} 2\ \text{pyruvate} + 2\ ATP + 2\ NADH + 2\ H^+$$

4–9.

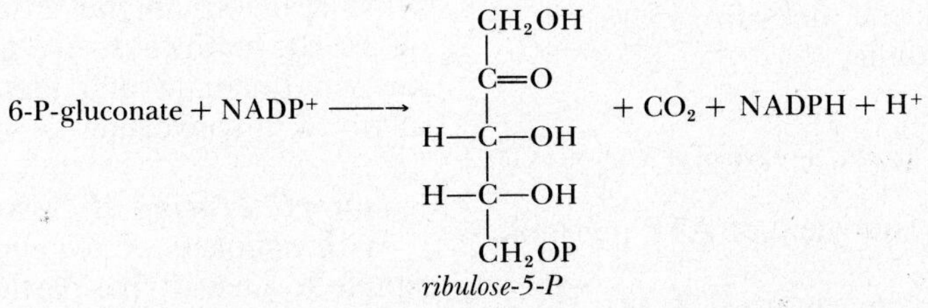

$$6\text{-P-gluconate} + NADP^+ \longrightarrow \begin{array}{c} CH_2OH \\ | \\ C{=}O \\ | \\ H{-}C{-}OH \\ | \\ H{-}C{-}OH \\ | \\ CH_2OP \\ \textit{ribulose-5-P} \end{array} + CO_2 + NADPH + H^+$$

4–10.

Pathway 2—Phosphoketolase

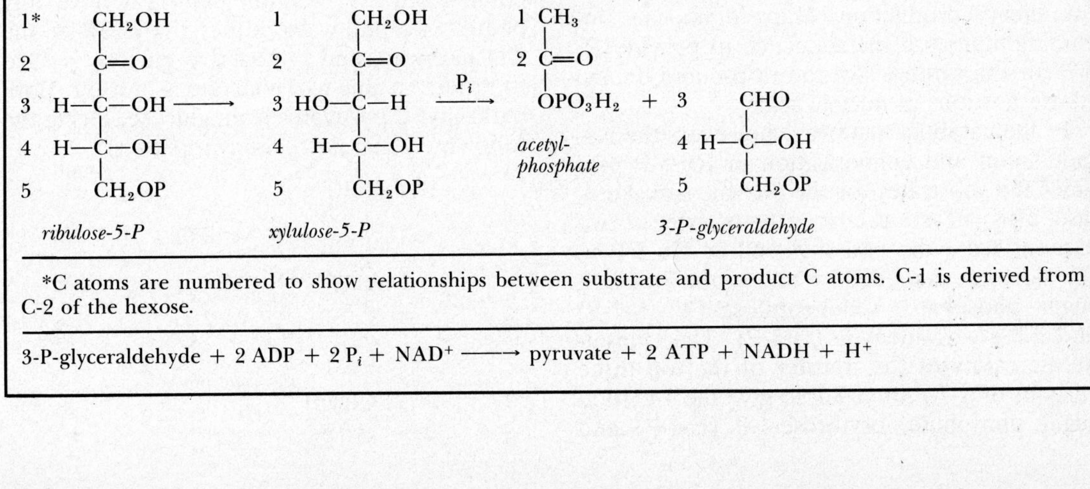

$$\begin{array}{cc} 1^* & CH_2OH \\ 2 & C{=}O \\ 3 & H{-}C{-}OH \\ 4 & H{-}C{-}OH \\ 5 & CH_2OP \end{array} \longrightarrow \begin{array}{cc} 1 & CH_2OH \\ 2 & C{=}O \\ 3 & HO{-}C{-}H \\ 4 & H{-}C{-}OH \\ 5 & CH_2OP \end{array} \xrightarrow{P_i} \begin{array}{c} 1\ CH_3 \\ 2\ C{=}O \\ OPO_3H_2 \\ \textit{acetyl-} \\ \textit{phosphate} \end{array} + \begin{array}{cc} 3 & CHO \\ 4 & H{-}C{-}OH \\ 5 & CH_2OP \end{array}$$

ribulose-5-P   *xylulose-5-P*   *3-P-glyceraldehyde*

---

*C atoms are numbered to show relationships between substrate and product C atoms. C-1 is derived from C-2 of the hexose.

$$3\text{-P-glyceraldehyde} + 2\ ADP + 2\ P_i + NAD^+ \longrightarrow \text{pyruvate} + 2\ ATP + NADH + H^+$$

high-energy phosphoanhydride bond, acetyl-phosphate. ATP can be made from acetyl-phosphate:

$$\text{acetyl} {\sim} P + ADP \rightarrow \text{acetate} + ATP$$

This reaction is important in microbial energy metabolism. In almost all cases of acetate accumulation as a product of energy metabolism, regardless of the mechanism of acetate production, the above acetyl-phosphate:ADP phosphotransferase is involved in the production of free acetate and ATP.

Pathway 2, however, is most prominent in the fermentation of hexoses by some members of the lactic acid family of bacteria, *i.e.*, certain lactobacilli and the genus *Leuconostoc*. These organisms normally use acetyl-phosphate as an electron sink to form ethanol (acetyl coenzyme A and acetaldehyde are intermediates; see p. 81 and **4–15**). Ethanol formation from acetyl-phosphate can use up the reducing equivalent of four H atoms formed during the fermentation (2 H = 1 NADH), but six H atom-equivalents are formed (four from hexose to pentose and two from glyceraldehyde-3-phosphate to pyruvate). The lactic acid bacteria use up the last pair of H atoms to make lactate from pyruvate (lactic dehydrogenase). The overall fermentation is

$$\text{glucose} + ADP + P_i \rightarrow$$
$$\text{lactate} + \text{ethanol} + CO_2 + ATP$$

Figure out why the net yield of ATP per mole glucose is 1.

Pathway 3. In pathway 3 (see **4–11**), Ru-5-P is converted to Xu-5-P, as in the second pathway. In addition, Ru-5-P is isomerized to ribose-5-phosphate (R-5-P). The formation of R-5-P by the sequence of glucose → 6-phosphogluconate → Ru-5-P → R-5-P is an extremely common sequence in nature even when the enzyme reactions are not essential for energy production. Many organisms, including man, use the sequence to provide R-5-P for the synthesis of the ribose and deoxyribose portions of nucleic acids.

In the catabolic pathway, however, the isomerization and epimerization of Ru-5-P provides the substrates for the enzyme transketolase. This enzyme catalyzes the transfer of two carbons from the carbonyl end of Xu-5-P to the aldehyde end of R-5-P to give the 7-carbon sugar phosphate, sedoheptulose-7-P (S-7-P) and 3-P-glyceraldehyde (G-3-P). The transaldolase catalyzes the transfer of the top three carbons of S-7-P to G-3-P to give the 4-carbon sugar phosphate, erythrose-4-P (E-4-P) and

fructose-6-P (F-6-P). Another transketolase reaction shuttles another two carbons from a second molecule of Xu-5-P to the aldehyde of E-4-P to yield F-6-P and G-3-P. Note that the acceptor compounds in the two transketolase reactions, R-5-P and E-4-P, are homologues.

At this stage of the pathway, the organism has accomplished the following:

$$3 \text{ glucose} + 3 ATP \rightarrow 2 \text{ F-6-P} +$$
$$\text{G-3-P} + 3 CO_2 + 12 \text{ [H]} + 3 ADP$$

The remaining reactions of the pathway are the same as those of the EMP scheme. The net yield of ATP per mole of glucose converted to pyruvate is 1⅔.

Other Pathways

A few other pathways for hexose breakdown are known, mainly slight modifications of one or another of the above. It is not clear why the several different pathways exist in nature. Whether they are survivors of different evolutionary attempts to obtain energy from hexoses or whether a particular organism obtains an advantage in its natural habitat from using a particular pathway is not known. The pathways differ, but there are many identical enzyme reactions in the different pathways. In all of the pathways, 3-P-glyceraldehyde is a key intermediate and identical enzymes are involved in converting G-3-P to pyruvate.

Isotopic Tracing of Pathways

With radioisotope techniques, it is relatively simple to identify the particular pathway used by a particular organism. Any carbon of a glucose molecule can be specifically labeled with radioactive ^{14}C. If an organism is fed labeled glucose, the location of the label in the product molecules provides an indication of the breakdown patterns. As an example, imagine that an organism ferments glucose to ethanol and CO_2. Assume that it can have only one of two pathways, either the EMP or the ED pathway, and radioactive glucose is used to provide a clue to which one is present. Both paths give 2 pyruvates from glucose, giving the following general breakdown pattern:

4–11.

Pathway 3—Transketolase-Transaldolase

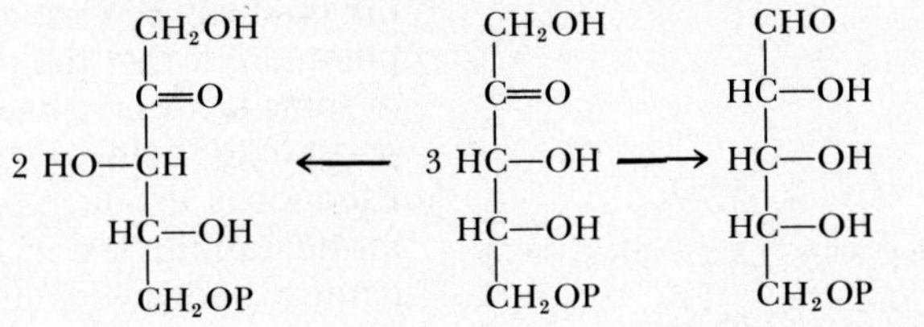

$$
\begin{array}{ccc}
\text{CH}_2\text{OH} & \text{CH}_2\text{OH} & \text{CHO} \\
| & | & | \\
\text{C}=\text{O} & \text{C}=\text{O} & \text{HC}-\text{OH} \\
| & | & | \\
2\ \text{HO}-\text{CH} \quad\longleftarrow\quad 3\ \text{HC}-\text{OH} \quad\longrightarrow\quad \text{HC}-\text{OH} \\
| & | & | \\
\text{HC}-\text{OH} & \text{HC}-\text{OH} & \text{HC}-\text{OH} \\
| & | & | \\
\text{CH}_2\text{OP} & \text{CH}_2\text{OP} & \text{CH}_2\text{OP}
\end{array}
$$

Xu-5-P   *Ru-5-P*   *R-5-P*

$$
\begin{array}{cccc}
& & \text{CH}_2\text{OH} & \\
& & | & \\
\text{CH}_2\text{OH} & \text{CHO} & \text{C}=\text{O} & \\
| & | & | & \\
\text{C}=\text{O} & \text{HC}-\text{OH} & \text{HO}-\text{CH} & \\
| & | & | & \\
\text{HO}-\text{CH} \quad+\quad \text{HC}-\text{OH} \quad\longrightarrow\quad \text{HC}-\text{OH} \quad+\quad \text{CHO} \\
| & | & | & | \\
\text{HC}-\text{OH} & \text{HC}-\text{OH} & \text{HC}-\text{OH} & \text{HCOH} \\
| & | & | & | \\
\text{CH}_2\text{OP} & \text{CH}_2\text{OP} & \text{CH}_2\text{OP} & \text{CH}_2\text{OP}
\end{array}
$$

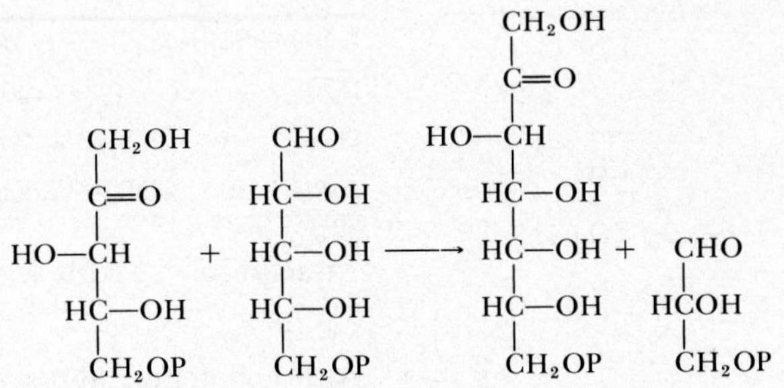

Xu-5-P   *R-5-P*   *S-7-P*   *G-3-P*

Transketolase

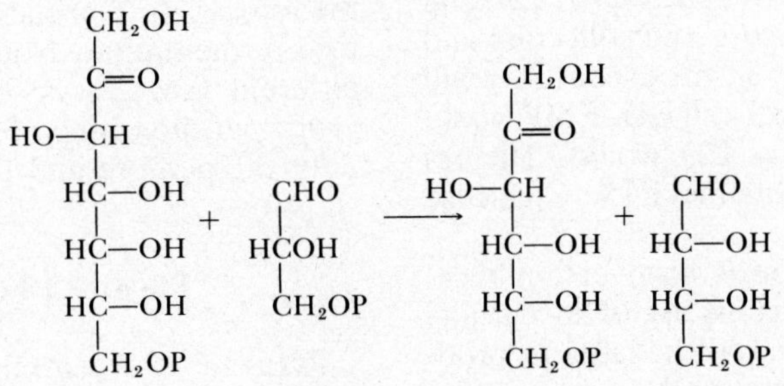

$$
\begin{array}{cccc}
\text{CH}_2\text{OH} & & \text{CH}_2\text{OH} & \\
| & & | & \\
\text{C}=\text{O} & & \text{C}=\text{O} & \\
| & & | & \\
\text{HO}-\text{CH} & & \text{HO}-\text{CH} & \\
| & \text{CHO} & | & \text{CHO} \\
\text{HC}-\text{OH} \quad+\quad \text{HCOH} \quad\longrightarrow\quad \text{HC}-\text{OH} \quad+\quad \text{HC}-\text{OH} \\
| & | & | & | \\
\text{HC}-\text{OH} & \text{CH}_2\text{OP} & \text{HC}-\text{OH} & \text{HC}-\text{OH} \\
| & & | & | \\
\text{HC}-\text{OH} & & \text{CH}_2\text{OP} & \text{CH}_2\text{OP} \\
| & & & \\
\text{CH}_2\text{OP} & & &
\end{array}
$$

S-7-P   *G-3-P*   *F-6-P*   *E-4-P*

Transaldolase

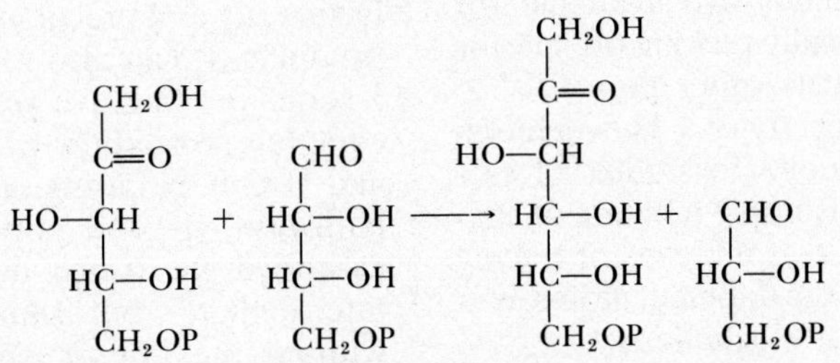

$$
\begin{array}{cccc}
& & \text{CH}_2\text{OH} & \\
& & | & \\
\text{CH}_2\text{OH} & & \text{C}=\text{O} & \\
| & \text{CHO} & \text{HO}-\text{CH} & \\
\text{C}=\text{O} & | & | & \\
| & \text{HC}-\text{OH} & \text{HC}-\text{OH} & \text{CHO} \\
\text{HO}-\text{CH} \quad+\quad \quad\quad \longrightarrow\quad \quad\quad +\quad \text{HC}-\text{OH} \\
| & \text{HC}-\text{OH} & \text{HC}-\text{OH} & | \\
\text{HC}-\text{OH} & | & | & \text{HC}-\text{OH} \\
| & \text{CH}_2\text{OP} & \text{CH}_2\text{OP} & | \\
\text{CH}_2\text{OP} & & & \text{CH}_2\text{OP}
\end{array}
$$

Xu-5-P   *E-4-P*   *F-6-P*   *G-3-P*

Transketolase

2 F-6-P + 2 ATP→2 fructose-1,6-biP (F-1,6-P) + 2 ADP
2 F-1,6-P→2 G-3-P + 2 dihydroxyacetone-P
2 dihydroxyacetone-P→2 G-3-P
5 G-3-P + 10 ADP + 10P$_i$ + 5 NAD$^+$→10 pyruvate + 10 ATP + 5 NADH + 5 H$^+$

The glucose molecule is conventionally numbered, and the question is, which C atoms will end up in which product C atoms with the two pathways?

EMP

$$
\begin{array}{cc}
1 & C \\
2 & C \\
3 & C \\
4 & C \\
5 & C \\
6 & C
\end{array}
\quad \longrightarrow \quad
\begin{array}{l}
3,4\ \mathrm{CO_2H} \\
2,5\ \mathrm{C{=}O} \\
1,6\ \mathrm{CH_3}
\end{array}
\quad \longrightarrow \quad
\begin{array}{l}
3,4\ \mathrm{CO_2} \\
+ \\
2,5\ \mathrm{CH_2OH} \\
1,6\ \mathrm{CH_3}
\end{array}
$$

ED

$$
\begin{array}{cc}
1 & C \\
2 & C \\
3 & C \\
4 & C \\
5 & C \\
6 & C
\end{array}
\quad \longrightarrow \quad
\begin{array}{l}
1,4\ \mathrm{CO_2H} \\
2,5\ \mathrm{C{=}O} \\
3,6\ \mathrm{CH_3}
\end{array}
\quad \longrightarrow \quad
\begin{array}{l}
1,4\ \mathrm{CO_2} \\
+ \\
2,5\ \mathrm{CH_2OH} \\
3,6\ \mathrm{CH_3}
\end{array}
$$

The numbers on the product carbons indicate the glucose carbons from which they were derived in the respective pathways. Feeding the organism $[1\text{-}^{14}C]$glucose and collecting and measuring radioactivity in produced CO_2 will distinguish between EMP and ED. EMP would yield no $^{14}CO_2$, whereas ED would. The reverse result would be obtained if $[3\text{-}^{14}C]$glucose were used.

The above illustration is an oversimplification. However, by judicious use of specifically labeled glucose and analysis of label in products, almost any pathway can be distinguished from any other, and the simultaneous operation of more than one pathway in an organism can be detected. Methods are available for chemically or enzymatically picking off specific carbon atoms of products other than CO_2 to determine their radioactivity. The general methodology is not unique to studies of carbohydrate catabolism; isotopic labeling of specific atoms of a molecule as a means of tracing the metabolic fate of the labeled atoms is a powerful general tool of biochemistry.

PENTOSE PATHWAYS

The only difference between the catabolism of a hexose and a pentose by either the transketolase-transaldolase sequence or the phosphoketolase sequence is in the overall O–R reactions. To form a pentose from a hexose,

the hexose aldehyde group has to be oxidized to a carboxyl which, in turn, is oxidatively decarboxylated to a pentose. Thus, more electron sink reactions are necessary for hexose breakdown. For example, it has already been pointed out that the phosphoketolase pathway of some lactic acid bacteria ends up with acetyl-phosphate being used as an electron sink. Ethanol is produced as a product of glucose fermentation. Using the same pathway for a pentose, however, eliminates the need to use acetyl-phosphate as an electron sink; if L-arabinose is fermented, for example:

$$\text{L-arabinose} + \text{ATP} \to\ \to \text{D-Xu} - 5 - \text{P}$$

$$\text{D-Xu} - 5 - \text{P} + \text{P}_i \to \text{acetyl} \sim \text{P} + \text{G} - 3 - \text{P}$$

$$\text{G} - 3 - \text{P} + 2\,\text{ADP} + \text{P}_i \to\ \to \text{lactate} + 2\,\text{ATP}$$

$$\text{acetyl} \sim \text{P} + \text{ADP} \to \text{acetate} + \text{ATP}$$

Sum:
$$\text{L-arabinose} + 2\,\text{ADP} + 2\,\text{P}_i \to$$
$$\text{lactate} + \text{acetate} + 2\,\text{ATP}$$

Although identical reactions are used once Xu-5-P is formed from the starting hexose or pentose, the elimination of the need to use acetyl-phosphate as an electron sink permits the formation of acetate and ATP during pentose fermentation. Not only are the products different (acetate vs. ethanol), but the ATP yields per mole sugar fermented are different: 2 for the pentose and 1 for the hexose.

PRODUCT FORMATION[37]

Pyruvate is a central intermediate between carbohydrate energy sources and the final carbon products of energy metabolism. It can serve as an electron sink, as a precursor of lactate, or as a precursor of other fermentation products. It can also serve as the beginning of a series of oxidative reactions that lead to the complete oxidation of carbohydrate to CO_2 and H_2O in respiring organisms. In the central pathways, a good portion (if not all) of the carbohydrate carbon flows into this important intermediate, but some products are made without the intermediate formation of pyruvate. In the pentose phosphate–based pathways, some product CO_2 is made from hexoses before pyruvate is formed. In the phosphoketolase pathway, the 2-carbon products, acetate (pentose fermentation) and ethanol (hexose fermentation), are made from acetyl-phosphate directly resulting from cleavage of Xu-5-P. Occasionally, microorganisms will use intermediates formed before pyruvate for electron sink reactions and excrete the products. An example of this is the formation of glycerol as a fermentation product:

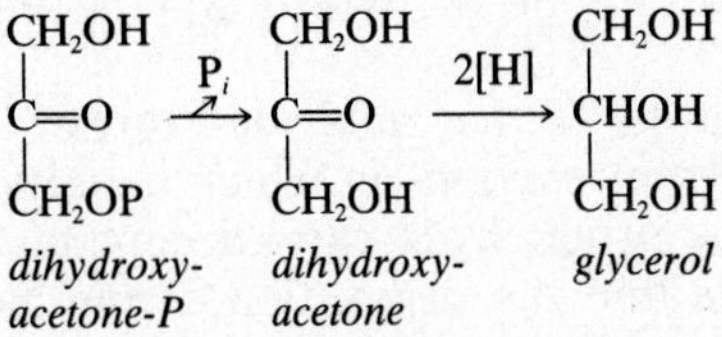

$$CH_2OH \mid C=O \mid CH_2OP \xrightarrow{P_i} CH_2OH \mid C=O \mid CH_2OH \xrightarrow{2[H]} CH_2OH \mid CHOH \mid CH_2OH$$

dihydroxy-acetone-P   *dihydroxy-acetone*   *glycerol*

The exceptions, however, do not detract from the central role of pyruvate.

Several important coenzymes are associated with pyruvate metabolism. Coenzymes are nonprotein organic compounds that are intimately associated with the chemistry of the transformation of substrates by certain enzymes. They are generally ubiquitous and generally related to the vitamins. They can be closely attached to enzymes (covalently linked or tightly bound) or participate in loose association by transferring a portion of the substrate to another enzyme. The coenzyme-attached chemical group is a substrate for the subsequent enzyme reaction. The mode of action of coenzymes in pyruvate metabolism illustrates how coenzymes function in intermediary metabolism.

One terminal electron sink reaction involving pyruvate (lactic dehydrogenase) has already been discussed. This reaction, a typical pyridine nucleotide coenzyme reaction, is written to show the specific portion of the pyridine nucleotide participating in the transfer of electrons (see **4-12**). The active portion of pyridine nucleotides is the nicotinamide ring which is derived from the vitamin niacin (nicotinamide). A hydride ion ($H^- = H^+ + 2 e^-$) is transferred to and from the fourth position of the ring in all pyridine nucleotide-linked oxidations and reductions. The major role of pyridine nucleotides is the shuttling of electrons from electron donor to electron acceptor substrates. The complete structures of NAD and NADP are shown in **4-12**.

Decarboxylation of Pyruvate

Several important pyruvate reactions result in the decarboxylation of pyruvate. All decarboxylations appear to involve thiamin pyrophosphate (TPP) as a coenzyme. The different

4-12.

Pyridine Nucleotide Reactions

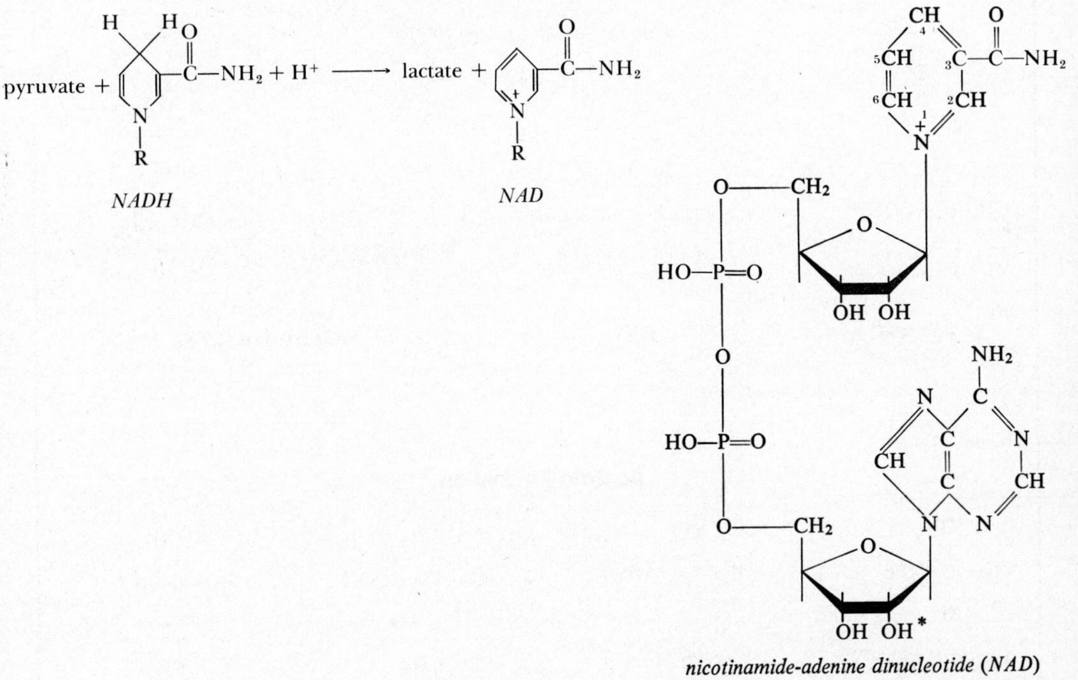

$$pyruvate + \text{(NADH)} + H^+ \longrightarrow lactate + \text{(NAD)}$$

NADH   *NAD*

nicotinamide-adenine dinucleotide (NAD)

* Position of third NADP phosphate group.

enzymes all initiate catalysis by forming α-hydroxyethyl-TPP as an enzyme-bound intermediate (see **4–13**). Yeast carboxylase proceeds in this manner and its reaction terminates with a split of the α-hydroxyethyl-TPP to acetaldehyde:

pyruvic acid + TPP-enzyme →
$\qquad$ α-hydroxyethyl-TPP-enzyme + CO_2
α-hydroxyethyl-TPP-enzyme →
$\qquad$ acetaldehyde + TPP-enzyme

The acetaldehyde produced by yeast is used as an electron sink substrate for ethanol formation:

$$CH_3CHO + NADH + H^+ \rightarrow CH_3CH_2OH + NAD^+$$

Ethanol is a fairly common bacterial fermentation product, and it is always produced from acetaldehyde by reduction with reduced pyridine nucleotide. In only one bacterial species, however, is acetaldehyde produced by a yeast carboxylase mechanism. Most bacterial acetaldehyde formation comes from reduction of acetyl–coenzyme A, which will be discussed later.

TPP is an "active aldehyde" carrier in all of the enzyme reactions in which it participates. The type of aldehyde carried depends on the substrate and the disposition of the aldehyde depends on the particular enzyme. Thiamin is the vitamin related to the coenzyme.

Another hydroxyethyl-TPP reaction important in the formation of fermentation products involves the condensation of the "active acetaldehyde" with a second molecule of pyruvate to give α-acetolactic acid (see **4–13**). The α-acetolactate never accumulates as a product; it is always decarboxylated to acetoin, which can accumulate as a product (see **4–13**). Some-

4–13.

Thiamine Pyrophosphate and Pyruvate Decarboxylation

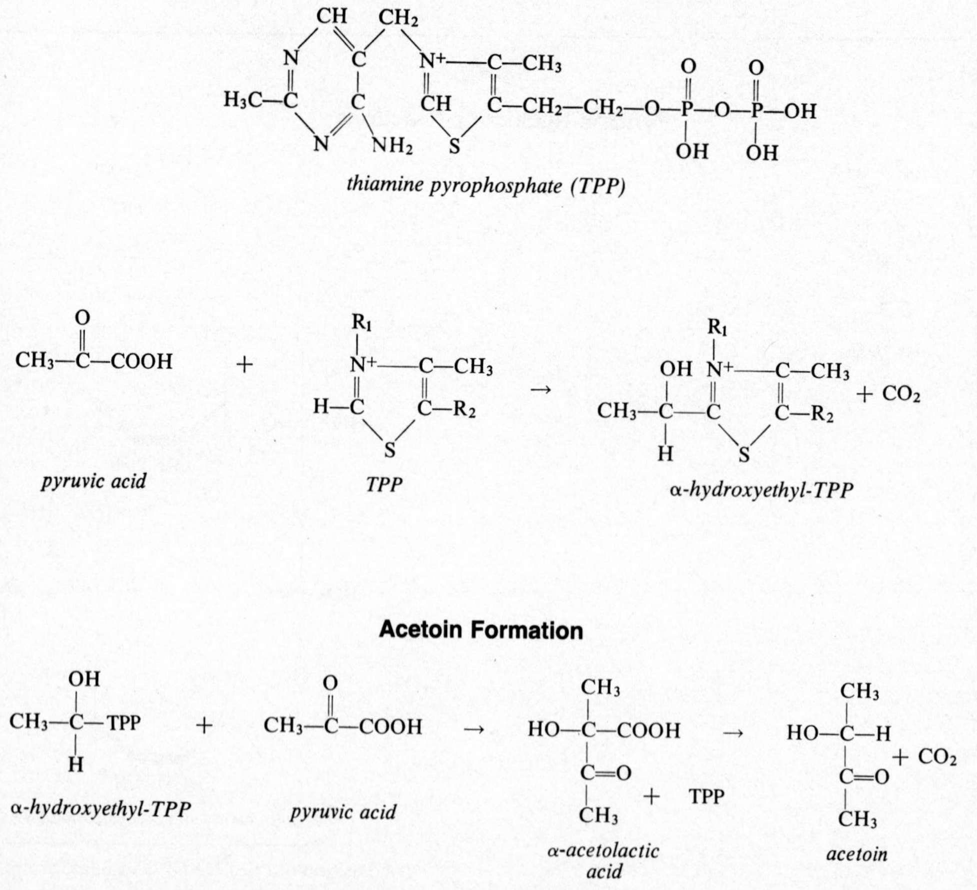

thiamine pyrophosphate (TPP)

pyruvic acid *TPP* *α-hydroxyethyl-TPP*

Acetoin Formation

α-hydroxyethyl-TPP *pyruvic acid* *α-acetolactic acid* *acetoin*

4-14.

Oxidation of α-Hydroxyethyl-TPP

(a) Transfer to Exogenous Electron Acceptor

$$CH_3CHOH—TPP + CoASH \longrightarrow CH_3CO \sim SCoA + 2 [H]$$

(b) H_2 Gas Formation

$$CH_3CHOH—TPP + CoASH \longrightarrow CH_3CO \sim SCoA + H_2 \uparrow$$

(c) Formic Acid Formation

$$CH_3COCO_2H + Enzyme\text{-}TPP \longrightarrow Enzyme\text{-}TPP$$

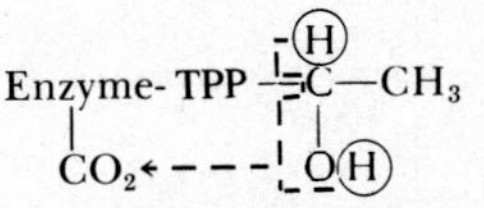

enzyme-CO₂-hydroxyethyl-TPP intermediate

$$intermediate + CoASH \longrightarrow CH_3CO \sim SCoA + HCO_2H + Enzyme\text{-}TPP$$

formic acid

---

times acetoin is further reduced to 2,3-buta-nediol,

$$CH_3CHOHCOCH_3 + 2[H] \rightarrow CH_3CHOHCHOHCH_3$$

or oxidized to diacetyl,

$$CH_3CHOHCOCH_3 \rightarrow CH_3COCOCH_3 + 2 [H]$$

Bacterial fermentation by good butanediol producers has been used commercially. Butanediol is important in making butadiene for synthetic rubber production. Diacetyl is an important aromatic component of bacterial fermentation–based foods like cheeses and butter.

The most important bacterial systems for decarboxylating pyruvate involve the oxidation of the α-hydroxyethyl group on TPP to an acetyl group. The acetyl group formed is almost always acetyl–coenzyme A (coenzyme A = CoASH), and the electrons are disposed of in one of three different ways:

1. Transfer to an exogenous electron acceptor
2. Formation of H_2 gas
3. Formation of formic acid

The three methods for oxidizing the hydroxyethyl group are shown in **4–14**. Method 3 is different from all the other pyruvate cleavage reactions because CO_2 is not a product nor is it a free intermediate. Although the mechanism has not been completely elucidated, the formulation shown in **4–14** is consistent with present information. This formulation suggests that a typical decarboxylation of pyruvate occurs with the production of enzyme-bound CO_2. Hydroxyethyl-TPP is oxidized to acetyl–coenzyme A with simultaneous reduction of the CO_2 to formate.

Formate and H_2 are common fermentation products of bacteria. The anaerobic spore-formers, members of the genus *Clostridium*, produce H_2 by reaction 2. Members of the family Enterobacteriaceae, the enteric bacteria, produce formate by reaction 3. In addition, some of the enteric bacteria (*e.g., Escherichia coli*) have an enzyme system called the formic hydrogenlyase system, which produces H_2 and CO_2 from formate:

$$HCO_2H \rightarrow H_2 + CO_2$$

Thus, there are two major bacterial systems for production of H_2 from carbohydrates, system 2 and a combination of system 3 with the hydrogenlyase system.

Product Formation from Acetyl–Coenzyme A

Acetyl–coenzyme A (acetyl-CoA) is an important precursor of the products of carbohydrate energy metabolism. It is also an example of an extremely important class of compounds of intermediate metabolism, the thioesters of coenzyme A. The vitamin pantothenic acid is part of the coenzyme A structure (see **4–15**). Coenzyme A, through its terminal thiol group, participates in the formation and transfer of

4-15.

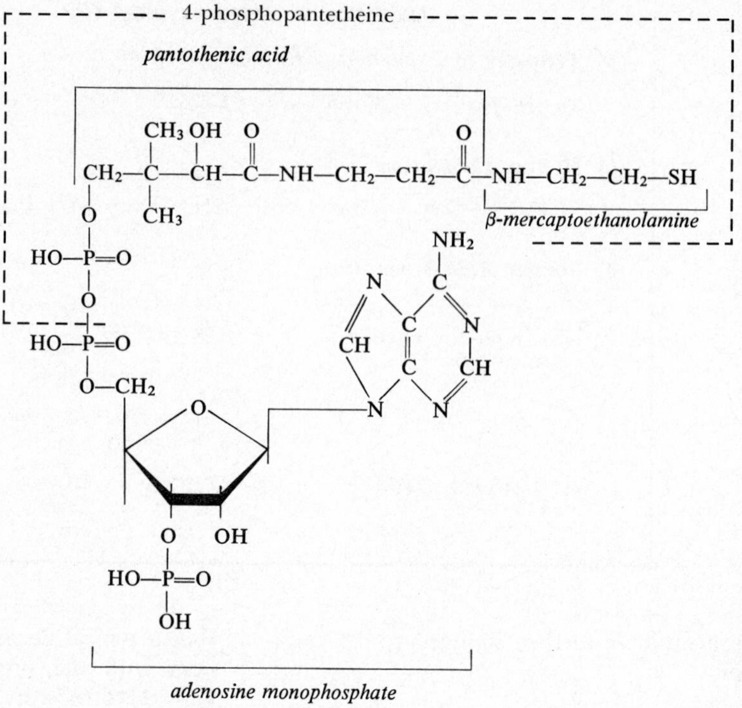

Coenzyme A (CoA)

(a)

$$CH_3-\overset{O}{\overset{\|}{C}}-S-CoA + H_3PO_4 \rightleftharpoons CoA + CH_3-\overset{O}{\overset{\|}{C}}-O-\overset{O}{\underset{OH}{\overset{\|}{P}}}-OH$$

acetyl-CoA　　　　　　　　　　　　　　　　　　*acetyl-phosphate*

(b)

acetyl-phosphate + ADP → acetic acid + ATP

acyl thioesters. A thioester bond is a high-energy bond, and the bond energy can be used for ATP synthesis. Acetyl-CoA can be converted to acetylphosphate, which can be converted to acetate and ATP. Acetyl–coenzyme A:orthophosphate acetyl transferase (phosphotransacetylase) is a common bacterial enzyme (see **4–15**). Acetyl-CoA, formed directly from pyruvate or from acetylphosphate (phosphoketolase pathway), is also reduced to acetaldehyde in most ethanol-forming bacteria:

$$H^+ + NADH + CH_3CO{\sim}SCoA \rightarrow$$
$$CH_3CHO + HSCoA + NAD^+$$

Note that the energy of the thioester bond is not made available as ATP when acetaldehyde is formed. The thioester bond energy is essentially excreted by the organism in the product ethanol.

Acetyl-CoA is also used to form acetoacetyl-coenzyme A, a precursor of several important bacterial fermentation products:

$$2\ CH_3CO{\sim}SCoA \rightarrow CH_3COCH_2CO{\sim}SCoA + CoASH$$
acetoacetyl-CoA

Acetoacetyl-CoA is used to form butyric acid, *n*-butyl alcohol, acetone, and isopropanol, important bacterial fermentation products (see **4–16**). The fermentation products derived from acetoacetyl-CoA are fairly common among members of the genus *Clostridium* but by no means restricted to this genus. Industrial production of the solvents acetone and butanol by clostridial fermentation was significant at one time and is still carried out. Interest in the fermentation has been stimulated because of the possibility of decreasing the amount of petroleum resources used in the chemical syn-

---

4–16.

Products from Acetoacetyl-CoA

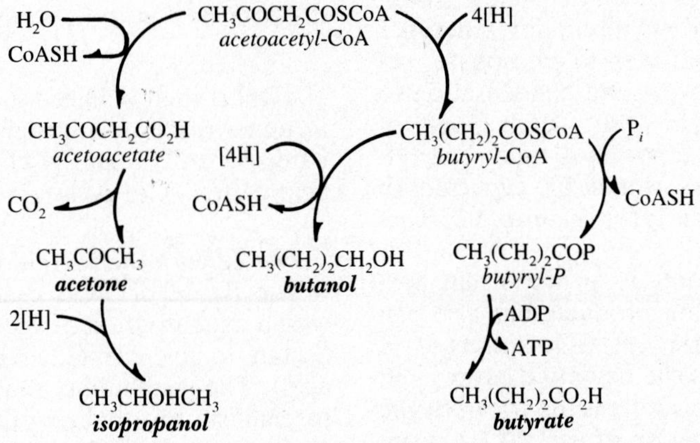

$$CH_3COCH_2COSCoA$$
$$\text{acetoacetyl-CoA}$$

H_2O , CoASH , $4[H]$

$$CH_3COCH_2CO_2H$$
acetoacetate

$[4H]$, CoASH

$$CH_3(CH_2)_2COSCoA$$
butyryl-CoA

P_i , CoASH

CO_2

$$CH_3COCH_3$$
acetone

$$CH_3(CH_2)_2CH_2OH$$
butanol

$$CH_3(CH_2)_2COP$$
butyryl-P

ADP , ATP

$2[H]$

$$CH_3CHOHCH_3$$
isopropanol

$$CH_3(CH_2)_2CO_2H$$
butyrate

---

thesis of the solvents. Starch and molasses have been used as carbohydrate substrates for the clostridial fermentation. The fermentation is also of some historical importance because Chaim Weizmann, a Russian-born British microbiologist, patented the use of the organism *Clostridium acetobutylicum*, which had been used for acetone production during World War I. Acetone was the solvent utilized in the manufacture of cordite, an important World War I explosive. Weizmann used both the prestige and money gained from his patent toward the promotion of the Balfour Declaration and the eventual establishment of the State of Israel, of which he became the first president.

4–17.

Lipoic Acid and Pyruvate Oxidation

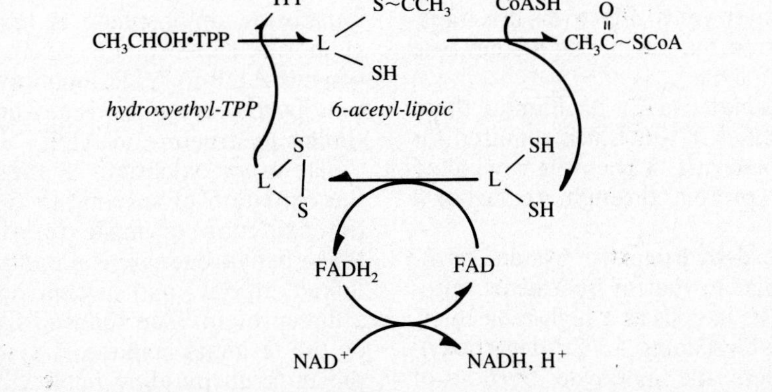

$$CH_2$$
$$CH_2 \quad CH-CH_2CH_2CH_2CH_2CO_2H$$
$$S——S$$
oxidized (disulfide) form

$$CH_2$$
$$CH_2 \quad CHCH_2CH_2CH_2CH_2CO_2H$$
$$SH \quad SH$$
reduced (sulfhydryl) form

α-Lipoic Acid

TPP , $S\sim\overset{O}{\overset{\|}{C}}CH_3$, CoASH

$$CH_3CHOH·TPP$$ L , $CH_3\overset{O}{\overset{\|}{C}}\sim SCoA$

hydroxyethyl-TPP , SH , *6-acetyl-lipoic*

$$S$$
$$L \quad |$$
$$S$$

$$SH$$
$$L$$
$$SH$$

$FADH_2$, FAD

NAD^+ , $NADH, H^+$

The enzymology of butyric acid and butanol formation from butyryl-CoA is completely analogous to the enzymology of acetic acid and ethanol formation from acetyl-CoA. The coenzyme derivative of a particular chemical group, *e.g.*, acetyl-CoA, participates in different types of reactions, *e.g.*, transfer to phosphate, reduction to acetaldehyde, and condensation to acetoacetyl-CoA. Coenzyme derivatives of homologues, *e.g.*, acetyl-CoA and butyryl-CoA, and analogues would be expected to participate in similar types of enzyme reactions.

Acetyl-CoA not only is an important precursor of fermentation products but also can be completely oxidized to CO_2 and H_2O in respiring organisms. The oxidative pathway in carbohydrate-using bacteria is the tricarboxylic acid cycle. The formation of acetyl-CoA from pyruvate in these respiring organisms is by system 1 (see **4–14**). The best studied of these systems is the pyruvate dehydrogenase system of *Escherichia coli*.[22] In the *E. coli* system the aldehyde group of the "active aldehyde" hydroxyethyl-TPP is oxidized to an acyl group to one of the sulfur atoms of the coenzyme (see **4–17**), oxidized lipoic acid:

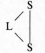

The electrons of the aldehyde are used to reduce one of the sulfurs to a sulfhydryl group. Acetyl-lipoic acid is a high-energy thioester. The acetyl group is transferred to CoA. Lipoic acid is then oxidized back to its oxidized form.

The oxidation is catalyzed by a flavoprotein, lipoic dehydrogenase. A flavoprotein is an enzyme that contains a coenzyme form of the vitamin riboflavin as a prosthetic group. The most common coenzyme forms are flavin mononucleotide (riboflavin phosphate) and flavin adenine dinucleotide, and they are usually tightly bound to enzymes. Electrons are transferred to and from the flavin ring system (see **4–18**).

Lipoic acid is not usually a vitamin; there are only a few cases in which it is required for growth. As a coenzyme, it is covalently linked to the enzyme protein through its carboxyl group.

The pyruvate dehydrogenase system of *E. coli* is very similar to that of beef heart mitochondria. It exists in cells as a high-molecular-weight complex containing a TPP-decarboxylase that transfers the aldehyde portion of

pyruvate to oxidized lipoic acid bound to the acetyl-lipoic:acetyl-CoA transacetylase. Lipoic dehydrogenase is also part of the multienzyme complex. The overall reaction accomplished is

$$CH_3COCO_2H + NAD^+ + CoASH \rightarrow$$
$$CH_3CO{\sim}SCoA + NADH + H^+$$

NADH is then oxidized to $NAD + H_2O$ by the terminal respiratory system and acetyl-CoA is oxidized to CO_2 and H_2O by the tricarboxylic acid cycle (TCA cycle).

The Tricarboxylic Acid Cycle

The Krebs or TCA cycle (see **4–19**) starts with a condensation of acetyl-CoA with oxaloacetate to give citrate, a 6-carbon tricarboxylic acid. The remaining reactions constitute a mechanism for oxidizing the condensed acetyl unit of acetyl-CoA to CO_2 and H_2O with regeneration of the oxaloacetate necessary for initiating the cycle.

Four reactions of the cycle involve the oxidation of intermediates. Isocitric dehydrogenase oxidizes isocitrate to oxalosuccinic acid with the reduction of pyridine nucleotide. The oxidation of α-ketoglutarate to succinic acid and CO_2 proceeds through succinyl-CoA. The mechanism of succinyl-CoA formation from α-ketoglutarate is identical to the pyruvate dehydrogenase mechanism discussed above and involves TPP, lipoic acid, NAD, and a flavin coenzyme. Pyruvate and α-ketoglutarate are both α-keto acids, and the overall reactions can be generalized as follows:

$$R{-}COCO_2H + CoASH + NAD^+ \rightarrow$$
$$R{-}CO{\sim}SCoA + CO_2 + NADH + H^+$$

where R is CH_3—in the case of pyruvate and $HO_2C(CH_2)_2$—in the case of α-ketoglutarate. The α-ketoglutarate dehydrogenase system exists as a multienzyme complex separate from, but analogous to, the pyruvate dehydrogenase complex. The high-energy bond of the succinyl-CoA is used to form ATP (see **4–20**). Guanosine diphosphate is first converted to guanosine triphosphate, which is then used to convert ADP to ATP. Guanosine diphosphate is a purine ribonucleoside diphosphate very similar in structure to ADP.

The other oxidations of the TCA cycle are the oxidation of succinic to fumaric acid and the oxidation of malic to oxaloacetic acid. Malic dehydrogenase is a pyridine nucleotide–linked enzyme, and succinic dehydrogenase is a flavoprotein. The reduced flavin is oxidized by the terminal respiratory system, as is all of the reduced pyridine nucleotide of the three

4–18.

Flavin Coenzymes

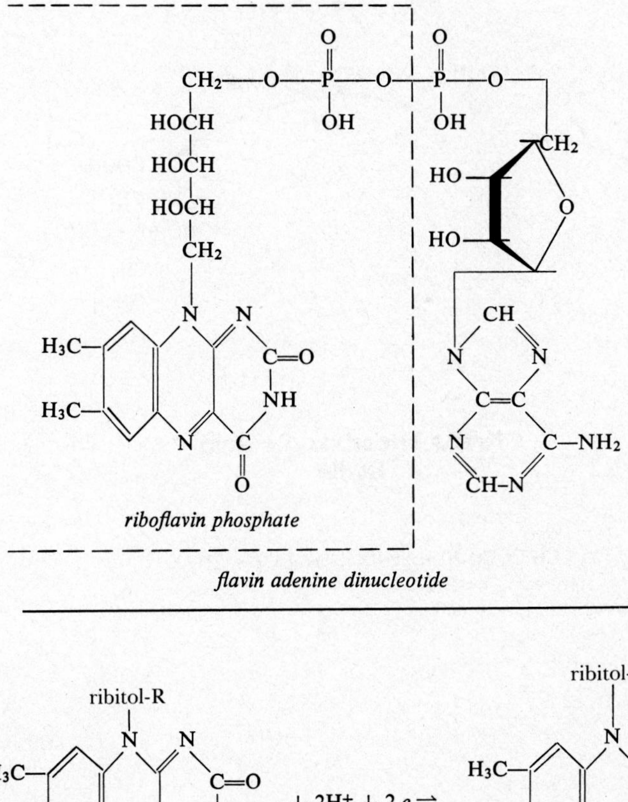

riboflavin phosphate

flavin adenine dinucleotide

$$+ 2H^+ + 2\,e \rightleftharpoons$$

oxidized form

reduced form

4–19.

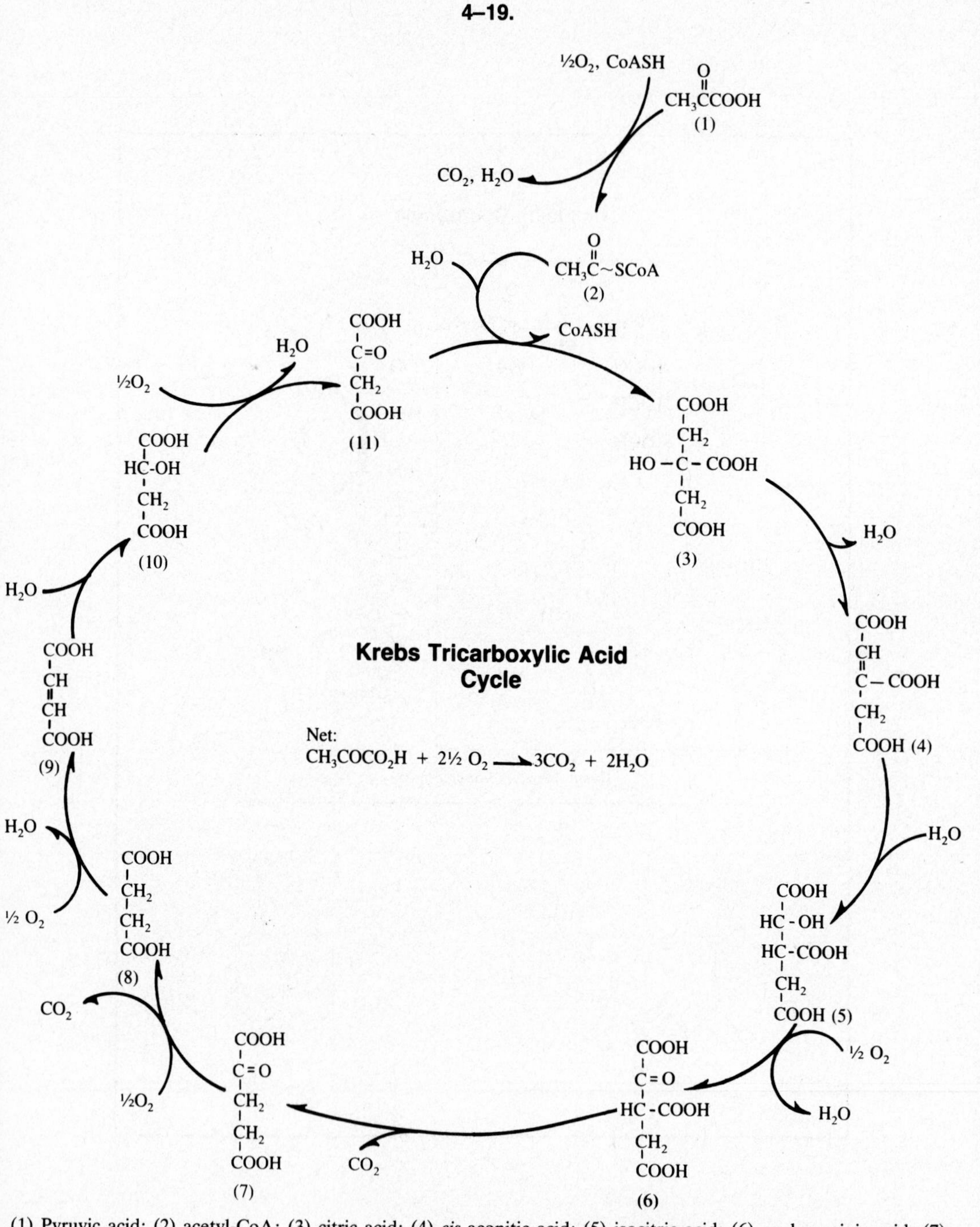

(1) Pyruvic acid; (2) acetyl-CoA; (3) citric acid; (4) *cis*-aconitic acid; (5) isocitric acid; (6) oxalosuccinic acid; (7) α-ketoglutaric acid; (8) succinic acid; (9) fumaric acid; (10) malic acid; (11) oxaloacetic acid.

4–20.

$$\text{succinyl} \sim \text{SCoA} + P_i + \text{guanosine diphosphate (GDP)} \longrightarrow \text{succinic acid} + \text{guanosine triphosphate (GTP)}$$

$$\text{GTP} + \text{ADP} \longrightarrow \text{ATP} + \text{GDP}$$

---

pyridine nucleotide–linked oxidations. As was pointed out previously, a great deal of ATP becomes available to the cell through phosphorylations coupled to these terminal oxidations. The only substrate phosphorylation of the TCA cycle is in the step from succinyl-CoA to succinate.

Succinate and Propionate Formation

Two important microbial fermentation products are formed from pyruvate in reactions that involve the carboxylation of pyruvate to oxaloacetate. These products are succinic acid and propionic acid. There are several known enzyme reactions for forming oxaloacetate from pyruvate or phosphoenolpyruvate. The specific CO_2-fixation reaction used by succinate-excreting bacteria is phosphoenolpyruvate carboxykinase (see **4–21**). Some of these bacteria use GDP rather than ADP as a substrate. After oxaloacetate is formed it is reduced to malate, which is then dehydrated to fumarate, which is reduced to succinate. The formation of large amounts of succinic acid as a fermentation product requires a large amount of fixation of CO_2. Bacteria that use a succinic acid fermentation as the sole means of generating energy for growth have to be supplied with high concentrations of CO_2 in natural or artificial environments.

Propionic acid formation has been intensively studied in the genus *Propionibacterium*.[36] Species of this genus are important in the commercial production of Swiss cheese,

where they are responsible for producing the holes (from CO_2) and propionic and acetic acid as odor and flavor components. It is difficult to describe the reaction sequence (see **4–22**) by simply starting with the initial reaction, since the initial reaction involves one of the terminal products of the sequence, methylmalonyl-CoA (MM-CoA). A carboxyl group from MM-CoA is transferred to pyruvate to give propionyl-CoA and oxaloacetate in a transcarboxylase reaction (see **4–23**). The transcarboxylase uses biotin as a coenzyme. Biotin is a CO_2 carrier in a variety of enzyme reactions (see **4–23**). It is always covalently linked to enzymes.

Oxaloacetate is then converted to succinate by reactions identical to those of the succinate fermentation pathway. Succinyl-CoA is next formed by a transacylation with propionyl-CoA produced in the transcarboxylase reaction,

$$\text{succinate} + \text{propionyl-CoA} \rightarrow$$
$$\text{succinyl-CoA} + \text{propionate}$$

Succinyl-CoA is then isomerized to methylmalonyl-CoA. The isomerase has a tightly bound vitamin B_{12} coenzyme (see **4–24**). The coenzyme is a deoxyadenosyl derivative of vitamin B_{12} with the deoxyadenosyl group attached to the cobalt of the vitamin. The commercially available form of vitamin B_{12} has a cyano group attached to the cobalt.

The isomerase reaction is depicted in **4–25**. The function of the coenzyme appears to be

---

4–21.

$$\underset{\textit{phosphoenolpyruvate}}{\overset{\overset{\displaystyle O \sim P}{|}}{CH_2{=}C{-}CO_2H}} + ADP + CO_2 \longrightarrow \underset{\textit{oxaloacetate}}{HO_2CCH_2COCO_2H} + ATP$$

$$\underset{}{HO_2CCH_2COCO_2H} + 2\,[H] \longrightarrow \underset{\textit{malate}}{HO_2CCH_2CHOHCO_2H}$$

$$\underset{}{HO_2CCH_2CHOHCO_2H} \longrightarrow \underset{\textit{fumarate}}{HO_2CCH{=}CHCO_2H} + H_2O$$

$$\underset{}{HO_2CCH{=}CHCO_2H} + 2\,[H] \longrightarrow \underset{\textit{succinate}}{HO_2CCH_2CH_2CO_2H}$$

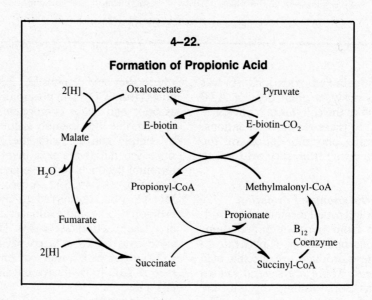

4–22.

Formation of Propionic Acid

4–23.

Biotin and Transcarboxylation

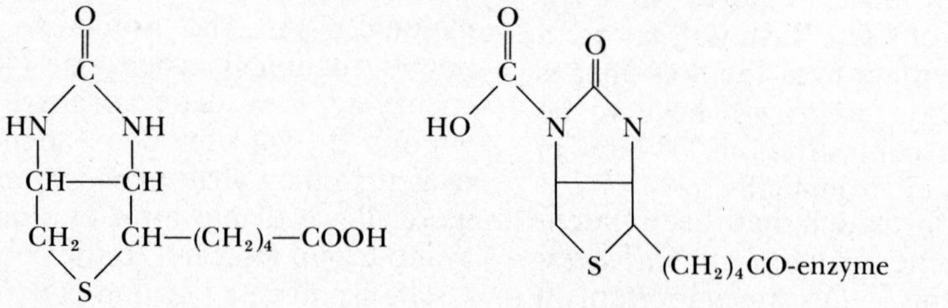

biotin

carboxybiotin-enzyme

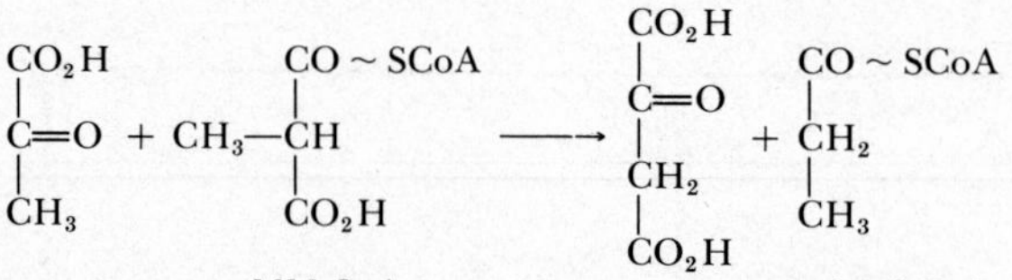

MM-*CoA*

propionyl-CoA

methylmalonyl-CoA + E-biotin $\xrightarrow{\text{transcarboxylase}}$ propionyl-CoA + E-biotin-CO_2

E-biotin-CO_2 + pyruvic acid → oxaloacetic acid + E-biotin

4–24.

Vitamin B$_{12}$ and Coenzyme B$_{12}$

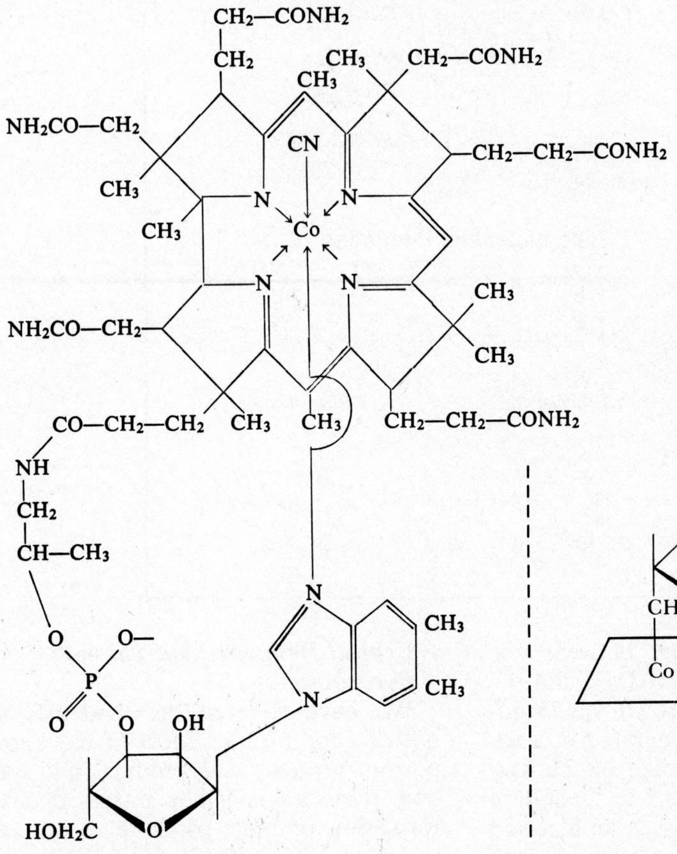

cyanocobalamin (vitamin B$_{12}$)

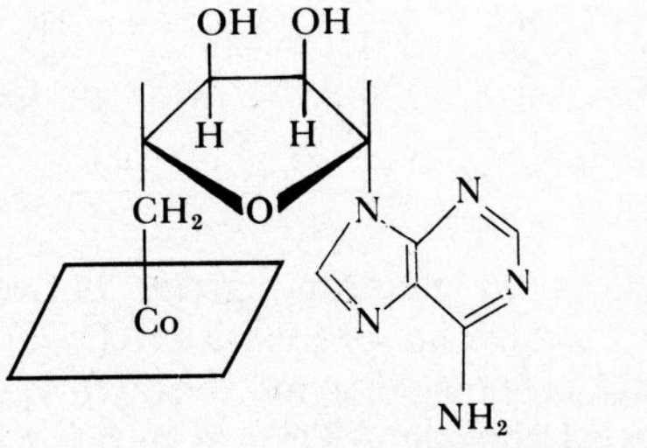

*5–deoxyadenosyl ligand
of B$_{12}$ Coenzyme*

one of labilizing a hydride ion of the substrate to allow the intramolecular rearrangement chemistry to proceed. Vitamin B$_{12}$ coenzyme participates in several fundamentally different types of enzyme reactions. The coenzyme usually acts as a donor and acceptor of hydride ions (H$^-$, a proton plus 2 electrons). For example, it is the coenzyme for a bacterial enzyme that converts glycerol to β-hydroxypropionaldehyde:

CH$_2$OH   CHO
CHOH   →   CH$_2$
CH$_2$OH   CH$_2$OH
glycerol   *β-hydroxy-
propionaldehyde*

This is an internal oxidation-reduction and contrasts markedly with the succinyl-CoA to methylmalonyl-CoA isomerization. There is a common denominator, however, because the chemistry of both reactions appears to require labilization of a hydride ion.

Possibly the most important B$_{12}$ coenzyme reaction is in the reduction of ribonucleotides to deoxyribonucleotides in some organisms. This is an important exception to the usual B$_{12}$ coenzyme reaction because it involves the oxidation of a disulfhydryl compound with reduction of the hydroxyl group of ribose to deoxyribose. It is likely, however, that a hydride transfer is involved (see **4–25**).

After methylmalonyl-CoA is formed by the isomerase, it is used in the transcarboxylase to form proprionyl-CoA and another molecule of oxaloacetate is produced for conversion to propionate (see **4–22**).

In propionibacteria, the reduction of fumarate to succinate involves the use of a cyto-

4–25.

Coenzyme B$_2$ and Isomerase

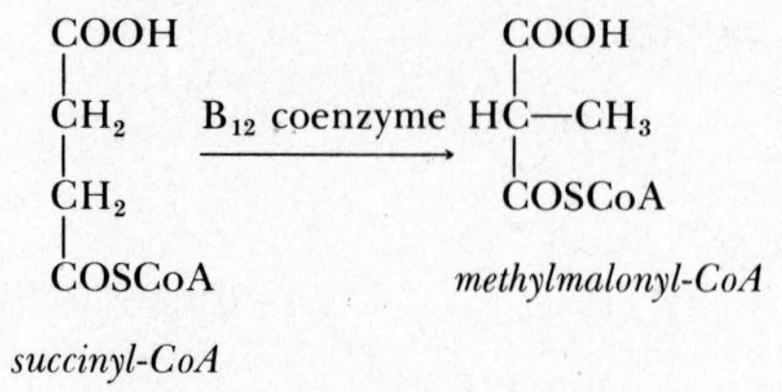

$$
\begin{array}{ccc}
\text{COOH} & & \text{COOH} \\
| & & | \\
\text{CH}_2 & \xrightarrow{\text{B}_{12}\text{ coenzyme}} & \text{HC—CH}_3 \\
| & & | \\
\text{CH}_2 & & \text{COSCoA} \\
| & & \\
\text{COSCoA} & & \textit{methylmalonyl-CoA} \\
\end{array}
$$

succinyl-CoA

Ribonucleotide Reduction

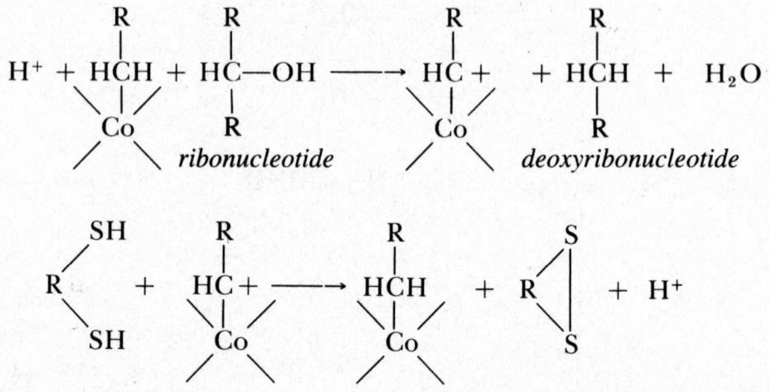

$$
\text{H}^+ + \underset{\text{Co}}{\text{HCH}} + \text{HC—OH} \longrightarrow \underset{\text{Co}}{\text{HC}} + \text{HCH} + \text{H}_2\text{O}
$$

ribonucleotide   *deoxyribonucleotide*

$$
\text{R} \underset{\text{SH}}{\overset{\text{SH}}{<}} + \underset{\text{Co}}{\text{HC}} \longrightarrow \underset{\text{Co}}{\text{HCH}} + \text{R} \underset{\text{S}}{\overset{\text{S}}{<}} + \text{H}^+
$$

chrome as an electron carrier between the primary reductant, probably NADH, and the fumarate-reducing enzyme. Growth yield studies suggest that an ATP is generated in association with this reduction. Some of the bacteria that produce succinate as a fermentation product also use a cytochrome as an electron carrier in the electron transfer step. At one time it was believed that cytochromes were restricted to organisms that respire in the presence of O$_2$. There are, however, several anaerobic processes and several strictly anaerobic bacteria that have upset this belief. We have already discussed the importance of cytochromes in phototrophic energy generation, a strictly anaerobic process in bacteria. Some of the phototrophs cannot grow at all in the presence of oxygen.

There are other bacteria that form propionic acid using pathways that are similar to the *Propionibacterium* pathway, *i.e.*, they use oxaloacetate, succinyl-CoA, and methylmalonyl-CoA as intermediates. There may be differences in detail. There is, however, a completely independent pathway for propionate formation that doesn't even use pyruvate as an intermediate. This pathway proceeds from lactic acid, either formed by the bacterium itself from carbohydrates, or formed by other bacteria. The pathway involves a dehydration of lactic acid to acrylic acid with reduction of acrylate to propionate (see **4–26**).

Central Pathways and Thiamin Pyrophosphate

We have covered the strategies used by bacteria for forming most of the known, important fermentation products and have seen how pyruvate is a key intermediate for the formation of most of these reactions. Using pyruvate as a starting point, we have surveyed the types of reactions carried out by several coenzymes. Some of these reactions will be referred to again with respect to other degradative or synthetic reactions. As far as carbohydrate breakdown is concerned, the only coenzymes we have been concerned with before pyruvate is formed (in the central pathways) are the pyridine nucleotides. There is one other of these coenzymes, however, that is important in two of these central pathways, thiamin pyrophosphate, and its role in these pathways will now be discussed.

The two pathways are the phosphoketolase and the transketolase-transaldolase pathways. The substrate of interest is xylulose-5-phosphate. An "active aldehyde" intermediate is formed in analogy with the pyruvate reactions. The top two carbons of Xu-5-P are transferred to TPP to give dihydroxyethyl-TPP, an analogue of the α-hydroxyethyl-TPP formed in the pyruvate reactions. Just as hydroxyethyl-TPP represents an "active acetaldehyde" (CH$_3$CHO), dihydroxyethyl-TPP represents an "active glycolaldehyde" (CH$_2$OHCHO). Phos-

---

4–26.

Acrylate Pathway for Propionate Formation

$$2 \text{ CH}_3\text{CHOHCO}_2\text{H} \longrightarrow 2 \text{ CH}_2{=}\text{CHCO}_2\text{H} + 2 \text{ H}_2\text{O}$$
$lactate$ $\qquad\qquad\qquad$ $acrylate$

$$\text{CH}_3\text{CHOHCO}_2\text{H} \longrightarrow \text{CH}_3\text{COCO}_2\text{H} + 2 \text{ [H]}$$
$\qquad\qquad\qquad\qquad$ $pyruvate$

$$\text{CH}_3\text{COCO}_2\text{H} \longrightarrow \text{CH}_3\text{CO}_2\text{H} + 2 \text{ [H]} + \text{CO}_2$$
$\qquad\qquad\qquad$ $acetate$

$$2 \text{ CH}_2{=}\text{CHCO}_2\text{H} + 4 \text{ [H]} \longrightarrow 2 \text{ CH}_3\text{CH}_2\text{CO}_2\text{H}$$
$\qquad\qquad\qquad\qquad\qquad\qquad$ $propionate$

Sum:
$$3 \text{ lactate} \longrightarrow 2 \text{ propionate} + \text{acetate} + \text{CO}_2$$

---

phoketolase transfers the "active glycolaldehyde" to phosphate with rearrangement to give acetyl phosphate. Transketolase transfers the "active glycolaldehyde" to an appropriate aldehyde acceptor to give an addition product. These reactions of dihydroxyethyl-TPP are summarized in **4–27**.

REGULATION[1, 34]

All of the general mechanisms for regulating microbial metabolism operate to regulate carbohydrate metabolism. These mechanisms include regulation at the level of repression and induction of the synthesis of enzymes, and feedback regulation. The latter includes **positive** and **negative feedback** in which small molecular weight compounds stimulate or inhibit the activity of existing enzymes independently of any role of the small molecules in the specific chemical reaction catalyzed by the enzyme. Energy charge regulation is a specific type of feedback regulation. In feedback regulation, the low-molecular-weight compounds (effectors) somehow change the three-dimensional structure of the enzyme to make it more or less effective in the conversion of substrate to product. Feedback regulation controls the rates of existing enzymes and is like the foot on a gas pedal controlling the speed of a car. Induction and repression are like the hand on the ignition key giving a "go–no go" type of signal.

The classic system that is the basis of our knowledge of the induction and repression of any protein synthesis is the β-galactosidase system of *Escherichia coli*. The enzyme cleaves lactose to glucose and galactose. *Escherichia coli* DNA contains the information for synthesizing β-galactosidase, but a repressor protein on the DNA prevents this particular portion of the genome from being transcribed into the messenger RNA that codes for the synthesis of β-galactosidase. When lactose is present, it interacts with the repressor protein and moves it off the DNA, thus inducing the synthesis of β-galactosidase messenger RNA and the eventual synthesis of β-galactosidase.

Similar induction systems regulate the metabolism of a large variety of carbohydrates and other nutrients. If no induction is necessary for metabolism, *i.e.*, no repressor is ever made, the system is called constitutive. Glucose catabolism is constitutive in *E. coli* and in many other bacteria.

Another type of all-or-none repression regulation is called **catabolite repression**. If lactose and glucose are simultaneously available to *E. coli*, lactose will not induce β-galactosidase formation until all of the glucose is used. Catabolite repression appears to be related to the levels of cyclic adenosine-3′,5′-monophosphate (cyclic AMP) in cells. Cyclic AMP is necessary for the lactose-induced synthesis of β-galactosidase. Glucose metabolism somehow prevents the accumulation of sufficient cyclic AMP for induction of β-galactosidase. The mechanism of regulation of cyclic AMP concentration is not completely clear, but the depletion of glucose permits cyclic AMP accumulation and switching on of β-galactosidase formation. A variety of energy substrates other than glucose can cause catabolite repression and a variety of enzymes are subjects to catabolite repression regulation.

Oxygen can act as a repressor or inducer. The formation of the photosynthetic apparatus of nonsulfur purple bacteria is repressed by oxygen. Synthesis of mitochondria in yeast is

4–27.

Dihydroxyethyl-TPP

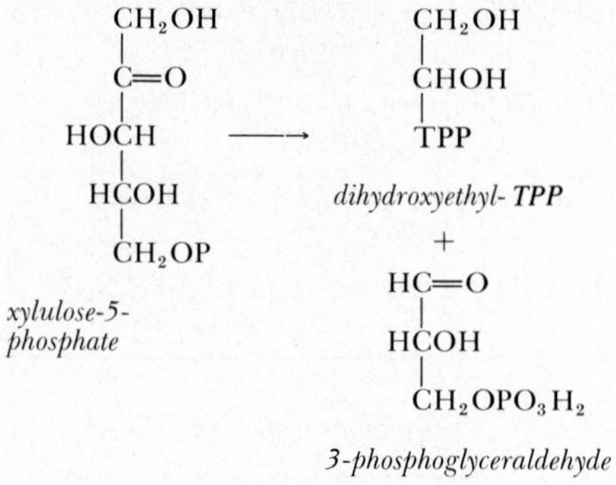

$$
\begin{array}{ccc}
\mathrm{CH_2OH} & & \mathrm{CH_2OH} \\
| & & | \\
\mathrm{C{=}O} & & \mathrm{CHOH} \\
| & \longrightarrow & | \\
\mathrm{HOCH} & & \mathrm{TPP} \\
| & & \\
\mathrm{HCOH} & & \textit{dihydroxyethyl-TPP} \\
| & & \\
\mathrm{CH_2OP} & & + \\
\end{array}
$$

xylulose-5-phosphate

$$
\begin{array}{c}
\mathrm{HC{=}O} \\
| \\
\mathrm{HCOH} \\
| \\
\mathrm{CH_2OPO_3H_2}
\end{array}
$$

3-phosphoglyceraldehyde

Phosphoketolase

$$
\mathrm{CH_2OHCHOH-TPP} + \mathrm{P}_i \longrightarrow \mathrm{TPP} + \mathrm{CH_3CO} \sim \mathrm{P}
$$
$$
\textit{acetyl} \sim P
$$

Transketolase

$$
\mathrm{CH_2OHCHOH-TPP} + \mathrm{RCHOHCHO} \longrightarrow \mathrm{TPP} + \mathrm{RCHOHCHOHCOCH_2OH}
$$

ribose-5-P	*sedoheptulose-7-P*
or	*or*
erythrose-4-P	*fructose-6-P*

induced by oxygen. Induction and repression by O_2 is not limited to these examples. The mechanism(s) by which O_2 acts as a regulator is unknown.

Other physiological parameters, such as pH and temperature of growth, can influence the expression of enzyme activity in bacteria. In most cases the mechanism has not been investigated sufficiently to show if the influence is at the level of enzyme synthesis or the regulation of the activity of existing enzymes. *Streptococcus faecalis* produces mainly lactic acid from glucose if the pH of the medium is allowed to drop as acid is produced. If the pH is controlled at neutrality by addition of alkali to neutralize produced acids, a considerable amount of ethanol, acetate, and formate is produced from glucose. Nutritional factors can also regulate enzyme activity. Although the pyruvate dehydrogenase system of *S. faecalis* is constitutive, the activity cannot be expressed unless lipoic acid is added to the medium, because the cells cannot synthesize lipoic acid. The formation of butyric and acetic acids and H_2 from glucose by some clostridia is significantly diminished when iron is limited in the growth medium. A shift to lactic acid formation occurs on low-iron mediums. The effect of iron would appear to be on the expression

of the pyruvate to acetyl-CoA, H_2 and CO_2 reaction in these organisms. The electron carrier required for the reaction, ferredoxin, is an iron-containing protein.

Feedback regulation of enzymes of bacterial carbohydrate metabolism has been studied in a few cases. Several lactic acid bacteria have lactic dehydrogenases that specifically require a small amount of fructose-1,6-bisphosphate to turn on enzyme activity. Feedback regulation is often complex, with several effectors operating on a single enzyme. Pyruvate dehydrogenase of *E. coli* (pyruvate + NAD^+ + CoASH → acetyl-CoA + NADH + CO_2 + H^+) is influenced by energy charge, acetyl-CoA, $NADH/NAD^+$ ratios and phosphoenolpyruvate. A low energy charge and phosphoenolpyruvate stimulate activity, and acetyl-CoA and a high $NADH/NAD^+$ ratio inhibit it. The concentrations of these effectors in the cell serve to modulate the activity of the pyruvate dehydrogenase.

Biosynthetic pathways, *e.g.,* amino acid and purine synthesis, are also regulated by repression and feedback control systems. The end product of a pathway usually acts as a corepressor for synthesis of enzymes of a pathway. It and a repressor protein are necessary for repressing messenger RNA synthesis.

When the end product is in short supply, no repression occurs, and synthesis of pathway enzymes provides a supply of the end product. Feedback control is usually by the end product which acts to inhibit the first irreversible step of the biosynthetic pathway.

Regulation is a complex subject, and this discussion can only touch its surface. Recognition of the importance of metabolic regulation should act as a psychological inhibitor of dogmatic extrapolations from experimental studies of test tube metabolism, carried out under only a few experimental conditions, to the activities of the same bacteria in distinctly different milieux, including the natural environment. Present knowledge of bacterial metabolism provides an excellent guide to the metabolic potential of individual species, but does not define the expression of this potential for all environmental conditions.

THE CARBON CYCLE

Carbohydrates are degraded to organic products by some bacteria in the absence of oxygen and oxidized to CO_2 and H_2O by other bacteria. The other major natural organic compounds—proteins, lipids, and nucleic acids—are also degraded to organic products under anaerobic conditions and oxidized to CO_2, H_2O, and ammonia (from the nitrogen-containing compounds) in aerobic environments. Bacteria have direct access to these cell constituents and also to waste products of their metabolism in animals. Allantoin and uric acid, for example, are excreted breakdown products of purine metabolism in animals that become available to bacteria. The gamut of pathways for the degradation of all of these compounds will not be considered here (as were those of the carbohydrates). Instead, it may be more useful to state a few principles (using carbohydrate degradation as an example) to outline the general strategy of catabolism and its biological significance.

Bacteria have hydrolytic enzymes to digest proteins, lipids, and nucleic acids to low-molecular-weight compounds that can enter the cell. Proteases hydrolyze proteins to peptides and, eventually, to amino acids; lipases hydrolyze lipids to glycerol and fatty acids; and nucleases hydrolyze nucleic acids to purines, pyrimidines, ribose, and deoxyribose. Once monomers are formed, anaerobic fermentation and respiration as well as aerobic respiration processes operate to provide energy for growth.

Consider, for example, the decomposition of a protein in an anaerobic environment. Some species of the genus *Clostridium* have extremely active proteolytic enzymes, and these species obtain energy for growth from metabolism of the resulting amino acids. A protein may have 16 to 20 different amino acids, however, and the *Clostridium* species has enzymatic machinery to nourish itself on many of these amino acids through an anaerobic respiration system called the **Stickland reaction.**[2] Amino acid pairs are used in a coupled oxidation-reduction system in which one amino acid is oxidized and the other is reduced:

(*1*) $RCHNH_2CO_2H \rightarrow RCOCO_2H + NH_3 + 2[H]$
(2) $RCOCO_2H \rightarrow RCO_2H + CO_2 + 2[H]$
(3) $4[H] + 2 R'CHNH_2CO_2H \rightarrow$
$$2 R'CH_2CO_2H + 2 NH_3$$

Sum:
$$RCHNH_2CO_2H + 2 R'CHNH_2CO_2H \rightarrow$$
$$RCO_2H + 2 R'CH_2CO_2H + CO_2 + 3 NH_3$$

In reaction *1*, the electron donor amino acid is oxidized to its corresponding keto acid and ammonia. The keto acid is oxidatively decarboxylated to a fatty acid and CO_2 (reaction 2). Reaction 2 is essentially the same reaction pattern previously described for the oxidative decarboxylation of pyruvate, and energy can be derived via acyl-CoA intermediates as in the pyruvate example. In reaction *3*, the electron acceptor reaction, a second, different amino acid is reductively deaminated to the corresponding fatty acid and NH_3.

There are many cases in which bacteria can obtain energy from the fermentation of single amino acids[2] derived from proteolysis. Formation of keto acids and energy generation from acyl-CoA intermediates is important in many of these fermentations, and fatty acids are the usual products. A special case of energy generation is associated with arginine breakdown. Here energy can be obtained by a nonoxidative pathway, an exception to the general use of O–R reactions for energy generation. Arginine catabolism leads to the formation of carbamyl-phosphate (see **4–28**). Carbamyl-phosphate contains a phosphoanhydride bond whose energy is used for ATP formation. Several *Streptococcus* species can obtain energy for growth from the arginine to ornithine conversion. Carbamyl-phosphate is a high-energy intermediate in the decomposition of allantoin and is probably an intermediate in pyrimidine breakdown.

Purine decomposition[2, 33] is another exception to the association of energy generation

4–28.

Arginine Breakdown

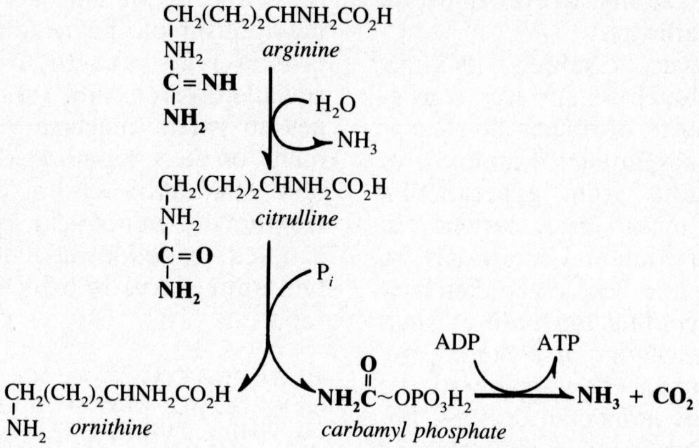

CH$_2$(CH$_2$)$_2$CHNH$_2$CO$_2$H
|
NH$_2$ *arginine*
|
C=NH
|
NH$_2$

H$_2$O
↳ NH$_3$

CH$_2$(CH$_2$)$_2$CHNH$_2$CO$_2$H
|
NH$_2$ *citrulline*
|
C=O
|
NH$_2$

P$_i$

CH$_2$(CH$_2$)$_2$CHNH$_2$CO$_2$H   ADP   ATP
|
NH$_2$ *ornithine*   NH$_2$C~OPO$_3$H$_2$ ⟶ NH$_3$ + CO$_2$
                          carbamyl phosphate

O
‖

4–29.

Folic Acid Coenzymes

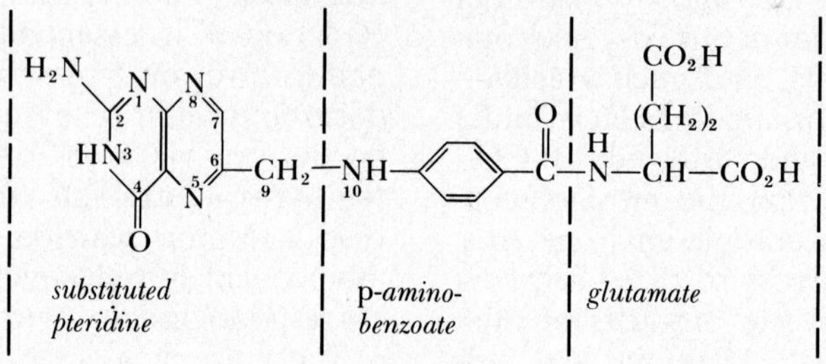

substituted   p-amino-   glutamate
pteridine   benzoate

Folic Acid

tetrahydrofolic   N^{10}-*formyl-THFA*
acid (THFA)

N^5-*formimino-THFA*   N^5, N^{10}-*methenyl-THFA*

N^5, N^{10}-*methylene-THFA*   N^5-*methyl-THFA*

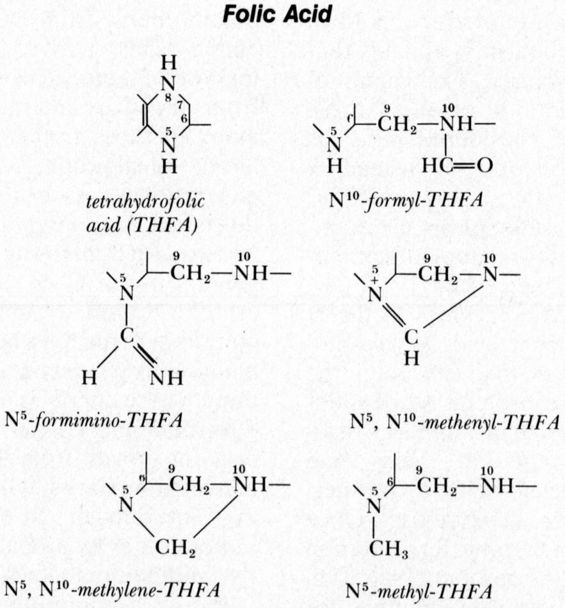

with O–R reactions and also illustrates the function of coenzyme forms of the vitamin folic acid in biochemical reactions. The coenzyme form of folic acid is the reduced vitamin tetrahydrofolic acid (THFA). Folic acid is composed of a substituted pteridine linked to a glutamic acid moiety and ρ-aminobenzoic acid (see **4–29**).

The various 1-carbon derivatives of THFA (see **4–29**) represent different oxidation states of the 1-carbon unit as follows:

1. N^5—CH_3(methyl)—THFA; oxidation state equivalent to that of methanol or a methyl group.

2. N^5,N^{10}—CH_2(methylene)—THFA; oxidation state equivalent to that of formaldehyde or a hydroxymethyl or methylene group.

3. N^5,N^{10}=CH(methenyl)—THFA, N^5—CH=NH-(formimino)—THFA, and N^{10}—CHO(formyl)—THFA; oxidation state equivalent to that of formate or methenyl, or formimino or formyl groups.

N^5-methyl-THFA is involved in methyl group transfer reactions, such as the formation of methionine from homocysteine:

$$N^5—CH_3—THFA + HSCH_2CH_2CH_2\overset{\overset{\displaystyle NH_2}{|}}{C}HCO_2H \rightarrow$$

homocysteine

$$CH_3SCH_2CH_2CH_2\overset{\overset{\displaystyle NH_2}{|}}{C}HCO_2H + THFA$$

methionine

N^5,N^{10}-methylene-THFA is involved in hydroxymethyl group transfer reactions, such as in the formation of serine from glycine:

$$N^5,N^{10}—CH_2—THFA + H_2O + \overset{\overset{\displaystyle NH_2}{|}}{C}H_2CO_2H \rightarrow$$

glycine

$$HO—CH_2\overset{\overset{\displaystyle NH_2}{|}}{C}H_2CO_2H + THFA$$

serine

Methylene-THFA is also used in the synthesis of the pyrimidine thymidine deoxyribonucleotide monophosphate (dTMP) from uridine deoxyribonucleotide monophosphate (dUMP). The methylene unit is transferred and the THFA portion of the molecule is simultaneously oxidized to dihydrofolic acid. This is the only known one carbon transfer reaction in which THFA is oxidized (see the formula at the bottom of the page).

In the accompanying purine decomposition pathway (see **4–30**) THFA is involved in formimino and formyl group transfer reactions. Formiminoglycine is formed from xanthine by a series of hydrolyses. The formimino group is transferred to THFA, and formimino-THFA is converted to N^{10}-formyl-THFA. The energy-yielding step in the pathway is the conversion of N^{10}-formyl-THFA, ADP, and P_i to formate, THFA, and ATP.

These few examples of anaerobic attack on organic substrates other than carbohydrates illustrate that microorganisms can obtain energy from substrate phosphorylations associated with the transformation of most organic substrates. Most of the substrates dealt with thus far can be used as energy sources by fermentative decompositions, by nonfermentative decompositions which do not involve pairing with an added electron acceptor, or by respiratory mechanisms. In aerobic decomposition, substrate transformations lead to substrate phosphorylations, but oxidative phosphorylation predominates as the energy-generating system.

Contemporary anaerobic energy generation is probably a reflection of those systems that evolved before photochemical systems had developed for introducing O_2 into the earth's atmosphere. In the early anaerobic environment, some anaerobic respiratory mechanisms developed along with some primitive oxidative phosphorylation systems. But the only major nonsubstrate phosphorylation system that could have existed in the anaerobic environment was that of the anaerobic phototrophic bacteria, because the only high-potential electron acceptor in the environment was the tran-

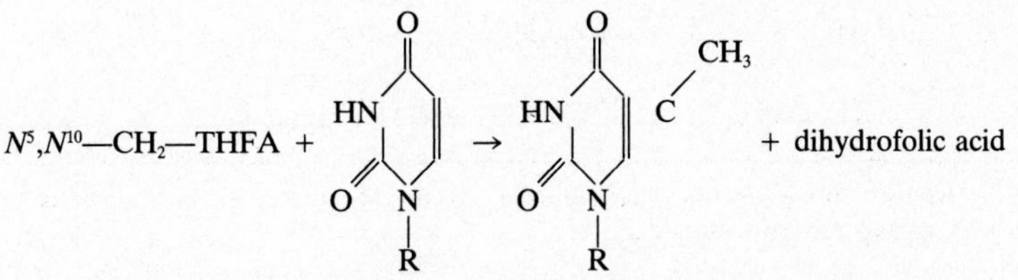

$$N^5,N^{10}—CH_2—THFA +$$ dUMP $$\rightarrow$$ dTMP $$+ \text{ dihydrofolic acid}$$

4–30.

Purine Decomposition*

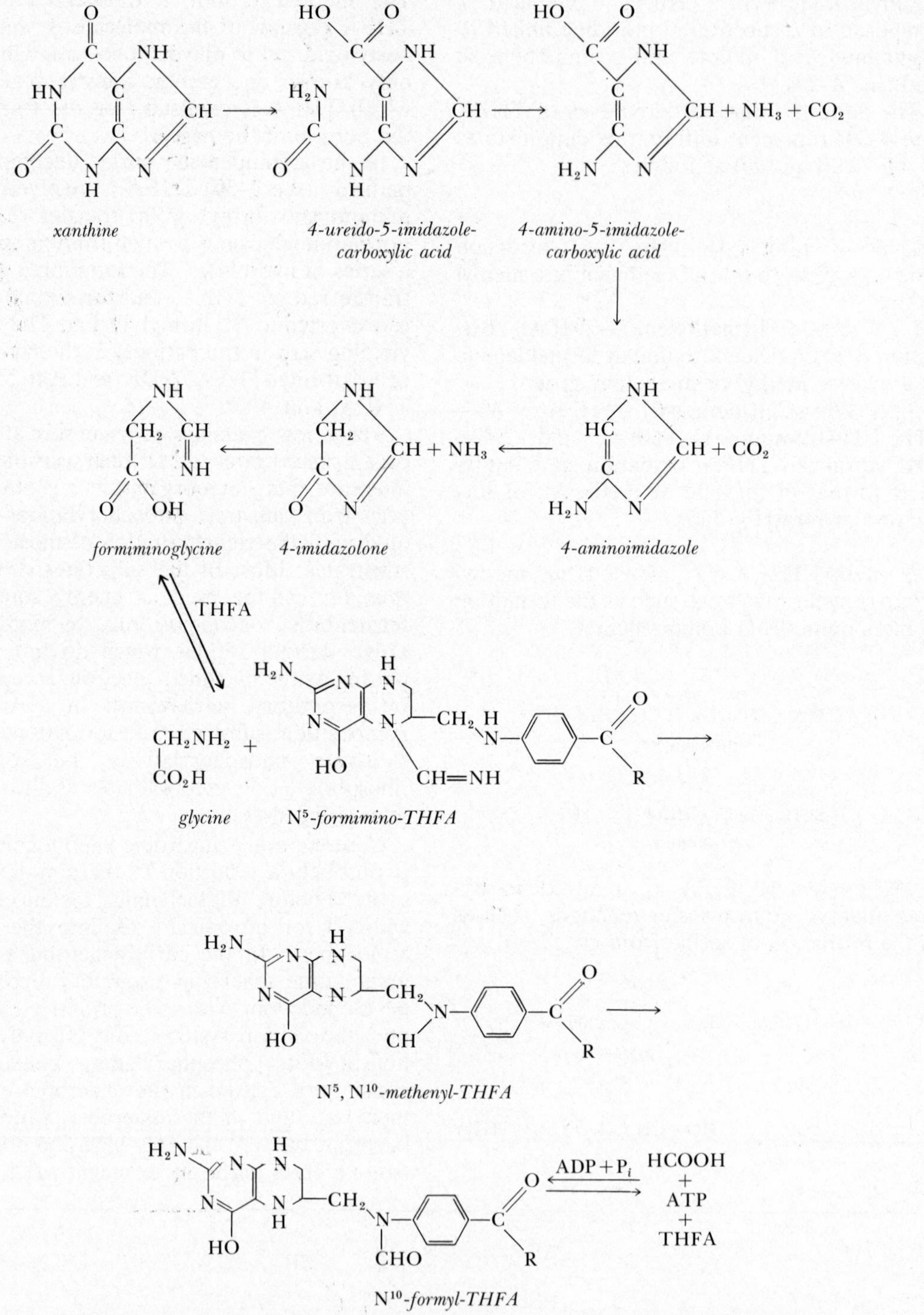

*Enzymatic reactions in the conversion of xanthine to glycine, formate, carbon dioxide, and ammonia by *Clostridium cylindrosporum.* (Adapted from Barker.[2])

sient oxidized chlorophyll produced by light quanta.

Most of the anaerobic decomposition mechanisms that have developed subsequently (and are contemporary) eventually lead to the accumulation of short-chain fatty acids and H_2 in the environment. We have seen that formate, acetate, propionate, and butyrate are common fermentation products. The other common fermentation products, *e.g.*, alcohols, lactate, and succinate, can be converted to the fatty acid end products and H_2 in anaerobic environments. The short-chain fatty acid products and H_2 are all eventually converted to methane[35] and CO_2. Known pure cultures of methane bacteria produce methane from four substrates—H_2, CO_2, formate, acetate—as follows:

$$4 H_2 + CO_2 \rightarrow CH_4 + 2 H_2O$$
$$4 HCO_2H \rightarrow CH_4 + 3 CO_2 + 2 H_2O$$
$$CH_3CO_2H \rightarrow CH_4 + CO_2$$

Conversions of other fermentation products to methane involve either mixed culture fermentations or unknown methane bacteria. The main point is that, given enough time in an anaerobic environment, almost all organic matter is converted to CH_4 and CO_2 by a mixture of diverse species. A single compound like glucose can be transformed by a variety of bacteria to a variety of organic products. Further metabolism of the products converges on the terminal point of CH_4 and CO_2.

There are some natural organic compounds that appear to be difficult to break down anaerobically. These include aromatic rings (such as those of the aromatic amino acids tyrosine, phenylalanine, and tryptophan) and hydrocarbons found in natural waxes. These accumulate in the anaerobic environment and, in fact, it is believed that natural gas and petroleum deposits are derived from the residue of anaerobic decomposition of organic matter that was locked into permanent anaerobic niches below the earth's surface.

In the aerobic environment everything eventually converges on CO_2, and H_2O, including the residue of anaerobic decomposition, *i.e.*, methane, hydrocarbons, and aromatic rings. As with anaerobic decomposition, many different tracks are used to get to the ultimate products. All organic matter is, however, eventually converted to CO_2 which is then converted back to organic matter by photosynthesis.

There is a tendency to overlook the importance of anaerobic decomposition in this cycle because of the apparent ubiquity of oxygen on the surface of the earth. The ubiquity of oxygen is, however, more apparent than real as far as microbial environments are concerned. These environments are aqueous, and the solubility of O_2 in water is low. If the organic load is high, the oxygen in the aqueous environment is quickly used up by microbial oxidations. Since the rate of dissolution of oxygen from the air is slow, anaerobic processes quickly take over. The predominant normal flora of the oral cavity and intestinal tract of man are either obligate anaerobes or organisms that obtain energy from anaerobic processes (although they may survive in the presence of oxygen). The intestinal tract microbial environment is definitely anaerobic, and the microenvironments where bacteria grow in the oral cavity become anaerobic quickly after colonization, even with the considerable entry of air into this cavity. Many important pathogens obtain energy for growth only by anaerobic decomposition, and those that can carry out anaerobic and aerobic energy-generating processes are probably often using anaerobic systems during infection. The surface of the skin is the only portion of the body that supports the growth of flora with significant aerobic metabolisms, and there are only a few pathogens that depend strictly on aerobic metabolism for growth.

NITROGEN AND SULFUR CYCLES

When microorganisms mineralize the carbon of biosynthesized organic compounds, they also mineralize the other elements of organic cellular constituents. Organic phosphate is converted to inorganic phosphate, organic nitrogen to ammonia, and organic sulfur to hydrogen sulfide.

The Nitrogen Cycle

In order to return nitrogen to the food chain, ammonia is converted to nitrate, the major stable form of nitrogen in the soil. Ammonia can be used as a nitrogen source by plants, but the stability of ammonia in the ecosystem is tenuous because ammonia disappears when the pH is alkaline. Nitrate formation assures the presence of a stable form of nitrogen that can be directly used by green plants. Nitrate formation from ammonia is carried out by chemolithotrophic, autotrophic bacteria in two stages:

(1) $NH_3 + 1\frac{1}{2} O_2 \rightarrow H^+ + NO_2^- + H_2O$
(2) $NO_2^- + \frac{1}{2} O_2 \rightarrow NO_3^-$

The overall process is called **nitrification**. Stage *1* is carried out by members of the genera *Nitrosomonas* and *Nitrosococcus* and stage *2* by the genus *Nitrobacter*.

Some bacteria compete with this process of nitrification. A portion use nitrate just like green plants, reducing it to ammonia, which then is incorporated into cellular organic nitrogen compounds. This still keeps the nitrogen in the ecosystem cycle. However, there are other bacteria (already discussed) that carry out "nitrate respiration," *i.e.,* they reduce nitrate to N_2. The gas, N_2, leaves the ecosystem. Reduction of nitrate to N_2 is called **denitrification**.

A replenishment process of extreme importance in nature is the fixation of N_2 gas into NH_3 by microorganisms.[20] This replaces N_2 lost by denitrification and nitrogen lost by natural leaching of nitrates. The NH_3 is used by N_2-fixing bacteria for synthesis of cellular N compounds by bacteria or plants. NH_3 is directly provided to plants by symbiotic microorganisms. The most prominent of these are members of the genus *Rhizobium*. Rhizobia infect roots of legumes (*e.g.,* soybeans, alfalfa) and elicit the formation of a nodule. The nodule contains a differentiated form of the free-living rhizobia that fixes N_2 into NH_3. A variety of free-living bacteria, *e.g., Clostridium, Bacillus, Klebsiella, Azotobacter,* phototrophic genera, and blue-green algae fix N_2. The latter are very important in providing fixed N_2 in rice paddies.

Nitrogenase, an enzyme complex of two proteins, has been purified from several bacteria. In the presence of a source of electrons and ATP, nitrogenase becomes a powerful reducing agent and reduces N_2 to NH_3:

$$6\,H^+ + 6\,e^- + N_2 \rightarrow 2\,NH_3$$

Although this is a 6-electron reduction, no intermediates have been identified. The role of ATP is not clear. It is broken down to ADP and P_i during N_2 fixation and approximately 5 ATPs are used per N_2 fixed. Whatever the mechanism, nitrogenase is a remarkable enzyme. Chemical synthesis of fixed nitrogen compounds from N_2 requires extremely high temperatures and pressures along with appropriate catalysts. Bacteria have no trouble doing this at 25° C. and 1 atm. pressure.

These processes of synthesis of organic N from NH_3, ammonification, nitrification, denitrification, and nitrogen fixation constitute the nitrogen (N) cycle (see **4–31**).

The Sulfur Cycle

The sulfur cycle is very similar (see **4–31**).[23] H_2S produced by decomposition of organic matter is fixed into sulfate by chemolithotrophic thiobacilli and phototrophic purple and green sulfur bacteria. Green plants and many bacteria use sulfate to synthesize cell sulfur compounds (*e.g.,* cysteine, methionine). A counteracting reaction is the reduction of sulfate to sulfide during the anaerobic respiration of sulfate-reducing bacteria. These bacteria (*e.g., Desulfovibrio*) use sulfate reduction to H_2S as an energy-generating process.

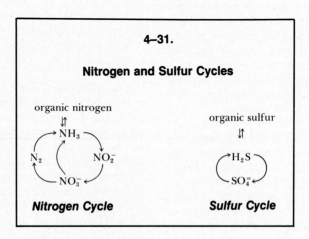

4–31.

Nitrogen and Sulfur Cycles

Nitrogen Cycle

Sulfur Cycle

Biosynthesis of Molecules

SYNTHESIS OF SMALL MOLECULES[3, 30]

Microorganisms differ considerably in their ability to synthesize the low-molecular-weight precursors of cell macromolecules and vitamins. Some bacteria, including many pathogens, have little synthetic ability and require preformed amino acids, vitamins, and purines and pyrimidines for growth. The specific requirements vary. Lack of synthetic ability, or the requirement for these low-molecular-weight compounds, indicates that these compounds are always abundant in the organism's natural environment. If an organism's ancestors ever possessed this missing synthetic capability, it was probably lost during evolution.

At the other end of the biosynthetic spectrum are organisms that synthesize all of their cell carbon compounds from carbon dioxide. These organisms, called autotrophs. include phototrophic bacteria, chemolithotrophic bacteria, and even a few chemoorganotrophs. There are a few bacteria that obtain energy by oxidizing organic compounds like formic acid or methane to CO_2 and H_2O, and are, therefore, chemoorganotrophs, but they synthesize all cell carbon from carbon dioxide. Bacteria that use preformed organic compounds directly for biosynthesis of cell macromolecules and vitamins are called heterotrophs.

Although there are exceptions, the specific pathways for the synthesis of specific low-molecular-weight compounds are very similar in all organisms. A simple example is the synthesis of alanine. Pyruvate is always the precursor of alanine and alanine is made by reductive amination of pyruvate.

$$CH_3COCO_2H + NH_3 + NADPH + H^+ \rightarrow$$
$$CH_3CHNH_2CO_2H + NADP^+ + H_2O$$
alanine

or by a transaminase reaction,

$$CH_3COCO_2H + HO_2C(CH_2)_2CHNH_2CO_2H \rightarrow$$
glutamate

$$CH_3CHNH_2CO_2H + HO_2C(CH_2)_2COCO_2H$$
α-ketoglutarate

The latter reaction requires that the organism has glutamic acid available to it or that it can synthesize glutamic acid, but we can conclude that all organisms that make alanine will first make pyruvate.

There are differences, however, in the way different bacteria enter the alanine pathway, *i.e.,* differences in how they make pyruvate from the starting carbon source. These entry differences exist for all the specific pathways for synthesis of all low-molecular-weight compounds. The major questions about the biosynthesis of small molecules are, therefore

1. What are the specific pathways of biosynthesis?
2. How are the specific pathways entered from the variety of carbon sources used by bacteria?
3. How is synthesis regulated?

Question 3 was already considered in the discussion of the regulation of carbohydrate breakdown.

Rather than providing a catalogue of specific pathways and the manner in which these pathways are entered from a variety of carbon sources, we will focus on the biosynthesis of a uniquely bacterial cell macromolecule, **peptidoglycan** (also called murein and mucopeptide).[25, 27, 29] Peptidoglycan is the polymer responsible for the rigidity of the bacterial cell wall and the shape of bacteria. It is found in almost all procaryotes except the *Mycoplasma,* which are bacteria without rigid cell walls, and a few bacteria that have rigid cell walls without peptidoglycan.

Peptidoglycan is a heteropolymer consisting of a backbone of a polysaccharide containing alternating units of *N*-acetylglucosamine and muramic acid (see **4–32**). Muramic acid is *N*-acetyl-glucosamine with an ether-linked acid attached to its 3-position (it is the ether that would be formed if lactic acid were joined to the 3-position of *N*-acetyl-glucosamine with the removal of a molecule of water). The carboxyl group of the acid substituent is available for forming an amide bond with L-alanine. The alanine is then attached to other D- and L-amino acids to give a short peptide side chain. Bacterial peptidoglycans differ with respect to (a) the specific amino acids in the side chain, (b) substituents on the polysaccharide backbone, and (c) cross linking between the peptide side chains. Two different peptidoglycans are shown in **4–33**, that of *Staphylococcus aureus* and that of *Escherichia coli*. We will be concerned with the synthesis of the basic structure, exemplified by the *E. coli* peptidoglycan, to illustrate biosynthetic principles. It is the cross linking between the adjacent polysaccharide chains that forms the rigid macromolecular sac around the bacterial cell.

4–32.

Disaccharide Backbone of Peptidoglycan

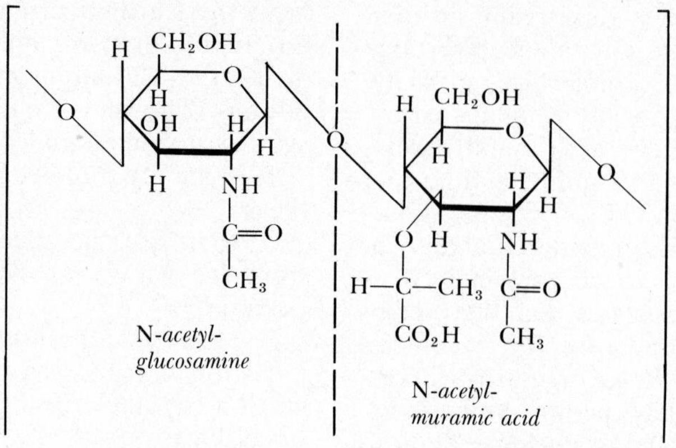

N-*acetyl-glucosamine*

N-*acetyl-muramic acid*

Synthesis from Glucose

Escherichia coli grows on glucose as its sole carbon and energy source. How does it make peptidoglycan components from the glucose? The *N*-acetyl-glucosamine moiety will be considered first. *Escherichia coli* makes fructose-6-phosphate by reactions discussed above (see **4–4**) and then it makes *N*-acetyl-glucosamine-6-phosphate from fructose-6-phosphate, glutamine, and acetyl-CoA (see **4–34**). We also have reviewed how acetyl-CoA is made from glucose (see **4–14**), but where did the glutamine come from? Glutamic acid is first made from α-ketoglutarate generated through TCA cycle reactions (see **4–19**), and glutamine from glutamate, ATP, and NH_3 (see **4–35**).

Reductive amination of α-ketoglutarate to glutamate and pyruvate to alanine are of general importance. Other amino acids are formed by transamination of keto-acid precursors. These transaminations depend on the prior incorporation of ammonia into glutamate or alanine, both of which become key amino donors in the transaminations. The amide group of glutamine is also of general importance as a participant in a variety of essential amidation reactions.

ATP is formed from ADP by energy-yielding reactions already discussed and used here for the energy-requiring synthesis of an amide bond. We have to be concerned, however, with how *E. coli* makes the purine nucleoside phosphate from glucose as well as how it makes the high-energy bonds.

Again *E. coli* has a starting point in carbohydrate metabolism in the formation of ribose-5-phosphate from glucose-6-phosphate. Ribulose-5-phosphate formed by oxidative decarboxylation of 6-phosphogluconic acid is isomerized to ribose-5-phosphate (see **4–7, 4–9,** and **4–11**), the foundation for construction of a purine molecule. The general pathway for purine biosynthesis is shown in **4–36**. The nitrogen of the purine ring derives from the amide nitrogen of glutamine and the amino groups of aspartic acid and glycine. The carbons came from glycine, 1-carbon derivatives of tetrahydrofolic acid, and CO_2.

To return to glucose to see how *E. coli* makes glycine and the 1-carbon tetrahydrofolate derivatives: glycine is made from serine, which in turn is made from 3-phosphoglyceric acid, an intermediate in the conversion of glucose to pyruvate (see **4–4**). The serine to glycine conversion involves tetrahydrofolic acid. The pathway from 3-phosphoglycerate to glycine is shown in **4–37**. The N^5, N^{10}-methenyl-THFA resulting from the conversion of serine to glycine can be oxidized to N^5, N^{10}-methylene-THFA. N^{10}-formyl-THFA, formed from N^5, N^{10}-methylene-THFA, is then available for the formylation reactions of the purine pathway. The basic portion of the purine pathway ends at inosinic acid (inosine monophosphate). Aspartic acid is necessary to convert inosinic acid to adenylic acid in an amino group donation reaction analogous to that used in the purine pathway itself. (see **4–38** for formation of adenosine and guanosine monophosphates from inosine monophosphate.) As-

4–33.

Peptidoglycan of Staphylococcus aureus

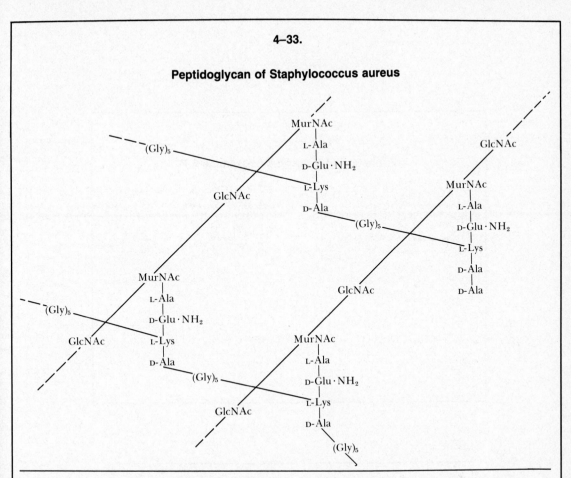

Abbreviations: GlcNAc, *N*-acetyl-glucosamine; MurNAc, *N*-acetyl-muramic acid; Ala, alanine; Glu-NH₂, isoglutamine; Lys, lysine; and Gly, glycine.

Peptidoglycan of Escherichia coli

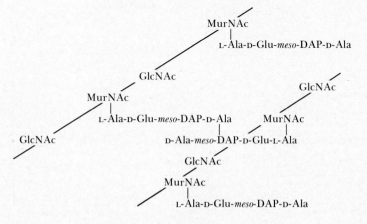

Abbreviations: See above; also Glu, glutamate; and DAP; diaminopimelate.

4–34.

Formation of *N*-acetyl-glucosamine-6-P

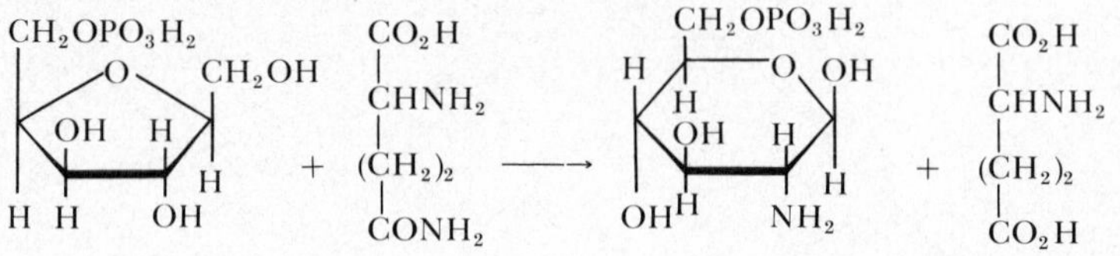

$$
\text{fructose-6-P} + \text{glutamine} \longrightarrow \text{glucosamine-6-P} + \text{glutamate}
$$

$$
R-NH_2 + CH_3CO \sim SCoA \longrightarrow R-N-\overset{\overset{\displaystyle O}{\parallel}}{C}-CH_3 + CoASH
$$

glucosamine-
6-P

N-acetyl-
glucosamine-
6-P

4–35.

Formation of Glutamine

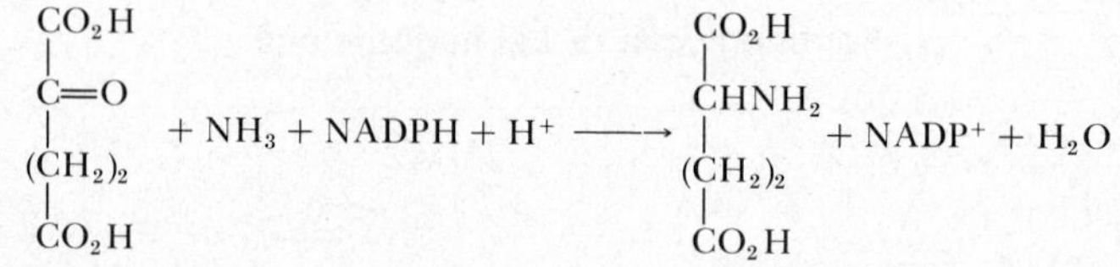

$$
\alpha\text{-keto-glutarate} + NH_3 + NADPH + H^+ \longrightarrow \text{glutamate} + NADP^+ + H_2O
$$

$$
\text{glutamate} + ATP + NH_3 \longrightarrow \text{glutamine} + ADP + P_i
$$

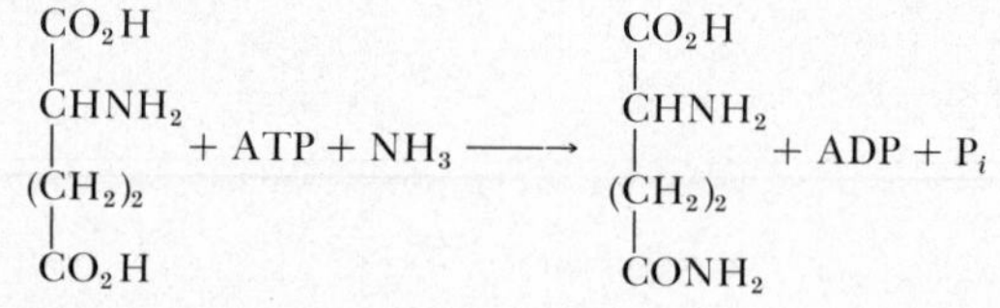

4–36.

Synthesis of Purines

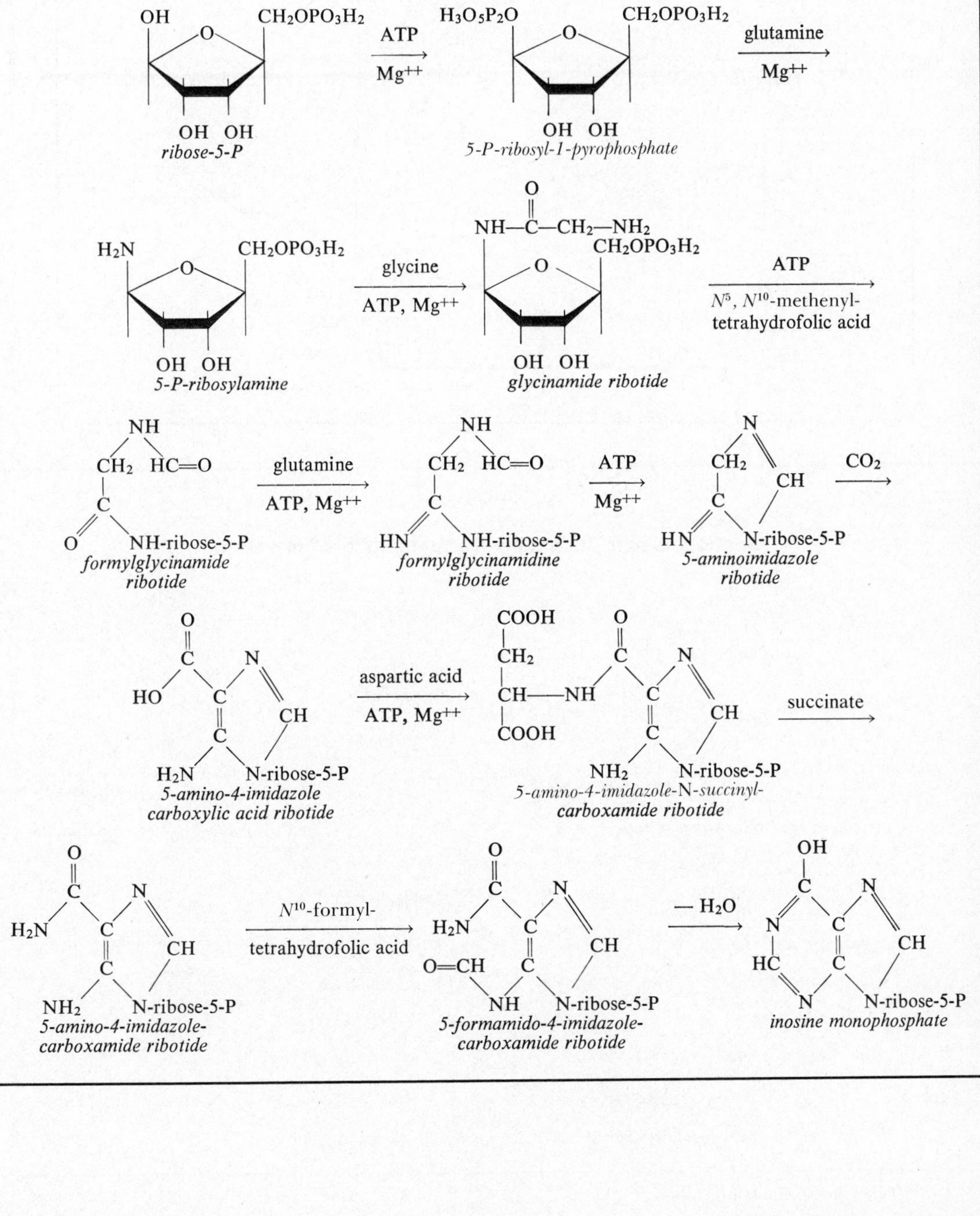

OH $CH_2OPO_3H_2$ $\xrightarrow[\text{Mg}^{++}]{\text{ATP}}$ $H_3O_5P_2O$ $CH_2OPO_3H_2$ $\xrightarrow[\text{Mg}^{++}]{\text{glutamine}}$

OH   OH
ribose-5-P

OH   OH
5-P-ribosyl-1-pyrophosphate

H_2N $CH_2OPO_3H_2$ $\xrightarrow[\text{ATP, Mg}^{++}]{\text{glycine}}$

OH   OH
5-P-ribosylamine

$$NH\!-\!\overset{\displaystyle O}{\overset{\|}{C}}\!-\!CH_2\!-\!NH_2$$

$CH_2OPO_3H_2$ $\xrightarrow[\substack{N^5, N^{10}\text{-methenyl-}\\ \text{tetrahydrofolic acid}}]{\text{ATP}}$

OH   OH
glycinamide ribotide

NH
CH_2 HC=O
C
O   NH-ribose-5-P
formylglycinamide ribotide

$\xrightarrow[\text{ATP, Mg}^{++}]{\text{glutamine}}$

NH
CH_2 HC=O
C
HN   NH-ribose-5-P
formylglycinamidine ribotide

$\xrightarrow[\text{Mg}^{++}]{\text{ATP}}$

N
CH_2 CH
C
HN   N-ribose-5-P
5-aminoimidazole ribotide

$\xrightarrow{\text{CO}_2}$

O
‖
C
HO   C   N
C   CH
H_2N N-ribose-5-P
5-amino-4-imidazole carboxylic acid ribotide

$\xrightarrow[\text{ATP, Mg}^{++}]{\text{aspartic acid}}$

COOH   O
CH_2 C   N
CH—NH   C   CH
COOH   C
NH_2 N-ribose-5-P
5-amino-4-imidazole-N-succinyl-carboxamide ribotide

$\xrightarrow{\text{succinate}}$

O
‖
C
H_2N C   N
C   CH
C
NH_2 N-ribose-5-P
5-amino-4-imidazole-carboxamide ribotide

$\xrightarrow[\text{tetrahydrofolic acid}]{N^{10}\text{-formyl-}}$

O
‖
C
H_2N C   N
C   CH
O=CH   C
NH   N-ribose-5-P
5-formamido-4-imidazole-carboxamide ribotide

$\xrightarrow{-\ H_2O}$

OH
|
C
N   C   N
HC   C   CH
N   N-ribose-5-P
inosine monophosphate

4–37.

Serine and Glycine Formation

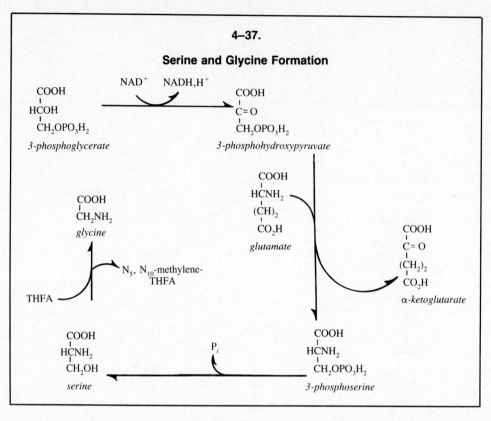

4–38.

Adenosine and Guanosine Monophosphate Formation

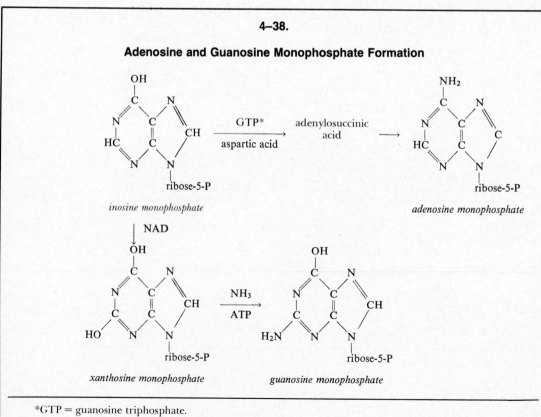

*GTP = guanosine triphosphate.

4–39.

Synthesis of UDP-N-acetyl-glucosamine

N-acetyl-glucosamine-6-P ⟶ N-acetyl-glucosamine-1-P (N-Ac-Gn-1-P)

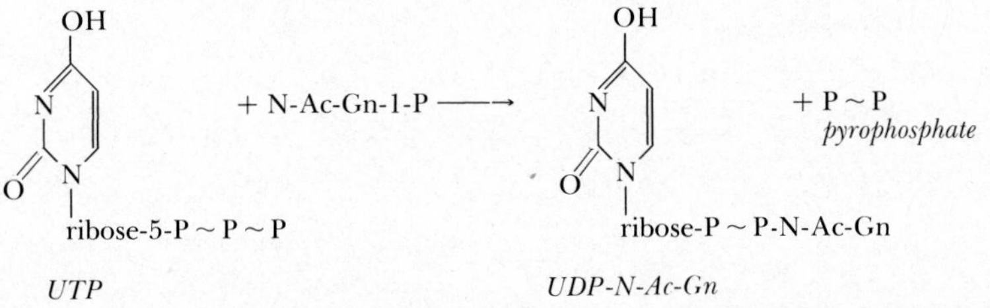

+ N-Ac-Gn-1-P ⟶   + P ~ P
     pyrophosphate

ribose-5-P ~ P ~ P   ribose-P ~ P-N-Ac-Gn

UTP   *UDP-N-Ac-Gn*

---

partic acid is made from oxaloacetate by a transamination reaction:

oxaloacetate + glutamate →
              aspartate + α-ketoglutarate

With all the ingredients from glucose *E. coli* can make AMP and then,

AMP + ATP → 2 ADP

Finally, *E. coli* has made glutamine and now can make *N*-acetyl-glucosamine-6-phosphate. To make muramic acid, the cell adds a nucleoside diphosphate handle to the hexosamine. In almost all sugar polymerization reactions, sugar nucleotides rather than free sugars are handled by enzymes. Other types of enzymatic manipulations of sugars also involve sugar nucleotides, *e.g.*, the previously mentioned conversion of galactose to glucose. Uridine-diphosphate-*N*-acetyl-glucosamine, formed from uridine triphosphate (UTP) and *N*-acetyl-glucosamine-1-phosphate, is the precursor of muramic acid (see **4–39**). The link between the phosphate and the sugar in all of the sugar nucleotides is always on the first carbon of the sugar:

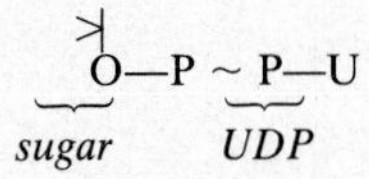

$$\overset{}{\underset{sugar}{\underbrace{O}}}-P \sim \underset{UDP}{\underbrace{P-U}}$$

Escherichia coli has to return to glucose to fashion a pyrimidine, uracil, for its cell wall factory. The first reaction in pyrimidine synthesis uses CO_2, NH_3, and ATP to make carbamyl-phosphate:

$$NH_3 + CO_2 + ATP \rightarrow H_2N\overset{O}{\overset{\|}{C}}O \sim P + ADP$$
                         carbamyl-phosphate

The synthesis of arginine begins with the formation of carbamyl-phosphate from CO_2, NH_3, and ATP. As with many other compounds, carbamyl-phosphate is a key intermediate in biosynthesis as well as in energy metabolism. In pyrimidine synthesis, carbamyl-phosphate condenses with aspartic acid, and the pathway is shown in **4–40**. Formation of uridine and cytidine triphosphates from uridine monophosphate is also shown in **4–40**. (See **4–36** for the formation of 5-P-ribosyl-1-pyrophosphate from ribose-5-phosphate.)

Now *E. coli* uses phosphoenolpyruvate and 2 [H] to make UDP-*N*-acetyl-muramic acid, as shown in **4–41**. (See **4–4** for phosphoenol pyruvate formation). The UDP derivatives, UDP-*N*-acetyl-glucosamine and UDP-*N*-acetyl-muramic acid, are the substrates for the final polymerization reactions in peptidoglycan formation.

For the peptide, *E. coli* has to construct from glucose: L-alanine (already discussed), D-alanine, *meso*-diaminopimelic acid, and D-glutamic acid. D-Amino acids are formed from L-amino acids by specific amino acid racemases, *i.e.*, a specific enzyme interconverts the D and L isomers:

L-alanine ⇌ D-alanine
L-glutamic acid ⇌ D-glutamic acid

Diaminopimelic synthesis remains to be carried out, and here *E. coli* starts with aspartic acid and pyruvate and uses the reaction sequence shown in **4–42** to make diaminopimelic acid. The same pathway is used to make lysine. The succinyl-CoA used in the pathway is made via TCA cycle reactions (see **4–19**).

This is how *E. coli* makes all the ingredients for peptidoglycan from glucose. Many of the ingredients are used for making other macro-

4–40.

Synthesis of Pyrimidines

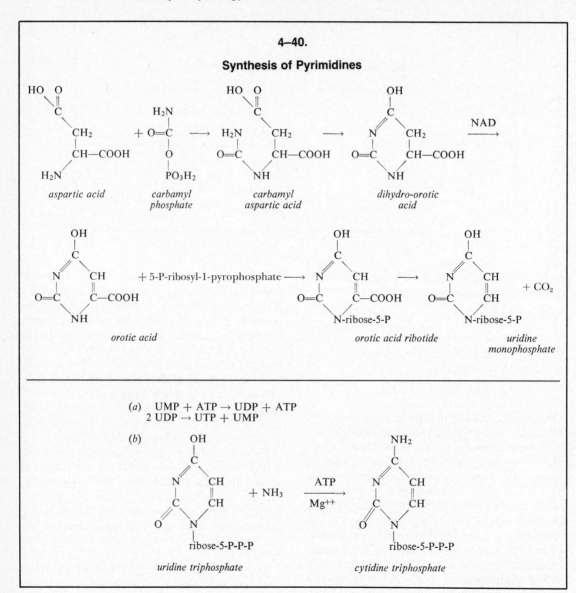

(a) UMP + ATP → UDP + ATP
2 UDP → UTP + UMP

(b)

uridine triphosphate   cytidine triphosphate

4–41.

Formation of UDP-N-acetyl-muramic acid

UDP-N-Ac-Gn   UDP-N-Ac-muramic acid

4–42.

Diaminopimelic Acid and Lysine Synthesis

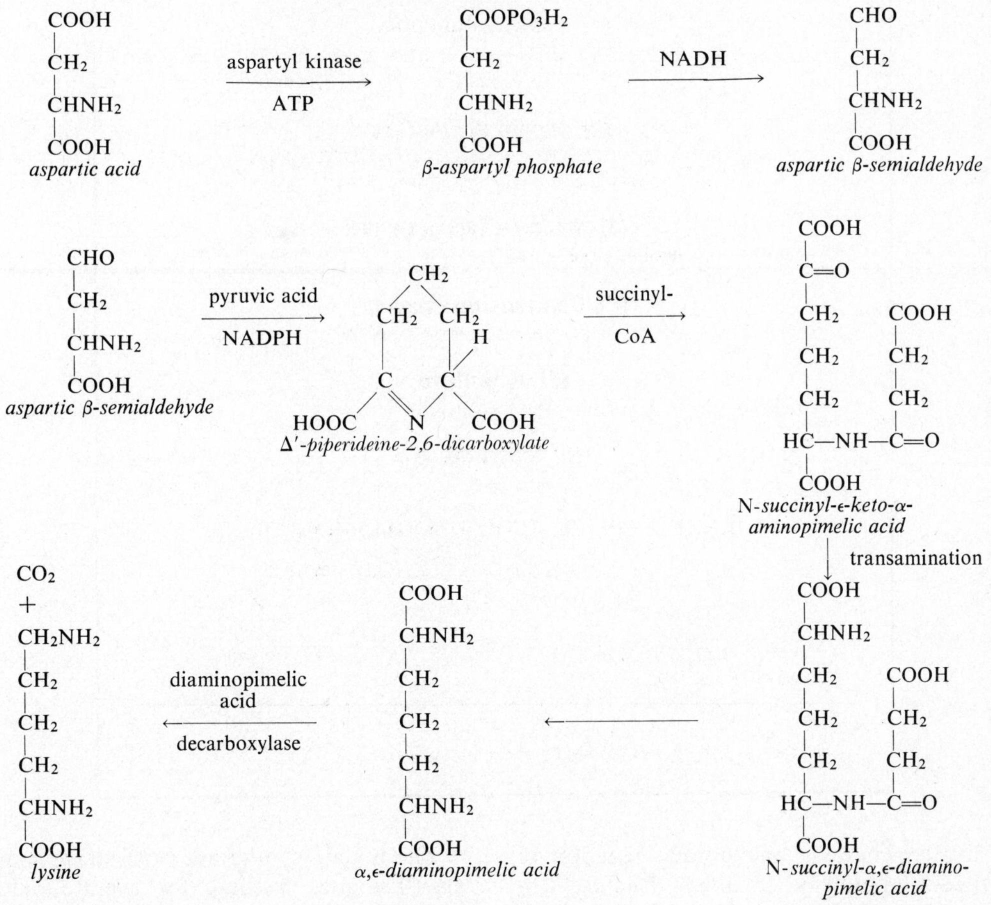

COOH
|
CH$_2$
|
CHNH$_2$
|
COOH
aspartic acid

→ aspartyl kinase / ATP →

COOPO$_3$H$_2$
|
CH$_2$
|
CHNH$_2$
|
COOH
β-aspartyl phosphate

→ NADH →

CHO
|
CH$_2$
|
CHNH$_2$
|
COOH
aspartic β-semialdehyde

CHO
|
CH$_2$
|
CHNH$_2$
|
COOH
aspartic β-semialdehyde

→ pyruvic acid / NADPH →

Δ'-*piperideine-2,6-dicarboxylate*

→ succinyl-CoA →

COOH
|
C=O
|
CH$_2$ COOH
| |
CH$_2$ CH$_2$
| |
CH$_2$ CH$_2$
| |
HC—NH—C=O
|
COOH
N-*succinyl-ε-keto-α-aminopimelic acid*

| transamination

COOH
|
CHNH$_2$
|
CH$_2$ COOH
| |
CH$_2$ CH$_2$
| |
CH$_2$ CH$_2$
| |
HC—NH—C=O
|
COOH
N-*succinyl-α,ε-diamino-pimelic acid*

CO$_2$
+
CH$_2$NH$_2$
|
CH$_2$
|
CH$_2$
|
CH$_2$
|
CHNH$_2$
|
COOH
lysine

← diaminopimelic acid decarboxylase ←

COOH
|
CHNH$_2$
|
CH$_2$
|
CH$_2$
|
CH$_2$
|
CHNH$_2$
|
COOH
α,ε-diaminopimelic acid

←

---

molecules: UTP and ATP for nucleic acids, and the L-amino acids and glutamine for proteins. These compounds are also used for other biosynthetic reactions. Diaminopimelic acid is used for peptidoglycan formation and as a precursor of lysine. The D-amino acids are found mainly in peptidoglycan but also in a few other cell surface polymers of bacteria. The pathways for synthesis of orotidine-5-phosphate and inosinic acid are fundamental pathways used for synthesis of all pyrimidines and purines.

Synthesis from Acetate[10]

Escherichia coli can grow aerobically on acetate as a sole carbon and energy source and, therefore, make peptidoglycan from acetate. Acetate carbon has to enter the pathways just reviewed. The key to the entry of acetate

is the series of reactions shown in **4–43**. A net synthesis of a 4-carbon compound, succinate, from two 2-carbon acetate units provides a starting point for forming pyruvate:

succinate → fumarate + 2 [H]

fumarate + H$_2$O → malate

malate → oxaloacetate + 2 [H]

oxaloacetate → pyruvate + CO$_2$

Pyruvate is then phosphorylated to phosphoenolpyruvate:

CH$_3$COCO$_2$H + ATP →

$$CH_2=\overset{O \sim P}{\underset{}{C}}-CO_2H + AMP + P \sim P$$

Reversal of the EMP scheme (see **4–4**) is used to form hexose phosphates from phosphoen-

---

4–43.

Synthesis of Succinate via Malate Synthetase and Isocitratase

(1) Acetate Activation

$$2 \text{ acetate} + 2 \text{ ATP} + 2 \text{ CoASH} \longrightarrow 2 \text{ acetyl-CoA} + 2 \text{ AMP} + 2 \text{ P} \sim \text{P}$$
adenylic acid

(2) Malate Synthetase

$$CH_3COSCoA + HO_2CCHO \longrightarrow HO_2CCH_2CHOHCO_2H + CoASH$$
glyoxylic acid   *malic acid*

(3) Malic Dehydrogenase

$$\text{malate} \longrightarrow \text{oxaloacetate} + 2 \text{ [H]}$$

(4) Condensing Enzyme

$$\text{acetyl-CoA} + \text{oxaloacetate} \longrightarrow \text{citrate} + \text{CoASH}$$

(5) Aconitase

$$\text{citrate} \longrightarrow \textit{cis}\text{-aconitate} \longrightarrow \text{isocitrate}$$

(6) Isocitratase

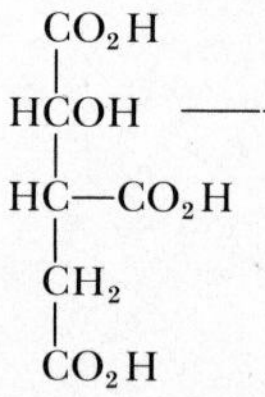

$$\begin{matrix} CO_2H \\ | \\ HCOH \\ | \\ HC-CO_2H \\ | \\ CH_2 \\ | \\ CO_2H \end{matrix} \longrightarrow HO_2CCHO + HOOCCH_2CH_2CO_2H$$

isocitrate   *glyoxylate*   *succinate*

Sum:

$$2 \text{ acetate} + 2 \text{ ATP} + 2 \text{ CoASH} \longrightarrow \text{succinate} + 2 \text{ AMP} + 2 \text{ P} \sim \text{P} + 2 \text{ [H]}$$

---

olpyruvate. There is one unique reaction in the reversal pathway, involving fructose-1,6-bisphosphate phosphatase:

$$\text{F-1,6-P} \rightarrow \text{F-6-P} + \text{P}_i$$

This enzyme pulls the EMP scheme in the direction of hexose-phosphate synthesis because the dephosphorylation is irreversible. This is an important metabolic control point along with phosphofructokinase (F-6-P + ATP → F-1,6-P + ADP). When *E. coli* is using a carbohydrate as an energy source, it has to have some mechanism for accenting the activity of phosphofructokinase relative to F-1,6-bisphosphate phosphatase, The reverse is true when it grows on acetate. We will not discuss the details of the regulation mechanism, but it is important to recognize that the EMP scheme has to be modified with F-1,6-bisphosphate phosphatase to allow hexose synthesis, and a regulation mechanism has to be introduced to permit the use of the EMP enzymes for either synthesis or breakdown of carbohydrates.

The malate synthetase-isocitratase sequence also provides a route for acetate oxidation when *E. coli* is grown on acetate. Although the TCA cycle could conceivably be used, the TCA cycle demands a continuous replenishment of oxaloacetate. This is because the TCA cycle is a so-called amphibolic pathway, *i.e.*, its functions are to provide both energy (catabolic) and precursors for synthesis of cell material (anabolic). The anabolic routes drain carbon from the TCA cycle, preventing the regeneration of the catalytic amounts of oxaloacetate necessary for the catabolic function. When carbohydrate is the energy source, carboxylation of pyruvate to oxaloacetate replenishes oxaloacetate. When acetate is the energy source, however, an alternative replenishment route is necessary because no continuous source of pyruvate from carbohydrate is available. The malate synthetase-isocitratase pathway provides a replenishment route for oxaloacetate. Replenishment reactions are called anaplerotic reactions. The operation of the reactions of acetate oxidation by acetate-grown *E. coli*, the glyoxylate cycle, is shown in **4–44**.

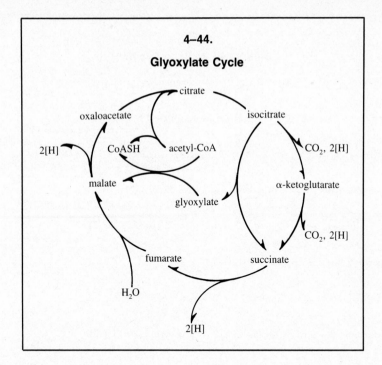

4–44.

Glyoxylate Cycle

Synthesis from CO_2

The synthesis of hexose phosphate, pyruvate, and TCA cycle intermediates from acetate by the malate synthetase-isocitratase sequence provides entry into those general paths for synthesis of peptidoglycan components already discussed. We will now examine a different entry sequence, that used by all autotrophic organisms. These include all the green plants as well as the autotrophic bacteria. The question here is how organisms using CO_2 as the sole source of cell carbon feed CO_2 into the major biosynthetic pathways. The answer is the reductive pentose cycle, which permits the synthesis of fructose-6-phosphate from CO_2. The reactions of the cycle are shown in **4–45**.

It is a pentose cycle because the key reaction used to fix CO_2 into an organic compound is the carboxydismutase reaction, in which ribulose-1,5-diP and CO_2 are converted to 2 moles of 3-P-glyceric acid (see **4–46**). In order for CO_2 fixation to continue, the sequence must operate to regenerate the CO_2 acceptor, ribulose-1,5-diP. Reducing power (NADPH) and ATP for reductive biosynthesis come from metabolism of the chemical energy source of chemolithotrophs and from light and the exogenous electron donors used by phototrophs. Most of the reactions of the cycle are similar or identical to reactions already discussed in connection with the catabolism of glucose via the transketolase-transaldolase pathway (see

4–11) and the synthesis of carbohydrate from acetate. The phosphorylation of ribulose-5-P to ribulose-1,5-diP (see **4–46**) is similar to the phosphofructokinase reaction of the EMP pathway (see **4–4**), and the fructose-1,6-diP and sedoheptulose-1,7-diP phosphatases are similar to the fructose-1,6-diP phosphatase we discussed in connection with hexose-P synthesis from acetate. These three reactions are irreversible and pull the sequence in the direction of synthesis. Synthesis of sedoheptulose-1,7-diP from erythrose-4-P and dihydroxyacetone-P (see **4–46**) is completely analogous to the formation of fructose-1,6-diP from glyceraldehyde-3-P and dihydroxyacetone-P, and the reaction is catalyzed by aldolase (see **4–4**).

Once net synthesis of fructose-6-P occurs, conventional heterotrophic reactions are used to get to the entry points for synthesis of the low-molecular-weight precursors of peptidoglycan. From the fructose-6-P on, the autotroph is essentially like *E. coli*.*

This review of peptidoglycan synthesis from three different carbon sources, carbohydrate, acetate, or CO_2, does not cover all possible entry points from all carbon sources. Discussion of the synthesis of peptidoglycan precur-

---

*This is not meant to imply that the peptidoglycan of autotrophs is identical to that of *E. coli*. The variations in peptidoglycan structure previously discussed would be found among various autotrophic bacteria.

4–45.

Reductive Pentose Cycle

6 ribulose-1,5-diP + 6 CO_2 + 6 H_2O → 6[intermediate] → 12 glycerate-3-P

carboxydismutase

12 glycerate-3-P + 12 ATP ⇌ 12 glycerate-1,3-diP + 12 ADP

phosphoglycerate kinase

12 glycerate-1,3-diP + 12 NADPH ⇌ 12 glyceraldehyde-3-P + 12 $NADP^+$ + 12 P_i

D-*glyceraldehyde phosphate dehydrogenase*

5 glyceraldehyde-3-P ⇌ 5 dihydroxyacetone-P

triosephosphate isomerase

3 glyceraldehyde-3-P + 3 dihydroxyacetone-P ⇌ 3 fructose-1,6-diP

aldolase

3 fructose-1,6-diP + 3 H_2O → 3 fructose-6-P + 3 P_i

phosphatase

2 fructose-6-P + 2 glyceraldehyde-3-P ⇌ 2 erythrose-4-P + 2 xylulose-5-P

transketolase

2 erythrose-4-P + 2 dihydroxyacetone-P ⇌ 2 sedoheptulose-1,7-diP

aldolase

2 sedoheptulose-1,7-diP + 2 H_2O → 2 sedoheptulose-7-P + 2 P_i

phosphatase

2 sedoheptulose-7-P + 2 glyceraldehyde-3-P ⇌ 2 ribose-5-P + 2 xylulose-5-P

transketolase

2 ribose-5-P ⇌ 2 ribulose-5-P

phosphopentose isomerase

4 xylulose-5-P ⇌ 4 ribulose-5-P

phosphoketopentose epimerase

6 ribulose-5-P + 6 ATP → 6 ribulose-1,5-diP + 6 ADP

phosphopentokinase

Sums:
6 ribulose-1,5-diP + 6 CO_2 + 18 ATP + 12 NADPH →
6 ribulose-1,5-diP + fructose-6-P + 18 ADP+ 17 P_i + 12 NADP + (H_2O not shown)

sors obviously excludes a discussion of the synthesis of all of the small molecular weight precursors of cell macromolecules, but illustrates the general features of the biosynthesis of small molecules. In addition to differences in pathways used to enter common biosynthetic schemes, it is clear that biosynthesis requires the ATP and reducing power made available through energy metabolism. Details about the synthesis of most other small molecules can be found in a comprehensive biochemistry text.[3, 30]

Coenzymes
Although the role of coenzymes in biosynthesis has not been stressed, they are just as important in biosynthesis as they are in catabolic pathways. Folic acid coenzymes are important in purine synthesis as well as degradation, and thiamin pyrophosphate is as important in a transketolase working to synthesize carbohydrate as it is in a transketolase of a catabolic pathway.

One coenzyme not considered before, pyridoxal phosphate, will now be discussed in connection with three reactions of peptidoglycan synthesis, transaminase, amino acid racemase, and glycine formation from serine. Pyridoxal phosphate (see **4–47**), which is related to the vitamin pyridoxal, has a major role in amino acid metabolism. Its magic is in the formation of a Schiff base (see **4–47**) with

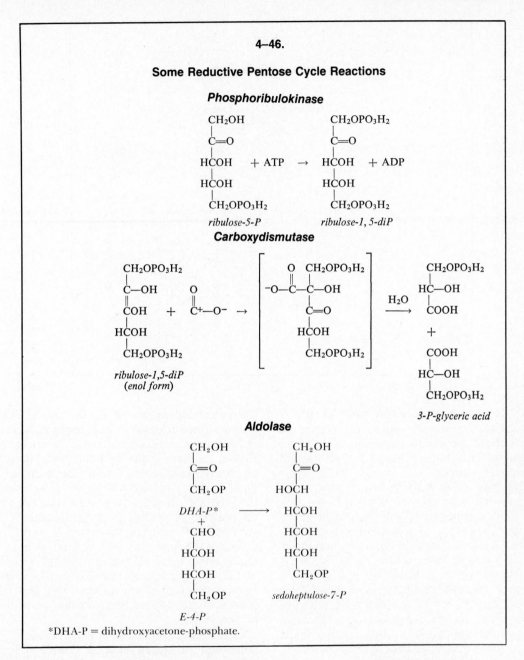

4–46.

Some Reductive Pentose Cycle Reactions

DHA-P = dihydroxyacetone-phosphate.

amino acids in the presence of a metal ion. Depending on the specific enzyme to which it is bound, this Schiff base can undergo a variety of reactions, such as transamination, racemization, and glycine formation. Many bacteria have specific amino acid decarboxylases that decarboxylate amino acids to CO_2 and amines:

$$RCHNH_2CO_2H \rightarrow RCH_2NH_2 + CO_2$$

These are, generally, pyridoxal phosphate enzymes. Their function is still somewhat obscure, although their suggested role is that of pH controllers, since their action will tend to raise the pH of the environment.

SYNTHESIS OF MACROMOLECULES

DNA Synthesis[9, 34]

All bacteria contain the two classes of nucleic acids, deoxyribonucleic acid (DNA) and ribonucleic acid (RNA). DNA serves as a template for replication of itself and for the synthesis of RNA. One type of RNA, called messenger RNA (mRNA) serves as the template for translation of the genetic information into the specific amino acid sequences of enzymes and structural proteins. DNA is also a template for the synthesis of transfer RNA

4–47.

Pyridoxal Phosphate

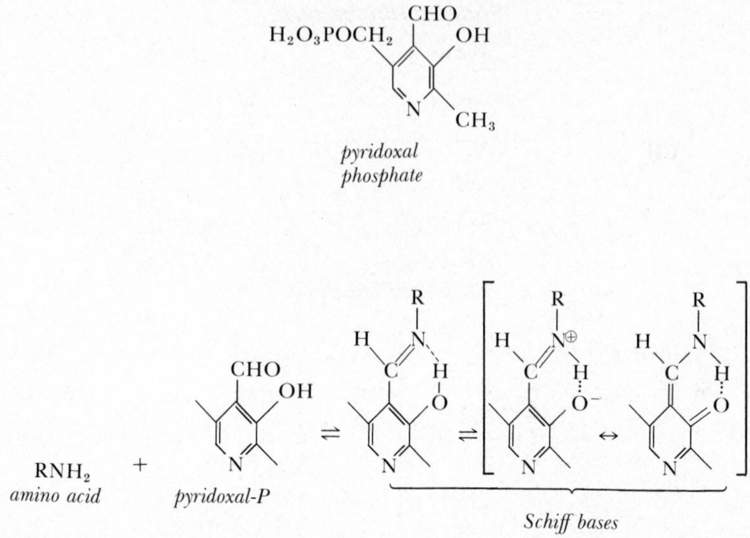

pyridoxal phosphate

RNH_2 + *pyridoxal-P* ⇌ ... ⇌ [... ↔ ...]

amino acid

Schiff bases

(tRNA) and ribosomal RNA (rRNA). tRNA becomes charged with amino acids prior to assembly of the amino acids into proteins on ribosomes, which are composed of rRNA and ribosomal proteins.

Bacterial DNA contains two strands of polydeoxyribonucleoside monophosphates that are held together by specific hydrogen bonds between opposing complementary bases: adenine (A) always with thymine (T), and guanine (G) always with cytosine (C) (Fig. 4–1). The bases within a strand are joined to one another through phosphodiester bonds between the 3′ and 5′ positions of adjacent deoxyribose moieties of nucleotides. The two strands run antiparallel to one another. That is, the sugar-phosphate backbone of one strand is oriented in the 5′ to 3′ direction, and the complementary strand is oriented in the 3′ to 5′ direction. The two strands of the DNA molecule are twisted about one another to form a right-handed, double helical structure (Fig. 4–2). The sugar-phosphate backbones of the two strands are on the outside and the hydrogen bonded base pairs are stacked perpendicular to the helical axis on the inside of the molecule.

The precursors of DNA are deoxyribonucleoside triphosphates (dNTP). With the exception of thymine, the deoxyribonucleoside phosphates are synthesized from the ribonucleoside diphosphates of A, G, and C. The enzyme ribonucleoside diphosphate reductase catalyzes the reduction of the 2′ hydroxyl of ribose, resulting in the formation of 2′ deoxyribose as the sugar moiety of the nucleoside diphosphate. The deoxyribonucleotide of uridine (dUMP) is reductively methylated at the C5 position of uridine to form thymine. The enzyme that catalyzes the reaction is thymidylate synthetase and the methyl donor is methylene-THFA. There are various specific and nonspecific kinases that participate in the interconversions of the mono-, di-, and triphosphate derivatives of deoxyribo- and ribonucleotides.

In probably all bacteria, the chromosome is composed of closed circular double helical DNA. The stages of DNA replication are

1. Recognition of a replicating origin.
2. Unwinding of short segments of the helix and strand separation to provide single stranded templates.
3. Initiation of synthesis of new complementary strands.
4. Elongation of the strands.
5. Termination of elongation.

Both strands serve as templates for synthesis of separate, new DNA strands. Because of the specificity of hydrogen bonding between A and T and G and C, the nucleotide sequence of the template strand dictates the order of ad-

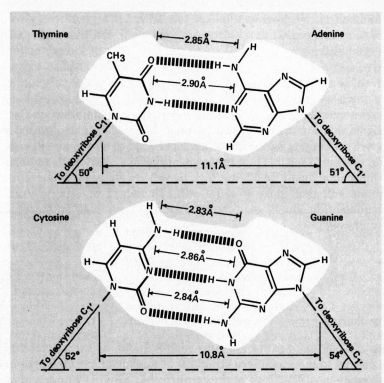

Figure 4–1. Hydrogen-bonded base pairs. Interatomic distances and angles are nearly the same for AT and GC pairs. (A. Kornberg, DNA Replication. W. H. Freeman and Co., San Francisco, 1980. Copyright 1980 by W. H. Freeman and Company. All rights reserved.)

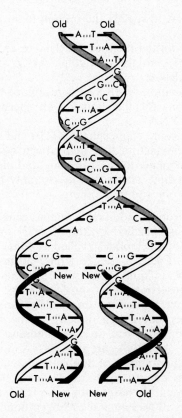

Figure 4–2. The replication of DNA. (J. D. Watson, Molecular Biology of the Gene, 3rd ed. W. A. Benjamin, Inc., Menlo Park, Calif., 1976.)

$$5' \quad \overset{A}{\underset{\diagdown}{P}} \quad \overset{G}{\underset{\diagdown}{P}} \quad \overset{C}{\underset{\diagdown}{P}} \quad \overset{}{\underset{3'}{OH}} + P{\sim}P{\sim}P \overset{T}{\underset{3'}{OH}} \rightarrow 5' \quad \overset{A}{\underset{\diagdown}{P}} \quad \overset{G}{\underset{\diagdown}{P}} \quad \overset{C}{\underset{\diagdown}{P}} \quad \overset{T}{\underset{\diagdown}{P}} \quad \overset{}{\underset{3'}{OH}} + PP_i$$

dition of dNTP to the new strands. The direction of synthesis of the new strand is always from the 5′ to 3′ direction of the sugar-phosphate backbone of the growing strand. After hydrogen bonding of the incoming dNTP to its complementary base in the template strand, DNA polymerase catalyses the formation of the phosphodiester bonds between adjacent deoxyribonucleotides in the new strand (see above). DNA synthesis is discontinuous. Small segments of about 1000 bases are polymerized and then joined to a previously synthesized segment by a ligating enzyme. The result of replication is two chromosomes, each containing one old (template) and one new complementary DNA strand. Genetic information is organized on chromosomes as genes. Genes consist of discrete segments of nucleotides that have recognition and termination regions that delineate the portion of the gene to be used as a template for RNA synthesis. If the gene codes for a protein, specific sequences of triplet nucleotides ultimately specify the order of amino acids in the polypeptide product.

RNA Synthesis[34]

RNAs are composed of single polyribonucleotides containing A, uracil (U), G, and C. All RNA is synthesized on DNA templates and only one strand of the chromosomal gene serves as a template. The monomeric precursors of RNA are ATP, UTP, GTP, and CTP. The precursors form hydrogen bonds with the bases in the template: A with T, U with A, G with C, and C with G. Thus, the sequence of the RNA strand is complementary to the DNA template. Synthesis of the RNA strand proceeds in the 5′ to 3′ direction of the elongating sugar phosphate backbone. The formation of the phosphodiester bonds between the 3′ and 5′ positions of the ribosyl moieties of adjacent nucleotides is catalyzed by RNA polymerase. It is a noncovalently bound aggregate of different polypeptide subunits: one each of β, β′, and σ and 2 of α. The stages of RNA synthesis are (Fig. 4–3):

1. Initial binding of the σ subunit of the RNA polymerase to a recognition site on the DNA template (usually an AT-rich region), and localized unwinding and hydrogen bond disruption of the DNA strands.

2. Diffusion of the polymerase to another AT-rich region called the binding site, where it becomes more tightly bound to the template.

3. Initiation of RNA synthesis. In *E. coli*, the RNA chains start with GTP or ATP at the 5′ end of the polyribonucleotide. The σ subunit then dissociates from the RNA polymerase:DNA complex.

4. Elongation of the chain continues with localized unwinding and hydrogen bond disruption of the template and reforming of the hydrogen bonds between the two DNA strands as the polymerase continues adding ribonucleoside triphosphates to the chain.

5. Termination of chain elongation occurs when the RNA polymerase reaches a GC-rich region followed by an AT-rich region of the DNA. With some genes, termination of RNA synthesis may also involve proteins called termination factors.

Protein Synthesis[4, 34]

Protein synthesis is a complex, assembly-line process that takes place on the ribosomes of the cell. For the synthesis of proteins, the ribosomes need the following materials:

1. mRNA to specify the protein to be made.
2. tRNA
   a. N-formyl-methionyl-tRNA to recognize the initiation codon, AUG, in the mRNA.
   b. Amino-acyl-tRNA to recognize the codons for the amino acids specified by mRNA.
3. Guanosine triphosphate (GTP) and soluble protein factors that help attach necessary components to the ribosome and move intermediate stages of the assembly process from one site to another.

The order of addition of amino acids in the protein is specified by the 5′ to 3′ order of triplets of nucleotides (called **codons**) in the mRNA. Each of the 20 amino acids has at least one unique triplet sequence that codes for its insertion into a protein. Some amino acids have more than one codon. An amino acid does not attach directly to the mRNA template, but is first activated and attached to a tRNA. All tRNAs are single RNA molecules which have regions of double-stranded helical structure due to hydrogen bonding between complementary bases within the RNA strand. The overall folding and hydrogen bonding result in a cloverleaf structure of single-stranded

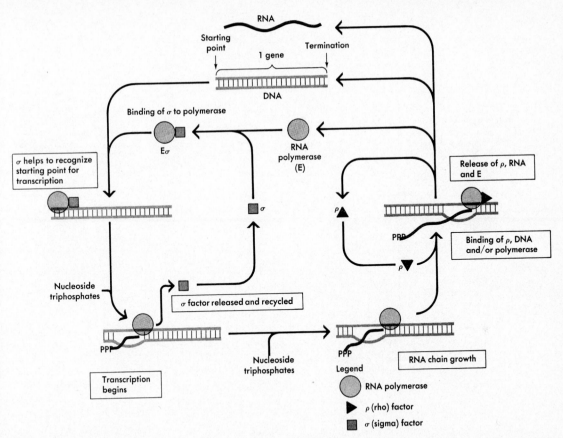

Figure 4–3. RNA synthesis. Here is illustrated a case in which chain termination requires a termination factor, called ρ factor. In many other situations, RNA polymerase by itself can read the terminating signal. (J. D. Watson, Molecular Biology of the Gene, 3rd ed. W. A. Benjamin, Inc., Menlo Park, Calif., 1976.)

loops. In all tRNAs, the 3′ terminal end of the molecule is 3′ ACC. One loop of the cloverleaf structure contains a triplet nucleotide sequence, called an **anticodon,** that is complementary to a codon for a given amino acid. Each tRNA molecule contains only one particular anticodon, and only one amino acid attaches to the specific tRNA that contains its anticodon.

There is a specific amino acyl synthetase for each amino acid that catalyzes a reaction between the carboxyl group of the amino acid and ATP:

$$AA + ATP \rightarrow AMP \sim AA + PP_i$$

The activated amino acid remains bound to the enzyme until the tRNA molecule specific for that amino acid binds to the enzyme. Then the enzyme catalyzes the transfer of the amino acid to the 3′ terminal adenine of the tRNA:

$$AMP \sim AA + tRNA \rightarrow AA \sim tRNA + AMP$$

Although there may be more than one tRNA for a given amino acid, they all bind to the same specific amino acyl synthetase.

The ribosome undergoes assembly and disassembly as it participates in manufacturing a protein. There are two subunits of the bacterial ribosome: a 30 S and 50 S subunit (see Chapter 2). They come together as the protein is being made from the mRNA template and fall apart as the product is finished. The individual subunits have both specific and integrated functions in protein synthesis.

Protein synthesis on ribosomes can be divided into stages (Fig. 4–4):

1. **Initiation** involves the 30 S subunit, mRNA, N-formyl-methionyl-tRNA (fmet-tRNA), GTP and proteins called **initiation factors**. After attachment of mRNA and fmet-tRNA to the 30 S subunit, the 50 S subunit binds to the 30 S subunit. The hydrolysis of GTP to GDP and Pi is required for these steps. After ribosomal assembly, the fmet-tRNA moves to a site called the **donor** or **peptidyl** site. Bacterial polypeptide synthesis starts with fmet-tRNA. Since the amino group is blocked, all polypeptide growth is from the N-terminal to the carboxy-terminal end of the polypeptide.

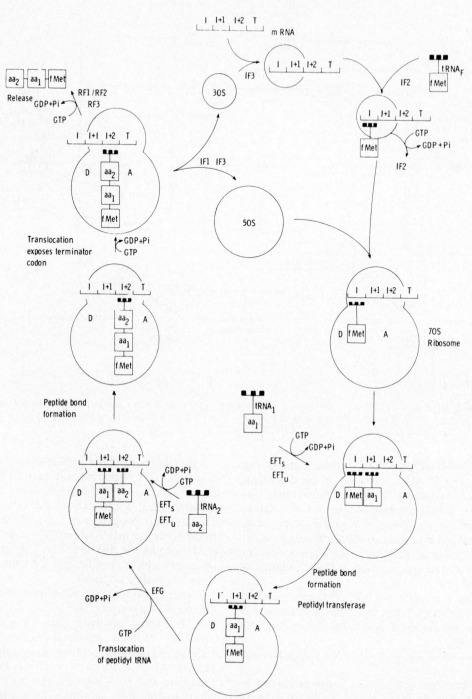

Figure 4–4. Diagrammatic scheme of major steps in polypeptide formation on a 70S ribosome. The scheme should be read clockwise starting at the top center. I, I + 1, I + 2 represent initiator and successive codons and T a terminator codon on mRNa; fMet, aa₁, and aa₂ represent N-formylmethionine and two other amino acids; and tRNA_F, tRNA₁, and tRNA₂ their specific transfer RNAs. A and D are the acceptor and donor sites. IF1, IF2, and IF3 are initiation factors; EFT_s and EFT_u are elongation factors; and RF1, RF2, and RF3 are release factors. (Modified from T. J. Franklin and G. A. Snow, Biochemistry of Antimicrobial Action, 3rd ed. Chapman and Hall, London and New York, 1981.)

2. The mRNA codon of the next AA-tRNA is exposed at a site called the **acceptor** site. The appropriate AA-tRNA attaches to the site in a step that requires the hydrolysis of GTP to GDP and Pi and proteins called **elongation factors.**

3. **Transpeptidation** is catalyzed by peptidyl transferase, a constituent of the 50 S subunit. A peptide bond is formed between the carboxyl group of the initiator fmet-tRNA at the donor site and the amino group of the AA-tRNA attached to the acceptor site.

4. **Translocation** involves the movement of the fmet-AA-tRNA (and subsequent peptidyl-tRNAs) from the acceptor to the donor site with release of the tRNA left at the donor site. Translocation requires elongation factors and the hydrolysis of GTP to GDP and Pi. Translocation frees the acceptor site for the binding of the next AA-tRNA. Peptidyl transferase then catalyzes transpeptidation between the carboxyl group of the peptidyl-tRNA on the donor site with the amino group of the AA-tRNA on the acceptor site. This frees the donor site for a repeat of the translocation reaction and sets the stage for the attachment of the next AA-tRNA to the acceptor site. Transpeptidation and translocation continue until the last amino acid is added to the polypeptide chain.

5. **Termination** involves the recognition of a termination or "nonsense" codon, UAA, UAG, or UGA, on the mRNA. Proteins called **release factors** and GTP hydrolysis cause the release of the polypeptide product and dissociation of the 70 S ribosome from the mRNA. In all bacterial proteins, the N-terminal formyl group is removed by an enzyme, and in some cases the N-terminal methionyl residue is also removed from the polypeptide.

The 30 and 50 S subunits can then participate in another round of protein synthesis. Any given mRNA usually acts as a template for the synthesis of multiple molecules of the polypeptide product. Once a 70 S ribosome has initiated protein synthesis and vacated the initiator codon, it becomes available for the formation of another 70 S ribosomal complex and initiation of synthesis of another polypeptide product. An mRNA containing multiple 70 S ribosomal units is called a **polysome.**

Lipid Synthesis[21, 32]

Although the path of lipid synthesis is essentially the same in bacteria and higher organisms, we will discuss lipids briefly for two reasons. The first is that the details of the pathway of fatty acid synthesis are clearer for bacterial synthesis. In bacteria the enzymes are in a soluble state, whereas in higher organisms the reactions leading to formation of long-chain fatty acids are associated with high-molecular-weight, multicomponent complexes. It has been difficult to unravel the details of synthesis with the complex fatty acid synthetases.

The second reason is related to the fact that almost all bacterial lipids are structural components of cell membranes and in some cases, part of the cell wall structure. An important area of contemporary biology is the unraveling of the structure-function relationships of membranes and cell surfaces and the elucidation of how the synthesis of surface components is integrated with the synthesis of all other cell components. The latter question is fundamental to complete understanding of cell growth and cell division, and the former question is concerned with such important processes as transport of nutrients into cells, electron transport, oxidative- and photophosphorylation, synthesis of surface structures, and excretion of extracellular products (including proteins). Aside from the implications of such studies of bacterial systems for microbiology, bacteria are proving to be as useful a tool for elucidating general biochemical principles about membranes as they have been in elucidating principles of intermediary metabolism and genetics.

The monomeric precursors of the long-chain fatty acids of lipids are acetyl-CoA and malonyl-CoA. Malonyl-CoA is formed from CO_2 and acetyl-CoA in a biotin-requiring reaction (see **4–48**). The polymerization of acyl units and the reduction and desaturation reactions of fatty acid synthesis all take place on a carrier protein containing a portion of the CoA molecule, 4′-phosphopantetheine (see **4–15**), which is covalently linked to the protein as a prosthetic group. The carrier protein is called **acyl carrier protein** (ACP). Malonyl-ACP loses a carboxyl group as it participates in the addition of an acetyl unit to a previously formed acyl-ACP unit. The process continues until the long-chain saturated acyl-CoA derivatives are synthesized (see **4–48**, which shows butyryl-CoA synthesis as an example, but C_{14} to C_{18} fatty acids are the common ones in bacterial lipids). These are then used for phospholipid synthesis (see **4–49** for the synthesis of two common phospholipids, phosphatidylserine and phosphatidylethanolamine). Almost all bacterial lipids are in the form of membrane

---

4–48.

Fatty Acid Synthesis

$$CO_2 + ATP + E\text{-biotin} \xrightleftharpoons[]{Mn^{++}} CO_2\text{-E-biotin} + ADP + P_i$$

$$CO_2\text{-E-biotin} + CH_3COSCoA \rightarrow E\text{-biotin} + HOOCCH_2COSCoA$$
$$\textit{malonyl-CoA}$$

---

(1) $CH_3COSCoA + ACP\text{-SH} \xrightleftharpoons[\text{transacetylase}]{\text{acetyl}} CH_3COS\text{-ACP} + CoA\text{-SH}$

(2) $HOOCCH_2COSCoA + ACP\text{-SH} \xrightleftharpoons[\text{transacylase}]{\text{malonyl}} HOOCCH_2COS\text{-ACP} + CoA\text{-SH}$

(3) $CH_3COS\text{-ACP} + HOOCCH_2COS\text{-ACP} \xrightleftharpoons[\text{synthetase}]{\beta\text{-ketoacyl-ACP}} CH_3COCH_2COS\text{-ACP} + ACP\text{-SH} + CO_2$
$$\textit{(acetoacetyl-)}$$

(4) $CH_3COCH_2COS\text{-ACP} + NADPH + H^+ \xrightleftharpoons[\text{reductase}]{\beta\text{-ketoacyl-ACP}} CH_3CHOHCH_2COS\text{-ACP} + NADP^+$
$$\textit{(β-hydroxybutyryl-)}$$

(5) $CH_3CHOHCH_2COS\text{-ACP} \xrightleftharpoons[\text{hydrase}]{\text{enoyl-ACP}} CH_3CH{=}CHCOS\text{-ACP} + H_2O$
$$\textit{(crotonyl-)}$$

(6) $CH_3CH{=}CHCOS\text{-ACP} + NADPH + H^+ \xrightarrow[\text{reductase}]{\text{enoyl-ACP}} CH_3CH_2CH_2COS\text{-ACP} + NADP^+$
$$\textit{(butyryl-)}$$

(7) $CH_3CH_2CH_2COS\text{-ACP} + CoASH \xrightarrow{\text{transacylase}} CH_3CH_2CH_2COSCoA + ACP\text{-SH}$
$$\textit{butyryl-CoA}$$

---

pnospholipids. Unsaturated fatty acid-CoA thioesters are formed from saturated acyl-CoA thioesters by oxidation and used for phospholipid synthesis. A variety of different lipids are found in the membranes of bacteria, usually several different fatty acids in several different phospholipids within a given species. Once phospholipids are formed, they are integrated with a variety of different proteins to produce the procaryotic membrane.

Synthesis of Surface Macromolecules[15, 21, 25]

Most of the unique macromolecules associated with bacterial cells are surface macromolecules, and most of them are polysaccharides or derivatives of polysaccharides. These include structures like peptidoglycan (see **4–33**), the lipopolysaccharides of gram-negative bacteria (see **4–50**), the teichoic acids of gram-positive bacteria (see **4–51**), and a large array of different polysaccharides found on cell surfaces, such as the type-specific polysaccharides of pneumococci.

Lipopolysaccharide consists of a lipid attached to a core polysaccharide which has attached to it polysaccharide chains that are the O antigen determinants of the Enterobacteriaceae.[12] The lipid, called lipid A, contains glucosamine, 3-deoxy-D-manno-octulosonic acid, fatty acids, and phosphate. The core polysaccharide contains ethanolamine, phosphate, the octulosonic acid, L-glycero-D-mannoheptose, glucose, galactose, and N-acetyl-glucosamine. The sugars of the O antigen chain vary with serological type. In the *Salmonella typhimurium* example (see **4–50**), the sugars are abequose (3,6-dideoxy-D-xylohexose), mannose, rhamnose, and galactose. The lipopolysaccharide is part of the endotoxin of these organisms.

Teichoic acids are polymers containing either ribitol or glycerol phosphates. Most of the teichoic acids have backbones of repeating units of the polyols linked to one another by phosphodiester bridges. Sugars, usually glucose or N-acetyl-glucosamine, are glycosidically linked to the polyol. D-Alanine is also

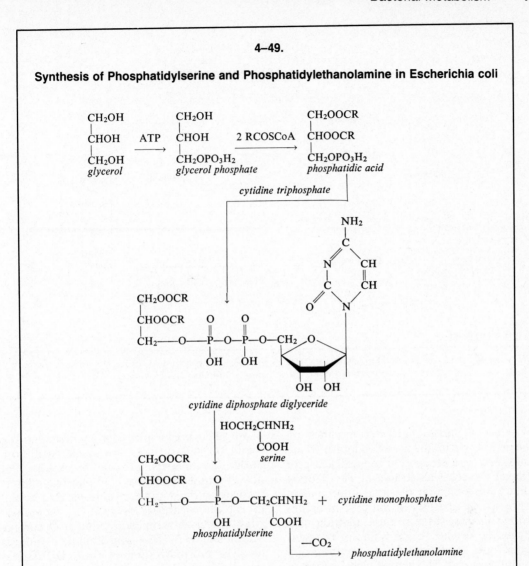

4–49.

Synthesis of Phosphatidylserine and Phosphatidylethanolamine in Escherichia coli

linked to the polyol by an ester linkage. The polymers occur either attached to cell walls (ribitol or glycerol polymers) or in intracellular association with membranes (glycerol polymers).

Except for peptidoglycan, the function of most of these substances in bacterial growth and division is unknown, even though the properties of some of these molecules as immunological determinants, as binding sites for bacteriophage, and as determinants of pathogenicity are known. The polysaccharide portions of these molecules are synthesized from nucleoside-diphosphate-sugars or their derivatives, and the enzymes of polymerization are generally found in cell membranes.

To initiate peptidoglycan synthesis, a uridine –diphosphate – muramyl – pentapeptide (see **4–52**) is synthesized by sequential addition of amino acids to muramic acid. The formation of the peptide bonds requires ATP and specific enzymes. Polymerization is initiated on the membrane through the mediation of a muramyl pentapeptide lipid intermediate. The lipid carrier in the membrane is a monophosphate of a C_{55} polyisoprenoid alcohol:

$$H_2O_3P—O—(CH_2—CH=\overset{\overset{\displaystyle CH_3}{|}}{C}—CH_2)_{11}\, H$$

After synthesis of the disaccharide unit on the lipid intermediate through interaction with

4–50.

Lipopolysaccharide of *Salmonella typhimurium*

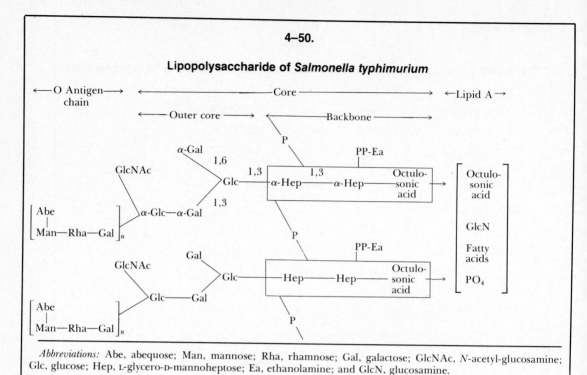

Abbreviations: Abe, abequose; Man, mannose; Rha, rhamnose; Gal, galactose; GlcNAc, *N*-acetyl-glucosamine; Glc, glucose; Hep, L-glycero-D-mannoheptose; Ea, ethanolamine; and GlcN, glucosamine.

UDP-*N*-acetyl-glucosamine and modification of the peptide chain, the modified intermediate is transferred to a preexistent cell wall acceptor to extend the cell wall structure. The peptide modifications occur on the lipid intermediate and are species-specific. In the case of *Staphylococcus aureus*, these include addition of a pentaglycine residue to the lysine of the pentapeptide and amidation of the carboxyl group of D-glutamic acid. The pentaglycine is formed by sequential addition of glycine from glycyl-tRNA. Amidation of glutamic acid leads to the formation of an isoglutamine, $HO_2C-(CH_2)_2CHNH_2CONH_2$, residue. The final reaction in *S. aureus* is the formation of cross-bridges by transpeptidation between adjacent peptidoglycan chains. The carboxyl group of D-alanine of the pentapeptide of one chain is linked to the amino group of the terminal glycine of the pentaglycine moiety of the adjacent chain. The terminal D-alanine of the pentapeptide is released in the transpeptidation reaction. The antibiotic activity of penicillin is exerted by inhibition of cell wall synthesis through inhibition of the transpeptidation reaction.

Synthesis of the lipopolysaccharides of gram-negative bacteria and teichoic acids by gram-positive bacteria also involves lipid phosphate intermediates derived from nucleoside-diphos-phate-sugar precursors. Many polysaccharides found on cell surfaces are synthesized from nucleoside-diphosphate-sugar precursors, but not all syntheses involve lipid phosphate intermediates. For example, hyaluronic acid, found in capsular material of group A hemolytic streptococci, is a repeating unit of glycuronic acid linked to *N*-acetyl-glucosamine. Synthesis involves polymerization of the UDP derivatives of both sugars without lipid phosphate intermediates. The type-specific substances of pneumococci are similarly synthesized from nucleoside-diphosphate-sugars.

There is such a large variety of distinct macromolecules that it is impossible to go into detail about them in this chapter. In addition to polysaccharides or polysaccharide derivatives, some bacteria (like *Bacillus anthracis*) have capsules composed of a polypeptide of D-glutamic acid. Special proteins, such as the M type proteins of group A streptococci, are also found on cell surfaces.

The bacterial cell surface is a mosaic of compounds built around, or attached to, the peptidoglycan sac. The surface is the interface between the bacterium and its environment, the place where antigen-antibody reactions occur, and a determinant of attraction or rejection by phagocytes. Both the unique nature of peptidoglycan and its essentiality for the integ-

4–51.

Teichoic Acids

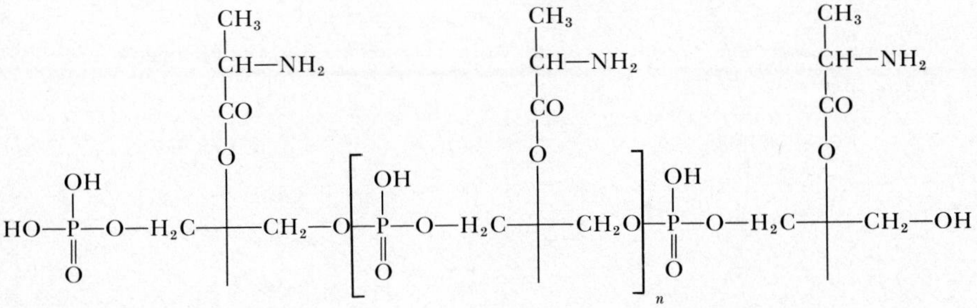

Lactobacillus casei (intracellular)

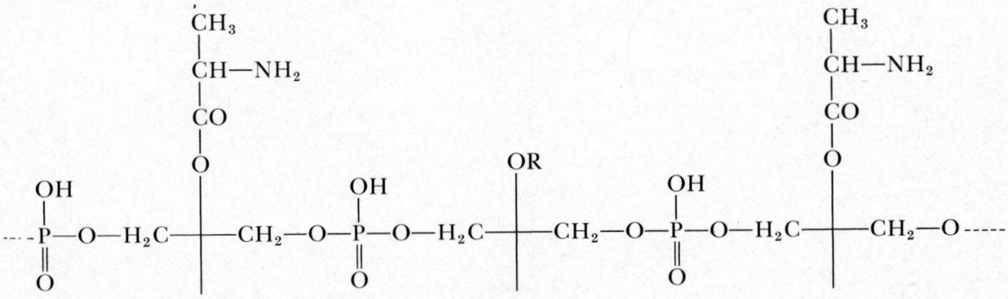

Lactobacillus plantarum (intracellular: R = α-glucosyl)

Glycerol Teichoic Acids

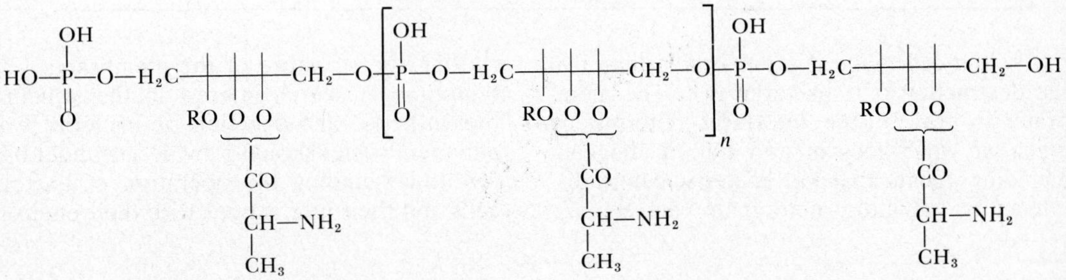

Bacillus subtilis (R = β-glucosyl; $n = 7$)
Staphylococcus aureus H (R = α- and β-N-acetylglucosaminyl; $n = 6$)

Ribitol Teichoic Acids

4–52.

Synthesis of Peptidoglycan of Staphylococcus aureus

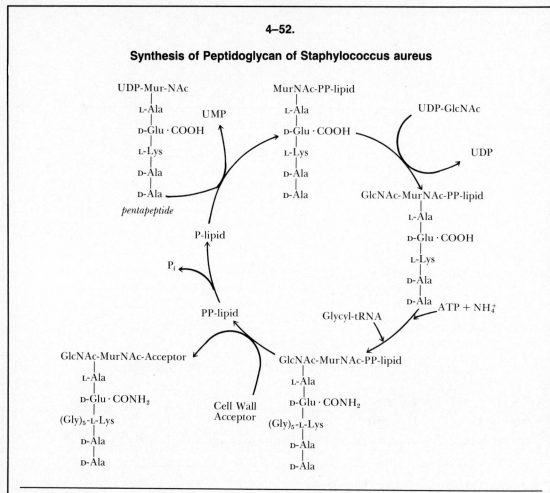

Abbreviations: MurNAc, *N*-acetyl-muramic acid; Ala, alanine; Glu·CO₂H, glutamic acid; Lys, lysine; Glu·CONH₂, isoglutamine; GlcNAc; *N*-acetyl-glucosamine; gly, glycine; and tRNA, transfer RNA.

rity of the cell make it a vulnerable target in the destruction of a bacterial cell. The membrane is part of the interface, determining much of what goes in and out of the cell, including agents that kill bacteria. Many disinfectants (alcohols, detergents) act by disrupting the structure of the membrane. Contemporary research interest in the structure, biosynthesis, and function of bacterial walls and membranes should provide a sounder basis for understanding the operation of bacterial cells and their interactions with their environs.

Nutrition of Bacteria

In order to synthesize the many components of their protoplasm and thus to grow and multiply, bacteria must be supplied with a medium containing the proper chemical constituents for supporting the necessary biosynthetic reactions. The chemical substances which must be furnished to bacteria in order that they may grow and multiply are known as their nutritional requirements. These nutritional factors are usually classified as:

1. Compounds required as energy sources.
2. Compounds required as building blocks for the synthesis of new cell material.
   a. Compounds required as carbon sources.
   b. Compounds required as nitrogen sources.
   c. Organic compounds required in their intact form as growth factors.
3. Inorganic ions required for metabolism and growth.

Given these necessary factors, bacteria will grow in the proper physicochemical environment (favorable temperature, pH, O_2 tension, etc.). Different kinds of bacteria have widely varying growth requirements, and even the same bacterium may have variable nutritional needs, depending upon the conditions of growth and the presence or absence of other substances in the medium.

Many aspects of bacterial nutrition have already been treated in terms of the metabolic functioning of the various nutritional factors. Much has also been said about the metabolic function of growth factors, so the chief object of this section will be to collect and summarize the basic information about the role of growth factors in bacterial nutrition.

GROWTH FACTORS

A growth factor may be defined as an organic compound which a bacterium needs for growth yet cannot synthesize. Since all cells have essentially the same chemical make-up, it follows that bacterium A, which does not need a growth factor required by bacterium B, lacks this requirement because it can synthesize the factor in question. Thus, *Lactobacillus casei* requires folic acid, while *E. coli* does not because it makes its own folic acid.

Growth factors are of two main types: (1) those required in minute amounts and which function catalytically as portions of enzyme systems: the B vitamins are the principal representatives of this type; and (2) those required in substantially large quantities and which are incorporated directly or with only minor modifications into cell material: the amino acids, purines, and pyrimidines are the chief examples of this kind of growth factor.

The Vitamin B Group
The B-complex vitamins, or the vitamin B group, are low-molecular-weight, water-soluble organic compounds which are constituents of almost all living cells, in which they function as coenzymes or portions of coenzymes. It is customary to designate as the vitamin the simplest compound which, when supplied to the cell, allows it to synthesize the coenzyme. Thus, pantothenic acid is a B vitamin whose coenzyme form is CoA.

Since the B vitamins function catalytically, they promote bacterial growth in very low concentrations. The B vitamins are usually supplied to bacteria in concentrations of about 10^{-6} to 10^{-10} M or 10^{-4} to 10^{-8} mg. per ml. of medium. Vitamin B_{12} and biotin are generally required in the smallest and nicotinic acid and riboflavin in the largest amounts. The table in **4–53** summarizes the metabolic functions of the B vitamins.

Thiamin. Thiamin is one of the most frequently required bacterial growth factors. It is synthesized by condensation of the thiazole portion and the pyrimidine portion of the molecule (see **4–54**). As expected from the way thiamin is synthesized, various bacteria require the thiazole alone, the pyrimidine alone, both thiazole and pyrimidine, or intact thiamin. So far, no microorganism has been found with a requirement for the whole coenzyme, TPP.

Nicotinic Acid (Niacin). Nicotinic acid and nicotinamide are the growth factors usually required by bacteria for the synthesis of NAD and NADP (see **4–12** for the

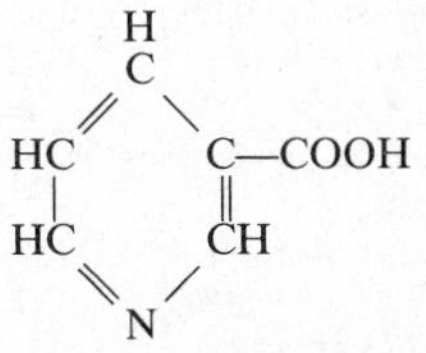

nicotinic acid 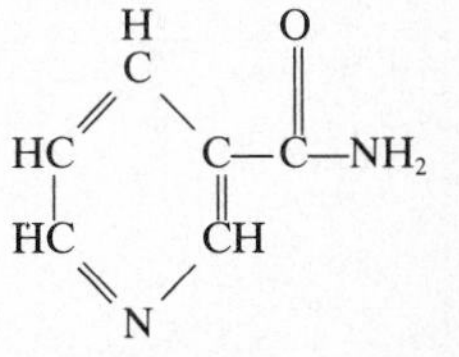   nicotinamide

structural formulas). However, many species of the genus *Haemophilus* cannot utilize nicotinic acids or its amide for the synthesis of NAD and NADP and must be supplied with the intact coenzymes or with nicotinamide riboside. The probable metabolic pathway from nicotinic acid to NAD and NADP is shown in **4–55**.

Riboflavin. Riboflavin as a growth factor resembles nicotinic acid, not in structure but in the functioning of its coenzyme in hydrogen transfer. Riboflavin has the structure shown in **4–56**. It is composed of a nitrogenous base, 6,7-dimethylisoalloxazine (flavin) and ribitol, the sugar alcohol corresponding to ribose. Its coenzyme forms are riboflavin-5-phosphate and flavin adenine dinucleotide (see **4–18** for structures). The riboflavin coenzymes are synthesized as shown in **4–56**.

Vitamin B_6. Vitamin B_6 is a collective term for several closely related factors (structural formulas in **4–57**). Of these, pyridoxal phosphate and pyridoxamine phosphate are the coenzyme forms. For higher animals, yeasts, and molds, pyridoxine, pyridoxal, and pyridoxamine are of equal activity as growth factors; but for most bacteria, either pyridoxal or pyridoxamine is required. Some, such as *L. casei*, respond only to pyridoxal, while a few

4–53.

Metabolic Functions of the Vitamin B Group

B Vitamin	Typical Organisms Requiring It	Coenzyme Form	Metabolic Functions
Thiamin	*Staphylococcus aureus* *Lactobacillus fermenti*	TPP	Activation of keto acids and keto sugars; transfer of 2-carbon units
Nicotinic acid	*Lactobacillus plantarum* *Proteus vulgaris*	NAD and NADP	Hydrogen transfer
Riboflavin	*Lactobacillus casei* *Streptococcus lactis*	Riboflavin-5-P Flavin-adenine-dinucleotide	Hydrogen transfer
Vitamin B$_6$ pyridoxal pyridoxal or pyridoxamine	*Lactobacillus casei* { *Clostridium perfringens* { *Streptococcus faecalis*	Pyridoxal-P Pyridoxamine-P	Decarboxylation, deamination, transamination, and racemization of amino acids
Pantothenic acid	*Brucella abortus* *Proteus morgani*	CoA 4'-Phosphopantetheine	Acyl activation and transfer Fatty acid synthesis
p-Aminobenzoic acid	*Clostridium acetobutylicum* *Acetobacter suboxydans*	Tetrahydrofolic acid	1-carbon-transfer
Folic acid	*Lactobacillus casei* *Clostridium tetani*	Tetrahydrofolic acid	
Biotin	*Leuconostoc mesenteroides* *Clostridium tetani* *Lactobacillus plantarum*	Biotin-CO$_2$	CO$_2$ fixation, fatty acid synthesis
Vitamin B$_{12}$	*Lactobacillus leichmannii* *Lactobacillus lactis*	5'-deoxyadenosyl-B$_{12}$	1-carbon transfer Synthesis of deoxyribosides Isomerization

4–54.

Synthesis of Thiamin

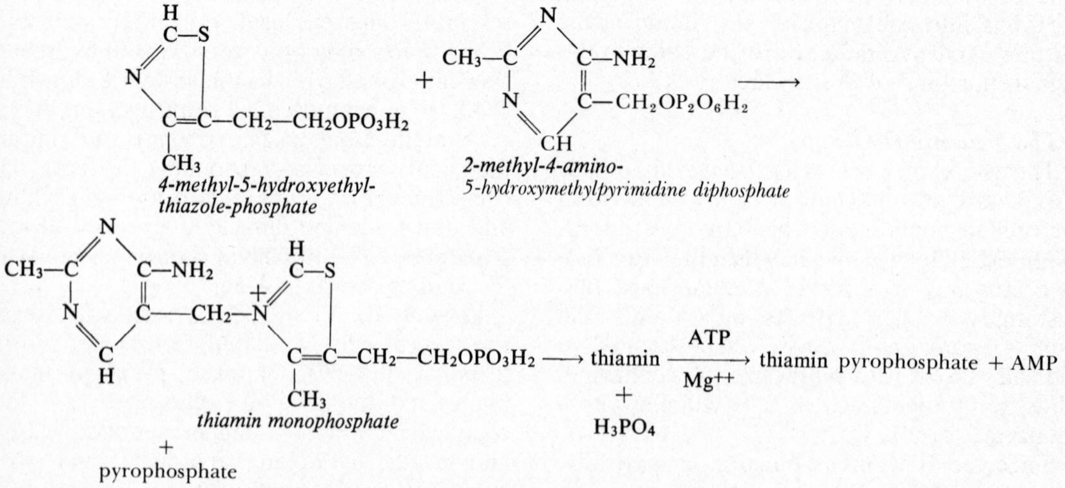

4–55.

Synthesis of NAD, NADP

(*1*) nicotinic acid + 5-P-ribosyl-1-pyrophosphate $\longrightarrow$ nicotinic acid ribonucleotide + pyrophosphate

(*2*) nicotinic acid ribonucleotide + ATP $\longrightarrow$ desamido-NAD + pyrophosphate

(*3*) desamido-NAD + NH_3 (or glutamine) + ATP $\longrightarrow$ NAD + (glutamate) + ADP + P_i

(*4*) NAD + ATP $\longrightarrow$ NADP + ADP

4–56.

Synthesis of Riboflavin-P and FAD

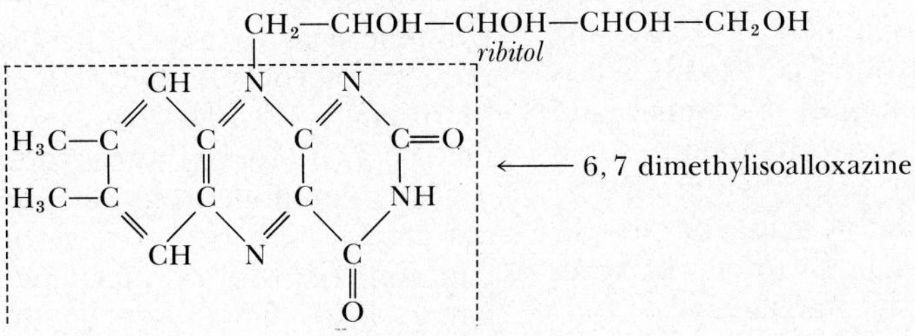

$$CH_2-CHOH-CHOH-CHOH-CH_2OH$$
ribitol

$\longleftarrow$ 6, 7 dimethylisoalloxazine

riboflavin + ATP $\rightarrow$ riboflavin-5-P + ADP
riboflavin-5-P + ATP $\rightarrow$ flavin adenine dinuclcotide + P-P

4–57.

The Vitamin B_6 Family

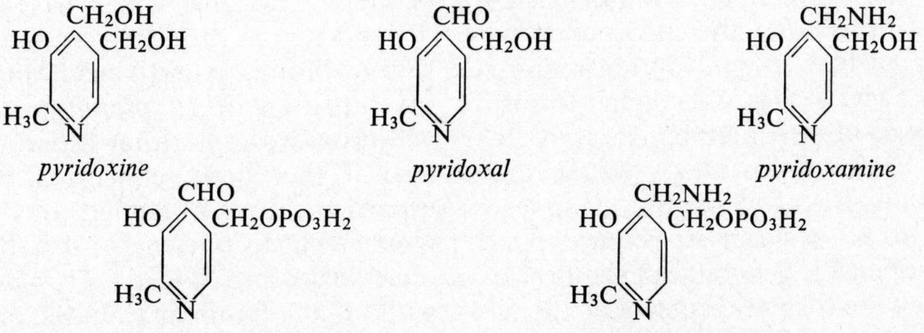

pyridoxine   *pyridoxal*   *pyridoxamine*

pyridoxal phosphate   *pyridoxamine phosphate*

4–58.

Synthesis of Pantothenic Acid

$H_2N—CH_2—CH_2—COOH$
β-alanine

+

$\quad\quad\quad\quad\quad\quad\quad\quad$ CH_3
$\quad\quad\quad\quad\quad\quad\quad\quad$ |
$\longrightarrow$ $\quad$ $CH_2OH—C—CHOH—CO—NH—CH_2—CH_2—COOH$
$\quad\quad\quad\quad\quad\quad\quad\quad$ |
$\quad\quad\quad\quad\quad\quad\quad\quad$ CH_3
$\quad\quad\quad\quad\quad\quad\quad\quad$ *pantothenic acid*

$\quad\quad\quad$ CH_3
$\quad\quad\quad$ |
$CH_2OH—C—CHOH—COOH$
$\quad\quad\quad$ |
$\quad\quad\quad$ CH_3
$\quad\quad\quad$ *pantoic acid*

+
AMP

+
pyrophosphate

+
ATP

strains of lactobacilli require either pyridoxal phosphate or pyridoxamine phosphate.

Pantothenic Acid. Pantothenic acid is required for the growth of many bacteria. Its principal function is as a part of CoA, the coenzyme of acyl transfer (see **4–15**). It is synthesized by the union of β-alanine and pantoic acid (see **4–58**). As with thiamin, some organisms require only one portion of the vitamin (β-alanine or pantoic acid) for growth, but the lactobacilli and many other bacteria can utilize only intact pantothenic acid.

One lactobacillus, *L. bulgaricus*, requires a higher form of pantothenic acid, pantetheine, 4'-Phosphopantetheine is the coenzyme of fatty acid synthetase (see **4–17**). CoA is not an absolute growth requirement for any microorganism, but it is a stimulatory factor for *Acetobacter suboxydans*.

p-Aminobenzoic Acid and the Folic Acid Group. The role of folic acid in 1-carbon transfer has already been discussed. Each member of the folic acid group contains *p*-aminobenzoic acid and a pteridine nucleus (see **4–29**).

p-Aminobenzoic acid is incorporated into folic acid, and the sulfonamides inhibit bacterial growth by preventing the incorporation. Many bacteria, such as *E. coli*, do not require *p*-aminobenzoic acid or any of its higher forms, but its importance in their metabolism is easily demonstrated by its ability to overcome the growth inhibition produced by sulfonamides. Others, such as *L. plantarum*, require preformed *p*-aminobenzoic acid but can synthesize the remainder of the folic acid coenzyme themselves. However, certain lactobacilli and clostridia also lack the ability to synthesize other portions of the folic acid molecule as well. Thus, *S. faecalis* requires a growth factor of at least the complexity of pteroic acid, in which the bond between *p*-aminobenzoic acid and the pteridine nucleus has already been formed. *L. casei* lacks, in addition, the ability to join glutamic acid to pteroic acid and, therefore, requires pteroylglutamic acid as a growth factor. Finally, *Pediococcus cerevisiae* needs folinic acid (N^5-formyl-tetrahydrofolic acid).

The *p*-aminobenzoic acid or folic acid requirement may be reduced or abolished by addition of the purines, pyrimidines, and amino acids which are synthesized in folic acid–requiring reactions. These same substances will also counteract the growth-inhibiting action of sulfonamides on organisms which require neither *p*-aminobenzoic acid nor folic acid.

Biotin. Biotin is a growth factor for many different types of microorganisms and for higher animals. In combination with a specific enzyme protein, biotin reacts with CO_2 to form an enzyme-biotin-CO_2 complex (see **4–23**, **4–48**). The biotin requirement of microorganisms, like that for the other B vitamins, is markedly affected by the presence of substances which are synthesized in biotin-dependent reactions. The best example of this dependency is furnished by the interrelationship of biotin, aspartic acid, and oleic acid in the nutrition of *L. plantarum*. The bacteria will grow without either aspartic acid or oleic acid if the biotin concentration is high. If aspartic acid is also added, the biotin requirement is cut to one-tenth; if both aspartic and oleic acids are added, *L. plantarum* grows without any biotin at all in the medium. Biotin is the coenzyme for fatty acid synthesis (oleic acid) and for the fixation of CO_2 on to pyruvate to give oxaloacetate, a precursor of aspartic acid.

Vitamin B₁₂. This vitamin is a large and complex molecule consisting of (1) a complex ring system, the corrin moiety, closely related to the porphyrins of the cytochromes, chlorophyll, and hemoglobin and synthesized by similar mechanisms; (2) an atom of trivalent cobalt bound to the porphyrin-like structure in much the same fashion as is the iron in hemoglobin; (3) a cyanide ion linked to the cobalt ion; (4) a nucleotide containing a substituted benzimidazole as the base; and (5) a molecule of an amino alcohol which is bonded to both the nucleotide phosphorus and a side chain of the corrin moiety (see **4–24**).

Although perhaps the greatest interest in vitamin B_{12} stems from its ability to combat certain human anemias, it is required by many lactobacilli, and numerous enzymatic reactions in bacteria are dependent on coenzyme forms of vitamin B_{12}. For example, the previously discussed conversion of methylmalonyl-CoA to succinyl-CoA and the reduction of ribonucleoside diphosphates to their deoxyribonucleoside counterparts require the participation of 5′-deoxyadenosyl-B_{12} in which the CN^- of vitamin B_{12} has been replaced with a 5′-deoxyadenosyl group derived from ATP.

Amino Acids

Many bacteria can synthesize all their amino acids themselves (as *E. coli*) or can synthesize all but one or two (*Salmonella typhi* requires only tryptophan). In general, the gram-negative organisms are potent amino acid synthesizers and require no preformed amino acids or only a limited number. The ability of gram-positive bacteria to synthesize amino acids is much more limited, particularly among the lactic acid bacteria. *Leuconostoc mesenteroides* requires, for example, 17 different amino acids. Amino acids are required in substantially higher concentrations than are the B vitamins, roughly about 10^{-4} M or about 0.01 mg. per ml. of medium.

Purines and Pyrimidines

Many bacteria, especially the lactobacilli, are unable to synthesize the purine and pyrimidine bases which they need as constituents of their nucleic acids, nucleotides, etc. In general, the synthetic block appears to be in the formation of the purine or pyrimidine nucleus, and the majority of nitrogen base–requiring organisms are still capable of some interconversion of the bases. Thus, *L. plantarum* can utilize adenine, guanine, hypoxanthine, or xanthine as its sole purine source. Other organisms are more exacting and respond much more to one purine than to another. The classic example of a pyrimidine requirement is that of *S. aureus* for uracil for anaerobic growth. The oxidation of dihydroorotic acid (see **4–40**) is oxygen-dependent in *S. aureus*. Uracil can be synthesized under aerobic but not anaerobic conditions.

Microbiological Assay

An important practical application of the elucidation of the growth factor requirements of bacteria has been the development of methods for quantitative determination of vitamins and amino acids in terms of the growth response of microorganisms. The high degree of specificity and sensitivity attainable in microbiological assay has made this technique an invaluable tool in many fields of biological research.

THE INORGANIC ELEMENTS

The elementary constituents of the bacterial cell other than the carbon, hydrogen, oxygen, and nitrogen present in organic compounds must also be supplied in an adequate nutritional medium. It is customary to include in bacteriological mediums phosphate, sulfate, potassium, calcium, magnesium, manganous, and ferric ions. The need for these ions in metabolism is obvious. Organic phosphate compounds play a role in almost every phase of intermediary metabolism, and, as phospholipids and nucleic acids, are a part of the structural framework of the cell. Sulfate, or some form of sulfur, is needed for synthesis of the sulfur amino acids. Potassium, calcium, magnesium, and manganous ions are cofactors or activators in many enzyme systems.

Some organisms also have more specific inorganic requirements. Thus, the diphtheria bacillus gives optimum toxin production with an iron concentration of about 0.00014 mg. per ml. of medium. Higher or lower concentrations inhibit toxin production without affecting growth. *Azotobacter* specifically requires molybdenum for nitrogen fixation.

Other inorganic ions also appear in bacterial protoplasm and, therefore, must be present in the medium. However, it is very hard to show clearly that a particular ion is absolutely required for growth. This is because the inorganic ions are universal contaminants of all types of materials, so that it is difficult to free mediums of the last traces of an ion.

REFERENCES

1. Atkinson, D. E. 1969. Regulation of enzyme function. Ann. Rev. Microbiol. **23**:47–68.
2. Barker, H. A. 1961. Fermentations of nitrogenous compounds. pp. 151–207. *In* I. C. Gunsalus and R. Y. Stanier (Eds.): The Bacteria, Vol. 2. Academic Press, New York.
3. Cohen, G. N. 1967. Biosynthesis of Small Molecules. Harper and Row, New York.
4. Franklin, T. J., and G. A. Snow. 1981. Biochemistry of Antimicrobial Action, 3rd ed. Chapman and Hall, London.
5. Haddock, B. A., and C. W. Jones. 1977. Bacterial respiration. Bacteriol. Rev. **41**:47–99.
6. Harold, F. J. 1977. Ion currents and physiological functions in microorganisms. Ann. Rev. Microbiol. **31**:181–203.
7. Kaback, H. R. 1970. Transport. Ann. Rev. Biochem. **39**:561–598.
8. Klotz, I. M. 1967. Energy Changes in Biochemical Reactions. Academic Press, New York.
9. Kornberg, A. 1980. DNA Replication. W. H. Freeman and Co., San Francisco.
10. Kornberg, H. 1965. The co-ordination of metabolic routes. pp. 8–31. *In* M. R. Pollack and M. H. Richmond (Eds.): Function and Structure in Microorganisms. Cambridge University Press, Cambridge, England.
11. Lehninger, A. L. 1971. Bioenergetics, 2nd ed. W. A. Benjamin Inc., Menlo Park, Calif.
12. Luderitz, O., A. M. Staub, and O. Westphal. 1966. Immunochemistry of O and R antigens of *Salmonella* and related *Enterobacteriaceae*. Bacteriol. Rev. **30**:192–255.
13. McBee, R. H., C. Lamanna, and O. B. Weeks. 1955. Definitions of bacterial oxygen relationships. Bacteriol. Rev. **19**:45–47.
14. Olson, J. M. 1970. The evolution of photosynthesis. Science **168**:438–446.
15. Osborne, M. J. 1969. Structure and biosynthesis of the bacterial cell wall. Ann. Rev. Biochem. **38**:501–538.
16. Payne, W. J. 1970. Energy yield and growth of heterotrophs. Ann. Rev. Microbiol. **24**:17–52.
17. Payne, W. J., and W. J. Wiebe. 1978. Growth yield and efficiency in chemosynthetic microorganisms. Ann. Rev. Microbiol. **32**:155–183.
18. Peck, H. D., Jr. 1968. Energy-coupling mechanisms in chemolithotrophic bacteria. Ann. Rev. Microbiol. **22**:489–518.
19. Pfennig. N. 1967. Photosynthetic bacteria. Ann. Rev. Microbiol. **21**:285–324.
20. Postgate, J. R. (Ed.). 1971. The Chemistry and Biochemistry of Nitrogen Fixation. Plenum Press, New York.
21. Raetz, C. R. H. 1978. Enzymology, genetics and regulation of membrane phospholipid synthesis in *Escherichia coli*. Microbiol. Rev. **42**:614–659.
22. Reed, L. J., and D. J. Cox. 1966. Macromolecular organization of enzyme systems. Ann. Rev. Biochem. **35**:57–84.
23. Roy, A. B., and P. A. Trudinger. 1970. The Biochemistry of Inorganic Compounds of Sulphur. Cambridge University Press, Cambridge, England.
24. Saier, M. H., Jr. 1977. Bacterial phosphoenolpyruvate:sugar phosphotransterase systems: structural, functional, and evolutionary relationships. Bacteriol. Rev. **41**:856–871.
25. Salton, M. R. J. 1964. The Bacterial Cell Wall. Elsevier, New York.
26. Scherp, H. W. 1971. Dental caries: prospects for prevention. Science **173**:1199–1205.
27. Schleifer, K. H., and O. Kandler. 1972. Peptidoglycan types of bacterial cell walls and their taxonomic implications. Bacteriol. Rev. **36**:407–477.
28. Sokatch, J. R. 1969. Oligosaccharide catabolism. pp. 55–66. *In* J. R. Sokatch: Bacterial Physiology and Metabolism. Academic Press, New York.
29. Strominger, J. L. 1962. Biosynthesis of bacterial cell walls. pp. 413–470. *In* I. C. Gunsalus and R. Y. Stanier (Eds.): The Bacteria, Vol. 3. Academic Press, New York.
30. Stryer, L. 1981. Biochemistry, 2nd ed. W. H. Freeman and Co., San Francisco.
31. Thauer, R. K., K. Jungermann, and K. Decker. 1977. Energy conservation in chemotrophic anaerobic bacteria. Bacteriol. Rev. **41**:100–180.
32. Volpe, J. J., and P. R. Vagelos. 1976. Mechanisms and regulation of biosynthesis of saturated fatty acids. Physiol. Rev. **56**:339–417.
33. Vogels, G. D., and C. Van Der Drift. 1976. Degradation of purines and pyrimidines by microorganisms. Bacteriol. Rev. **40**:403–468.
34. Watson, J. D. 1976. Molecular Biology of the Gene, 3rd ed. W. A. Benjamin, Inc., Menlo Park, Calif.
35. Wolfe, R. S. 1971. Microbial formation of methane. Adv. Microbiol. Physiol. **6**:107–146.
36. Wood, H. G., and R. L. Stjernholm. 1962. Assimilation of carbon dioxide by heterotrophic organisms. pp. 41–117. *In* I. C. Gunsalus and R. Y. Stanier (Eds.): The Bacteria, Vol. 3. Academic Press, New York.
37. Wood, W. A. 1961. Fermentation of carbohydrates and related compounds. pp. 59–149. *In* I. C. Gunsalus and R. Y. Stanier (Eds.): The Bacteria, Vol. 2. Academic Press, New York.

5

Physical Agents, Disinfectants, and Chemotherapeutic Agents

M. J. Wolin, Ph.D.
T. L. Miller, Ph.D.

A variety of physical and chemical agents are available for killing bacteria or at least preventing their multiplication. Killing agents are called **bactericidal agents.** When they are entirely removed from the environment, the target bacteria are obviously no longer capable of multiplication. **Bacteriostatic agents** are those that prevent multiplication of the target bacteria only when in contact with the microorganisms. Removal of a bacteriostatic agent leads to resumption of microbial growth if the bacteria are placed in a suitable environment. **Sterilization** is a bactericidal process because the object is to kill all of the bacteria in the treated substance.

Bactericidal agents irreversibly inactivate essential cell functions. For example, if all the proteins of a cell are coagulated by heat, the cell dies. Penicillin inhibits the synthesis of cell walls, and cell growth without a wall produces death because of lysis. Bacteriostatic agents exert a potentially reversible inhibition of cell functions. Sulfonamides, for example, inhibit the synthesis of folic acid and prevent tetrahydrofolic acid enzyme reactions from occurring. Cell growth and multiplication cease, but no permanent damage is done. Upon removal of the sulfonamide, the cell will start making folic acid and new cells.

The killing of cells and the prevention of

cell multiplication is important in the treatment and prevention of disease. More generally, it is a way for man to exert some influence over the microbial population of an environment. If spoilage bacteria could not be controlled by sterilization methods, the modern food processing industry would be nonexistent and outer space would be contaminated with earthly organisms carried by space vehicles. This chapter reviews some of the more important physical and chemical methods used for controlling populations by killing and preventing multiplication of cells.

Physical Agents

Temperature[4, 6]

Bacteria survive and even grow over a wide range of temperatures. At the optimum temperature, they attain their maximal growth rate. Growth rate slows below the optimum, usually not very sharply at first, but finally a sharp minimum growth temperature is achieved. Growth rate decreases rapidly above the optimum, as heat inactivation begins, until a maximum growth temperature is achieved. Above the maximum, heat denaturation cannot be compensated by biosynthesis, and death ensues.

Bacteria are categorized as psychrophiles, mesophiles, or thermophiles to indicate the temperatures at which they like to grow. **Mesophiles** like moderate temperatures. Mammal-loving mesophiles have growth optima of body temperatures, *e.g.,* 37° C. for human parasitic or commensal bacteria. Those living in nature usually have lower optima of about 25° to 30° C. **Psychrophiles** like cold temperatures. Although their optimum temperatures are not much lower than those of the outdoor mesophilic species, their minimum growth temperatures are much lower. Some psychrophiles can grow below 0° C. if water is kept from freezing by the addition of solutes, *e.g.,* sugars. **Thermophiles** are heat lovers with optimal growth temperatures of about 55° to 65° C. Most can grow at higher temperatures. Recently, a bacterium was isolated that could grow at a temperature of up to 98° C. Some thermophiles are obligate thermophiles, *i.e.,* they cannot grow in the mesophilic range. Some are facultative thermophiles and can grow from the mesophilic through the thermophilic ranges. There are no hard and fast correlations between temperature characteristics and genera, but thermophiles appear to be more common in the spore-forming genera, *Clostridium* and *Bacillus*, and psychrophiles are common in the genus *Pseudomonas.*

Cold temperatures (just above freezing) are generally bacteriostatic except for psychrophiles. The chemical reactions of life and death slow down considerably at low temperatures. There are exceptions, *e.g.,* gonococci and meningococci die out faster at refrigerator temperatures than at 37° C., but most bacteria can be stored for weeks or months in a viable, dormant state in a refrigerator.

Lethal Effects of Heat. Cooking kills bacteria. All vegetative cells are killed by moist heat, *i.e.,* water or steam, after exposure for a few minutes to a temperature somewhat higher than their maximum growth temperature. The rate of killing is both time- and temperature-dependent. The higher the temperature, the shorter the killing time. The tubercle bacillus is killed in 30 minutes at 58° C., 20 minutes at 59° C., and 2 minutes at 65° C. One can determine the thermal death time of bacteria, *i.e.,* the time it takes to kill them at a given temperature. The thermal death point can also be measured and is the temperature at which death occurs when time is held constant.

The temperature and time of practical heat killing are determined by the kinds of organisms to be killed and the effect of heating on the material the organisms are in. If absolute sterilization is required, and it is required in preparing canned foods and almost all bacteriological mediums, the most resistant microbial form dictates the time and temperature of treatment. Vegetative cells are not the prime concern in sterilization; bacterial spores dictate the rules. Some of the more heat-resistant spores survive boiling for many hours, and it is necessary to make use of higher temperatures (under steam pressure) to kill them in a reasonably short period of time. Steam autoclaves operated at 121° C. for 15 minutes do an excellent job of killing if conditions for heat transfer are good. (For example, well-spaced test tubes containing small volumes of liquid are easily sterilized at 121° C. for 13 minutes in a conventional autoclave, but it takes a longer time to sterilize 15 liters of liquid in a 20-liter jug.) In canning, the pressure build-up in the cooked cans permits the development of high, sterilizing temperatures.

Sometimes complete sterility is not required. If the objective is to get rid of all possible pathogenic bacteria on a syringe, boiling for 10 to 15 minutes is sufficient because spores of pathogenic bacteria are not as heat-resistant as those of nonpathogenic bacteria.

Sometimes it is not necessary to consider spores. Milk is pasteurized by heat to kill milkborne pathogens, including brucellae, salmonellae, streptococci, and, most notably, the tubercle bacilli. None of these are spore-formers. **Pasteurization,** or heating at 62° C. for 30 minutes or 72° C. for 15 seconds, is a method for killing the vegetative cells of milkborne pathogens. Pasteurized milk is not a sterile product, as can easily be demonstrated by leaving an unopened container at room temperature for a day or two.

In addition to time, temperature, and bacterial cell or spore, other factors influence the rate of killing by heat. High or low pH levels increase the killing rate. Acid food products like tomatoes need less heat for sterilization than neutral products like corn. Addition of sodium carbonate to water for boiling surgical instruments increases the efficiency of heat kill (and reduces rusting). A very important factor is moisture itself. Dry heat is a much poorer killing agent than moist heat for a given amount of heat input. The relative efficiency of moist and dry heat in the killing of bacteria is similar to the effect of water content on the efficiency of coagulation of egg albumin.* Dry heat is very convenient for sterilizing certain types of material, *e.g.,* glass petri dishes and pipettes. Temperatures of 160° to 170° C. must be maintained for two to three hours to effect sterilization with dry heat.

Heat kills by causing denaturation of macromolecules. Proteins coagulate, nucleic acid base-pair interactions are disrupted, and lipids melt away from their normal associations with each other and proteins of cell membranes. Protein coagulation is probably the major cause of cell death. The rate of heat coagulation of proteins in solution closely parallels the rate of destruction of bacteria by hot water.

---

*Egg albumin in aqueous solution is coagulated at 56° C.; with 25 per cent water content at 74° to 80° C.; 18 per cent water content at 80° to 90° C.; with 6 per cent water content at 145° C. Anhydrous egg albumin may be heated to 170° C. without coagulation.

Freezing.[4, 19] Freezing can be lethal for bacteria, but in general, it is bacteriostatic. Because frozen bacterial cultures remain dormant and potentially viable, freezing is a valuable and practical method of preserving bacteria. Furthermore, freezing is used to prevent bacterial growth in materials susceptible to bacterial decomposition. This is the basis of preserving food in the frozen state.

Several variables influence what happens to a cell when it is frozen. These include the cell itself, the rate of freezing, the rate of thawing, the temperature of storage in the frozen state, and the medium in which the cells are suspended. When cells are cooled below the freezing point of cytoplasm, usually above $-1°$ C., they do not freeze immediately. They become supercooled down to $-10°$ to $-15°$ C. even when ice is present externally. The vapor pressure of water is, therefore, higher internally than externally. Two processes operate to equilibrate the internal and external vapor pressures. Either water freezes inside the cell or water moves out of the cell to the external medium. The former leads to dehydration through ice crystal formation, and the latter causes dehydration through disappearance of water from the cell. Intracellular ice crystal formation predominates when cooling is rapid, whereas a slow rate of cooling minimizes ice crystal formation. In both cases, solutes concentrate and precipitate intracellularly as water is removed. The cause of cell damage during freezing is still uncertain, but it is thought that the concentration of solutes during freezing leads to membrane damage and subsequent lysis during thawing. In addition, ice crystal formation is thought to disrupt cell membranes. In general, rapid cooling is more damaging to cells than slow cooling. As seen in Figure 5–1, the situation is complicated because optimal survival occurs at an optimal cooling rate. Intracellular freezing occurs above the optimal rate and not below it. The optimum is presumably a balance point where the cells are not damaged by ice crystals and are minimally exposed to high solute concentrations due to dehydration.

Slow thawing leads to more damage to a frozen cell population than fast thawing. The ice crystals that form when cells are rapidly frozen grow larger during slow thawing and presumably lead to more physical damage. Slow thawing is also usually bad for cells frozen slowly without ice crystal formation, but the reason is not completely clear.

Low-molecular-weight, nonelectrolyte, permeable solutes, *e.g.,* glycerol, sucrose, and

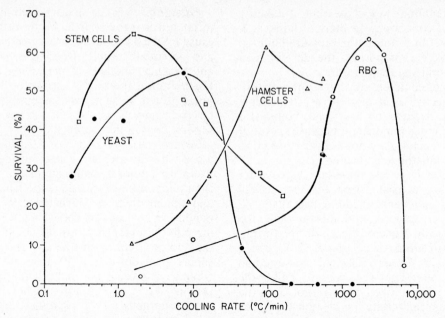

Figure 5–1. Comparative effects of cooling velocity on the survival of various cells cooled to −196° C. and thawed rapidly. The yeast and human red cells (RBC) were frozen in distilled water and blood, respectively. The marrow stem cells and hamster cells were suspended in balanced salt solutions containing 1.25 M glycerol. (Modified from Mazur *et al.* in G. E. Wolstenholme and M. O'Connor, The Frozen Cell, 1970, courtesy of J. & A. Churchill, London.)

dimethyl sulfoxide, protect cells against damage by freezing. They are probably able to do this by displacing intracellular electrolytes from the aqueous phase during cooling, and thereby preventing exposure of the cell to high concentrations of electrolytes. High-molecular-weight, impermeable substances, *e.g.,* serum albumin, dextran, and polyvinylpyrrolidone, also protect against freezing damage. The mechanism of such protection is not clear.

Preservation in the frozen state requires low-temperature storage. The lower the temperature, the better the preservation. Solid CO_2 (−78° C.) or liquid N_2 (−180° C.) refrigeration is generally used for storage. If any liquid water is left in the frozen cell, degenerative biochemical reactions will occur down to about −130° C. Low-temperature storage prevents or slows down these degenerative reactions. **Freeze-drying (lyophilization),** *i.e.,* drying in a vacuum from the frozen state, completely removes water from cells and is an excellent method for cell preservation.

Cryobiology, which is the study of the effects of freezing on biological materials, is a relatively new field of study. Cell destruction and preservation studies are only one aspect of cryobiology, but the practical use of freezing to preserve cells, tissues, and organs has been an important stimulus for research on the effects of freezing.

Drying

In contrast to freeze-drying, drying in air is lethal to vegetative cells of many bacteria. Perhaps the destructive action of high-solute concentrations produced by dehydration is accelerated when cells are dried at normal air temperatures. Bacteria differ in their sensitivity to drying. The tubercle bacillus is resistant and the cholera vibrio is very sensitive. Spores are highly resistant. Sensitivity to drying of pathogens of the upper respiratory tract is of particular interest. Respiratory infections are commonly transmitted by airborne droplets. The length of time a droplet remains infectious is a function of the resistance of the infectious agent to drying. Maximal death of microorganisms in droplets in air occurs at 50 per cent relative humidity. At lower humidities, rapid desiccation renders the organism resistant to concentrated solutes, and higher humidities retard the concentration of intracellular solutes.

Physical Disintegration of Cells

Because of their small size and the strength of the rigid cell wall, bacteria are relatively difficult to break up by physical methods. These methods are important, however, for obtaining subcellular fractions for biochemical studies and preparation of antigens, but they are not useful as sterilization procedures.

High-frequency ultrasonic waves, grinding with micrometer-sized abrasives such as glass beads, and rapid pressure changes of 500 to 600 atmospheres are methods commonly used to break open bacterial cells physically.

Filtration

Sterilization by filtration is becoming increasingly important as new filter materials are developed that permit rapid filtration of contaminated gases and liquids. Glass, porcelain, and asbestos fiber filters that can sterilize liquids are available, but advances in technology have made membrane filters the major filtration medium for sterilization. Membrane filters are usually made of cellulose nitrate and cellulose acetate. They are available with different pore sizes, to permit selective filtration of different particle sizes, and can be obtained in sheet and cartridge configurations. The latter are particularly suitable for sterilization of large volumes of materials. Some commercial beverages, e.g., cider and beer, are now being sterilized by filtration, as are heat-labile pharmaceutical solutions.

Radiation[5, 8, 27]

Sunlight has long been known to be bactericidal. Ultraviolet (UV) radiation is the major bactericidal agent supplied by the sun. Aromatic amino acids of proteins and the purine and pyrimidine bases of nucleic acids absorb UV radiation. Pyrimidine bases, in particular the thymine of DNA, are the main target compounds involved in the bactericidal action of UV radiation. The energy absorbed by thymine causes it to undergo a photochemical reaction with adjacent thymine molecules in the same DNA strand. DNA replication is blocked because the formation of thymine dimers prevents the base pairing required in replication of DNA daughter strands.

Some repair of the thymine dimer lesion can be effected by repair enzymes present in bacterial cells. DNA recombination events also take place that lead to nonlethal mutants. Most recombinations, however, lead to the formation of lethal mutations. Whether death occurs or not depends upon the balance between the amount of damage and the efficiency of the repair mechanisms in a given cell. As dosage increases, cytosine-thymine and cytosine-cytosine dimers can be formed to add to the lethality of UV radiation.

The lowest wavelength of UV light reaching the earth's surface from the sun is 290 nm. High-intensity UV light can be generated by low-pressure mercury vapor lamps. Their major emission is at 253.7 nm., which is close to the absorption maximum of DNA. These "germicidal" lamps are used for experimental studies of UV radiation on mutation and death. They are also of practical use for sterilization, mainly in decreasing airborne infection, and especially in hospital wards and animal rooms where close contact between individuals can be minimized. Since many materials including ordinary glass strongly absorb UV light, it is necessary for the bacteria to be exposed directly to UV radiation for the treatment to be effective.

The visible light of sunlight can also cause cell death by unknown photochemical processes.[11] Carotenoid pigments produced by some bacteria protect against visible light damage. However, it is usually not a good idea to expose bacterial cultures to light for long periods if they are to be preserved.

Ionizing Radiation. Ionizing radiations give cells a more powerful blast of energy per quantum of radiation than the radiation of UV or visible light. Ionizing radiations include α-rays (nuclei of helium atoms), β-rays (fast-moving electrons), γ-rays, and x-rays. The latter two are the most common sources used in studies of the effects of ionizing radiation on bacteria. Ionizing radiation has not achieved distinction as a sterilizing tool. It has been used to sterilize some materials, e.g., foods, but the amount of radiation needed to kill bacteria is often sufficient to damage the product, e.g., odors and off flavors develop in foods.

The killing effect of ionizing radiations is due to the nonspecific ionization of molecules in their path. The ionized molecules react chemically with other ionized or unionized molecules in their vicinity. As with UV radiation, the important site of destruction appears to be DNA.[8] So many chemical modifications of nucleic acids can be demonstrated after treatment with ionizing radiation that it is uncertain whether death is caused by a single change or several changes in the nucleic acid molecules. In dilute solution, DNA is destroyed mainly through interaction with H· and OH· free radicals produced by radiolysis of H_2O. These in turn interact with nucleic acids to produce free radicals (in the nucleic acid) that subsequently oxidize or cross-link. Phosphodiester bonds are broken, inorganic phosphate and bases are liberated, the deoxyribose is oxidized, bases are deaminated and dehydroxylated, and hydroperoxides are formed. It is probable, however, that the lethal effects are produced by direct hits of the ionizing radiation on the nucleic acid molecule, rather than indirectly through radiolysis of water. The major effect of direct hits is the nicking of the sugar-phosphate backbone of DNA. Scission of the DNA interferes with replication. Again, enzyme repair mechanisms exist as with UV radiation damage, and the lethal effects of ionizing radiation are the net result of the interaction of damage and repair.

Disinfectants[4, 9, 13]

Chemical agents that destroy pathogens are generally referred to as disinfectants. Sterilization may or may not result from the action of a disinfectant. Disinfectants are often toxic to human beings or other targets of pathogens; nevertheless, disinfectants are extremely valuable for destroying pathogens in the human or animal environment. Disinfectants that can be applied topically to body surfaces are usually referred to as **antiseptics.**

Acids and Alkalis

Both strong acids and strong alkalis, *i.e.,* those that are highly dissociated, exert a marked bactericidal effect. The lethal activity of mineral acids is proportional to the degree of their dissociation, but that of organic acids appears to be an effect of the whole molecule, for the degree of dissociation is, as a rule, not great. Fermentation acids, *e.g.,* lactic and acetic acids, help protect "sour" food products (pickles, sauerkraut, cheese, etc.) and silage from undesirable spoilage organisms. Undissociated, short-chain, volatile fatty acids (acetic, propionic, and butyric acids) are bacteriostatic and slightly bactericidal for enteric bacteria (*Escherichia, Salmonella, Shigella*). Since the volatile fatty acids are major products of the bacterial fermentation in the large intestine of monogastric animals, they may play a role in regulating the growth of the enteric bacteria in the intestinal tract. Benzoic acid is an antifungal and antibacterial agent that is used as a preservative in pharmaceuticals and food, as is sorbic acid, an antifungal agent. Acid douches, usually containing lactic or acetic acid (vinegar), are used to treat vaginal tract infections. The disinfectant action of alkalis such as sodium hydroxide is likewise proportional to the degree of dissociation. The germicidal activity of the hydroxides of the alkaline earths is, however, greater than can be accounted for on the basis of dissociation, for the metallic ion is often toxic in itself. Both acids and alkalis, in too low a concentration to kill bacteria rapidly, often enhance the activity of other disinfecting agents. For example, the germicidal activity of many salts is greater in the presence of acid or alkali, and, as noted above, bacteria are killed much more rapidly by heat in the presence of dilute acid or alkali than at neutrality.

Heavy Metals

The most active of the heavy metals are mercury, silver, and copper. Mercuric chloride is highly active in 0.1 per cent aqueous solution. Mercuric oxide is used in ointments to treat infections of the eyelid and conjunctiva. In general, relatively few mercury compounds have antibacterial activity, and those that do as a result of the presence of mercuric ion are primarily bacteriostatic rather than bactericidal. The silver salts, such as silver nitrate, although somewhat less active, are still highly efficient germicides. Silver nitrate solutions are used to treat eye infections and infected burns. Copper salts are still less active but are highly efficient in the destruction of algae and other chlorophyll-containing organisms.

The antibacterial activity of heavy metals is most probably due to the formation of poorly dissociable salts of the sulfhydryl groups of proteins, *e.g.,*

$$2 \text{ Protein} - \text{SH} + \text{Hg}^{2+} \rightarrow$$
$$\text{Protein} - \text{S} - \text{Hg} - \text{S} - \text{Protein} + 2 \text{ H}^+$$

The effects of heavy metals are reversed by treatment with high concentrations of sulfhydryl compounds. The above equation is, in effect, reversed when the heavy metal cation binds to the added sulfhydryl compound.

Some organic compounds containing mercury or silver have disinfectant properties and are not markedly toxic to body tissue. Thimerosal and nitromerosal (see **5–1**) are used to disinfect skin and mucous membranes, and the former is used to preserve some bacterial and viral vaccines. Silver protein complexes are also used to treat eye infections.

5–1.

C_2H_5HgS ⬡ COONa

thimerosal
(Merthiolate)

CH_3 ⬡ NO_2 ONa HgOH

nitromersol
(Metaphen)

Oxidizing Agents

Potassium permanganate and the sodium and calcium salts of hypochlorous acid (HOCl) show marked bactericidal activity owing to their properties as oxidizing agents. Mole for mole, hypochlorous acid is one of the most powerful germicides known, and its calcium salt (commonly known as bleaching powder) has a wide use in the treatment of private and small municipal water supplies. Chlorine gas reacts with water to form hypochlorous acid and is widely used to disinfect water supplies and swimming pools. Hypochlorous acid reacts with organic compounds containing an amide group with the formation of compounds known as chloramines. These compounds show strong disinfectant properties that are apparently associated with the presence of the $=NCl$ group. Free chlorine is slowly released from the chloramines. Two of these, chloramine-T and dichloramine-T, were used with considerable success in the disinfection of deep wounds in World War I.

Bromine and iodine are also potent germicides. In addition to acting as an oxidant, I_2 combines irreversibly with proteins by iodinating tyrosine. Iodine in the form of its tincture (2 to 7 per cent I_2 in aqueous alcohol containing KI) is an efficient skin disinfectant. Some nonionic surface active agents such as polyvinyl pyrrolidone are called iodophores because they dissolve I_2, which is slowly released from micelles upon dilution. Slightly acid solutions of I_2 in iodophores are effective, nonirritating disinfectants that have good wetting properties because of the presence of the detergent. Bromine has been used occasionally as a disinfectant for swimming pool water. Both hydrogen peroxide and ozone are bactericidal, but the former is rapidly decomposed by tissue catalase and has little penetrating power when applied to wounds and abrasions.

Oxidizing agents presumably act by irreversibly oxidizing essential molecules in the cell, *e.g.*, sulfhydryl groups of proteins oxidized to sulfoxides. Mild oxidation of proteins with performic acid, for example, leads to the formation of cysteic acid residues from cysteine, methionine sulfone from methionine, and destruction of tryptophan.

Phenols

Phenol and its derivatives are among the most useful of the antibacterial organic compounds. A 5 per cent aqueous solution of phenol rapidly destroys vegetative cells of bacteria and more slowly destroys spores. Antibacterial activity is not seriously reduced by the presence of organic matter. Phenol is used as the standard of comparison (called phenol coefficient) for other disinfectants, particularly those of similar chemical structure.

The activity of phenol is enhanced by substitution in the ring. The methyl phenols, ortho, meta, and para cresols, and halogenated phenols have greater activity than the parent compound. Resorcinol, hydroxyphenol, however, is only mildly bactericidal. In general, the substitution of aliphatic side chains in both phenol and hydroxyphenol increases antibacterial activity in direct proportion to the length of the side chain, but solubility in water is decreased and limits the practical value of such compounds.

The bisphenols have become the most useful of the phenolic disinfectants because of their relatively high bacteriostatic and fungistatic properties and relatively low toxicity. These compounds consist of two phenol rings attached carbon-to-carbon or through oxygen, sulfur, or alkalene, especially methylene, groups.

The most important of the bisphenols are orthohydroxydiphenyl and the chlorinated methylene and sulfur compounds. Hexachlorophene (see **5–2**) has the unusual and useful property of retaining substantially all its antibacterial activity when incorporated into soaps. An example of a sulfur chlorophene in common use is the thio bisphenol, bithionol (see **5–2**), a sulfur analogue of tetrachlorphene. These compounds are relatively insoluble in water, but are soluble in dilute alkali and in many organic solvents. The bisphenols, however, differ from phenol in their bactericidal activity. Although they are more active than phenol under the conditions of the phenol coefficient test (see p. 140), more prolonged exposure is required for maximal bactericidal activity. The bisphenols are also bacteriostatic in high dilutions.

Phenolic disinfectants precipitate proteins, but the minimal concentrations necessary for

5–2.

hexachlorophene	bithionol

killing cells are below the concentrations necessary for protein precipitation. There is accumulated evidence that interaction of phenolic disinfectants with proteins in the membrane causes disruption of membrane structure. The bactericidal action is probably related to destruction of membrane structure and membrane functions.

Detergents

The surface-active detergents fall into three groups: anionic, cationic, and nonionic (see **5–3**). The **anionic** group includes soaps, sodium and potassium salts of higher fatty acids, alkyl sulfates such as sodium lauryl sulfate, and alkylbenzenesulfonates. The **cationic** group consists of quaternary ammonium compounds, and the **nonionic** group includes polyethers and polyglycerol esters. Some of these compounds have antibacterial activity.

Soaps are not effective antiseptics or disinfectants because their antibacterial activity is limited. They are, nevertheless, useful agents for the mechanical removal of bacteria from the skin by emulsification of lipoidal secretions in which microorganisms are embedded. Thus, the number of bacteria present on the skin is markedly, but temporarily, reduced by washing with soap. The antibacterial activity of

soaps may be enhanced by combining them with disinfectant substances such as cresols, but, in general, the activity of the incorporated substance is reduced in combination with soap. Hexachlorophene is, as noted above, a significant exception to this general rule. The use of hexachlorophene-containing soaps results not only in an immediate reduction of the numbers of bacteria present on the skin, but the bacteriostatic activity of the residual hexachlorophene significantly inhibits the growth of bacteria on the skin.

Some of the alkyl sulfates have more antibacterial activity than soaps, inhibiting growth in relatively high (0.1 per cent) concentrations. Those that are active are markedly selective, affecting gram-positive bacteria but not gram-negative bacteria.

The **quaternary ammonium** compounds, often called "quats," are a group of amines that may be regarded as derivatives of ammonium chloride in which various radicals are substituted for the hydrogens. Ordinarily one is a long-chain (C_8 to C_{18}) alkyl group, and the others smaller alkyl groups, phenyl groups, etc. Very many, perhaps a thousand, of these compounds have been synthesized, and several, including Zephiran (alkyldimethylbenzylammonium chloride), Ceepryn (cetyl-

5–3.

Surface-Active (Detergent) Substances

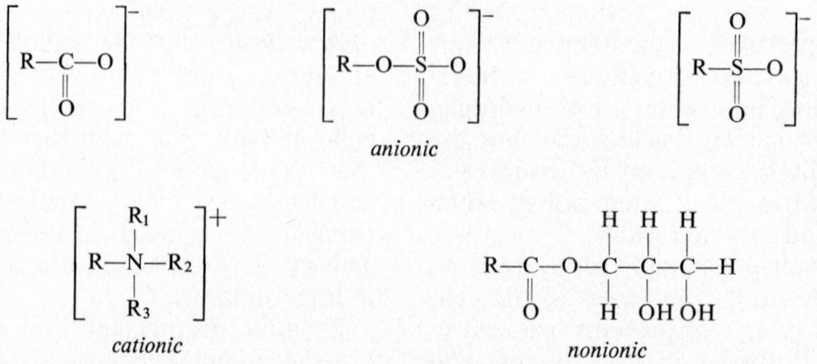

anionic

cationic

nonionic

5–4.

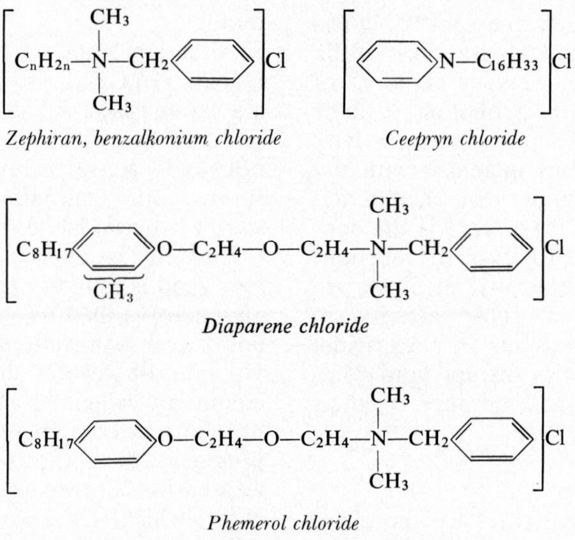

$$\left[C_nH_{2n}-\overset{\overset{\displaystyle CH_3}{|}}{\underset{\underset{\displaystyle CH_3}{|}}{N}}-CH_2\!\!\left\langle\!\!\bigcirc\!\!\right\rangle \right] Cl$$

Zephiran, benzalkonium chloride

$$\left[\left\langle\!\!\bigcirc\!\!\right\rangle\!\!N-C_{16}H_{33} \right] Cl$$

Ceepryn chloride

$$\left[C_8H_{17}\!\!\left\langle\!\!\underset{\underline{CH_3}}{\bigcirc}\!\!\right\rangle\!\!O-C_2H_4-O-C_2H_4-\overset{\overset{\displaystyle CH_3}{|}}{\underset{\underset{\displaystyle CH_3}{|}}{N}}-CH_2\!\!\left\langle\!\!\bigcirc\!\!\right\rangle \right] Cl$$

Diaparene chloride

$$\left[C_8H_{17}\!\!\left\langle\!\!\bigcirc\!\!\right\rangle\!\!O-C_2H_4-O-C_2H_4-\overset{\overset{\displaystyle CH_3}{|}}{\underset{\underset{\displaystyle CH_3}{|}}{N}}-CH_2\!\!\left\langle\!\!\bigcirc\!\!\right\rangle \right] Cl$$

Phemerol chloride

pyridinium chloride), Phemerol (diisobutyl-phenoxyethoxyethyldimethylbenzyl ammonium chloride), and Diaparene (diisobutylcresoxy-ethoxyethyldimethylbenzyl ammonium chloride) have gained general acceptance (**5–4**). The cationic detergents are equally effective against gram-positive and gram-negative bacteria.

There is a marked incompatibility between anionic and cationic detergents. When these two types of detergents are mixed, antibacterial activity disappears. The nonionic detergents do not have this effect; for example, quaternary ammonium compounds may be mixed with nonionic detergents having good solubilizing activity to give an antibacterial cleansing agent.

Detergents are bactericidal because they destroy the integrity of the cell membrane by disrupting the interactions between membrane proteins and lipids. Since the bacterial surface is normally negatively charged, the cationic detergents are probably more effective because of the attraction of the detergent molecule to the membrane surface.

Chlorhexidine

The gluconate of the bisguanide chlorhexidine (see **5–5**) is extensively used for preoperative skin disinfection, wound irrigation, and treatment of burns. Chlorhexidine is bactericidal to gram-positive and gram-negative cells, but it is not effective against mycobacteria, spores, or viruses. The gluconate is freely water soluble, and cationic and nonionic detergents can be added to solutions to improve wetting and cleansing properties. Because of its low toxicity and irritancy, chlorhexidine has been used in oral hygiene to reduce caries and periodontal disease. The disinfectant binds to mucous membranes and is slowly released, with continued antibacterial action. Chlorhexidine appears to interfere with membrane permeability. It inhibits membrane adenosine triphosphatase and, the uptake of potassium, and causes leakage of cytoplasmic solutes.

5–5.

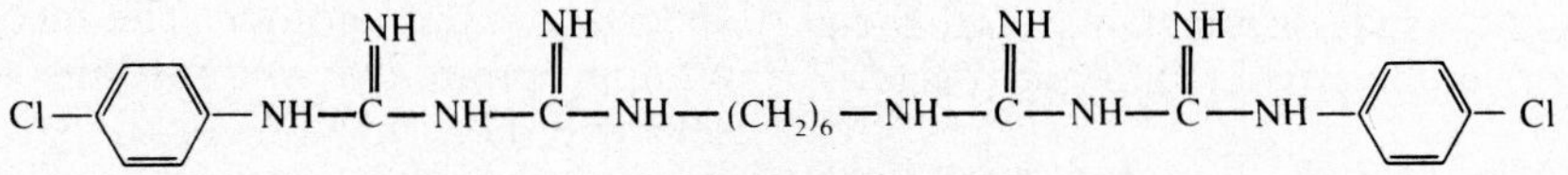

$$Cl\!-\!\left\langle\!\!\bigcirc\!\!\right\rangle\!-\!NH\!-\!\overset{\overset{\displaystyle NH}{\|}}{C}\!-\!NH\!-\!\overset{\overset{\displaystyle NH}{\|}}{C}\!-\!NH\!-\!(CH_2)_6\!-\!NH\!-\!\overset{\overset{\displaystyle NH}{\|}}{C}\!-\!NH\!-\!\overset{\overset{\displaystyle NH}{\|}}{C}\!-\!NH\!-\!\left\langle\!\!\bigcirc\!\!\right\rangle\!-\!Cl$$

chlorhexidine

Alcohol and Ethers

Ethyl alcohol and ethyl ether, often used as skin disinfectants, are not very good germicides. Their limited effectiveness probably lies in the solution of the lipoidal secretions of the skin and consequent mechanical removal of microorganisms. Absolute alcohol has little or no germicidal activity. The bactericidal activity of alcohol-water solutions increases with the addition of water, but 50 per cent alcohol and less has little activity; 70 per cent is the concentration usually used for skin disinfection. Absolute propyl and isopropyl alcohols are likewise ineffective but show activity in aqueous solution. Alcohols may be bactericidal because of their ability to disrupt lipid complexes in membranes and because of their ability to denature proteins.

Gaseous Disinfectants

The use of bactericidal gases for the disinfection of rooms, dwellings, and the like (fumigation or terminal disinfection) has declined markedly in recent years with no coincident increase in the prevalence of infectious disease. The commonly used gas, sulfur dioxide (generated by burning flowers of sulfur), is probably not bactericidal as a gas but is bactericidal in aqueous solution; it is effective, therefore, only in the presence of adequate amounts of moisture (a relative humidity of 60 per cent or higher). Sulfur dioxide, added as a gas or as sulfite or metabisulfite, is an effective antifungal and antibacterial agent for the preservation of foods and beverages. Other gases such as hydrogen cyanide have little or no effect on bacteria. Although the value of terminal disinfection is open to serious question, that of disinfestation is well established and the gases, hydrocyanic acid in particular, are widely used for the destruction of rats aboard ship, and like purposes.

Alkylating Agents. Certain alkylating agents have been found to be highly effective bactericides in gaseous form, both on solid objects and solutions, and on bacteria suspended in air. These include ethylene oxide, propylene oxide, ethylene amine, methyl bromide, and formaldehyde. These substances have the unusual property of being relatively more effective in the destruction of bacterial spores than the usual disinfectants, and their activity seems to be irreversible and bactericidal.

Formaldehyde has been used for many years, but is often unsatisfactory because it penetrates poorly and requires a relatively high humidity. It has been used more recently in combination with low-temperature steam-vacuum sterilization for textiles and similar materials.

Although not a gas, glutaraldehyde, $OHC(CH_2)_3CHO$, is similar in action to the alkylating gases. A 2 per cent aqueous solution buffered at pH 7.5 to 8.5 with sodium bicarbonate is active against vegetative bacteria, spores, fungi, and viruses, and can be used to sterilize thermolabile materials.

Ethylene oxide is a more recent development and is similarly highly effective. It forms an explosive mixture with air, but the attendant danger is prevented by mixing with 7 to 10 volumes of carbon dioxide; the mixture is commonly called carboxide. It may be applied to fabrics or equipment of various kinds under pressure; the objects to be sterilized are treated in the dressing-sterilizer type of autoclave, which is evacuated to 14 pounds, and ethylene oxide is run in to 20 to 23 pounds of pressure and left overnight.

Another alkylating agent that has been of particular interest is β-propiolactone. Unlike ethylene oxide, it is not flammable, but requires a high humidity (80 per cent) to be effective, and has only limited penetrating power so that it functions most effectively as a surface disinfectant. It is highly bactericidal and virucidal in concentrations of 1 to 5 mg. per liter and is considered to be about 25 times more effective than formaldehyde. While lacking the general utility of ethylene oxide, it is especially effective in the decontamination of enclosed spaces such as rooms and buildings and may also be used for the sterilization of heat-labile materials.

Alkylating agents are highly reactive with a variety of functional groups of nucleic acids and proteins, i.e., $-NH_2$, $-OH$, $-CO_2H$, and $-SH$. Bactericidal activity presumably results from the alkylation of these functional groups in essential macromolecules.

Dyes

The dyes are widely used in bacteriology both for staining purposes and as indicators. In addition, many of them show a marked bacteriostatic and bactericidal activity that is often specifically directed against one bacterial species and not another. The incorporation of an appropriate dye in a medium will render it selective; i.e., it will favor the growth of some species of bacteria and inhibit that of others. In general, this specificity is correlated with the Gram reaction; the gram-negative organisms are, for the most part, much less sensitive to dyes than are the gram-positive species. The activity of these compounds is affected by pH. The toxicity of the acid dyes increases with acidity and that of the basic dyes increases with alkalinity.

A number of the triphenylmethane dyes are inhibitory in high dilutions. The bacteriostatic properties of the triamino-triphenylmethane dyes, the so-called rosanilins, are apparently associated with the substitution of alkyl groups in the amido side chains. Basic fuchsin, a mixture of the unsubstituted simple dyes rosanilin and pararosanilin, is a relatively weak bacteriostatic agent. Acid fuchsin, a mixture of various sulfonated derivatives of basic fuchsin, is also only weakly bacteriostatic. Methyl violet,* a mixture of tetra-, penta-, and hexamethyl pararosanilin, is markedly bacteriostatic and completely inhibits the growth of bacteria such as staphylococci and diphtheria bacilli in dilutions of 1:1,000,000 to 1:5,000,000. The gram-negative bacilli such as the colon and typhoid bacilli are less sensitive to methyl violet and require approximately 150 times as much dye to suppress growth.

The acridine dye proflavine was introduced during the First World War as a topical disinfectant, but other agents have since proved to be more satisfactory. The related compounds mepacrine and chloroquine are used for treating malaria and trypanosome infections, respectively. These compounds bind to DNA and inhibit its synthesis.

Factors Influencing Disinfection

Several factors influence the velocity of the chemical reactions that result in disinfection. The most important factor is the concentration of the reacting substances, *i.e.,* the concentration of disinfectant and the numbers of bacteria present. The effective concentration of a disinfectant is, in turn, dependent upon two other factors: first, the presence of water, and second, the presence of extraneous organic matter. Water makes coagulation by heat and ionization of the bactericidal salts possible. It acts as a solvent and suspending medium in which intimate contact between the disinfectant and the microorganism is achieved.

Several disinfectants act by combining with the protein of the cell. If extraneous organic matter is present, it too will react with the

disinfectant, thereby reducing the effectiveness of the process of disinfection. Disinfectants vary widely in the degree to which their bactericidal activities are affected by organic matter. The salts of heavy metals, for example, are rapidly precipitated by organic matter, whereas phenol and the cresols are only slightly affected. The rate of destruction by heat is also affected by organic matter. When bacteria are embedded in a mass of fecal matter, it takes longer to destroy them with heat. Other factors that influence the rate of destruction by bactericidal agents or heat are temperature and pH. A rise in temperature increases the rate of destruction. Increases or decreases in pH above or below pH 7.0 also increase the rate of destruction. Although other factors such as the presence of salts affect the rate of disinfection, these are not of practical importance.

The time of exposure of bacteria to a given disinfectant is of considerable practical significance and bears an inverse relation to the rapidity of killing. The time allowed for the destruction of bacteria is determined not only by the factors discussed above but also by the kinds of bacteria that are to be killed. In certain cases the specificity of a disinfectant may be so marked that it must be taken into consideration. For example, the relative atoxicity of hypochlorite for the tubercle bacillus precludes its use in the disinfection of tuberculous sputum. Bacterial spores are much more resistant to heat and chemical disinfectants than are the vegetative cells, and considerably more time must be allowed for their destruction. The vegetative cells of some bacteria may be more resistant than those of others, but, for the most part, such differences are too small to be of practical significance.

The Dynamics of Disinfection

Quantitative studies on the rate at which microorganisms are killed by lethal agents have indicated that in many instances the organisms die at a logarthmic rate; *i.e.,* if the logarithms of the numbers of viable organisms are plotted against time, the points tend to fall on a straight line (see Fig. 5–2). This phenomenon has been observed in the death of both spores and vegetative cells under the influence of chemical disinfectants or moist heat and also occurs in the death of bacteria in old cultures. The velocity of the reaction, the slope of such a line, depends upon the concentration and kind of disinfectant, the nature of the organisms—whether spores or vegetative cells—and

---

*Gentian violet is a more or less impure mixture of methyl violet and dextrin. Crystal violet, hexamethyl-*p*-rosanilin, is one of the constituents of methyl violet.

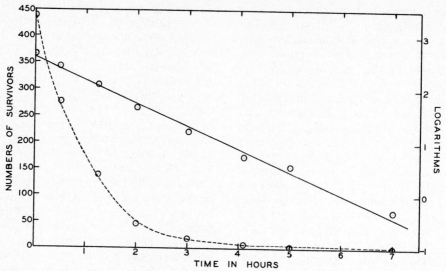

Figure 5-2. Death rate of anthrax spores treated with 5 per cent phenol. The dotted line is the arithmetic plot and the solid line the logarithmic plot. The negative logarithm was obtained by taking samples of several times the unit volume. (After Chick.)

other factors that influence the process of disinfection.

Plots of the logarithm of the time it takes to kill standard populations of bacteria against the logarithm of the concentration of disinfectant yield slopes that provide concentration exponents or dilution coefficients that indicate the effectiveness of disinfectants with dilution. Mercuric chloride has a dilution coefficient of 1, which means that a threefold decrease in concentration increases disinfection time by threefold. Phenol has a dilution coefficient of 3, and a threefold dilution causes a 729-fold decrease in its activity. The temperature coefficient, usually expressed as the ratio of the time it takes to kill a standard population at a particular temperature to the killing time obtained when the temperature is raised to 10° C., is characteristic of particular disinfectants. The effectiveness of formaldehyde is increased more than that of phenol when temperature is increased.

Of practical importance is the fact that in disinfection by chemicals and by heat there is a minority of cells, possibly more resistant, that survive long after the majority have perished. The small number of resistant cells must be destroyed in order to obtain complete sterilization. The determination of antiviral activity poses special technical problems because of the necessity of measuring residual viable virus by infectivity titrations.[14] These assays are complicated by the effects of autointerference

when a large number of viruses have been inactivated near the end point (Chapter 38).

In any case, it is not possible to extrapolate the exponential death rate to zero and assume that the indicated time of exposure insures sterility. Such an assumption resulted in incomplete inactivation of poliovirus by formalin in the preparation of vaccines.[25]

The Standardization of Disinfectants

The value of a quantitative method for the determination of the killing power of germicides was recognized early in the development of bacteriology. Standardized techniques were developed that make it possible to determine the bactericidal power of a given chemical compound relative to that of phenol. The numerical value obtained is called the **phenol coefficient** and indicates whether, and to approximately what extent, the compound is a better or poorer bactericide than phenol. The phenol coefficient of a disinfectant used against the typhoid bacillus is calculated as follows (see Table 5-1):

Divide the greatest dilution of the disinfectant capable of killing *Salmonella typhi* in 10 minutes but not in five minutes by the phenol dilution that so kills and divide these figures one into another. In order not to convey a false idea of the accuracy of the method the coefficient is calculated to the nearest 0.1 point if under 1, to the nearest 0.2 point if between 1 and 5, to the nearest 0.5 point if between 5 and 10, and to the nearest 1.0 point if

Table 5-1. **Determination of the Phenol Coefficient***

Disin- fectant	Dilution	Time in Minutes		
		5	10	15
Unknown	1:300	0	0	0
	1:325	+	0	0
	1:350	+	0	0
	1:375	+	+	0
	1:400	+	+	+
Phenol	1:90	+	0	0
	1:100	+	+	+

The test is satisfactory only when the resistance of the test organisms, here *S. typhi,* gives one or another of the following reactions:

1:90	+ or 0	+ or 0	0
1:100	+	+	+ or 0

$$\text{phenol coefficient} = \frac{350}{90} = 3.89 = 3.9$$

*From L. S. Stuart, *in* G. F. Reddish: Antiseptics, Disinfectants, Fungicides, and Chemical and Physical Sterilization, 2nd ed. Lea & Febiger, Philadelphia, 1957. In the table, 0 means no growth and + means growth of *S. typhi* after the indicated times of exposure to the disinfectant.

between 10 and 20. The conditions regarded as standardized in the United States, the FDA phenol coefficient, have been defined by the Food and Drug Administration.

The effect of extraneous organic matter on the bactericidal power of a disinfectant is commonly taken into consideration by carrying out the test with and without added organic matter. Three per cent of dried fecal matter or dried yeast may be added to the bacterial suspension or the organisms may be suspended in 50 per cent serum. It is important to recognize that bacteria differ considerably in their

resistance to phenol; staphylococci, for example, are much more resistant than the typhoid bacillus, so that in strict accuracy it is necessary to specify "typhoid phenol coefficient," "pneumococcus phenol coefficient," etc.

The phenol coefficient criterion of antimicrobial activity has many defects, including failure to evaluate concentration effects, temperature coefficients, etc. In addition, the validity of a phenol coefficient determined for a nonphenolic disinfectant is open to serious question. Consequently, many variations of the procedure have been used. For example, the germicidal equivalent concentration test has been developed for the evaluation of the lethal activity of unstable substances such as hypochlorites. Survival is measured after frequent short intervals of exposure to hypochlorite and the unknown disinfectant. Concentrations giving the same killing pattern as those of a reference compound are determined. This kind of test is illustrated in the example in Table 5-2; here the activity of the unknown disinfectant in a concentration of 10 ppm is equivalent to that of the reference standard, NaOCl, in a concentration of 50 ppm.

Assay of the antimicrobial activity of detergents is difficult because of the tendency of the test bacteria to adsorb to the walls of the test tube as a consequence of altered charge in the presence of the disinfectant. So-called use dilution tests have been employed for these substances in which a suspension of the test microorganism is dried on the surface of a carrier such as glass rods or rings, immersed in the disinfectant for varying periods, and subsequently cultured. Such methods are not new but were used many years ago by Koch and others who dried anthrax spores on silk threads, glass beads, etc., for testing bactericidal activity.

Table 5-2. **The Germicidal Equivalent Concentration Test***

Disinfectant	Concentration (in ppm)	Subculture Series†									
		1	2	3	4	5	6	7	8	9	10
Unknown	10	0	0	+	+	+	+	+	+	+	+
	20	0	0	0	0	+	+	+	+	+	+
	25	0	0	0	0	0	+	+	+	+	+
NaOCl control	50	0	0	+	+	+	+	+	+	+	+
	100	0	0	0	+	+	+	+	+	+	+
	200	0	0	0	0	0	0	+	+	+	+

*From L. S. Stuart, *in* G. F. Reddish: Antiseptics, Disinfectants, Fungicides, and Chemical and Physical Sterilization. 2nd ed. Lea & Febiger, Philadelphia, 1957.
†The time interval for exposure may vary from 30 seconds to 2 minutes between each transfer to the 10 subculture tubes.

The Chemotherapeutic Drugs[7, 9, 10, 13]

The feasibility of using antibacterial substances *in vivo* as chemotherapeutic agents is dependent primarily upon the specificity of action of such substances. The objective is to kill microorganisms without significant harmful effects on the host. This idea is by no means new. It was the basis of Ehrlich's search, begun in 1904, for a "magic bullet," a compound strongly germicidal for a given micoorganism yet sufficiently nontoxic that it could be injected in a suitable amount to give effective concentrations in the tissues. His work, originally directed toward the therapy of African sleeping sickness of trypanosome etiology, attempted to retain the antimicrobial activity of arsenic compounds and at the same time reduce toxicity for the host. It culminated in the synthesis of salvarsan.

Prior to 1940 the approach to chemotherapy of infectious diseases was fundamentally the same trial-and-error approach used by Ehrlich. The demonstration of a chemical antimicrobial activity *in vivo* was followed by determination of the active portion of the molecule. A great number of related compounds were then tested with the hope of retaining or enhancing the antimicrobial activity with coincident reduction in toxicity to the host. For example, the small but significant antimalarial activity of the substituted thionine, methylene blue, was exploited by the German workers in the development of Atabrine. A general practice, then, has been the routine testing of synthetic organic chemicals, especially dyestuffs and dye intermediates, for antimicrobial activity *in vivo*. This procedure led Domagk in 1935 to the observation of the marked chemotherapeutic activity of the dye Prontosil in experimental streptococcus infections. Routine procedure led to identification of the active portion of the molecule, *p*-aminobenzene sulfonamide (sulfanilamide), and the synthesis of a great number of related compounds known as the sulfonamides. Domagk's observation was of great practical significance. The sulfonamides were the first chemotherapeutic agents found to be effective in bacterial infections.

The 1940s began the era of antibiotics. Penicillin, discovered by Fleming in 1929, was the first microbial product to be used as a significant chemotherapeutic agent. Although the trial-and-error search for therapeutic synthetic chemicals continues, it has been largely overshadowed by the trial-and-error search for antibiotics. The latter are produced by molds and bacteria, the most important bacterial producers being the actinomycetes.

Testing of Agents

Whether for a synthetic chemical or an antibiotic, the trial-and-error procedure involves testing for antimicrobial activity, mainly *in vitro* against known pathogens. Promising agents are tested for toxicity and efficacy in controlling *in vivo* experimental animal infections. Continued promise results in the eventual testing of the agents in treatment of diseases of man. With antibiotics, purification and chemical characterization are important adjuncts to biological testing procedures. It is necessary to remove extraneous, potentially toxic material and to show that the antibiotic is different from existing antibiotics. The mode of action of the chemotherapeutic agent is also investigated. Studies of the mode of action have been useful in unraveling the mysteries of cell metabolism and in providing a rational approach to designing or finding new chemotherapeutic agents.

Modes of Action

Effective chemotherapeutic agents work because they inhibit essential metabolic reactions of the target organism and are relatively innocuous to the host. This selective toxicity can be due to distinct differences between the metabolism of the host and that of the target organism. For example, penicillin inhibits bacterial cell wall synthesis, an anabolic process peculiar to bacteria, and, except for allergic reactions, is harmless as far as animals are concerned. Selective toxicity can also be due to selective binding to grossly similar metabolic structures. Chemotherapeutic agents that act by selective binding to and disruption of membranes of sensitive organisms are known. Finally, selective toxicity could be due to differences in permeability of cells to chemotherapeutic agents.

It is important to know whether a chemotherapeutic agent is bactericidal or bacteriostatic and whether it acts on growing or nongrowing cells. A practical illustration of the importance of these parameters is the antagonism by sulfonamides to penicillin action. Sulfonamides are bacteriostatic. Penicillin is bactericidal but kills only growing cells. Since sulfonamides stop growth, they inhibit the action of penicillin. Whether a drug is bactericidal or bacteriostatic can easily be tested by examining the viability of cells after treatment and removal of the chemotherapeutic agent.

With some chemotherapeutic agents, it is possible to describe the site of inhibition of bacterial growth and the reason for their bactericidal or bacteriostatic action. With other agents, information about modes of action is still incomplete. The chemotherapeutic agents are considered here in terms of modes of action as they are presently understood. An important feature of chemotherapy, the development of resistance of pathogens to chemotherapeutic agents, will also be discussed.

INHIBITORS OF FOLIC ACID SYNTHESIS[7, 12, 24]

Sulfonamides

The structural similarities between the vitamin *p*-aminobenzoic acid and *p*-aminobenzene sulfonamides (see **5–6**) suggested to Woods and to Fildes that sulfonamides interfered with the use of *p*-aminobenzoic acid by microorganisms. It is now known that sulfonamides are inhibitors of the synthesis of folic acid, and *p*-aminobenzoic acid is part of the folic acid molecule. Sulfonamides do not inhibit organisms that cannot synthesize folic acid, including man and those bacteria that require preformed folic acid for growth. Inhibition is also offset in organisms that synthesize folic acid from *p*-aminobenzoic acid but are still capable of using preformed folic acid available in tissues of the host. *Escherichia coli* synthesizes folic acid from *p*-aminobenzoic acid but appears to be impermeable to exogenous folic acid and, therefore, is particularly susceptible to inhibition by sulfonamides.

Inhibition is also offset by the availability of products of biosynthetic pathways that require folic acid coenzymes. These products include methionine, purines, and thymidine. In other words, if there is no need for folic acid coenzymes because of the availability of the products the coenzymes are helping to manufacture, inhibition of folic acid synthesis by sulfonamides will not be detrimental to the cell. There is one folic acid coenzyme reaction in bacteria, however, that results in a product, N^{10}-formyl-tetrahydrofolic acid, that is not found exogenously. This coenzyme is necessary for synthesis of formyl-methionyl-tRNA. Formyl-methionyl-tRNA is necessary for initiation of protein synthesis.

Sulfonamides are competitive inhibitors of the synthesis of folic acid from *p*-aminobenzoic acid, substituted pteridine, and glutamic acid. On the enzyme level, they are competitive with *p*-aminobenzoic acid. Inhibition depends,

5–6.

Para-aminobenzoic Acid and Sulfonamides

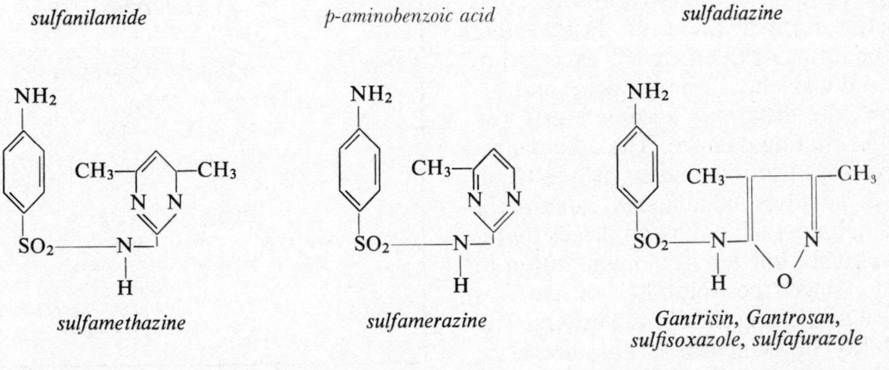
NH2
SO2—NH2
sulfanilamide
NH2
CO2H
p-aminobenzoic acid
NH2
H
C
N
CH
CH
SO2—N—C
H
N
sulfadiazine
NH2
CH3
CH3
N N
SO2
N
H
sulfamethazine
NH2
CH3
N N
SO2
N
H
sulfamerazine
NH2
CH3
CH3
SO2
N
N
H
O
Gantrisin, Gantrosan, sulfisoxazole, sulfafurazole

therefore, on the relative affinities of the enzyme site for sulfonamides and p-aminobenzoic acid and the relative concentration of the two competitors. As previously indicated, noncompetitive reversal of sulfonamide inhibition of bacteria can be effected by folic acid and end products of folic acid coenzyme pathways.

Sulfonamides are bacteriostatic. Taking the sulfonamide away or even loading up the medium with p-aminobenzoic acid will permit the restoration of growth of the sensitive organism. The latter is used as a practical method of culturing sulfonamide-sensitive organisms from the blood of individuals receiving sulfonamide therapy, i.e., to overcome the inhibitory action of a blood sample that contains sulfonamide in addition to the bacteria of interest.

Despite the possibilities for overcoming sulfonamide inhibition, sulfonamides have been remarkably useful agents. They are cheap and relatively nontoxic. Inhibition obviously depends on a complex of interacting factors: the bacterium's ability to synthesize folic acid, its permeability to folic acid, and the presence of noncompetitive reversing compounds in the environment. Because of natural and acquired resistance of bacteria, side-effects of sulfonamides, and the availability of antibiotics, sulfonamides alone are now used for treatment of a limited number of infections.

The term sulfonamide is generally taken to include the parent compound sulfanilamide and its derivatives. Several thousand sulfonamides have been prepared, usually by substitution in the amido group attached to the sulfone radical (see 5–6). There appears to be little qualitative difference among sulfonamides so far as antibacterial activity is concerned, but they differ with respect to solubility, rates of absorption and excretion, and other factors. In general, they are only sparingly soluble in water, but their solubility increases with alkalinity. On absorption a portion of the drug is inactivated by combination with plasma protein, and a portion acetylated to an inactive form in the liver. Both active and inactive forms of the drug are excreted in the urine. When the urine is acid and its volume low, the drug may accumulate in the kidney with resulting damage. The administration of mixtures of sulfonamides, such as triple sulfa, which contains sulfadiazine, sulfamethazine, and sulfamerazine, has no direct therapeutic advantage, but reduces precipitation in the kidney, since the solubility of each is independent of the presence of the others. The high solubility of Gantrisin is also useful in overcoming the problem of precipitation in the kidney.

Aminohydroxybenzoic Acids

These are synthetic drugs that are also p-aminobenzoic acid analogues, and their mode of action is the same as that of sulfonamides. Para-aminosalicylic acid (see 5–7) has been the most commonly used of this group of chemotherapeutic agents. They are particularly useful against the tubercle bacillus and are not effective inhibitors of other bacteria. The reason for the restricted activity spectrum is not known.

Sulfones

Some of these synthetic compounds have a chemical relationship to the sulfonamides, and their mode of action may be similar. Like the hydroxybenzoates, they have a highly selective activity spectrum. One of the sulfones, diaminodiphenylsulfone or Dapsone (see 5–7), is used to treat leprosy.

Inhibitors of Dihydrofolate Reductase

The coenzyme form of folic acid is tetrahydrofolic acid (see p. 94, 4–29). Biochemical reduction of folic acid produces dihydrofolic acid, which is then further reduced to tetrahydrofolic acid. Inhibitors of the reduction of dihydrofolic to tetrahydrofolic acid have been synthesized. Two examples are methotrexate and trimethoprim (see 5–8). Mammalian and bacterial cells differ in their permeability to these inhibitors and in the sensitivities of their dihydrofolate reductases to the inhibitors. Mammalian cells are sensitive to methotrexate but relatively insensitive to trimethoprim, but

5–7.

Sulfones

p-aminosalicylic acid

diaminodiphenylsulfone

5–8.

Dihydrofolic Reductase Inhibitors

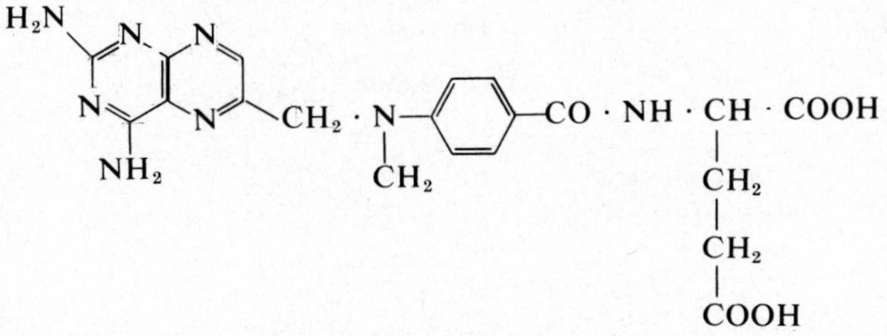

methotrexate

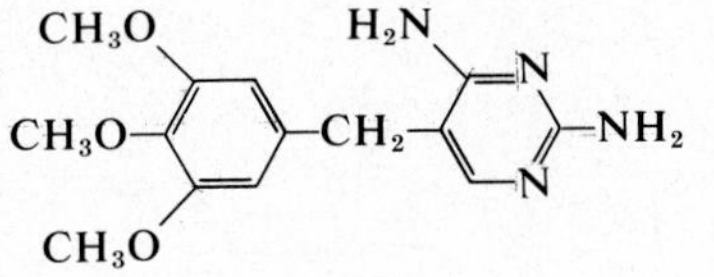

trimethoprim

bacteria are very sensitive to trimethoprim. Trimethoprim has been combined with a sulfonamide, sulfomethoxazole, to yield a chemotherapeutically effective mixture. Bacterial growth is inhibited by the synergistic inhibition of the synthesis of folic acid from *p*-aminobenzoic acid and the synthesis of tetrahydrofolic from dihydrofolic acid.

INHIBITORS OF PEPTIDOGLYCAN SYNTHESIS[1, 7, 9, 21, 22, 27]

Several antibiotics are inhibitors of bacterial peptidoglycan synthesis. Almost all are bactericidal and the bactericidal action is on growing cells. Continued growth of the cell without synthesis of the rigid, structural layer of peptidoglycan leads to lysis of the cells. Peptidoglycan normally acts as a force opposing the high osmotic pressure of the inside of a bacterial cell. Most bacteria live in environments that are hypotonic relative to the cell interior and need a peptidoglycan girdle to prevent them from bursting. If *Escherichia coli* is treated with penicillin, an inhibitor of peptidoglycan synthesis, the bacterium does not explode in a hypertonic environment, *e.g.*, 2.5 M sucrose. Instead, round spheroplasts are formed from growing rod-shaped cells. The spheroplasts contain little peptidoglycan on their surface, but they can grow to a limited extent. They cannot divide and they lyse if exposed to a hypotonic environment.

It is probable that enzymes in the cell membrane capable of hydrolyzing portions of the peptidoglycan participate in the disruption of the peptidoglycan after inhibition of its synthesis. It is thought that these enzymes normally participate in the growth of cell walls and in the cell division process. When peptidoglycan synthesis stops, the hydrolytic enzymes continue to be synthesized and may start to digest existing peptidoglycan. It is known that continued protein synthesis is necessary for penicillin to exert its killing action.

Inhibitors of cell wall synthesis include the penicillins, vancomycin, ristocetin, bacitracin, and novobiocin. The sites of inhibition of peptidoglycan synthesis by these various antibiotics are shown in Figure 5–3 (see Chapter 4 for a discussion of peptidoglycan synthesis). Except for cycloserine, the antibiotics inhibit the membrane-associated assembly of peptidoglycan from uridine nucleotide precursors.

Cycloserine
This agent inhibits the formation of one of the uridine nucleotide precursors, the uridine diphosphate muramyl pentapeptide. The pentapeptide terminates with two D-alanine molecules,

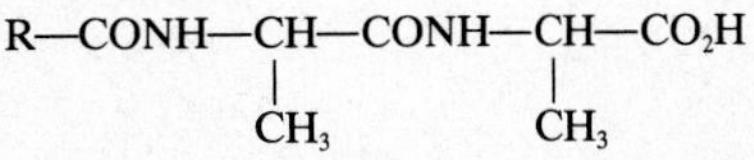

$$R—CONH—CH—CONH—CH—CO_2H$$
$$\quad\quad\quad\quad CH_3 \quad\quad\quad CH_3$$

Cycloserine is structurally related to alanine (see **5–9**). It was discovered as an actinomycete

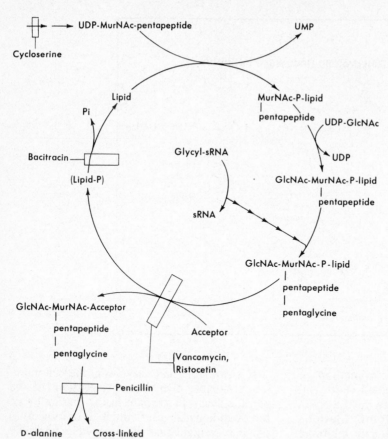

Figure 5–3. Sites of inhibition of peptidoglycan synthesis. (B. D. Davis, *et al.*, Microbiology, 1967, courtesy of Harper & Row; after Matsuhashi *et al.*)

product, but is now produced by chemical synthesis. It inhibits the formation of the pentapeptide by inhibiting two early reactions leading to pentapeptide synthesis, the conversion of L-alanine to D-alanine and the formation of a dipeptide from 2 molecules of D-alanine. Cycloserine is mainly used in treatment of tuberculosis when more suitable agents are contraindicated because of patient sensitivity or microbial resistance.

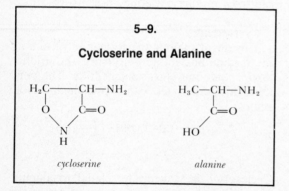

Penicillins

The penicillins (see **5–10**) are by far the most famous and most useful of all the antibiotics. They are produced by strains of the mold *Penicillium,* and have in common a 6-aminopenicillanic acid moiety. Different penicillins have different acyl side chains on the 6-amino group. The side chains are necessary for penicillin action and are introduced either biologically or chemically. The enzymes responsible for introduction of the acyl side chain are relatively nonspecific. If excess phenylacetic acid is added to the production medium, the mold makes benzyl penicillin (penicillin G). By changing the acid added to the medium, other substituted penicillins can be made. Phenoxymethyl penicillin (penicillin V) is made this way. The phenoxymethyl group gives greater protection against acid hydrolysis of the four-membered β-lactam ring in the stomach.

Penicillin Resistance. Hydrolysis of the lactam ring by enzymes—penicillinases—of bacteria is the basis of most of the resistance to penicillin by strains of otherwise susceptible

5–10.

Penicillin

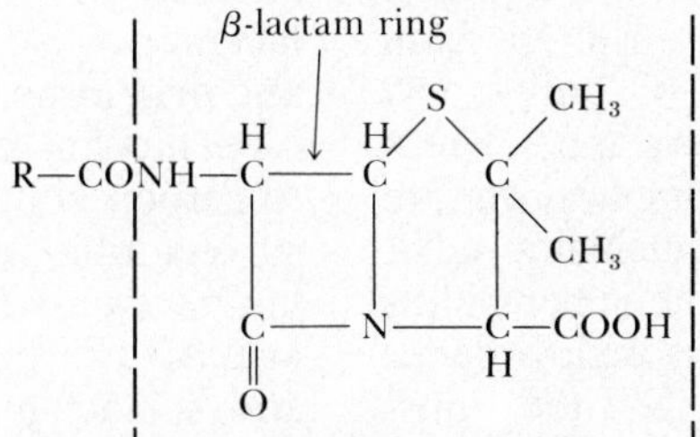

Penicillin general structure showing β-lactam ring, R—CONH— side chain, S, CH_3, CH_3, C—N, C—COOH, and 6-aminopenicillanic acid.

Penicillins

Penicillin	Prosthetic Group (R)	Penicillin	Prosthetic Group (R)
Ampicillin	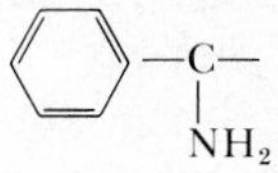 ring—C— with NH_2	Nafcillin	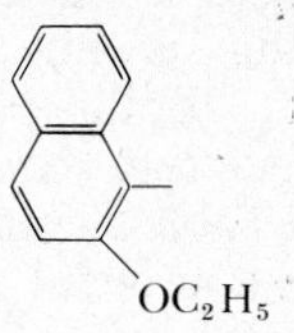 naphthalene ring with OC_2H_5
Benzyl (Penicillin G)	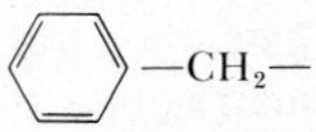 ring—CH_2—		
Cloxacillin	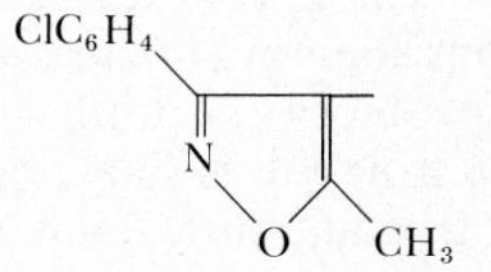 ClC_6H_4 isoxazole with CH_3	Oxacillin	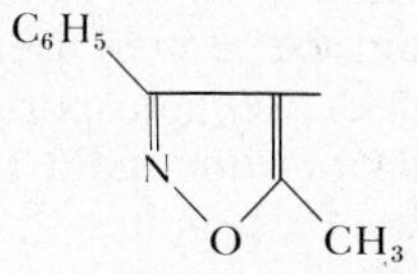 C_6H_5 isoxazole with CH_3
Dicloxacillin	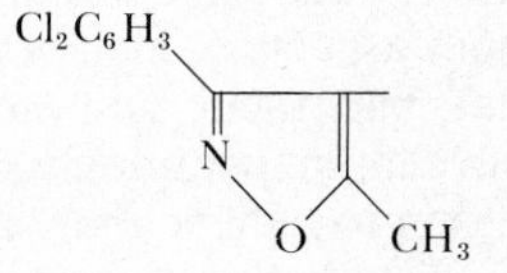 $Cl_2C_6H_3$ isoxazole with CH_3	Phenethicillin	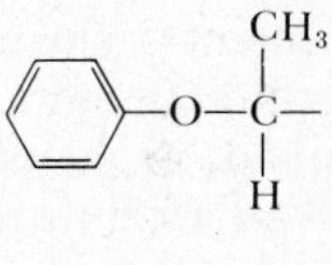 ring—O—C— with CH_3 and H
Methicillin	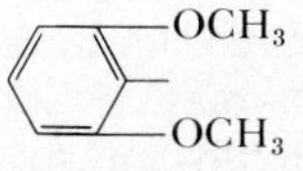 ring with OCH_3, OCH_3	Phenoxymethyl (Penicillin V)	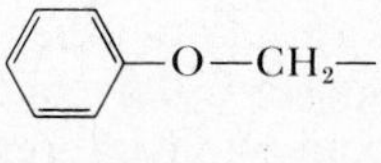 ring—O—CH_2—
Methylthioallyl (Penicillin O)	$CH_2{=}CH{-}CH_2{-}S{-}CH_2$—	Quincillin	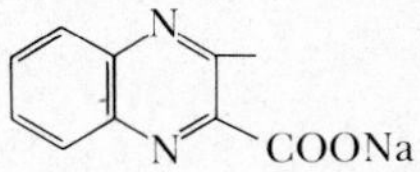 quinoxaline ring with N, N, COONa

species. The staphylococci are classic examples of how penicillin treatment can wipe out penicillinase-negative strains and permit the takeover of the environment by penicillinase-positive strains. Penicillin-resistant strains of *Staphylococcus aureus* were uncommon when penicillin was first introduced, but antibiotic selection over the years has produced populations of staphylococci with a high frequency of penicillinase-positive strains.

Studies of the specificity of penicillinases suggested the possibility that modification of the naturally introduced acyl side chains could lead to production of penicillinase-resistant penicillins. Attempts to remove the side chain of naturally produced penicillins by hydrolysis also hydrolyzed the essential β-lactam ring and inactivated the molecule. Two solutions to this problem were found. One was the discovery that the medium for production of penicillin could be controlled such that only 6-aminopenicillanic acid without a side chain could be produced and isolated. Side chains could then be added chemically. In addition, microbial enzymes, amidases, were found that would cleave off preexisting side chains of naturally produced penicillins. These were then applied to the production of 6-aminopenicillanic acid from natural penicillins for chemical introduction of new side chains.

Semisynthetic Penicillins. Several useful semisynthetic penicillins have resulted from these advances. Introduction of bulky acyl groups leads to penicillinase resistance. These groups are introduced by reacting appropriate acyl chlorides with 6-aminopenicillanic acid. Another advantage of semisynthetic penicillins is the construction of penicillins with broader antibiotic spectra. Penicillin G, the most widely used penicillin, is much more active against gram-positive than against gram-negative bacteria. Ampicillin, a semisynthetic penicillin with an alpha-aminobenzyl group instead of a benzyl group, is much more active against gram-negative bacteria than is penicillin G. Ampicillin is not, however, penicillinase-resistant. Both penicillinase-resistant and broad-spectrum semisynthetic penicillins are listed in Table 5–3, and some of the structures are shown in detail in **5–10**.

A related use of the semisynthetic procedures is in the construction of a useful antibiotic from the almost useless antibiotic cephalosporin C. Cephalosporin C is produced by a *Cephalosporium* mold and has a structure and mode of action like those of penicillin, but it lacks the potency of penicillin. Chemical replacement of the natural side chains of cephalosporin C permitted construction of a useful compound, cephalothin (see **5–11**). Although limited to administration by injection, cephalothin has a broad spectrum of activity.

A variety of other useful derivatives of cephalosporin C have been synthesized. In addition to continued interest in the synthesis of new cephalosporins and penicillins, new compounds that contain the β-lactam ring are under active investigation as new antibiotics or as precursors of antibiotics. These are **monobactams** in which the C—N bond of the β-lactam ring is not part of a second ring system, and **penems** in which the sulfur-containing ring of penicillins contains an unsaturated carbon to carbon bond. Mixtures of penicillinase-sensitive antibiotics and nonantibiotic β-lactamase inhibitors have been developed as therapeutic agents. The inhibitors include clavulanic acid and sublactam. These inhibitors, and others under investigation, will no doubt contribute to extending the usefulness of the antibiotics that are destroyed by β-lactamases of resistant strains of pathogens.

Other Inhibitors of Cell Wall Synthesis

Vancomycin and ristocetin are actinomycete products and appear to be similar compounds, but their structures are not completely known. They are composed of amino acids and sugars. Bacitracin is produced by a strain of *Bacillus subtilis*. It is a mixture of cyclic polypeptides consisting of D- and L-amino acids (see **5–12**). Novobiocin is produced by an actinomycete. Its structure is shown in **5–13**.

In addition to inhibiting peptidoglycan synthesis, vancomycin and ristocetin may inhibit other aspects of metabolism. There is evidence that bacitracin and novobiocin also inhibit more than peptidoglycan synthesis. There is reason to believe that vancomycin and bacitracin disturb the integrity of the bacterial membrane, and inhibition of peptidoglycan synthesis may be one aspect of the disruption of membrane structure and function. There is no

Table 5–3. **Semisynthetic Penicillins***

Generic Name	Side Chain
Penicillinase-stable	
Ancillin	(2-biphenylcarboxamido)
Cloxacillin	6-[3-(o-chlorophenyl)-5-methyl-4-isoxazolecarboxamido]
Dicloxacillin	6-[3-(2,6-dichlorophenyl)-5-methyl-4-isoxazolecarboxamido]
Methicillin	6-(2,6-dimethoxybenzamido)
Nafcillin	6-(2-ethoxy-1-naphthamido)
Oxacillin	6-(5-methyl-3-phenyl-2-isoxazoline-4-carboxamido)
Quinacillin	3-carboxy-2-quinoxalinyl
Broad-spectrum	
Adicillin	(D-4-amino-4-carboxybutyl)
Ampicillin	6-[D(-)-α-aminophenylacetamido]
Carbenicillin	6-(α-carboxyphenylacetamido)
Hetacillin	6-(2,2-dimethyl-5-oxo-4-phenyl-1-imidazolidinyl)

*Modified from Grollman and Grollman[10]

5–11.

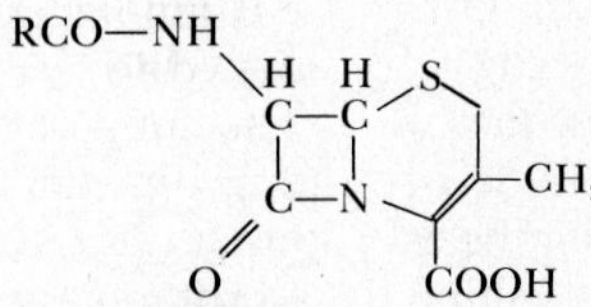

RCO—NH

cephalosporin nucleus

Cephalosporins

Cephalosporin	Rco	R′
Cephalosporin C	H_3N^+ $\,^-OOC$ $CH(CH_3)_3 \cdot CO$	$OCOCH_3$
Cephalothin	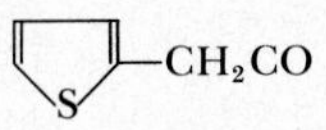 $-CH_2CO$	$OCOCH_3$

5–12.

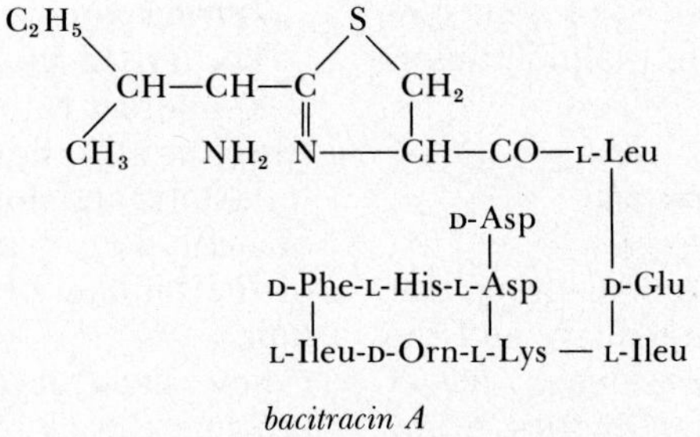

C_2H_5 CH_3 NH_2 N—CH—CO—L-Leu

D-Asp

D-Phe-L-His-L-Asp   D-Glu

L-Ileu-D-Orn-L-Lys — L-Ileu

bacitracin A

5–13.

$OCONH_2$ OH   NHCO

CH_3O OH CH_3

H_3C CH_3

H_3C OH CH_3

CH_3

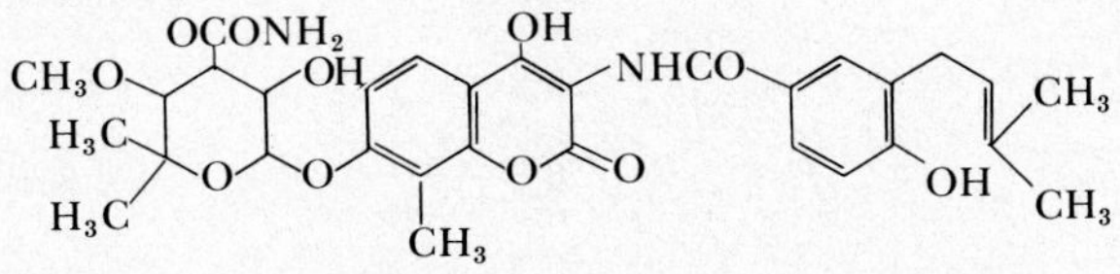

novobiocin

requirement that antibiotic inhibitions be restricted to effects on single sites or one specific enzyme reaction.

Novobiocin is the only one of the inhibitors of cell wall synthesis that is bacteriostatic or only very slowly bactericidal. The latter fact is not completely inconsistent with the mode of attack of inhibitors of peptidoglycan synthesis because novobiocin also appears to inhibit DNA and RNA synthesis. Novobiocin would, therefore, indirectly inhibit protein synthesis, which is known to be necessary for the bactericidal action of penicillin.

Compared to the penicillins, these other inhibitors of peptidoglycan synthesis are of more limited practical value because of host toxicity or limited spectra of action or both.

INHIBITORS OF PROTEIN SYNTHESIS[7, 9, 16, 23]

A variety of antibiotics have been found to be inhibitors of protein synthesis (see Chapter 4 for a discussion of protein synthesis). Table 5–4 shows that a variety of antibiotics inhibit protein synthesis in procaryotes. The table also shows whether functions attributable to the 30 S or 50 S subunit are inhibited. Inhibitors have been studied in a variety of ways to localize their effects on specific stages of protein synthesis. The effects of the more useful antibiotics are summarized in Table 5–4.

Aminoglycoside Aminocyclitols (AGAC)

The first antibiotic of the AGAC group was streptomycin. Because of ototoxicity and the rapid development of resistance, newer AGAC are more important antibiotics. Some of the newer AGAC are gentamicin, spectinomycin, amikacin, tobramycin, and kanamycin (Fig. 5–4). Except for amikacin, these compounds and streptomycin are produced by actinomycetes. Amikacin is a semisynthetic AGAC that is produced from kanamycin A. All of the AGAC contain a substituted aminocyclitol as part of the antibiotic molecule. The aminocyclitol in streptomycin is streptidine, in amikacin it is actinamine, and in the other AGAC mentioned above it is deoxystreptamine. Except for spectinomycin, they contain amino sugars that are glycosidically linked to the aminocyclitol. All of the AGAC are bactericidal except for spectinomycin, which is bacteriostatic. All bind with the 30 S subunits of ribosomes and inhibit protein synthesis (see Table 5–4).

Streptomycin now has only a limited role in the treatment of tuberculosis. Spectinomycin is used for treating gonorrhea, especially when penicillin-resistant *Neisseria gonorrhoeae* cause the infection. Gentamicin is effective against many gram-negative bacilli, as are most of the AGAC. The choice of a particular AGAC for use against a particular infection depends on the relative susceptibility of the pathogen to the different AGAC, the prevalence of resistant strains to a particular AGAC, and the significance of side effects of an individual AGAC, particularly its ototoxicity and nephrotoxicity.

Tetracyclines

The broad-spectrum tetracyclines (see Fig. 5–5) interact with 30 S subunits. In contrast to streptomycin, however, tetracyclines are bacteriostatic and not bactericidal. Their main site of inhibition of protein synthesis is inhibition of the binding of AA-tRNA to the 30 S subunit.

Several tetracyclines are known, all of which are very closely related structures produced by streptomyces. They all have identical, broad antibacterial spectra, and development of bacterial resistance to one results in resistance to

Table 5–4. **Inhibitors of Protein Synthesis**

Antibiotic	Ribosomal Subunit Site	Stage of Inhibition
Aminoglycoside aminocyclitols	30 S	Initiation, codon recognition*
Tetracyclines	30 S	Codon recognition
Chloramphenicol	50 S	Transpeptidation
Erythromycin	50 S	Translocation
Lincomycin	50 S	Transpeptidation

*Except spectinomycin and kasugamycin.

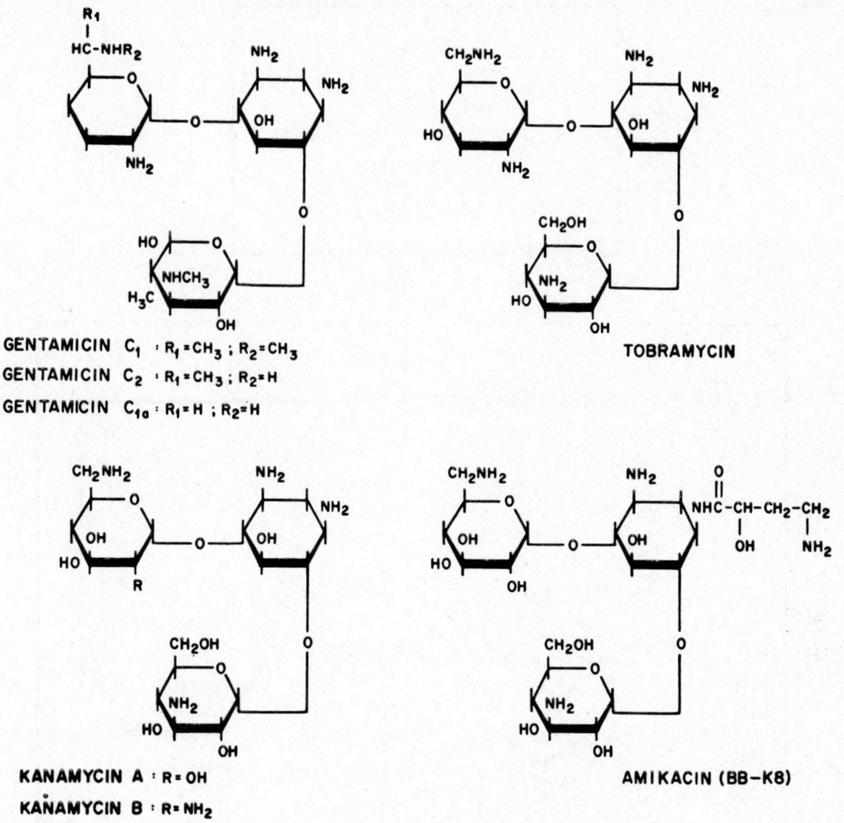

Figure 5–4. Structures of aminoglycoside aminocyclitols. The middle ring compound is the aminocyclitol moiety. (R. C. Moellering[20])

all the tetracyclines. There are, however, some differences in the stability of the various tetracyclines and possible other minor differences in absorption and excretion rates.

Other Inhibitors of Protein Synthesis

Chloramphenicol (see **5–14**) is another bacteriostatic, broad-spectrum antibiotic, but it

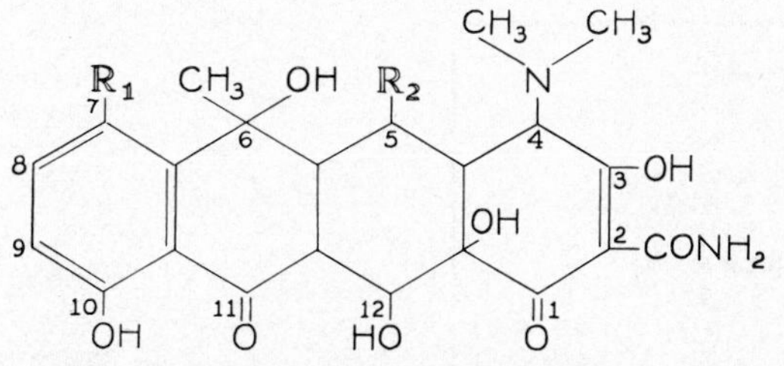

Figure 5–5. Structural formula and numbering system of the tetracycline nucleus. In chlortetracycline R_1 = Cl and R_2 = H; in oxytetracycline, R_1 = H and R_2 = OH; in tetracycline, both R_1 and R_2 = H. Demethylchlortetracycline resembles chlortetracycline but lacks the CH_3 group at C-6. In doxycycline, R_1 = H, R_2 = OH, and H is substituted for the OH at C-6. (Grollman and Grollman.[10])

affects the 50 S rather than the 30 S subunit and inhibits the transpeptidation stage of protein synthesis. Binding to the 50 S subunit is reversible. Although originally isolated as a product of a streptomyces, it is now produced by chemical synthesis. Chloramphenicol may cause serious blood dyscrasias.

Macrolides also act on the 50 S subunit. Erythromycin (see **5–15**) is the most important practical therapeutic agent in this group of antibiotics. Macrolides typically contain large lactone rings (macrolides) linked glycosidically to sugars or dimethylamino sugars. The macrolides are produced by actinomycetes. Erythromycin inhibits the translocation stage of protein synthesis. The macrolides are bacteriostatic at concentrations near the minimum necessary for growth inhibition, but they are bactericidal at tenfold higher concentrations. Gram-positive bacteria are sensitive to macrolides but gram-negatives are insensitive because of impermeability.

Lincomycin (see **5–16**) is another actinomycete antibiotic with an antibacterial spectrum similar to that of the macrolides, but with an

5–14.

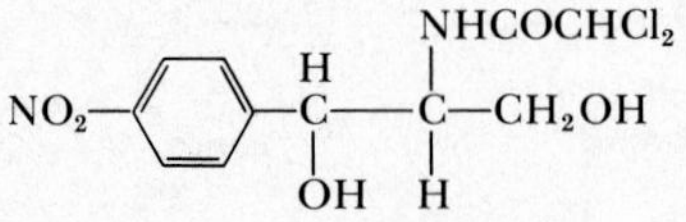

chloramphenicol

5–15.

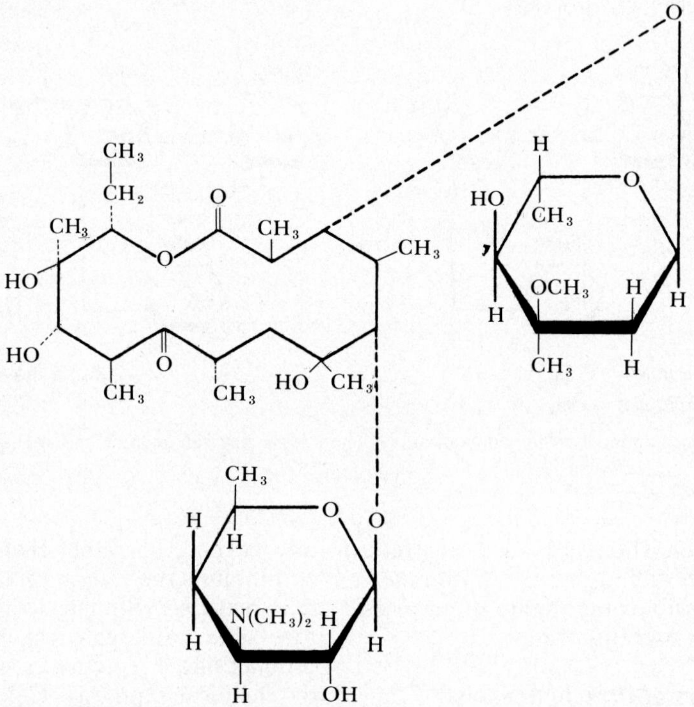

erythromycin

5–16.

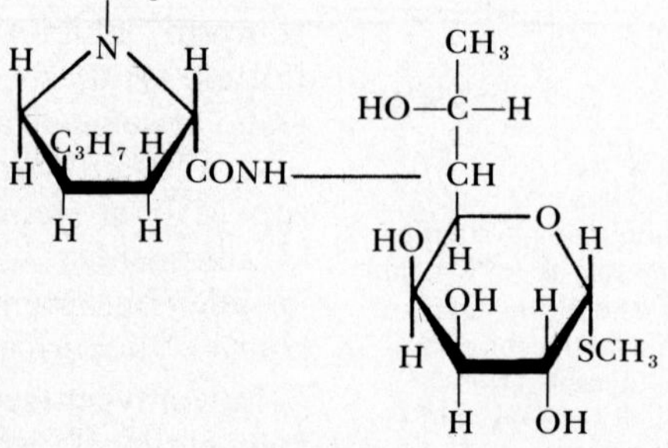

lincomycin

entirely different structure. Lincomycin may act by interference with the attachment of mRNA to ribosomes, by inhibiting initiation, or both. Clindamycin, a clinically useful analogue, is chemically synthesized from lincomycin.

INHIBITORS OF NUCLEIC ACID FUNCTION[7, 9, 26]

Antibiotics are known that inhibit nucleic acid function in one of three ways:

1. Interaction with DNA and sometimes RNA templates, causing interference with transcription or replication.
2. Interaction with polymerases involved in transcription or replication.
3. Some nucleoside antibiotics are analogues of nucleic acid components and interfere with nucleic acid synthesis or are incorporated into a nucleic acid with subsequent alteration of structure and function.

Actinomycin and mitomycin are examples of type 1, rifamycin and streptovaricin are examples of type 2, and cytosine arabinoside is an example of type 3. The only important bacterial chemotherapeutic agents are of type 2 because they are the only ones that are selectively toxic to bacteria.

Rifamycins

These are actinomycete products (see **5–17**). Rifamycin B, the first rifamycin isolated, has no antibacterial activity. However, it is rapidly degraded to rifamycin S, which is a very potent antibiotic and is formed by oxidation and hydrolysis of rifamycin B. Rifamycin S can also easily be reduced to rifamycin SV. Since these antibiotics can not be administered orally, derivatives have been prepared that are orally active and vastly increase the clinical usefulness of the rifamycins. Rifampin is the genetic name used in the United States and rifampicin is the generic name used elsewhere for the most common derivative.

5–17.

Rifamycins

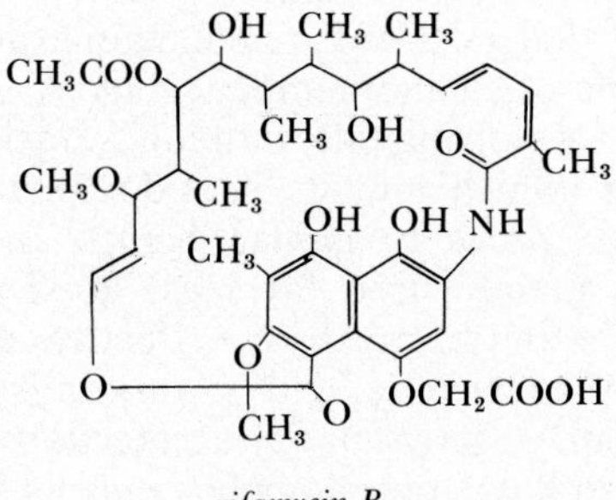

rifamycin B

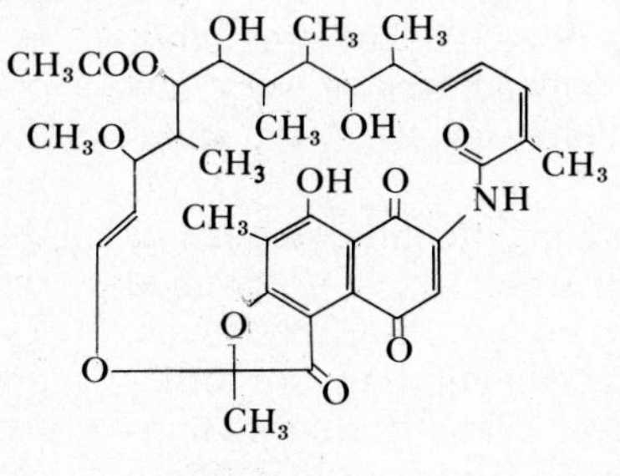

rifamycin S

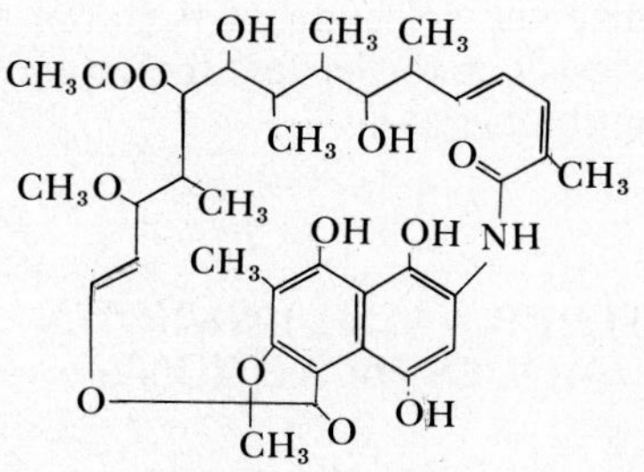

rifamycin SV

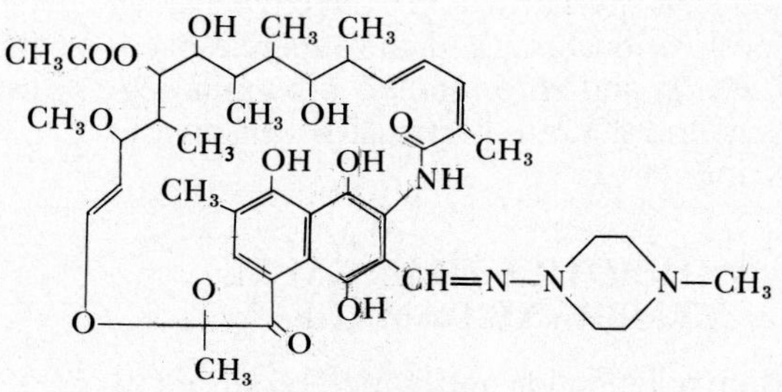

rifampicin

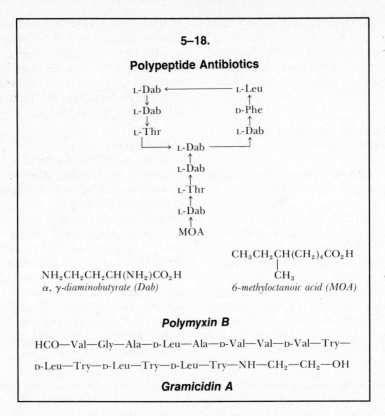

5–18.

Polypeptide Antibiotics

α, γ-diaminobutyrate (Dab)

$NH_2CH_2CH_2CH(NH_2)CO_2H$

6-methyloctanoic acid (MOA)

$CH_3CH_2CH(CH_2)_4CO_2H$
CH_3

Polymyxin B

HCO—Val—Gly—Ala—D-Leu—Ala—D-Val—Val—D-Val—Try—

D-Leu—Try—D-Leu—Try—D-Leu—Try—NH—CH₂—CH₂—OH

Gramicidin A

Rifamycins specifically inhibit DNA-dependent RNA polymerase by blocking the initiation of synthesis of RNA. The drug binds tightly to bacterial polymerases at very low concentrations that have no effect on mammalian polymerases.

The rifamycins contain a naphthoquinone or naphthohydroquinone ring which is spanned by a long aliphatic bridge. Streptovaricins, tolypomycins, and geladanamycin are other antibiotics which have aromatic ring systems spanned by an aliphatic bridge. All of these compounds are called ansa compounds, and it has been proposed that the whole group of antibiotics be called ansamycins. Streptovaricins and tolypomycins also inhibit initiation of RNA polymerization and bind to the same site of the polymerase as does rifamycin.

Rifamycins are particularly effective against gram-positive bacteria and the tubercle bacillus. *Neisseria* and *Haemophilus* are gram-negative bacteria that are particularly sensitive to rifamycins.

barrier. Tyrothricin, which is a mixture of gramicidin (see **5–18**) and tyrocidine, as well as polymyxin (see **5–18**) are the main examples of this type of chemotherapeutic agent. All of the bacterial polypeptide antibiotics, including bacitracin (which inhibits peptidoglycan synthesis), are toxic to human beings and are therefore mainly used for local application. Tyrothricin and bactracin are effective against gram-positive bacteria, and polymyxin is effective in gram-negative bacterial infections. It is common to have topical applications like ointments prepared from a mixture of some of the toxic antibiotics, *e.g.*, bacitracin, polymyxin, and neomycin, to provide a combination with broad-spectrum activity. Utilizing these more toxic antibiotics where their toxic properties are of little consequence to the patient helps to minimize the selection of bacterial strains that are resistant to the less toxic (and more useful) antibiotics.

ANTIBIOTICS THAT CAUSE MEMBRANE DAMAGE[7, 9]

Certain polypeptide antibiotics[3] produced by members of the *Bacillus* genus appear to kill bacteria primarily by damaging the cell membrane and destroying the cell's permeability

OTHERS WITH UNKNOWN MODES OF ACTION[7, 9]

Isoniazid
Isoniazid (isonicotinic acid hydrazide) is effective in treating tuberculosis, but at this time

---

5–19.

Isoniazid and Analogues

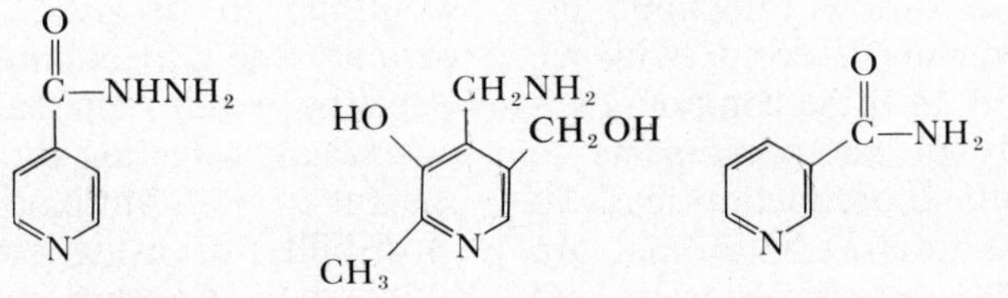

isoniazid   pyridoxamine   nicotinamide

---

the mode of action is not clear. This synthetic drug resembles both nicotinamide and pyridoxamine (see **5–19**). In contrast to the folic acid inhibitors, it is bactericidal. Enzymes that incorporate nicotinamide into nicotinamide adenine dinucleotide can also make the isoniazid analogues (isoniazid also inhibits enzymes that require pyridoxal phosphate as a coenzyme). Whether interference with the function of pyridine nucleotide or pyridoxal phosphate enzymes or both is the cause of isoniazid's lethality is not clear. It may be that the important site of action is still unknown. The reason for the selective action of isoniazid on the tubercle bacillus and not on other bacteria is also unclear.

Nitrofurans and Metronidazole
Furfural and related compounds have long been known to have antibacterial activity. The activity is greatly increased by substitution of a nitro group in the 5-position, and a great many derivatives have been prepared by substitution of various sidechains in the 2-position (see **5–20**). The first of these to show promise as a synthetic chemotherapeutic agent was 5-nitro-2-furaldehyde semicarbazone, or nitrofurazone (Furacin). Other nitrofurans include N-(5-nitro-2-furfurylidene)-1-amino hydantoin, or nitrofurantoin (Furadantin), and N-(5 - nitro - 2 - furfurylidene) - 3 - amino - 3 - oxalolidone, or furazolidone (Furoxone). As a group, these compounds have a broad antimicrobial spectrum, affecting certain fungi and protozoa as well as bacteria. Nitrofurazone has been used as a topical application in man in the therapy of burns, etc. Nitrofurantoin is excreted in the urine following oral administration and is an effective chemotherapeutic agent in urinary tract infections. Furazolidone

---

5–20.

Nitrofurans and Metronidazole

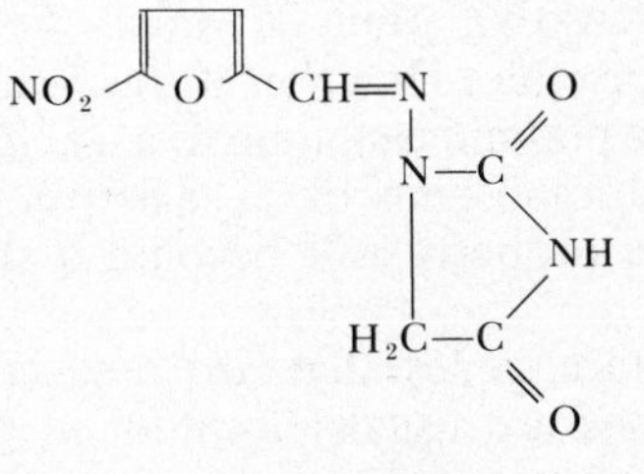

nitrofurantoin

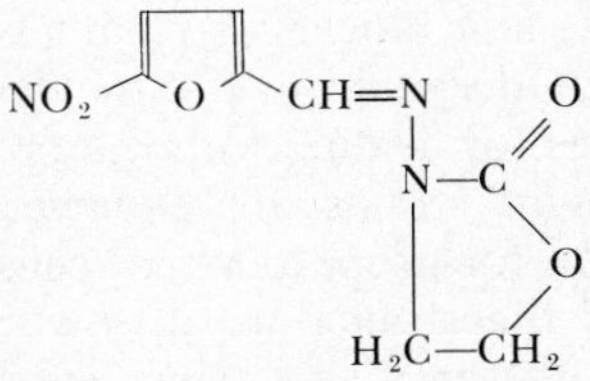

furazolidone

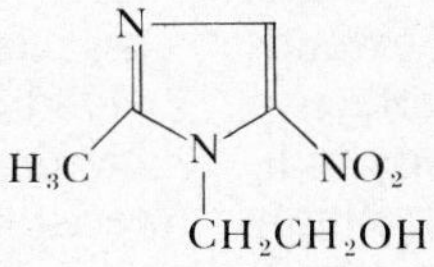

metronidazole

remains in the intestinal tract following oral administration and is used in the treatment of enteric infections of bacterial etiology, such as *Salmonella* and *Shigella,* and is also a trichomonacide. These and other nitrofurans are also used in the therapy of various infectious diseases of domestic animals. Recent evidence suggests that sensitivity to these compounds is related to the ability of microorganisms to reduce the nitro group. Bioreduction leads to formation of reactive intermediates that are believed to interact with deoxyribonucleic acid to inhibit its synthesis or cause lethal mutations. Metronidazole (**5–20**) is a synthetic compound that is extremely effective against parasite infections such as amoebic dysentery and trichomoniasis and against infections caused by anaerobic bacteria,[2] and its mechanism of action is probably similar to that of the nitrofurans.

THE APPLICATION OF CHEMOTHERAPEUTIC AGENTS

Development of Resistance[7, 17]

Soon after the introduction of penicillin, resistant strains of previously sensitive pathogens were isolated from infections. The same story has been repeated every time a new antibiotic has been introduced. Sometimes the emergence of resistant strains follows soon after the introduction of an antibiotic, as was the case with penicillin-resistant staphylococci. However, almost 30 years elapsed after the introduction of penicillin before penicillin-resistant gonococci became significant. The development of resistant strains of bacteria is obviously an extremely important practical problem. Fortunately, studies of the ecology, genetics, and biochemistry of resistance have contributed significantly to the development of strategies for dealing with the problem.

Resistant strains are endowed with genes that code for properties that cause resistance. Even if the strains are in low concentration relative to sensitive strains, resistance will be selected for by the exposure of sensitive strains to chemotherapeutic agents. Therefore, as the use of a chemotherapeutic agent increases, the frequency of occurrence of resistant strains increases. Judicious use of antibiotics extends the length of time they can be used for effective treatment. Using antibiotics without any indication that they might be beneficial simply increases the probability that resistant strains will increase in the environment. Whenever possible, an antibiotic that is effective against strains that are resistant to another antibiotic should be used only when resistance to the latter is encountered. For example, spectinomycin should be reserved for penicillin-resistant strains of gonococci, and penicillin should continue to be used for penicillin-sensitive strains. Using spectinomycin to treat penicillin-sensitive strains increases the probability of eventually selecting for gonococci that are resistant to both antibiotics and eliminating the possibility of using either for treatment of gonorrhea. Another important factor that increases the frequency of resistance is the existence of mechanisms that allow the transport of DNA between bacteria. If the transported DNA codes for a resistance property, a sensitive cell will become resistant when it receives and incorporates the DNA into its own DNA. Resistance properties would be restricted to daughter cells of resistant strains if it were not for the movement of resistance genes between strains.

The most significant features of bacterial genetics that influence transfer of DNA and resistance properties are plasmids and transposons. **Plasmids** are extrachromosal elements composed of DNA that are transported with relative ease between cells of the same species and even between different species and genera. Genes that determine resistance are usually contained in plasmids. **Transposons** are particular sequences of DNA that have the property of being able to move very easily from one DNA element to another, i.e., from plasmid to plasmid, from plasmid to chromosome, and from chromosome to plasmid. Therefore, transposons increase the facility with which resistance genes can be incorporated into the genetic material of sensitive strains. For example, a plasmid in a resistant strain might enter a sensitive strain in which the plasmid itself is unstable. However if the genes on the resistance plasmid can jump to a stable plasmid or the chromosome of a sensitive cell, the resistance property will become a stable entity.

Resistance genes that are associated with transposons are usually located on plasmids. All resistance genes are transferred between cells by direct transfer of plasmids or by bacteriophage vectors. The discovery of plasmid-associated resistance and transposons has provided an explanation for the almost explosive increase in the frequency of occurrence of resistant strains after the introduction of treatment with a variety of agents, *e.g.,* tetracycline, streptomycin, ampicillin, and sulfonamides.

Resistance to only a few antibiotics, *e.g.*, methicillin and rifampicin, is restricted to chromosomal genes. Of those resistance genes that are mainly associated with plasmids, some are not yet known to be associated with transposons, *e.g.*, genes for resistance to cephalosporins and nitrofurantoins. Some resistance genes, such as those for resistance to chloramphenicol, are located in plasmids without any association with transposons and also are found associated with transposons either singly or together with genes that code for resistance to other antibiotics. For example, a multiple resistance transposon is known that is associated with resistance to tetracycline, erythromycin, and chloramphenicol. The practical importance of particular locations of genes and the development of new locations, *e.g.*, from chromosome to plasmid, is influenced by the frequency of use of chemotherapeutic agents and the facility with which genes are transferred between particular resistant and sensitive pathogens.

Resistance genes code for different mechanisms of resistance, depending on the antibiotic, and in some instances, there are different mechanisms for the same antibiotic (Table 5–5). As has already been mentioned, resistance to penicillins and cephalosporins involves the production of β-lactamases that destroy those antibiotics. Enzyme inactivation is also the basis of resistance to most of the aminoglycoside aminocyclitol antibiotics, but here the situation is more complicated. There are different enzyme modifications that can lead to inactivation, including acetylation of amino

groups and phosphorylation and adenylation of hydroxyl groups of the antibiotics. There are actually families of inactivating enzymes that have different spectra of activities against different aminoglycoside aminocyclitols, depending on whether or not the group attacked is present and on the effect of other parts of the different molecules on the ability of a common group to undergo attack. For example, there are three different enzyme groups that acetylate three different hydroxyl groups present in one or another of the aminoglycoside aminocyclitols, and several distinct enzymes are known for each group. Another mechanism of resistance involves decreased ability to transport these antibiotics into the cell. Finally, resistance to streptomycin has also been associated with changes in the structure of the target site of action, the 30 S ribosomal subunit.

Acetylation and permeability changes are two mechanisms that also apply to resistance to chloramphenicol. Methylation of ribosomal RNA is responsible for resistance to macrolide antibiotics, and permeability changes are responsible for resistance to tetracycline. Resistance to sulfonamides and trimethoprim is due to changes in the enzymes that are the targets for these agents. Folic acid synthesis and thymidylate synthesis can then take place even in the presence of sulfonamides and trimethoprim, respectively.

Information about resistance mechanisms provides guidelines for seeking new agents that are not susceptible to these mechanisms. This has already been discussed for the semisyn-

Table 5–5. **Mechanisms of Plasmid- and/or Transposon-Mediated Resistance***

Antibiotic	Resistance Mechanism	Action on Drug
Aminoglycoside aminocyclitols	(a) Enzymatic modification n-acetylation o-phosphorylation o-nucleotidylation (b) Transport block	Direct inactivation
Penicillins and cephalosporins	Enzymatic hydrolysis of β-lactam ring	Direct inactivation
Chloramphenicol	(a) Enzymatic o-acetylation (b) Permeability	Direct inactivation No effect on drug
Erythromycin and lincomycin	Enzymatic methylation of 23 S ribosomal RNA	No effect on drug
Sulfonamides and trimethoprim	Substitute drug-resistant enzyme	No effect on drug
Tetracyclines	Permeability	Drug efflux, energy dependent

*Adapted from Levy.[17]

thetic penicillins and cephalosporins in which antibiotics have been synthesized that are resistant to β-lactamases. Semisynthetic aminoglycosides have also been produced that are less susceptible to enzyme inactivation. Although the emergence of resistant strains is an ongoing problem, the continual effort to develop agents that are active against resistant strains and the judicious use of chemotherapeutic agents help to keep the problem under control.

Assay of Activity[18]

Measurements of the activity of chemotherapeutic agents are performed in either liquid or solid mediums. With liquid mediums, serial twofold dilutions of the agent are prepared in a standard culture medium. The mediums are inoculated with a constant number of bacteria, incubated, and then examined for growth. Activity is measured as the smallest concentration that inhibits growth, which is termed the **minimum inhibitory concentration (MIC).** Assays are carried out on a macro scale in test tubes or on a micro scale in microtiter trays. Wells in the trays usually contain 0.1 ml. of medium with different concentrations of chemotherapeutic agents. They are inoculated with about 5 μl. of a bacterial culture. Automated equipment for filling and inoculation of the trays is available. Completely automated systems are also now available that add liquid medium, antibiotics, and inoculum to growth cuvettes and then automatically monitor growth by turbidometric methods. These new developments in automation should help facilitate the rapid typing of the sensitivity of clinical isolates, which is immensely important for rational therapy.

Assays using solid mediums are performed with either dilution or diffusion of the antimicrobial agent in the medium. Agar is generally the solidifying agent. In principle, dilution tests are similar to dilution tests in liquid mediums. Different dilutions of the agent are added to melted standard agar mediums, which are then solidified in Petri plates. Mechanical replicating devices are available that are used to spot standard volumes (usually 1 μl) of different bacterial cultures to a single Petri plate. A large number of plates with different concentrations and different agents can be inoculated to determine MICs. Diffusion tests are run by inoculating a standard medium in a Petri plate with a single strain. Different concentrations of antimicrobial agents are placed on the plates as impregnated filter paper discs or as solutions placed either in cylinders placed on the solid surface or in wells cut out of the solid medium. During incubation, the agent diffuses into the solid medium as the inoculum begins to grow. If the bacterial strain is sensitive, a zone without growth will appear as a clear area in the diffusion zone that surrounds the point where the agent was applied. The diameter of the zone is related to the concentration of the agent and can be used to quantitate the potency of a compound.

Body Fluids. Measurement of concentrations of chemotherapeutic agents in body fluids is becoming increasingly important. Information about concentrations allows dosages to be varied to provide optimum concentrations in the blood and at the site of infection. Undesirable side effects can be minimized by controlling dosages. Some of the methods for determining the concentration of agents in body fluids are modifications of the procedures used to detect activity against bacteria. Standard strains that are sensitive to particular agents are used, and the inhibitory activity of serum or other body fluids is compared to that of different concentrations of the agent of interest. Agar diffusion, liquid medium tests using microtiter trays, and automatic turbidometric tests are suitable methods for measuring activity against the standard bacterium. A variety of other different kinds of methods are available for measuring concentrations in body fluids. Sensitive chemical tests are used for some compounds, *e.g.,* trimethoprim. A fluorescence quenching method can be used to detect gentamycin. A fluorescent derivative of gentamycin is mixed with a specimen and antigentamycin sera. The antiserum decreases the fluorescence of the derivative. Gentamycin in the specimen binds to the antibody and prevents the decrease in fluorescence in proportion to the amount of nonfluorescent gentamycin in the specimen. Radioimmunoassay techniques are also available for detecting antibiotics. Specific enzyme methods are used for measuring aminoglycoside aminocyclitols and chloramphenicol. These take advantage of the adenylating and acetylating enzymes present in bacteria that are resistant to AGAC and acetylating enzymes in bacteria resistant to chloramphenicol. Either radioactive ATP, the adenylating substrate, or acetyl-CoA, the acetylating substrate, is incubated with the specimen in the presence of a specific enzyme. After incubation, the adenylated or acetylated antibiotic is separated from the mixture and the amount of radioactivity provides a measure of the concentration of the antibiotic in the specimen.

Combined Therapy[15]

In view of the selective action of antimicrobial substances, their administration in combination was inevitable. Theoretically, combinations could broaden the antimicrobial activity of the therapy in the absence of precise diagnosis of the etiological agent and in treatment of mixed infections, could minimize secondary infections occurring during intensive therapy, and could reduce the probability of the development of resistance by the microorganisms.

Despite the theoretical possibilities, combined therapy has been of practical use in only a few special clinical situations. This is probably due to the following: the development of broad-spectrum antibiotics which can be used when precise diagnosis is difficult, the improvement of diagnostic procedures, the interference and antagonism between drugs (see below), and the complexity and vagaries of the development of resistance of bacteria to chemotherapeutic agents. When antibiotics were first introduced, it was thought that the development of resistance would be a simple expression of natural mutation frequencies. Thus, if there is a mutation frequency of 1×10^{-7} for resistance to drug A and a similar mutation frequency for drug B, then the possibility for developing simultaneous resistance to both drugs is 1×10^{-14}. Combined therapy would appear to have the potential of essentially eliminating the development of resistance. In most cases, however, development of resistance is a selection for existing resistant strains in natural populations and not a selection for mutants of a sensitive population.

Until recently, the combination of streptomycin, isoniazid, and p-aminosalicylic acid was routinely used in the treatment of tuberculosis. The disease requires prolonged therapy, which favors the development of bacterial resistance. More potent oral antibiotics, e.g., rifampin, have largely replaced streptomycin, but multiple drug therapy for the treatment of tuberculosis is still recommended.

Synergism and Antagonism. The effect of a combination of two substances on a single species of microorganism can be additive, synergistic, or antagonistic. If the effect of the combination is equal to the sum of the effects of the individual agents, the combined effect is additive. If the sum of the effects is significantly greater than the independent effects, the combined effect is synergistic, and if the sum is significantly less, the combined effect is antagonistic. Figure 5–6 illustrates these effects in a disc diffusion assay with two antibiotics,

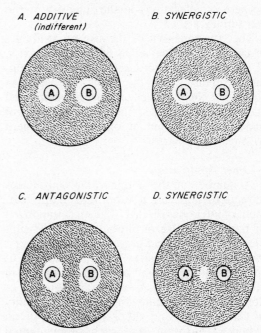

Figure 5–6. Assessment of antimicrobial combinations by the disc diffusion technique. *Shading* indicates bacterial growth, and clear zones around discs indicate inhibition of growth. (D. C. Krogstad and R. C. Moellering.[15] Copyright 1980, the Williams & Wilkins Co., Baltimore.)

labeled A and B, and a single bacterium. Figure 5–6D illustrates a case in which neither drug alone is inhibitory, but the combination produces a zone of inhibition where the two drugs have diffused into the same region.

Synergism against a wide range of bacteria has been demonstrated with the combination of a sulfonamide with trimethoprim. The combination has been extensively used for therapy. The synergistic effect is probably due to the fact that the agents inhibit the synthesis of tetrahydrofolic acid at two different sites. Synergism also occurs when β-lactam antibiotics are combined with β-lactamase inhibitors, e.g., cloxacillin and ampicillin. Cloxacillin is a β-lactamase–inhibiting, semisynthetic penicillin. Synergism occurs only with bacteria that produce β-lactamase. Chloramphenicol acts synergistically with β-lactam antibiotics because it prevents the synthesis of inducible β-lactamases by resistant bacteria. Combinations of cell-wall synthesis inhibitors, e.g., vancomycin and cephalosporins or penicillins, result in synergism presumably because of inhibition of different stages of cell-wall synthesis by the different antibiotics. Cell-wall synthesis inhibitors also act synergistically with aminoglycoside aminocyclitols where the former antibiotic appears to cause increased uptake of the latter because of alterations in the integrity of the cell surface.

The consequences of the use of combined drugs are dependent upon the mode of action of the drugs, the microorganism, and the conditions under which the drugs are used. As with other chemotherapeutic agents, combined agents should be used judiciously to prevent unnecessary enrichment of the environment with resistant strains.

Other Applications

A number of the antimicrobial substances have useful applications other than in the treatment of infectious disease. The most important of these is the use of antibiotics as feed supplements and in food preservation. In the first instance it is established that the inclusion of small amounts (2 to 50 ppm) of antibiotics in animal feeds results in more rapid growth of domestic meat animals, increased hatchability of fertile eggs, and other indications of an enhanced nutrition, and such supplemented feeds are widely used. There is controversy about these nontherapeutic uses of antibiotics because of their potential for contributing to the selection of antibiotic-resistant organisms in the general environment. There is also the possibility of the occasional occurrence of a sensitivity reaction to residual antibiotics in food.

The treatment of freshly dressed meats such as fish and fowl in dilute solutions of broad-spectrum antibiotics has a preservative effect such that they stay fresh appreciably longer, and these substances may have application in food preservation.[29] Chlortetracycline has been approved for this purpose in a concentration of 7 ppm; it is destroyed when the food is cooked.

REFERENCES

1. Ball, A. P. 1982. Clinical uses of penicillins. Lancet **2**:197–199.
2. Bartlett, J. G. 1982. Anti-anaerobic antibacterial agents. Lancet **2**:478–481.
3. Bodanszky, M., and D. Perlman. 1969. Peptide antibiotics. Science **163**:352–358.
4. Block, S. S. 1977. Disinfection, Sterilization, and Preservation. Lea & Febiger, Philadelphia.
5. Doudney, C. O. 1976. Mutation in ultraviolet light-damaged microorganisms. pp. 309–374. In S. Y. Wang (Ed.): Photochemistry and Photobiology of Nucleic Acids, Vol. 2. Academic Press, New York.
6. Farrell, J., and A. Rose. 1967. Temperature effects on microorganisms. Ann. Rev. Microbiol. **21**:101–120.
7. Franklin, T. J., and G. A. Snow. 1981. Biochemistry of Antimicrobial Action. 3rd ed. Chapman and Hall, London.
8. Ginoza, W. 1967. The effects of ionizing radiations on nucleic acids of bacteriophages and bacterial cells. Ann. Rev. Microbiol. **21**:325–368.
9. Goodman, A. G., L. S. Goodman, and A. Gilman. 1980. The Pharmacological Basis of Therapeutics. 6th ed. Macmillan, New York.
10. Grollman, A., and E. F. Grollman. 1970. Pharmacology and Therapeutics. Lea & Febiger, Philadelphia.
11. Harrison, A. P., Jr. 1967. Survival of bacteria. Ann. Rev. Microbiol. **21**:143–152.
12. Hitchings, G. H., and J. J. Burchall. 1965. Inhibition of folate biosynthesis and function as a basis for chemotherapy. Adv. Enzymol. **27**:417–468.
13. Hugo, W. B., and A. D. Russell. 1977. Pharmaceutical Microbiology. Blackwell Scientific Publications, Oxford.
14. Isaacs, A. 1957. Particle counts and infectivity for animal viruses. Adv. Virus Res. **4**:112–158.
15. Krogstad, D. J., and R. C. Moellering. 1980. Combinations of antibiotics, mechanisms of interaction against bacteria. pp. 298–341. In V. Lorian (Ed.): Antibiotics in Laboratory Medicine. Williams & Wilkins Co., Baltimore.
16. Kugers, A. 1982. Chloramphenicol, erythromycin, vancomycin, tetracyclines. Lancet **2**:425–429.
17. Levy, S. B. 1982. Microbial resistance to antibiotics. Lancet **2**:83–88.
18. Lorian, V. 1980. Antibiotics in Laboratory Medicine. Williams & Wilkins, Co., Baltimore.
19. Mazur, P. 1970. The freezing of biological systems. Science **168**:939–949.
20. Moellering, R. C., Jr. 1977. Microbiological considerations in the use of tobramycin and related aminoglycosidic aminocyclitol antibiotics. Med. J. Australia Spec. Suppl. **2**:4–8.
21. Neu, H. C. 1982. Clinical uses of cephalosporins. Lancet **2**:252–255.
22. Osborne, M. J. 1969. Structure and biosynthesis of the bacterial cell wall. Ann. Rev. Biochem. **38**:501–538.
23. Phillips, I. 1982. Aminoglycosides. Lancet **2**:311–314.
24. Reeves, D. 1982. Sulphonamides and trimethoprim. Lancet **2**:370–373.
25. Timm, E. A., et al. 1956. The nature of the formalin inactivation of poliomyelitis virus. J. Immunol. **77**:444–452.
26. Wehrli, W., and M. Staehelin. 1971. Actions of the rifamycins. Bacteriol. Rev. **35**:290–309.
27. Wise, R. 1982. Penicillins and cephalosporins: antimicrobial and pharmacological properties. Lancet **2**:140–143.
28. Witkin, E. M. 1976. Ultraviolet mutagenesis and inducible DNA repair in Escherichia coli. Bacteriol. Rev. **40**:869–907.
29. World Health Organization. 1962. The Public Health Aspects of the Use of Antibiotics in Food and Feedstuffs. Report of an Expert Committee. World Health Organization, Geneva.

6

Gene Expression and Evolution in Bacteria: Genetic and Molecular Bases

Dennis J. Kopecko, Ph.D. and
Louis S. Baron, Ph.D.

For a long period in the history of bacteriology, the idea prevailed that the laws governing inheritance in sexually reproducing organisms were not applicable to bacteria. Bacteria reproduced asexually and possessed no known system of genetic exchange; it was doubted even that they contained a nuclear apparatus. Thus, the fields of bacteriology and genetics went their separate ways, neither seemingly having anything to contribute to the other. But as bacteriologists became increasingly concerned with the problem of explaining the commonly observed variability of bacterial populations, some recognized that the answers had to be found in the same genetic principles which applied in higher organisms. It was

within this framework of thought that the discipline of bacterial genetics originated in the mid-1940s. Despite the facts that bacteria contain no organized nucleus and that they reproduce asexually, some of the basic rules and mechanisms governing gene expression in bacteria have been found to apply directly to more developed organisms. Because bacteria are easy to grow and manipulate, they have served as a major source of molecular genetic studies. Thus, the basic concepts reviewed in this chapter should aid in understanding at a molecular level the various states of more developed cells (*e.g.*, hereditary defects, repressed or induced synthetic pathways).

With the recognition that bacteria possess

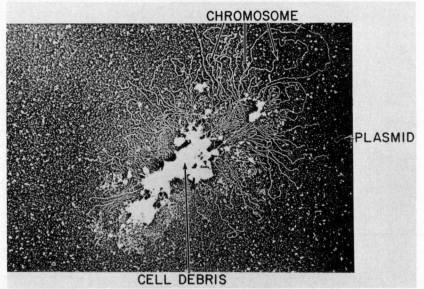

Figure 6–1. The hereditary material of a typical bacterium. Electron micrograph of an *Escherichia coli* cell in the process of being lyzed. The normal rod-shaped cell has spewed out spaghetti-like strands of broken chromosomal DNA from the structural debris of the collapsed cell. Genetic studies have revealed that *E. coli* as well as many other bacteria contain a single large, circular, double-stranded DNA chromosome. In addition to chromosomal hereditary material, many bacteria carry accessory genetic information extrachromosomally. For example, the above *E. coli* cell has released during lysis a small circular extrachromosomal DNA element, or plasmid. Bacteria commonly carry one or more different plasmids, which offer important genetic diversity and evolutionary potential to a cell. (Micrograph courtesy of C. Garon.)

the same hereditary material that exists in higher organisms, and with the discovery and elucidation of bacterial gene transfer mechanisms, the microbe soon became the focus of intensive genetic study (Fig. 6–1). The genetic approach revealed the nature of bacterial variation and provided new knowledge of the capacity for genetic exchange among bacteria, both in the laboratory and in their native habitats. Bacterial systems have provided fundamental knowledge concerning both the chemical nature of genetic information in the cell and the regulatory processes controlling the metabolism of this genetic material. More recently, knowledge of the biochemistry of nucleic acids has been utilized to define the molecular bases of genetic mechanisms in bacteria. On the applied side, genetic analyses have revealed key steps in the pathogenesis of certain bacterial diseases, and genetic manipulations of bacteria have been employed to construct bacterial vaccine strains and to develop industrially useful organisms. Also, the recent recombinant DNA technology, which allows for the specific isolation in bacteria of prokaryotic and eukaryotic DNA segments, represents a momentous practical application of bacterial genetic knowledge. For both bacteriology and genetics, which had seen fit to avoid each other for so many years, the merger has proved most beneficial.

The present chapter will show how gene expression and bacterial evolution are currently understood in terms of their underlying genetic and biochemical mechanisms. With this view, many of the concepts derived from studies in bacterial genetics and its companion science, molecular biology, will be presented. It should be recognized, however, that the presentation of these concepts within a single chapter cannot adequately cover the subject matter of those sciences, and it is not intended to do so. For the interested reader, a comprehensive treatment of these scientific areas and new developments in those fields of study may be obtained in several excellent general reference works and in the more specific publications referred to in sections of this chapter.

The Nature of Bacterial Variation

It has been recognized for many years that the various attributes of any bacterial population—morphological characteristics, biochemical characteristics, antigenic makeup, virulence, and so forth—are subject to change among the members of that population. However, this so-called "variability" of bacterial populations was, for a long time, simply observed and reported; few serious efforts were made to subject it to critical experimentation. Descriptions of bacterial variations as being slow or abrupt, reversible or irreversible, spontaneous or induced were, for the most part, dependent upon the conditions under which the particular variation happened to be observed. Under those circumstances, and in view of the then prevalent belief that bacterial cells contained no genetic apparatus comparable to that of higher organisms, it is not surprising that the underlying causes of these diverse changes remained obscure for many years. Indeed, even after the genetic nature of bacterial variations had been demonstrated, acceptance among some microbiologists came about slowly.

MUTATION

The chance that any given bacterial gene will undergo a spontaneous inheritable alteration (**mutation**) varies, depending upon the gene, the host cell, and the mutational mechanism, from approximately one in every 10^2 to 10^9 bacterial cell generations. Normally, in a population one out of every 10^6 to 10^9 new daughter cells will be mutated in a given gene; however, several recently described mutational mechanisms can lead to higher mutation frequencies under certain circumstances. Inasmuch as bacteria are studied usually as populations and rarely as single cells, it is evident that a single mutant cell will not be detected unless its progeny become a substantial proportion of the population. This situation occurs when the bacteria are placed in an environment which is favorable to a mutant cell that happens to be present, but adverse to the growth of the nonmutant population. The mutant, because of its resistance to the adverse environmental effect, will have a selective advantage over the majority of the population

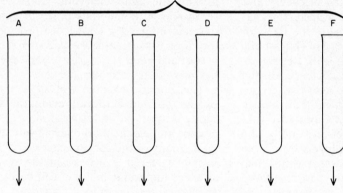

BROTH CULTURES OF VIRUS SENSITIVE BACTERIA

(NUMBER OF COLONIES ARISING ON VIRUS–COATED AGAR MEDIUM)

SAMPLE NUMBER	A	B	C	D	E	F
1	46	30	10	183	57	173
2	56	—	—	—	—	—
3	52	—	—	—	—	—
4	48	—	—	—	—	—
5	44	—	—	—	—	—

Figure 6–2. Fluctuation test, a statistical analysis of *E. coli* mutation to resistance to infection by the bacterial virus T1. Broth cultures were each inoculated with 10^3 cells/ml of virus-susceptible cells and incubated to full growth, *i.e.*, about 5×10^9 cells/ml. Identical small aliquots of each culture were then incubated on virus-coated agar medium to detect the number of resulting virus-resistant bacterial colonies. The fluctuation in number of mutant cells/aliquot was much greater among independent cultures (*i.e.*, tubes B–F) than among multiple samples from the same culture (*i.e.*, tube A). (Data from Luria, S. E., and Delbrück, M., Genetics *28*:491, 1943.)

and will rapidly outgrow it. In liquid culture, the speed with which this population change can come about, often 12–24 hours, is such that many early bacteriologists believed that the cells of the original population had changed or "adapted" in direct response to a new environment; *e.g.*, exposure to streptomycin was thought to cause all of the sensitive cells to adapt and become resistant. The two experimental procedures described below put an end to this line of reasoning and demonstrated that bacterial mutations occur randomly. Today it is understood that the function of such an environment is not to induce a specific mutation, but rather to select for those mutants which occur spontaneously within the population. It should be noted, of course, that induction or repression of an enzymatic process in the presence of substrate or product, respectively, is an entirely separate phenomenon, and it is discussed elsewhere in this chapter.

The Fluctuation Test

The first critical experimental evidence that bacterial mutations occur independently of a selective environment was provided in 1943 by the fluctuation test of Luria and Delbrück.[55] These workers chose for their study the acquisition of resistance to a virulent bacterial virus (see section on transduction later in this chapter for description of virulent bacterial viruses) as the mutable property of the bacterial population. They reasoned that if mutation to virus resistance were a spontaneous event unasso-

ciated with exposure to the virus, then a large number of independent bacterial cultures, each grown from a small inoculum, should show a marked fluctuation in the number of virus-resistant mutants present. In other words, in those cultures in which the mutation occurred early in the growth of the culture, plating of a sample of that culture on virus-coated agar would reveal many mutant cells, whereas, in those cultures in which the mutation occurred late, similar plating would reveal few or no mutant cells. Conversely, if a large number of samples were plated from a single bacterial culture inoculated under similar conditions, the numerical distribution of virus-resistant mutants should be much more homogeneous. Carrying out this test with the bacterium *Escherichia coli*, these are exactly the results which Luria and Delbrück observed (Fig. 6–2). The fluctuation in numbers of mutant cells among the samples plated from the single culture was slight and within the range expected from sampling error; the fluctuation among samples from the independent cultures, however, was as much as several hundred-fold.

Replica Plating

Although furnishing indirect, statistical proof of the spontaneous nature of bacterial mutation, the fluctuation test did have the disadvantage of requiring contact between the bacterial population and the agent (virus) required for selection of the mutation. Some still argued that the agent induced the mutation.

This problem was overcome in 1952 by J. and E. M. Lederberg with a simple but ingenious procedure called replica plating[50] (Fig. 6–3). A bacterial population, growing confluently over the surface of a nutrient agar plate, is pressed gently against a pad of sterile velvet or similar material. The projecting fibers of the velvet act as tiny inoculating needles, sampling the **clones** (*i.e.*, groups of cells that arose from a single cell) making up the cell lawn. If this velvet imprint of the original population is then impressed on virus-coated agar, the existence of any virus-resistant clones on the original, or master, plate will be revealed. Several virus-coated agar plates can be imprinted from the same velvet replica to control the experiment, as virus-resistant clones may appear on these plates as a consequence of mutations which arise shortly after the cells are transferred. However, a virus-resistant **colony** (*i.e.*, physically separate population of cells on solid media) appearing at the same location on each of the replica plates will indicate the position of a virus-resistant colony on the master plate. By carefully picking cells from the indicated location on the master plate, an inoculum enriched in virus-resistant cells may be obtained. Successive respreadings of the progeny of this inoculum on nutrient agar can then be carried out to isolate single, virus-resistant mutant colonies. The significant feature of this procedure is that the cells from the virus-free master plate are always subcultured in virus-free medium, the mutants being isolated from a cell population that is never directly exposed to the virus (also termed bacteriophage). Replica plating thus provides a direct demonstration of the spontaneous occurrence of bacterial mutations in the absence of a selective agent.

EFFECTS OF GENE MUTATION ON THE PHENOTYPE

Certain cellular functions, such as some events involved in DNA replication, RNA and protein synthesis, and cell division, are indispensable for cell survival. Mutations that inactivate any of the genes determining those functions are lethal regardless of the cellular environment. Thus, lethal mutations are, in essence, undetectable and of no use in determining the nature of the affected cell function.

Little of our present knowledge of bacterial genetics would be available were it not for the fact that many bacterial properties and functions are dispensable, that is, not essential for cell survival under appropriate environmental conditions. In addition to growth factor genes, other dispensable functions that have been mutated include genes controlling antigenic makeup, virulence, and susceptibility to viruses or chemicals. Therefore, mutations which affect these properties and functions can be genetically analyzed to study the altered traits. The total genetic complement of a cell is commonly referred to as its **genotype**. In contrast, the observable characteristics of a cell are referred to as its **phenotype** (*e.g.*, lactose nonutilizing or sucrose utilizing). One cannot deduce the cell's genotype without detailed genetic analyses. For example, a mu-

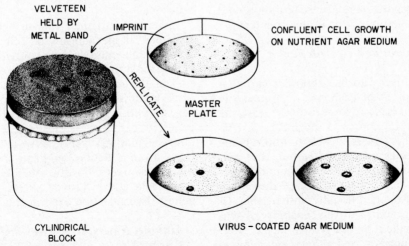

Figure 6–3. Replica plate procedure. Virus-sensitive cells ($\approx 10^5$) were spread onto the surface of nutrient agar medium and grown to a density of $\approx 10^{10}$ cells/plate. Sterile velvet or similar material, firmly attached to the flat end of a cylindrical block, was pressed lightly against the master plate. The inoculated velveteen was then replicated by pressing successively on the surface of two plates of virus-coated agar medium. By marking each plate for orientation (see vertical marks), the resulting virus-resistant mutant colonies appeared in coincident positions on each replica plate.[50]

tated cell which cannot metabolize a compound may be deficient in an intracellular enzyme responsible for degradation of the compound and/or an enzyme required for transport of the compound into the cell. Thus, many different genotypic alterations can be expressed as the same phenotype. Some examples of mutations involving dispensable as well as indispensable functions are described in the following sections with respect to their effect on the bacterial phenotype.

Conditionally Lethal Mutants

The genetic study of indispensable cellular functions was made possible by utilizing conditionally lethal mutations—*i.e.,* genetic alterations that are lethal only under certain conditions. For example, some mutations which affect necessary cell functions cause the mutant protein to be temperature sensitive at elevated temperatures (42° C.; the lethal condition), whereas the affected protein is functional at lower temperatures (30° C.; the permissive condition). Conversely, other mutations which affect indispensable functions have been found that are expressed phenotypically only at lower temperatures; such mutants grow normally at elevated temperatures. Another class of conditionally lethal genetic alterations that have been extremely useful in genetic analyses are termed nonsense mutations. These mutations involve a particular alteration in the genetic code causing premature termination of protein synthesis. There are certain bacterial strains which carry "suppressor" genes that are capable of alleviating the effect of these mutations and allowing continuation of protein synthesis (see sections on nonsense mutations and suppressor mutations later in this chapter).

Carbon Source and Growth Factor Mutants

A cell's capacity to use different carbohydrates as sources of carbon is a dispensable property (provided, of course, that at least one utilizable carbon source is available). *Escherichia coli,* for example, is able to utilize many carbohydrates as sources of carbon, but mutants are obtainable that are phenotypically nonutilizing with respect to any of the carbohydrates. Also conditionally dispensable (if supplied exogenously) is the capability of synthesizing specific required growth factors, *i.e.,* amino acids, purines, pyrimidines, or vitamins. Mutations affecting these essential nutritional properties are called **auxotrophic** (Gr. *auxo,* increased; *trophic,* nutrition), and the mutant

organism is termed an *auxotroph,* as distinguished from the growth factor–independent, wild-type organism, the **prototroph** (Gr. *proto,* original; *trophic,* nutrition). Auxotrophic mutants are recognized by their inability to grow in a chemically defined medium lacking the required growth factor which is not synthesized. Thus, wild-type *Escherichia coli,* which is capable of synthesizing all of its growth factors, will grow in a defined (commonly referred to as minimal) medium consisting of an inorganic nitrogen source, salts, water, and a utilizable carbon source, such as glucose; auxotrophic mutants of *E. coli* will grow in this medium only after addition of the required amino acid, purine, pyrimidine, vitamin, or other supplement.

As described in Chapter 4, the various growth factors are synthesized from elementary precursors by a series of discrete steps, and each of these steps is mediated by a specific enzyme. Therefore, auxotrophic mutations may be further characterized biochemically in terms of the specific enzyme affected in an anabolic or catabolic pathway. Auxotrophs carry out synthesis or degradation up to that step of the pathway which is mediated by the affected enzyme, and thus accumulate this intermediate product. If the next intermediate product in the sequence is supplied exogenously, synthesis/degradation continues along the pathway, and cell growth is resumed. Thus, auxotrophic mutants which are "genetically blocked" at different steps of a biosynthetic pathway can be utilized to yield information regarding the number, order, and nature of the intermediate products and enzymes involved.

In addition to their role in elucidating the biochemical mechanisms of cell metabolism, auxotrophic mutants have provided the necessary tools for our examination of gene function at the molecular level. Genetic analyses of many different auxotrophic mutations have revealed both the existence and the nature of genetic regulatory systems (see section on genetic regulation). Also, as will be discussed later in the section on gene transfer, such mutations make possible the recognition of newly inherited wild-type alleles, or traits, in genetic hybridization experiments.

Mutants Resistant to Virus and Chemicals

Falling also into the category of dispensable cellular functions is resistance to bacteriophages and to inhibitory chemical agents such as streptomycin, chloramphenicol, azide, or nalidixic acid. Generally, these agents are specifically transported into the bacterial cell and affect some essential cellular machinery. Mutation to virus resistance can involve an alteration of the virus receptor site on the bacterial surface, so that the virus is no longer able to adsorb to the cell and inject its DNA. However, it may also involve a change in some internal host mechanism which is essential for the replication of the injected virus genome. Resistance to antimicrobial agents may come about as the consequence of a loss of cell membrane permeability to the agent, or it may reflect a change in the cell's ability to handle the agent internally, *i.e.*, to modify or degrade it chemically. In contrast to the above examples, some mutations can result in increased sensitivity to an environmental condition or chemical compound, and others can render an organism dependent on a particular compound, such as streptomycin. This antibiotic normally inhibits protein synthesis by altering the typical conformation of a ribosomal subunit. Streptomycin-dependent mutations result in altered ribosomes that regain their active conformation in the presence of the antibiotic.

Antigenic Alteration

It is from those bacterial structures external to the cell membrane, *i.e.*, the outer membrane–lipopolysaccharide layer, capsule, pili (fimbriae), and flagella, that the cell derives its antigenic character (Chapter 2). Mutations in the genes governing the biosynthesis of these structures will result in their loss or alteration, and, therefore, in a change in antigenic make-up. The major portion of a cell's antigenic character is accounted for by the outer membrane–lipopolysaccharide layer, which is the site of the somatic antigens. In terms of their chemistry, these antigens have been studied most extensively in the gram-negative bacteria, especially the genus *Salmonella*, whose members exhibit a wide variety of different serological specificities, and whose antigenic specificity resides in the lipopolysaccharide portion of the outer membrane.

The core structure of the *Salmonella* lipopolysaccharide consists of an inner region containing 3-deoxy-D-*manno*-octulosonate, ethanolamine, phosphate, and lipid, and an outer part consisting of short chains comprising glucose, galactose, heptose, phosphate, and *N*-acetylglucosamine (Fig. 6–4). Attached to the short chains of the core (whose structure is common to all members of the genus) are the

long, O-specific side chains composed of repeating oligosaccharide units. The kinds of sugars present in these side chains and their arrangement in the repeating units determine the different O-antigenic specificities among the various *Salmonella* serotypes. Mutations in the genes governing the various steps in the biosynthesis of either the core structure or the attached antigenic side chains can result phenotypically in the loss of the particular O-antigen specificity. Such mutants are termed rough (because of their unusual autoagglutinability in saline and altered colonial morphology), in contrast to the antigen-synthesizing wild-type, which is referred to as smooth due to the homogeneous appearance of its colonies. The use of rough mutants has greatly

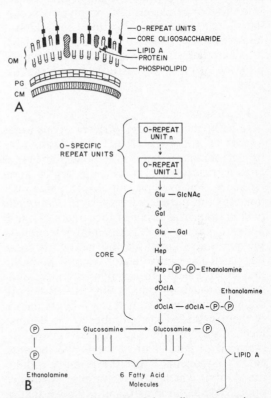

Figure 6–4. Structure of the *Salmonella* outer membrane lipopolysaccharide components. *A*, The location and composition of the outer membrane *(OM)* are shown in relation to the underlying peptidoglycan layer (PG) and the inner cell membrane (CM). *B*, The specific chemical organization of lipid *A*, the oligosaccharide core structure, and the O-specific repeat units are demonstrated. In core biosynthesis from bottom to top, a specific enzyme adds each sugar residue in a $1 \rightarrow 4$ linkage towards lipid *A*. The O-repeat units consist of from two to six sugars in a linear or branched configuration attached to the core in repeating blocks ranging up to 40 repeat units. *Hep*, L-glycero-D-mannoheptose; *dOclA*, 3-deoxy-D-manno-octulosonate (formerly abbreviated KDO); *Glu*, glucose; *Gal*, galactose; *GlcNAc*, , *n* = acetylglucosamine.

facilitated analysis of outer membrane–polysaccharide biosynthesis, illustrating again the potential value of mutations which involve a dispensable cell function. Thus, the outer lipopolysaccharide layer can undergo substantial modification from a variety of mutations (each involving a particular step in its biosynthesis) without affecting the viability of the organism (unlike, for example, the peptidoglycan or murein wall component, whose synthesis is critical for cell survival).

Flagella, pili, and capsules are, of course, dispensable cell surface structures, and their loss as a consequence of mutation also is reflected in the loss of antigenicity which resides in their structure. The loss of flagella, as a consequence of mutation in the genes determining the polypeptide subunits which constitute these appendages, also produces a secondary phenotypic change in the cell, which is loss of motility. However, mutations also occur in genes that affect motility, causing flagellar paralysis without concurrent loss of the flagella.

Virulence

In pathogenic bacteria, virulence constitutes a series of properties, each of which is alterable by gene mutation. Some mutations of the types already described also have an effect upon virulence. For example, an auxotrophic mutation affecting purine biosynthesis in *Salmonella typhimurium* will result in the organism's inability to mount an experimental infection in the peritoneal cavity of the mouse, because this particular growth factor is not supplied in that environment. In a similar manner, antigenically rough mutants of the virulent smooth organism will be avirulent, as a consequence of their increased susceptibility to the defense mechanisms of the host. Clearly, however, synthesis of purines or of the O-specific antigenic components is not the primary cellular function(s) which confers mouse virulence upon *S. typhimurium*. It is now known that *S. typhimurium* cells encode functions that enable them (1) to attach to intestinal epithelial cells, (2) to invade the epithelial mucosa, (3) to disseminate throughout the host's blood and tissues, and (4) to multiply in the host's blood and tissues and cause mouse typhoid. In this case, as with most pathogenic organisms, the chromosomal location and specific nature of those genes directly concerned with the determination of virulence is unknown. However, our ignorance of the number and exact function of the genes involved does not change their susceptibility to mutation.

In theory, virulence should be as amenable to genetic study as any other dispensable cell property. In practice, however, such studies are complicated by a number of factors. Among these are (1) the above-mentioned situation in which the altered gene controls a function which is not primarily involved with virulence but, nevertheless, results in the avirulent phenotype, (2) the polygenic nature of virulence, (3) the availability of a suitable experimental genetic system in the case of the particular pathogen studied, and (4) the availability of inexpensive, quick assays for virulence traits. Despite these problems, genetic studies of bacterial virulence traits have met with some success. For example, the abilities to colonize the surface of the small intestine and to elaborate an enterotoxin are two primary virulence traits, identified by mutation, of both *Vibrio cholerae* and enterotoxigenic *E. coli*. In contrast, dysentery (an invasive intestinal infection limited to the colonic epithelium) is caused by organisms that have the abilities (defined by genetic studies) to attach to, penetrate, and multiple within the colonic mucosa.

THE MOLECULAR BASIS OF MUTATION

The structure of DNA, elegantly deduced by Watson and Crick in 1953, is now well known.[80] Its salient features are two complementary polynucleotide chains, each composed of repeating nucleotide units of four different bases, organized into a regular double helix, as shown in Figure 6–5. The two chains are cross-linked by hydrogen bond base pairing; two bonds between the complementary bases adenine (A) and thymine (T) and three bonds between the complementary bases guanine (G) and cytosine (C). Finally, the stereochemical result of this specific base pair cross linking between DNA strands is that the polynucleotide chains run in opposite directions with respect to the sugar-phosphate linkages within each chain (Fig. 6–5).

Genetic information, stored in DNA, is transcribed into messenger RNA (mRNA), ribosomal RNA (rRNA) and amino acid–carrying transfer RNAs (tRNAs). Messenger RNA molecules are then translated into proteins (Fig. 6–6). Genetic information is encoded in the sequence of the nucleotides in the DNA molecule, every three successive nucleotides providing the "code" for a single amino acid (see Table 6–1). Thus, a **gene** may be defined in molecular terms as a specific segment of the DNA molecule in which the nucleotide base sequence determines: (1) the synthesis of a rRNA or tRNA molecule, (2) a functionally active site on DNA, or (3) the amino acid sequence of a polypeptide chain. As an average polypeptide is generally composed of 200 to 600 amino acids, each encoded by a three-base sequence, it follows that the determining gene will contain from 600 to 1800 nucleotides. On the other hand, tRNA molecules range from 80 to 100 nucleotides in size, and some regulatory sites on DNA are only 20 base pairs in length. Through the intensive study of many types of different mutations, geneticists have developed our present concepts of the molecular bases of mutation and the organization of information in DNA.

Having defined the gene in molecular terms, it is now possible to define mutation as any alteration in DNA nucleotide sequence. These alterations in double-stranded DNA may be grouped into three categories: (1) those which involve insertion of an additional base pair or pairs into the normal DNA base pair sequence; (2) those which result in a deletion of one or more base pairs from the normal sequence; and (3) those in which a substitution of one base pair for another occurs. Despite their normal low frequency of spontaneous occurrence, most mutations can be induced at a relatively high frequency by chemical or physical agents (see section on induction of mutation).

Base Pair Substitution

The transcription of genetic information by RNA polymerase to form an RNA message occurs along one strand of the DNA molecule. The base sequence of this polyribonucleotide message is determined by and is complementary to the corresponding DNA base sequence, except that RNA contains the base uracil in place of thymine. Transcription can take place on both DNA strands, but for any given gene only one strand is transcribed and RNA chain elongation proceeds in the 5' to 3' direction. Each group of three successive messenger RNA bases forms a codon, defined as the genetic code for a specific amino acid (Table

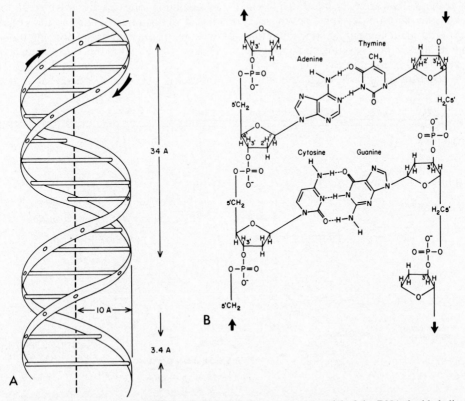

Figure 6–5. The stereochemical structure of bacterial DNA. *A,* Diagrammatic model of the DNA double helix. Bacterial DNA is composed of two polynucleotide chains organized in a regular, right-handed, double helix, with a diameter of 20°A. There are ten base pairs for each turn of the helix, which corresponds to a length of 34°A. *B,* Segment of a DNA duplex showing the antiparallel nature of the complementary chains. The stereochemical consequence of hydrogen bond base pairing between adenine and thymine or between guanine and cytosine is that the two chains must run in opposite directions with respect to the 3' → 5' sugar-phosphate linkages within each chain.

Table 6–1. **Degeneracy of the Genetic Code**

5′ End	Middle Nucleotide				3′ End
	U	**C**	**A**	**G**	
U	phe	ser	tyr	cys	U
	phe	ser	tyr	cys	C
	leu	ser	TERM	TERM	A
	leu	ser	TERM	trp	G
C	leu	pro	his	arg	U
	leu	pro	his	arg	C
	leu	pro	gln	arg	A
	leu	pro	gln	arg	G
A	ile	thr	asn	ser	U
	ile	thr	asn	ser	C
	ile	thr	lys	arg	A
	met	thr	lys	arg	G
G	val	ala	asp	gly	U
	val	ala	asp	gly	C
	val	ala	glu	gly	A
	val	ala	glu	gly	G

The 64 possible triplet ribonucleotide codons. Each of the 20 amino acids specified is listed by the appropriate codon. Abbreviations for the amino acids correspond to those currently used in *E. coli* genetic nomenclature.[6] The codons UAA, UAG, and UGA, signals for the termination of polypeptide chain elongation (labeled TERM), are now referred to as terminator codons. Although these codons were identified mainly in *E. coli,* they appear to apply universally to most organisms. However, some animal mitochondrial DNA's have recently been determined to have quite different genetic codes. Degeneracy in the code (*i.e.,* the use of 61 codons to encode 20 amino acids) allows for the occurrence of viable mutations and the sequential selection of increasingly useful proteins (*i.e.,* evolution).

6–1). As these codons are translated in a linear fashion on the ribosomes, they result in a linear, ordered arrangement of specific amino acids linked into a polypeptide chain by the protein synthesizing machinery (Fig. 6–6). A base pair substitution in DNA has the effect of changing one of the mRNA codon bases that it determines. Thus, as the consequence of substituting cytosine for guanine in the DNA triplet TAG, the normal corresponding RNA codon AUC becomes AUG, and methionine will replace isoleucine at that point in

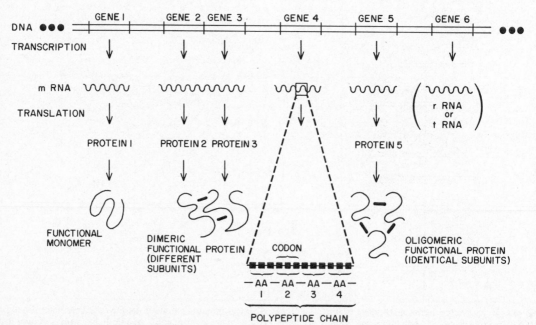

Figure 6–6. Schematic diagram of the flow of genetic information from DNA to RNA to protein. Transcription of the encoded DNA generates mRNA, tRNA, or rRNA. Resulting mRNA is then translated into amino acids (AA), which are linked tgoether into polypeptide chains (Modified from Davis, Dulbecco, Eisen, Ginsberg, and Wood's "Microbiology-3rd Ed.", p. 185, 1980, with permission).

the peptide chain. Substitution mutations are called transitions when a purine (A or G) is replaced by a different purine, or a pyrimidine (T or C) by the opposite pyrimidine; they are called transversions when a purine is replaced by a pyrimidine, and vice versa.

A single base pair substitution can change the consequent amino acid and result in a functionally altered protein, as happens, for example, in sickle cell anemia. However, base pair substitutions cannot always be detected. For instance, there are many places in a polypeptide chain in which one amino acid may be substituted for another without any loss of biological function. Also, the genetic code is redundant or degenerate (*i.e.*, in many instances two or more codons determine the same amino acid) and an altered codon may yield the same amino acid as the wild type codon. Nevertheless, when loss of biological activity does occur as a consequence of base pair substitution, it can be restored simply by a reverse mutation resulting in the wild-type codon sequence. However, reversion to the original phenotype does not always require restoration of the original genotype. For example, a substitution at the same codon site, but involving a different base from that in the wild type (AUC) or the initial mutant (AUG) may result in an alternate codon (AUU) for the wild-type amino acid, or it may specify a new, but functionally equivalent amino acid. Additionally, restoration of the original phenotype may result from a suppressor mutation (see below), which affects a genetic site other than that of the primary mutation and cancels the effect of the primary mutation.

Frame-Shift Mutations[68]

Mutations can occur by the insertion or the deletion of a DNA base pair or pairs. When such insertion or deletion mutations involve changes unequal to multiples of three base pairs, the normal reading frame of the triplet RNA codons is shifted from the point of the mutation. Hence, all the following codons in that message are changed, and such mutants are termed "frame-shift." For example, if a wild-type RNA message is transcribed and translated in the order

DNA Sequence   3'. . . Ⓣ C A G G T A G T G A A T T A . . . 5'

RNA Sequence   5'. . . A G U C C A U C A C U U A A U . . . 3'

Polypeptide Product   . . . Ser — Pro — Ser — Leu — Asn . . .
(Wild–Type)

deletion of the circled DNA base would result in a RNA message lacking the initial adenine

(see below). The mRNA triplet codon reading frame will shift one nucleotide rightward causing a new translational product.

Altered
RNA Sequence   5'. . . G U C C A U C A C U U A A U . . . 3'
                          ↑ deleted base

Polypeptide Product   . . . Val — His — His — Leu — Ile . . .
                                                          or
                                                          Met

The effect of a base pair deletion may be counteracted by a base pair insertion, and vice versa. Thus, in the example above, a second mutation resulting in the insertion of an additional base, say guanine, immediately following the first mutant codon (GUC) will subsequently restore the original reading order to the message

Restored
RNA Sequence   5'. . . G U C G C A U C A C U U A A U . . . 3'
                              ↑ inserted base

Polypeptide Product   . . . Val — Ala — Ser — Leu — Asn . . .

If, as in this example, only one or two codons remain changed, the resulting protein may retain its biological activity despite the replaced amino acids. A secondary insertion or deletion mutation within the mutant gene which thus compensates for a primary frame-shift mutation is referred to as an intragenic suppressor. Recently, mutations have been described that lie outside of the affected genes and can effectively suppress several different primary frame-shift mutations (see section on suppressor mutations).

It should be noted that, in certain instances, frame-shift mutations can affect the expression of adjacent genes. As described in a later section on genetic regulation, clusters of related genes are often transcribed as single units. Thus, if three genes are unidirectionally transcribed on a single messenger RNA, a frame-shift mutation at the beginning of the first gene could cause the production of three nonfunctional proteins (*i.e.*, the mutation would exert a polar effect on more distal genes in a coordinately transcribed unit).

Mutations can arise by the addition or deletion of multiples of three base pairs. Though not considered frame-shift mutations, these alterations would result in the addition or deletion of one or more amino acids to a protein, which may or may not affect protein function. Deletion as well as insertion mutations may also involve a large number of base pairs. Sometimes, hundreds of nucleotides may be deleted or added and, in some cases, numerous genes may be lost or gained. Following such large deletions, reverse mutations to the normal nucleotide arrangement are virtually impossible and the original gene function cannot be restored by suppressor mechanisms.

Nonsense Mutations[25]

Generally, the effect of both substitution and frame-shift mutations is to produce altered codons which are translated into amino acids different from those of the wild type. This type of codon alteration is referred to as a missense mutation. Three codons, UAG, UAA, and UGA, have been found which are not translated into any amino acid, but, instead, cause termination of polypeptide chain elongation, and release of the incomplete polypeptide from the ribosome. These codons are referred to as termination or nonsense codons, and mutations which produce them are called nonsense mutations. Before the nature of these mutations was understood they were assigned the names amber (now known to produce the UAG codon) and ochre (mutations producing the codon UAA), and these names have remained in use. There is no corresponding name for the UGA codon. Mutations resulting from a base pair substitution that creates a termination codon usually cause a moderate decrease in the expression of distal genes. These mutations can revert to wild type or can be suppressed by secondary mutations, as discussed below.

Besides their appearance in those mutations causing premature termination of polypeptide chain elongation, the UAG, UAA, and UGA codons appear to exist in the wild-type organism as its normal mechanism for polypeptide chain termination. They do not stimulate the binding of any transfer RNA, but appear to be read by specific proteins termed release factors. Thus, terminator codons are protein synthesis (*i.e.,* translational) "stop" signals.

Suppressor Mutations

There are several mutational mechanisms which may compensate for the presence of an altered codon, or codons, resulting from a primary mutation. These suppressor mutations are classed as intragenic when they occur at a different site within the same gene and extragenic when they occur in a different gene. The restorative effect of one type of intragenic suppressor mutation, namely, a base pair insertion or deletion near the site of a primary frame-shift mutation, was described above. Intragenic suppression may also occur as the consequence of a second missense mutation in the same gene, when the appearance of a second missense amino acid in the polypeptide restores, in some way, the original stereochemical configuration around the functional part of the molecule.

Unlike the intragenic suppressors, extragenic suppressor mutations do not work by altering mRNA codons; instead, they change the way these codons are read by the cell's translation machinery. They affect the amino acid or anticodon specificity of transfer RNA (tRNA) molecules. For example, instead of a wild-type tRNA translating the primary mutant codon with a missense amino acid, the secondary (or suppressor) mutant may encode a suppressor tRNA that now carries a different amino acid, but one which is functionally "correct" for that place in the polypeptide. Such a mutant tRNA, however, will be carrying the "wrong" amino acid for all of the cell's wild-type codons that are similar to the suppressible mutant codon. It follows, therefore, that suppression generally results in a low level of gene expression. This mechanism must operate with low efficiency because the suppression of large numbers of wild-type codons would be lethal. Certain mutant minor tRNA species, however, are highly efficient suppressors, but are nonlethal because their corresponding wild-type codon does not occur very often in mRNA. Although one can easily see how extragenic suppression of both missense and nonsense mutations occurs, extragenic frame-shift suppressors were thought to be nonexistent. Recently, however, mutant tRNAs that suppress frame-shift mutations have been isolated and characterized. These tRNA mutants were found to contain an extra nucleotide in the anticodon and to suppress only insertion mutations.

Mutations Caused By Transposable Elements[44, 77]

The mutations described above result from nucleotide changes of from one to a few base pairs and can be induced by chemical and physical agents, as described in the next section. However, until fairly recently there were no experimental facts through which the insertion, deletion, inversion, or transposition of relatively large DNA segments could be explained. Yet these large chromosomal rearrangements often occur at frequencies higher than smaller mutations. Evidence obtained over the past 10 years has revealed a group of elements, termed transposable elements, that appear to be responsible for many of these large DNA rearrangements. **Transposable elements** are discrete multinucleotide DNA units that do not exist in a physically autonomous state but rather are normal constituents of the bacterial **genome** (*i.e.,* the total genetic makeup of bacteria including the chromosome, plasmids, and viruses). Transposable elements fall into two classes: (1) **insertion sequence** (*IS*) elements, which vary in size from 750 to approximately 2000 base pairs in length and do not encode any phenotypically detectable properties, and (2) large transposable elements, known as **transposons** (abbreviated Tn's), which range from 2000 to as large as 80,000 base pairs (*i.e.,* comparable in size to 2 per cent of the *E. coli* chromosome) and which encode phenotypically identifiable traits such as genes specifying antibiotic resistance. All transposable elements consist of a central group of sequences bracketed by inverted repeat DNA termini (Fig. 6–7). These terminal DNA sequences are recognized by specialized recombination enzymes, as described in a later section on specialized recombination systems, which mediate the transposition, inversion, or deletion events. Mutations caused by transposable elements result from specialized recombination events and are not the typical consequence (*i.e.,* small nucleotide alteration) of chemical or physical mutagenic agents on DNA metabolism.

Transposable elements were first detected following their spontaneous transposition as discrete units to different positions in the same chromosome or to another chromosome. The resulting insertion often produced a strongly polar mutation or resulted in the acquisition of a new phenotype (*e.g.,* antibiotic resistance). Further studies have revealed at least five different *IS* elements (*IS1* · · · *IS5*) in the *E. coli* chromosome, some of which exist as multiple copies per chromosome and which together comprise 1 to 2 per cent of the total chromosomal DNA. Besides the involvement of *IS* elements in insertion mutations, *IS* units can promote specific multinucleotide deletions immediately adjacent to their insertion site. Also, identical *IS* units can cause the specific inversion, deletion, or transposition of any chromosomal sequence that they bracket. Larger transposable elements, which were first detected on bacterial plasmids, have also been detected on bacterial chromosomes and appear to carry out the same DNA rearrangements as the smaller *IS* elements. Certain Tn's encode the enzymatic machinery for their own transposition and some are bracketed by the simple *IS* units at their termini; thus, the larger Tn's appear to be structurally and evolutionarily more complex than the simpler *IS* units. The most complex bacterial Tn characterized to date is bacteriophage Mu, which is a 25-megadalton DNA molecule that has inverted repeat termini and can behave as a complex Tn or can exist as a virus. Functionally similar *IS* and Tn units have been found in other gram-negative and gram-positive bacteria as well as in several eucaryotic systems; these elements appear to be heavily involved in the evolution of these genomes.

Why are transposable elements so impor-

TRANSPOSABLE DNA ELEMENT

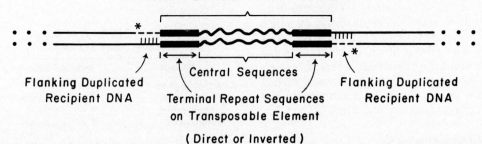

Flanking Duplicated
Recipient DNA

Central Sequences

Terminal Repeat Sequences
on Transposable Element

Flanking Duplicated
Recipient DNA

(Direct or Inverted)

Figure 6–7. The structure of transposable elements. This unscaled diagram illustrates a transposable DNA element, which is delineated by the rectangles and wavy line, inserted within a recipient molecular DNA sequence, which is depicted by the thin continuous or broken lines. Both *IS* elements and the larger *Tn* units are composed of a central DNA segment (wavy line) flanked by terminal sequences (rectangles) that are repeated in either direct or inverted order. However, all transposable elements contain short inverted repeat sequences at their ends. Apparently, during insertion, staggered single-strand cleavage occurs at the sites marked by the asterisks, and the extended single-strand ends of the recipient molecule are joined to the transposable element. Subsequent gap-filling DNA synthesis (broken lines) and ligation create duplicated recipient molecular sequences at the ends of the inserted transposable element (From Kopecko, D. J., Specialized Genetic Recombination Systems in Bacteria: their involvement in gene expression and evolution. *In* F. Hahn (Ed.), Progress in Molecular and Subcellular Biology, Vol. 7, Springer-Verlag Press, Heidelberg, 1980, pp. 135–234, with permission.)

tant? First, the transposition process does not involve loss of the donor DNA sequences, but rather duplication and transposition of a copy of these sequences to a new site (see later section on specialized recombination). Thus, this process offers a means of disseminating blocks of genes from one chromosome to another or from one site to another. Second, mutations caused by transposable elements occur at frequencies ranging from 10^{-2} to 10^{-7}; *i.e.*, these large DNA rearrangements can occur at frequencies 10,000-fold higher than smaller mutations. It is now thought that transposable elements promote a major fraction of all spontaneous mutations in bacteria. In addition to mediating these functions, discrete *IS*-like, invertible DNA segments have been shown to act as novel regulatory switches that can control operon expression (see section on other types of bacterial variation and their regulation). Finally, in contrast to small mutations, which usually affect one or a few genes, transposable elements mediate the insertion, deletion, or inversion of large DNA segments that can encode hundreds of genes. Thus, transposable elements appear to be heavily involved in bacterial evolution. There have been several recent reviews of this topic.[10, 43, 44, 71, 77]

THE INDUCTION OF MUTATION[19, 20, 35]

The usefulness of mutants in genetic and molecular analyses of bacteria has stimulated much research on defining the different kinds of mutations (described in the previous section). In addition, considerable effort has been made to understand the mechanisms by which mutagenic agents (mutagens) promote DNA changes. The mutagenic mechanisms of some agents commonly employed in the laboratory are discussed below, as well as those of certain metabolic events likely to contribute to the normal spontaneous mutation rate in bacteria.

Chemical Mutagenesis
Knowledge of the molecular basis of gene mutation has come about mainly through studies of the mutagenic effects of certain groups of chemicals, which are known to interact in specific ways with the purine and pyrimidine bases of DNA. For example, chemicals that are close analogues of normal nucleic acid bases can become incorporated into DNA during replication. Two potent mutagens among

the base analogues are 5-bromouracil, an analogue of thymine, and 2-aminopurine, which is similar to adenine. As 5-bromouracil sometimes pairs with guanine instead of with adenine, and 2-aminopurine can pair also with cytosine instead of thymine, the effect of both base analogues (once incorporated) is to produce on subsequent rounds of replication base pair transitions of AT→GC and TA→CG.

Unlike the base analogues whose action depends upon their incorporation into replicating DNA, some chemical mutagens act directly on resting DNA to alter its bases. Nitrous acid, for example, acts by oxidatively deaminating adenine to hypoxanthine (which pairs with cytosine rather than thymine) and by deaminating cytosine to uracil (which pairs with adenine). Thus, nitrous acid produces AT↔GC and TA↔CG base pair transitions. Other chemical mutagens, such as the alkylating agent ethyl ethanesulfonate, act to alkylate a DNA base—in this instance, guanine. Mutagenesis takes place by direct mispairing of the alkylated guanine with any of the other three nucleotide bases, producing both transitions and transversions (Table 6–2).

Acridine dyes, such as proflavin and 5-amino acridine, produce mutants of the frame-shift type.[19] These mutants revert spontaneously, and their reversion at a higher rate can be induced by acridine dyes, but never by base analogues or nitrous acid. Reversions of acridine dye–induced mutations are usually the consequence of second site mutations within the same gene. The insertion or deletion of DNA bases by acridine dyes is apparently related to their ability to intercalate between these bases. Thus, as depicted below, the in-

Table 6–2. **Effects of Some Common Mutagens on DNA**

Mutagen	Induced DNA Alteration
Chemical Agents	
5-Bromouracil	T → C transition
2-Aminopurine	A → G transition
Nitrous acid	A → G transition
	C → T transition
Ethyl ethanesulfonate	Transition or transversion
Mn^{++}	Transition or transversion
Acridine dyes	Frame-shift
Physical Agents	
Ultraviolet irradiation	Frame-shift, transversion
	C → T transition,
	deletion
Visible light	Transition, transversion,
	frame-shift
Heat	Transition or transversion

tercalation of an acridine molecule between two adjacent bases of the template strand will produce during DNA replication a gap at that point in the new strand, which may be filled by the insertion of an extra base. Occasionally,

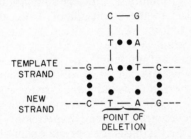

base mispairing occurs in a DNA molecule, creating a looped-out region in the template strand. Complementary strand synthesis on a template with a looped-out region would result in a base pair deletion.

The divalent cation, Mn^{++}, is strongly mutagenic in bacteria, producing both transitions and transversions. Since Mn^{++} can induce DNA polymerase to make errors *in vitro,* it has been proposed that the mutagenic effect of this cation is exerted during DNA polymerization.[19]

Radiation and Heat as Mutagens

Due to their relative specificity and ready availability, chemical mutagens have tended to replace radiation for routine investigational mutagenesis (Table 6–2). Nonetheless, ultraviolet (UV) mutagenesis has been used to reveal key steps in DNA repair, recombination, and replication processes. In addition, heat and visible light have been found to possess mutagenic abilities.

Ionizing radiations, such as x-rays, cause both single- and double-strand DNA breaks and are a source of mutations, but little is understood of the mutagenic mechanisms of these radiations. In contrast, many of the chemical alterations induced by exposure of bacteria to nonionizing radiation, such as UV light, have been studied. UV light causes frame-shift mutations, the transition C→T, transversions, and deletions. Chemical changes resulting from UV irradiation involve the pyrimidine bases, which become hydrated at their 4:5 double bonds, cytosine being more susceptible than thymine nucleotides. Apparently, the hydration of cytosine alters its pairing affinity, resulting in the C→T transition. A second UV-induced effect is the formation of pyrimidine dimers (*i.e.,* a cyclobutane ring formed between adjacent pyrimidines within the same DNA strand). Thymine-thymine di-

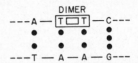

mers appear most often, although dimers of other combinations of pyrimidines are also observed. Frame-shift mutations seem likely to be an indirect consequence of pyrimidine dimer formation. During excision repair of DNA containing pyrimidine dimers (see section on DNA repair), single-strand gaps are created. Mutations are thought to be produced by the aberrant repair of these gaps, a general phenomenon now termed **misrepair mutagenesis**. Unlike mutagens that induce specific DNA alterations, such as a specific transition, agents that cause misrepair ultimately produce a variety of mutational types including transitions, transversions, frame-shifts, and deletions.

Intense visible light can be lethal or mutagenic—inducing transitions, transversions, and frame-shift mutations. This light-induced activity has been termed photodynamic mutagenesis and its effectiveness is enhanced by the presence of certain dyes, such as methylene blue or psoralen. The fact that many pyrimidine dimers are formed during exposure to intense visible light indicates that mutant formation may result from misrepair mechanisms.[19]

Although mutation frequencies have been observed to vary at different temperatures, until recently these effects were assumed to have arisen from disturbances of normal DNA repair and replication enzymes. However, heat is now known to cause mutations. At 0° C., mutations have been found to develop in free bacterial virus particles, and the mutation frequency greatly increases at 37° C. and above. Both heat-induced transitions and transversions have been observed, but only GC base pairs seem to be affected. Despite the fact that heat mutagenesis has received little attention to date, it appears to be an important phenomenon.

Spontaneous Mutation

Somewhat of a misnomer, this term serves to cover our present ignorance of the specific causes of mutations that occur in the absence of any known mutagenic agent(s). The frequency of spontaneous mutation (usually one in 10^6 to 10^9 cells for mutation in almost any specific gene) can be affected by environmental conditions (*e.g.*, heat, light, growth medium), by the genetic composition of the bacterial host, as well as by mutagenic products or intermediates of cell metabolism. Errors introduced into DNA during faulty replication or recombination events, if improperly repaired, are also mutagenic. These errors in normal DNA metabolism probably account for many of the mutants observed at this low frequency level. However, as mentioned previously and discussed further in the section on recombination, *IS* elements and other discrete transposable DNA units can promote insertion, deletion, or inversion mutations, sometimes at frequencies as high as one per 10^2 cells. Recent studies of enterobacteria indicate that *IS* elements exist in multiple copies in the chromosome and comprise anywhere from 1 to 5 per cent of the total chromosomal DNA. It now appears that *IS* units and other transposable DNA segments cause a significant fraction of all spontaneous mutations in bacteria.[44, 77]

Initially observed in *Salmonella typhimurium,* mutations in specific genetic loci termed "mutator" genes have been shown to increase the spontaneous mutation rate of many genes by as much as 100,000-fold.[15] The original *Salmonella* **mutator locus** affects a gene that normally codes for the synthesis of a purine base, but in the mutant state determines the synthesis of a mutagenic base analogue that at high frequency subsequently causes transition mutations. At present, in *E. coli* K-12, more than six separate mutant genes exist that exhibit various degrees of mutator activity. Some of these mutator genes cause an increased frequency of transversion and others result in increased frequencies of both transition and frame-shift mutations, while one gene, *mutD*, increases the frequencies of formation of all mutant types. Oddly, besides increasing the frequencies of specific mutant types, some mutator genes actually cause a decrease in the frequencies of other mutant types (*i.e.*, have antimutator activity). Other mutations in *E. coli* that result in an increased mutation rate are known to affect the genes determining DNA adenine methylation, and DNA polymerases I, II, and III. In bacteriophage T4, mutator and antimutator activities have been shown to result from mutations in the phage genes coding for DNA polymerase or DNA unwinding protein, strengthening the argument that an increased mutation rate occurs by the introduction of copy errors during DNA synthesis.[15] Mutations produced by mechanisms that are similar, if not identical, to those described above must certainly account for a large proportion of spontaneous genetic alterations in bacteria.

GENETIC REGULATION

Before the mutational nature of bacterial variation was understood, some viewed population variability as a direct adaptation of the organism to the environment. Ironically, this interpretation was reinforced by the finding that certain enzymes are, in fact, synthesized in significant amounts only in the presence of their substrate. The study of this phenomenon, now referred to as inducible enzyme synthesis, has led to our present conceptualization of the genetic control of gene expression. Besides providing the basis for our understanding of a wide variety of inducible bacterial enzyme systems, these concepts have also furnished us a means for comprehending—in terms of genetic and molecular mechanisms—certain bacterial variations which are not explainable by mutation or inducible enzyme synthesis.

Obviously, a cell would self-destruct if it could not regulate both genetic transcription and translation so that sufficient but not excessive quantities of many different proteins are made at the required time. When one considers that, for example, the *E. coli* chromosome codes for 4000 ± 1000 proteins, most of which are needed in differing quantities, the magnitude of the regulatory system becomes apparent. Some enzymes that are needed continuously by the cell, such as those involved in the TCA cycle or in the electron transport system, are probably synthesized **constitutively** (*i.e.*, maintained at fairly constant levels). However, many gene products are made only when necessary (*i.e.*, are **inducible**). The manner in which both the cell environment and internal genetic mechanisms function to regulate phenotypic expression in bacteria is discussed in detail below. Variation of enzyme activity can be regulated at two different levels: (1) regulation of activity of preformed enzyme, and (2) regulation of enzyme synthesis. Enzymes, being allosteric proteins whose biological activities can be changed by binding small effector molecules, can be activated in the presence of the proper cofactor or can be inhibited by binding the end product of the respective pathway (*i.e.,* feedback inhibition). Though bacteria successfully utilize regulation of preformed enzymes as a fine-tuning adjustment to control gene expression (see Chapter 4), this section is directed at defining the relatively coarse regulatory controls of gene activity at the transcriptional level. Most of the intensive genetic studies of bacteria have been conducted in *E. coli* because of readily available genetic exchange systems with which to manipulate this organism. However, the basic genetic concepts developed in *E. coli* apply also to other gram-negative and gram-positive organisms and, in some instances, to higher organisms.

The Lactose Operon of E. coli[7]

Analysis of the gene system controlling lactose utilization in *E. coli,* the regulation of which was intuitively deduced by Jacob, Monod, and colleagues, laid the foundation for our current understanding of how enzyme induction and repression operate at the genetic level. In wild-type *E. coli* K-12, lactose *(lac)* fermentation is inducible; that is, it takes place only in the presence of an inducing β-galactoside substrate such as lactose or a nonmetabolizable synthetic β-galactoside (called a gratuitous inducer) in the culture medium. A mutational study of the lactose gene region of *E. coli* K-12 has indicated that there are three enzymes involved: mutants altered in the *lacY* gene are deficient in a galactoside permease required for lactose uptake; a β-galactosidase, encoded at a locus called *lacZ,* is needed to degrade lactose to its monosaccharide moieties; and a transacetylase, coded for at the *lacA* locus, of unknown function in lactose utilization is coordinately induced along with the other two enzymes. However, other mutants, regulatory in nature, are found in which the synthesis of all three enzymes becomes constitutive so that synthesis can take place with or without inducer in the medium.

The employment of many different lactose fermentation mutants in genetic analyses has established the presence of two distinct types of genes in this system: structural genes that code for structural components (in this case, cellular enzymes such as β-galactosidase); and regulatory genes that encode allosteric proteins involved in regulation (*e.g.,* repressors), or contain specific DNA sequences that act as protein recognition sites for genetic regulation (*e.g.,* operator and promoter genes). In addition, fine structure mapping of the lactose genes, through exhaustive complementation and recombination studies (see section on genetic analysis by conjugation), indicated that most of these genes function as a single integrated transcriptional unit now termed an operon.

Figure 6–8 is a simple diagram of the lactose operon as deduced from genetic and molecular analyses. The regulatory gene, *lacI,* determines the constitutive production of a diffusible cytoplasmic repressor or negative effector protein; generally, there are 10 tetrameric molecules of repressor per cell. This repressor normally binds at a specific DNA site called the operator *(lacO),* another type of regulatory gene, and reduces transcription and expression of the structural genes (*i.e.,* negative control) to about 0.1 per cent of fully induced wild-type levels. Induction occurs when a β-galactoside inducer enters the cell and combines with the repressor molecule, causing inactivation and release of repressor from the operator, and allowing transcription to take place. All of the structural genes are transcribed as a single polygenic messenger RNA molecule; thus, the **operon** forms a genetic unit of coordinated transcription. Mutations to constitutive synthesis of the enzymes occur either by alteration of the *lacI* gene (*e.g.,* I⁻ mutation which blocks repressor production) or by a change in *lacO* (operator constitutive or Oᶜ mutation) so that it cannot bind repressor. Finally, mutations in a separate area of the operon have defined yet another regulatory gene, the promoter or *lacP,* which contains the RNA polymerase binding site. Evidently, operator-bound repressor overlaps the promoter region and effectively covers the RNA polymerase binding site. The nucleotide sequences in both *lacP* and *lacO* have been determined and, together with genetic data, they indicate that these two regions overlap slightly. The relative length and location of each of the *lac* genes is given in Figure 6–8.

Originally, the *lac* operon was thought to be regulated by negative control (*i.e.,* repression) alone. However, an additional positive control of *lac* gene expression has now been defined. The existence of a positive control or activator protein was first indicated by the observation that during growth in the presence of both lactose and glucose the *lac* operon was expressed only at about 2 per cent of the level observed during growth in lactose alone. Sim-

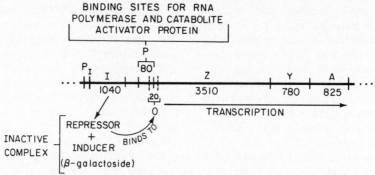

Figure 6–8. The *E. coli* K-12 lactose operon and its associated regulatory locus. This diagram represents an *E. coli* genome segment which carries the genes determining lactose fermentation. Purposefully not drawn to scale, the linkage map gives the location and size, in base pairs, of the various *lac* operon associated genes.[79] The *lacI*, or repressor, gene is constitutively regulated by an adjacent promoter (labelled P_I) and both of these genes are closely linked to the *lac* operon. The *lac* operon comprises two regulatory genes with overlapping sequences, the promoter *(lacP)* and the operator *(lacO)*, as well as three structural genes which code for β-galactosidase *(lacZ)*, β-galactoside permease *(lacY)*, and a transacetylase *(lacA)*. In the absence of inducer, the repressor binds to *lacO*, effectively preventing polymerase binding and transcription. The β-galactoside inducer, when present, complexes with, induces an allosteric change in, and inactivates *lac* repressor protein, which frees the *lacO* sequences. *Lac* operon transcription begins when an RNA polymerase molecule attaches to *lacP*, and it proceeds from *lacZ* through *lacA*. Recent results indicate that RNA polymerase binding is greatly enhanced by the prior binding of catabolite activator protein to the first half of the *lacP* sequences.

ilarly, glucose was found to block the normal expression of the catabolic enzymes for several other sugars (*e.g.*, galactose, arabinose, and maltose). Investigations into this glucose effect, also termed **catabolite repression**, have led to the following interpretation. During *lac* operon induction in the absence of glucose, the repressor-inducer complex is released from the *lac* operator. A molecule called the catabolite activator protein (CAP) combines with cyclic adenosine monophosphate (cyclic AMP); the composite structure, which can bind at a very specific site on *lacP* or on several other promoters such as the galactose promoter, greatly enhances RNA polymerase attachment to the promoter. However, during glucose catabolism, the intracellular level of cyclic AMP is somehow drastically lowered, thereby blocking the CAP-mediated RNA polymerase binding and subsequent *lac* gene expression. Catabolite repression ensures the preferential utilization of the most efficient source of carbon and energy (glucose, in this case).

Extension of the Operon Concept

An understanding of genetic regulation of the lactose utilization genes and, as noted above, the observed negative effect that glucose exerted on the utilization of arabinose, maltose, or galactose soon led to the extension of the operon concept. The inducible galactose utilization system of *E. coli* involves three contiguous structural genes that are coordinately controlled in a manner identical to the *lac* operon, except that the cytoplasmic repres-

sor is produced by a gene that is located at a relatively great distance from (*i.e.*, it is genetically unlinked to) the operon it controls. The genes involved in arginine biosynthesis in *E. coli* are distributed in three unlinked operons, all of which are under the control of the same repressor; this system is termed a **regulon**. In contrast, the histidine biosynthetic pathway contains 10 genes in one coordinately controlled operon.

As opposed to the negative control systems described above, the inducible fermentations of arabinose and rhamnose are each mediated by coordinately controlled adjacent genes, but the regulatory mechanism is one of positive control, as exemplified in Figure 6–9. For example, the arabinose operon contains three structural genes *(araD, araA, araB)*, a promoter region *(araP)*, and an operator/initiator sequence *(araO)*. Additionally, a regulatory gene *(araC)* located immediately adjacent to the *ara* operon codes for the production of a repressor/activator protein. Full induction requires both the CAP–cyclic AMP–mediated RNA polymerase binding to the promoter as well as activator-inducer enhanced transcription through the operator/initiator gene region.

An example of, perhaps, a more important extension of the operon concept is found in the *E. coli* K-12 tryptophan biosynthetic operon. Here, the end product, tryptophan, when in excessive quantities, acts as a corepressor by binding to an inactive form of the repressor, thus enabling it to bind to the tryptophan operator and prevent transcription, as demonstrated in Figure 6–10. Most of the biosyn-

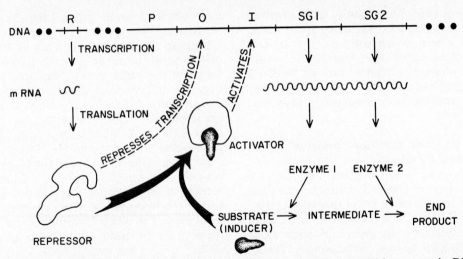

Figure 6–9. Schematic diagram of a positively controlled inducible enzyme system. Essential features on the DNA would include a regulatory gene *(R)*, which may be be genetically unlinked to the operon that consists of a promoter *(P)*, an operator *(O)*, an initiator *(I)*, and two structural genes *(SG)*. The regulatory gene specifies the constitutive production of an active repressor that normally binds to the operator gene and inhibits transcription. In the presence of the substrate inducer, the repressor is not just inactivated, but rather takes on a new conformation and becomes a positive activator that enhances transcription. RNA polymerase does not easily proceed through the initiator gene unless activator facilitates its movement (Modified from ref. 28 with permission).

thetic systems characterized to date (including the arginine and histidine pathways mentioned above) utilize coordinate repression of enzyme synthesis by the end product of a biosynthetic pathway. Derepressed mutants, in which enzyme synthesis continues even with excess end product present, occur by mutations in the corepressor gene, which prevent active corepressor synthesis, or in the operator, so that active repressor is not bound. These basic variations of the original operon concept appear to be largely responsible for regulating cell growth. The physical location, gene order, and direction of transcription of some of the above-mentioned operons are diagrammatically depicted on the *E. coli* chromosomal map (see Fig. 6–21).

It should be noted again that certain en-

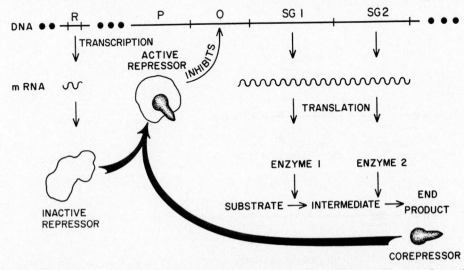

Figure 6–10. Diagrammatic representation of an end product–controlled repressible biosynthetic pathway. Essential features on the DNA include a regulatory gene *(R)*, which may be genetically unlinked to the operon that consists of a promoter *(P)*, an operator *(O)*, and two structural genes *(SG)*. The regulatory gene constitutively encodes (inactive) aporepressor molecules. It is the product of the biosynthetic pathway, not the substrate, which when present in sufficient quantities binds to and activates the aporepressor. Active repressor binds to the operator gene and prevents transcription (Modified from ref. 28 with permission).

zymes in *E. coli*—for example, those involved in glucose catabolism—remain at relatively constant levels, which suggests that at least some protein synthesis is constitutive. Also, certain nongenetic systems, such as feedback inhibition of enzyme activity, are used by bacteria to prevent unnecessary synthesis (see Chapter 4).

Other Types of Bacterial Variation and Their Regulation

Certain reversible antigenic and colonial morphological variations in bacteria have been observed to occur with such rapidity (*i.e.*, 10^{-2} to 10^{-4} frequency) that these changes were not readily explainable by either mutation alone or by simple operon induction/repression. Nonetheless, the predictability of these antigenic changes suggests that some form of regulation is involved. For instance, many bacterial serotypes of the genus *Salmonella* may express alternatively one or the other of two antigenically different flagellar types, termed phase 1 and phase 2. The structural genes determining phase 1 antigen production occupy the same chromosomal location, labeled H_1, in all of these organisms, even though the phase 1 flagella of many serotypes are antigen-

ically distinct from the phase 1 flagella of other serotypes. These genetic determinants of phase 1 flagellar antigen production are said to comprise a series of **allelic** genes (*i.e.*, alternative forms of the same gene). Similarly, phase 2 flagellar antigens from different serotypes are antigenically distinct, but occupy a common chromosomal locus, designated H_2. The H_2 locus is physically quite distant from (*i.e.*, not genetically linked to) the H_1 locus. In any given *Salmonella* strain, when the H_2 genes are active in the synthesis of phase 2 flagella, the activity of the H_1 genes is repressed, and vice versa. The frequency at which variation occurs from phase 1 to phase 2, or the reverse, differs from strain to strain, but can be as high as 10^{-3}.

The mechanism controlling flagellar antigen phase variation has been defined on three levels; genetic, biochemical, and DNA sequence. The H_2 locus is an operon in which the regulatory control region contains a reversibly invertible 970 base pair DNA segment (*i.e.*, comparable to an *IS* element) that regulates the transcription of this operon which encodes not only phase 2 antigen but also a repressor that acts on the H_1 operon (Fig. 6–11).[72, 73] In this case, the invertible DNA

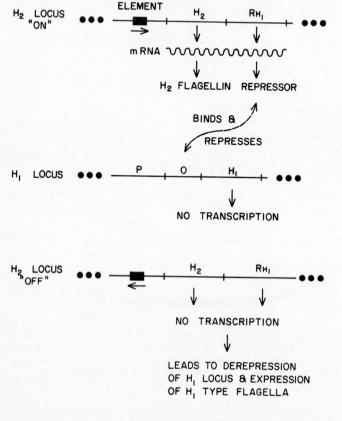

Figure 6–11. Schematic model of genetic mechanism controlling *Salmonella typhimurium* flagellar antigen-phase variation.[72, 73]

segment contains a genetic promoter encoded on one DNA strand. When the invertible DNA segment exists in one orientation (*i.e.,* H_2 "on") at the beginning of the H_2 operon, the invertible segment promotes H_2 operon transcription, allowing for phase 2 antigen expression and the formation of an H_1 operon repressor. In the opposite orientation (*i.e.,* H_2 "off"), the invertible segment prevents transcription and expression of the H_2 operon, which results in derepression of the H_1 locus and expression of the H_1 flagellar antigen. This novel system demonstrates how specific recombinational inversion, within an operon, of a discrete regulatory DNA segment is involved in controlling certain types of bacterial behavior. Why have bacteria evolved such elaborate genetic regulatory schemes? One important consequence of regulatory switching of surface antigen expression is that the altered bacterium is not susceptible to antibody specific for the primary antigen. In a related but more complex system, the protozoan trypanosomes have evolved a phenomenal surface antigen switching mechanism that allows them to express interchangeably one of 50 to 100 different surface antigens; this system permits these organisms to defeat the host immune defense system.

Because of their striking similarity to the well-studied *Salmonella* phase variation, there is good reason to believe that many other types of bacterial antigenic variation are regulated by similar systems. Two examples of such variations are the rapid, reversible transition between production and nonproduction of capsular polysaccharide in *E. coli*, which results in the formation of mucoid or nonmucoid colony forms,[57] and a similar transition between Vi capsular antigen production and nonproduction in *Salmonella typhi* and in certain serotypes of *Citrobacter*.[76] These regulatory switches may serve to conserve cell energy; *i.e.,* capsular polysaccharide may be consistently synthesized only when needed.

In addition to existing as normal components of bacterial chromosomes, similar invertible DNA segments have been found on bacterial virus chromosomes. For example, a virus called Mu has an invertible DNA segment that is involved in controlling its host range. One strand of the invertible DNA segment encodes one set of virus coat adsorption proteins and the opposite strand encodes an analogous but different set of proteins. When the invertible segment is in one orientation, a specific set of virus adsorption coat proteins are made and the resulting mature viral particles can infect certain bacterial species. Inversion of this DNA segment occurs at an easily detectable frequency, and the opposite orientation of the invertible DNA segment results in mature viruses that have a different host range. Thus, this specific DNA inversion event gives the virus a broad host range capability but allows for energy conservation; *i.e.,* the virus doesn't have to synthesize all host range coat proteins at once.[38]

Finally, some bacteria appear to encode certain genes that usually are silent (*i.e.,* not expressed) but which can be expressed occasionally. For example, many *E. coli* isolates do not utilize salicin but when 10^9 *E. coli* cells are spread onto a minimal salts agar medium containing salicin as sole carbon source, 10 to 100 stable salicin-utilizing colonies will appear. Molecular characterization of these mutants has revealed that an *IS* element encoding a genetic promoter has inserted in front of the nontranscribed salicin locus, resulting in salicin utilization. Thus, *IS* elements can transpose to new chromosomal sites and, in addition to inhibiting gene activity, can induce gene expression.

The DNA inversion and transposition events described here now represent important mechanisms whereby bacteria regulate gene expression. Only a few examples of these types of phenomena have been well characterized, due to inherent experimental difficulties and lack of genetic knowledge of the involved genes. However, similar transposable regulatory DNA elements have now been found in several eukaryotic systems and also appear to be important in genetic regulation of higher organisms.[71]

The Nature of Gene Transfer in Bacteria

The employment of genetic analyses, which have been mentioned in the preceding sections, was essential in establishing the organization of information in DNA and consequently the nature of bacterial variation. Any genetic analysis must involve an experimental system for the mixing of two different genotypes. For instance, the presumed dominance (*i.e.,* expression) of the wild-type β-galactosidase gene in the presence of the mutant (β-galactosidase nonproducing) allele can be tested only by experimental introduction of both wild-type and mutant alleles into the same system. In addition, genotypic mixing can allow mapping of the specific chromosomal location of a gene and determination of its linear distance relationship (gene linkage) to other genes of interest, such as those involved in a related biochemical pathway.

Reproduction of the unicellular bacteria, as opposed to that of multicellular organisms, does not require the genetic interchange between two gametes, but simply results from the growth, chromosomal duplication, and finally division of a single bacterial cell into two daughter cells (*i.e.,* akin to mitotic reproduction in eucaryotes). Thus, genetic exchange is not involved in bacterial propagation. Nevertheless, bacteria have several prominent systems for accomplishing genotypic mixing between organisms. Three general mechanisms of bacterial genetic exchange have been found to exist. The specifics of these mechanisms, termed transformation, conjugation, and transduction, are briefly summarized in Table 6–3 and detailed below. A fourth mechanism, cell fusion, is also briefly described.

TRANSFORMATION[61, 75]

In 1928, a medical microbiologist named Griffith, while engaged in a study of pneumococcal infections, discovered a phenomenon which later led to the identification of DNA as the hereditary material of the cell.[29] The pneumococcus (*Streptococcus pneumoniae*), in the encapsulated state, is an extremely virulent microorganism. This high virulence level is due primarily to its polysaccharide capsule, which protects the bacterium from the natural defenses of the infected host. Mutant pneumococcal strains that have lost their ability to synthesize this immunologically specific (*i.e.,* causing the production of specific antibodies) capsular polysaccharide arise spontaneously, however. Such rough or R mutants exhibit a flat, rough look on agar medium compared with the smooth, shiny colonial appearance of the encapsulated or S form of the pneumococcus. More importantly, having lost its protective capsule, the R mutant is no longer virulent.

In Griffith's classic experiment, depicted in Figure 6–12, mice were subcutaneously injected with avirulent R cells (previously isolated from virulent S cells with type II capsular polysaccharide specificity), plus a heat-killed and seemingly innocuous preparation of type III S cells (containing an immunologically different capsule). Neither the sample of viable R cells nor the heat-killed type III S cell preparation, when injected alone, killed any mice. However, a considerable proportion of the mice died after being injected jointly with R cells and the heat-killed preparation of type III S cells. Encapsulated organisms isolated from the mice upon autopsy were found to have acquired the type III capsular specificity as a stable trait. These results indicated that an inheritable genetic trait responsible for synthesis of a specific polysaccharide capsule had been transferred from the heat-killed type III S cells to the viable, but avirulent, R cells.[29] The avirulent R cells had been changed to the virulent state by the genetic exchange process that is now commonly called **transformation**.

DNA as the Transforming Principle

Griffith's experimental results were quickly confirmed by other workers, and transformations were soon being accomplished by the mixed *in vitro* cultivation of different bacterial strains. Shortly thereafter, *in vitro* transformation experiments were performed using filtered, soluble bacterial cell transforming extracts, but the chemical nature of the hereditary material or transforming principle was unknown. In 1944, Avery, MacLeod, and McCarty were able to purify chemically the transforming material and identify it as highly polymerized DNA.[5] Their inability to detect demonstrable protein, lipid, or polysaccharide in this purified DNA led them to propose that the genetic inheritance of a cell is biologically contained within the structure of its DNA. Several years later, when deoxyribonuclease (DNase) became available, Hotchkiss and others[61] demonstrated that the transforming ability of DNA is specifically destroyed by DNase, but not by RNases, proteases, or lipases. Finally, many other bacterial traits, such as genes determining penicillin resistance or the biosynthesis of different amino acids, were found to be transferred by the transformation process, using as little as 0.01 to 0.001 µg. of purified DNA. Today, a variety of bacterial genera (*e.g., Streptococcus, Bacillus, Haemophilus, Neisseria,* and *Moraxella*) have been shown to be capable of genetic exchange through the mechanism of transformation. Additionally, other organisms (*e.g.,* the enterobacteria, *Staphylococcus, Pseudomonas, Rhizobium,* and *Streptomyces*) can be artificially induced to undergo transformation.

Table 6–3. Comparison of DNA Transfer Systems in Bacteria

DNA Exchange Process	Mechanism	DNA Amount Transferred Per Event	Probable Relative Importance in Nature
Conjugation	Specific DNA exchange process occurring between two cells.	From < 1% to 100% of bacterial chromosome; entire plasmids of any size.	Major; widespread among Gm(−) bacteria and also found in Gm(+) genera; can occur at high frequency.
Transformation	Specific uptake of DNA by a competent cell.	Usually 1–5% of chromosome; or plasmids of < 70 megadaltons.	Minor; relatively few genera have known efficient transformation systems.
Transduction	Mistaken incorporation of bacterial DNA into a virus particle and virus-mediated transfer of this DNA.	Usually 1–2% of bacterial chromosome; or plasmids of < 70 megadaltons.	Minor; relatively few genera have known transducing viruses; low frequency event.
a. Generalized	Virus mistakenly incorporates only bacterial DNA.	Usually 1–2% of chromosome; or plasmids of < 70 megadaltons	Any bacterial gene can be transferred.
b. Specialized	Virus capsid incorporates phage plus some bacterial DNA.	Usually < 1% of chromosome.	Only prophage associated bacterial genes can be transferred.
Cell fusion	Membrane intermixing of two protoplasted cells.	Entire cellular DNA content.	Minor; probably a rare event.

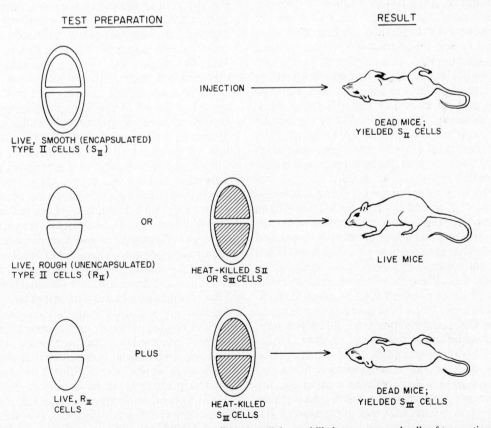

Figure 6–12. Griffith's transformation of pneumococci.[29] Various living or killed pneumococcal cells of two antigenically different capsular polysaccharide types were used in single or mixed preparations to determine if, upon injection, they would cause mouse lethality. Dead mice were autopsied to assess the presence of living pneumococci.

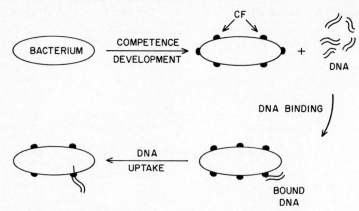

Figure 6–13. The transformation process. During growth a bacterial cell reaches a transient physiological state, termed competence. Competence factors *(CF)* appear to be protein cell surface receptors for the binding of DNA. Random collisions occur between DNA and cells; the DNA is bound to the cell surface receptors. During DNA uptake in the pneumococci, the energy derived from the nucleolytic digestion of one DNA strand is employed to transport the complementary strand into the cell, as shown. However, other bacterial genera can assimilate linear and/or circular, double-stranded DNA, by as yet uncharacterized means.

Transformation Mechanisms

A compilation of facts describing the transformation process has been obtained from studies on many different bacterial genera.[61, 75] Although experimental transformation procedures and resulting transformation frequencies differ among the various genera, there are definite overall similarities among these systems. In brief, transformation is accomplished by the adsorption and uptake of DNA into recipient cells that are in a competent state (a transient physiological condition which predisposes cells to assimilate naked nucleic acid), as depicted in Figure 6–13. Following uptake by the cell, the incoming DNA can genetically recombine with (*i.e.*, become physically integrated into) the host chromosome, and is subsequently expressed (Fig. 6–36).

DNA molecules between 1.0 and 100 megadaltons (1.5 to 150 kilobase pairs) have been successfully transformed. The mean chemical composition of DNA is commonly expressed as moles per cent guanine plus cytosine (%GC) and the mean chromosomal composition among the different bacterial genera varies from 25 to 75 per cent GC. In general, similarity in mean DNA base composition between donor DNA and recipient cell DNA is a minimum requirement for transformation. Undenatured double-stranded DNA is the most active structure for transformation, but some bacteria have a less efficient system for the uptake of single-stranded DNA. Also, there are several reports that transformation of *Bacillus* or streptococcal cells can be effected by RNA instead of DNA.[61]

The conditions required to produce or maintain competence for transformation have been found to differ among the various genera. Some bacteria (*e.g.*, *Bacillus, Streptococcus, Haemophilus,* and *Neisseria*) are natural transformers and can attain competence simply under the proper growth conditions. Other bacteria, notably the *Enterobacteriaceae*, are normally not transformable, probably due to their natural impermeability to DNA. However, this latter group of bacteria, when properly mutated and/or grown under appropriate conditions to induce competence and subsequently exposed to $CaCl_2$ to cause spheroplast formation (partial loss of cell wall), can be artificially induced to transform at a relatively low frequency (10^{-4} to 10^{-6}). For *Bacillus subtilis* or *Haemophilus*, competence develops near the end of the period of exponential growth. By contrast, competence in *Rhizobium* or *E. coli* is maximally expressed in early or mid-log phase cultures, respectively. Whereas *Haemophilus* and *Streptococcus* cells require complex growth media to develop maximum competence, this physiological state in *Bacillus* is achieved best in a minimal medium. The competence factors of streptococci and *Bacillus* are sensitive to proteolytic enzymes, are inactivated by heat, and appear to be cell surface components that are easily lost by washing. In addition, these competence factors (molecular weight of 5 to 10,000 daltons) are positively charged at physiological pH. The acquisition of competence in all natural transformation systems is sensitive to protein synthesis inhibition, even when saturating concentrations of competence factor are added to incompetent cells, suggesting the participation of another protein(s) in the establishment and maintenance of the competent state. Mutants that are blocked at different stages of transformation have been isolated and may increase our understanding of the different factors involved in competence, as well as other aspects of this DNA exchange process.[61]

The sequence of probable events that occurs during transformation in natural transformers is schematically illustrated in Figure 6–13. Analysis of the kinetics of transformation shows that DNA molecules (which are negatively charged) interact by random collisions with receptor sites on the recipient cells, initially binding by weak ionic, reversible association. The number of DNA binding sites per cell has been estimated at 30 to 80 in pneumococci and as low as 1 to 4 in *Haemophilus*. Competence factor has the cationic properties expected of a DNA binding protein and all the facts are compatible with competence factor's being the DNA receptor site. Within minutes of reversible binding, DNA becomes irreversibly bound and insensitive to the action of added DNase, presumably due to the fact that the DNA is being transported into the cell (uptake step). Because only single strands of incorporated DNA were observed after the uptake step in pneumococci and half of the incoming DNA was converted to acid-soluble material, Lacks proposed that the energy released during the nucleolytic digestion of one DNA strand allows for the entry into the cell of the complementary strand.[48] However, double-stranded DNA does not appear to be similarly degraded during transformation in *Haemophilus*, and the mechanism(s) for double-stranded DNA uptake is still speculative.[61] Recent studies in *Haemophilus* indicate that DNA segments must contain a specific ~10 bp transformation recognition sequence in order to be transformed. The general nature of such a recognition phenomenon in other transformation systems is unknown.[75]

Detection of transformed cells is possible only if the incoming DNA is expressed, which, in most instances, necessarily follows integration into the recipient chromosome of some of the donor DNA. In the majority of transformation systems studied to date, the incoming DNA which has been assimilated by the cell undergoes recombination with the host cell chromosome shortly after penetration. Though the exact joining mechanism(s) remains unclear, several possible models are discussed in the section on recombination (Fig. 6–36). The actual sizes of integrated DNA segments resulting from transformation have been estimated to be between 2000 and 5000 nucleotide pairs.[61, 75] This represents 2 to 5 genes, if one assumes that the average protein is encoded in a DNA sequence of 1000 nucleotide pairs. Although transformation frequencies in *Bacillus* or *Haemophilus* are usually 1 to 5 per cent, for unknown reasons, *E. coli* K-12 cells are transformed at a much lower frequency (10^{-5}).

Transformation studies with *Bacillus subtilis* have resulted in the determination of a large number of linked chromosomal genes, and in the construction of a partial genetic map of this organism. However, notwithstanding some notable achievements in the *B. subtilis* system, gene mapping over an entire linkage group is extremely difficult to accomplish with a mechanism such as transformation that is severely limited with respect to the size of the DNA segments it can exchange.

Adaptations of Transformation

As will be discussed in later sections, purified DNA that is isolated from bacteriophage can be introduced into bacteria by a process called **transfection**, which has competence requirements similar to transformation. Among other advantages, this process permits one to study viruses that are defective in normal infection (cannot inject DNA into the host cell). Similarly, the DNA of extrachromosomal genetic elements (plasmids), which exist as circular, double-stranded DNA molecules, can participate in the transformation process.[14] These adaptations have proved to be of great value in analyzing the molecular nature of bacterial plasmids and viruses. Note that transformation of plasmid DNA is a requisite method of the powerful new recombinant DNA technology (described in the section on applied genetic engineering).

CONJUGATION[2, 35, 53, 82]

Experimental utilization of transformation as a method for genetic exchange resulted in the identification of DNA as the material of genetic inheritance and in the empirical demonstration of physically linked genetic traits. Although the amount of DNA per cell could be estimated by chemical analysis, the molecular organization of DNA within the cell still remained a mystery. The momentous discovery by Lederberg and Tatum,[51] in 1946, of the existence of a bacterial process called conjugation has led to our present concept of bacterial genome organization.

Conjugation (so named because the process

involves the conjugal union of two cells) is a genetic exchange mechanism whereby a sexually differentiated donor (or male) cell may transfer its genetic material to a recipient (or female) bacterium. The process of conjugation was originally described in a strain of *E. coli* called K-12, and has been extensively studied in that strain. In this system, sexual differentiation and conjugal ability are dependent upon the intracellular presence of an extrachromosomal genetic element called the sex or fertility (F) factor. Similar extrachromosomal genetic elements, generally referred to as conjugative plasmids, have subsequently been found to promote conjugation in a wide variety of gram-negative and in some gram-positive bacteria, and the F plasmid has become the prototype with which all other sex factors are compared. The conjugal transfer mechanism mediated by the F plasmid, as opposed to other conjugation systems, is well understood. Consequently, the majority of work described in the following sections is aimed at defining our current understanding and illustrating the importance of the F conjugal transfer system.

Of the four mechanisms of bacterial gene transfer summarized in Table 6–3, conjugation is by far the most important system. Many different bacterial genera can undergo conjugal DNA transfer. Second, large amounts of DNA containing hundreds or thousands of genes can be transferred, at a relatively high frequency, *en bloc* between cells via this process. Considering the fact that conjugation can even occur between cells of different bacterial genera, this gene transfer mechanism must be largely responsible for the evolutionary flexibility of many bacteria.

Fertility of E. coli K-12

In the initial experiments on conjugation,[51] two *E. coli* K-12 strains, each containing triple but different auxotrophic mutations (abcJKL × ABCjkl; in which each letter represents a different gene and the lower-case letters denote recessive auxotrophic mutant alleles) were mixed and grown. Neither strain alone could grow on a nutritionally minimal medium, demonstrating that multiple mutational reversion to wild type could not occur. However, when the two strains were cultured together and then plated on minimal medium, one per 10^6 to 10^7 parental bacteria formed colonies. Subsequent cloning of these colonies ruled out any effects such as cross feeding between nutritionally complementary cells and demonstrated that stable prototrophic recombinants

(ABCJKL) had been formed. Somehow, one of these bacterial strains had transferred the appropriate wild-type genes to the other bacterium.

An important concept in understanding the nature of conjugation was the finding that recombinant formation is mediated by the unilateral transfer of genetic material from the donor cell to a recipient bacterium. Additional studies demonstrated that the donor state is conferred by the intracellular presence of the F plasmid, and this plasmid is readily transmitted to recipient cells at frequencies of 5 to 95 per cent after one hour of mixed cultivation. The extremely rapid transfer, to recipient cells, of the donor state from a small number of F^+ donor cells indicated that the sex factor can proliferate autonomously and can do so much faster than once per cell generation. Finally, conjugal transfer of the F plasmid, which normally occurs independently of bacterial chromosome transfer, requires cell-to-cell contact, as cell-free filtrates or donor cell extracts are insufficient for conjugal transfer.

The data obtained from extensive studies of the conjugal transfer of many *E. coli* genetic traits were consistent with the presence of a single, unique linkage group (*i.e.*, one set of unique traits on one chromosome) in this organism. However, in most conjugal mating studies, only chromosomal DNA fragments of limited size appeared to be transferred to recipient cells. It was later learned that these donor DNA fragments result from random physical breakage of the single large chromosome due to lability of the conjugal union. Experimental support of these interpretations was augmented by the chance isolation of a new type of donor strain that promoted chromosome transfer at a higher frequency (10^{-2} to 10^{-1}) and that is called an Hfr donor. The recombinants produced at high frequency from these Hfr genetic crosses were always found to receive a particular segment of the donor chromosome, but did not generally inherit the donor state. However, a very small proportion of the recombinant types from Hfr crosses did inherit donor ability along with chromosomal traits, and behaved in subsequent crosses identically to the Hfr donor strain. These and other facts led to the conclusion that, in Hfr donors, the F plasmid had stably integrated into the chromosome at a specific site, promoting the ordered unidirectional transfer of chromosomal genes from the F plasmid insertion site. Only if conjugal transfer was effected without chromosome breakage, a relatively rare event, was the entire chromosome (including its most distal portion, the integrated sex factor conjugal transfer genes) transferred to the recipient, subsequently resulting in a cell that behaves like the original Hfr parent. Hfr donors were found to generate autonomous F plasmids occasionally, due presumably to the precise excision of the original integrated plasmid sequences. Very infrequently, however, the integrated F sequences in an Hfr chromosome are excised along with some adjacent chromosomal sequences, creating a conjugally transmissible F plasmid that contains some attached bacterial genes (referred to as an *F-prime* or *F'* plasmid). The F$^+$, Hfr, and F' states of the F plasmid are diagrammatically depicted in Figure 6–14.

Before further discussion of the types of F-promoted genetic exchange or of the application of conjugation in genetic analyses, we will

first consider the current knowledge on the molecular and genetic nature of the F plasmid. Complete descriptions of the genetic characterization of conjugation in *E. coli* can be found elsewhere, and only the most pertinent aspects of these analyses are given here.[1, 2, 16, 35, 53, 82]

The F Plasmid

The fertility plasmid, F, is an obligately intracellular genetic element that can mediate conjugal transfer and is capable of autonomous replication. Though inherited as a stable trait, the F plasmid is not required for normal cell functioning and is lost spontaneously on occasion. In the extrachromosomal state the F plasmid is a covalently sealed, circular, double-stranded DNA molecule that has a molecular mass of 63 megadaltons (Mdal.; or 94.5 kilobase pairs) and is about 1/40 the size of the *E.*

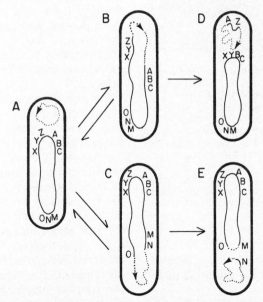

Figure 6–14. The molecular states of the F plasmid in *E. coli* K-12. The various donor states of the F plasmid are illustrated (not drawn to scale). Each cell is shown harboring a circular chromosome (thin continuous line) which contains an ordered set of genes that are depicted alphabetically. The F plasmid DNA sequence (dotted line) contains a site known as the transfer origin (indicated by the arrowhead). *A, F$^+$ cell,* which contains a physically autonomous F plasmid that can be transferred conjugally to an F$^-$ cell, or which can be lost spontaneously, creating an F$^-$ recipient cell. Occasionally, the F plasmid can integrate at different sites on the bacterial chromosome in either of two orientations to form Hfr cells (see *B* and *C*). *B, Hfr cell.* The F plasmid sequences are integrated linearly between the chromosomal genes Z and A, in an orientation that would effect chromosome transfer in the order ZYX···ONM···CBA·F plasmid. The integrated F sequences can revert to the autonomous, or F$^+$ state, as shown in *A,* or after imprecise excision, can give rise to an F' (F-prime) plasmid (see *D*). *C, Hfr cell.* Same as *B* above except that integration occurred at a different chromosomal site and the F sequences are inserted in opposite polarity; the gene transfer order would be (O···XYZABC···MN·F plasmid). *D, F' cell.* Imprecise excision of F sequences has resulted in a plasmid that carries bacterial genes from both sides of the *F* integration site plus all of the F sequences. *E, F' cell.* Abnormal excision of F sequences has created a plasmid that has lost some F sequences and gained some adjacent bacterial DNA. The chromosome now carries a small segment of the F plasmid, which has a high affinity for the wild-type F sequence and promotes high-frequency F integration. Conjugal recipients of an F' plasmid become F' donors. Also, the chromosomal sequences on the F' plasmid potentiate Hfr formation in a secondary host, and some cells are transiently converted to the Hfr state.

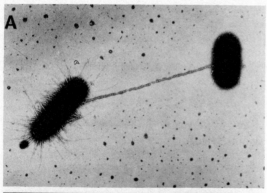

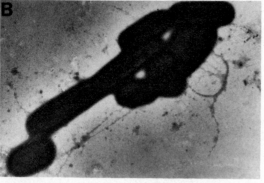

Figure 6–15. *A,* Electron micrograph of a conjugal mating pair after initial contact. The *E. coli* K-12 donor cell, on the left, contains numerous short, hairlike type I or common pili, in addition to the single long sex pilus. Shown here surrounded by adsorbed, spherical male-specific phage paticles, the F sex pilus forms the initial conjugal bridge between donor and recipient cells. The recipient *E. coli* cell is easily identified by its "bald" (pili-free) state. (Courtesy of C. C. Brinton, Jr.) *B,* Light microscopic photograph of a mating aggregate. After initial contact, mating cells form multicellular aggregates. (From Achtman, M., et al. J. Bacteriol. **135**:1053–1061, 1978 with permission).

coli chromosome. There are 1 to 2 copies of the F plasmid molecule per chromosome in *E. coli* K-12 cells.

Phenotypic sexual differentiation in donor cells is due mainly to the presence of a specific surface appendage, referred to as the sex-pilus or F-pilus, that is coded for by the F plasmid. This thin cylindrical, hair-like appendage, extruded through the cell membrane, has a diameter of about 8.5 nm. and grows to a length of 1–20 μm. It is composed of two entwisted parallel rods, each consisting of repeating 11,800 dalton subunits of the F pilin protein.[8] In contrast to the relatively short common pili, or fimbriae, of *E. coli,* which are present in large numbers on the cell surface, there is only one or a few F pili per cell (Fig. 6–15*A*). Interestingly, the F-pilus has been shown to be the receptor site for a class of bacteriophage

known as male-specific phage (discussed in section on genetic properties of extrachromosomal elements). Known to be essential for the formation of an effective conjugal union, the F-pilus is thought to mediate the initial attachment between donor and recipient cells (Fig. 6–15*A*). Next, the mating cells are drawn close together in aggregates (Fig. 6–15*B*), and the DNA transfer process is triggered. Conjugal DNA transfer is initiated by cleavage at a distinct site on the F DNA molecule, called the transfer origin, resulting in a single break in one DNA strand. The 5′ end of this unique strand of the F plasmid is then specifically transferred to the recipient cell, as illustrated in Figure 6–16. Although DNA replication is not absolutely required for conjugal transfer, the single-stranded F molecule transferred to the recipient cell undergoes subsequent complementary strand synthesis, as does the remaining single-stranded donor DNA. Finally, following separation of the conjugal pair (Fig. 6–16*C*), both cells now have a copy of the same plasmid and can behave as donors. Most importantly, conjugal transfer results in the dissemination of large blocks of DNA without the actual loss of any information from the donor cell.

Despite the fact that a molecule as large as F could code for between 50 and 100 proteins, only about 25 genes have been detected and the exact functions of only a few of these genes are known. Genetic analyses of a series of transfer-deficient mutants have defined about 15 transfer genes that are clustered on half of the F molecule. Further studies have resulted in the identification of two other closely linked transfer genes, an operator and a co-repressor locus, that regulate the expression of the 15 clustered transfer genes which apparently form one large operon. Several other loci, including the transfer origin, have also been mapped. Very recently, by means of restriction enzyme and electron microscope heteroduplex techniques, molecular analyses of F and many F′ derivative plasmids have resulted in a relatively detailed structural understanding of the F plasmid; the more pertinent details are shown in Figure 6–17. An important development from these studies was the identification of *IS* elements at various but specific locations on the F molecule. From molecular determinations of the sites and probable events involved in chromosomal DNA insertions within F′ molecules, Davidson and co-workers deduced that each *IS* element acts as the recognition site at which the F molecule inserts into or excises from an identical site on the *E. coli* K-12 chromosome

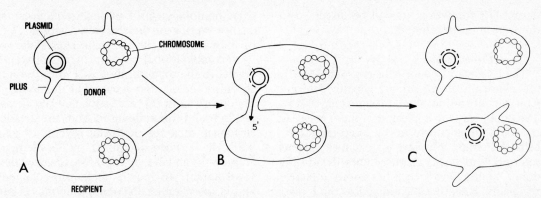

Figure 6–16. The process of bacterial conjugation. This schematic illustration depicts the conjugal transfer of a bacterial plasmid. *A,* The donor bacterial cell contains its single circular, supercoiled chromosome as well as a conjugative plasmid which encodes the mating pilus. Although normally supercoiled like the chromosome, the plasmid is depicted here as a relaxed duplex DNA circle, for ease of illustration. *B,* Following initial contact, the mating cells are drawn together in close approximation. The plasmid undergoes specific, single-strand DNA cleavage at the transfer origin (arrowhead) and the free 5'-end of the plasmid DNA single strand is transferred to the recipient cell. During DNA transfer, complementary strand synthesis occurs in the donor to maintain a double-stranded plasmid copy. *C,* The incoming DNA strand in the recipient cell is duplicated and circularized. Both donor and recipient cells have copies of the same conjugative plasmid and both cells can act as donors.

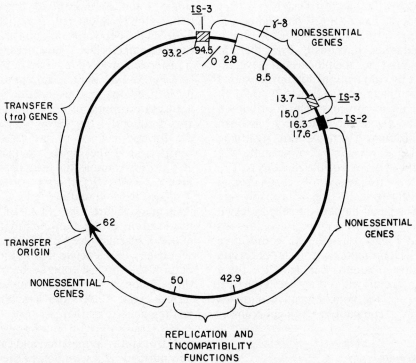

Figure 6–17. Structural map of the F (sex) plasmid.[17, 39, 74] In this scaled map, the locations of various functions, constructed from published data are physically positioned through the use of a kilobase (kb.) coordinate mapping system devised by Davidson and co-workers.[17] The map order of 15 genes that determine the necessary functions for conjugal transfer *(tra)* plus two associated regulatory genes is known, and these genes occupy the last one-third of the total 94.5-kb. pair length of the F plasmid. The origin of conjugal transfer (denoted by the arrowhead) has recently been mapped at kilobase coordinate 62. By the use of restriction enzyme procedures, construction and study of large deletion mutants of F has led to the conclusion that all functions necessary for self-replication and incompatibility (a locus responsible for the inability of two similar plasmids to coexist within the same cell) are encoded on a small 7.1-kb. long DNA segment.[74] The regions labeled as nonessential genes have been genetically deleted without observed consequences on either F self-replication or transfer ability. Additionally, locations are given for *IS-2, IS-3,* and the gamma-delta sequences, all of which are separate integration sites for Hfr formation, and which also participate in F plasmid recombinational rearrangements.[17]

during Hfr formation, as will be discussed in the section on Hfr donors.[17]

Gene Transfer by F⁺ Strains

The F⁺ state of donor cells is propagated by the physically independent, genetic determinant of conjugation, the F plasmid (Fig. 6–14). The donor state or F plasmid of these cells can be lost spontaneously or by exposure of F⁺ cells to certain physical or chemical agents referred to as **curing** agents. Other than losing donor ability and becoming more effective recipients, bacteria which have lost the F plasmid are unchanged. The donor state can be restored to these F⁻ cells by reintroduction of the sex factor by conjugation.

Although only one in every 10^4 to 10^6 cells of an F⁺ population transfers some chromosomal genes to recipients, from 5 to 95 per cent of recipient bacteria become F⁺ within one hour of mixed incubation with F⁺ donors. Two separate processes apparently account for the above observations: first, the F plasmid promotes its own conjugal transfer at a very high frequency; second, the F plasmid causes the relatively infrequent transfer of donor chromosomal traits. Statistically, then, the rare transconjugants (*i.e.,* recipients that have received DNA by conjugation) for chromosomal genes will also have received the F plasmid by the high frequency process. The F-promoted transfer of host genomic characters has been called **mobilization**, a general term signifying the ability of a sex factor to promote the transfer of chromosomal or plasmid DNA. The relatively low frequency of chromosomal marker transfer from F⁺ cells is probably due entirely to the small number of cells in which F integrates to form Hfr donors. Recent results indicate that F and other known conjugative plasmids, which promote the transfer of certain nonconjugative plasmids, can mobilize these small linkage groups without apparent physical integration (*i.e.,* the nonconjugative plasmids must contain a compatible conjugal transfer origin).

The Hfr Donor

The F plasmid in the Hfr state (depicted in Fig. 6–14) has been integrated into the chromosome by a relatively infrequent recombinational event. As a consequence, the sex factor DNA exists as a linear insertion within the chromosomal linkage group, forming a single integrated unit of replication and/or transfer. There appear to be a number of loci on the *E. coli* K-12 chromosome which share some homology with F plasmid sequences; the chance pairing of the sex factor with any one of these specific chromosomal sites, followed by recombinational crossing over, apparently results in the incorporation of F into the host chromosome at that locus. The homologous regions on both the sex factor and the *E. coli* K-12 chromosome, deduced from the detailed structural analyses of F and several F' plasmids, have been identified as *IS* elements (Figs. 6–17 and 6–18). Therefore, besides their involvement as genetic regulatory elements and in insertion or deletion mutations, *IS* segments appear to act as recombinationally active "hot spots" for Hfr formation.[17]

The sites for F integration into the chromosome as well as the orientation in which F is inserted are predetermined by the positions and polarity of the homologous *IS* regions on both of these molecules. During conjugal transfer from an Hfr donor, a single-strand cleavage is made at the transfer origin in the F DNA sequences, and the resulting donor single-strand is transferred linearly, 5' end first, to the recipient cell, as depicted in Figure 6–19. Thus, depending upon the orientation of the integrated F DNA sequences, chromosome transfer can proceed in either of two directions (see Fig. 6–14B and C), but the transfer polarity is fixed for any given Hfr. Since spontaneous interruption of the conjugal process occurs frequently, the chromosomal traits that are located nearest to the free 5' end are transferred at the highest frequency (10^{-2} to 10^{-1}). For example, in the Hfr illustrated in Figure 6–14B, the transfer order would be ZYX···ONM··· and in Figure 6–14C the Hfr lead markers are O···XYZABC···. Due to the location of the transfer origin of an integrated F plasmid (see Fig. 6–16), the sex factor sequences that encode the conjugal transfer operon are the last traits to be transferred to the recipient from an Hfr donor and are transferred about 10,000-fold less often than the leading genetic markers.

Hfr strains develop at a frequency of about 10^{-5} from an F⁺ population and can be isolated and purified by a variation of the replica plating technique. All cells of a cloned Hfr strain transfer their genetic markers in the same order; for instance, ABC···XYZ. However, when many different Hfr strains were analyzed, it became obvious that different chromosomal segments were transferred, sometimes with reverse polarity (*e.g.,* XWV···BAZ), at high frequency from different donors. The composite picture derived

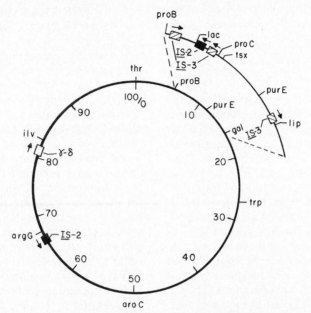

Figure 6–18. Insertion sequences act as recombinational "hotspots" for Hfr formation. The circular linkage map of *E. coli* K-12 is schematically divided into 10 minute length segments and the chromosomal locations of various genes and insertion sequences are shown.[6,17] The genetic markers listed include those that affect the synthesis of threonine *(thr)*, proline *(proB, proC)*, adenine *(purE)*, tryptophan *(trp)*, chorismic acid *(aroC)*, arginine *(argG)*, and isoleucine-valine *(ilv)*; those that affect utilization of lactose *(lac)* or galactose *(gal)*; and those that affect the requirement for lipoate *(lip)* or the resistance to phage T6 *(tsx)*.[6] Through an intensive study of the molecular relationships among F and several F′ plasmids, N. Davidson and co-workers have deduced the identities and physical orientations of the insertion sequence elements that are actively involved in Hfr formation (indicated by shaded blocks in the figure) at six different locations on the *E. coli* genome.[17,77] Although the *E. coli* K-12 chromosome was estimated, by DNA–DNA hybridization studies, to carry five copies of *IS-2*, the locations of only two such sequences are known.[77] To create an Hfr strain the autonomous F plasmid apparently integrates into the chromosome after complementary pairing between an insertion sequence region in the F plasmid and a homologous sequence in the chromosome. Thus, Hfr polarity (indicated by the arrows in the figure) would be a direct consequence of the orientations of the homologous sequences on each parental molecule. Twenty-seven different Hfr strains are thought to have been formed by F integration at one of the sequences mapped above.[17] It is likely that other known Hfr strains were constructed by F integration at other insertion sequences located on the chromosome which have not yet been mapped.

from these studies was that the *E. coli* genetic material is organized on a single circular haploid linkage group. Linked marker transfer frequency, then, is dependent on the F integration site, F orientation, genetic linkage between the chromosomal traits, and the proba- bility of spontaneous breakage of the chromosome during conjugation. Finally, the integrated sex factor DNA segment can be observed to excise from the host genome at the same low frequency with which it integrated. Although in most instances the result-

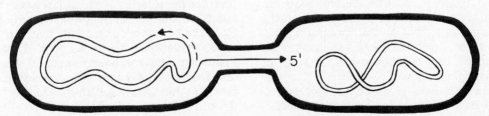

Figure 6–19. Schematic illustration of the process of Hfr-mediated conjugal transfer of the bacterial chromosome. Following contact of the donor (on left) and recipient cells during conjugal mating, a single-strand DNA cleavage occurs at the transfer origin (designated by the arrowhead) of the integrated F plasmid and the free 5′-end of the chromosome is transferred in an ordered, linear manner to the recipient cell. The incoming DNA can be recombined into an homologous region of the recipient bacterial chromosome. It takes 100 min. for the entire chromosome to be transferred from one *E. coli* cell to another, but this event is rare, since the conjugal union is increasingly subject to breakage with time.

ing cells become F$^+$, abnormal excision of the F sequences, which is observed very rarely, gives rise to F-prime (F′) plasmids (see Fig. 6–14).

The F-prime State

During removal of the F plasmid from the integrated state, an abnormal recombinational event causes the infrequent release of the sex factor along with some of the adjacent bacterial genes, creating an F′ or substituted sex factor (see Fig. 6–14D and E). Abnormal excision events can give rise to two types of F′ sex factors: the first type has all of the F sequences plus some bacterial genes from both sides of the chromosomal integration site, as shown in Figure 6–14D; and the other type has lost some F DNA sequences from one end of its integrated linear configuration, but has gained some of the adjacent bacterial genes at the opposite end as depicted in Figure 6–14E. Both types of F′ elements have been shown to exist as covalently closed, double-stranded circular DNA molecules. As a consequence of the latter type of imprecise F plasmid excision from an Hfr strain, a small segment of F remains in the host chromosome, creating a specific affinity locus which has been found to promote a high frequency of subsequent F integration.[16]

In the original or primary host strain, the F′ sex factor carries a few bacterial genes for which the chromosome bears a corresponding deletion. Thus, only one full set of host chromosomal genes is harbored and the cell is referred to as haploid. The F′ plasmid, and the associated bacterial traits, is transferred at high frequency to F$^-$ cells, whereas chromosomal markers not carried on the F′ are mobilized at low frequencies (10^{-5} to 10^{-4}) and without specific orientation. Transconjugants for the F′ plasmid are partially diploid with respect to those bacterial genes that are carried on the F′ plasmid. The considerable sequence homology between the bacterial alleles on the F′ plasmid and those on the chromosome results in the rapid chromosomal integration/excision of this sex factor; i.e., a state of dynamic equilibrium.

F′ plasmids have provided a useful experimental means of performing genetic complementation tests and of determining the dominance or recessiveness of various alleles. Furthermore, molecular characterization of various F′ elements was essential to the recent discovery that certain IS elements act as Hfr integration sites.

THE TRANSFER OF THE BACTERIAL CHROMOSOME[35]

Essentially, conjugation between bacteria of the same species results in the pooling of some or all of the DNA of two parental cells within a single cell, which becomes genetically diploid (carries two similar sets of genes) or partially diploid. Subsequent recombinational events promote the incorporation of some of the transferred donor chromosome into the complete circular recipient chromosome, producing a haploid recombinant that carries one full set of genes. In contrast to other systems of bacterial genetic transfer, conjugation can generate complete or nearly complete diploid zygotes (Gr. *zugon* = yoke, *i.e.*, union of two cells) so that widely separated as well as adjacent genes on a chromosome can be mapped.

The preceding section was devoted to an examination of the properties of the F plasmid and the different donor states in which it can exist. Chromosome transfer from any given Hfr was shown to provide only a linear picture of the bacterial linkage group. However, the comparative behavior of several different Hfr strains demonstrated that all bacterial genes are situated on a single circular linkage group. This section includes a brief description of the experimental utility of conjugation in examining the genetic and structural properties of the chromosome, as well as a presentation of certain specific *E. coli* K-12 genome properties. Also, the employment of F and other sex plasmids in the genetic analysis of the chromosomes of other bacterial genera is described.

Interrupted Mating[35]

Genetic analyses of many different Hfr × F$^-$ crosses has shown that for any given Hfr strain a particular group of linked genes is transferred at high frequency. For instance, consider the transfer of the ordered set of Hfr donor prototrophic chromosomal genes, A, B, C, D, and E, to recipient cells that carry the recessive deficient alleles a, b, c, d, and e. Following sufficient mating time and selection for proximal (closer to transfer origin) gene A function, the unselected distal (further from the transfer origin) donor genes B, C, D, and E can be detected in the transconjugant population at respective frequencies of 90, 75, 45, and 25 per cent. Although all of these traits are transferred at high frequencies, one can easily detect the gradient of decreasing transmission frequencies that presumably results from an increased distance between the transfer origin and any particular marker. As indicated previously, there is an increasing probability with time that the mating pairs will separate, causing chromosome breakage and termination of the transfer process. The consequent gradient of conjugal transmission frequencies provided the initial means by which chromosomal genes could be linearly ordered. Although of obvious benefit, gradients of transfer frequencies did not allow for accurate quantitative mapping of distances between gene loci.

In an attempt to define the kinetics of conjugal transmission, Wollman and Jacob[83] conducted their famous interrupted mating studies. These experiments involved mixing donor Hfr cells with recipient F⁻ cells in a broth culture at time zero, removing samples at various mating intervals, and, most importantly, interrupting the mating pairs in these samples by immediate, vigorous agitation in a mechanical blender. The agitated samples were then plated on various supplemented minimal media to determine which donor markers had been inherited by the recipients after various mating times. The kinetics of interrupted mating in a mixed broth culture between an Hfr H donor and an F⁻ recipient are illustrated in Figure 6–20. Transfer of the proximal markers, *thr⁺-leu⁺*, was not observed until after 8 min. of mating and the number of *thr⁺-leu⁺* recipients continued to increase for about 30 min. until a maximum frequency was reached. The entry of the *gal⁺* and *trp⁺* markers in transconjugants began at later respective times and continued until a constant frequency was established for each. In addition to demonstrating different marker entry times, Figure 6–20 shows the gradient of maximum transfer frequencies observed for the different traits that were examined. The probability of chromosomal breakage increases with distance from the transfer origin; this is factually shown by a comparison of the respective maximum transfer frequencies of the *thr⁺-leu⁺*, *gal⁺*, and *trp⁺* loci. More recently, the probability of spontaneous interruption of mating, reported to be independent of temperature or growth medium, has been estimated at 6.4 per cent per minute of transfer time; thus, only 1 of 100 initial conjugal unions would remain after about 70 min. of mating.[84] These results and those obtained in similar experiments demonstrated that genetic markers enter the recipient after different, but specific, mating times. The genetic marker most proximal to the transfer

origin is observed first in transconjugants, followed by adjacent donor chromosomal genes in a linear sequence. Another extremely useful finding was that under standard mating conditions at 37° C., the difference in the time of entry between any two particular markers is highly reproducible even when different Hfr strains are employed. Thus, the physical distance between genes can be expressed as differences in times of entry. Therefore, during conjugation a single strand of the normally circular, double-stranded DNA chromosome is mobilized, at a relatively constant rate, as a linear molecule which is spontaneously broken at a low probability or can be mechanically severed to examine specific marker entry times.

Data obtained from a multitude of different genetic studies which include interrupted conjugal matings with many different Hfr donor strains and P1 transductional analyses (see section on transduction) have recently been used to conclude that the contiguous circular

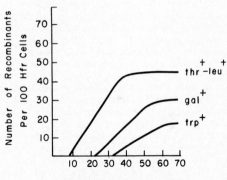

Figure 6–20. Kinetics of interrupted mating in *E. coli* K-12. The number and type of recombinants formed after various mating times are represented graphically. The Hfr H donor strain is prototrophic and sensitive to streptomycin, which is a distal marker; the streptomycin-resistant recipient strain requires threonine *(thr)*, leucine *(leu)*, and tryptophan *(trp)*, and does not ferment galactose *(gal)*. Broth cultures of the parental strains were mixed at a donor to recipient ratio of 1:20 and incubated at 37° C. Samples were removed at intervals, agitated in a blender, diluted, and then plated. Recombinants were scored on minimal agar containing streptomycin, which prevents growth of the donor cells, plus one or more required nutrients. Transfer of the genetically linked *thr* and *leu* loci were selected for simultaneously, and *thr⁺-leu⁺* recombinants were observed after 8 minutes of mating. The X-axis intercepts on the above graph are the transfer entry times for the *thr⁺-leu⁺*, *gal⁺*, or *trp⁺* markers. Maximal transfer frequencies for all markers examined were obtained within 70 minutes of mating time.[35] (Redrawn from Hayes. W.: The Genetics of Bacteria and their Viruses. 1968, J. Wiley and Sons, New York, p. 681, with permission.)

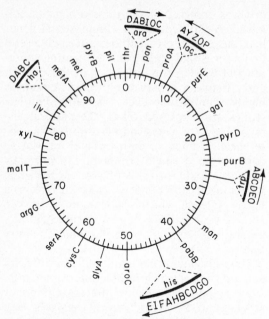

Figure 6–21. Chromosomal map of *E. coli* K-12. Representative genetic loci, distributed around the circular genome, are shown in this map, which is divided into 100 segments of one minute each, based on interrupted mating studies. However, the complete map contains over one thousand different genetic determinants that have been mapped by a variety of genetic procedures.[6] The genetic determinants shown above affect either the biosynthesis or utilization of adenine (*purB, purE*), aminobenzoate (*pabB*), arabinose (*araD, araA, araB, araI, araO, araC*), arginine (*argG*), chorismic acid (*aroC*), cysteine (*cysC*), galactose (*gal*), glycine (*glyA*), histidine (*hisE, hisI, hisF, hisA, hisH, hisB, hisC, hisD, hisG, hisO*), isoleucine-valine (*ilv*), lactose (*lacA, lacY, lacZ, lacO, lacP*), maltose (*malT*), mannose (*man*), melibose (*mel*), methionine (*metA*), pantothenate (*pan*), pili (*pil*), proline (proA), rhamnose (*rhaD, rhaA, rhaB, rhaC*), serine (*serA*), threonine (*thr*), tryptophan (*trpA, trpB, trpC, trpD, trpE, trpO*), uridine (*pyrB, pyrD*), and xylose (*xyl*). As shown in the expanded portions of the map, the location of genes as well as the directions of transcription (indicated by arrows) within each of five different operons is indicative of the complexity of the chromosome. For example, in the arabinose operon, *araC* is transcribed in one direction, while *araI* through *araD* are transcribed in the opposite direction and by necessity on the complementary DNA strand.

map length of the *E. coli* K-12 chromosome is 100 ± 2 minutes, enough information to encode approximately 4000 ± 1000 genes. To date, about 1000 different genes have been mapped on this chromosome.[6] Although only a relatively few loci evenly distributed around the genome were chosen for the map illustrated in Figure 6–21, several map segments have been expanded to show the complexity of a few operons. The unit of map distance used at present is the minute, and the location of a gene is determined by the time of entry difference between that gene and a known

marker in interrupted mating studies conducted at 37° C. On the basis of length measurements, obtained by electron microscopy, of large chromosomal segments on various F' plasmids, the total 100 minute genome length was extrapolated to be 4.1×10^6 base pairs (2.7×10^9 daltons), which corresponds to 41 kilobase pairs per minute. Assuming that the average gene contains 1000 base pairs, for simplicity, then each map minute corresponds to about 40 genes. The circularity of both F⁻ and Hfr chromosomes had earlier been demonstrated by autoradiographic techniques and the previously estimated length agrees well with the newer, more accurate determinations.

Initially, it seemed as if all Hfr strains mobilized the genome at relatively similar and constant rates, and that different conjugal pairs formed equally stable unions. However, certain Hfr strains have been isolated which transfer the chromosome faster than other Hfr donors. Also, a few Hfr strains have been isolated which appear to maintain more stable conjugal unions, resulting in an unusually high frequency of distal marker transfer. Significant differences in transfer frequencies have also been detected when the same Hfr strain is crossed with different F⁻ recipients. In addition, it seems that the proximal half of the genome is transferred at a constant speed, while the latter portion is mobilized more slowly.[35] However, by carefully employing a series of Hfr strains, each transferring different but overlapping segments of the genome at a relatively constant rate, all known loci can be mapped. In fact, the currently available *E. coli* Hfr strains have transfer origins so situated that all genes lie within 20 minutes of one or more Hfr origins.

Genetic Analysis by Conjugation

Several other facets of the conjugal process that are pertinent to its use in genetic analyses have been characterized. Since marker transfer is usually detected by recombinant formation, the use of the interrupted mating technique to determine the linear relationships among a series of markers would only be valid if one could assume that all markers transferred to the recipient have both an equal chance and similar rates of integration. Jacob and Wollman[41] rather convincingly demonstrated that the widely spaced *gal⁺*, *trp⁺*, and *his⁺* markers of Hfr H all have the same probability (0.5) of being integrated following transfer; also, the high degree of similarity for gene order obtained by either conjugation or transduction studies has resulted in the assumption that the integration rates for different chromosomal segments must be similar. However, there is one exception, at least. Markers that lie within the first 4 to 5 minutes of the Hfr transfer origin are inherited at a much lower than expected frequency, this effect being the greatest for the leading marker.

As illustrated above, both the interrupted mating procedure and gradients of conjugal transmission are useful in specifying the linear relationships among well-spaced (at least 2 minutes apart) loci. However, there must be some more refined method for determining the order of the 40 to 80 genes that reside within 2 minutes on either side of a known marker. The distance (or time of entry difference) between two genomic traits has been shown to determine the frequency of coinheritance of these two markers. Though all donor chromosomal traits are physically linked on a single DNA molecule, each one of any two given traits that are separated by more than 5 minutes of transfer time recombines, at a probability of 0.5, with the recipient chromosome as if each existed on a separate DNA fragment; these traits are considered to be genetically unlinked. Since the probability of integration for any transferred trait is 0.5, it follows that two genetically unlinked traits would be randomly coinherited 50 per cent of the time or less. Thus, relationships among genetically linked traits can be determined from an examination of marker coinheritance frequencies among the recombinants. For example, if recombinants are selected for the presence of a distal donor gene and subsequently examined for the presence of more proximal unselected markers, all unselected genes that lie within several minutes of the selected marker are coinherited at frequencies of between 50 and 100 per cent, the frequency being higher for more closely linked traits. Any unselected genes that lie further than several minutes from the selected trait are randomly coinherited at a 50 per cent frequency. The converse experiment, in which recombinants selected for the presence of a proximal donor marker are then scored for the unselected inheritance of distal donor genes, can also be employed in the construction of genetic linkage maps. These procedures are termed mapping by recombinational analysis, and the donor DNA segment to be recombined can be introduced into the recipient by conjugation, transduction, or transformation. Usually in a fine structure genetic analysis the unknown gene is mapped in relation to two genetically linked genes of known map positions. Briefly, both mapped

traits are separately employed as the selected marker in different experiments. The coinheritance frequency for either or both of the two remaining unselected markers, of which the location of one is known, with the known selected trait, can be used to map the unknown linked trait.[35]

Occasionally, it is important to know if a mutant allele is dominant (such as $lacO^C$ mutants) or recessive (such as $lacI^-$ mutants) to the wild-type genes. Also, it is necessary to know if two different, but phenotypically similar, mutations are located within the same gene, like $lacY1$ and $lacY3$, or in separate genes that normally complement one another to perform a single function such as $lacY$ and $lacZ$. These questions can be answered by allelic complementation studies with cells that are made diploid for the characters in question. Suffice it to say that F' plasmids that carry many differet chromosomal sequences have been extremely useful in genetic complementation tests. For example, a mutation in a different location in each $lacY$ allele of a strain made diploid for the lac operon would, in the absence of recombination, result in the Lac⁻ phenotype. However, if one lac operon was $lacZ^-$ while the other was $lacY^-$, the diffusible enzymes of the functional $lacZ$ and $lacY$ genes would create a Lac⁺ phenotype. These gene products are said to function in $trans$ (L. $trans$ = across—i.e., they are mediated by diffusible proteins). In contrast, an operon containing the $lacO^C$ and $lacZ^-$ mutations (causing constitutive synthesis of functional $lacA$ and $lacY$ enzymes, but phenotypically Lac⁻), in the presence of a wild-type operon, would not result in the constitutive Lac⁺ phenotype. The $lacO^C$ mutation is said to function in cis (L. cis = on this side—i.e., a mutation in a recognition sequence that functions only on the DNA molecule in which the alteration is located). For the interested reader, many excellent experimental protocols for genetic analysis of both bacteria and bacteriophage have been assembled into lab manuals.[18, 59, 70] Also, it should be noted that the proposal of Demerec and co-workers for the uniform nomenclature of bacterial mutants has been invaluable in organizing the mass of available data on bacterial mutants into understandable genetic and physical maps.[6]

The Intergeneric Transfer of E. coli K-12 Genes

In addition to interspecific gene transfer, male cells of *E. coli* K-12 have been shown to form conjugal unions with related genera of the family Enterobacteriaceae (*e.g., Salmonella, Shigella, Serratia,* and *Proteus*). In fact, in some cases, large segments of the *E. coli* genome can be conjugally transferred intergenerically at reasonably high frequencies. This gene transfer, though reduced by host DNA restriction systems (see later section on DNA restriction), must still play an important role in the overall evolution of these bacteria.

Conjugal Transfer in Bacteria Other than E. coli K-12

The transfer of the *E. coli* K-12 sex factor, F, to other strains of *E. coli, Shigella,* and *Salmonella* has resulted in the isolation of Hfr type donors in those strains. Generally speaking, these donors behave in a manner similar to their K-12 counterparts. The isolation of such donors has made possible the creation of intrastrain mating systems other than that of *E. coli* K-12, which has led to the construction of genetic maps of these other bacterial chromosomes. In addition, these donors have greatly broadened the scope of intergeneric and interspecific gene transfer.

Conjugal transfer systems in many different organisms, involving sex factors other than F, have been exploited more recently (see next section on plasmids). Utilizing the FP sex plasmids of *Pseudomonas* and interrupted mating procedures using *Pseudomonas* Hfr derivatives, a partial genetic map of *Pseudomonas aeruginosa* strain PAO has now been constructed.[37] Despite the unusual difficulties encountered in studying bacteria like *Streptomyces*, which exist as vegetative multicellular filaments that are coenocytic (*i.e.*, have incomplete walls separating adjacent cells, thus allowing protoplasmic mixing), a conjugal mating system has been detected. Apparently, a sex plasmid can form Hfr-like derivatives, which cause high-frequency ordered gene transfer, or can form elements comparable to F′ plasmids. A fairly detailed circular genetic linkage map of *Streptomyces coelicolor* has resulted from intensive genetic analyses. In addition, chromosomal gene transfer within other bacterial genera, like *Rhizobium, Klebsiella, Citrobacter,* and *Vibrio,* has been reported. It should also be noted that conjugative plasmids have been found in a wide variety of gram-positive and gram-negative bacterial genera (Table 6–4), and it seems reasonable to predict that these elements occasionally promote both interspecific and intergeneric chromosomal gene transfer.

The observed dissimilarities among gene products of similar function from these differ-

Table 6–4. Host Range of Bacterial Plasmids

Gram-negative Genera

Facultatively anaerobic rods: *Escherichia, Shigella, Salmonella, Citrobacter, Edwardsiella, Proteus, Klebsiella, Enterobacter, Serratia, Yersinia, Aeromonas, Haemophilus, Pasteurella, Erwinia, Providencia, Legionella*
Anaerobic rods: *Bacteroides, Campylobacter*
Anaerobic/aerobic cocci: *Veillonella, Neisseria*
Aerobic rods: *Pseudomonas, Rhizobium, Agrobacterium, Xanthomonas, Vibrio*
Aerobic coccobacilli: *Alcaligenes, Bordetella, Francisella*

Gram-positive Genera

Cocci: *Staphylococcus, Streptococcus, Micrococcus*
Aerobic endospore–forming rods: *Bacillus*
Anaerobic endospore–forming rods: *Clostridium*
Aerobes: *Arthrobacter*
Non–spore-forming rods: *Lactobacillus*

Other Genera

Actinomycetales: *Streptomyces, Mycobacterium*
Mycoplasmas: *Mycoplasma*
Phototrophic bacteria: *Rhodopseudomonas,* cyanobacteria
Budding/appendaged bacteria: *Caulobacter*
Obligate halophile: *Halobacterium*
Rickettsias: *Coxiella*

ent bacteria, as well as the different map distance interrelationships among specific genes within these bacterial genomes, indicates that these bacterial chromosomes are not appreciably homologous to each other or to the more closely interrelated enteric genera, *Escherichia, Salmonella,* and *Shigella.* However, for each genome analyzed to date, it appears as if genes involved in a common biochemical pathway are usually closely linked, often within a single operon. For those interested, a compilation of available bacterial chromosome maps has been published.[49]

Genotypic Mixing By Cell Fusion

Though not related directly to conjugation or transformation, it is notable that a new type of genotypic mixing process has recently been described. In this process, termed bacterial cell fusion, protoplasts (cell wall–less forms) of different auxotrophic *Streptomyces* or *Bacillus* cells were apparently fused to form large diploid protoplasts which could produce prototrophic recombinant cells. Cell fusion may provide a means for studying large segments of the chromosomes of bacteria for which conjugal transfer systems are inadequate or have not been found. Cell fusion probably occurs to a limited extent in nature and most likely represents a minor natural means for genetic exchange between bacteria.

EXTRACHROMOSOMAL GENETIC ELEMENTS[9, 23, 33, 52, 53]

Plasmids, often referred to as extrachromosomal genetic elements, are self-replicating units of inheritance that are conserved in an extrachromosomal state, through successive bacterial cell divisions. Considered dispensable, plasmids are nonessential for cell survival under normal conditions. Despite their dispensability, however, plasmids play a role in both host virulence and resistance of their bacterial host to most clinically employed antibacterial agents such as antibiotics and heavy metal cations. Thus, the presence of certain plasmids can be selectively advantageous to their host in special environments. It appears that the ability of bacteria to vary in response to their environment is largely due to the plasmids that they carry and the facility with which plasmids can evolve and be disseminated.

To date, more than 40 widely diverse bacterial genera (Table 6–4) have been found to harbor a variety of plasmids that mediate the expression of many different phenotypes; it is likely that plasmids exist universally among bacteria. Notwithstanding this variability in genetic constitution, plasmids can be divided into two broad categories: (1) **conjugative** plasmids (formerly called transfer factors), exemplified by the F plasmid, which encode the genes necessary for the conjugal transfer of DNA; and (2) **nonconjugative** plasmids which cannot promote conjugal DNA transfer. Certain plasmids like F, which can exist either autonomously or integrated within the host chromosome, have previously been termed episomes. The usefulness of this term is limited, however, in that F can integrate into the *E. coli* genome, for example, but behaves only as an autonomous element in *Proteus*. Instead, F and similar elements are now considered as plasmids with the potential for existing in the integrated state. Similarly, increased knowledge of plasmids has necessitated other changes in terminology; the newcomer is directed to a recent working proposal on plasmid nomenclature.[62]

Historical Perspective and Medical Significance

The introduction of each new antibiotic over the past 50 years has raised the hopes of both human and veterinary clinicians. However, as clearly documented in numerous studies, shortly after the introduction of each new antimicrobial agent, bacteria resistant to that compound have been isolated. In fact, the frequency of isolation of drug-resistant bacteria from clinical sources is now alarmingly high. What is the cause of this bacterial drug resistance?

It was noted during the initial years of antibiotic usage that bacteria could become drug-resistant through a single spontaneous chromosomal mutation; such a mutation occurs in about one per every 10 million cells in a population and causes the resulting bacteria to become resistant to a single antibiotic or a single chemical class of antibiotics. This type of drug resistance remains an important obstacle to chemotherapy. However, combined drug therapies were instituted to overcome this problem. In 1959, Japanese scientists observed multiply drug-resistant bacterial strains that were concomitantly resistant to four or more chemically distinct antibiotics. More importantly, this resistance was found to exist on extrachromosomal DNA elements and to be conjugally transferable between different bacteria. The responsible agents were termed drug-resistance or R plasmids. During the past 25 years, R plasmids have been isolated worldwide and now appear to be responsible for the majority of bacterial drug resistance encountered today.

Genetic studies of bacterial plasmids have revealed that a single plasmid can mediate concomitant resistance to as many as 10 different antibiotics as well as express other important phenotypic properties. For example, plasmids have been identified that are essential for bacterial virulence, that can alter a bacterium's diagnostic biochemical characteristics, or that can enable bacteria to degrade disinfectant compounds (*i.e.,* hexachlorophene). Thus, plasmids are medically significant accessory genetic elements to the bacterial host. These facts, together with the knowledge that plasmids can evolve relatively rapidly via specialized recombination systems and can be disseminated efficiently to other bacteria, make these genetic entities extremely important in bacterial evolution.

Plasmid Detection

How are plasmid-borne traits initially detected? Though generally conserved by both daughter cells following division, plasmids are characteristically and spontaneously lost at a low frequency (10^{-2} to 10^{-8}) from cells that harbor them. This frequency can be enhanced 100- to 100,000-fold by certain **curing** agents (*e.g.,* acridine orange, sodium dodecyl sulfate, ethidium bromide, heat) that affect plasmid replication and/or segregation of the daughter plasmid molecules at cell division. Thus, spontaneous or induced curing of genetic traits is indicative of plasmid-borne characters and is commonly employed in establishing the non-chromosomal nature of the genetic trait in question. Reintroduction of suspected plasmid-borne traits into the cured host strain, accomplished either by their own transmissibility or through mobilization promoted by a conjugative plasmid, further substantiates the extrachromosomal state of these characters. Procedures for bacterial transformation using purified plasmid DNA can also be used to establish specific traits as being plasmid determined. Plasmid DNA isolation techniques have often revealed the presence of plasmids for which no phenotypic properties can yet be ascribed; these have been termed **cryptic** plasmids.

Plasmid Classification

The first plasmid discovered was the conjugative F plasmid, as described previously. Subsequently, the extrachromosomal nature of bacteriocin production (bacteriocins are secreted, bacterial proteins with antibiotic properties) and then multiple antibiotic resistance was noted. More recently, many other plasmid-borne traits, as listed in Table 6–5, have been observed. Historically, plasmids have been named on the basis of the initial associated traits. For example, if the determinants for antibiotic resistance, lactose utilization, or virulence were located extrachromosomally, the respective plasmid would be designated as a drug-resistance (or R) plasmid, a lactose plasmid, or a virulence plasmid. Although initially useful, this classification system now has limited value because many single plasmids have been observed that simultaneously mediate several different functions (*e.g.*, bacteriocin production, antibiotic resistance, and virulence traits); and many plasmids of a characteristic type, like different R plasmids, are often genetically unrelated. Aside from their classification on the basis of conjugal ability and regardless of the phenotypic properties encoded, plasmids can be grouped very specifically on the basis of the general property of incompatibility. Plasmid incompatibility can be defined as the inability of two related plasmids to coexist in the same host cell in the absence of selective pressure (see next section for possible mechanism). Genetically related plasmids (*i.e.*, having related replication functions) are incompatible; on this basis, plasmids are arbitrarily classified in a specific incompat-

Table 6–5. Phenotypic Functions Mediated by Plasmids

*Autonomous replication
*Incompatibility
Conjugation functions (transfer genes)
Entry exclusion
Resistance to antibiotics (*e.g.*, streptomycin, ampicillin, tetracycline, sulfonamide, and chloramphenicol)
Resistance to heavy metals (*e.g.*, divalent Cd, Hg, Pb, Co, and Ni)
Resistance to ultraviolet light
Resistance to specific phages (*e.g.*, T1, λ)
DNA restriction and modification (*e.g.*, EcoR1 system)
Antibiotic production
Bacteriocin production (*e.g.*, colicins E, V, K, and B)
Toxin production (*e.g.*, enterotoxin, tetanus)
Production of virulence enhancing factors and cell surface antigens (*e.g.*, K88 antigen, plant crown gall tumor formation)
Gas vacuole formation (*e.g.*, certain halobacteria)
Production of hemolysin, coagulase, or H₂S
Substrate catabolism (*e.g.*, degradation of octane or naphthalene, or fermentation of lactose or sucrose)
Specialized recombination system(s) (*e.g.*, RTF-r-determinant dissociation and association, and drug resistance transpositions)

Descriptions of some of the above functions are given in the text, while the remainder have been described elsewhere.[9, 23, 33, 53] Entry exclusion or surface exclusion is the phenomenon whereby certain resident plasmids interfere with the entry of an incoming compatible plasmid, but not with the hereditary stability of the incoming plasmid once it has entered the cell. The two functions marked by asterisks are common to all plasmids.

ibility group. At present, there are at least 25 different incompatibility groups among the thousands of plasmids isolated from the Enterobacteriaceae alone. Additionally, there are at least 11 incompatibility groups for the *Pseudomonas* plasmids and 7 for *Staphylococcus* plasmids. As will be discussed later, plasmids within an incompatibility group appear closely related by DNA sequence homology, and this classification system has contributed significantly to the study of plasmids.

Genetic Properties

As listed in Table 6–5, all plasmids encode genes necessary for autonomous replication and incompatibility. Additionally, some plasmids have been observed to carry genes necessary for conjugal DNA transfer, genes that enable the host to resist normally lethal doses of chemical or physical agents, genes for resistance to specific virus infection, genes involved in an organism's pathogenicity, genes necessary for catabolism of a variety of substrates, genes involved in gas vacuole formation (*i.e.*, regulates buoyancy of aquatic bacteria for efficient photosynthesis), or genes essential for rapid evolution of plasmids. Genetic studies of all of these properties have revealed the biochemical bases of many of the responsible mechanisms. For example, the genes involved in conjugal DNA transfer of the F plasmid have been identified (see Fig. 6–17), as described in an earlier section, and the conjugal transfer mechanism has been deciphered (see Fig. 6–16). The most important evolutionary consequence of conjugal plasmid transfer is that plasmid traits are disseminated to new bacteria without being lost from the parent strain.

During the early studies of plasmids in enteric bacteria, several important genetic aspects of plasmids were uncovered. Many R plasmids (previously termed R factors) were observed to transfer at relatively low frequencies (10^{-5} to 10^{-8}), whereas the conjugal transfer of F occurred at a high frequency (10^{-1}). In fact, certain R plasmids were found to repress the conjugal ability of the F plasmid when coharbored by the same cell. These R plasmids, originally termed fertility inhibition positive (fi^+), are now referred to as F-like plasmids. Both the F plasmid and F-like plasmids determine the production of antigenically related sex pili, which are encoded within an homologous transfer operon consisting of 15 structural genes, negatively controlled by a two-component repressor. These F-like R plasmids are now known to make both general and plasmid-specific corepressor components which together repress transfer operon transcription. However, the F plasmid codes only for the F-specific corepressor component and can not repress its own transferability except in the presence of the R plasmid–encoded general corepressor component. Though many conjugative plasmids have repressed transfer operons, the infrequent initial recipients for the plasmid become derepressed for conjugal transfer for several generations until sufficient repressor levels accumulate. A second large group of enteric R plasmids, termed I-like, have been found to specify sex pili that are antigenically distinct from F pili but similar to the donor pili specified by the colicin (Col) I plasmid.

Notwithstanding the fact that many enteric conjugative plasmids specify either F-like or I-like sex pili, other plasmids that determine the production of different donor pili, which are antigenically unrelated to F or I pili, are no longer uncommon among the enterobacteria. In addition, distinct conjugative plasmids have been observed in a variety of other bacteria (*e.g., Pseudomonas, Vibrio, Campylobacter, Streptococcus faecalis, Bacteroides fragilis, Neisseria gonorrhoea,* and *Clostridium perfringens*). These conjugation systems promote plasmid transfer at frequencies ranging from 10^{-8} to 10^{-1} and can often mobilize nonconjugative plasmids or chromosomal genes. The mechanistic nature of these latter transfer systems is largely unknown, but the conjugal mating system of *S. faecalis* appears to be unique; it involves a recipient cell-mediated sex pheromone that triggers donor cells to modify their cell surface and aggregate with recipient cells.[21]

Although plasmids have been isolated from many diverse bacterial genera, intergeneric conjugal transfer of most plasmids usually occurs only between bacteria with close genetic relationships. Despite this general tendency, some plasmids, such as certain *Pseudomonas* plasmids, are conjugally promiscuous and, for example, can transfer from *Pseudomonas* to *E. coli, Rhizobium,* or *Neisseria.* Recently, *Bacillus subtilis* cells, following transformation with staphylococcal plasmid DNA, have been found to be capable of stably maintaining and expressing staphylococcal plasmids.[22]

Certain bacteriophages, referred to as donor-specific or male-specific, have been found that only infect cells carrying a conjugative plasmid of a specific incompatibility group. These virulent phages, which enter the cell via the sex pilus, have been useful experimentally in classifying plasmids, but their biological significance is unknown. Another useful genetic finding was that cells carrying a conjugative plasmid—for example, the F or an R plasmid—are much poorer donors in the stationary phase than in the exponential phase of growth. In fact, these stationary phase donor cells appear to behave phenotypically as if they were F^- or R^- and are now termed F^- or R^- phenocopies, and they can even act as good recipients for related plasmids. Two incompatible plasmids can be forced experimentally into the same cell by using an F^- or R^- phenocopy recipient, thus permitting genetic complementation analyses between related plasmids.

Analyses of antibiotic resistance in both gram-negative and gram-positive organisms have revealed that plasmids are oftentimes responsible and can specify resistance to one or more of the agents listed in Table 6–6. Plasmids have not yet been shown to mediate resistance to the nitrofurans, the polymyxins, nalidixic acid, bacitracin, vancomycin, rifampicin, or the cycloserines. Plasmids mediate antibiotic resistance through one of the five mechanisms summarized in Table 6–7. For example, normally the MLS antibiotics bind to

Table 6–6. **Plasmid-Specified Resistance to Antimicrobial Agents**

Amikacin	Neomycin
Cephalosporins	Penicillins
Chloramphenicol	Spectinomycin
Clindamycin-lincomycin	Streptomycin
Erythromycin	Tobramycin
Fusidic acid	Sulfonamides
Gentamicin	Tetracyclines
Kanamycin	Trimethoprim
Lividomycin	

23S rRNA and inhibit protein synthesis. Resistance plasmids specifically methylate the target site, which prevents the binding of the MLS antibiotics but allows for normal protein synthesis. Alternative plasmid-mediated resistance mechanisms include plasmid-encoded functions that render a cell impermeable to an antibiotic, that chemically detoxify the compound, or that are drug-insensitive and replace the affected enzyme. Other genetic studies have revealed the mechanisms by which plasmids mediate resistance to the toxic ions of various heavy metals, including silver, arsenic, cadmium, mercury, lead, cobalt, nickel, tellurium, bismuth, and zinc. Plasmid-mediated resistance to ultraviolet irradiation has been defined, in one case, to be due to a plasmid-encoded repair DNA polymerase.

Studies of plasmid-borne antibiotic resistance traits have shown that 30 to 50 per cent of all *E. coli* from healthy humans and animals contain conjugative R plasmids and as many as 90 per cent of all pathogenic *E. coli* strains carry self-transmissible plasmids. Considering that *E. coli* exist in large numbers in the intestinal flora, these data strongly indicate the tremendous potential for plasmid dissemination in nature.[23]

Recently, plasmids have been found to en-

Table 6–7. **Plasmid-Mediated Mechanisms of Drug Resistance**

1. Alteration of the target site; *e.g.,* methylation of 23S rRNA causes macrolide-lincosamide-streptogramin (MLS) resistance in Gm(+) bacteria.

2. Altered cell permeability to the agent; *e.g.,* tetracycline resistance in both Gm(−) and Gm(+) cells.

3. Hydrolysis of the agent; *e.g.,* beta-lactamases inactivate beta-lactam antibiotics.

4. Chemical modification of the antibiotic; *e.g.,* phosphorylation or adenylation of aminoglycosides.

5. Enzyme replacement; *e.g.,* synthesis of a drug-resistant replacement dihydrofolate reductase in trimethoprim resistance.

code a series of important virulence-enhancing properties of diverse pathogenic bacteria. In some instances, these plasmid-borne traits are essential to pathogenicity (Table 6–8). Plasmid-mediated toxin production has now been demonstrated for: (1) the heat-labile and stable enterotoxins of *E. coli*, (2) the anthrax toxin of *Bacillus anthracis*, (3) the tetanus toxin of *Clostridium tetani*, (4) the exfoliative toxin of staphylococci, and (5) several other toxins. Specific cell surface structures that allow enteric bacteria to colonize humans or animals or that enable agrobacteria to colonize certain plants have now been defined as plasmid-encoded. Also, the genes for production of hemolysins, long implicated in disease, and for factors that make bacteria more resistant to the normal inhibitory effects of serum (*e.g.,* the conjugal transfer protein *traT*) have been shown to exist on plasmids. Organisms that invade the blood and tissues must be able to accumulate approximately 10^{-5}M iron in order to continue multiplying, but the free iron concentration is about 10^{-22}M due to the iron-binding proteins lactoferrin and transferrin. Although some bacteria encode these iron accumulation functions chromosomally, other bacteria have been shown to maintain these genes on plasmids that are essential to the organisms' pathogenicity. Similarly, both *Shigella* and *Salmonella typhimurium* contain plasmids that encode an essential virulence trait; *i.e.,* the ability to penetrate intestinal epithelial cells. Also, plasmids can code for synthesis of lipopolysaccharide O-side chains (*e.g., S. sonnei*) or for unspecified functions that enable

Table 6–8. **Plasmid-Mediated Virulence Properties**

1. Toxin production; *e.g., E. coli* enterotoxin.

2. Colonization antigen synthesis; *e.g.,* animal, plant, or human colonizing factors.

3. Hemolysin production; *e.g.,* alpha and beta.

4. Serum resistance factor production; *e.g., traT* protein.

5. Iron chelation and transport system; *e.g.,* invasive organisms.

6. Tumor induction in plants; *e.g.,* tumor-inducing plasmid of *Agrobacterium tumefaciens.*

7. Attachment/invasion of epithelial cells; *e.g.,* intestinal penetration by *Shigella* and *Salmonella typhimurium.*

8. Intracellular survival function(s); *e.g.,* undefined ability of *Yersinia* plasmids.

9. Somatic antigen synthesis; *e.g., Shigella sonnei.*

bacteria to survive intracellularly (*e.g., Yersinia*). Finally, certain plasmids have been shown to cause neoplastic growth in plants. The best studied example is the tumor-inducing plasmid of *Agrobacterium tumefaciens* that, through the insertion of specific plasmid sequences into the plant chromosome, causes crown-gall tumors in certain dicotyledonous plants. Also, strains of *Agrobacterium rhizogenes* have been shown to contain a plasmid that provokes an extensive proliferation of root tissue, termed hairy root disease, in certain plants. Thus, plasmids now appear to be heavily involved in determining the virulence properties of a wide variety of pathogenic bacteria.

Although not yet studied intensively, plasmids also encode a variety of metabolic properties. Plasmid genes for H_2S or urease production as well as catabolic genes for the utilization of sugars (*e.g.,* lactose, raffinose, sucrose, citrate) have been found in enteric bacteria. Also, *Pseudomonas* strains have been shown to carry plasmids that determine the degradation of complex hydrocarbons such as naphthalene, octane, xylene, salicylate, hexachlorophene, or even the highly toxic chlorinated biphenyls. Some of these properties are of direct medical importance: (1) the ability to degrade and utilize a disinfectant solution as a sole carbon and energy source, (2) certain bacteria can be misidentified owing to their carriage of plasmids specifying atypical key diagnostic biochemical properties, such as urease production or lactose utilization.

Molecular Nature

Genetic and molecular studies of many different plasmids have revealed that these elements share certain general properties (Table 6–9). However, a large amount of additional molecular information about plasmids has been obtained through intensive investigations, which followed the development of techniques for isolating purified plasmid molecules in their native intracellular form. This section reviews briefly some of the experimental techniques employed in molecular plasmid analyses and summarizes the more pertinent molecular properties of plasmids.

Plasmids, and the bacterial chromosome, are now thought to exist in the host predominantly as covalently closed, circular, double-stranded DNA molecules with four to six negative superhelical twists per megadalton of DNA (*i.e.,* the supercoiled state; Figure 6–22). Most plasmid DNA purification procedures have successfully exploited the small size and supercoiled nature of plasmids to separate these molecules from the chromosome. During most gentle cell lysis procedures the large circular host chromosome is broken, while the much smaller supercoiled plasmid molecules remain intact. Cesium chloride (*i.e.,* a salt which upon

Table 6–9. General Properties of Bacterial Plasmids

1. Can exist in physically autonomous state within a cell.
2. Consist of double-stranded, circular, supercoiled DNA.
3. Contain genes for self-replication as well as accessory properties.
4. Probably are attached to cell membrane maintenance site for replication and segregation.
5. Generally are 0.1 to 10 per cent of the size of the bacterial chromosome.
6. Considered to be nonessential for cell survival.

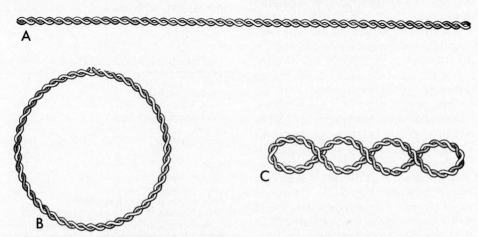

Figure 6–22. Three typical forms of double-stranded DNA. *A,* Linear double-stranded DNA in standard α helix; *B,* Relaxed circular duplex molecule with cleavage in one strand; *C,* α-helical, covalently sealed and negatively supertwisted (*i.e.,* supercoiled), circular duplex DNA. Conversion of relaxed to supercoiled DNA is catalyzed by DNA gyrase; this process keeps DNA in a compact form within the cell. (From Clowes, R. C.: The molecules of infectious drug resistance. Sci. Am. April, 1973, p. 21.)

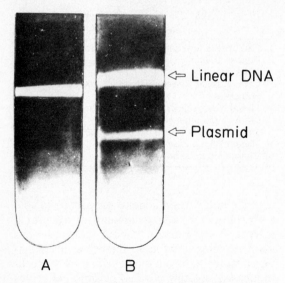

⇐ Linear DNA

⇐ Plasmid

A   B

Figure 6–23. Cesium chloride-ethidium bromide gradients of total cellular DNA obtained from plasmid-free cells (left) and plasmid-containing cells (right). The DNA bands are illuminated by UV-fluorescence. Both tubes show a chromosomal or linear DNA band. The lower DNA band (on right) represents purified plasmid DNA. (From Elwell, L. et al., Infect. Immun. **12**:404–410, 1975, with permission.)

dissolution and centrifugation has the special property of generating a linear density gradient) gradient separation of plasmid from host chromosomal DNA is readily effected in the presence of the dye ethidium bromide, which intercalates between bases on the same DNA strand; this results in unwinding and a consequent decrease in density of the unconstrained linear DNA to a much greater extent than covalently closed circular plasmid DNA (Fig. 6–23). Plasmid DNA, purified and separated as shown in Figure 6–23, can be fractionated, dialyzed, and used for molecular analysis. Accurate plasmid size determinations can now be obtained within hours by agarose gel electrophoretic analysis, as exemplified in Figure 6–24. Moreover, different plasmids can be compared with one another for total intermolecular DNA sequence homology by DNA-DNA hybridization procedures, or more directly through the analysis of specific heteroduplex DNA molecules (*i.e.,* hybrids containing one strand each from different molecules) by electron microscopy (Fig. 6–25). More recently, rapid plasmid comparisons have been conducted by analyzing the set of specific fragments of a plasmid that are generated by cleavage with a specific restriction endonuclease (*i.e.,* recognizes a specific DNA sequence of from 4 to 8 base pairs; see later

section) and by electrophoresis on slab gels. Finally, new technology has brought us to an era in which the nucleotide sequence of from 300 to 500 base pairs of DNA can be determined by an investigator in one day. In fact, the entire nucleotide sequence of certain small plasmids of about 5000 base pairs total size has been determined.

The results of physical analyses of many different plasmids have demonstrated that these elements generally fall into two size groups, as summarized in Table 6–10. Most small plasmids generally range from about 1 to 10 Mdal. in size. These DNA molecules are characteristically nonconjugative and exist in a multicopy state in which there are 5 to 10 or more plasmid molecules per host chromosome. Though small, these plasmids, owing to their multicopy nature, can comprise from a few per cent to greater than 50 per cent of total cellular DNA. The second size class of plasmids are often conjugative and range from 1 to 10 per cent of the size of the host chromosome. These larger plasmids contain sufficient DNA to encode hundreds of accessory genes. As shown in Figure 6–24, it is common for many bacteria to carry concomitantly both small and large plasmids; strains carrying as many as 12 different plasmid species have been reported.

The average chemical composition of different plasmid DNAs has been found to range from 30 to about 70 per cent guanine plus cytosine. However, most bacteria carry plasmids with average compositions similar to the host chromosome.

Early studies of plasmid-borne antibiotic resistance produced seemingly contradictory results as to the molecular nature of these elements. Extrachromosomally mediated multiple antibiotic resistance in some bacteria was con-

Table 6–10. **Molecular Classes of Plasmids**

Small
  Nonconjugative
  1–10 Mdal.
  Multiple copies/chromosome
  Could encode 1–15 average-size proteins
  Are less than 0.5% of the size of the host chromosome

Large
  Usually conjugative
  25–300 Mdal.
  One or few copies/chromosomes
  Could encode 50–500 average-size proteins
  Usually are 1–10% of the size of the host chromosome

For comparison purposes, the *E. coli* chromosome is 2500 Mdal. in size, *i.e.,* enough information to encode about 3750 average sized proteins. One megadalton (Mdal.) equals 1500 base pairs.

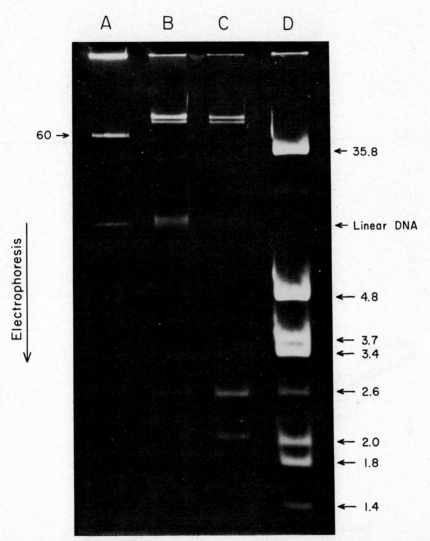

Figure 6–24. Agarose gel electrophoretic analysis for plasmid size determination.[70] Small quantities of fairly pure plasmid preparations are added to wells at the top of a vertical slab agarose gel. During electrophoresis, from top to bottom, supercoiled DNA molecular species separate and migrate with a linear relationship between $\log^{10}$ of the molecular size and the $\log^{10}$ of the distance migrated. The resulting DNA bands, stained with ethidium bromide and illuminated by UV light, can then be recorded by photography. Well A, 60-Mdal. plasmid species, specifying sucrose utilization, obtained from an atypical salmonella. Wells B and C, plasmid preparations from two colonial morphological types of *Shigella flexneri*. Though difficult to see, both strains contain 2 small plasmids of about 2.0 and 2.6 Mdal. as well as two large plasmids of ≈ 140 and ≈ 105 Mdal. Well D represents a plasmid preparation obtained from an atypical citrate-utilizing clinical isolate of *E. coli*. This single strain was found to harbor nine separate plasmid species ranging in size from 1.4 to ≈ 36 Mdal. Linear, chromosomal contaminating DNA migrates at the position indicated above. Relaxed circular molecules migrate differently. (From Kopecko, D. et al., Infect. Immun. **24**:580–582, 1979, with permission.)

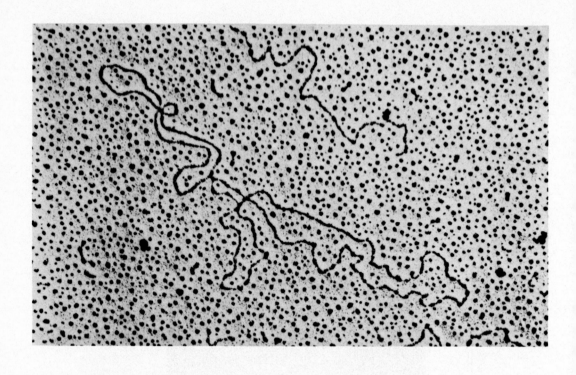

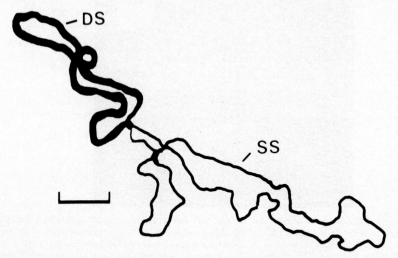

Figure 6–25. Direct visualization by electron microscope heteroduplexing procedures of the nucleotide sequences shared by two DNAs. In this technique, complementary single strands from each of two different molecules are allowed to reanneal; the resulting partially duplex structure, called a heteroduplex molecule, is examined in the electron microscope. This electron micrograph and corresponding tracing represent a heteroduplex molecule formed between the plasmid pSC101 and a recombinant plasmid called pSC120 that was constructed by the insertion of a large DNA segment into pSC101. In this example, all of pSC101 DNA sequences (9.1 kilobases) are homologous with pSC120 and form a circular double-stranded structure, labeled DS, recognized by its thicker appearance as compared to the less even or spotty lines representative of the remaining pSC120 sequences which form a single-stranded addition loop, labeled SS. The bar scale on this photograph represents 0.25 μm. (From Kopecko, D. J., Specialized genetic recombination systems in bacteria: their involvement in gene expression and evolution. *In* F. Hahn (Ed.), Progress in Molecular and Subcellular Biology, Vol. 7, Springer-Verlag Press, Heidelberg, 1980, pp. 135–234. Used with permission.)

jugally transferred as a single genetic linkage group, whereas certain other bacteria appeared to harbor multimolecular plasmid aggregates which could transfer the different antibiotic resistance markers separately. Molecular analyses have confirmed both of these observations. To date, plasmid-mediated drug resistance in many bacteria has been found to exist on a single molecular DNA species, referred to as a cointegrate plasmid, which encodes the functions necessary for its replication, conjugal transfer, and drug resistance. However, some instances of plasmid-borne multiple drug resistance have been shown to result from multimolecular DNA species or plasmid aggregates.[23] In the latter cases, coexisting small nonconjugative R plasmids, which determine resistance to various antibiotics, are separately mobilized by a larger conjugative plasmid.

Molecular studies have now revealed that conjugative plasmids can mobilize (*i.e.,* promote the transfer of) nonconjugative plasmids through cointegration of the two molecules. Alternatively, the nonconjugative plasmid can be mobilized as a physically independent entity if it contains a DNA sequence that is recognized as a compatible origin of transfer.

Plasmid Replication[47]

All current models of plasmid **replication** (*i.e.,* linear assemblage of nucleotides to form an exact replica of the original molecule) encompass the intuitive ideas reported in 1963 by Jacob and co-workers on the regulation of DNA replication.[40] Accordingly, a plasmid, virus, or bacterial chromosome constitutes a unit of replication, or **replicon,** which codes for at least two specific genetic determinants: a regulatory DNA sequence termed the replicator (now termed a replication origin); and a structural gene that determines the limited synthesis of a diffusible protein, the initiator, which acts on the replicator locus, allowing a DNA polymerase to commence replication. Thus, regulation of replication was postulated to be under positive control, analogous to positive control of transcription. However, some experimental results cannot be explained by positive control alone, and it is likely that a repressor is involved in replication control, and perhaps incompatibility, of some plasmids.[65]

To explain hereditary conservation of a DNA species in all cells during successive cell divisions, it was proposed that replicons are attached to a specific cell membrane site, which at cell division would partition the daughter molecules equally to each cell. The above hypotheses are supported by experimental facts and serve as one plausible explanation for plasmid incompatibility. For example, incompatibility between two similar conjugative plasmids would be due to competition for a single specific attachment-replication membrane site and would result in loss of one of the plasmids at cell division. Unrelated or compatible plasmids are assumed to have separate, distinct membrane attachment-replication sites and would coexist stably within a single cell.

Plasmid replication involves the same basic enzymatic events as described in a subsequent section on chromosome replication. There are three overall steps: (1) initiation of polymerization at the origin of replication, an event which is controlled by the limited synthesis of a consumable initiator protein or by a repressor; (2) elongation can occur in either one or both directions from the origin, depending upon the plasmid. The parental DNA strands are separated and each acts as a template for a nascent complementary strand; and (3) synthesis ceases at the replication terminus and the two daughter molecules are separated and supercoiled. As discussed above, plasmids fall into two classes with respect to regulation of their DNA synthesis. Large plasmids generally preserve a nearly 1:1 plasmid-to-host chromosome copy number ratio during all phases of cell growth. These larger plasmids, which require DNA polymerase III for replication (see later section on replication), are termed stringently regulated. In striking contrast, replication of the smaller multicopy nonconjugative plasmids, some of which require DNA polymerase I for replication, is termed relaxed. In certain cases, plasmids under relaxed replication control are found to increase in copy number several-fold during stationary phase or many times over in the presence of a protein synthesis inhibitor like chloramphenicol; *e.g.,* 3000 copies (80 per cent of total cellular DNA) of the colicin plasmid, Col E1, can be present per cell after growth in chloramphenicol.[13, 47]

Through the use of recombinant DNA technology[11] (see later section), it has become possible to cleave various plasmids into smaller self-replicating fragments and introduce these fragments into bacterial recipients. Under these circumstances, a 9.0 kb fragment of the 94.5 kb F plasmid was found to be capable of autonomous replication, was incompatible with F, and existed as 1 or 2 copies per host chromosome in *E. coli*. These data indicate that essential replication and incompatibility functions are clustered on a small region of these larger plasmids and that replication control is a function of the specific replicon, not of plasmid size.[74]

Nucleotide Sequence Interrelationships

Sequence homologies among a variety of different plasmids have been examined mainly by DNA-DNA hybridization techniques. The results of these studies show that plasmids within an incompatibility group are highly homologous in nucleotide sequence, usually 75 per cent homology or greater. Conversely, plasmids of different incompatibility groups generally share very few common sequences (less than 10 per cent).[31]

Notwithstanding the usefulness of hybridization as described above, which gives an estimate of total homology, heteroduplexing techniques have been developed which permit the direct visualization with the electron microscope of the homologous sequences shared by two DNAs (Fig. 6–25). As mentioned earlier, heteroduplex analyses of the homologous DNA sequences among F and several different F' plasmids resulted in the finding that IS elements behave as recombinationally active loci for the chromosomal integration or excision of the F plasmid. Further studies of the sequence relationships between F and several F-like R plasmids demonstrated that the transfer gene region is clustered on the F molecule and that these same DNA sequences associated with conjugal ability have been preserved as a discrete DNA segment with common endpoints in each of the different F-like R plasmids examined. These results suggested that plasmids may have evolved by recombination between discrete DNA segments.

Certain F-like R plasmids, or cointegrate molecules, are known to dissociate under certain conditions into two physically and functionally distinct molecular components: a large resistance transfer factor (RTF) which carries the genes for conjugal transfer, self-replication, and incompatibility; and a smaller, circular DNA species carrying the drug resistance determinants. In addition to demonstrating that at least some R plasmids are recombinational assemblages of a transfer replicon and clustered drug resistance determinants, this dissociation-association phenomenon again suggests the involvement of specific DNA loci. In fact, the RTF component sequences in these different cointegrate plasmids are now known to be bracketed by identical IS-1 DNA sequences; and dissociation and association of these discrete components occurs by a recombinational event involving these IS-1 sequences (Fig. 6–26A).

During molecular studies of antibiotic resistance plasmids, it was noted that discrete DNA segments, encoding drug-resistance genes, could transpose from one plasmid molecule to another. For example, the DNA insertion in plasmid pSC101 that generated plasmid pSC120 (see Fig. 6–25) is a discrete transposable segment, termed Tn4 (Table 6–11), that specifies resistance to streptomycin, the sulfonamides, and ampicillin. Similar analyses have revealed that most of the phenotypic properties carried by plasmids exist on discrete multinucleotide DNA units which range from 2000 to 80,000 base pairs in length (for characteristic properties of Tn's, see Figure 6–7 and earlier section on transposable elements). Although only a few representative Tn elements are listed in Table 6–11, virtually all plasmid-mediated antibiotic resistance genes, as well as many other properties including virulence and metabolic determinants, are located on Tn units. These Tn elements transpose at frequencies which range from 10^{-2} to 10^{-7}; and transposition does not involve loss of the donor sequences but rather their duplication and recombination into a new chromosomal site (see later section on specialized recombination). When plasmids isolated from a variety of different bacteria are compared at a molecular level, it appears that plasmids evolve rather rapidly by the physical exchange of transposable DNA segments. In fact, mapping of the drug-resistance transposons on several related F-like R plasmids has demonstrated that the different Tn units are situated directly adjacent to one another (Fig. 6–26B), indicating that the termini of these transposons act as recombinationally active sites for the insertion of other transposons. Thus, plasmids are now considered to be constantly evolving, recombinational assemblages of various replicons with assorted transposable determinants.[44, 45]

Evolution of Plasmids: Causes and Consequences

The origin of plasmids has been debated for years with no definitive answers; plasmids could be vestiges of bacterial viruses. Evidence clearly shows that antibiotic-resistance plasmids existed long before the commercial employment of antibiotics. One popular theory is that antibiotic-resistance genes could have arisen as self-protective mechanisms for antibiotic-producing organisms, and then these genes may have been disseminated to other bacteria via plasmids. Regardless of their ori-

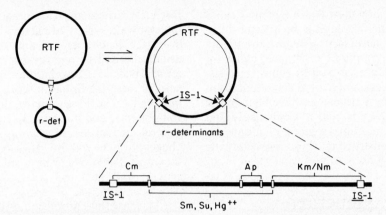

Figure 6–26. Sequence relationships within cointegrate R plasmids. *A,* Schematic representation of the dissociation-association phenomenon of cointegrate R plasmids whereby the large DNA segment carrying the determinants of conjugal transfer, the resistance transfer factor (RTF), separates from or recombines with the smaller drug resistance determinants component (r-determinants). The joining and separation occur at homologous *IS*-1 sequences. *B* The r-determinants region of an R plasmid has been diagrammatically expanded for examination of sequence relations with this DNA segment. The example shown is that of the R1–19 plasmid. Between the *IS*-1 sequences that border this region, the r-determinants component comprises a series of discrete transposable DNA segments determining resistance to various agents. Most of these transposable sequences were observed by heteroduplex procedures to be bordered by some type of repeat DNA sequences (indicated by open boxes) and be situated immediately adjacent to one another. The ampicillin resistance (Ap) gene lies on a transposable segment that is inserted in a larger transposable segment determining resistance to streptomycin (Sm), sulfonamides (Su), and Hg.[++] The Ap gene can be translocated either alone or together with the larger transposon. The closely linked determinants for resistance to chloramphenicol (Cm) and kanamycin/neomycin (Km/Nm) are also independently transposable.[45, 69]

gin, however, it is likely that the present tremendous worldwide usage of antibiotics, in medicine, as food preservatives, and as animal growth promotants, has served as a major selective force for the current population of bacteria that carry multiple plasmid species. How can we reduce the incidence of plasmid-borne antibiotic resistance? A decrease in total antibiotic deployment as well as the use in animal feeds of antibiotics that are chemically dissimilar to the antibiotics presently used in human medicine might reduce the overall incidence of antibiotic-resistance plasmids.

As detailed in the preceding sections, plasmids encode many medically important properties, *e.g.,* genes for antibiotic resistance, conjugal transfer, virulence, specialized recombination systems (Tn), resistance to UV light or disinfectant solutions, and key diagnostic biochemical properties. Plasmids now appear to play major roles in the antibiotic resistance and increased virulence of many typical pathogenic bacteria. In addition, certain opportunistic gram-negative organisms have emerged as the predominant offending pathogens in hospital-acquired (nosocomial)

Table 6–11. **Representative Plasmid-Associated Transposable Elements**

Tn Element Designation	Tn-Encoded Properties	Total Tn Length (bp)	Transposition Frequency (events/cell)
Tn*3*	Ap^R	~ 4,500	10^{-2}–10^{-5}
Tn*4*	Ap^R, Su^R Sm^R, Hg^{++R}	~20,500	10^{-6}–10^{-7}
Tn*5*	Km^R	~ 5,200	10^{-2}–10^{-3}
Tn*7*	Tp^R, Sm^R	~12,750	10^{-4}
Tn*9*	Cm^R	~ 2,500	10^{-6}–10^{-7}
Tn*10*	Tc^R	~ 9,300	10^{-6}–10^{-7}
Tn*1681*	Heat-stable enterotoxin	~ 2,060	~10^{-7}
Tn*551*	Em^R	~ 5,200	10^{-4}–10^{-5}
Tn*951*	Lactose catabolism	~16,600	10^{-4}
Tn*(Tol)*	Toluene/xylene catabolism	~52,500	—

The Tn-encoded properties include resistance to ampicillin (Ap), sulfonamides (Su), streptomycin (Sm), mercuric ions (Hg^{++}), kanamycin (Km), trimethoprim (Tp), chloramphenicol (Cm), tetracycline (Tc), and erythromycin (Em), as well as to various catabolic enzymes and production of enterotoxin. Tn sizes are given in nucleotide base pairs.[44]

infections. An organism can adapt to various hospital or other ecological niches by accumulating the necessary genetic equipment (*e.g.,* genes for antibiotic resistance, genes for increased virulence, as well as genes for resistance to or degradation of disinfectant solutions). All of these properties have been found on bacterial plasmids, and it seems likely that these extrachromosomal genetic elements are involved in constructing these nosocomially adapted pathogens.

TRANSDUCTION[54, 58]

Bacterial viruses (also called bacteriophages; Gr. *phagein,* to eat) were initially discovered around the beginning of the twentieth century, although the involvement of some viruses in the intercellular transfer of bacterial DNA was not demonstrated until 1952.[86] In contrast to the previously discussed systems of bacterial gene transfer, which require either cell-to-cell contact or the cellular uptake of naked DNA, bacteriophage-mediated transfer of genetic material (referred to as **transduction**) results from the infection of a cell with a virus particle that mistakenly contains bacterial DNA. A variety of bacterial viruses that can transduce bacterial DNA, termed transducing phages, are now known. Furthermore, transduction has been reported in a limited but diverse group of bacterial genera; *e.g., Escherichia, Salmonella, Shigella, Pseudomonas, Proteus, Bacillus, Klebsiella,* and *Staphylococcus.*[35]

Following a brief description of some general properties of bacterial viruses and their life cycles, the mechanisms by which transducing phages mediate the transfer of bacterial DNA are discussed. Examples of the utility of transduction in fine structure genetic analysis, mentioned earlier, are presented briefly. In addition, the virus-mediated phenomena of lysogenic conversion and zygotic induction, though not directly related to transduction, have been included here.

General Properties of Bacterial Viruses

Bacteriophages are obligate intracellular parasites that consist simply of a protein coat, the capsid, surrounding a central nucleic acid core (Fig. 6–27A). The viral nucleic acid encodes the phage structural coat proteins and other phage-related functions. The capsid protects the viral nucleic acid when the virus exists outside of a cell and sometimes provides for specific attachment to the proper host cell.

Bacterial viruses are widespread in nature and infect a wide variety of bacterial genera. However, the host range of any specific virus is usually limited to one or several related bacterial species. Considerable diversity exists among bacterial viruses in both physical structure (*e.g.,* capsid geometry, absence of tail components) and nucleic acid content. Certain general properties of several representative phages, which will be described below, are shown in Table 6–4. The results of extensive genetic and chemical analyses of bacteriophages and the use of viruses in genetic analyses of bacterial chromosomes have helped to shape our present concepts in molecular genetics. The interested reader can find detailed genetic maps of λ and other viruses as well as current descriptions of phage functions and their experimental utilities in the recent literature.[36, 53, 54, 58]

Bacterial viruses can be grouped into two broad categories based on whether their life cycles are virulent or temperate. Infection of bacteria with a virulent bacteriophage invariably results in virus replication and the subsequent release of new viral particles (also called **virions**) causing death and cell lysis of the host bacterium. As shown in Table 6–12, virulent viruses can be relatively large, like the T-even DNA viruses, or very small, like the R17 RNA phage. Male-specific viruses, mentioned previously, that only infect male bacterial cells (those which contain sex pili) are virulent viruses. In addition to being able to follow a lytic pathway similar to virulent viruses, an infecting temperate bacterial virus can alternately persist in the host cell in a quiescent state (*i.e.,* **prophage** state) as an inheritable genetic entity, a host condition termed **lysogeny**.

The Life Cycle of Virulent Viruses

Bacteriophage T4 is a typical virulent virus. As diagrammed in Figure 6–27A, the mature virion consists of a head linked to the complete tail assembly. The head contains the nucleic acid packed within the coat protein, the subunits of which are arranged in a hexagonal shape. The tail structure is composed of a rigid core surrounded by a sheath to which is attached a base plate and tail fibers. The tail fibers recognize specific receptor sites on the surface of susceptible bacterial cells and mediate viral attachment (Fig. 6–27B). Following virus attachment to the bacterial cell surface, the tail sheath contracts, pushing the rigid tail core through the bacterial cell envelope. The viral nucleic acid is then injected through the

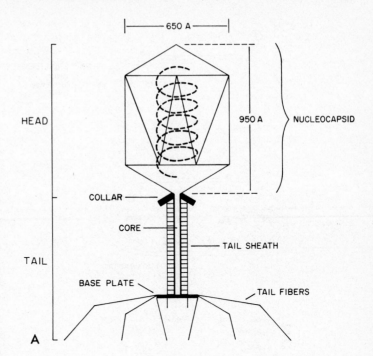

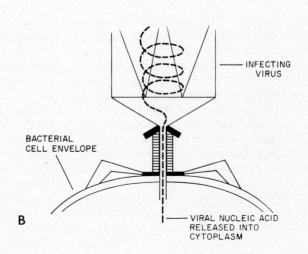

Figure 6–27. Schematic illustration of the T4 bacteriophage component structure and the mechanism of viral attachment/DNA injection into a bacterial cell. *A,* The T4 virus consists of a hexagonal nucleocapsid (nucleic acid tightly packed within the protein capsid head) linked to the tail assembly. The tail is comprised of a collar and a central rigid core surrounded by a flexible, helical sheath. Distal to the capsid, the tail contains a base plate to which tail fibers are attached. *B,* During viral attachment, the virus tail fibers recognize appropriate bacterial cell surface receptors. Following initial attachment, the sheath contracts, forcing the rigid core through the bacterial cell envelope. Finally, the viral nucleic acid is injected into the cytoplasm. (Modified from Luria, Darnell, Baltimore, and Campbell's "General Virology," 3rd ed., 1978, John Wiley and Sons, N.Y., p. 159, with permission.)

Table 6–12. **General Properties of Selected Bacterial Viruses**[54, 58]

Virus	Normal Host	Nucleic Acid Content (Mdal.)	Type of Nucleic Acid	Type of Virus	Normal Transduction Capability
T2, T4, T6	*E. coli*	110–120	Duplex DNA	Virulent	—
λ	*E. coli*	30	Duplex DNA	Temperate	Specialized
fd	*E. coli*	1.7	Simplex DNA	Virulent	—
φX174	*E. coli*	1.6	Simplex DNA	Virulent	—
T7	*E. coli*	24	Duplex DNA	Virulent	—
P1	*E. coli*	60	Duplex DNA	Temperate	Generalized
P22	*S. typhimurium*	26	Duplex DNA	Temperate	Generalized
R17	*E. coli*	1.1	Simplex RNA	Virulent	—

The male-specific phages fd and R17 infect only male or donor *E. coli* cells. Phage DNA content is described in terms of size in megadaltons (Mdal.), and as simplex (single-stranded) or duplex (double-stranded) in nature.

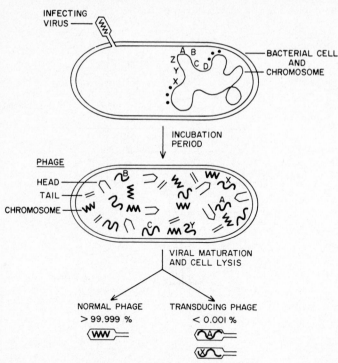

Figure 6–28. Scheme of lytic viral growth and generalized transduction. An infecting virus enters a susceptible bacterial cell which contains its large circular chromosome. Viral replication and expression occur, resulting in the synthesis of viral heads, tails, and chromosomes, and in the fragmentation of the bacterial chromosome. During viral maturation, the phage chromosomes are loaded into phage heads, which are then linked to tails. Occasionally, however, a piece of the fragmented bacterial chromosome, instead of phage DNA, is mistakenly loaded into the phage head; the resulting defective transducing virus, which carries no phage DNA, can infect a new susceptible cell. Virtually any piece of the bacterial chromosome has an equal chance of being transduced by generalized transduction. (Modified from Davis, Dulbecco, Eisen, Ginsberg, and Wood's "Microbiology-3rd Ed.", p. 142, 1980, with permission.)

core into cytoplasm. The injected virus chromosome is expressed and replicated, generating many copies of the viral chromosome as well as incomplete head and tail structures (Fig. 6–28). Maturation enzymes then are involved in loading the phage heads with nucleic acid and attaching the complete tail assembly. Finally, the new virions (usually from several to several hundred/cell) are released by viral-induced lysis of the bacterial cell. The resulting normal phage particles can exist extracellularly for varying periods of time and are fully capable of repeating this lytic/propagation process, which generally requires from one to several hours for completion.

Temperate Viruses: The Lytic or Lysogenic Pathway

Temperate viruses, upon infection, can either (1) multiply lytically, or (2) lysogenize the host cell, *i.e.*, persist as a quiescent, inheritable genetic entity (provirus). The viral chromosome contains genes organized into several operons, some of which function in lytic viral reproduction and others that function in host lysogenization. One of the genes involved in lysogenization codes for a protein repressor which prevents transcription of the operon(s) controlling the lytic response. The major factor that controls which pathway the infecting virus will take is how fast repressor protein is made to prevent expression of the virus lytic/replication machinery. If repressor is not made fast

enough, the virus will replicate and proceed through the lytic pathway like a virulent virus. However, if sufficient repressor is formed before virus replication occurs, the lytic machinery becomes repressed, the lysogenic machinery is expressed, and the virus will become converted to the prophage (or provirus) state. In the lysogenic state, a bacterial host can carry the prophage in one of two diffferent physical forms, depending upon the specific phage. During lysogenization, *E. coli* phage lambda (λ) and *Salmonella* phage P22 are each integrated by phage-encoded specialized recombination mechanisms as a single linear insertion at a specific site on the bacterial chromosome, as exemplified in Figure 6–29A–C. Though many proviruses are inserted into a unique site on the host bacterial chromosome, some viruses can insert into more than one site (*e.g.*, P2 has two preferred but 9 total insertion sites, and Mu phage can insert into any site within the host chromosome). Other viruses, like P1, do not integrate but rather exist as autonomous provirus plasmids in lysogenic cells (*i.e.*, a viral-encoded repressor molecule prevents expression of the lytic functions and limits proviral plasmid replication to once per cell division so that each daughter cell maintains one copy of the proviral plasmid).

Maintenance of the lysogenic state requires continuous repressor synthesis. When the repressor level becomes subminimal, which oc-

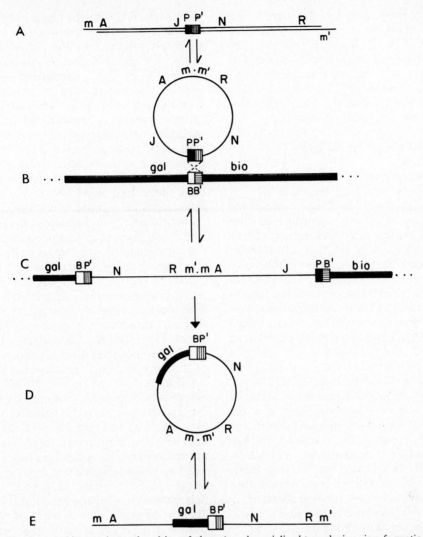

Figure 6–29. Chromosomal integration and excision of phage λ and specialized transducing virus formation. This diagram (not drawn to scale) depicts various molecular states of the temperate bacteriophage λ. The phage chromosome is represented by a thin line(s), while the thicker lines correspond to segments of the bacterial chromosome. The rectangles labeled *PP'* and *BB'* represent the analogous attachment/DNA recognition sites on the phage and bacterial chromosomes, respectively. The DNA sequences marked with *A, J, N,* and *R* are phage structural genes, while *m* and *m'* are single-stranded, 12 nucleotide long complementary 5' ends of λ DNA that circularize during lytic infection or before integration. The only bacterial genes shown are those for utilization of galactose of galactose *(gal)* and the synthesis of biotin *(bio)*.

A, The linear λ genome, show as a double-stranded DNA molecule with cohesive ends. This is the form in which λ DNA is packaged in the virion. For ease of illustration, in steps *B–E* the single thin or wide lines represent double-stranded DNA. *B,* Phage circularization and lysogenization. Once injected intracellularly, linear λ circularizes by annealing at the complementary cohesive termini, *m* and *m'*. In most cells, the circularized λ DNA usually undergoes lytic replication. However, in 1 to 10 per cent of the infected cells, repressor is made fast enough to ensure establishment of the provirus state. During lysogenization phage integration occurs, after pairing of the analogous attachment regions on both λ *(PP')* and the host *(BB')* genomes, by a specific recombinational crossover mediated by the λ-coded integration *(int)* protein. *C,* λ Prophage. The normal, ordered linear arrangement of the λ prophage genome within the host chromosome is shown. This integration process is reversible, and upon induction, excision of the λ genome is effected by both *int* and the excision *(xis)* proteins, resulting usually in the production of normal λ phage (see *B*). Occasionally, however, the excision is inexact and creates a defective specialized transducing phage (*i.e.,* one defective per every 10^5 to 10^6 normal phage: see *D*). *D,* Circular λ d*gal*. During excision of the λ prophage, the recombinational crossover took place between a site within λ and a site in the *gal* region of the chromosome, giving rise to a defective phage particle that has lost a set of phage genes but gained a corresponding length of bacterial DNA, in this case the *gal* genes. Although not shown, a similar abnormal excision involving the opposite end of the λ prophage can create λ d*bio* transducing phage. *E,* Linear λ d*gal*. λ d*gal* is packaged into the phage head as a linear structure, opened at the cohesive ends *m* and *m'*.

curs spontaneously at a low frequency, the prophage switches to the lytic or replicative state (Fig. 6–29A–C). For experimental purposes, prophage induction can be effected at high frequency by various treatments (e.g., exposure to ultraviolet light, mitomycin C, or thymine starvation), although the mechanisms of induction are not totally understood.

Generalized Versus Specialized Transduction

During lytic growth of some viruses (e.g., P1 and P22) or following induction of a λ lysogen, fragments of the host chromosome are sometimes mistakenly incorporated into phage coats during viral maturation. These defective phage particles act as genetic transfer vectors by mediating the transfer of bacterial DNA from one cell to another. Transduction of a DNA fragment is usually detected following its recombination with an homologous region of the chromosome (see Fig. 6–36). Transducing viruses fall into two classes, generalized or specialized, as defined below.

Zinder and Lederberg[86] showed in 1952 that spontaneously induced *Salmonella* P22 phages, separated by filtration from their bacterial hosts, could transduce bacterial genes at a low frequency (10^{-6}) upon infection of auxotrophic bacteria. Furthermore, the transduction phenomenon, unlike transformation, was totally insensitive to both DNase and RNase treatment. More recent studies have shown that this type of transduction is **generalized** (i.e., virtually any chromosomal region can be transduced). As exemplified in Figure 6–28, generalized transduction is the result of a phage packaging error during maturation, in which a bacterial DNA fragment is mistakenly incorporated into a phage coat. Although nearly any gene of the donor bacterium can be transduced, only closely linked markers can be cotransduced by the same phage particle because the length of the incorporated chromosomal fragment is limited by the size of the phage head. Thus, each defective transducing virus generally carries from 45 to 90 kilobase pairs of bacterial DNA, corresponding to 1 to 2 minutes of the host chromosome. Furthermore, there is no association of phage genes and bacterial genes in generalized transducing phage particles, so that virions are either completely defective and carry only bacterial DNA, or normal and carry active phage genomes.

Compared with generalized transduction, some temperate viruses, such as the well-studied *E. coli* K12 lambda phage, can transduce only specific chromosomal genes located immediately adjacent to the phage attachment site on the chromosome, as illustrated in Figure 6–29C–E. Thus, **specialized transduction** involves the transduction of specific chromosomal genes and requires viral integration. In further contrast to generalized transduction, specialized transducing virions can be generated only upon induction of the integrated prophage and never result from phage replicative/lytic growth. Lambda phage, the prototype specialized transducing virus, normally integrates into a single site within the *E. coli* chromosome. Upon induction, prophage excision is usually precise, resulting in the production of normal phage. Occasionally, however, prophage excision is inexact and the adjacent galactose (*gal*) or biotin bacterial genes are incorporated into the excised DNA segment, eventually creating a hybrid transducing phage that can transduce only those specific bacterial genes (Fig. 6–29). Specialized transducing phage chromosomes always contain a portion of the normal phage chromosome linked to a small piece (i.e., about 5 to 10 Mdal.) of the adjacent bacterial chromosome. Expression of the transduced gene (e.g., galactose) can occur as a result of lysogenization of the recipient cell with the transducing λ*gal* phage or via normal general recombination (see Fig. 6–36). Most specialized transducing phages are considered to be defective phage; i.e., they have deleted essential phage functions. Thus, production of high titer lysates of specialized transducing phages requires the participation of a "helper phage" that can supply the missing functions.

Transductional Analysis

The transduction frequency (usually about 10^{-6}) is low enough to eliminate statistically the possibility of two genetically unlinked markers (i.e., two separate transduction events) appearing in the same transductant. This means that the frequency of cotransduction of two or more linked determinants becomes quite important for chromosomal mapping and relative ordering of gene loci by recombinational analysis, as discussed in a previous section.

With the P22 generalized transductional system available for genetic analysis of *S. typhimurium,* fine structure studies of various genetic loci were undertaken. In the histidine operon, for example, the order of nine adjacent genes, which control the formation of all of the enzymes responsible for the biosynthesis of L-histidine, were determined by transductional mapping.[34] Phage P1 and similar viruses have been used extensively in transductional analyses of *E. coli* and *Shigella*. An excellent example of such an analysis was presented by Yanofsky and Lennox in their study of the K-12 tryptophan *(trp)* operon. They were able to order the cluster of five genes involved in tryptophan biosynthesis and to orient these loci in relation to the cysteine B *(cysB)* marker on the K-12 genome. In this study, a number of mutant strains, each containing a characterized genetic lesion in the *trpA* gene, were later correlated with the exact location of the improper amino acid(s) inserted within the mutant polypeptide chain of the *trpA* protein. Thus, these workers established that the linear array of nucleotides in the *trpA* gene coincided with the sequence of amino acids making up the polypeptide chain. This finding provided unequivocal evidence for the widely held concept of the **colinearity** of the structure of the gene with the protein it encodes.[85]

Specialized transduction systems have also been very useful in the isolation and genetic mapping of specific genetic regions of enteric bacterial chromosomes. During the 1960s and early 1970s, these special transducing viruses were extremely valuable in the study of operon regulation.

Abortive Transduction

Although some transduced bacterial DNA segments, following generalized transduction, become stably incorporated into the recipient cell chromosome, an appreciable number of transduced fragments are unstably inherited. In these transductants, termed abortive, the transduced gene fragment does not integrate into the host genome, is incapable of autonomous replication, and is, therefore, segregated to one daughter cell at each cell division, essentially becoming diluted during cell growth. This abortive DNA fragment must circularize in order to avoid being degraded by nucleases. The phenomenon of abortive transduction was first seen in experiments involving the transduction of genes determining motility in *Salmonella*, where trails of colonies occasionally occurred in semisolid agar.[78] These trails were interpreted to be due to the fact that in the presence of the abortively transduced fragment controlling motility, the previously nonmotile recipient cell is motile until, at cell division, this fragment is passed to one daughter cell. Since the other daughter cell is not motile, it grows *in situ* and forms a colony. At each successive cell division the same process occurs, eventually resulting in a series of close colonies that form a trail, the motile abortive transductant cells being at the tip of the trail. Abortive transductants for fermentation or nutritional markers, which appear as minute colonies, have also been observed. The abortive state can persist for many generations, only rarely giving rise to stable recombinants.

Zygotic Induction

Though not directly related to transduction, the phenomenon of zygotic induction deserves mention. This phenomenon is observed during conjugation when that portion of the male chromosome containing a prophage enters a nonimmune female recipient. The zygote thus formed, lacking specific phage repressor, is unable to prevent the newly acquired prophage from being induced to yield a lytic or vegetative response. Moreover, zygotic induction does not take place when the recipient cells are lysogenic for a homologous virus. Inasmuch as prophage genes after conjugal transfer to a nonimmune recipient are expressed without a recombination event, zygotic induction proved to be a useful tool in developing the initial concepts of time of gene entry and unlinked coinheritance frequencies.

Lysogenic Conversion

Virulent strains of *Corynebacterium diphtheriae* release a toxin responsible for the pathogenicity of this microorganism. In 1951, Freeman[24] showed that avirulent, nontoxigenic strains of *C. diphtheriae* are sensitive to a temperate phage known to be carried by all toxigenic *C. diphtheriae*. When avirulent strains are lysogenized with this phage, named β, they are converted to the toxigenic or virulent state (*i.e.,* the phage encodes the diphtheria toxin gene). Thus, the alteration of the state of a bacterium (*e.g.,* from nontoxigenic to toxigenic) by the presence of a lysogenic phage has been termed lysogenic conversion. Conversion of some *Clostridium botulinum* strains to toxin production also involves lysogenic conversion.

A similar involvement of lysogenic bacterial viruses in the expression of certain cell surface antigens has been demonstrated in various *Salmonella* and *Shigella* species. This phage conversion phenomenon has been termed antigenic conversion.

Processes Affecting Gene Expression, Duplication, Integrity, and Evolution

Continued intracellular existence and expression of either preexisting or newly transferred genetic traits necessarily involves constant exposure of these DNA molecules to a variety of metabolic processes. Transcription of the encoded DNA sequences and translation of the resulting mRNA molecules lead to the production of the many proteins required for cell growth as well as for other DNA metabolic events. For instance, stable inheritance of newly transduced genes would require, at a minimum, recombination with the bacterial chromosome, which must then be faithfully replicated and passed to both daughter cells at cell division. Despite the fact that the metabolic processes of restriction, replication, repair, and recombination differ in overall purpose, these phenomena are very much interrelated. As an example, DNA repair sometimes requires recombination mechanisms, and certain enzymes involved in these pathways are also employed in replication. At present, the molecular aspects of these metabolic events are better understood than the nature and regulatory control of their genetic determinants, even though the chromosomal locations of some of these genes have been mapped. Finally, it is now apparent that many DNA metabolic events contribute to the overall evolution of bacteria. The following sections are intended to give a brief review of our current general understanding of these processes affecting gene expression, duplication, integrity, and evolution.

GENE EXPRESSION[27, 28]

Transcription
Transcription is the process whereby the information encoded within DNA is rewritten into mRNA, rRNA, or tRNA. Bacteria contain a DNA-dependent RNA polymerase which requires the four ribonucleotides, GTP, CTP, ATP, and UTP (uracil occurs in RNA

instead of thymine), as substrates. Transcription begins at specific DNA sequences, termed **promoters,** and the single RNA chain polymerization proceeds in the 5′ to 3′ direction; *i.e.,* only one DNA strand is transcribed. Sequence analyses of many different promoters (popularly called **Pribnow boxes**) has revealed that bacterial promoters are approximately 40 base pairs in length and contain two conserved regions involved in RNA polymerase binding (Fig. 6–30). As mentioned previously, only genes containing promoters that are not repressed will be transcribed. Transcription is initiated when the two major components of RNA polymerase, the core enzyme and the sigma factor, bind to a promoter sequence. Following initiation, the sigma factor is released and the core enzyme polymerizes RNA until it reaches a transcription stop signal (*i.e.,* a short discrete termination sequence). Of the three major classes of RNA, only mRNA has a short half-life (averaging 3 min. in *E. coli*). Transcription is largely regulated by the affinity of a promoter for RNA polymerase, by the levels of transcriptional repressors, and sometimes by the requirement for activators of RNA-polymerase binding or for stabilization of the traveling core enzyme.

Translation
This process converts the structural information contained in mRNA (see Table 6–1) into a polypeptide chain. mRNA molecules usually contain from a few to a hundred or so untranslated bases at each end. The untranslated bases at the 5′ end of mRNA contain a ribosome-binding sequence (popularly called a Shine-Dalgarno sequence) which has sequences complementary to 16S rRNA. This is the site at which the 30S and 50S ribosomal components are joined to the message. tRNA molecules are cloverleaf-shaped structures (Fig. 6–31) that carry a specific amino acid at one end and have a specific anticodon region at the opposite end that is complementary to

$$R\sigma \qquad\qquad Rc \qquad\qquad I$$

-A C A A C T G T T A A A - (12-14 bp)-A T A Py T A Py - (5 6 bp)-Py

Figure 6–30. Nucleotide sequence of an ideal genetic promoter. This consensus sequence contains the base pairs that are found most often in more than 20 known promoters. The promoter can be divided into three regions: *Rσ*, which is responsible for sigma factor binding; *Rc*, which is the region recognized by the RNA polymerase core component; and *I*, the site at which transcription is initiated. There are two spacer regions of 12 to 14 bp and 5 to 6 bp in length. The sequence shown is that of the transcribed strand.[28] bp = base pairs, py = pyrimidine.

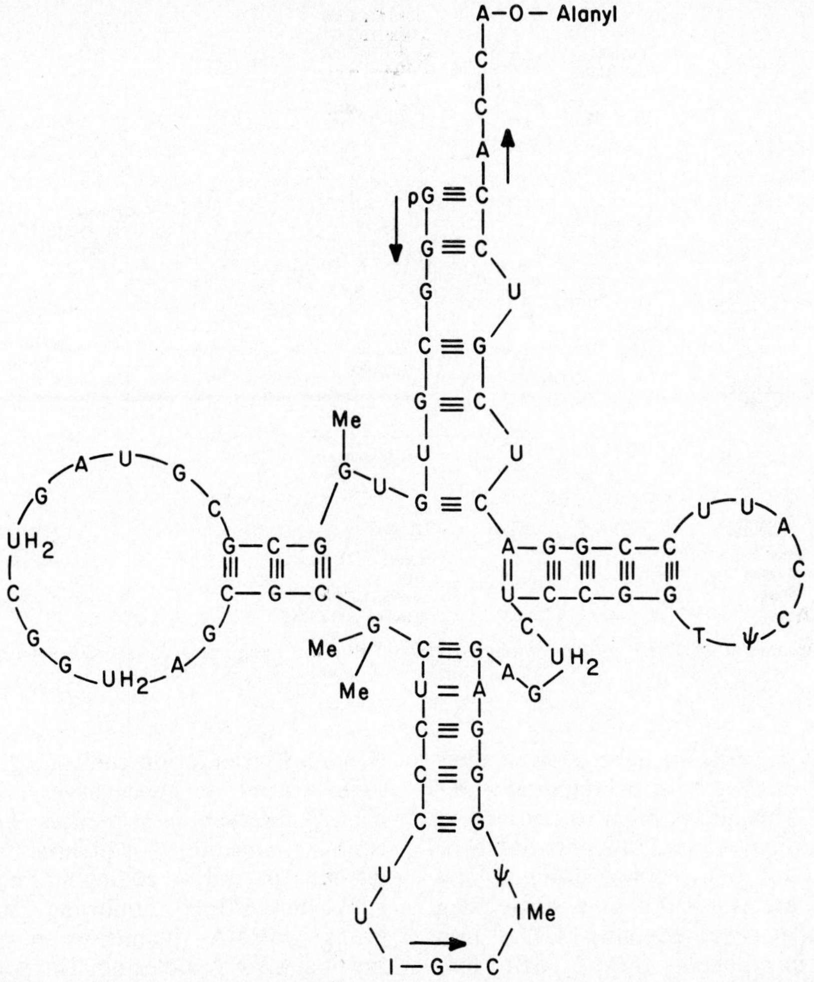

Figure 6–31. Typical secondary structure of a tRNA molecule. The sequence shown here is that of yeast alanine tRNA. In addition to the normal ribonucleotides, this tRNA contains methylated *(Me)* nucleotides, pseudouridine *(ω)*, inosine, and dihydrouridine *(UH₂)*. The arrows denote the 5′ to 3′ direction.

a specific mRNA codon; there are about 60 different tRNA species per cell. Initiation of translation begins at the AUG start codon and *n*-formyl methionine begins the polypeptide chain (Fig. 6–32). As the ribosome moves from codon to codon, a new amino acid is joined to the existing polypeptide chain. The ribosome contains two regions for binding tRNA molecules, the active (A) site and the peptidyl (P) site. A charged aminoacyl tRNA recognizes the appropriate codon and binds to the A site. During elongation, the growing polypeptide chain is translocated from the tRNA at the P site and is linked to the charged tRNA at the A site. Next, the ribosome moves one codon along the message, the uncharged tRNA is released from the P site, the peptidyl tRNA (*i.e.*, carrying the nascent peptide chain) is shifted to the P site, and a new specific tRNA enters the A site. Translation stops at one of

the three termination codons, the polypeptide chain is released from the complex via a variety of termination factors, and the ribosome is disassembled back to its basic components. Thus, in addition to the 3 rRNA species and more than 50 ribosomal proteins, there are a series of initiation, elongation, and termination factors that are involved in protein synthesis. Aside from the availability of the various cofactors and the short half-life of mRNA, translation is regulated by the strength of the ribosome binding sites.

Gene Expression: Variations on the General Theme

Though most bacterial genes are expressed as uninterrupted, single transcription units or as members of an operon, several important conceptual variations to typical bacterial gene expression have been noted (Fig. 6–33). Cer-

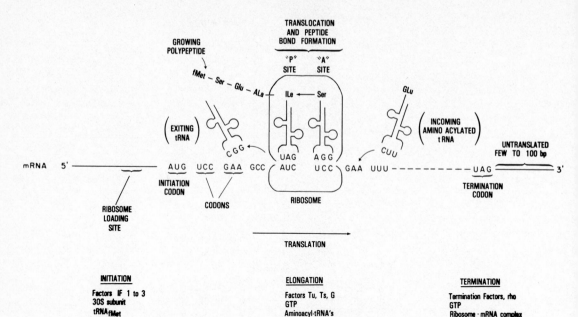

Figure 6–32. Scheme of bacterial protein synthesis. (Modified from Lehninger, A. L., *Biochemistry,* 1970, with permission.)

tain viruses (*e.g.,* φX174) have evolved their genomes so that they have overlapping genes (Fig. 6–33*A*). This allows them to carry more structural information per unit length of DNA. In other systems (*e.g.,* polio virus) several genetic traits are translated as a single long polypeptide that is subsequently cleaved into its functional components (Fig. 6–33*B*). This system alleviates the need for certain transcrip-tional and translation control signals. Finally, some eucaryotic genes have been found to contain intervening sequences; *i.e.,* the gene contains noncoding sequences (now termed **introns**) as well as coding (termed **exon**) re-gions (Fig. 6–33*C*). Following synthesis of the primary mRNA, the introns are spliced out of the final mRNA molecule. This splicing system is a critical feature of the genes that encode

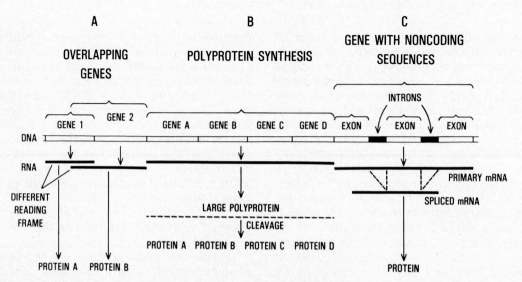

Figure 6–33. Variations on the normal theme of gene organization and expression. Though not necessarily observed in the bacterial chromosome, these important variations from typical bacterial gene organization have been observed. (Modified from Davis, Dulbecco, Eisen, Ginsberg, and Wood's "Microbiology-3rd Ed.," p. 186, 1980, with permission.)

immunoglobulin synthesis where a common determinant gene region is spliced to one of various different variable determinant regions.

REPLICATION

Since the elucidation of the chemical structure of DNA, many studies have been conducted to explain how the information in chromosomal DNA is duplicated and segregated equally to each daughter cell at cell division. The following description of bacterial chromosome replication is meant to convey the concept of how this process occurs in *E. coli*, the system in which most data have been obtained. Most of the biochemical and stereochemical details of this and other replication systems can be found elsewhere.[47, 81, 83]

Bacterial Chromosome Replication

The replicon theory[40] (described in the section on extrachromosomal elements), introduced as a simple model for the regulation of chromosomal replication and subsequent equal partitioning of the newly synthesized molecules, still fulfills its original purpose. The replication process can be divided into three steps: (1) **initiation,** which involves the priming of DNA at the replication origin to begin nucleotide polymerization, (2) **elongation** of the primed DNA to generate two nearly complete daughter molecules, and (3) **termination,** which involves separation of the daughter molecules, gap-filling synthesis, and the introduction of superhelical twists. Initiation of replication in *E. coli* requires the action of several proteins at the replication origin, located at minute 74 on the chromosome map. The two helical strands at the replication fork are catalytically separated by the action of a DNA helicase. This action permits DNA single-strand binding proteins to separate the complementary strands. Subsequently, the synthesis of a short complementary primer RNA sequence on each template DNA strand is required for the action of DNA polymerase III, which is the main replication polymerase and one of three enzymes in *E. coli* that can catalyze the synthesis of polydeoxyribonucleotides. Replication proceeds bidirectionally from the replication origin in *E. coli*, by the joining of nucleotides in the 5' to 3' direction from the primer. Thus, the chromosome begins replicating with a small eye-shaped bubble at the origin which expands in both directions, giving rise to an intermediate structure shaped like the Greek letter theta (θ), and finally to

two complete duplex DNA chromosomes. Following replication each daughter DNA molecule is composed of one entire conserved parental strand plus a newly synthesized complementary strand. This duplication process has been dubbed semiconservative replication. These events are diagrammatically described in Figure 6–34. Okazaki and co-workers[63] found at each growing point newly synthesized DNA comprising relatively short polynucleotide chains (now referred to as Okazaki fragments) of about 1000 units covalently linked to short RNA primer segments. It is now known that DNA polymerization, which proceeds in the 5' to 3' direction from an RNA primer, occurs continuously on one DNA strand in each replication fork while polymerization on the opposite strand occurs discontinuously between short oligonucleotide RNA primers that are laid down about every 10^3 base pairs. Following the synthesis of Okazaki fragments, DNA polymerase 1 serves to fill the gaps between these fragments while the RNA primer segments are simultaneously removed by the exonucleolytic ability of this bifunctional enzyme. Covalent closure is accomplished by the enzyme polynucleotide ligase, which catalyzes the synthesis of a phosphodiester bond between two adjacent but unlinked nucleotides in the same DNA strand. Finally, supercoiling of the completed chromosomes is carried out by DNA gyrase, and the two resulting chromosomes are segregated to each daughter cell at cell division. Replication of the *E. coli* chromosome requires 40 minutes, representing the polymerization of about 1000 nucleotides per second.

DNA REPAIR[30, 32, 47]

Bacterial cells possess, in addition to replication and recombination machinery, enzymes that function in the repair of DNA damaged by various radiations, chemicals, and metabolic events. Perhaps the simplest repair system, termed **photoreactivation,** can be observed following exposure of bacteria to lethal doses of ultraviolet (UV) light. The main UV-induced photoproduct in DNA, a pyrimidine dimer, is enzymatically converted back to normal linked monomers in the presence of strong visible light.

An excision and resynthesis repair mechanism which depends upon the double-stranded structure of DNA has been found that is responsible for removing from either DNA strand structural alterations caused by UV

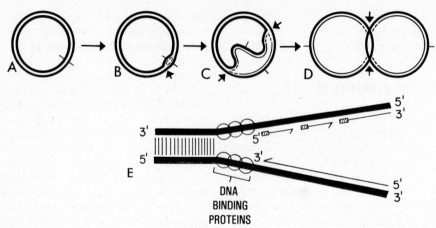

Figure 6–34. Chromosome replication in *E. coli*. This diagram illustrates the bacterial chromosome in various stages of replication. Parental or template DNA strands are represented by thick lines, while thin lines correspond to newly synthesized complementary DNA strands. The two tick marks on each molecule shown in steps *A* to *D* indicate the replication origin, and the small arrows in steps *B* to *D* point to the replication where active DNA synthesis is occurring (indicated by dashed lines). *A,* Upon initiation, the normally supertwisted chromosome is conformationally relaxed at the origin and RNA primers are added to each separated template strand. *B,* Following this primary reaction DNA polymerase catalyzes complementary strand synthesis on both of the parental (*i.e.,* template) strands. Replication proceeds bidirectionally from the origin creating two replication forks (indicated by arrows). At this stage, the replicating area appears as a small eye-shaped bubble. *C,* Replicative intermediate in which the chromosome is approximately half-replicated. *D,* As a result of the semiconservative replication of the chromosome, the two nearly complete daughter DNA molecules each contain one conserved parental DNA strand and a newly synthesized complement. Subsequent to complementary strand synthesis, the new daughter chromosomes are supercoiled and segregated to each daughter cell. *E,* Diagrammatic expansion of a chromosomal replication fork. Subsequent to separation of the parental strands by DNA helicase and the attachment of DNA bnding proteins, short complementary RNA primer sequences (indicated by small hatched boxes), required for the action of DNA polymerase, are synthesized on the template strand. DNA polymerization occurs in the 5′ to 3′ direction from the RNA primer. Because the DNA strands run in opposite directions, DNA polymerization occurs continuously on one DNA template strand and discontinuously (*i.e.,* in short stretches of about 1000 nucleotides) on the opposite template strand at each replication fork. Finally, the RNA primer segments are removed and the single-strand gaps are filled by the bifunctional enzyme, DNA polymerase I.[47, 81]

light, alkylating agents, mitomycin C, and similar agents. Repair is initiated by a damage-specific endonuclease (an enzyme that breaks internal phosphodiester DNA linkages) that mediates one break in the structurally altered strand at a point close to the damaged area. Next, an exonuclease (a phosphodiesterase that degrades DNA beginning at the terminus of a strand) degrades an oligonucleotide (6 to 7 nucleotides) segment containing the structural alteration. Using the unaltered strand as a template, a DNA polymerase synthesizes the correct oligonucleotide complement and the final covalent closure is made by DNA ligase. A similar mechanism of excision and resynthesis appears to be involved in the repair of a variety of different single-strand interruptions caused by exposure of DNA to x-rays and gamma rays.

Occasionally, both DNA strands are damaged at the same site and no unaltered DNA strand remains to serve as the template for repair synthesis. These structural alterations can be replaced through a recombinational exchange with an undamaged homologous DNA segment. The recombinational repair mechanism depends upon the bacterial general recombination system (see section on recombination).

RESTRICTION AND MODIFICATION[4, 35, 60, 67]

The process by which bacterial cells recognize and degrade entering "foreign" DNA, such as bacteriophage or plasmid molecules, was first characterized in the early 1950s. In these studies, bacteriophages grown on any specific bacterial strain were typically stunted in their ability to infect other strains of the same species. The molecular bases of this phenomenon, now called restriction and modification, are as follows: (1) most bacterial strains contain a restriction-modification system comprising two different enzymes, both of which recognize an identical specific short double-stranded DNA sequence; (2) one enzyme, the modification methylase, modifies the DNA sequences so that they are no longer substrates for endonucleolytic attack by the corresponding restriction enzyme; and (3) the second enzyme, a restriction endonuclease, catalyzes a double-stranded cleavage of unmodified DNA by the process termed **restriction.** Thus, in the presence of a restriction enzyme unmodified ("foreign") DNA, but not modified bacterial DNA, would be enzymatically cleaved to linear fragments, which subsequently would be further digested by intracellular exonucleases. Such systems that participate in the selective elimination of unmodified DNA may be partially responsible for maintaining the genetic integrity of bacterial species.

Molecular and Genetic Characterization

Approximately 200 restriction-modification systems coded for by a variety of bacterial, phage, or plasmid genomes are known.[67] These systems are divided into two classes for both functional and structural reasons. Restriction enzymes of *E. coli* K-12 and B, representatives of the Class I enzymes, are large molecules (300,000 daltons) that have several stringent cofactor requirements. Though activated by recognition of a specific DNA sequence, Class I restriction enzymes nonspecifically cause one double-stranded cleavage at some site outside the recognition sequence. All other restriction enzymes (Class II) cleave within the specific DNA recognition sequence, are lower in molecular weight ($<100,000$ daltons) than Class I enzymes, and have simple ionic cofactor requirements. In all systems examined to date, modification is dependent only upon the cofactor S-adenosylmethionine and results in nucleotide methylation.

Genetic analyses of many nonrestricting mutants of *E. coli* K-12 and B have revealed three closely linked genes, designated *hsdR*, *hsdM*, and *hsdS*, which, respectively, control production of a protein involved in restriction, a component of the modification enzyme, and a common sequence-recognition subunit used by both the restriction and modification proteins. The genetic bases of Class II enzyme systems are, as yet, not very well established.

Palindromic DNA Sequences

All Class II restriction enzymes (Table 6–13) recognize specific sequences of four to eight nucleotides in length, that display twofold rotational symmetry about an axis (*i.e.*, palindromes, or inverted repeat DNA sequences which upon analysis look identical

Table 6–13. Representative Class II Restriction Endonucleases

Enzyme	Originally Isolated From	Nucleotide Recognition Site
*Bam*H1	*Bacillus amyloliquefaciens* H	G↑GATCC
*Eco*R1	*E. coli* R1	G↑AATTC
*Hind*II	*Haemophilus influenzae* Rd	GTPy↑PuAC
*Hind*III	*Haemophilus influenzae* Rd	A↑AGCTT
*Sma*1	*Serratia marcescens*	CCC↑GGG
*Hae*III	*Haemophilus aegypticus*	GG↑CC

The nucleotide recognition sequences are written from 5′ to 3′ and only one strand is shown. Some of the above enzymes produce staggered cleavages (*e.g.*, *Bam*H1), while others produce a flush-ended, double-strand cleavage (*e.g.*, *Sma*1).[67]

from either end due to the antiparallel complementary nature of DNA), as exemplified in Figure 6–35. Many of these enzymes cleave each DNA strand at staggered but symmetrically identical locations within the recognition sequence, resulting in fragments with termini containing overlapping complementary sequences. This special property of certain restriction enzymes has been used to construct recombinant plasmid molecules containing DNA segments from either bacteria or higher organisms (see Figure 6–39 and last section on applied genetic engineering). Following transformation of bacterial hosts, such cloned recombinant DNA molecules can be used to study the organization and expression of isolated gene segments.

It is worth noting that palindromic DNA sequences are highly specific protein-DNA interaction sites for a variety of proteins, including various endonucleases and repressor molecules. Intrastrand annealing of the complementary sequences of a DNA palindrome, shown in Figure 6–35B, has been proposed as the stereochemical structure involved in specific protein recognition.[42]

RECOMBINATION[12, 35, 44, 66]

The term genetic recombination refers to various processes in different organisms that promote new linkage relationships of genes or parts of genes. In addition to physical exchange, or crossing over, of DNA segments between largely homologous regions of similar chromosomes, recombination processes encompass such diverse events as the chromosomal integration of plasmids or bacteriophage (*e.g.*, F and λ), chromosomal duplications

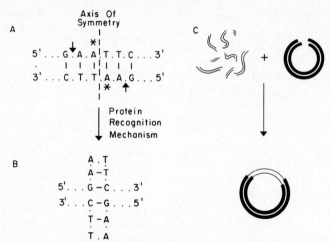

Figure 6–35. Protein recognition at palindromic DNA sequences and the molecular cloning of DNA fragments. *A,* Double-stranded polynucleotide sequence illustrating a DNA palindrome. Because of the antiparallel and complementary nature of duplex DNA, the sequence on either side of the symmetrical axis is identical. The specific sequence shown is the recognition site for a class II restriction-modification system called *Eco*R1. The modification enzyme normally methylates two adenine nucleotides (marked by asterisks); unmodified sequences are specifically cleaved at staggered but symmetrically identical sites (marked by small arrows) within the recognition sequence, creating overlapping ends with complementary nucleotides. *B,* Within a single strand of a DNA palindrome, complementary nucleotides from both sides of the symmetrical axis can anneal. Such intrastrand self-annealed stuctures have been proposed to be specific protein recognition sites for DNA interacting proteins such as endonuclease and repressor molecules.[42] *C,* Diagram depicting a commonly employed procedure for the molecular cloning of DNA fragments. As shown in the top of this illustration, the DNA to be cloned (represented by thin lines) is fragmented by a specific endonuclease as described in *A.* Also, a self-replicating identifiable cloning vehicle (indicated by thick lines), such as plasmid, containing only one endonuclease specific recognition site, is cleaved. Following mixing, foreign DNA is inserted into the cloning vehicle (see lower half of illustration). The overlapping complementary ends of this *in vitro* constructed recombinant plasmid are covalently closed by DNA ligase, and these molecules are inserted into bacterial cells by transformation.

(–ABAB–), inversions (–ABDC–), and deletions (–ABD–), as well as the transposition of drug resistance transposons and *IS* elements. Albeit varied, these events can be organized into two categories: (1) **general recombination** mechanisms mediate genetic exchanges at random points between largely homologous DNA segments, such as the chromosomal integration of transduced bacterial DNA, and these processes require certain host general recombination functions; and (2) **specialized recombination** processes catalyze specific (*i.e.,* nonrandom) exchanges of genetic information between DNA segments that share little or no sequence homology; *e.g.,* λ integration into the *E. coli* chromosome, or transposition of Mu phage or an *IS* element. Different types of recombination (*i.e.,* general versus specialized) appear to be mediated by separate overall processes, but may share common biochemical components of DNA metabolism, such as DNA unwinding enzymes, polymerases, and various nucleases.

Genetic Analysis of General Recombination[12]

Recombination-deficient (Rec⁻) bacterial mutants have been detected following muta-

genesis by screening **clones** (*i.e.,* groups of cells derived from the same parent) for inability to form hybrids in matings with Hfr strains, or for their pleiotropic sensitivity to radiation or radiomimetic agents. In *E. coli,* approximately 10 different *rec* genes have been located. Mutations in the *recA* gene, chromosomally located at map minute 50, are the only mutations known to prevent all detectable chromosomal general recombination. The *recB* and *recC* genes, both located at 54 minutes on the *E. coli* map, encode separate moieties of the recombination enzyme, exonuclease V. The functions of most other *rec* genes remain uncharacterized, although molecular cloning techniques have recently permitted the isolation of several *rec* genes and their corresponding proteins.

Through complementation analysis of various Rec⁻ mutations, Clark[12] has deduced the existence of two general recombination pathways, both of which require *recA* gene function. One pathway that utilizes the *recB, recC* exonuclease system accounts for almost all general recombination. In the absence of the *recB, recC* enzyme, a second pathway involving the uncharacterized *recF* gene mediates recombination at about 1 per cent of wild-type levels, but, under certain conditions, the *recF* pathway can function equally well.

No *rec* function has been detected that is absolutely essential for cell survival, but the *recA*, *recB*, or *recC* mutations each normally cause a decrease in cell viability. Thus, these gene products are very important to DNA metabolism. In addition, studies similar to that described above have revealed phage-specified general recombination systems in λ and T4.

Molecular Mechanisms of General Recombination[47, 66]

Little is factually known about the molecular events involved in recombination. However, based on studies of bacterial, phage, and plasmid recombinant DNA molecules, it is currently thought that general recombination accompanies breakage of parental molecules and reunion of exchanged DNA segments. Molecular models for general recombination are necessarily speculative and those included here are used only to generate a general concept of events likely to be involved in recombination.

Figure 6–36, based on a number of experimental findings, diagrammatically illustrates events likely to be involved in the integration of a single linear DNA strand, acquired by conjugation or transformation, into the bacterial chromosome. The exchange of a single strand between two duplex DNA molecules, as shown in Figure 6–36E, could occur by a minor variation of the scheme for single-strand integration. Although more involved, double-strand exchange between two duplex DNA molecules might follow a similar course of events—*i.e.*, pairing, extension, and recombinational exchange. Because of the complexity of double-strand exchange models, only the end product of a single reciprocal (*i.e.*, an event in which all DNA ends created by recombinational cleavage are rejoined to new sequences) double-strand exchange is shown in Figure 6–36F. It is important to note that one crossover event between two circular molecules sharing some homology (*e.g.*, an *IS* element) would produce one larger circular molecule, a product observed not only in plasmid-plasmid recombi-

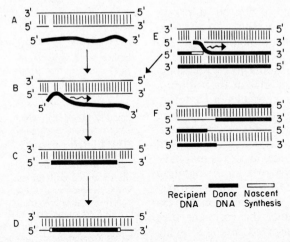

Figure 6–36. Molecular models for genetic recombination. Interacting DNA strands are indicated by horizontal lines; hydrogen bonds between complementary nucleotides are shown as short vertical lines. Steps *A* to *E* describe events likely to occur during the integration of a single DNA strand into a recipient double-stranded molecule (*i.e.*, nonreciprocal exchange of DNA). *A*, Entering single-stranded donor DNA quickly pairs with a homologous region of the chromosome. Genetic exchange is initiated on the recipient genome at a single-strand gap created by a recombination enzyme(s) or some other DNA metabolic activity. *B*, Extension of the exchanged region (see wavy arrow) follows displacement of degradation, or both, of the corresponding recipient strand. *C*, Termination of the genetic exchange may occur at a gap introduced by a specific recombination enzyme or by some other event. Unincorporated donor sequences are removed exonucleolytically. *D*, The gaps on each side of the incorporated DNA segment are repaired by DNA polymerase and ligase. Any differences (base mispairings, nucleotide additions or deletions) between the strands of these recombinant DNA molecules are either corrected by DNA repair processes or expressed following replication. *E*, The exchange of a single DNA strand between two double-stranded DNA molecules could occur in a manner similar to that described above, except that exchange between paired regions would require, at least, single phosphodiester bond cleavages in corresponding strands of both donor and recipient molecules. Incorporation of the exchanged DNA segment would occur as shown in steps *B* to *D*. Complementary donor strand synthesis could occur subsequent to or simultaneously with displacement of the donor single strand. Alternatively, (not shown) a single strand from each molecule could exchange with the opposite molecule, giving rise to a reciprocal exchange of single DNA strands. *F*, This diagram depicts the products expected from a reciprocal, double-stranded exchange between two DNA molecules. It should be noted that chromosomal integration of the F plasmid or phage λ occurs by a specific, reciprocal, double-stranded exchange.[66]

nation (see Fig. 6–26) but also in the chromosomal integration of phage (see Fig. 6–29) or plasmids (see Fig. 6–14).

Specialized Recombination Systems[44]

The distinct behavior of this group of systems (*i.e.*, independence from known general recombination systems and the lack of a requirement for extended homology between interacting DNA regions) allows them to be categorized as **specialized.** Specialized recombination systems include the processes involved in temperate phage integration into and excision from the bacterial chromosome (*e.g.*, λ, P22, or Mu) or the transposition of transposable elements (*IS* or Tn units). The λ phage specialized recombination system has been described earlier (Fig. 6–29); it allows λ to integrate into or excise from a specific attachment region on the *E. coli* chromosome. Similar specialized recombination systems allow P22 to recombine with a limited number of specific attachment/recognition regions on the *Salmonella* chromosome and Mu phage to integrate as a discrete provirus unit into virtually any site in the bacterial chromosome.

The physical exchange of discrete transposable genetic elements represents another example of specialized recombination. For example, in order for these elements to be transposed from chromosome to chromosome as discrete units, distinct sites at their termini must be enzymatically recognized (see Fig. 6–7). All transposable elements studied to date are bracketed by characteristic inverted repeat, or palindromic, DNA sequences which can form intrastrand annealed complexes that have been proposed as DNA-protein recognition structures (see Fig. 6–35*B*). Even though transposable elements are recombinationally exchanged as discrete units, the recipient sites into which they are inserted are not highly specific, but are nonrandomly situated (*i.e.*, the recipient sites are clustered). Though transposition of the simple *IS* units must employ chromosomally encoded specialized recombination systems, some of the larger Tn elements (*e.g.*, Tn3) have been demonstrated to encode certain transposition functions. The mechanism of transposition for several of the large Tn elements has been defined in genetic and molecular detail and is diagrammatically illustrated in Figure 6–37. The total number of different Tn specialized recombination systems or mechanisms of transposition, if different from that shown in Figure 6–37, is not known.

Recent data indicate that *IS* elements and their associated specialized recombination sys-

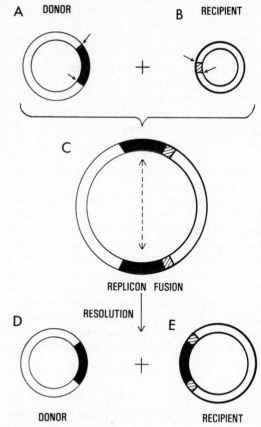

Figure 6–37. Mechanism of transposition. The model shown below, first proposed by J. Shapiro (reviewed in refs. 44 and 71) depicts the manner in which several transposable elements apparently undergo transposition. *A*, The donor plasmid carries a transposable element (shaded in black), which during transposition is single-strand cleaved on opposite strands at opposing ends (see arrows); *B*, the recipient replicon (denoted by thick lines) is apparently cleaved at staggered sites (see arrows) on opposing strands to generate short overlapping ends; *C*, the extended ends of the two molecules are recombined with one another and gap-filling synthesis creates a replicon fusion structure that contains two copies of the transposable element and two copies of the recipient site sequence (marked by diagonal lines). The replicon fusion structure undergoes an enzymation resolution event in which a site in the middle of the transposable element recombines (see dashed line) with the same site in the other copy of this element. The result of this resolution event is that the original donor sequences, *D*, are regenerated and the recipient molecule, *E*, now carries a copy of the transposable element between a directly repeated, short recipient site duplication.

tems are responsible for many large chromosomal deletion, inversion, and transposition mutations. In addition, *IS* elements have been observed to act as the homologous DNA regions during general recombination dependent reactions such as Hfr formation (Fig. 6–14) and the association/dissociation phenomenon exhibited by certain R plasmids (Fig. 6–26*A*).

These latter two examples show that although *IS* elements are transposed by special enzymes, general recombination systems can promote DNA insertion, deletion, inversion, or transposition reactions between homologous *IS* units. The fact that transposable elements are involved in both general and specialized recombination events points out the complex interrelationships between these systems.

EVOLUTION

Definition

Bacterial evolution, until recently, was thought by many to occur by a very slow process encompassing the induction of a small mutation (Fig. 6–38*B*), environmental selection for all desirable mutations, and the accumulation of beneficial mutations through intercellular genetic exchange and general recombination (Fig. 6–38*C*). It seems appropriate to refer to these mutational events, which involve the addition, deletion, or substitution of only one or a few nucleotides, as **microevolutionary.** Within the past 10 to 15 years, however, it has become apparent that large chromosomal rearrangements (*e.g.,* duplications, deletions, inversions, and transpositions of large DNA segments; Fig. 6–38*D* and *E*) occur in bacteria, often at relatively high frequencies. These events, involving the loss, gain, or rearrangement of large DNA segments, can accordingly be described as **macroevolutionary** and certainly must account for a major proportion of bacterial evolution. It now appears that bacterial evolution results from the temporal accumulation of both micro- and macroevolutionary DNA alterations (Fig. 6–38*F*).

Evolutionary Considerations

Although all mutagens, DNA recombination processes, and intercellular DNA transfer mechanisms influence the overall evolution of bacteria, three factors (plasmids, transposable elements, and conjugal DNA transfer systems) would appear to have the most significant evolutionary impact. Transposable elements carry large blocks of genes and cause macroevolutionary chromosomal DNA rearrangements, often at high frequencies. Plasmids, which appear to be recombinational assemblages of various transposable elements, can be conjugally transferred both interspecifically and intergenerically among many diverse bacterial genera. Thus, evidence indicates that bacterial genomes are constantly undergoing both micro- and macroevolutionary alterations. Despite these observations, bacterial species have remained remarkably stable in a genetic sense. Perhaps most regions of the

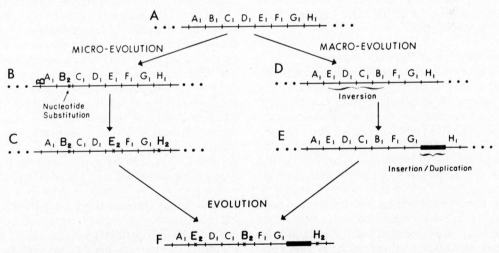

Figure 6–38. Diagrammatic representation of evolution. The horizontal lines represent a portion of the bacterial chromosome, and arbitrary genes are labeled A, B, ⋯ and H. The subscript, 1 or 2, after each gene designates an allelic form of that gene. The chromosomal segment shown in *A* can undergo small single nucleotide base changes or microevolutionary events, such as that shown in *B* and *C*. The mutated genes are indicated by a subscript 2 and bold-faced print, and the mutations are located by an X. In addition, large chromosomal or macroevolutionary rearrangements such as the inversion of a DNA segment *D*, the deletion of a DNA segment (not shown) or the insertion of a DNA sequence *E* can occur. Overall bacterial evolution appears to result from the accumulation, via genetic recombination, of both micro- and macroevolutionary chromosomal alterations, as shown in *F*. (From Kopecko, D. J., Specialized genetic recombination systems in bacteria: their involvement in gene expression and evolution. *In* F. Hahn (Ed.), Progress in Molecular Biology, Vol. 7. Springer-Verlag Press, Heidelberg, 1980, pp. 135–234. Used with permission.)

bacterial chromosome have reached a thermodynamically stable state with their neighboring DNA regions. If so, many spontaneous DNA alterations, large or small, might upset this stability, would not be advantageous (or might even be deleterious) to the cell, and eventually would be selected against. Following this logic, plasmids (which could be lost without affecting cell viability) and transposable elements may often offer the fastest and safest means of transiently adapting to new environmental forces.

Practical Applications of Bacterial Genetics

Aside from gaining a fundamental knowledge of how various bacterial properties are encoded in DNA and what events control gene expression and evolution, the information reviewed briefly in this chapter has been directly applied to the solution of some important practical problems that, because of their medical importance, bear mentioning here.

Mutagenesis in Industry

Selection of industrially useful bacterial mutants has been employed for many years. Bacteria are mutated in steps using a variety of different mutagens to select for an organism that produces more of an important cell metabolite. For example, the strain of *Penicillium notatum* used to produce penicillin commercially has been mutated in more than 55 steps, so that it now makes 10,000-fold more antibiotic than the initial isolate. Similarly, many other industrially useful strains have been improved by mutations that increase expression of a desirable gene or decrease expression of an undesirable trait.

Construction of Vaccine Strains

Mutagenesis techniques have been useful in constructing attenuated strains of both bacteria and viruses. A debilitated strain can be used as a live vaccine, which generally stimulates higher levels of immunity than a killed vaccine, but will not cause overt disease. For example, typhoid fever has been an important disease for hundreds of years. Various killed vaccine preparations of the causative agent, *Salmonella typhi*, have been used for more than 50 years and have provided significant immunity. Unfortunately, most recipients develop significant adverse reactions to these vaccines (*i.e.,* extremely sore arm at site of injection, fever, malaise, and nausea). Using mutagenic techniques, Germanier and co-workers[26] have developed an attenuated *S. typhi* oral vaccine strain, Ty 21a, which has proven in large field trials to provide long-term protection against infection by *S. typhi*. More importantly, Ty 21a was found to be safe (*i.e.,* nonreverting to

virulent) and was not associated with the untoward side effects of the killed vaccines. Several attenuated virus vaccines have also been developed using similar genetic technology.

Ames Test for Carcinogenicity of Chemical Compounds[3]

Noting the strong correlation between the mutagenicity and carcinogenicity of various compounds, Ames and collaborators developed a group of specially mutated bacterial strains which could be used to test compounds for their carcinogenicity. These strains were mutagenically modified in three ways: (1) the cell wall of tester bacterial strains was mutated so that they became highly permeable to organic compounds, (2) the strains were mutated to inhibit DNA repair activity so that visualization of mutations could be maximized, and (3) each tester strain received a different, well-characterized histidine auxotrophic mutation (*e.g.,* frame-shift, transversion, transition).

The test is conducted by separately exposing tester cell populations, each containing a different histidine auxotrophic mutation, to the suspected agent. Then the exposed cell groups are each enumerated, versus an unexposed control cell population, on a minimal agar medium lacking histidine; only histidine-independent revertant strains will grow. Using a series of defined histidine mutants, one can assess if a compound increases the normal reversion mutation frequency and also what type of mutations the compound stimulates.

The Ames test, which is heavily used in industry today, offers a simple, rapid, and very inexpensive way to screen large numbers of compounds for potential carcinogenicity. Some potential carcinogens need to be activated by liver microsomal enzymes before testing. Also, some compounds that are thought to be carcinogenic may not be mutagenic in this assay (*e.g.,* asbestos fibers).

Applied Genetic Engineering[11, 56, 64]

Recombinant DNA technology is an extremely important application of bacterial ge-

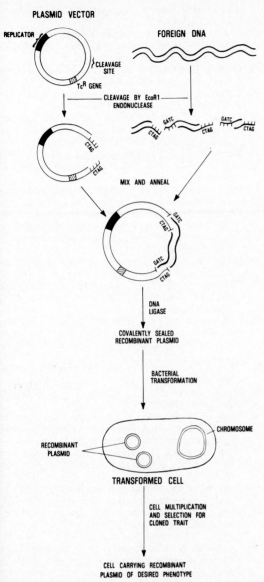

Figure 6–39. Diagram showing the essential steps for constructing a recombinant DNA molecule and inserting it into a bacterial host. Note that there are alternative techniques for constructing recombinant molecules and also alternative recipient cells.

netic knowledge. The essential ingredients of this technology, outlined in Figure 6–39, are as follows: (1) a self-replicating plasmid or virus vector that is relatively small, contains one or more easily detectable phenotypic properties (*e.g.,* tetracycline resistance), and has one or more unique sites susceptible to Class II restriction endonuclease cleavage; (2) highly polymerized foreign DNA containing a gene(s) of interest; (3) a method for linking foreign DNA to the vector; (4) a means of introducing the recombinant DNA molecule into a recipient host cell; and (5) some method for detect-

ing the cloned foreign trait(s) of interest. As shown in Figure 6–39, the vector plasmid and the foreign DNA are separately cleaved by the same restriction endonuclease, which creates short complementary single-strand tails at each fragment end. Upon mixing these DNA's at the appropriate concentration and ratio, the reaction favors the recircularization of the single vector fragment with a foreign DNA fragment. The hybrid molecule, which is held together by a few hydrogen bonds, can be covalently sealed with DNA ligase. The covalently sealed recombinant molecule then can be used to transform competent bacterial cells. Selection of the desired recombinant clone can be performed directly (*e.g.,* examine for acquisition of the appropriate phenotype) or indirectly (*e.g.,* by radioimmunoassay). Note that there are many variations to the above basic scheme for cloning a specific DNA fragment.

Recombinant DNA technology allows one to isolate genes of interest from virtually any organism and to insert them into a variety of different systems (*i.e.,* yeast, many bacteria, and higher organisms). Applied genetic engineering encompasses the use of recombinant DNA technology together with many other procedures (*e.g.,* genetic, biochemical, immunological) to construct highly useful strains of bacteria, yeast, plants, etc. For example, genetic engineering procedures have been used to construct bacteria that overproduce human insulin, human growth hormone, various interferons, and blood clotting factors, all of which were heretofore available only in small quantities. Recently, major surface antigenic components of various viruses (*e.g.,* foot and mouth disease virus, hepatitis virus) have been cloned, via recombinant DNA techniques, in efforts aimed at making purified component vaccines. In addition to these direct medical applications, genetic engineering technology has opened the door to the detailed study of genes of higher organisms.

REFERENCES

1. Achtman, M., G. Morelli, and S. Schwuchow. 1978. Cell-cell interactions in conjugating *Escherichia coli:* role of F pili and fate of mating aggregates. J. Bacteriol. **135**:1053–1061.
2. Achtman, M., and R. Skurray. 1977. A redefinition of the mating phenomenon in bacteria. pp. 233–279. *In* J. L. Reissig (Ed.): Microbial Interactions, Receptors, and Recognition, Ser. B. V3. Chapman and Hall, London.
3. Ames, B. N. 1979. Identifying environmental chemi-

cals causing mutations and cancer. Science **204**:587–593.

4. Arber, W. 1974. DNA modification and restriction. Progr. Nucleic Acid Res. Molec. Biol. **14**:1–37.

5. Avery, O. T., C. M. MacLeod, and M. McCarty. 1944. Studies on the chemical nature of the substance inducing transformation of pneumococcal types. J. Exptl. Med. **79**:137–158.

6. Bachman, B. J., and K. B. Low. 1980. Linkage map of *Escherichia coli* K-12, Edition 6. Microbiol. Rev. **44**:1–56.

7. Beckwith, J., and D. Zipser (Eds.). 1970. The Lactose Operon. Cold Spring Harbor Laboratory, Cold Spring Harbor, N.Y.

8. Brinton, C. C. 1971. The properties of sex pili, the viral nature of "conjugal" genetic transfer systems, and some possible approaches to the control of bacterial drug resistance. Crit. Rev. Microbiol. **1**:105–160.

9. Broda, P. 1979. Plasmids. W. H. Freeman, San Francisco.

10. Calos, M. P. and J. H. Miller. 1980. Transposable elements. Cell **20**:579–595.

11. Chakrabarty, A. M. (Ed.). 1978. Genetic Engineering. CRC Press, Inc., Boca Raton, Florida.

12. Clark, A. J. 1973. Recombination deficient mutants of *E. coli* and other bacteria. Ann. Rev. Genet. **7**:67–86.

13. Clewell, D. B. 1972. Nature of colE$_1$ plasmid replication in *Escherichia coli* in the presence of chloramphenicol. J. Bacteriol. **110**:667–676.

14. Cohen, S. N., A. C. Chang, and L. Hsu. 1972. Nonchromosomal antibiotic resistance in bacteria: genetic transformation of *Escherichia coli* by R-factor DNA. Proc. Natl. Acad. Sci. USA **69**:2110–2114.

15. Cox, E C. 1976. Bacterial mutator genes and the control of spontaneous mutations. Ann. Rev. Genet. **10**:135–156.

16. Curtiss, R. 1969. Bacterial conjugation. Ann. Rev. Microbiol. **23**:69–136.

17. Davidson, N., et al. 1975. Electron microscope studies of sequence relations among plasmids of *Escherichia coli*. p. 56. In D. Schlessinger (Ed.): Microbiology—1974. American Society for Microbiology, Washington, D.C.

18. Davis, R. W., D. Botstein, and J. R. Roth. 1980. Advanced Bacterial Genetics. Cold Spring Harbor Laboratory, Cold Spring Harbor, N.Y.

19. Drake, J. W. 1969. Mutagenic mechanisms. Ann. Rev. Genet. **3**:247–268.

20. Drake, J. W., and R. H. Baltz. 1976. The biochemistry of mutagenesis. Ann. Rev. Biochem. **45**:11–37.

21. Dunny, G. M., B. L. Brown, and D. B. Clewell. 1978. Induced cel aggregation and mating in *Streptococcus faecalis*: Evidence for a bacterial sex pheromone. Proc. Natl. Acad. Sci. USA **75**:3479–3483.

22. Ehrlich, S. D. 1977. Replication and expression of plasmids from *Staphylococcus aureus* in *Bacillus subtilis*. Proc. Natl. Acad. Sci. USA **74**:1680–1682.

23. Falkow, S. 1975. Infectious Multiple Drug Resistance. Pion Ltd., London.

24. Freeman, V. J. 1951. Studies on the virulence of bacteriophage-infected strains of *Corynebacterium diphtheriae*. J. Bacteriol. **61**:675–688.

25. Garen, A. 1968. Sense and nonsense in the genetic code. Science **160**:149–159.

26. Germanier, R. and E. Furer. 1975. Isolation and characterization of *galE* mutant Ty21a of *Salmonella typhi*: a candidate strain for a live, oral, typhoid vaccine. J. Infect. Dis. **131**:553–558.

27. Glass, R. E. 1982. Gene Function—*E. coli* and Its Heritable Elements. University of California Press, Los Angeles.

28. Goldberger, R. F. (Ed.). 1979. Biological Regulation and Development. Vol. 1, Gene Expression. Plenum Press, New York.

29. Griffith, F. 1928. The significance of pneumococcal types. J. Hygiene **27**:113–159.

30. Grossman, L., et al. 1975. Enzymatic repair of DNA. Ann. Rev. Biochem. **44**:19–43.

31. Guerry, P., and S. Falkow. 1971. Polynucleotide sequence relationships among some bacterial plasmids. J. Bacteriol. **107**:372–374.

32. Hanawalt, P. C., Friedberg, E. C., and C. F. Fox (Eds.). 1978. DNA Repair Mechanisms. Academic Press, New York.

33. Hardy, K. 1981. Bacterial Plasmids. American Society for Microbiology, Washington, D.C.

34. Hartman, P. E., J. C. Loper, and D. Serman. 1960. Fine structure mapping by complete transduction between histidine-requiring *Salmonella* mutants. J. Gen. Microbiol. **22**:322–353.

35. Hayes, W. 1968. The Genetics of Bacteria and Their Viruses. 2nd ed. John Wiley & Sons, New York.

36. Hershey, A. D. (Ed.). 1971. The Bacteriophage Lambda. Cold Spring Harbor Laboratory, Cold Spring Harbor, N.Y.

37. Holloway, B. W. 1975. Genetic organization of *Pseudomonas*. pp. 133–161. In Genetics and Biochemistry of Pseudomonas. John Wiley & Sons, New York.

38. Howe, M. M. 1978. Invertible DNA sequences. Nature **271**:608–610.

39. Hu, S., et al. 1975. αβ sequence of F is *IS*3. J. Bacteriol. **123**:687–692.

40. Jacob, F., S. Brenner, and F. Cuzin. 1963. On the regulation of DNA replication in bacteria. Cold Spring Harbor Symp. Quant. Biol. **28**:329–348.

41. Jacob, F., and E. L. Wollman. 1961. Sexuality and the Genetics of Bacteria. Academic Press, New York.

42. Jovin, M. 1976. Recognition mechanisms of DNA-specific enzymes. Ann. Rev. Biochem. **45**:889–920.

43. Kleckner, N. 1981. Transposable elements in prokaryotes. Ann. Rev. Genet. **15**:341–404.

44. Kopecko, D. J. 1980. Specialized Genetic Recombination Systems in Bacteria: Their Involvement in Gene Expression and Evolution, pp. 135–234. In F. Hahn (Ed.): Progress In Molecular and Subcellular Biology. Vol. 7. Springer-Verlag Press, Heidelberg.

45. Kopecko, D. J., J. Brevet, and S. N. Cohen. 1976. Involvement of multiple translocating DNA segments and recombinational hotspots in the structural evolution of bacterial plasmids. J. Molec. Biol. **108**:333–360.

46. Kopecko, D. J., J. Holcombe, and S. B. Formal. 1979. Molecular characterization of plasmids from virulent and spontaneously occurring avirulent colonial variants of *Shigella flexneri*. Infect. Immun. **24**:580–582.

47. Kornberg, A. 1980. DNA Replication. W. H. Freeman & Co., San Francisco.

48. Lacks, S. 1962. Molecular fate of DNA in genetic transformation of Pneumococcus. J. Molec. Biol. **5**:119–131.

49. Laskin, A. I., and H. A. Lechevalier (Eds.). 1974. Handbook of Microbiology. CRC Press, Cleveland, Ohio.

50. Lederberg, J., and E. M. Lederberg. 1952. Replica plating and indirect selection of bacterial mutants. J. Bacteriol. **63**:399–406.

51. Lederberg, J., and E. L. Tatum. 1946. Novel geno-

types in mixed cultures of biochemical mutants of bacteria. Cold Spring Harbor Symp. Quant. Biol. **11**:113–114.

52. Levy, S. B., R. C. Clowes, and E. L. Koenig (Eds.). 1981. Molecular Biology, Pathogenicity, and Ecology of Bacterial Plasmids. Plenum Press, New York.

53. Lewin, B. 1977. Plasmids and Phages. Vol. 3, Gene Expression. John Wiley & Sons, New York.

54. Luria, S. E., *et al.* 1978. General Virology. 3rd ed. John Wiley & Sons, New York.

55. Luria, S. E., and M. Delbrück. 1943. Mutations of bacteria from virus sensitivity to virus resistance. Genetics **28**:491–511.

56. Maniatis, T., E. F. Fritsch, and J. Sambrook. 1982. Molecular Cloning. A Laboratory Manual. Cold Spring Harbor Laboratory, Cold Spring Harbor, New York.

57. Markovitz, A. 1964. Regulatory mechanisms for synthesis of capsular polysaccharide in mucoid mutants of *Escherichia coli* K-12. Proc. Natl. Acad. Sci. USA **51**:239–246.

58. Mathews, C. K. 1971. Bacteriophage Biochemistry. Van Nostrand Reinhold Co., New York.

59. Miller, J. 1972. Experiments in Molecular Genetics. Cold Spring Harbor Laboratory, Cold Spring Harbor, N.Y.

60. Nathans, D., and H. O. Smith. 1975. Restriction endonucleases in the analysis and restructuring of DNA molecules. Ann. Rev. Biochem. **44**:273–293.

61. Notani, N. K., and J. K. Setlow. 1974. Mechanism of bacterial transformation and transfection. Vol. 14. p. 39. *In* J. N. Davidson and W. E. Cohn (Eds.): Progress in Nucleic Acid Research and Molecular Biology. Academic Press, New York.

62. Novick, R. P., *et al.* 1976. Uniform nomenclature for bacterial plasmids: a proposal. Bacteriol. Rev. **40**:168–189.

63. Okazaki, R., *et al.* 1968. *In vivo* mechanism of DNA chain growth. Cold Spring Harbor Symp. Quant. Biol. **33**:129–142.

64. Old, R. W., and S. B. Primrose. 1980. Principles of Gene Manipulation. University of California Press, Los Angeles.

65. Pritchard, R. H., P. T. Barth, and J. Collins. 1969. Control of DNA synthesis in bacteria. Symp. Soc. Gen. Microbiol. **19**:263–297.

66. Radding, C. M. 1978. Genetic recombination: strand transfer and mismatch repair. Ann. Rev. Biochem. **47**:847–880.

67. Roberts, R. 1976. Restriction endonucleases. Crit. Rev. Biochem. **4**:123–164.

68. Roth, J. R. 1974. Frameshift mutations. Ann. Rev. Genet. **8**:317.

69. Rownd, R. H., *et al.* 1977. Dissociation, reassociation and replication of composite R plasmid DNA. *In* D. Schlessinger (Ed.): Microbiology—1978. American Society for Microbiology, Washington, D.C.

70. Schleif, R. F. and P. C. Wensink. 1981. Practical Methods in Molecular Biology. Springer-Verlag, New York.

71. Shapiro, J. (Ed.). 1983. Mobile Genetic Elements. Academic Press, New York.

72. Silverman, M., *et al.* 1979. Phase variation in *Salmonella*: genetic analysis of a recombinational switch. Proc. Natl. Acad. Sci. USA **76**:391–395.

73. Simon, M., *et al.* 1980. Phase variation: the evolution of a controlling element. Science **209**:1370–1374.

74. Skurray, R. A., *et al.* 1976. Replication region fragments cloned from F-*lac* are identical to *Eco*R1 fragment f5 of F. J. Bacteriol. **127**:1571–1575.

75. Smith, H. O. and D. B. Danner. 1981. Genetic transformation. Ann. Rev. Biochem. **50**:41–68.

76. Snellings, N. J., *et al.* 1981. Genetic regulation of variable Vi antigen expression in a strain *Citrobacter freundii*. J. Bacteriol. **145**:1010–1017.

77. Starlinger, P., and H. Saedler. 1976. *IS*-elements in microorganisms. Curr. Topics Microbiol. Immunol. **75**:111.

78. Stocker, B. A. D. 1956. Abortive transduction of motility in *Salmonella*, a non-replicated gene transmitted through many generations to a single descendant. J. Gen. Microbiol. **15**:575–598.

79. Watson, J. D. 1976. The Molecular Biology of the Gene. 3rd ed. W. A. Benjamin, New York.

80. Watson, J. D., and F. H. C. Crick. 1953. The structure of DNA. Cold Spring Harbor Symp. Quant. Biol. **18**:123–131.

81. Wickner, S. H. 1978. DNA replication proteins of *Escherichia coli*. Ann. Rev. Biochem. **47**:1163–1191.

82. Willetts, N., and R. Skurray. 1980. The conjugation system of F-like plasmids. Ann. Rev. Genet. **14**:41–76.

83. Wollman, E. L., and F. Jacob. 1958. Sur les processus de conjugaison et de recombinaison chez *E. coli*. V. Le mécanisme du transfect de matériel génétique. Ann. Inst. Pasteur **95**:641–666.

84. Wood, T. H. 1968. Effects of temperature, agitation and donor strain on chromosome transfer in *Escherichia coli* K-12. J. Bacteriol. **96**:2077–2084.

85. Yanofsky, C., *et al.* 1964. On the colinearity of gene structure and protein structure. Proc. Natl. Acad. Sci. USA **51**:266–272.

86. Zinder, N., and J. Lederberg. 1952. Genetic exchange in *Salmonella*. J. Bacteriol. **64**:679–699.

Immunology

Introduction to Immunology

Gary R. Pearson, Ph.D.

Immunology arose from studies directed at determining the mechanisms of resistance to infectious diseases. The fact that individuals were resistant to second attacks of the same disease was noted even in ancient times. Some 2500 years ago, during the plague in Greece, Thucydides recorded observations indicating that people who recovered from the disease were generally resistant to reinfection. The concept of immunity was first established by Edward Jenner following his classical experiments with smallpox. Jenner observed that individuals who had acquired cowpox, a benign disease in cows, were generally resistant to the development of smallpox in subsequent epidemics. To test his belief that prior exposure to cowpox protected against smallpox, in 1796 Jenner successfully immunized against smallpox with the cowpox agent. This was the first recorded attempt at what is now known as "active immunization." Almost 100 years later Jenner's findings were extended by Pasteur, who successfully employed weakly virulent strains of anthrax bacillus to protect chickens against highly virulent forms of this organism. The term "immunity" (Latin *immunis*, free of) was used to describe this protection against infectious agents and was subsequently broadened to include foreign substances other than infectious agents.

One of the important features noted in the early studies on resistance to infection was the "specificity" of this protection. That is, individuals exposed to a specific organism were protected against reinfection with the same organism but not others. The basis of this specificity was postulated by von Behring and Kitasato and by Paul Ehrlich in the latter part of the nineteenth century as due to the presence of circulating factors in the body fluids which specifically reacted with the inciting agent. In support of this hypothesis, von Behring and Kitasato reported that serums from individuals immunized with tetanus were capable of neutralizing the tetanus toxin and that the capacity to neutralize this toxin could be successfully transferred with serums from these people to nonimmune or susceptible individuals. The foreign substance that elicited the formation of the serum factors was termed **antigen,** while the circulating serum or humoral factor produced in response to the antigen was subsequently defined as **antibody.** Ehrlich envisioned the reaction between antibody and antigen as a "lock and key" arrangement in which the antigen was inserted into a crevice in the antibody, and specificity was determined by complementariness between the antigen and its corresponding antibody. In addition, he believed that this was a chemical reaction and that the antibody combined with the antigen in definite proportions. Later studies by Avery, Heidlelberger, and Kendall using pneumococcal polysaccharides led to the isolation of pure antibody from antigen-antibody reactions and opened the door for detailed studies on the nature of these reactions.

An alternative hypothesis to explain immunity to infectious agents was advanced by the Russian zoologist Metchnikoff in the late nineteenth century. This hypothesis attributed immunity to a cellular rather than a humoral mechanism and emphasized the role of phagocytic cells which could engulf and destroy toxic substances. Although this was initially greeted with much controversy, it is now apparent that cellular components of the reticuloendothelial system play a major role in the development of the immune response to antigens and also constitute important effector mechanisms in the destruction of certain kinds of bacteria, viruses, parasites, and eucaryotic cells. In addition, such cells are major elements in delayed hypersensitivity or allergic responses to certain antigens. Thus it became apparent that the immune system was composed of both humoral and cellular components functioning individually or together in the development of immunity. The major component of the humoral response is antibody, while the cellular response to antigens involves the induction of immune cells capable of reacting with antigen in the absence of antibody or other humoral factors.

There has been an explosion of knowledge in immunology over the past 20 years, and it is now recognized that the development of an immune response to an antigen involves a complex array of events controlled by genetic and molecular mechanisms. This boom is largely attributed to developments and advances in molecular biology and genetics. This and the following four chapters will focus on some of these points, including the nature of the participants in both humoral and cellular immune responses, methods for accurately measuring the antigen-antibody reactions, the genetic control of the immune response encompassing what is now known about immune response genes and cellular interactions in antibody synthesis, cellular immunity and hypersensitivity, and effector mechanisms important in resistance to different types of diseases. In addition, diseases with an immunological basis, such as autoimmune or immune complex diseases, will be discussed in Chapter 11, which focuses on more clinically oriented immunological phenomena. This section is directed toward the beginning immunology and medical student. For detailed information on specific subjects, the reader is referred to the references listed at the end of each chapter.

Components of the Immune Response

ANTIGENS: NATURE, IMMUNOGENICITY, AND SPECIFICITY[2, 3, 4, 21, 23, 25, 31, 59, 61]

Antigens are classically defined as **foreign** (nonself) substances capable of provoking an immune response in the inoculated or exposed host. Two major properties of antigens are the ability to induce this response, *i.e.,* induction of antibody synthesis or specifically immune lymphoid cells, and the capacity to specifically react with these newly synthesized immune factors. It has become fashionable recently to refer to substances capable of provoking or inducing an immune response as being **immunogenic,** instead of antigenic, and those substances as **immunogens,** instead of antigens. A number of macromolecules can act as antigens; these include proteins, polysaccharides, lipoproteins, nucleoproteins, and many smaller molecules when coupled to a suitable carrier (see below). Proteins are generally considered the most potent antigens, while most purified nucleic acids and lipids by themselves are not antigenic.

Molecules of high molecular weight are generally better antigens than smaller molecules; the most potent antigens generally have molecular weights greater than 100,000. Molecules of molecular weight less than 10,000 daltons are generally poor antigens, with some exceptions, unless they are coupled to a larger carrier molecule. Such molecules are referred to as **haptens,** a name given by Landsteiner in 1921 to describe substances not capable of provoking an immune response by themselves.

Large molecular weight substances such as proteins and polysaccharides generally contain more than one chemical structure or site capable of provoking an antibody response. Each of these sites on an antigen is referred to as an **antigenic determinant** or **epitope.** The number of determinants on an antigen, which constitutes the **valence** of that molecule, varies and is a property not only of the size of the molecule but also of its shape or configuration. For example, some determinants are only present when a protein is in its native form (secondary or tertiary structure) and are not detected after the protein is denatured by heat or chemical treatment. This can be readily demonstrated by **absorption** experiments. Since antibody produced against an antigen will specifically and under optimal conditions irreversibly react with only that antigen or one closely related, it is possible to remove this antibody by incubating the serum containing the antibody (**antiserum**) with antigen and then removing the antigen-antibody complexes that form in this mixture. This can be repeated until the specific antibody has been completely removed from the antiserum. For example, if the native form of a protein, such as bovine serum albumin (BSA), is used for absorption of anti-BSA antibodies, it is possible to selectively and completely remove all antibody to this protein from the antiserum. However, if the BSA is first denatured by heat and then used in the absorption experiments, it will not be possible to remove all of the anti-BSA

antibodies from the absorbed serum, showing that some of the antigenic determinants that serve as targets for anti-BSA antibodies are dependent on the native form of the protein. Similarly it is possible by this approach to show that an antigen expresses multiple determinants. For example, if an antiserum containing antibodies to BSA is tested against both BSA and human serum albumin (HSA), it will react with both, indicating that HSA contains some antigenic determinants closely related to those present on BSA. On the other hand, if the antiserum is first absorbed with HSA, the absorbed antiserum will still react with BSA but not with HSA, *i.e.,* absorption with HSA removes all antibodies reactive with antigenic determinants shared by BSA and HSA. Therefore, by this simple approach, it is possible to state conclusively that BSA contains at least two antigenic determinants, one that is shared by BSA and HSA and one that is only present on BSA. Thus, when an individual is immunized with a complex antigen such as a bacterium or virus, antibodies will be produced against the different macromolecules that compose that agent and also against different antigenic determinants expressed on individual molecules, resulting in a multitude of antibodies to that particular agent.

The size of antigenic determinants on different antigens has been determined by inhibition studies. Such studies employ appropriate oligosaccharides or polypeptides of varying sizes to determine the number of sugars or amino acid residues required to completely inhibit the reaction between an antibody and the appropriate polysaccharide or protein antigen. The size of different antigenic determinants, as estimated by this approach, is shown in Table 7–1. Approximately 6 sugar residues can act as an antigenic determinant for a polysaccharide molecule, 5 to 7 amino acid residues for a protein, and 5 nucleotides for nucleic acids.

The first precise determination of the entire antigenic structure of a protein was that of myoglobin, which took approximately 11 years to complete. The antigenic structure of lyso-

Table 7–1. **Size of Different Antigenic Determinants**

Antigen	Composition of Antigenic Determinants	Approximate Maximum Size (Å)
Hapten	1 small molecule	5–15
Polysaccharide	6 sugar residues	35
Nucleic acid	5 nucleotides	20
Protein	5–7 amino acids	19–30

zyme was next determined following 10 years of research. It was shown by these determinations that myoglobin, which has a molecular weight of approximately 17,000, has 5 antigenic determinants, while lysozyme, with a molecular weight of 14,000, has 3 distinct antigenic determinants. A schematic diagram showing the structure of myoglobin and the position of its antigenic determinants is shown in Figure 7–1. This work on the structure of myoglobin also revealed the interesting finding that all the antigenic determinants are located on the outer surface of the molecule and not internally. For both myoglobin and lysozyme, it was also found that the configuration of the antigenic sites played an important role in their reactivity with their respective antibodies.

Factors other than size, shape, or chemical composition influence the immunogenicity of a macromolecule. The more important of these are listed here:

1. Species of animal used for the production of antibody. Some guinea pig strains respond well to diphtheria toxoid, while others are poor responders. This response is controlled by antigen specific immune response (Ir) genes in the host, as discussed in Chapter 9.

2. Routes of immunization. The most common routes of immunization are intravenous, subcutaneous, intraperitoneal, intramuscular, and intradermal. In addition, some antigens are effectively administered by the oral route. The route of immunization also influences the primary site for antibody production, *i.e.*, spleen or regional lymph nodes.

3. Antigen concentration. Generally, a few micrograms of antigen are sufficient for the induction of an immune response. In contrast, a large concentration of antigen is sometimes ineffective in inducing an immune response and, in fact, can induce a refractory state called immunological intolerance, as discussed in Chapter 10. A classical example of this dose effect is the response of mice to the purified polysaccharide of pneumococcus. Doses as small as 5×10^{-4} mg. will induce optimal antibody production, whereas relatively large doses (0.5 mg. or greater) are ineffective. Effects of concentration vary depending on the nature of the antigen and is an important consideration in the development of vaccines.

4. The amino acid composition of the protein. The presence of aromatic amino acids appears to enhance the immunogenicity of proteins. This was initially reported by Sela, who demonstrated that the attachment of tyrosine residues to gelatin greatly increased its immunogenicity in the guinea pig and rabbit, whereas glutamic acid, alanine, proline, serine, lysine, and cysteine had no apparent effect. It is now believed that this increase in immunogenicity is due to the increased rigidity of the antigenic determinants caused by the creation of side chains through aromatic amino acids.

5. Adjuvants. The immunogenicity of weak antigens can sometimes be enhanced through the use of adjuvants. These nonspecifically enhance the immune response to an antigen when mixed with the antigen before inoculation. A common adjuvant is **Freund's adjuvant,** a water-in-oil emulsion generally employing lanolin or Aralacel A (mannide mono oleate) as the emulsifying agent. This form of the adjuvant is commonly referred to as **incomplete Freund's adjuvant.** In some preparations, killed mycobacteria are added to yield **complete Freund's adjuvant.** Other adjuvants commonly used include corynebacterial species and *Bordetella pertussis,* endotoxins prepared from gram-negative bacteria, and, more recently, inducers of interferon formation, such as synthetic polyribonucleotides. In addition, some mineral salts such as aluminum hydroxide, calcium phosphate, silica, and iron oxide have adjuvant activity. Adjuvants are particularly effective for enhancing the immunogenicity of soluble proteins or other antigens that are degraded by tissue enzymes and eliminated quickly. Adjuvants such as mineral salts en-

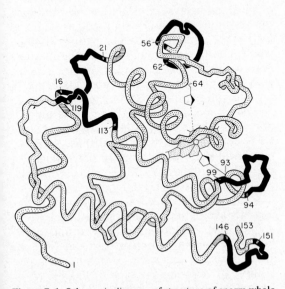

Figure 7–1. Schematic diagram of structure of sperm whale myoglobin showing location of four major antigenic determinants (outlined in black). (Reprinted with permission from Atassi, M. Z., Antigenic structure of myoglobin: the complete immunochemical anatomy of a protein and conclusions relating to antigenic structure of proteins. Immunochemistry **12**:423, 1975. Copyright 1975, Pergamon Press, Ltd.)

hance immunogenicity by the formation of relatively insoluble precipitates from which the antigen is released slowly, thereby prolonging its *in vivo* lifespan. Adjuvants such as Freund's form deposits from which antigen is released slowly to the immune system. The resultant effect is antibody production extending over a period of months, as opposed to a few weeks when adjuvant is not included, and generally results in higher antibody levels in the serum.

Some adjuvants influence cellular immunity as well as antibody production. Complete Freund's adjuvant, in particular, is an effective vehicle for inducing delayed hypersensitivity responses to soluble antigens or simple haptens. It also nonspecifically enhances macrophage activity, which is important for the processing of certain antigens. In complete Freund's adjuvant, the component responsible for activing cellular immunity is a muramyl dipeptide of the mycobacterial cell wall, *N*-acetyl-muramyl-L-alanyl-D-isoglutamine. Because of its effect on cellular immunity, adjuvants containing mycobacteria have been used for immunotherapy against cancer, but with equivocal results. Some corynebacteria, such as *Corynebacterium parvum,* have also been used as adjuvants because of their nonspecific effect on cellular immunity. Similarly, activation of certain arms of the cellular immune system by interferon or interferon-inducers may increase resistance to infections or certain diseases such as cancer.

CLASSES OF ANTIGENS

Haptens[4, 6, 55, 56]

Haptens have been instrumental in studies directed at understanding the nature of factors involved in the development of immune response against specific antigenic determinants. As mentioned earlier, these chemicals (generally with molecular weights less than 10,000 daltons) will not provoke an immune response by themselves, *i.e.,* are not immunogenic, but will do so when coupled to a suitable protein carrier. In this case, the generated response is largely directed against the specific hapten portion of the hapten-carrier immunogen and the hapten acts, therefore, as a new antigenic determinant on the carrier molecule.

The first step in producing antibodies to a haptenic group involves the coupling of the hapten to an appropriate carrier; this is generally a large molecule, immunogenic in itself. Coupling agents produce stable, covalent bonds between the hapten and reactive sites on the carrier molecule, including amino, carboxyl, or thio groups. Commonly, diazonium salts are employed to couple the hapten to amino acids such as tyrosine, histidine, lysine, tryptophan, and cysteine residues. This method causes minimal denaturation of the protein carrier. Other methods utilize isocyanate, isothiocyanate, or amide bonds for conjugating a hapten to protein or organic halogenic compounds. A widely used coupling agent of this type is toluene 2,4-diisocyanate.

Anti-hapten antibodies are produced by immunization of an appropriate animal with the conjugate. The resultant antiserum is then tested for antibodies reactive with the unconjugated hapten determinant. Alternatively, the antiserum may be reacted with the hapten that has been coupled to a second carrier protein that does not share antigenic determinants with the original carrier. This is essential, since immunization with the hapten-carrier conjugate will result in the production of antibodies specific not only to the haptenic group, but also to other determinants on the carrier molecule. For example, if 2,4-dinitrophenol (DNP) is coupled to bovine serum albumin to form a DNP–BSA conjugate, antibodies to DNP and to other natural determinants on BSA will be produced following immunization. Anti-DNP antibodies can be specifically identified by one of several methods. In inhibition or blocking assays, free DNP is used to block the reaction of anti-DNP antibodies with the DNP–BSA conjugate by competing with the whole conjugate for antibody reaction sites. Alternatively, the antiserum can be reacted with a conjugate prepared with DNP and a protein unrelated to BSA, such as keyhole limpet hemocyanin (KLH). The antiserum will not react with native KLH by itself, since the KLH determinants differ from those of BSA, but it will react with the DNP determinant of the DNP-modified KLH, demonstrating the existence of anti-DNP antibodies.

Antibodies produced against hapten determinants are extremely discriminating. For example, such antibodies will discriminate between the D- and L-isomeric forms of different amino acids, between different charged groups, or between the type of linkage (α or β) in different polysaccharides. This approach for producing highly specific antibodies to normally nonimmunogenic substances has been very useful for producing antibodies to synthetic polypeptides of defined structure and against polynucleotide sequences; it has also been valuable for elucidating the size of antibody sites directed against specific determinants.

There is also evidence that the carrier, in some instances, contributes to the specificity of the antibody response to some haptens. This was established largely through the eloquent studies of Mitchison and co-workers. These investigators observed that animals immunized with a specific hapten-carrier immunogen responded vigorously with the production of anti-hapten antibodies when rechallenged with the homologous conjugate, but sometimes only weakly when inoculated with the same hapten coupled to another carrier. For example, animals immunized with DNP coupled to bovine gamma globulin (BGG) produce high levels of anti-DNP antibodies when inoculated a second time with DNP–BGG but only respond weakly when inoculated with DNP coupled to KLH, indicating that the carrier participated in the specificity of the immune response to that antigen. This contribution of the carrier to specificity, which is referred to as the **carrier effect,** appears to occur at the site of coupling between the hapten and carrier and presumably involves specific amino acid residues at this site.

Carbohydrate Antigens

Polysaccharides participate as major antigenic determinants on many bacterial and mammalian cells. This has been established primarily through the use of the polysaccharide capsule of pneumococcus and through the analysis of blood group antigens. Some carbohydrate antigens express their immunogenic properties as a complex with lipid and protein, as in the cell walls of gram-negative bacteria, while others are immunogenic by themselves. Polymers composed of one type of sugar such as dextran, a high-molecular-weight polymer of glucose, are generally efficient immunogens, rivaling heteropolymers in this respect; specificity is influenced by the type of linkage (α or β) between sugars. Some sugars, however, may be more dominant than others in influencing antigenic specificity. For example, in inhibition studies directed at a pure polysaccharide, all sugar units generally inhibit the antigen-antibody reaction to some degree, but one sugar might inhibit more than others. This has given rise to the **dominant sugar concept** for polysaccharide immunogenicity. The evidence suggests that the dominant sugar is usually located at the end of polymer chains and represents the major component of the antigenic determinant interacting with the antibody binding site. As already mentioned and shown in Table 7–1, inhibition studies have established that the polysaccharide antigenic determinant generally is composed of 6 to 7 sugar residues, since inhibition of antigen-antibody reactions with different size oligosaccharides increased through hexosaccharides, then remains relatively constant with larger molecules.

Lipid Antigens[53]

Lipids alone are generally poor immunogens but when coupled artificially or naturally to an appropriate carrier they can act as haptens. Thus it is possible to generate antibodies to lipid molecules. In nature, the specificity of antibodies generated against a lipid-protein or lipid-polysaccharide complex is primarily directed against the polysaccharide or protein unit and not against the lipid moiety. There is some evidence, however, that the lipid component can contribute to the immunogenicity of these lipid-containing complexes. It has been reported that a reduction in fatty acid chain length reduces the ability of glycolipid haptens to react with antibody directed against such artificially prepared haptens.

Nucleic Acid Antigens[51]

Nucleic acids are also poor immunogens, although individuals with certain diseases do produce antibodies to DNA. This is particularly notable in patients with autoimmune diseases, such as systemic lupus erythematosus, rheumatoid arthritis, and some forms of cancer. Serum from many individuals with these diseases contain a variety of antibodies to nuclear components, including DNA. It has also been reported that the DNA from T_4 bacteriophage, which contains glycosylated 5-hydroxymethyl cytosine, also induces antibodies in rabbits. The specificity of the antibody in this instance appears to be directed against the glycosylated base. Reactivity between the phage DNA and antibody requires denatured DNA, however, indicating that nucleotides are also involved in the reaction with antibody. Similarly, success has been reported in the production of antibodies to ribonucleoproteins, with results indicating that nucleotides were part of the antigenic determinants. This suggests that it is indeed possible to produce antibodies to nucleotides if they are attached naturally to a carrier protein. This was substantiated by Pleisca and co-workers, who demonstrated that DNA strands act as haptens when artificially coupled to methylated bovine serum albumin and that the antibodies generated with such conjugates are directed against base sequences. Inhibition studies with different size polynucleotides indicate that 5 to 7 nucleotides are necessary to compose an antigenic determinant. Therefore, it is now accepted that nucleic acids can serve as immunogens when coupled to an appropriate carrier molecule.

Blood Group Antigens[18, 42]

A description of these antigens is included in this chapter to illustrate how subtle changes in the carbohydrate or protein moiety of an antigen can radically alter its antigenic specificity. The blood group systems identified so far have been designated ABO, Rh, I, Lewis, Mn, P, Kell, Duffy, and Kidd (Table 7–2). All of these can be antigenically distinguished from each other. The ABO and Rh systems are the major blood group antigens and are the focus of this discussion.

ABO blood group antigens were originally identified by Landsteiner, who observed that red blood cells from some individuals were agglutinated by serum from others. By systematically studying these agglutination patterns, four major groups of antigens were defined and designated, A, B, AB, and O. In other words, individuals express the A antigen, B antigen, both A and B, or neither (O) on their red blood cells. Serums from individuals contain natural antibody (isoagglutinins) directed against the antigen missing from their own red blood cells, but not against the one expressed. For example, individuals expressing A antigens on their red blood cells possess anti-B antibodies in their serum and vice versa; individuals expressing both antigens on their red blood cells (AB) do not contain antibody to either antigen in their serum, while those that do not express either antigen (O) contain antibodies to both A and B (Table 7–3). Because of this, individuals with O type blood are considered universal donors, since their cells, lacking both

Table 7–2. **List of Major Human Blood Group Antigens**

ABO
Rh
Kell
Lewis
Duffy
Kidd
Mn
P
I

Table 7–3. **ABO Blood Groups**

Antigen	Genotypes	Natural Serum Antibodies
A	A/A A/O	Anti-B
B	B/B B/O	Anti-A
O	O/O	Anti-A Anti-B
AB	A/B	None

A and B antigens, will be accepted by all individuals with the different blood types. Similarly, individuals with AB blood type will accept all other blood types, since their serum does not contain antibodies to A or B. The expression of antigens A and B is under genetic control, with the expression of each antigen controlled by two alleles. The A and B alleles are both dominant to O (Table 7–3).

The antigenic specificities of A and B reside in small oligosaccharides bound to sphingolipids. The only difference in the chemical composition of blood group antigens A and B is the carbohydrate unit attached to the terminal galactose on the oligosaccharide chain, and this accounts for the difference in specificity. For blood group A, this carbohydrate is N-acetylgalactosamine, while for group B, it is galactose (Fig. 7–2). The addition of these different sugars to the backbone oligosaccharide chain is under genetic control and is performed by transferase enzymes. Red blood cells of the O type contain a nonantigenic substance on their surface, called the H substance. This is a necessary precursor for the formation of A or B antigens; the formation of H substance is also under the control of a gene, designated the H gene. The addition of fucose to the oligosaccharide chain by a fucosyl transferase, encoded by the H gene, results in the formation of the H substance. The A antigen is then formed by the addition of N-acetylgalactosamine to the terminal galactose residue on the H chain by an enzyme coded for by the A gene, while the B antigen is formed by addition of galactose to the terminal residue of the H chain by an enzyme encoded by the B gene. The sequence of events can also be shown by enzymatic removal of the terminal sugar from A or B antigens, resulting in the appearance of H substance. Therefore, by the addition of one sugar moiety to an oligosaccharide chain, it is possible to convert

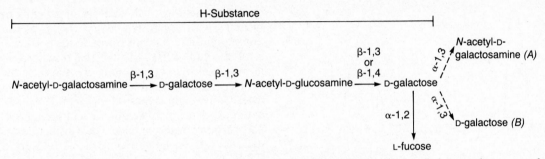

Figure 7–2. The carbohydrate structure of blood group A and B antigens showing the terminal sugars that account for the antigenic differences between these two groups. Structure of H substance; β-1,3; β-1,4; α-1,2; α-1,3 are linkages between different sugar moieties.

a nonimmunogenic substance (H substance) to an immunogen and to alter the specificity of the antigen by replacing this terminal sugar. A third antigen, Lewis (Le), has also been identified on some red blood cells; it is under the control of a separate gene, the Le gene. The Le antigen differs from A and B by the addition of fucose at the next to the last sugar residue.

Blood group antigens are also found in secretions of some individuals, e.g., saliva. The antigens, however, appear as glycoproteins in secretions and not as glycosphingolipids. The presence or absence of blood group antigens in saliva is also under genetic control by a secretor (Se) gene. Approximately 80 per cent of normal individuals are secretors.

Rh System[20, 36]

This system was initially identified by Landsteiner and Weiner, who observed that a rabbit antiserum prepared against rhesus monkey red blood cells agglutinated erythrocytes from 80 per cent of normal humans. This red blood cell system, designated Rh, has subsequently been shown to be composed of a large number of antigens under genetic control. The chemical nature of the antigens is, however, still largely unknown.

It was proposed by Fisher and Race that the expression of the Rh antigen was controlled by three pairs of closely linked genes, designated Cc, Dd, and Ee. However, because of the identification of a number of subgroups for each locus, the exact genetics of the Rh system still remains somewhat uncertain. The antigen controlled by the D locus is the strongest immunogen and therefore is considered to be the antigen of clinical importance in hemolytic diseases and transfusion reactions. This antigen, expressed only in the membranes of red cell, is therefore used to determine whether an individual's red blood cells are Rh antigen

positive or negative. An immune response is elicited only when an Rh-negative individual is exposed to red blood cells from an Rh-positive individual. In contrast to the ABO system, there are no natural antibodies against this antigen.

The Rh antigen is the cause of a hemolytic disease of newborns called **erythroblastosis fetalis.** This disease commonly occurs in Rh-positive babies born of Rh-negative mothers. The disease is normally not noted during the first pregnancy in that the first fetus is not affected, but can become a major complication during subsequent pregnancies. If, during the first pregnancy, maternal and fetal blood should mix, the Rh-positive red blood cells of the fetus induces an antibody response in the Rh-negative mother. This commonly occurs at delivery or abortion. These antibodies are capable of crossing the placenta, so that in subsequent pregnancies, maternal antibodies destroy red blood cells of Rh-positive babies, resulting in severe anemia which is often fatal to the child. It has recently been found that the initial immunizing event can be prevented by treating the mother, before delivery, with gamma globulin containing high levels of anti-Rh antibodies. Such antibodies neutralize the Rh antigen, thereby preventing active immunization of the mother. This is now common practice in hospitals in cases where an Rh factor mismatch between child and mother is suspected; it has resulted in a very significant decrease in the incidence of the disease.

ANTIBODIES: NATURE AND STRUCTURE[13, 15, 24, 33, 34, 41, 48, 49, 52, 57]

Antibodies are serum proteins produced in response to a specific antigen. They are found in the globulin fraction of serum and are frequently known as **immunoglobulins.** The glob-

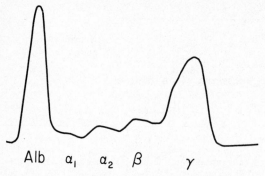

Figure 7–3. Densitometric tracing of the electrophoretic mobilities of the different human serum proteins (α,β,γ) following electrophoresis. Alb, albumin; α_1,α_1-globulin; α_2,α_2-globulin; β,β-globulin; γ,γ-globulin.

ulin fraction is a heterogeneous group of proteins accounting for approximately 20 per cent of the total serum proteins. The globulin fraction of serum can be divided into subclasses based primarily on the electrophoretic mobility of the proteins. If a mixture of proteins is subjected to an electrical field, the different proteins will migrate at different rates, depending on their various charge groups (Fig. 7–3). By this technique, called **electrophoresis,** it was possible to identify three major categories of globulin proteins, designated alpha, beta, and gamma. In 1939, Tiselius and Kabat localized antibody activity to the gamma fraction of the plasma proteins. Later it was realized that some antibodies migrated in a fast gamma fraction, while others migrated in a slow fraction. Similarly, there were differences in the sedimentation of antibody molecules in the ultracentrifuge. The concept of a family of proteins with antibody activity known as immunoglobulins, was not formulated, however, until the late 1950s. As will be discussed in more detail below, immunoglobulins can now be placed into different subclasses, based on molecular weight, types of polypeptide chains, antigenic determinants, amino acid sequences, and carbohydrate content. The various designations of these immunoglobulins are listed in Table 7–4.

All immunoglobulins are glycoproteins in nature, and the individual types contain different amounts of carbohydrate. The biological activity of antibody molecules resides in their protein structure. Antibody molecules generally have two combining sites capable of specifically reacting with the antigen that stimulates their production, although monovalent antibodies are also produced under some circumstances. In the case of naturally occurring bivalent antibodies, both combining sites are directed against the same antigenic determinant. However, antibodies have been produced experimentally with one site directed against one determinant and the other reacting with a different antigenic determinant.

The bivalency of antibody molecules has been established using simple chemical haptens acting as single antigenic determinants. With such substances, it is possible to determine the number of molecules required to saturate all available antibody sites specific for that particular haptenic component. At saturation, the number of haptenic components bound per antibody molecule is the **valence** of the anti-

Table 7–4. Classification of Immunoglobulins of Normal Human Serum*

Immunoglobulin	IgG	IgA	IgM	IgD	IgE
Synonyms	γ, 7Sγ, γ_2, γG	βx, β_2A, γ_1A, γA	γ_1, 19Sγ, β_2M, γ_1M, γM	γD	γE
Heavy-chain Classes Subclasses	Gamma, γ IgG1, IgG2, IgG3, IgG4	Alpha, α IgA1, IgA2	Mu, μ —	Delta, δ ?Ja, La	Epsilon, ϵ —
Light-chain types	Kappa, κ Lambda, λ	κ λ	κ λ	κ λ	κ λ
Molecular formula	$\gamma_2 \kappa_2$ $\gamma_2 \lambda_2$	$\alpha_2 \kappa_2$† $\alpha_2 \lambda_2$†	$(\mu_2 \kappa_2)5$ $(\mu_2 \lambda_2)5$	$\delta_2 \kappa_2$ $\delta_2 \lambda_2$	$\epsilon_2 \kappa_2$ $\epsilon_2 \lambda_2$
Designation	IgG κ IgG λ	IgA κ IgA λ	IgM κ IgM λ	IgD κ IgD λ	IgE κ IgE λ

*From R. A. Kyle and E. D. Bayed, The Monoclonal Gammopathies, 1976. Courtesy of Charles C Thomas, Publisher, Springfield, Ill.

†May form polymers.

body. Using a method called **equilibrium dialysis**, antibody and free hapten are separated by a membrane permeable to small molecular weight molecules, but not to soluble antibody. The hapten will, therefore, freely diffuse through the membrane until the concentration of free hapten is the same in both chambers. If no antibody is present in either chamber, equilibrium is reached when the concentration of hapten is the same in both chambers. However, if antibody is present in one of the chambers, it will bind the hapten until all available antibody sites are saturated. Therefore, when equilibrium is finally reached, the amount of hapten in the antibody chamber will exceed that present in the other. This difference represents the amount of hapten bound to antibody. If the antibody concentration is known, it is possible to compute the ratio of haptenic molecules bound per antibody molecule, yielding the valence of the antibody molecule. By this approach, the majority of antibody preparations exhibit a ratio of 2, indicating that each antibody molecule has 2 identical binding sites. However, larger anti-

body molecules of the immunoglobulin M class (see below) have up to 10 binding sites per antibody molecule as determined by equilibrium dialysis.

Immunoglobulins are divided into a number of different subtypes or **isotypes** based primarily on size and their antigenic properties, which reflect amino acid differences in the peptide chains composing the immunoglobulin molecule. Some of the distinguishing properties among the different immunoglobulins are listed in Table 7–5.

Immunoglobulin G (IgG or γG) is the predominant immunoglobulin fraction that contains antibody activity. Immunoglobulin G has a molecular weight of approximately 150,000 and a sedimentation coefficient of 7S; approximately 2 to 3 per cent of this immunoglobulin is carbohydrate. As discussed in more detail below, IgG is divided further into four subclasses designated IgG1, IgG2, IgG3, and IgG4. One distinguishing characteristic of IgG immunoglobulins is their ability to cross the placenta, which results in the protection of the fetus from adventitious agents. IgG represents

Table 7–5. **Properties of Immunoglobulins of Normal Human Serum***

	IgG	IgA	IgM	IgD	IgE
Electrophoretic mobility	Gamma to alpha-2	Gamma to beta	Gamma to gamma-2	Gamma to beta	Gamma to beta
Sedimentation coefficient	6.7S	7–15S†	19S	7S	8S
Molecular weight	150,000	150,000–400,000†	900,000	180,000	200,000
Carbohydrate, %	2.6	5–10	9.8	10–12	11
Serum half-life (T½), days	23	5.8	5.1	2.8	2.3
Serum concentration, mean mg/ml	11.4	1.8	1.0	0.03	0.0003
Total serum immunoglobulin, %	74	21	5	0.2	0.002
Total body pool in intravascular space, %	45	42	76	75	51
Intravascular pool catabolized per day, % (normal)	6.7	25	18	37	89
Normal synthetic rate, mg/kg/day	33	24	6.7	0.4	0.02
Fixes complement	Yes (IgG₄ via alternate pathway)	Alternate pathway	Yes	No	Alternate pathway
Crosses placenta	Yes	No	No	No	No

*From J. L. Fahey and R. A. Kyle, Tests for Humoral Components of the Immunological Response. *In* N. R. Rose and H. Friedman (Eds.): Manual of Clinical Immunology, 2nd ed. American Society for Microbiology, Washington, D.C., 1980.
†Tends to form polymers of the monomer form.

70 to 80 per cent of the normal serum immunoglobulins and has a half-life of 23 days *in vivo.*

A second major category is designated **immunoglobulin M** (IgM or γM). These are macroglobulins with molecular weights between 900,000 and 1 million daltons and sedimentation coefficients of 19S. Approximately 10 per cent of this globulin is carbohydrate. This class is characterized by a pentamer structure composed of five subunits, each with molecular weights of approximately 180,000, linked by disulfide bonds. IgM antibodies readily fix a lytic serum component, called complement, and generally represent the first class of antibodies produced following primary exposure to an antigen. In contrast to IgG, IgM antibodies do not cross the placenta. This immunoglobulin component constitutes 5 to 10 per cent of the total serum immunoglobulins and has a half-life of approximately 5 days. Many so-called natural antibodies, such as blood group isoagglutinins, are of the IgM class.

A third major immunoglobulin class is **immunoglobulin A** (IgA or γA). It has been studied extensively and is important in immunity, particularly to infectious agents. This immunoglobulin is not only found in serum, but is the predominant antibody-containing immunoglobulin species found in secretions, *e.g.,* saliva, tears, bronchial and vaginal secretions, and secretions from the mucosal membranes lining the intestines. Serum IgA has a molecular weight of approximately 150,000 to 160,000 and a sedimentation coefficient of 7S; its half-life is approximately 6 days. In contrast, secretory IgA has a molecular weight of approximately 400,000 and a sedimentation coefficient of 11S. The larger size of the secretory IgA molecule is caused by the presence of a **secretory component** linked to the IgA molecule. The nature of this component is still largely unknown, but it appears to be linked to immunoglobulin A molecules through disulfide bridges (see below). There are two known subclasses of IgA molecules designated IgA1 and IgA2, which constitute 5 to 10 per cent of the total serum immunoglobulins.

Two other immunoglobulin classes that have been identified in serum are **immunoglobulin D** (IgD or γD) and **immunoglobulin E** (IgE or γE). IgD immunoglobulins constitute 0.2 to 0.3 per cent of the total serum immunoglobulins, while the serum concentration of IgE is less than 0.1 per cent. Both have molecular weights of approximately 180,000, sedimentation coefficients of 7 to 8S, and contain 10 to 12 per cent carbohydrate. The half-life of both

immunoglobulins is only 2 to 3 days. The functions of IgD molecules in immunity are largely unknown, although recent evidence indicates that IgD molecules are present in the membranes of cells involved in antibody synthesis and therefore might act as antigen receptors on such cells. In contrast, IgE antibodies, sometimes referred to as **reagins,** play a major role in allergies or in immediate hypersensitivity reactions to some antigens. These antibodies have the capacity to bind to certain specialized cells, such as mast cells, at high concentrations. This binding can trigger the release of pharmacological agents, *e.g.,* histamines, from these cells to result in the wheal and flare reactions that characterize allergic responses (Chapter 10). The binding characteristic of IgE is heat labile and is destroyed by heating at 56°C. for 30 minutes.

Structure of Immunoglobulin G[11, 16, 17, 19]

The elaboration of the basic structure of the IgG molecule was pioneered by Porter on rabbit gamma globulin and by Edelman on human myeloma proteins in the years between 1959 and 1964. In 1959, Porter and colleagues reported that treatment of rabbit IgG with papain resulted in the production of three separate fragments as identified by ion exchange chromatography. Two of these fragments contained the antigen-binding sites and were referred to as **Fab fragments** or **antigen-binding fragments.** Further studies demonstrated that the two antigen-binding sites were identical. The third fragment, which crystallized easily, did not bind to antigen but contained other sites important in antibody reactions. These include the site for binding complement and a second site that allows antibodies to bind to specific cell receptors. This piece was designated **Fc fragment** (for crystallizable fragment). Approximately two-thirds of the papain-digested material contained the Fab fragments with molecular weights of approximately 45,000 each, while one-third was composed of the Fc fragment with a molecular weight of approximately 50,000. This led to the development of a model of the antibody molecule in which two Fab fragments were attached to one Fc fragment. Further evidence supporting this model was provided from experiments using pepsin for cleaving the antibody molecule. This resulted in the production of a fragment with a molecular weight of approximately 100,000 containing two antigen-binding sites, which was designated (Fab)$_2$, and one Fc fragment. Thus, the antibody was visualized as a structure composed of two Fab units attached to one Fc unit by chemical bonds susceptible to enzymatic digestion.

The second major breakthrough in the elaboration of the structure of the antibody molecule was reported by Edelman in 1959. He showed that, following reduction of disulfide bonds, two subunits could be isolated with molecular weights of 23,000 and 50,000 daltons. The 23,000 dalton component was referred to as the **light chain** (L chain) of the antibody molecule while the 50,000 dalton component was referred to as the **heavy chain** (H chain). This led to the visualization of the antibody molecule as being composed of four chains—two heavy chains and two light chains—joined by interchain disulfide bond linkages. In this model, the Fc fragment was composed of the H chains, the Fab fragments were composed of both H and L chains, and the antibody combining sites involved both the H and L chains in the Fab fragment. The portion of the heavy chain in the Fab fragment was designated the **Fd region**. This model is schematically shown in Figure 7–4.

Further elaboration of the structure of antibody was hampered because of the heterogeneity of such molecules in normal serum. This obstacle was largely overcome through the use of serum from patients with a disease called multiple myeloma, a malignancy involving antibody-producing cells. The serum of such patients contains a high level of a homogeneous immunoglobulin class, known as **myeloma pro-**

tein, which is produced by the individual tumor. In addition, it has long been known that such individuals secrete in their urine proteins referred to as **Bence-Jones proteins.** These proteins were known to be related to the myeloma proteins detected in serum, although their exact nature was not determined until the 1960s. It has subsequently been shown that Bence-Jones proteins are composed of the light chains of the myeloma protein and, therefore, serve as good sources of homologous L chains for immunological and biochemical characterization.

A second more recently developed method for producing homologous immunoglobulins for antigenic and biochemical studies was reported by Kohler and Milstein in 1975. Hybrid cells, called **hybridomas,** are produced in tissue culture by cell fusion of antibody-producing spleen cells and myeloma cells. Some of these hybrid cells will produce monoclonal antibodies, or antibodies of one specific type directed against one antigenic determinant as specified by the spleen donor. Clones of these hybrid cells can be grown in the peritoneum of mice with the production of ascites fluid containing a very high level of these antibodies. This material serves as an excellent source of homologous immunoglobulin protein for various analyses.

Immunological analysis of the human light chains using rabbit antiserums prepared against Bence-Jones protein revealed that there were two antigenic classes, or isotypes, of L chains, designated **kappa** (κ) and **lambda** (λ). Furthermore, each Bence-Jones protein was composed of either kappa or lambda chains, but not both, indicating that the specific myeloma protein contained only one of the two classes of chains. Immunological analysis of the heavy chains present in myeloma proteins revealed the presence of five major heavy chain isotypes. These H chains were designated γ for IgG, μ for IgM, α for IgA, δ for IgD, and ε for IgE. The antigenic markers characterizing the different H chain isotypes were localized on the Fc fragment of the immunoglobulin molecule. Thus different immunoglobulin classes are distinguished by immunological isotypic markers on the H chains that compose each of the different classes. The same L chains, either kappa or lambda, are found to be present in all the immunoglobulin classes, so that the distinguishing antigenic markers between different immunoglobulin classes are associated solely with the H chains and not with the L chains. More detailed immunological analysis of the various human

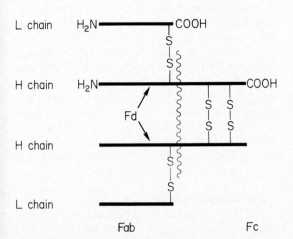

Figure 7–4. Schematic representation of IgG molecule, showing the cleavage region by papain (wavy line), which results in the production of Fab and Fc fragments (Fahey, J. L., and Kyle, R. A. *In* N. R. Rose and H. Friedman [Eds.], Manual of Clinical Immunology, 2nd ed. American Society for Microbiology, Washington, D.C., 1980, pp. 102–108.)

heavy chains, discussed later in this chapter, revealed that there are four subclasses for the γ chain (designated γ_1, γ_2, γ_3, γ_4), one subclass of the μ chain, and two subclasses of the α chain (α_1, α_2). Each myeloma protein of a specific type is composed of only one of these H chains and not a mixture of the different subclasses, *i.e.,* is homogeneous for both the H and L chains.

Biochemical analysis of homogeneous IgG heavy and light chains has resulted in the detailed definition of these chains from different immunoglobulin classes and has identified the basis for antigenic differences between different molecules. Amino acid analyses were first performed on Bence-Jones light chains. Analysis of two different kappa chain preparations by Hilschmann, both of which contained 212 amino acid residues, revealed that the amino acid residues in the carboxyl terminal half of these chains were identical, while there were many differences in the amino terminal portions. This was subsequently shown to be true for all H and L chains. The gamma chain was determined to be composed of 440 amino acid residues. This led to the designation of a **variable,** or **V,** region at the amino terminal half of the chain and a **constant,** or **C, region** at the carboxyl terminal half of each chain. For IgG, the variable regions of kappa or lambda chains and of the gamma chain involves approximately 107 amino acids. The remainder of the amino acid sequences in these different chains are constant.

Amino acid sequences of H and L chains and examination of the tertiary structure of the IgG molecule revealed linear repeating units of 110 to 120 amino acids on each chain, referred to as **domains.** Four of these domains are in the H chain. Three are in the constant region and are designated C_H1, C_H2, and C_H3, and one in the variable region is designated V_H. The two domains on the L chains, one variable and one constant, are designated V_L and C_L, respectively. The H chain constant domains, each extending 101 to 107 residues, are homologous in sequence to one another as well as to the constant domain on the L chain. Each domain forms a loop on the appropriate chain stabilized by intrachain disulfide bonds. These domains are genetically determined (Chapter 9), and have been linked to specific biological activity. For example, the C_H2 domain, composed of constant region 2 of the heavy chain, is associated with the fixation of complement, while the V_H and V_L domains are associated with antibody specificity. This dem-

onstration of domains led to the formulation by Edelman of the **domain hypothesis.** According to this hypothesis, each domain has a specific function and exists as structurally stable sections of the polypeptide chain. This is supported by the finding that proteolysis of intact polypeptide chains results in the release of domains that maintain their structural and functional conformations. A hinge region of 15 amino acids has been identified between C_H1 and C_H2 that corresponds to the linkage between Fab and Fc fragments. Differences in the molecular weights of H chains of the different immunoglobulin classes are caused by the presence of different numbers of domains composing the constant regions of these chains.

In the variable regions of both H and L chains there are **hypervariable regions,** in which great variation occurs in the amino acid residues between different chains of one class. The less variable residues in the V regions have been designated **framework residues,** thought to be important in keeping the hypervariable regions in their proper configuration. Three hypervariable areas within the V region of human L chains have been identified and mapped. These are L1 from residues 23 to 36, L2 from 52 to 58, and L3 from 91 to 99. Corresponding hypervariable regions have been found in the H chain from residues 31 to 36 (H1), 49 to 66 (H2), and 99 to 104 (H3). It has been proposed that the antibody binding site resides in the hypervariable section of the V regions of L and H chains. This is supported by the finding that mouse myeloma proteins produced in different mice have been identified that bind to the same antigenic determinant. Such proteins have remarkably similar amino acid content in their hypervariable regions. Analysis by crystallography has revealed that the amino acids that come in contact with an antigenic determinant are located in the hypervariable region. The carbohydrate moiety on IgG is located mainly on the C_H2 domain, although some sugar has also been identified on the Fab fragment. A schematic diagram of this immunoglobulin is shown in Fig. 7–5.

Immunoglobulin M[19, 39]

The IgM molecule is a pentamer composed of five 7S subunits, each with two heavy (μ) chains and two light chains (κ or λ) (Fig. 7–6). Each subunit has a molecular weight of approximately 180,000. An extra chain has been identified in this molecule, designated **J chain** or **joining chain.** This chain, with a molecular weight of approximately 15,000 and

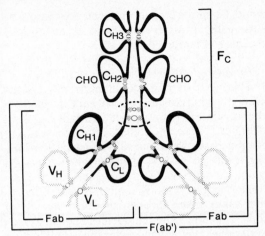

Figure 7–5. Schematic representation of the complete IgG molecule showing the different domains. (Courtesy of Dr. David McKean, Department of Immunology, Mayo Foundation and Mayo Medical School, Rochester, Minn.). C_{H1}–C_{H3}, domains in the heavy chain constant region; C_L, domain in light chain constant region; V_H, domain in heavy chain variable region; V_L, domain in light chain variable region.)

composed of 106 amino acids, is thought to serve as the link for joining the five subunits into a pentameric structure through disulfide bonds to the μ chains. The H chain from monoclonal IgM has been sequenced. It differs from the IgG heavy chains in that it lacks the hinge region between the Fab and Fc regions identified in IgG and has an extra domain of about 130 amino acid residues in the constant region. Therefore, IgM H chains have four domains instead of three in the constant region. Two of the C domains are in the Fc

fragment, one in the hinge region, and one in the Fd region. The domain in the hinge region appears to be one that has been lost in the IgG molecule. Five different carbohydrate moieties are attached to the heavy chain, all in the constant region.

By electron microscopy, the IgM molecule has a star-like appearance with five points equally distributed around a central ring. Theoretically, this molecule would be expected to have 10 antigen-binding sites. However, with some antigens, only five binding sites have been identified. The reasons for this remain unclear, but might be related to the need for some type of interaction among the different subunits on the intact molecule.

Antibodies of the IgM class contain a complement receptor on the Fc fragment and are considered to be more efficient than IgG antibodies in mediating lysis of cells in the presence of this lytic component. These antibodies are produced early in the primary immune response and then disappear, being replaced by IgG antibodies. Consequently, the presence of IgM antibodies in a serum specimen is a useful diagnostic tool, since its presence denotes an acute phase of the disease. Many natural antibodies, such as those directed against blood group antigens, are IgM antibodies. In addition, IgM molecules are frequently expressed in the membranes of antibody-precursor cells and are believed to function as antigen receptors in the initiation of the immune response, as discussed in Chapter 9.

Immunoglobulin A[19, 26, 35]

This is the major immunoglobulin class present in secretions and exists in both monomeric and polymeric forms. The basic molecule is composed of two H (α) chains and two L chains similar to the other immunoglobulin molecules and has a molecular weight of approximately 170,000 (Fig. 7–7). In the poly-

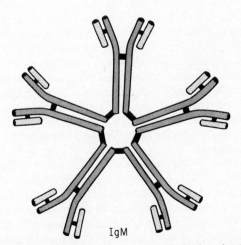

Figure 7–6. Schematic diagram of the IgM molecule. (Fahey, J. L., and Kyle, R. A. *In* N. R. Rose and H. Friedman (Eds.), Manual of Clinical Immunology, 2nd ed. American Society for Microbiology, Washington, D.C., 1980, pp. 102–108.)

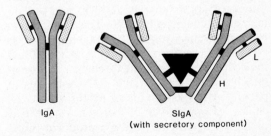

Figure 7–7. Schematic drawing of monomeric IgA and secretory IgA showing position of the secretory component (Fahey, J. L., and Kyle, R. A. *In* N. R. Rose and H. Friedman (Eds.), Manual of Clinical Immunology, 2nd ed. American Society for Microbiology, Washington, D.C., 1980, pp. 102–108.)

meric form, IgA monomers are linked by disulfide bridges to a J chain, identical to the analogous J chain in IgM molecules; linkage occurs between the J chain and the Fc fragment of the H chain. Each dimer or polymer of IgA is associated with only one J chain. As with IgG, the H chain of IgA is composed of four domains—one V_H and three C_H.

In secretions, IgA appears primarily as a dimer with a molecular weight of approximately 400,000 and a sedimentation coefficient of 11S. This 11S IgA molecule is designated **secretory IgA** (sIgA) and contains an additional component attached to the J chain, the **secretory piece** (Fig. 7–7). The secretory piece is a glycoprotein of 60,000 molecular weight and is found both free and bound to IgA in mucous secretions. It is composed of two polypeptide chains linked by disulfide bonds and becomes associated with the H chain of IgA molecules through both covalent and disulfide linkages. The secretory piece is synthesized in mucosal epithelial cells, and it has been postulated that the formation of sIgA takes place in these same cells, following entry of the IgA monomer that has been synthesized and secreted from plasma cells. The major role of the secretory piece appears to be protection of IgA from digestion by proteolytic enzymes. Experimental studies have shown that sIgA is more resistant than serum IgA to digestion by papain, pronase, trypsin, and pepsin. The sIgA immunoglobulin is thought to represent an important first line of defense against antigens entering through the oral or respiratory route because of its presence in secretions.

Immunoglobulin D[19, 58]

This immunoglobulin was first identified in 1965 by Rose and Fahey, who isolated a myeloma protein with H chains that differed antigenically from the corresponding chains on other known immunoglobulins. The structure of IgD is similar to IgG, with a molecular weight of approximately 180,000 and a sedimentation coefficient of 7S. The H (δ) chain has a molecular weight of 70,000 and there is an overrepresentation of the proportion of IgD molecules containing L (λ) chains. Approximately 80 per cent of the IgD molecules in patients with IgD-producing myelomas have λ chains, as opposed to 30 per cent of the IgG molecules in patients with IgG-producing myelomas. The reason and significance of this observation are unknown. Although IgD concentration in serum is low, it is frequently detected in membranes of cells involved in antibody synthesis. Therefore, like IgM, it

could be important in antigen recognition by such cells, possibly by acting as an antigen receptor (Chapter 9).

Immunoglobulin E[5, 19, 29]

This class of immunoglobulins was discovered by Ishizaka and co-workers in 1966, in the serum of patients with certain types of allergies. These antibodies, also referred to as **reagins,** have the unusual characteristic of fixing firmly to tissues, thereby sensitizing such tissue to participate in hypersensitivity reactions (Chapter 10). This binding to cell receptors takes place through the Fc fragment of the H chain. The characterization of such antibodies was advanced by the identification of patients with IgE-producing myelomas. Using such myelomas, it has been determined that this immunoglobulin has a molecular weight of 200,000 and a sedimentation coefficient of 8S. As mentioned earlier, IgE has a short half-life of 2 to 3 days; this, coupled with a low synthetic rate, results in the low serum concentrations of this protein. In common with other immunoglobulins, IgE is composed of two H (ϵ) chains and two L chains. IgE mediates hypersensitivity reactions by attaching to histamine-containing cells, *e.g.,* mast cells or basophils. Vasoactive material is released from such cells, following reaction of the allergin with the fixed IgE antibody, and is responsible for the characteristic wheal and flare reaction.

IMMUNOGLOBULIN ANTIGENIC DETERMINANTS[10, 11, 22, 28, 48]

As already indicated in this chapter, immunoglobulins themselves are immunogens when inoculated into a foreign species and can be antigenically distinguished from each other. Their individual constituents can also be distinguished using immunological techniques. Three types of immunological determinants have been identified on immunoglobulin molecules—isotypic, allotypic, and idiotypic.

Isotypic determinants are common to or shared by all members of the same animal species. They are expressed on the different L chains and on H chains of the different immunoglobulin classes in a given species and are recognized by antiserums against H or L chains, prepared in another animal species. The isotypic markers on H chains distinguished the different H chain classes, *i.e.,* H(α), H(γ), H(δ), H(μ), H(ϵ). L(κ) and L(λ) chains are also distinguished through isotypic markers.

Allotypic specificities distinguish polymorphic forms of immunoglobulins not present in all members of a given species, *i.e.*, they are individual-specific determinants, which distinguish immunoglobulin molecules between different individuals of the same species. These are identified by alloantibodies produced in members of the same animal species. For example, immunization of individual A with an immunoglobulin fraction from individual B will result in the production of antibodies to antigens on B that are not expressed on the corresponding immunoglobulin fraction in A. These markers or antigenic determinants are expressed on H and L chain constant regions and are expressed as alternative forms of a single genetic locus which segregates in the population according to simple Mendelian genetics. The allotypic determinants, located on the H(γ) chain of human IgG, are referred to as Gm markers and are found on the Fc and Fd segments of the H(γ) chain. Over 20 defined Gm markers on IgG molecules have been identified. Two H chain allotypes have also been identified in the IgA2 subclass and have been designated $A_2M(1)$ and $A_2M(2)$.

Polymorphic forms of human immunoglobulins were first recognized by Grubb in 1956 while examining serums from patients with rheumatoid arthritis. These investigators found that Rh^+ erythrocytes, when coated with anti-Rh antibodies that did not clump or agglutinate these cells, could be agglutinated by serums from some rheumatoid patients. These results suggested that there might be antigenic differences between anti-Rh antibodies from different individuals. Two allotypes were subsequently defined using this Rh indicator system and were designated $GM(a^+)$ and $Gm(a^-)$. Genetic studies demonstrated that $Gm(a^+)$ was inherited as a dominant Mendelian trait that was not sex-linked. The Gm loci have now been identified as structural genes from amino acids of the constant regions of the H chain. The expression of Gm determinants is complex and a single H chain often expresses more than one Gm determinant, all located in the C_H regions. If it is assumed that one gene encodes the entire C_H region, a single gene must also be capable of expressing more than one Gm specificity. This is now supported by experimental findings.

Three different allotypes have been identified on kappa L chains. These were originally designated Inv markers, but are now called Km(1), Km(2), and Km(3). The differences between these allotypes are due to amino acid substitutions in two positions, amino acid residues 153 and 191 in the C domain. In Km(1), the amino acids at these two positions are valine and leucine, respectively; in Km(2), alanine and leucine; and in Km(3), alanine and valine. The Km allotypes for human kappa chains are encoded on chromosome number 6. No allotypes have so far been identified on lambda L chains. Allotypes similar to human Gm and Km have been found on rabbit and mouse immunoglobulins.

Immunoglobulin allotypes are codominantly expressed. This means, for example, that an individual heterozygous for Km(1) and Km(2) will synthesize both Km(1) and Km(2) kappa L chains and both will be present in the serum. Individual antibody-producing cells, however, will synthesize only one of the two possible kappa allotypes, *i.e.*, both Km(1) and Km(2) will not be synthesized by the same cell. Therefore, some cells will synthesize Km(1) and others Km(2). This phenomenon is referred to as **allelic exclusion,** *i.e.*, the expression of one allele in an individual cell excludes the expression of the other and is unique to immunoglobulin gene-containing alleles.

Idiotypic determinants are serologically defined antigenic determinants involving the hypervariable regions of the immunoglobulin molecule. These determinants are unique to individual antibody molecules and are sometimes used as an identifying marker for specific antibodies produced by a single clone of cells. The existence of such determinants was shown by Kunkel and co-workers, who prepared antibody against human myeloma proteins. All antibodies directed against the constant regions of one myeloma protein were removed by absorption with other myeloma proteins of the same isotypes and allotypes, but antibodies still remained which reacted only with the immunizing protein; these were directed mainly against the hypervariable regions of the molecule. The antiserum bound strongly to the myeloma protein used for immunization, but not to other immunoglobulins even of the same class, *i.e.*, the antibodies were specific for the immunizing protein. These antibodies were subsequently shown to be directed against a determinant in the hypervariable region of the myeloma protein. Idiotypic antibodies are now produced by immunizing genetically identical individuals, naive for a particular antigen, with antibody-containing serum from another individual exposed previously to the specific antigen. Antiserums generated by this method, in effect containing antibody produced against another antibody, effectively block the ability of the immunizing antibody to bind to its specific antigen. This blocking effect on antigen binding is due to steric hindrance, but indicates that the idiotype determinant is physically near, if not a part of, the antigen binding site of the antibody molecule. This can be most effectively shown using antibody to a single hapten determinant. All idiotypes are in the variable regions of the H and L chains, and both chains are required for this expression. Thus, anti-idiotypic antibodies appear to be directed against specific amino acid sequences in the hypervariable region composing the antibody binding site. Antibodies of the same or different class share the same idiotype only if they are produced against the same antigenic determinant. There is also some evidence, however, for the existence of **public idiotypic** markers shared by antibodies with closely related amino acid sequences in the variable domains. Interestingly, naturally occurring anti-idiotypic antibodies have been identified in the serum of some individuals. This has led to speculation that such antibodies might be involved in the regulation of the immune response, since idiotypic determinants are also present on different lymphocyte populations involved in antibody production and are considered to be important in the initial phases of antibody synthesis.

CELLULAR CONSTITUENTS OF THE IMMUNE SYSTEM

A number of cell types participate in the different arms of the immune response to antigenic stimuli. These include macrophages; different categories of lymphocytes; plasma cells; and, in the case of allergies and other immediate hypersensitivity reactions, eosinophils, basophils, and mast cells. One or more of these cells may interact in the development of the immune response, depending largely on the nature of the antigen. For example, some antigens, especially those of a particulate nature, require the participation of macrophages and cells derived from both the thymus and bone marrow for the initiation of antibody synthesis. In these situations, removal of the thymus gland at birth abrogates the ability of the mature animal to produce antibody to this type of antigen following immunization. Antibody responses to such antigens are said to be **thymus-dependent.** With other antigens, including many soluble proteins, antibodies can be induced even in the absence of an intact thymus, indicating that cells originating in the thymus are not required for the initiation of

antibody synthesis. This is **thymus-independent** antibody synthesis and involves only cells derived from the bone marrow. Generally these antibodies are of the IgM class.

Lymphocytes constitute the major category of immunological effector cells. In the chicken, mature lymphocytes arise from a precursor or stem cell which originates in fetal life in the yolk sac and is found subsequently in the liver and bone marrow. The stem cells can then differentiate in two different directions. Some migrate to the thymus where, in the presence of the thymic epithelium and hormonal influences, the cells acquire certain markers and functional characteristics that separate them from other lymphocyte subpopulations. These lymphocytes are referred to as **thymus-derived** or **T lymphocytes** and are active in cellular immune functions, *e.g.,* graft rejection and delayed hypersensitivity, as well as initiation of antibody synthesis. Mice deprived of an intact thymus at birth do not develop mature T cells and are incapable of mounting T cell–dependent immune reactions. Other stem cells may stay in the bone marrow or, in the chicken, migrate to an organ called the bursa of Fabricius. In these environments, the cells differentiate into **B lymphocytes** (bursa-derived or bone marrow–derived lymphocytes), and acquire surface markers that differentiate them from T lymphocytes. This differentiation phase is under the control of factors in the bursa and bone marrow environment, including hormonal factors. These cells subsequently differentiate into **plasma cells,** the mature, antibody-producing cells, and represent the end product of B cell differentiation.

The important role of the bursa of Fabricius in antibody synthesis was initially determined in bursectomized chickens. Such chickens failed to produce antibody, although they maintained an intact cellular immune system mediated by T cells. An organ equivalent to the bursa has not been conclusively demonstrated in mammals, but it is believed that the bone marrow, and possibly the liver and spleen, probably function in the maturation of B lymphocytes. Following maturation, T and B lymphocytes migrate to peripheral lymphoid organs, such as the spleen and lymph nodes, where they can initiate and participate in immune responses to foreign substances. The thymus and bursa are often referred to as **primary lymphoid organs,** since this is where antigen-independent maturation of lymphocytes takes place, while the spleen and lymph nodes are designated **secondary lymphoid organs.** It is in the secondary organ that antigen is concentrated and processed and specific immune responses are initiated.

ORGANS OF THE IMMUNE SYSTEM

Thymus Gland[40]

The thymus gland is a bilobed structure derived from the endoderm of the third and fourth brachial pouches. It increases in size during fetal development, reaching a maximum at birth and gradually decreasing in size with aging. The cells that compose the thymus are mainly epithelial and lymphoid (thymocytes). The thymus gland is composed of a medulla and cortex. The cortex, constituting the major part of the thymus, is composed mainly of epithelial cells and lymphocytes of varying sizes. The stellate-shaped epithelial cells are in close contact with each other, established through desmosomes. Thymocytes are usually more dense in the periphery of the cortex and are largely immature, lacking certain markers that are characteristic of mature T lymphocytes, and are not capable of responding to antigen stimulation. Thymocytes mature in the cortex, acquiring surface characteristics of the T lymphocytes and then migrate into the medullary region of the thymus. Mature thymocytes comprise approximately 5 to 10 per cent of the total lymphocyte population in this gland. These thymocytes are capable of responding to immune stimuli in a manner analogous to T cells present in secondary lymphoid organs. The nature of the factors responsible for differentiation of immature into mature thymocytes is largely unknown, although it has been postulated that this differentiation step is under control of hormonal factors synthesized by epithelial cells. This is largely indicated by the finding that extracts prepared from thymus glands will support the partial differentiation of immature thymocytes to the mature state *in vitro*. A polypeptide hormone has now been isolated from such extracts that mimics the action of the whole extract. From the medulla, the mature thymocytes exit through the peripheral blood circulation and become seeded into the secondary lymphoid organs.

Bursa of Fabricius

This organ in the chicken is located near the cloaca and develops from lymphocytic infiltration of an epithelial outpouching from the cloaca. It is composed of lymphoid centers similar to the thymus, but these centers contain immunoglobulin-producing B cells. Like the thymus, this organ atrophies during the first six months of life. The factors involved in the maturation of B lymphocytes are also largely unknown but probably involve hormonal factors. However, it is clear that this organ is necessary for the maturation of B cells, since bursa-negative chickens have low B cell numbers, low immunoglobulin levels, and lack plasma cells.

Spleen

The spleen is the largest of the secondary lymphoid organs and is a major site for antibody synthesis. It is composed of a cortex and medulla similar to the organs just discussed. The organ functions largely to trap or concentrate foreign substances carried in the blood and is the main site of antibody production against bloodborne substances. The spleen is further divided into red pulp and white pulp regions. The white pulp is rich in lymphoid tissue, while the red pulp is abundant in sinuses and contains large quantities of red blood cells. The white pulp is located mainly around small arteries. The periarterial region of the white pulp is composed primarily of T lymphocytes and is called the **thymus-dependent** area, since it is depleted of lymphocytes in thymectomized animals. The external lymphoid area surrounding this periarterial section is a **thymus-independent** region, and the presence of lymphocytes that compose this area is not affected by thymectomy. Approximately 30 to 40 per cent of the cells in the spleen contain T cell markers as opposed to approximately 50 per cent with B cell markers. Following antigenic stimulation, germinal centers are produced in the white pulp that are composed of large numbers of rapidly dividing cells. These dividing cells differentiate into plasma cells and replace the bulk of the T cells in the periarterial region. Plasma cells are also found in the red pulp and in the marginal regions between the red and white pulp areas.

Lymph Nodes

Lymph nodes are small, round, or ovoid-shaped organs found in various regions throughout the body. They are generally located in close proximity to major lymphatic tracts that connect to the thoracic duct. This duct then passes lymphocytes and lymph to the large vein connected to the heart. As with the other organs, lymph nodes are composed of a medulla with many sinuses and cortex surrounded by a connective tissue capsule. The cortex is further subdivided into the external cortex, located just below the capsule, and a deep cortex, also called the paracortical or diffuse cortex. The external cortex contains aggregates of lymphocytes in regions called **follicles**; this is where the **germinal centers** develop following antigenic stimulation. These are areas of intense mitotic activity, leading to the accumulation of numerous dividing cells. As in the spleen, the external cortex region is composed largely of B cells and is considered a thymus-independent region; the deep cortex is a thymus-dependent region. Macrophages are also scattered throughout both regions and are primarily responsible for trapping antigen in the lymph nodes. This trapping event is an important step in immune recognition by cells in the lymph nodes. In the resting lymph nodes, approximately 75 per cent of the cells have T cell markers, while 15 per cent have B cell markers. The medullary region of the activated lymph node contains large numbers of plasma cells actively secreting antibody; plasma cells are carried from the cortex to the medulla through lymphatic channels connecting these two regions.

CELLS OF THE IMMUNE SYSTEM

B Lymphocytes[1, 12, 14, 32, 37, 50, 60]

B lymphocytes are classified primarily by the presence of immunoglobulins on the surface or in the membranes of viable cells. This is true for B lymphocytes isolated from most mammalian species. Surface immunoglobulin is a differentiation marker for B cells, since immature B cells express cytoplasmic but not surface immunoglobulins. The immunoglobulin expressed in the membranes of these cells is generally IgM, but other immunoglobulin types have also been identified on B lymphocytes, including IgG, IgD, and IgA. Immunoglobulins are generally not expressed in the membranes of other categories of lymphocytes, including T lymphocytes, so that this is a useful identifying marker for this subclass of lymphocytes. Generally, only one immunoglobulin class is expressed by an individual B lymphocyte. However, there have been instances in which both IgM and IgD were identified on the same lymphocyte. The appearance of different immunoglobulin classes on the same B lymphocyte appears to be related to the process of B cell differentiation. Interestingly, when this happens each immunoglobulin has the same idiotype. Experiments on the differentiation of B cells to antibody-producing plasma cells indicate that cells with surface IgM differentiate into IgM antibody-producing cells during the primary immune response. On the other hand, cells with surface IgD develop into IgG or IgA antibody-producing cells. Both classes of light chains can also be detected in the membranes of B lymphocytes, although not on the same cell, suggesting that surface immunoglobulin markers are complete immunoglobulin molecules. The presence of immunoglobulin markers on the surface of B cells also permits separation and purification of these cells from other populations through the use of antibody-coated columns. For example, if a column is prepared with beads coated by antibody to IgM and a mixture of lymphocytes passed over this column, those lymphocytes with surface IgM will attach to the antibody on the beads, while IgM-negative cells will pass through. Subsequently, the attached cells can be eluted from the column to yield a pure population of B lymphocytes with surface IgM.

Surface IgG as well as other membrane antigens can participate in a phenomenon known as **capping** when cells are reacted with antibody against the surface immunoglobulin. This is a metabolically active process that occurs at an optimal rate at 37°C. and can be readily observed by a variety of immunological tests. First, there is a redistribution of the antigen, called **patching,** following reaction with the antibody; this is followed by movement of the antigen to one pole of the cells, or the capping event. Capping is followed by a process similar to pinocytosis, resulting in the disappearance of antigen from the cell. These events demonstrate the fluidity of the membrane surface, but its biological significance remains unclear.

Immunoglobulins on the B cell surface are antigen receptors of a specific idiotype that are responsible for triggering the antibody response by one lymphocyte to a specific antigen. This has been shown by a number of methods. One approach is to follow the binding of labeled antigens to B lymphocytes. It has been observed that only a small number of lymphocytes will specifically bind to the labeled antigen. If an animal is now immunized with this same antigen, and the lymphocytes from the immune animal are reacted with the labeled antigen, the number of reactive B lymphocytes binding antigen will increase from 10- to 100-fold. This binding of specific antigen can be blocked with antibody to immunoglobulin, providing further evidence for the receptor specificity of the surface immunoglobulin. Another approach for showing that the surface immunoglobulins on B lymphocytes are receptors for specific antigens is by depletion experiments as reported by Wigzell and co-workers. If B lymphocytes are passed over an antigen such as BSA, some lymphocytes will bind to this protein, while the remainder are nonreactive. If the nonreactive population is then treated with radiolabeled BSA, no binding will be noted. In addition, attempts to induce antibody production to BSA from this depleted population will not be successful. Results of this kind indicate that a subpopulation of B lymphocytes, capable of reacting with BSA, is removed from the whole population following this interaction with BSA. Therefore, membrane immunoglobulin markers on B lymphocytes are receptors for specific antigens and participate in the initiation of antibody synthesis (Chapter 9). Furthermore, the fact that each immunoglobulin isotype on a specific cell expresses the same idiotype receptor indicates that each cell is capable of producing antibody with a single antigen specificity, regardless of the immunoglobulin class.

A second major marker on the surface of most B lymphocytes is the Fc receptor. Cells bearing this receptor will bind antigen-antibody complexes or aggregated immunoglobulin. Binding takes place between the Fc receptor on the cells and the Fc fragment of the immunoglobulin molecule. Most B cells have receptors for the Fc fragment of IgG immunoglobulin molecules, although there is also evidence for separate Fc receptors for other immunoglobulin classes, including IgM and, possibly, IgG. It is now known that Fc receptors are also expressed on other cell types and, therefore, are not absolute markers for B lymphocytes. These other cell types include subpopulations of T lymphocytes, null (N) cells, and cells infected with certain herpesviruses.

Some B cells also express a complement receptor which binds certain activated components (mainly C3) of the complement pathway. This is commonly demonstrated by showing that red blood cells coated with IgM and complement will attach to these B cells, forming rosettes on the surfaces of the lymphocytes. Complexes that lack the activated complement components will not form rosettes. This receptor is not expressed on immature B cells and, therefore, is a product of the maturation process.

In addition to these receptors, membranes of B lymphocytes from mice contain an antigen referred to as **Ia antigen,** which is a product of the immune response genes in the H-2

complex (Chapter 9). These antigens are also present on macrophages but are not expressed in the membranes of most T lymphocytes. The Ia antigen is required for antigen recognition and the initiation of antibody synthesis. An antigen probably analogous to the mouse Ia antigen, encoded by the human DR locus, has also been recently identified in the membranes of human B lymphocytes. Other differentiation antigens on mouse B cells include a series of alloantigens designated Lyb 1, Lyb 2, Lyb 3, Lyb 5, and Lyb 7. The expression of these antigens varies depending on the strain of mouse, but when present they are expressed only on B cells. A listing of the different B cell antigens expressed on mouse and human cells is shown in Tables 7–6 and 7–7.

T Lymphocytes[7, 8, 9, 12, 27, 37, 54, 60]
Among the main surface markers of T lymphocytes that allow differentiation from B lymphocytes is a receptor for binding sheep red

Table 7–6. **Major B, T, and N Cell Markers on Mouse Lymphocytes**

Cell Type	Markers
B cell	Surface Ig (IgM, IgD) Fc receptor (IgG, IgM) Complement (C′3) receptor Ia antigen Lyb 1–7 antigen
T cell	Theta antigen (θ) Lyt 1, 2, 3 antigen Ia antigens on some subpopulations Fc receptor (IgG, IgM) on some subpopulations TL antigen, GIX antigen
N cell	Fc (IgG) Complement (C′3) receptor

Table 7–7. **Major T and B Cell Markers on Human Lymphocytes**

Cell Type	Markers
B cell	Surface Ig (IgM, IgD) Fc receptor (I, G, IgM) Complement (C′3) receptor HLA–DR antigen EBV receptor

T cell	Sheep red blood cell receptor
	  T cell–specific antigens identified with
	  monoclonal antibodies (OKT 1–OKT
	  11, Leu 1–Leu 3)
	HLA–DR antigen on some
	  subpopulations
	Fc receptor (IgM, IgG) on some
	  subpopulations

blood cells and an alloantigen designated theta (θ), occurring on mouse T cells (Tables 7–6 and 7–7). This same antigen is expressed in mouse brain cells and possibly some epidermal cells, but not on other cells of the mouse. In humans, theta-like antigen has also been detected in T lymphocytes, using an antiserum prepared against brain cells. Both of these T cell markers are expressed in immature (thymocytes) as well as mature T cells, although their expression generally increases following maturation. In mice, the expression of theta is under the control of a locus on chromosome 9 with two alleles; the antigenic specificities determined by these loci have been designated Thy 1.1 and Thy 1.2. The antigen has a molecular weight of 17,500 to 18,500 daltons and is heavily glycosylated.

A number of other alloantigens are useful for detecting murine T lymphocytes and are shown in Table 7–6. The **TL antigen** is expressed in immature T cells of certain strains of mice, but not in mature cells, and in some murine T cell leukemias; thus, the designation of TL for thymus-leukemic specific antigen. The expression of this antigen is under the control of four genes on chromosome 17. The GIX antigen, like TL, is expressed on some thymocytes and in T cell leukemias induced by the Gross murine leukemia virus. The significance of its expression is largely unknown. Lyt antigens, lymphocytic alloantigens in the mouse, have been detected by antiserums prepared against lymphocyte antigens expressed in different strains of mice. Three Lyt antigens, designated Lyt 1, Lyt 2, and Lyt 3, are found in the membranes of immature murine thymocytes and on approximately 50 per cent of murine peripheral T cells. These are important

markers for relating certain T cell subsets to specific immune functions. This has been accomplished by lysing cells with complement and antibody directed against one or a combination of these markers and then examining the depleted lymphocyte populations for functional properties characteristic of T cells. In this way, four functional T cell subsets have been identified (Table 7–8):

1. **Helper T cells** (T_H). Ly 1+ cells required for the induction of antibody synthesis and the generation of cytotoxic T cells.
2. **Suppressor T cells** (T_S). Ly 2,3+ cells that inhibit the immune functions of B and T effector cells.
3. **Cytotoxic T cells** (T_C) or **killer T cells** (T_K). Ly 2,3+ cells that lyse certain target cells. These last two subpopulations can be differentiated, since suppressor T cell, but not cytotoxic T cells, also express the Ia antigen, encoded by the immune response gene.
4. **Delayed hypersensitivity T cells** (T_{DTH}). Ly 1+ cells.

In addition, some T cells populations contain Fc receptors. Similar markers have recently been identified on human T cell populations using monoclonal antibodies prepared against such cells (Table 7–7).

Null Cells

A third population of lymphocytes is found in various animal species. These lack both major B and T cell markers, *e.g.,* surface immunoglobulin, sheep red blood cell receptors, etc., and are designated N or null cells. Although these cells do not express the major B or T cell surface markers, many of them have an Fc receptor for both IgG and IgM

Table 7–8. **Correlation of Cell Markers with Functional Properties of Mouse T Cell Subpopulations**

T-Cell Degeneration	Antigen Markers	Functions
T helper (T_H)	Ly 1+	Helper cell (a) Antibody production (b) Generation of cytotoxic T cells (c) Generation of suppressor T cells
T killer (T_K)	Ly 2, 3+, Ia−	Cytotoxic effector cell (a) Transplantation immunity (b) Tumor immunity (c) Graft versus host disease (d) Anti-viral immunity
T suppressor (T_S)	Ly 2, 3+, Ia+	Suppress antibody synthesis and generation of cytotoxic T cells
T delayed hypersensitivity (T_{DTH})	Ly 1+	(a) Moderate delayed hypersensitivity reactions (b) Produce lymphokines

immunoglobulins; thus, they bind IgG or IgM antibodies. Some also express the complement receptor. These cells appear to be effectors of a cytotoxic reaction known as **antibody-dependent cellular cytotoxicity** (ADCC). The effector cells referred to as K or killer cells mediate the destruction of antibody-coated target cells by attaching to the antibody through its Fc receptor. A second cytotoxic reaction, effecting natural or spontaneous cytotoxicity against a variety of tumor and virus-infected cells, is mediated by **natural killer** (NK) cells. These are also characterized by the lack of readily detectable B and T cell receptors and the presence of the Fc receptor. Whether K and NK cells are the same is still not clear, although Herberman and co-workers have suggested that they are indeed the same. These workers have also detected some T cell markers in this cell population, inferring that NK cells arise as part of the T cell lineage.

Macrophages

Mononuclear phagocytic cells are also important cells in the initiation of the immune response to some antigens. In addition, these phagocytic cells constitute an important defense mechanism against some infectious agents (Chapter 12). These phagocytic cells originate from precursor cells in the bone marrow and are present in the peripheral circulation as mononuclear cells or monocytes. In addition, tissue macrophages can be found which originate both from the blood and from local proliferation. Maturation to tissue macrophages is accompanied by an increase in the expression of certain macrophage surface markers, such as Fc and complement receptors and Ia determinants. Characteristics of macrophages include the capacity to adhere to glass or plastic surfaces and the ability to engulf particles of various sizes, a process known as **pinocytosis** for small (less than 0.1 nm.) particles and **phagocytosis** for larger particles. These processes involve the attachment of the particle to the cell membrane, followed by ingestion and subsequent intracellular degradation. Prior immunization of macrophage donors enhances the ability of these cells to ingest the specific antigen. Mononuclear cells from immunized animals are also cytotoxic to appropriate tumor cells. Macrophages are also necessary for the initiation or induction phase of the immune response as discussed in the next chapter. In fact, macrophage participation constitutes an absolute requirement for both the initiation and expression of B and T cell functions. Macrophages synthesize and secrete proteases, complement components, and other soluble factors, known as **lymphokines,** that inhibit or interfere with normal cell functions.

DIFFERENTIATION OF B AND T CELLS BY RESPONSE TO GENERAL MITOGENS

B and T lymphocytes can be distinguished by their response to general mitogens, substances that stimulate resting cells to synthesize DNA and form blast cells. This is monitored mainly by the incorporation of labeled DNA precursors into DNA. Various materials from plants and bacteria, mainly carbohydrates, can induce this proliferation of resting lymphocytes. These include phytohemagglutinin (PHA), derived from kidney beans; concanavalin A; pokeweed mitogen; and bacterial lipopolysaccharide components. Not all lymphocyte subpopulations respond to the same mitogens, as shown in Table 7–9. Some mitogens, such as PHA and concanavalin A, stimulate primarily T cells, and are, therefore, **T cell mitogens.** This applies to both mouse and human T lymphocytes; B cells respond weakly or not at all to these two mitogens. Other mitogens stimulate primarily B cells and are **B cell mitogens.** One of the most commonly used mitogens in this regard is bacterial lipopolysaccharide (LPS). Another effective B cell mitogen is the Epstein-Barr virus, responsible for infectious mononucleosis and a candidate for human cancer virus. This virus only infects B lymphocytes, resulting in the stimulation of DNA synthesis and the transformation of these cells into permanent lymphoblastoid cell lines. Other common mitogens, such as pokeweed mitogen, stimulate both B and T lymphocytes. Thus, different lymphocytic populations can be broadly categorized as B or T cells based upon their response to a variety of mitogens.

COMPLEMENT

Complement is a component of normal serum that, in concert with appropriate anti-

Table 7–9. **Response of B and T Cell Populations to Common General Mitogens**

Mitogen	Cell Response T	B
Phytohemagglutinin (PHA)	+	−
Concanavalin A (ConA)	+	−
Lipopolysaccharide (LPS)	−	+
Polkweed mitogen (PWM)	+*	+

*Helper T cells.

Table 7–10. Proteins of the Complement System*

Component	Serum Concentration (μg/ml)	Activation Products	Molecular Weight	Polypeptide Chains	Biological Function
			Classical Pathway (CP)		
C1q	150		410,000	6 × 24,000 (A) 6 × 23,000 (B) 6 × 22,000 (C)	Triggers classical pathway on binding to aggregated immunoglobulin. Binds C1r to collagen-like "tails"
C1r	50	C$\overline{1}$r	166,000	2 × 83,000 2 × 56,000 (H) 2 × 27,000 (L)	Zymogen of serine proteinase, autoactivates on binding to C1q. Active site of C$\overline{1}$r in L chain, cleaves C1s
C1s	50	C$\overline{1}$s	83,000	56,000 (H) 27,000 (L)	Zymogen of serine proteinase, activated by C$\overline{1}$r. Cleaves C2 and C4 to give CP C3 convertase, C$\overline{42}$
C4	400		210,000	95,000 (α) 80,000 (β) 33,000 (γ)	
		C4a	10,000		Anaphylatoxin
		C4b	200,000	85,000 (α') 80,000 (β) 33,000 (γ)	Binds covalently to immunoglobulin and to carbohydrate surfaces. Modulates C2 activity in C3 convertase
C2	15		100,000		Zymogen of novel type of serine proteinase
		C2a	70,000		Active site of CP C3/C5 convertase
		C2b	30,000		Binding site of C2 for C4
			Alternate Pathway (AP)		
Factor D	5		25,000		Active serine proteinase in plasma, cleaves Factor B complexes with C3b
Factor B	200		95,000		Zymogen of novel type of serine proteinase
		Ba	35,000		
		Bb	60,000		Active site of AP C3/C5 convertase
Properdin	25		200,000	4 × 50,000	Binds to C3 convertase, stabilizes enzyme

Table continued on opposite page

body, causes lysis of mammalian and bacterial cells and inactivation of viruses. In 1890, Pfeiffer showed that the lysis of bacteria by immune serum depended on the presence of both antibody and a heat-labile serum factor. The lytic activity was lost upon heating, but could be restored by the addition of fresh serum, indicating that the lytic component was present in normal serum. During the following 70 years it was determined that complement was not a single entity but composed of different components, then designated C1, C2, C3, and C4. In the past two decades, at least 18 chemically and immunologically distinct serum proteins have been identified as components of the complement system. The designation of these proteins and some of their characteristics are listed in Table 7–10. These individual proteins compose approximately 15 per cent of the serum globulin fraction and are normally present in the circulation as functionally inactive molecules. However, under certain stimuli, the components can be sequentially activated to produce an active lytic unit. Complement activation can take place through two pathways—**classical** and **alternative**—each having the same end result, *i.e.*, lysis of a target cell (Fig. 7–8). The classical pathway involves activation of complement by specific antigen-antibody reactions, while the alternative pathway can be initiated by nonimmunological means with substances such as zymosan (yeast cell wall), endotoxin, and other complex lipopolysaccharides and polysaccharide substances. This is sometimes referred to as the **properdin** pathway, as discussed later. Complement components involved in the classical pathway are designated C1, C4, C2, C3, and

Table 7–10. **Proteins of the Complement System** (*Continued*)*

Component	Serum Concentration (µg/ml)	Activation Products	Molecular Weight	Polypeptide Chains	Biological Function
			Common Components		
C3	1200		180,000	105,000 (α) 75,000 (β)	
		C3a	10,000		Anaphylatoxin
		C3b	170,000	95,000 (α) 75,000 (β)	Multifunctional; subunit of AP C3 convertase, CP and AP C5 convertases. Ligand for immune adherence reactions.
C5	80		180,000	105,000 (α) 75,000 (β)	
		C5a	11,000		Anaphylatoxin, potent leucocyte chemoattractant
		C5b	170,000	95,000 (α') 75,000 (β)	Binding site for membrane and for C6, leads to assembly of lytic complex
			Terminal Components		
C6	70	130,000			
C7	65	110,000			
C8	80	163,000		77,000 63,000 14,000	Terminal components forming lytic complex
C9	200	79,000			
			Control Proteins		
C1 INH	200	100,000			Typical serum protease inhibitor. Inhibits C̄1r and C̄1s (and plasmin) by tight binding
C3b/C4b inactivator	25	100,000		55,000 (H) 45,000 (L)	Regulatory proteolytic enzyme. Specificity directed by appropriate modulator
1H	700	150,000			Binds to C3b, directs specificity of inactivator to C3b
C4b-binding protein	100	550,000		8–10 × 60,000	Binds to C4b, directs specificity of inactivator to C4b

*Reprinted with permission from M. A. Kerr, The complement system, Biochemical Education. Copyright 1981, Pergamon Press, Ltd.

C5 through C9. These can be further grouped into three functional units: C1, the **recognition unit**; C4, C2, and C3, the **activation unit**; and C5–C9, the **membrane attack unit.** Most of the biologically significant activities of complement take place after the activation of the last six complement components. Immunoglobulins IgG1, IgG2, IgG3, and IgM are capable of initiating the classical pathway, while IgA, IgD, IgE, and IgG4 are ineffective. The complement factors involved in the alternative pathway have been designated Factors B, D, and P; the latter is also known as properdin. A bar placed over the letter or number indicates the enzymatically active form of the component, *e.g.*, C̄1, C̄3, D̄, while cleavage products are generally designated with lower-case letters, *e.g.*, C2a, C2b, C3a, C3b, etc. The steps for complement activation in both

pathways are schematically shown in Figure 7–9.

Classical Pathway[43–46]

The lytic activation of complement on cells has been used to develop a quantitative assay for the activity of whole complement or its individual components. Generally, sheep red blood cells coated with antibodies (IgG or IgM) and complement are utilized in this assay. The degree of hemolysis, reflected by the amount of hemoglobin released, is proportional to the amount of complement present. From the sigmoidal shape of the curve of this lytic system, it became apparent that the curve was steepest at 50 per cent hemolysis. Therefore, complement units are usually expressed in 50 per cent units and one unit is defined as that amount of complement that will lyse 50

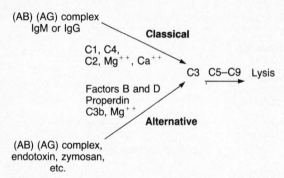

Figure 7–8. General outline of the activation of complement by the classical and alternative pathways.

per cent of the antibody-coated sheep erythrocytes. In this system, therefore, any single component can be assayed for its role in the lytic reaction by adding it in its purified form to a mixture containing the remainder of the complement components. In addition, since complement shows little species specificity, it is possible to compare complement from different animal species.

The initial step of the classical pathway is the activation of C1 by the antigen-antibody complex (Fig. 7–9). This takes place via binding of C1 to a site on the Fc fragment of the antibody molecule. C1 is the heaviest of the complement components with a molecular weight of 650,000 to 700,000 and is actually a complex of three proteins, C1q, C1r, and C1s, linked by calcium ions. C1q has a molecular weight of 410,000; C1r, a weight of 166,000; and C1s, a weight of 83,000. C1q consists of 18 polypeptide chains arranged into six triple helices as visualized by electron microscopy. It is rich in glycine, hydroxyproline, and hydroxylysine, with a composition that is similar to that of collagen. At the end of each helix is a globular portion that binds to a receptor, possibly on the C_H2 domain, of IgG or IgM. Activation of C1 requires the binding of C1q to two molecules of IgG antibody or one molecule of IgM; bound C1q then activates C1r by an unknown process. In turn, a bond is cleaved in C1s to result in $\overline{C1s}$ with proteolytic enzyme activity. Upon generation of $\overline{C1s}$, the initial phase of complement activation is completed.

The next phase of this complement pathway involves the activation of C4 and C2 by $\overline{C1s}$ to form $\overline{C42}$. Both C4 and C2 are β_1 globulins with molecular weights of 210,000 and 100,000, respectively. In the activation process, $\overline{C1s}$ cleaves a peptide bond in the longest (α) chain of the three peptide chains of C4, resulting in the loss of a fragment, C4a, with a molecular

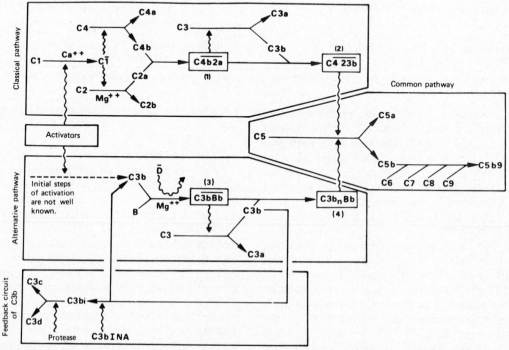

Figure 7–9. Detailed scheme of the activation of complement components by the classical and alternative activation pathways (Peltier, A. P. *In* J. F. Bach (Ed.), Immunology, 2nd ed. John Wiley & Sons, Inc., New York, 1982, pp. 252–284. Reproduced with permission of Flammarion Medécine-Sciences, Paris.)

weight of 8,000. The remaining fragment, C4b, then binds to a receptor on the cell surface where it is quite stable. $\overline{C1s}$ then cleaves C2, releasing fragment C2b with a molecular weight of 30,000. The larger fragment, C2a, binds to C4b in the presence of magnesium to form $\overline{C42}$, a proteolytic enzyme also termed **C3 convertase.** Fragment C2a is very labile and will decay with a half-life of 10 minutes if not bound to C4b.

The substrate for $\overline{C42}$ is C3, a β_1 globulin with a molecular weight of 180,000. Component C3 is pivotal, because of the many biological activities it generates and because of its important role in the alternative pathway. Fragment $\overline{C42}$ splits a small fragment from the N-terminal portion of the α chain of C3, fragment C3a of 10,000 molecular weight. The larger fragment, C3b (molecular weight of 170,000), then attaches to a cell membrane receptor near the antibody attachment site. Binding of C3b leads to the formation of $\overline{C423}$; this complex also has enzymatic activity and cleaves C5 into a small C5a (molecular weight of 11,000) and C5b (molecular weight of 170,000), which binds to the $\overline{C423}$ complex. C6, C7, and C8 now are capable of attaching to this complex in nonenzymatic fashion at a ratio of one molecule of each per molecule of C5. This complex can now bind up to six molecules of C9. C9 is inserted into the membrane in such a way as to form channels through which large and small molecules can freely traverse. Because of the high protein content of the cytoplasm of living cells, osmotic lysis will occur if the cells are placed in an isotonic environment free of protein. Thus, the classical complement pathway consists of a series of specific events leading to the sequential formation of several complement enzymes, with the end result being lysis of the cell.

Alternative Pathway[43, 47]

This pathway of complement activation is generally activated by nonimmunological mechanisms. However, IgA antibody and, possibly, some IgG, IgM, and IgE molecules can also activate this pathway as can a factor in cobra venom. The pathway was originally described as the **properdin system** by Pillemer in 1954 and involves a group of serum proteins, none of which are necessarily antibody, that appear to function in immunity against infectious agents. A number of these proteins have been purified and characterized. These include **properdin** (P), a glycoprotein with the mobility of a gamma globulin and a molecular weight

of 200,000. It has an isoelectric point of around 9.5 and is composed of four identical subunits each with a molecular weight of 50,000. **Factor B** is a thermolabile β-globulin with a molecular weight of approximately 100,000. **Factor D,** a globulin-like molecule, is a serine esterase with molecular weight of 25,000. The other major component of the properdin system, originally designated Factor A, is now known to be C3. Another factor, **initiating factor** (IF), participates in the alternate pathway and has a molecular weight of approximately 170,000. The end result of the protein interactions in the alternate pathway is the activation of C3 (Fig. 7–9).

The complete mechanism of the alternative pathway has still not been delineated, but a major step is the conversion of Factor B to an active form, $B\overline{b}$, capable of cleaving C3 in a manner similar to that of $\overline{C42}$ in the classical pathway. Factor D is responsible for cleaving B into $B\overline{b}$; this action requires the presence of native C3 and magnesium. Once C3 is converted to C3b, both C3b and $B\overline{b}$ form a complex (C3 convertase) on the surface of the initiator. C3b is a more efficient promoter of the conversion of B to $B\overline{b}$ than is native C3, so that the C3b generated by this mechanism accelerates the conversion of more B to $B\overline{b}$ and thus of C3 to C3b. Properdin participates in this pathway by binding to $\overline{C3bBb}$, thereby preventing the spontaneous decay of this complex. This complex can then activate the rest of the complement system.

The mechanism by which different substances activate this pathway is still not completely known. However, there are indications that "activators" do not really activate but function by preventing the shutdown of spontaneous activation that is probably continuously ongoing as a result of the activation of B by D in the presence of C3. It is known that once C3b is produced, it can be cleaved into an inactive form, designated C3d, by a β-globulin, C3 inactivator (C3INA). The efficiency of C3INA is enhanced by another β-globulin, B1H, that binds to $\overline{C3bBb}$ in such a way as to displace Bb, thereby inactivating this molecule and rendering C3b more susceptible to the action of C3INA. Activators are thought to function by protecting $\overline{C3bBb}$ from inactivation by B1H and C3INA.

Biological Activities Mediated by Complement

Besides mediating cytotoxic reactions, complement or C3 derivatives are also involved in a number of biological activities, as shown in

Table 7–11. **Other Immune Activities Associated with Complement Components**

Function	Component
Chemotaxis	C3a, C5a
Degranulation (release of histamine)	C3a, C5a, C4a
Mobilization of leukocytes	C3e
Phagocytosis (opsonization)	C3b
Immune adherence	C3b

Table 7–11. The C3a and C5a products generated during the activation of C3 and C5 can stimulate the release of histamine from mast cells, contraction of smooth muscle, increased vascular permeability, and edema. These and C4a are referred to as **anaphylatoxins.** In addition, both C3a and B5a have chemotactic activity and cause the migration of granulocytes, eosinophils, and macrophages into regions of antigen-antibody reactions. Both components have an arginine residue at their COOH terminal end that appears to be necessary for this activity. C3b is capable of binding to specific receptors on granulocytes and macrophages, thereby promoting phagocytosis. It can also bind to receptors on B lymphocytes, suggesting that C3b functions in the activation of lymphocytes participating in the immune response. This attachment of antibody-antigen-complement complexes through C3b is referred to as **immune adherence.** Other components believed to participate in immunological phenomena include C3d, which can attach to B lymphocytes and may play a role in the elimination of antigen-antibody complexes, and C3e liberated from C3c by trypsin. This component is capable of mobilizing leucocytes from bone marrow and, therefore, may play an important role in the initiation of inflammatory responses.

The major role of complement, however, appears to be as an effector mechanism by which antibodies help the host eliminate foreign substances, including infectious disease agents. This is accomplished largely through the release of products, such as C3a, C3b, and C5a, that contribute to the development of the inflammatory response. This is supported by the finding that congenital lack of complement is often associated with the development of certain diseases. Patients with deficiencies of C3 and C3INA are very susceptible to bacterial infections, as are patients lacking C6, C7, or C8. In addition, lack of certain complement components, such as C4 and C3, appears to be associated with a high frequency of lupus erythematosus. These observations implicate complement as an immune defense mechanism against the development of disease.

References

1. Abdou, N. I., and M. Richter. 1970. The role of bone marrow in the immune response. Adv. Immunol. **12**:201–270.
2. Amos, D. 1969. Genetic and antigenic aspects of human histocompatibility systems. Adv. Immunol. **10**:251–297.
3. Atassi, M. Z. 1975. Antigenic structure of myoglobulin. The complete immunochemical anatomy of a protein and conclusions relating to antigenic structures of proteins. Immunochemistry **13**:423–438.
4. Avrameas, S. 1969. Coupling of enzymes to proteins with glutaraldehyde. Use of the conjugate for the detection of antigens and antibody. Immunochemistry **6**:43–52.
5. Bennich, H., and S. G. O. Johansson. 1971. Structure and function of human immunoglobulin E. Adv. Immunol. **13**:1–55.
6. Boyden, S. V. 1951. The adsorption of proteins on erythrocytes treated with tannic acid and subsequent hemagglutination by antiprotein serum. J. Exptl. Med. **93**:107–120.
7. Cantor, H., and E. A. Boyse. 1975. Functional subclasses of T lymphocytes bearing different Ly antigens. I. The generation of functionally distinct T-cell subclasses as is a differentiation process independent of antigen. J. Exptl. Med. **141**:1376–1389.
8. Cantor, H., et al. 1975. Characterization of subpopulations of T-lymphocytes. Separation and functional studies of peripheral T cells binding different amounts of fluorescent anti Thy 1.2 antibody. Cellular Immunol. **15**:180–196.
9. Cantor, H., and I. Weissman. 1976. Development and function of subpopulations of thymocytes and T lymphocytes. Prog. Allergy **20**:1–64.
10. Capra, J. D. 1977. Idiotypy as a molecular and cellular probe. Fed. Proc. **36**:203–206.
11. Capra, J. D., and J. M. Kehoe. 1975. Hypervariable regions, idiotypy and the antibody-combining site. Adv. Immunol. **20**:1–40.
12. Chess, L., and S. F. Schlossman. 1977. Human lymphocyte subpopulations. Adv. Immunol. **25**:213–242.
13. Cohen, S., and C. Milstein. 1967. Structure and biological properties of immunoglobulins. Adv. Immunol. **7**:1–89.
14. Dickler, H. B. 1976. Lymphocyte receptors for immunoglobulin. Adv. Immunol. **24**:167–214.
15. Dorrington, K. J., and C. Tanford. 1970. Molecular size and conformation of immunoglobulins. Adv. Immunol. **12**:333–381.
16. Edelman, G. M., and J. A. Gally. 1962. The nature of Bence-Jones proteins: chemical similarities to polypeptide chains of myeloma globulins and normal γ-globulins. J. Exptl. Med. **116**:207–227.
17. Edelman, G. M., et al. 1969. The covalent structure of an entire G immunoglobulin molecule. Proc. Natl. Acad. Sci. **63**:78–85.
18. Fahey, J. L. 1970. Classes of blood-group antibodies. Ann. N.Y. Acad. Sci. **169**:164–167.
19. Fahey, J. L., and R. A. Kyle. 1980. Section B. Tests

for humoral components of the immunological response. pp. 102–108. *In* N. R. Rose and H. Friedman (Eds.): Manual of Clinical Immunology, 2nd ed. American Society for Microbiology, Washington, D.C.

20. Freda, V. J. 1971. The control of Rh disease. pp. 266–281. *In* R. A. Good and D. W. Fisher (Eds.): Immunobiology. Sinauer Associates, Stamford, Conn.

21. Freund, J., *et al.* 1948. Antibody formation and sensitization with aids of adjuvants. J. Immunol. **60**:383–398.

22. Gill, P. G., and A. S. Kelns. 1967. Anti-antibodies. Adv. Immunol. **6**:461–478.

23. Gill, T. J. 1972. The chemistry of antigens and its influence on immunogenicity. pp. 5–13. *In* F. Borek (Ed.): Immunogenicity. North Holland Publishing Co., Amsterdam.

24. Green, N. M. 1969. Electron microscopy of the immunoglobulins. Adv. Immunol. **11**:1–30.

25. Habir, E. 1969. Immunochemistry. Ann. Rev. Biochem. **37**:497–520.

26. Halpern, M. S., and M. E. Koshland. 1970. Novel sub-unit in secretory IgA. Nature **228**:1276–1285.

27. Haynes, B. F. 1981. Human T lymphocyte antigens as defined by monoclonal antibodies. Immunol. Rev. **57**:127–161.

28. Hopper, J. E., and A. Nisonoff. 1971. Individual antigenic specificity of immunoglobulins. Adv. Immunol. **13**:58–99.

29. Ishizaka, K. 1976. Cellular events in the IgE antibody response. Adv. Immunol. **23**:1–76.

30. Ishizaka, T., C. M. Sian, and K. Ishizaka. 1972. Complement-fixation by aggregated IgE through alternate pathway. J. Immunol. **108**:848–851.

31. Kabat, E. A. 1968. Structural Concepts in Immunology and Immunochemistry. Holt, Rinehart and Winston, New York.

32. Kincade, P. W. 1981. Formation of B lymphocytes in fetal and adult life. Adv. Immunol. **31**:177–246.

33. Kockwa, S., and E. H. Kunkel (Eds.). 1971. Immunoglobulins. Ann. N.Y. Acad. Sci. **190**:5–584.

34. Koshland, M. E. 1975. Structure and function of the J chain. Adv. Immunol. **20**:41–69.

35. Lamm, M. E. 1976. Cellular aspects of immunoglobulin A. Adv. Immunol. **22**:223–290.

36. Levine, P. 1970. Prevention and treatment of erythroblastosis fetalis. Ann. N.Y. Acad. Sci. **169**:234–240.

37. McKenzie, I. F. C., and T. Potter. 1979. Murine lymphocyte surface antigens. Adv. Immunol. **27**:181–338.

38. Metzger, H. 1970. The antigen receptor problem. Ann. Rev. Biochem. **39**:889–928.

39. Metzger, H. 1970. Structure and function of γM macroglobulins. Adv. Immunol. **12**:57–116.

40. Miller, J. F. A. P., A. H. E. Marshall, and R. G. White. 1962. The immunological significance of the thymus. Adv. Immunol. **2**:111–162.

41. Milstein, C., and A. J. Munro. 1978. Genetic basis of antibody specificity. Ann. Rev. Microbiol. **24**:335–358.

42. Morgan, W. T. J. 1970. Molecular aspects of human blood group specificity. Ann. N.Y. Acad. Sci. **169**:118–130.

43. Morrison, D. C., and L. F. Kline. 1977. Activation of the classical and properdin pathways of complement by bacterial lipopolysaccharides (LPS). J. Immunol. **118**:362–368.

44. Müller-Eberhard, H. J. 1971. Biochemistry of complement. pp. 553–565. *In* B. Amos (Ed.): Progress in Immunology. Academic Press, New York.

45. Müller-Eberhard, H. J. 1975. Complement. Ann. Rev. Biochem. **44**:697–724.

46. Müller-Eberhard, H. J. 1977. Chemistry and function of the complement system. Hospital Practice **12**:33–43.

47. Müller-Eberhard, H. J., and R. D. Schreiber. 1980. Molecular biology and chemistry of the alternative pathway of complement. Adv. Immunol. **29**:2–55.

48. Natvig, J. B., and H. G. Kunkel. 1973. Human immunoglobulins: classes, subclasses, genetic variants, and idiotypes. Adv. Immunol. **16**:1–60.

49. Nisonoff, A., J. E. Hopper, and S. B. Spring. 1975. The Antibody Molecule. Academic Press, New York.

50. Nussenzweig, V. 1974. Receptors for immune complexes on lymphocytes. Adv. Immunol. **19**:217–258.

51. Plescia, O. J., and W. Braun. 1967. Nucleic acids as antigens. Adv. Immunol. **6**:231–252.

52. Potter, M., and R. Lieberman. 1967. Genetics of immunoglobulins in the mouse. Adv. Immunol. **7**:92–146.

53. Rapport, M. M., and L. Graf. 1969. Immunochemical reactions of lipids. Prog. Allergy **13**:273–331.

54. Reinher, E. L., and S. F. Schlossman. 1980. The differentiation and function of human T-lymphocytes. Cell **19**:821–827.

55. Sela, M. 1966. Immunological studies with synthetic polypeptides. Adv. Immunol. **5**:30–129.

56. Sela, M. 1970. Structure and specificity of synthetic polypeptides. Ann. N.Y. Acad. Sci. **169**:23–35.

57. Spiegelberg, H. L. 1974. Biological activities of immunoglobulins of different classes and subclasses. Adv. Immunol. **19**:259–294.

58. Spiegelberg, H. L. 1977. The structure and biology of human IgD. Immunol. Rev. **37**:3–24.

59. Trentin, J. (Ed.). 1967. Cross-Reacting Antigens and Neoantigens. Williams & Wilkins Co., Baltimore.

60. Werner, N. L. 1974. Membrane immunoglobulins and antigen receptors on B and T lymphocytes. Adv. Immunol. **19**:67–216.

61. White, R. G. 1967. Antigen adjuvants. Mod. Trends Immunol. **2**:28–52.

CHAPTER 8

Humoral and Cellular Immune Reactions

Gary R. Pearson, Ph.D.

SEROLOGICAL REACTIONS	ANTIBODY-MEDIATED
QUANTITATIVE	CYTOTOXICITY
PRECIPITATION	NEUTRALIZATION
PRECIPITATION IN GELS	COMPLEMENT-FIXATION
IMMUNOELECTROPHORESIS	**CELLULAR IMMUNE**
AGGLUTINATION	**REACTIONS**
LABELED ANTIBODY ASSAYS	LYMPHOCYTE CYTOTOXICITY
Immunofluorescence	LYMPHOCYTE
Radioimmune Assays	TRANSFORMATION
ELISA Assays	LYMPHOKINE ASSAYS

Both antibody and cellular immune responses can be readily studied in the laboratory. Antigen-antibody reactions can be visualized and measured *in vitro* using a variety of different methods; the most common of these are precipitation, agglutination, and complement fixation. Other more sensitive procedures employ antigens or antibodies labeled with a radioactive or fluorescent marker. Other tests have as their basis the ability of antibody to block or neutralize infection processes, *e.g.,* virus or toxin neutralization, or to mediate a cytotoxic reaction in the presence of complement or certain subpopulations of lymphoid cells. This has made it possible to define the different phases of the reaction between these components, to determine the optimal conditions for forming antigen-antibody complexes, to identify factors that will inhibit or enhance the reaction of antibody with its corresponding antigenic determinant, and to develop immunological tests for the diagnosis and clinical management of patients with a variety of diseases. Some of these laboratory reactions, such as precipitation, have their counterpart in the whole animal and, in fact, are apparently involved in the mediation of some of the symptoms of diseases with an immunological basis (Chapters 10 and 11). Because antibodies are present in serum, the manifestations of the secondary phase of antigen-antibody reactions are classified as serological reactions and the general subject matter is designated as **serology.** The last serum dilution to cause a measurable effect, as discussed below, is designated the titer of the serum.

Similarly, cell-mediated immune responses can be studied in the laboratory. Such procedures generally test the ability of different lymphoid cell populations to mediate a recognizable and measurable event following interaction with the appropriate antigen. When the antigen is associated with the membranes of living cells, cellular immune responses can be detected by cytotoxic or growth inhibiting effects, mediated by lymphocytes, on antigen-positive target cells. Alternatively, following interaction of the antigen with an immune cell, soluble factors are often released that have a measurable effect on certain types of bystander cells. The macrophage migration inhibitory factor (MIF) is an example of one of these factors; it is released following the interaction of antigen with immune T cells. This chapter focuses on some of the major approaches for detecting and measuring antibody and cellular immune responses in the laboratory.

Serological Reactions[7, 15, 22, 45, 47]

The first phase of antigen-antibody reaction involves the interaction between the antigenic determinant and the hypervariable region of the antibody site. This reaction does not occur through covalent bonding, but involves electrostatic properties of the antigen and antibody molecules and is largely influenced by pH, temperature, and salt concentration. Most antigen-antibody reactions proceed optimally at 37°C. in isotonic salt at a neutral pH. These immunological reactions will also proceed at lower temperatures, such as 4°C., but at a slower rate. Exposure of antigen-antibody complexes to alkaline (pH 9.0 or above) or acidic (less than pH 4.0) conditions or to hypertonic salt solutions will disrupt the union between these two components and result in the release of free antigen and antibody. The second phase results in the visual reactions, such as precipitation, and only occurs when multivalent antigens and antibodies are the components involved. Because of their multivalent properties, lattices of the antigen and antibody complexes are built through crosslinking, resulting in a precipitate when lattice formation reaches an optimal size. This lattice formation is illustrated in Figure 8–1. Crosslinking results from the ability of one bivalent antibody molecule to react with two antigen sites. For obvious reasons, such lattice formation cannot take place with monovalent antigens such as small haptens or monovalent antibody. However, since monovalent reagents can combine with specific antigen or antibody sites, they can block further attachment of multivalent reagents with these specific sites, thereby blocking the secondary reactions. This type of inhibition or blocking has been useful for characterizing the immune response to single antigenic determinants.

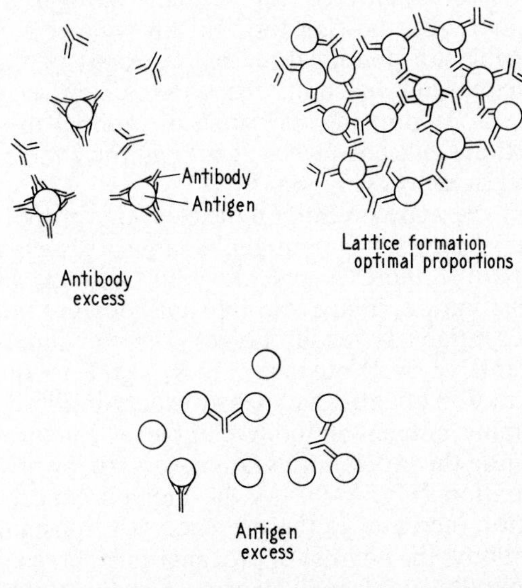

The primary reaction between antigen and antibody has been determined mainly through the use of simple hapten determinants and the method of equilibrium dialysis, as discussed in Chapter 7. It was shown that the initial reaction was reversible and could be written in the following way:

$$Ab + Ag \underset{K_2}{\overset{K_1}{\rightleftharpoons}} (Ab{\cdot}Ag)$$

where K_1 and K_2 are the association and dissociation constants of the reaction, Ab stands for the antibody binding site and Ag is the antigen concentration. The association constant, K, is determined by the following formula based on the law of mass action:

$$\frac{K_1}{K_2} = K = \frac{(Ab{\cdot}Ag)}{(Ab)(Ag)}$$

This association constant K is a measure of the strength of the interaction between a homogeneous antibody population and the corresponding monovalent antigenic determinant and is termed **antibody affinity.**

In measuring antibody affinity, more than one antigen concentration is tested in equilibrium dialysis and the concentrations of free and bound antigen are determined after reaching equilibrium. If the reciprocal of the bound antigen (1/r) is plotted against the reciprocal of free antigen (1/c) for each antigen concentration, under ideal conditions, a straight line will result with an intercept on the 1/r axis, designated 1/n (Fig. 8–2). The point of intercept is a measure of the number of antigen-binding sites per antibody molecule, or its valence (usually 2). The point on the graph at which one-half of the antibody combining sites are bound to antigen is the **intrinsic association constant** and is a measure of the binding strength of the antibody population. Since antibody populations are generally heterogeneous with respect to their binding sites to the same antigen determinant and, therefore, to their association constants, the intrinsic association constant is generally used to express affinity or binding strength of a heterogeneous antibody population to a monovalent antigen.

Figure 8–1. Diagrammatic representation of possible complexes between antigen and antibody.

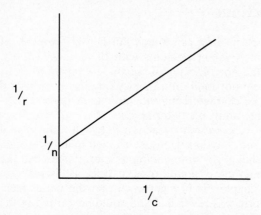

Figure 8–2. Ideal binding curve of univalent antigen by antibody as determined by method of equilibrium dialysis as shown by Langmuir plot. Reciprocal of bound hapten (1/r) is plotted against the reciprocal of free hapten (1/c). The point of intercept on the 1/r axis (designated 1/n) is a measure of the antibody valence.

The term **avidity** is also frequently used to describe the binding strength of an antibody population. This is because it is often difficult or impossible to determine the intrinsic association constant against multivalent antigens as opposed to monovalent antigens. With such antigens, the interaction of antigen and antibody is dependent not only on the intrinsic association constant of the reaction between the antibody and each determinant on the multivalent antigen, but on the number of sites as well as on nonspecific factors involved in the secondary reaction. For example, the intrinsic association constant can increase as much as 100,000-fold in the reaction of a given antibody molecule with a bivalent antigen as opposed to the reaction of the same antibody with a monovalent determinant because of these different variables. For this reason, avidity is normally used to describe the binding capacity, in a semiquantitative fashion, of an antibody population with a multivalent antigen. It is also useful for describing the binding strength of antibodies in biological systems such as viral or toxin neutralization, agglutination, and so forth. Affinity is reserved for reactions between monovalent antigens and corresponding antibodies.

Tests for measuring antigen-antibody reactions largely depend on the nature of both the antigen and the antibody, the ability of the antibody to fix complement, and the concentrations of the different components of the tests. Described below are some of the more common methods used for measuring antigen-antibody reactions.

QUANTITATIVE PRECIPITATION[23, 45]

The reaction between bivalent antibody and a multivalent, soluble antigen will result in precipitation of the reactant substances due to lattice formation by the multivalent participants; each antigen is linked to more than one antibody and each antibody to more than one antigen. This test can be performed in solution as the **precipitin test** or in agar gels as **gel precipitation,** in which lines of precipitate form following diffusion of the reactants. The simplest form of precipitation in liquid is the **ring test,** performed by layering increasing amounts of antigen over a constant amount of antibody. A ring of precipitate forms in the interphase layer as an indicator of a specific antigen-antibody reaction. This test has subsequently been modified extensively *e.g.,* by use of radiolabeled antigen, so that the precipitation test has become an ideal method for immunochemical studies.

The quantitative precipitation method was originally used by Heidelberger and associates to measure the amount of antibody present in an antiserum. This was accomplished using pneumococcal capsular polysaccharide antigen and a rabbit antiserum directed against it. Since the polysaccharide antigen does not contain nitrogen, it was possible in this system to measure the amount of antibody in the precipitate by measuring the nitrogen content. In order to obtain accurate measurements, it was first necessary to eliminate other serum proteins, such as complement, that participate in antigen-antibody reactions. In addition, the supernatants from each antigen-antibody mixture were analyzed for residual antigen or antibody by the ring test. In this way, it was possible to identify three major zones in the precipitation reaction: the zone of antibody excess, or prozone; the zone of optimal proportions, or equivalence zone; and the zone of antigen excess (Fig. 8–3).

In the zone of **antibody excess,** the proportion of antibody to antigen is large. In such a situation, there is only a small amount of precipitation, if any, and free antibody but not free antigen is readily detected in the supernatants of such mixtures. This is due to the saturation of antigenic sites by excess antibody, forming antigen-antibody complexes but preventing the lattice formation necessary for precipitation (Fig. 8–1). As the antigen concentration increases in the presence of a constant antibody, the amount of precipitation increases in parallel until **equivalence,** or **optimal pro-**

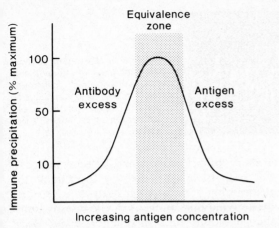

Figure 8–3. Illustration of the three major zones in the precipitation reaction.

portions, is reached. At this point, precipitation is maximum and it is no longer possible to detect free antibody or antigen in supernatants from such mixtures, *i.e.,* all antigen and antibody will have combined and precipitated (Fig. 8–1). The amount of antibody present in the antiserum can, therefore, be accurately determined by measuring the protein content of the precipitate formed at equivalence. With additional increases in antigen concentration, precipitates will decrease in size and free antigen but no free antibody is detectable in the supernatants. This is the zone of **antigen excess**; the decrease in the formation of precipitates in this zone is due to the saturation of antibody sites by excess antigen, again preventing lattice formation. By measuring the amount of antigen and antibody in the precipitates at different points of the precipitation curve, it is possible to determine the valence of both the antigen and the antibody by mathematical computations.

PRECIPITATION IN GELS[12, 31, 34, 47, 48]

Precipitation reactions can also be detected in gels or semisolid mediums as antigen and antibody molecules diffuse toward each other. The original method introduced by Oudin was a single diffusion method in agar. The antibody is mixed in an agar layer and antigen in solution is then allowed to diffuse into the agar. This results in the formation of bands of precipitation in the agar corresponding to the number of different antigenic specificities recognized by the antiserum, *e.g.,* with a single antigen-antibody system, only one precipitate line forms, as opposed to multiple bands in a heterogeneous system. Individual precipitation bands form when antibody and antigen for each antigen-antibody system are at optimal proportions (equivalence). This varies for the different antigen-antibody systems, depending on the individual concentrations, resulting in separate bands for each.

A modification of the Oudin method, known as **single radial immunodiffusion** was developed by Mancini and associates and has been useful for measuring antigen in the clinical laboratory. In this method, antibody monospecific for an antigen is mixed with agar, which is then poured into a plate to form a uniform layer. Wells are then cut in the agar and filled with a measured volume of antigen solution. Antigen diffuses out of the well, forming a halo or ring around the well when a precipitate is formed. This ring will expand until equivalence is reached. This is illustrated for IgG in Figure 8–4. It was determined by Mancini that a linear relationship exists between the square of the diameter of the ring and the concentration of antigen in the well. Therefore, if a series of known concentrations of an antigen are tested along with the unknown sample, a

Figure 8–4. Single radial immunodiffusion (Mancini method). Rings formed with three different known concentrations of IgG (STI, STII, STIII) are compared with those produced with three different whole serums. Based on the diameters of the rings, the concentrations of IgG in the three whole serum specimens can be calculated by comparison with the precipitation rings formed with the three known standard concentrations.

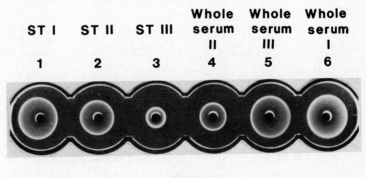

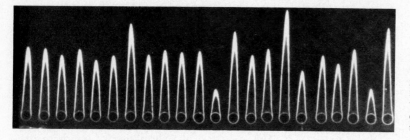

Figure 8–5. Illustration of rocket electrophoresis of different antigen concentrations electrophoresed through agar containing antibody. The area of the cones is directly related to antigen concentration.

standard curve can be prepared relating concentration to the square of the diameter of the precipitation ring. The concentration of the test antigen is then determined from the standard curve simply by knowing the diameter of the precipitation ring. Less than 0.1 to 0.2 μg. of antigen can be detected with single radioimmune diffusion. This method has been particularly important for the measurement of serum immunoglobulin concentrations in the clinical laboratory.

A more sensitive variation of this test is **rocket electrophoresis,** in which the antigen is electrophoresed through an agar gel containing an excess of antibody (Fig. 8–5). Initially, antigen-antibody complexes precipitate and form lines parallel to the antigen well. However, as antigen continues to migrate, the precipitin lines start to converge to form cone-like structures which cease to grow in the absence of free antigen. The area of the cone is directly related to the antigen concentration so that with this technique, it is possible to accurately determine the concentration of a single antigen in solution.

An immunodiffusion technique now used widely in immunological studies is the **double immunodiffusion** test described by Ouchterlony. Separate wells are prepared in an agar gel; antigen and antibody are placed in opposing wells and allowed to diffuse toward each other. Precipitation lines will form when the reactants for each antibody-antigen system are at their optimal proportions. The advantage of this assay is that it is possible to examine the relationship of different antigens to each other because multiple antigens can be tested against the same antiserum. In practice, a well is cut in the center of the gel with additional wells surrounding it. Antiserum is placed in the center well and antigens are placed in the surrounding wells. When the reactants are allowed to diffuse toward each other, several events can occur (Fig. 8–6). If the antigens are completely unrelated, the bands of precipitation formed by each separate antigen-antibody system will cross each other. This is referred to as a reaction of **nonidentity.** If the antigens are identical, the precipitation lines will fuse to form a line of **identity.** If the antigens are only partly related, the precipitation lines will partly fuse, but leave a spur. This represents a cross-reaction, or reaction of **partial identity.** Double immunodiffusion is a reliable and valuable test for examining similarities between different antigens and has been very useful, for example, in virology to determine the identity of new virus isolates. This assay can detect less than 0.1 μg. protein.

IMMUNOELECTROPHORESIS[2, 10, 18, 28]

Immunoelectrophoresis combines electrophoresis, or migration based on charge in an electrical field, with immunodiffusion. In this

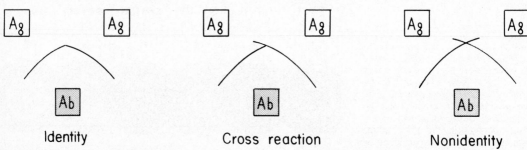

Identity   Cross reaction   Nonidentity

Figure 8–6. Diagrammatic representation of the Ouchterlony double diffusion technique with single bands of antigen-antibody precipitates. *Left,* The juncture of the bands indicates identity between the antigens; *Center,* Line of cross-reaction or partial identity (note spur); *Right,* Line of nonidentity as indicated by the lack of fusing between the lines. The antiserum (Ab) contains antibodies to both antigens.

system, a thin layer of agar is placed on a glass slide and wells cut in the agar layer. The antigen is then placed in the well and subjected to an electrical field. The antigen components migrate in this field and separate from each other according to their charge at a specific pH. Following electrophoresis, a trough is cut in the gel parallel to the direction of migration, filled with antiserum, and allowed to diffuse for an appropriate period of time. Precipitation bands then form where the antibodies encounter the appropriate antigen (Fig. 8–7). This technique is highly sensitive and is used extensively in clinical laboratories to identify and measure various serum immunoglobulins.

AGGLUTINATION[7, 8, 45, 47]

This serological test involves the interaction of antibody with insoluble or particulate antigens such as bacteria, mammalian cells, erythrocytes, or soluble antigens coupled to larger particles. The addition of antibody to such a multivalent antigen results in agglutination of the antigen-bearing particles through cross-linking. The antibody in this reaction is known as an **agglutinin**; when red blood cells are used as the antigen, the reaction is called **hemagglutination.** Agglutination tests are of two general types—slide and tube. The slide test is performed by mixing antiserum and antigen suspensions on a glass slide and observing for rapid clumping of the particles. Tube agglutination tests are semiquantitative, in that antigen suspension is added to a series of antiserum dilutions. After incubation, the particles agglutinate and fall out of suspension.

Agglutination proceeds in two steps, as in the precipitation reaction. The first step involves the binding of antibody to the antigenic determinant, while the second step involves cross-linking to adjacent particles until large, visible aggregates are formed. With very high levels of antibody, a prozone effect is sometimes noted as in the precipitation test. The prozone is due to the saturation of antigenic sites by antibody, thereby preventing cross-linking. Upon further dilution of the antiserum, the prozone effect is overcome and visible agglutination takes place. Agglutination does not require the presence of complement or other heat-labile serum factors. IgM antibodies appear to be more effective in agglutination than IgG antibodies.

When particulate substances coated with a soluble antigen are used as the source of antigen, the test is called passive agglutination. Common particles that serve as vehicles for soluble antigens are latex beads and red blood cells. Antigen attachment to the particles is by simple adsorption or by covalent linkage, using fixatives such as glutaraldehyde. A widely used method for attaching soluble antigens to red blood cells is through the treatment of the cells with dilute tannic acid. This treatment alters the cell surface in such a way that a number of different kinds of antigens bind firmly to the surface. The **passive hemagglutination test** is a relatively sensitive technique for measuring antibody, yielding titers 5 to 10 times higher than noted with conventional agglutination tests.

Some antigens are buried deep in the cell membrane so that antibody fails to agglutinate the particles. This is sometimes a major problem with red blood cell antigens. Further, univalent antibodies cannot be detected by routine agglutination tests, but they can be detected by the antiglobulin or **Coombs' test.** In this assay, red blood cells are first treated with the univalent antibody directed against

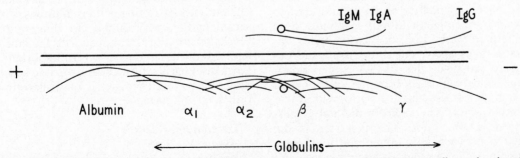

Figure 8–7. Diagrammatic representation of an immunoelectrophoretic pattern. In the upper well are placed purified preparations of human IgM, IgA, and IgG; in the lower well, whole human serum. Each protein on electrophoresis moves from the well according to its characteristic mobility under the conditions employed. After electrophoresis, antibody prepared against human serum is placed in the trough, and the pattern of precipitation between each protein and its specific antibody develops.

red cell antigens. In the second step, these globulin-coated cells are treated with an antibody against the globulin molecule. This second antibody causes agglutination by reacting with the IgG previously attached to the cell surface. The Coombs' test is used extensively for red blood cell typing, evaluation of hemolytic diseases, and diagnosis of autoimmune hemolytic anemia.

The agglutination method is routinely used in clinical laboratories to detect a group of antibodies, called cold agglutinins, that occur in the serum of patients with certain diseases, including hemolytic anemia, chronic lymphocytic leukemia, and certain infections such as infectious mononucleosis. These are monoclonal IgM antibodies that agglutinate homologous and heterologous red blood cells at 4°C. but not at 37°C. The antigenic specificity of cold agglutinins appears to be directed primarily against a red blood cell antigen, the I antigen, which is almost universally distributed. Cold agglutinins are present at low levels in the serum of most normal individuals, but are greatly elevated in patients with certain disease manifestations.

LABELED ANTIBODY ASSAYS

The use of antibodies labeled with specific markers has been extremely useful to detect antigens expressed in cells or components of soluble immune complexes. The most commonly used antibody marker is fluorescein isothiocyanate, which fluoresces when excited by ultraviolet light, making it possible to visualize the antigen-antibody complex by ultraviolet microscopy. This is termed **immunofluorescence.** In **radioimmune assays,** the antibody is labeled with radioactive substances, such as radioactive iodine (^{125}I or ^{131}I). Enzymes, *e.g.,* peroxidase or alkaline phosphatase, have recently been coupled to antibody and used to demonstrate antigen-antibody reactions; these are termed the **ELISA,** or **enzyme-linked immunosorbent assay**. All three assays are extremely sensitive; the ELISA and radioimmune assays can detect picogram quantities of protein. Each assay can be performed in two different ways. The **indirect method** is performed in two steps. The first step is the reaction between the antigen and its specific antibody, as in serological tests previously described, to form antigen-antibody complexes. In the second step, a second antibody, directed against the immunoglobulin component of the

immune complex, is labeled with one of the above markers and used to localize the antigen-antibody reaction. The second antibody is usually directed against the immunoglobulin isotype characteristic of the first antibody, *e.g.,* if the first antibody is of human origin, the second is an antihuman immunoglobulin. Thus, in the indirect test, the labeled second antibody reacts with the antibody component of the initial antigen-antibody reaction.

In contrast, the **direct test** is performed in one step. In this case, the specific label is coupled directly to the immunoglobulin fraction containing the antibody. This labeled antibody is then employed directly for detecting its specific antigen. The indirect technique has several advantages over the direct technique. The principal advantage is that one reagent can be used to detect a multitude of antigen-antibody reactions. The indirect technique is also more sensitive than the direct method, since several tagged anti-immunoglobulin molecules can react with a single antibody molecule. The direct method has an important advantage in that it can be readily used to screen large numbers of serums for antibody directed against a single antigenic determinant through **inhibition** or **blocking assays.** For example, if one has a labeled antibody directed against antigen A expressed on some cells and wishes to determine the frequency of antibody to this antigen in a specific disease population, this can be determined by first pretreating cells with the serum in question before reacting the cells with labeled antibody. If the pretreatment serum contains antibody to antigen A, it will react with this antigen on the target cells, thereby denying access to the labeled antibody. If the serum contains antibody directed against another antigen, the labeled antibody will still react with antigen A following the pretreatment step. It is also possible to determine the concentration, or inhibition titer, of this blocking antibody by testing various dilutions of the serum and identifying the last dilution that blocks reaction of the antigen with the labeled antibody. This approach is very important in those diseases in which antibody to one specific disease-associated antigen is of diagnostic or prognostic importance.

Immunofluorescence
Assay[3, 4, 11, 16, 25, 27, 38]

Immunofluorescence can be performed on fixed or viable cells. When viable cells are used, the antibody reaction is directed against membrane determinants, since antibody will

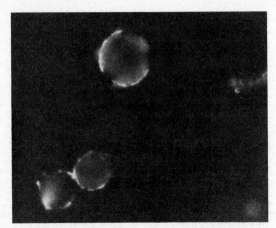

Figure 8–8. Demonstration of viral antigens in the membranes of viable cells infected with the Epstein-Barr virus by membrane immunofluorescence.

not penetrate intact membranes; these are **membrane immunofluorescence tests,** illustrated in Figure 8–8, and are commonly used to identify immunoglobulin-positive B lymphocytes.

Cytoplasmic or nuclear antigens can be identified if the cells are fixed to slides or coverslips with agents that disrupt the cell membrane, *e.g.,* acetone or methanol. This method is commonly used in clinical laboratories to detect antinuclear antibodies in the serum of patients with autoimmune diseases.

Careful control of experimental conditions is required when using immunofluorescence procedures. This is particularly true for the indirect test. When lymphoid cells are used as target cells, the anti-immunoglobulin reagent will react with immunoglobulin molecules in the membranes of such cells, as well as with the specific antibody used in the first step of the test. This sometimes causes great difficulty

in the interpretation of results. Similarly, when cells with Fc receptors are used as target cells, antibody can bind nonspecifically to such receptors through their Fc fragment, generating nonspecific fluorescence. This is a technical problem not only with lymphoid cells, but with cells infected with some herpesviruses and can result in false-positive reactions.

Some of these problems are minimized in the widely used **anticomplement immunofluorescence assay** (Fig. 8–9). Complement in the reaction mixture is fixed by some antigen-antibody reactions and is detected by an indicator system of fluorescein-conjugated antibodies to complement. This fluorescent antibody, therefore, reacts with the fixed complement components and not with the antibody itself. This assay is more sensitive than the routine immunofluorescent assays, possibly because complement contains a larger number of sites for binding the second antibody. For example, the nuclear antigen present in cells infected with the Epstein-Barr virus can be detected with the anticomplement, but not the anti-immunoglobulin immunofluorescence assay.

Radioimmune Assays[14, 17, 20, 29, 32]

As mentioned earlier, radioimmune assays employ radioactive markers coupled to antigen or antibody. The most common label is radioactive iodine coupled to protein through substitution of a hydrogen ion in the aromatic ring of tyrosine residues.

A number of different assays qualify as radioimmune assays. One method is to label antibody with ^{125}I or ^{131}I and to use such antibodies in indirect or direct tests against cell membrane antigens, as described above for the immunofluorescence test. The amount

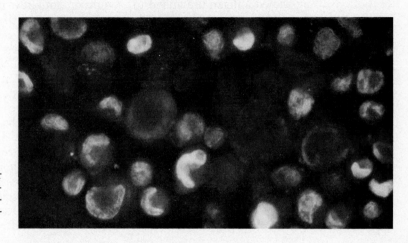

Figure 8–9. Detection of nuclear antigens in cells infected with cytomegalovirus using the anticomplement immunofluorescence procedure.

of antibody bound to the cells is an indicator of the antigen-antibody reaction and is measured by radioisotope counting methods. This assay has the same disadvantages enumerated for the immunofluorescent assays, but is more sensitive for detecting small amounts of antigen.

A more common application is to use purified antigen labeled with one of the radioactive substances. This assay requires highly specific antibody, purified antigen, and the necessary equipment for measuring radioactive substances. Its application is to detect low levels of antibody directed against a specific antigenic determinant or low levels of antigen by competition techniques.

Assays of this type depend upon the union of highly specific antibody with labeled purified antigen to produce immune complexes. These complexes must then be separated from the unbound labeled antigen. Several separation methods are used. In the Farr technique, the complexes are separated by precipitation with 50 per cent saturated ammonium sulfate, leaving free antigen in the supernatant. Alternatively, the complexes can be removed by reaction with a second antibody directed against the immunoglobulin in the immune complex. A third technique employs staphylococcal protein A to remove the complexes. Protein A possesses receptors for the Fc fragment of IgG molecules and readily binds antigen-antibody complexes. Thus, it is possible to determine the ratio of bound to free antigen for different concentrations of antigen in the presence of a constant amount of antibody.

Competition experiments to detect antigen in a test sample can be set by reacting the radiolabeled antigen with an antibody concentration that will precipitate about 70 per cent of the labeled antigen. Different known concentrations of unlabeled antigen are added to compete with the labeled antigen for antibody binding sites, thereby preventing or inhibiting precipitation. By determining the bound/free ratio of labeled antigen in the presence of different concentrations of unlabeled antigen, a standard curve can be constructed which is linear over a relatively limited range. Using this standard curve, the presence and concentration of the antigen in an unknown sample can be determined. This type of assay is routinely used in clinical endocrinology for measuring hormone levels; in cancer immunology for measuring tumor-associated antigens, such as carcinoembryonic antigen; and for measuring hepatitis antigen. A solid phase modifica-

tion, the **radioallergosorbent test** (RAST), has also been useful for detecting IgE antibodies to allergens.

ELISA Assay[1, 13]

The enzyme-linked antibody assay is one of the more recently developed methods for measuring antigen-antibody reactions. It can also be performed as a direct or indirect assay, depending on whether the enzyme (peroxidase, alkaline phosphatase) is conjugated to the primary or secondary antibody. It can be used with either cellular antigens or soluble antigens fixed to a plastic surface. Following attachment of the enzyme-labeled antibody to the specific antigen, an enzyme-specific substrate is added which undergoes a color change following enzymatic action. Thus, the antigen-antibody reaction may be measured photometrically. This is an easy assay, with sensitivity near that of radioimmune assays and can be readily used for large-scale screening often required in clinical laboratories.

ANTIBODY-MEDIATED CYTOTOXICITY[5, 19, 26, 36, 46]

Antibody to some cellular antigens is cytotoxic in the presence of either complement or certain types of lymphoid cells. Both IgG and IgM antibodies are capable of mediating these cytotoxic reactions. Damage to the cell membrane is monitored by the uptake of a strain, usually trypan blue, by damaged cells or through the release of radioactive level, such as sodium chromate (^{51}Cr), from such cells. Complement-dependent cytotoxic tests are used routinely in the clinical laboratory for tissue typing in transplantation programs.

A second type of cytotoxicity reaction requiring antibody is the **antibody-dependent cellular cytotoxicity reaction (ADCC).** It is mediated by the interaction of antibody to a membrane antigen and a lymphoid cell, designated killer (K) cell, bearing an Fc receptor. Antibody-coated cells are incubated for 3 to 4 hours with K cells and the resulting cytotoxicity measured by the release of ^{31}Cr from the labeled target cells. Antigen specificity is determined by the antibody, while the killing mechanism requires lymphoid cells; complement is not required. IgG is the principal antibody capable of mediating ADCC, although there is evidence that IgM antibodies can also trigger the reaction; IgA antibodies appear to be ineffective. This assay is a very efficient and sensitive method for measuring antibody activity. The significance of ADCC in immunity remains to be determined, although evidence indicates that ADCC is an active immunity mechanism against some virus-infected cells and, possibly, against some forms of cancer.

NEUTRALIZATION[30, 42]

Antibody directed against certain sites on an infectious agent, such as a virus, or on a toxin can block or neutralize activity of these agents. The infectivity of viruses is blocked by antiviral neutralizing antibodies directed against specific viral proteins. Not all antibodies against a virus can neutralize infectivity, but only those directed against certain virus antigens. Similarly, antibodies to specific determinants on a toxin molecule neutralize the toxic activity of that substance. These antibodies are very important in immunity to infectious disease.

Antibodies neutralizing virus infectivity can be demonstrated by a number of different methods. Neutralizing activity is shown by the capacity of virus-specific antibody to block or inhibit the viral cytopathic effect induced in a tissue culture system. Alternatively, neutralization can be shown in animals by pretreating virus with the antibody before inoculation. Effective antibody neutralization is indicated by protection from the specific virus disease. This reaction is very specific and does not necessarily require the participation of complement, although complement may enhance antibody neutralization of some viruses, such as the herpesviruses. Such antibodies are very useful for identifying viral isolates and for the diagnosis of viral infections. The mechanism of viral neutralization involves the inhibition of an early step in the virus replication cycle.

Neutralization is also applied to the detection of **antitoxins,** antibodies capable of neutralizing the effects of toxins produced by bacteria. Toxin is mixed with different dilutions of antitoxin and the mixtures injected into animals susceptible to the effects of the toxin. Generally, the titer of the antiserum is expressed as that amount of antibody required to protect 50 per cent of the animals from the lethal effects of the toxin, *i.e.,* LD_{50} (Chapter 12). The presence of antitoxins can also be demonstrated by skin tests. Intradermal injection of small quantities of a toxin, such as diphtheria toxin, into nonimmune individuals causes a localized erythematous reaction. This effect is neutralized if the individual is immune and contains antitoxins in the serum. This is the basis of the Dick test for showing immunity to diphtheria toxin.

Early in the study of toxin-antitoxin reactions, Danysz observed that toxin neutralization is greatly affected by the way in which the components are mixed. He found that a given amount of antitoxin would neutralize more toxin when added all at one time, as opposed to the addition of the same amount of toxin in increments. This is known as the **Danysz phenomenon** and is caused by the fact that antigen and antibody combine in multiple proportions. A multivalent antigen can, therefore, react with more antibodies than are needed for neutralization. Under these circumstances, a small amount of antigen can tie up a disproportionate share of antibody, leaving little free antibody available for neutralization of a second increment of toxin.

COMPLEMENT FIXATION[7, 45, 47]

The most widely used clinical test for measuring specific antigen-antibody reactions is the complement fixation test. Complement fixation is a sensitive method, detecting as little as 1 μg. of protein, and can be used with either particulate or soluble antigens. This test is limited, however, to those antibodies capable of fixing complement, primarily those of the IgG and IgM classes. Microcomplement fixation assays make possible the use of this test for large-scale screening.

The complement fixation test is performed by reacting an antigen with its antibody in the presence of an amount of complement sufficient to lyse 100 per cent of antibody-coated sheep red blood cells. In the presence of an antigen-antibody reaction, complement will be fixed by the original complexes, thereby reducing the amount of free complement remaining in the mixture. Therefore, when an indicator system of antibody-coated red blood cells is added, lysis will be less than 100 per cent. Fixation of C1 to C9 must occur to produce lysis of antibody-coated cells. To quantitate this test, lysis is usually measured by estimating the amount of the hemoglobin released from the sensitized red blood cells using spectrophotometric methods. Alternatively, the red blood cells can be labeled with ^{51}Cr before use in the test, lysis being measured by its release from lysed cells.

Before performing the complement fixation

assays, it is necessary to standardize all the reagents, including the antibody to sheep red blood cells called **hemolysin,** and complement, so that the reagents are present at optimal proportions to each other. The source of complement can be from a species differing from the antibody donor; rabbit, guinea pig, or human complement is normally used.

Standardization of complement involves the determination of the optimal amount of complement required to mediate lysis of a certain portion of the sensitized red blood cells. This is determined by testing different dilutions of the complement source in the presence of a standard concentration of red blood cells. This will result in an S-shaped curve. Since a linear relationship exists in the curve at around 50 per cent hemolysis, it is common to use this degree of hemolysis as an end point in the complement fixation reaction. In performing the test, it is first necessary to determine the dilution of complement that results in 50 per cent hemolysis, defined as one CH50 unit of complement. In most complement fixation assays, a minimum of two units are added to the mixtures. A serum titer is then calculated as the last dilution that will fix 50 per cent of the free complement.

A number of variables can cause difficulty in the interpretation of the complement fixation assay. Some antigen or antibody preparations have anticomplementary activity and can inactivate certain complement components by themselves. This is sometimes caused by the presence of antigen-antibody complexes in the serum or by aggregated immunoglobulins. Anticomplementary activity can result in false-positive results if not properly controlled.

Cellular Immune Reactions[6]

Cell-mediated immune responses to specific antigens are measured by a variety of *in vitro* techniques. These include cytotoxicity or growth inhibition assays against target cells expressing specific antigens; stimulation of DNA synthesis in lymphocytes following reexposure to an antigen; and the release of lymphokines following exposure of sensitized lymphocytes to the appropriate antigen. This latter technique is considered to be a good laboratory correlate of delayed hypersensitivity reactions. All of these assays are reliably used to demonstrate and measure specific cell-mediated immune reactions to different antigens.

LYMPHOCYTE CYTOTOXICITY[9, 24, 35, 37, 43]

This assay is used when the antigen is a membrane component of a cell, such as those responsible for the rejection of skin or tumor grafts. Cell membrane damage mediated by immune lymphocytes is measured either by using a dye, such as trypan blue, which will be taken up by cells with damaged membranes, or through the release of a radioactive chemical, such as sodium chromate, from cells previously labeled with the radioactive marker. Radioisotopes accumulate in the cytoplasm of living cells, but are released into the environment following damage to the cell membrane. Generally, an incubation period of 4 hours or longer is required to demonstrate cell-mediated cytotoxicity, as opposed to 1 to 2 hours required for antibody-complement mediated cytotoxicity. Over this incubation period, generally 1 to 2 per cent of the incorporated radioisotope will be released each hour, depending on the nature of the target cell. With some cells, the spontaneous release rate is even higher, thereby limiting the applicability of this method to those target cells that slowly release the radioactive substance. Typical results from this type of cytotoxicity assay are illustrated in Table 8–1.

Lymphocyte damage to cell membranes is also widely measured by the **colony inhibition assay.** It is normally used with tumor cell lines and measures inhibition of cell growth as determined by colony formation. Tumor cells will grow in a semisolid agar suspension or on a flat surface to produce visible colonies, each derived from a single cell. Normal lymphocytes do not form colonies under these circumstances. Therefore, it is possible to measure lymphocyte-mediated damage to different cells by the inhibition of colony formation either on a flat surface or in semisolid agar. Colony inhibition is most efficient with cell lines that have a high cloning efficiency; properly controlled, it can be employed to measure specific cell-mediated immune responses to viral, tumor, or different types of cellular antigens.

A variation of the colony inhibition assay is the **microcytotoxicity assay.** Small numbers of adherent target cells are seeded into wells in microtiter plates. After the cells have adhered to the surface of the wells, varying concentra-

Table 8–1. **Illustration of Cell-Mediated Immunity Based on
Release of Radioactive Substance**

Lymphocyte Donor	Target Cells	^{51}Chromium Released (Counts Per Minute)	Cytotoxicity*
None†	Tumor A	615	—
Immune to Tumor A	Tumor A	2400	31.3%
Immune to Tumor B	Tumor A	645	<1.0%
None	Tumor B	780	—
Immune to Tumor A	Tumor B	825	<1.0%
Immune to Tumor B	Tumor B	2750	29.3%

*Cytotoxicity calculated by dividing ^{51}chromium released in the presence of lymphocytes by total amount of ^{51}chromium incorporated by target cells after subtracting spontaneous release from each figure. Total ^{51}chromium incorporated by Tumor A was 6000 counts per minute and 7500 counts per minute for Tumor B.

†^{51}Chromium released over 4-hour period represents spontaneous release of radioisotope by target cells in the absence of lymphocytes.

tions of lymphocytes are added and the plates incubated for another 24 hours. The wells are then washed to remove dead cells and those remaining adherent to the wells are stained and counted. If the lymphocytes have mediated a cytotoxic effect, the number of target cells remaining will be significantly lower than the number present in control wells without added lymphocytes or in wells treated with nonimmune lymphocytes, as illustrated in Table 8–2. The advantage of this microassay is the small number of target cells and lymphocytes required, making it useful for large-scale screening. Direct contact between cells is required for cytotoxicity, although direct attachment may not be necessary. Kinetic studies have determined that one lymphocyte can attack more than one target cell. The exact mechanism of lymphocyte-mediated cytotoxicity remains unknown, although viable and metabolically active lymphocytes are required.

LYMPHOCYTE TRANSFORMATION[6]

Another experimental approach used extensively for measuring cellular immune responses to both cellular and soluble antigens is the lymphocyte transformation assay. This assay is made possible by the fact that resting or non-activated lymphocytes do not divide. Activated lymphocytes or those reexposed to a specific antigen are, however, stimulated to initiate DNA synthesis and to undergo mitosis. Morphologically, these cells change from small lymphocytes into large "blast-like" cells, changes that can be recognized and measured by histochemical staining. It is more common, however, to measure DNA synthesis as an indicator of the immune response to a specific antigen. This is accomplished by adding radioactive thymidine to a lymphocyte culture exposed to a specific antigen; thymidine is then incorporated into newly synthesized DNA. If the lymphocyte preparation is not activated following exposure to an antigen, DNA synthesis is not initiated and very little radioactive thymidine will be incorporated. However, if the lymphocytes are activated by exposure to an antigen, they rapidly incorporate measurable amounts of labeled thymidine into their DNA. This test has been employed as a measure of T cell immunity, since T lymphocytes are the cell type stimulated by second exposure to antigen.

A variation of this lymphocyte transformation assay, the **mixed leucocyte reaction** (MLR), is used to detect major or minor

Table 8–2. **Example of Cell-Mediated Immunity Using
Microcytotoxicity Assay**

Lymphocyte Donor	Target Cells	Viable Cells	% Reduction
None	Tumor A	235	—
Immune to Tumor A	Tumor A	15	93.6
Immune to Tumor B	Tumor A	240	0
None	Tumor B	285	—
Immune to Tumor A	Tumor B	280	0
Immune to Tumor B	Tumor B	12	95.8

histocompatibility differences between different cells. Peripheral lymphocytes from one individual are usually mixed with those of an unrelated individual. Generally, one of the lymphocyte preparations is rendered incapable of initiating DNA synthesis by irradiation or by treatment with mitomycin C; it is, therefore, possible to measure one responding lymphocyte population. The mixed culture is incubated for 5 to 7 days, followed by addition of radioactive thymidine to measure DNA synthesis or cell proliferation. The stimulation of DNA synthesis under these conditions occurs in the T lymphocytes and reflects the ability of these cells to recognize foreign histocompatibility antigens on the nonproliferating cell population. The MLR does not require prior sensitization and is believed to represent the initiation of an immune response to a foreign antigen. Cells activated in culture by this method are generally cytotoxic when added to new target cells expressing the same histocompatibility antigens present in the nonproliferating cells. This type of assay is used frequently in tumor immunology in efforts to detect the presence of new tumor-specific antigens in cancer cells (Chapter 10).

LYMPHOKINE ASSAYS[21, 33, 39–41, 44]

In addition to the above assays, T cell immunity can also be detected by measuring the release of different soluble factors, or lymphokines, following interaction of the cells with a specific antigen. A variety of lymphokines have been identified in the supernatants from antigen-exposed lymphocyte cultures; a current list of these is shown in Table 8–3. These include **chemotactic factors** that attract a variety of different cell types to the site of an immune reaction; **mitogenic factor,** released by sensitized T lymphocytes, which induces lymphocytes to proliferate; a factor that inhibits the adherence of leucocytes to a flat surface; **lymphotoxin,** which exerts a toxic effect on certain types of unrelated tumor cells; **inter-**

Table 8–3. **Major Lymphokines Released by Immune T Cells Following Reaction with Specific Antigens**

Macrophage migration
Chemotactic factors
Lymphotoxin
Mitogenic factor
Interferon
Leucocyte inhibitory factor

feron, the antiviral substance that also enhances the cytotoxic activity of NK cells; and **macrophage migration inhibitory factor** (MIF). This last substance is considered to be important in delayed hypersensitivity responses. It has been used more extensively than the other lympokines as an indicator of T cell immune response.

As early as 1932, it was observed that the migration of cells from spleen and lymph node explants from tuberculous guinea pigs was inhibited upon addition of tuberculin in the culture medium. Subsequent studies showed that if lymphoid cell preparations from immune guinea pigs were placed in capillary tubes bathed in fluid medium, the macrophages migrated from the tube. When tuberculin was added to the culture fluid, the macrophages failed to migrate. Further studies showed that this inhibitory effect on macrophage migration was mediated by supernatant fluids from cultures containing immune T cells along with the appropriate antigen, thereby establishing the soluble nature of MIF. It is now recognized that MIF is a product of T lymphocytes and that its production requires the interaction of immune T cells with specific antigen. This factor is present in culture fluids as early as 6 hours after exposure of the lymphocytes to a specific antigen and it continues to be produced over a period of 3 to 4 days. The production of MIF is a metabolically active process, blocked by inhibitors of RNA and protein synthesis. Once produced, MIF inhibits the migration of normal macrophages, as well as those from immune animals; *i.e.*, its action is nonspecific.

MIF is a heat-stable glycoprotein with a molecular weight between 20,000 and 60,000 daltons. It is susceptible to the action of proteolytic enzymes, such as trypsin and chymotrypsin; its glycoprotein nature is established by sensitivity to neuraminidase.

Routine laboratory assays for MIF employ two approaches. The first is the inhibition of normal macrophages from capillary tubes as discussed above and illustrated in Figure 8–10. The extent of migration can be accurately measured and a "migration index" calculated by comparing the migration of macrophages in the presence of a specific antigen to migration in its absence. A more recent technique replaces capillary tubes with agar droplets. Macrophages normally migrate from the agar but, as with the capillary tube technique, migration is inhibited in the presence of MIF.

T lymphocyte populations that produce MIF are present in peritoneal exudate, lymph

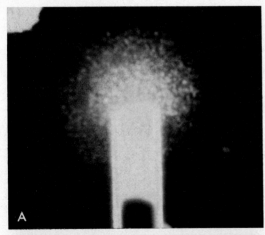

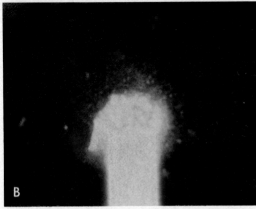

Figure 8–10. Demonstration of cell-mediated immunity to histoplasma with the capillary tube macrophage migration inhibition assay; migration of peripheral blood macrophages from an infected individual from a capillary tube in *(A)* the absence of histoplasmin and *(B)* in the presence of histoplasmin. Note the inhibition of macrophage migration in the presence of the sensitizing antigen. (Courtesy of Dr. H. Markowitz, Department of Laboratory Medicine, Mayo Foundation and Mayo Medical School, Rochester, Minn.)

nodes, peripheral blood, and spleen from sensitized animals. Generally, peripheral blood is used as the source of T cells in human studies that employ this assay to measure cellular immunity.

References

1. Avrameas, S. 1969. Coupling of enzymes to proteins with glutaraldehyde. Use of the conjugate for the detection of antigens and antibodies. Immunochemistry **6**:43–52.
2. Axelsen, N. H., J. Kroll, and B. Weeke (Eds.). 1973. A Manual of Quantitative Immunoelectrophoresis, Methods and Applications. pp. 37–46. Universitetsforlaget, Oslo.
3. Beutner, E. H. 1961. Immunofluorescent staining: the fluorescent antibody method. Bacteriol. Rev. **25**:49–76.
4. Beutner, E. H. 1971. Defined immunofluorescent staining. Ann. N.Y. Acad. Sci. **177**:5–529.
5. Biberfeld, P., *et al.* 1975. A plaque technique for assay and characterization of antibody-dependent cytotoxic effector (K) cells. Scand. J. Immunol. **4**:859–864.
6. Bloom, B. R., and J. R. David. 1976. In Vitro Methods in Cell-Mediated Immunity and Tumor Immunity. Academic Press, New York.
7. Boyd, W. C. 1966. Fundamentals of Immunology, 4th ed. Wiley-Interscience, New York.
8. Boyden, S. V. 1951. The adsorption of proteins on erythrocytes treated with tannic acid and subsequent hemagglutination by antiprotein sera. J. Exptl. Med. **93**:107–120.
9. Brunner, K. T., *et al.* 1968. Quantitative assay of the lytic action of immune lymphoid cells on ^{51}Cr-labelled allogeneic target cells *in vitro*: inhibition by isoantibody and drugs. Immunology **14**:181–196.
10. Cawley, L.-P. 1969. Electrophoresis and Immunoelectrophoresis. Little, Brown and Co., Boston.
11. Cherry, W. B., and M. D. Moody, 1965. Fluorescent antibody techniques in diagnostic bacteriology. Bacteriol. Rev. **29**:222–250.
12. Crowle, A. J. 1973. Immunodiffusion. Academic Press, New York.
13. Ervall, E., and P. Perlmann. 1971. Enzyme-linked immunosorbent assay (ELISA). Quantitative assay of immunoglobulin G. Immunochemistry **8**:871–874.
14. Gill, T. J., III. 1976. Principles of radioimmunoassay. pp. *In* N. R. Rose, and H. Friedman (Eds.): Manual of Clinical Immunology. American Society for Microbiology, Washington, D.C., pp. 169–171.
15. Goldberg, R. J. 1952. A theory of antibody-antigen reactions. I. Theory for reactions of multivalent antigen and bivalent and univalent antibody. J. Amer. Chem. Soc. **74**:5715–5725.
16. Goldwasser, R. A., and C. C. Shepard, 1958. Staining of complement and modification of fluorescent antibody procedures. J. Immunol. **80**:122–131.
17. Gorsky, Y., and D. Sulitzeanu, 1975. A radioactive antibody binding-inhibition assay for the detection of cell membrane related antigens in body fluids. J. Immunol. Methods **6**:291–300.
18. Grabar, P., and P. Burtin (Eds.). 1964. Immunoelectrophoresis Analysis. Elsevier, New York.
19. Harada, M., *et al.* 1973. Enhancement of normal lymphocyte cytotoxicity by sera with high antibody titers against H-2 or virus-associated antigens. Cancer Res. **33**:2886–2893.
20. Harder, F. H., and C. F. McKhann, 1968. Demonstration of cellular antigens on sarcoma cells by an indirect ^{125}I-labeled antibody technique. J. Natl. Cancer Inst. **40**:231–241.
21. Harrington, J. T., and P. Stastny, 1973. Macrophage migration from an agarose droplet: development of a microassay for assay of delayed hypersensitivity. J. Immunol. **110**:752–759.
22. Heidelberger, M. 1939. Quantitative absolute methods in the study of antigen-antibody reactions. Bacteriol. Rev. **3**:49–95.
23. Heidelberger, M., and F. E. Kendall, 1935. Precipitin reaction between type III pneumococcus polysaccharides and homologous antibody; quantitative study and theory of reaction mechanisms. J. Exptl. Med. **61**:563–591.
24. Hellström, I., *et al.* 1971. Demonstration of cell-

mediated immunity to human neoplasms of various histological types. Int. J. Cancer **7**:1–16.

25. Hinuma, Y., *et al.* 1962. Evaluation of the complement method of fluorescent antibody technique with myxoviruses. J. Immunol. **89**:19–26.

26. Humphrey, J. H., and R. R. Dourmashkin. 1969. Lesions in cell membranes caused by complement. Adv. Immunol. **11**:75–115.

27. Klein, G., *et al.* 1967. Membrane immunofluorescence reactions of Burkitt lymphoma cells from biopsy specimens and tissue cultures. J. Natl. Cancer Inst. **39**:1027–1044.

28. Laurell, C. B. 1966. Quantitative estimation of proteins by electrophoresis in agarose gel containing antibodies. Anal. Chem. **15**:45–52.

29. Lucas, Z. 1970. An assay for antibodies to histocompatibility antigens based on inhibition of radioiodine-labeled antibody binding. Transplantation **10**:512–521.

30. Mandel, B. 1960. Neutralization of viral infectivity: characterization of the virus-antibody complex including association, dissociation and host-cell interactions. Ann. N.Y. Acad. Sci. **83**:515–527.

31. Mancini, G., A.-O. Carbonara, and J. F. Heremans. 1965. Immunochemical quantitation of antigens by single radial immunodiffusion. Immunochemistry **2**:235–254.

32. Marchalonis, J. J. 1969. An enzymatic method for the trace iodination of immunoglobulins and other proteins. Biochem. J. **113**:299–305.

33. McCoy, J. L., J. H. Dean, and R. B. Herberman. 1977. Human cell-mediated immunity to tuberculin as assayed by the agarose micro-droplet leucocyte migration inhibition technique: comparison with the capillary tube assay. J. Immunol. Methods **15**:355–371.

34. Ouchterlony, O. 1968. Handbook of Immunodiffusion and Immunoelectrophoresis. Ann Arbor Science Publishers, Ann Arbor, Mich.

35. Pearson, G. R., R. J. Hodes, and S. Friberg, 1969. Cytotoxic potential of different lymphoid cell populations against chromium-51 labelled tumour cells. Clin. Exptl. Immunol. **3**:273–284.

36. Perlmann, P. 1976. Cellular immunity: antibody-dependent cytotoxicity (K cell activity), pp. 107–132. *In* F. H. Bach, and R. A. Good (Eds.): Clinical Immunology III. Academic Press, New York.

37. Perlmann, P., and G. Holm. 1969. Cytotoxic effect of lymphoid cells. Adv. Immunol. **11**:117–181.

38. Riggs, J. L., *et al.* 1958. Isothiocyanate compounds as fluorescent labeling agents for immune serum. Amer. J. Pathol. **34**:1081–1097.

39. Rocklin, R. 1974. Products of activated lymphocytes: leucocyte inhibitory factor (LIF) distinct from migration inhibitory factor. J. Immunol. **112**:1461–1466.

40. Rocklin, R. E., O. L. Meyers, and J. R. David. 1970. An *in vitro* assay for delayed hypersensitivity in man. J. Immunol. **104**:95–102.

41. Rosenberg, S. A., and J. R. David. 1970. Inhibition of leucocyte migration: an evaluation of this *in vitro* assay of delayed hypersensitivity in man to a soluble antigen. J. Immunol. **105**:1447–1452.

42. Svehag, S. E. 1968. Formation and dissociation of virus antibody complexes with special reference to the neutralization process. Prog. Med. Virol. **10**:1–63.

43. Takasugi, M., and E. Klein. 1970. A microassay for cell-mediated immunity. Transplantation **9**:219–227.

44. Thor, D., and S. Dray. 1968. A correlate of human delayed hypersensitivity: specific inhibition of capillary tube migration of sensitized human lymph node cells by tuberculin and histoplasmin. J. Immunol. **101**:51–61.

45. Weir, D. M. 1963. Antigen-antibody reactions. Mod. Trends Immunol. **2**:28–62.

46. Wigzell, H. 1965. Quantitative titrations of mouse H-2 antibodies using ^{51}Cr-labelled target cells. Transplantation **3**:423–431.

47. Williams, C. A., and M. W. Chase (Eds.). 1971. Methods in Immunology and Immunochemistry, Vol. 3. Academic Press, New York.

48. Vaerman, J. P., *et al.* 1969. Further studies on single radial immunodiffusion. I. Direct proportionality between area of precipitate and reciprocal of antibody concentration. Immunochemistry **6**:279–293.

9

Immunogenetics and Cellular Regulation of the Immune Response

Gary R. Pearson, Ph.D.

IMMUNOGENETICS[3–5, 11, 18–25, 31, 38]

The immune response to different antigens is governed by a set of genes located in or in close proximity to what has been described as the **major histocompatibility complex** (MHC). The MHC is a cluster of genes in higher vertebrates responsible for the synthesis of cell-surface antigens involved in the rejection of skin or other tissue grafts between two genetically distinct individuals of the same or different species. Until recently, the products of this genetic locus were of principal interest because of their role in the immunological rejection of transplanted tissue. Less attention was focused on genetic control, or regulation, of the immune response. Over the past 20 years, however, studies using genetically defined strains of animals and a variety of antigens have resulted in the identification of a set of **immune response** (Ir) genes that control immunological phenomena ranging from immune recognition to the formation of specific antibody. It has been demonstrated conclusively that these genes are located in the major MHC locus in a variety of species, including humans, and that these genes regulate the immune response to thymus-dependent anti-gens. The MHC-associated Ir genes are referred to as **regulatory** genes to distinguish them from the **structural** genes responsible for both the synthesis of antibody chains and the generation of antibody diversity. Current evidence suggests that these Ir genes function either by controlling the repertoires of T cell receptors or by controlling antigen presentation to T cells.

The existence of genetic control mechanisms for immune responses was first demonstrated in 1933 by Webster who showed, by genetic selection, that there were both good and poor antibody responders to diphtheria toxoid. The first definitive evidence showing that animals differ in their ability to respond to different antigens and that these differences are inherited according to Mendelian genetics came in 1963. Using randomly bred guinea pigs, Levine and Benacerraf showed that some animals produced specific antibodies and developed delayed hypersensitivity when immunized with the hapten 2,4-dinitrophenol conjugated to poly-L-lysine (DNP–PLL), while others were nonresponders. Crossbreeding experiments showed that the capacity to respond to this conjugate was controlled by a single dominant gene. It was subsequently shown that nonresponder animals could produce anti-DNP antibodies when the DNP–PLL conjugate was coupled to another carrier, such as bovine serum albumin. Thus, the defect in nonresponder animals was not due to the inability of the animal to produce anti-DNP antibodies, but was apparently at the antigen recognition stage and was related to the inability of T lymphocytes to recognize the carrier, PLL, as an immunogen.

Similar findings were reported in the mouse by McDevitt and Sela in 1969 while examining the immune response to a polypeptide composed of lateral chains of poly-DL alanine bound onto ε-amino groups of a long poly-L-lysine chain. Some strains of mice responded well to this synthetic polymer, while others were nonresponsive. Breeding experiments using genetically defined inbred strains of mice differing only at the MHC locus established that there was a close association between the ability of a mouse to respond immunologically to this antigen and its MHC type. Experiments of this kind revealed the existence of Ir genes in different species, closely linked to the MHC locus.

This chapter will focus on current knowledge of the genetic control of the immune response, including the cellular interactions required for the initiation and regulation of the immune response, and the genetic basis for antibody diversity. However, before discussing these topics, it is first necessary to describe the MHC in which Ir genes reside.

Major Histocompatibility Complex

H-2 COMPLEX[9, 20, 24, 34, 36]

The structural antigens responsible for inducing the rejection of tissues in genetically nonidentical individuals are termed **transplantation antigens.** In the mouse, the genes responsible for the expression of these antigens were designated by Snell and associated as **histocompatibility genes** (H-2) and were assigned to the IX linkage group on the basis of their association with the fused tail gene. This is the major histocompatibility locus in the mouse and consists of a series of genes. It is, therefore, generally referred to as the **H-2 complex.** Originally, immunologists were interested in the H-2 complex primarily because of its involvement in the expression of the major transplantation antigens. However, with progress in the characterization and definition of the gene products of this locus, it became apparent that the genes in this locus also controlled a remarkable array of immunological functions. Some of these are listed in Table 9–1 and are of great importance in regulating immune responses at several levels.

The identification and characterization of the major histocompatibility locus in the mouse was dependent on the development of genetically defined inbred strains of mice. These were developed by Snell and associates using various combinations of inbreeding and selection. Inbred strains are produced by brother-sister mating for at least 20 generations, with the result that nearly 99 per cent of the gene pairs (alleles) are homozygous.

With mice, this can be accomplished in a few years and has resulted in the production of several hundred inbred strains of mice. These mice will accept skin grafts from members of the same strain, but will reject grafts from other inbred strains. The production and utilization of such inbred strains of mice was critical for demonstrating existence of a major histocompatibility system controlling graft rejection and the location of responsible genes on the chromosome 17.

A further advance, accelerating the definition of the H-2 gene complex, was the development of congenic strains of mice. These were inbred in such a way that they differed only at the H-2 locus. The advantage of such strains is that the functions of single gene loci and their multiple alleles can be evaluated on an otherwise identical genetic background. Studies with congenic strains established that there are multiple alleles for each H-2 locus and that each allele controls the expression of

Table 9–1. **Different Immune Functions Associated With The Major Histocompatibility Complex**

Graft rejection
Graft versus host disease
Cellular interactions in antibody synthesis
Immune responses to specific antigens
Cytotoxic reactions against virus-infected and tumor cells
Mixed lymphocyte reaction
Levels of some complement components
Susceptibility to some autoimmune diseases

several antigens identifiable with appropriate antiserums. The H-2 phenotypes previously recognized as alleles have recently been designed **H-2 haplotypes.** Some H-2 specificities are limited to an independent haplotype and are termed **private,** while others exhibit cross-reactivity with several haplotypes and are, therefore, **public.** Private H-2 specificities are controlled by three closely linked loci designated H-2K, H-2D, and H-2L. Genes of each locus control the production of separate molecules, as shown by the independent antibody-induced capping of antigens encoded by the different genes, *e.g.,* H-2K antigens are capped by antibody to H-2K antigens, but not by antibodies to H-2D and vice versa. Therefore, each haplotype bears an H-2K, an H-2D, and H-2L allele; each allele is characterized by a particular antigenic specificity. In addition, it has been shown that differences at both D and K can lead to skin graft rejection. Histocompatibility antigens are controlled by codominant alleles. This has been shown by the fact that skin grafts from an F_1 hybrid, produced from a cross between members of two different strains, will be rejected by both parents. If some H-2 genes were recessive, their antigenic products would not be expressed in the F_1 hybrid and, therefore, the skin graft would be accepted by the appropriate parent. Minor histocompatibility systems exist which can provoke weak immunity to grafted tissue. These have been identified by skin grafting experiments between strains of mice identical at the major H-2 loci.

The gene products of H-2K and H-2D have been purified and are transmembrane, hydrophobic glycoproteins with molecular weights of approximately 45,000. They are associated in the membrane with a β_2 microglobulin with a molecular weight of 12,000, encoded by a gene not linked to the histocompatibility complex. A schematic model of this glycoprotein is shown in Figure 9–1. Besides serving as the major transplantation antigens, these antigens are believed to participate in the production of cytotoxic T lymphocytes. They also play a particularly important role in cytotoxic reactions directed against viral or tumor-associated antigens (Chapter 10).

A fourth region located in the major MHC complex is identified as the **I region** and contains the immune response or Ir genes. A number of loci, I–A, I–B, I–J, I–E, and I–C, have been identified in the I region of the MHC. The products of the I region have been designated **Ia antigens.** These membrane-associated antigens were detected by the use

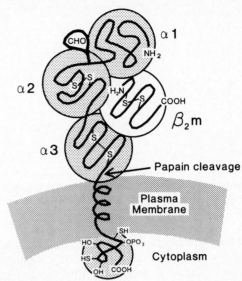

Figure 9–1. Schematic representation of the gene products of the H-2K and H-2D regions of the H-2 complex, which are composed of a 45,000 dalton glycoprotein associated with a β_2 microglobulin (β_2m) with a molecular weight of 12,000 daltons. α_1, α_2, and α_3 represent three domains identified on the 45,000 dalton glycoprotein. (Courtesy of Dr. Chella David, Department of Immunology, Mayo Foundation and Mayo Medical School, Rochester, Minn.)

of antiserums directed against I region incompatibilities between different congenic strains of mice and most of them mapped to the I–A subregion. The antigens are composed of two subunits, α and β chains, with respective molecular weights of 35,000 and 28,000; these are not covalently linked or associated with β_2 microglobulin (Fig. 9–2). Ia antigens are expressed in the membranes of most mature B cells, on macrophages, and on some T lymphocytes, in contrast to the antigens coded for by the H-2D and H-2K regions, which are distributed on most cell types. These antigens have also been detected on spermatozoa and

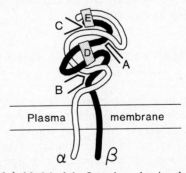

Figure 9–2. Model of the Ia antigen showing the location of five potential immunological interaction sites *(A–E)* on the two subunits (α,β) that compose this antigen. (Courtesy of Dr. David McKean, Department of Immunology, Mayo Foundation and Mayo Medical School, Rochester, Minn.)

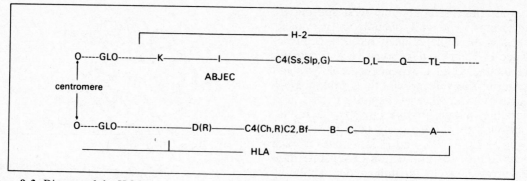

Figure 9–3. Diagram of the H-2 locus in the mouse and the human leucocyte antigen (HLA) locus in humans. (M. J. Owen and M. J. Crumpton, Immunol. Today **1**:117–122, 1980; reproduced with permission of Elsevier Biomedical Press B. V., Amsterdam.)

epidermal cells. Ia antigens play an important role in the initiation of antibody synthesis against thymus-dependent antigens (see below). Ia antigens are also important in the initiation of the mixed lymphocyte reactions (Chapter 8).

In addition to the four regions discussed above, a fifth region, S, has also been mapped in the H-2 region by recombinant experiments and is responsible for the synthesis of the C4 component of complement. This region maps between the I and D regions, so that the order of these regions (from left to right from the centromere) on chromosome 17 is K, I, S, D, L (Fig. 9–3).

In summary, the major histocompatibility region, or H-2 locus, in the mouse is responsible for the antigens involved in transplantation immunity. The genes in this region also control a large array of biological phenomena, including the ability to respond to a specific antigenic stimulus. The glycoproteins expressed by the genes in this complex are membrane associated and, therefore, are important antigens in the regulation of different phases of the immune recognition of thymus-dependent antigens (see below).

HUMAN LEUCOCYTE ANTIGEN COMPLEX[1, 37, 39, 41, 44]

The human counterpart of the H-2 system in the mouse is the human leucocyte antigen complex or HLA. As is true for H-2, HLA antigens function in the regulation of immune responses to thymus-dependent antigens, as well as serving as the major target antigens for graft rejection. The HLA loci have been mapped to the short arm of chromosome 6, which also contains the genes that control levels of the C2 and C4 components of com-

plement, erythrocyte glyco-oxidase, and phosphoglucomutase-3. These genes have been mapped in close proximity to the HLA complex by hybridization (Fig. 9–3).

HLA antigens have been identified mainly by testing serums from multiparous women, which commonly contain antibodies to the father's HLA antigens, and from individuals who have received multiple blood transfusions for antibodies reactive with peripheral blood lymphocytes from different donors. This has resulted in the identification of antibodies reactive with an array of antigenic specificities linked to the HLA loci. Results from studies on families with these antibodies established the existence of four genetic loci designated HLA–A, HLA–B, HLA–C, and HLA–D, inherited as codominant Mendelian tracts (Fig. 9–3). Multiple alleles exist for each locus and each allele can control the expression of an antigenic product. The HLA–A and HLA–B antigens have been purified and, like the mouse H-2 antigens, are membrane glycoproteins with molecular weights of approximately 45,000, and are associated with a β_2 microglobulin of approximately 12,000 daltons.

Antigens associated with the HLA–A, HLA–B, and HLA–C loci are generally detected using cytotoxicity assays mediated by antibody and complement, and are therefore called **serologically determined** antigens. These antigens are expressed on most cells and appear to be equivalent in function to the H-2K and H-2D antigens of the mouse. In contrast, the HLA–D–associated antigens are only recognized by the ability of lymphocytes from one individual to stimulate the lymphocytes of a second individual in the mixed leucocyte culture reaction (Chapter 8) and are not detected with antibody. These are, therefore, **lymphocyte-determined antigens.** Antigens controlled by a locus close to HLA–D have been identified on B lymphocytes by repeatedly absorbing serums from multiparous women with platelets to remove antibodies to HLA–A, HLA–B, and HLA–C antigens. Many serums still contain antibodies reactive with B lymphocytes and some macrophages as well as against epidermal cells and spermatozoa. This distribution is similar to that noted with mouse Ia antigens, suggesting that these antigens are the products of human Ir-like genes. The B cell antigens detected in this way are **D-related** (DR) antigens. Absorbed antiserums also frequently inhibit the mixed leucocyte culture reaction, however, suggesting that the HLA–D and HLA–DR loci are the same, but the issue is not resolved. Similarities in the properties of the DR antigen in human versus Ia antigens in the mouse indicate very strongly that the HLA–DR locus contains the human Ir genes.

Cellular Interactions in the Immune Response[2, 3, 5, 7, 18, 26, 30, 38]

The initiation of antibody synthesis involves a complicated interaction between the different cellular elements of the immune system and is under strict genetic control. The exact mechanisms are still largely unknown, although there has been extensive progress over the past few years in defining specific cell-to-cell interactions that appear to be critical for the initiation of antibody synthesis and in determining the regulatory role of Ir genes. The initiation of antibody synthesis to many antigens requires the active participation of macrophages and T cells working in concert with B cells. Animals in which T cells have been eliminated by neonatal thymectomy, by cytotoxic antibodies to T cells, or by the administration of cytotoxic drugs, generally are poor antibody producers when exposed to antigenic stimuli.

Conclusive proof for the requirement for both thymus and bone marrow cells for optimal antibody synthesis to sheep red blood cells was provided by Claman and co-workers in 1966. Lethally irradiated mice were reconstituted with thymus or bone marrow cells or with a mixture containing both. These mice were then immunized with sheep red blood cells and monitored for antibody production. Only mice that had received both types of lymphocytes produced specific antibody, leading to the postulate, later substantiated, that bone marrow contained the antibody precursor cells, while the thymus provided helper cells.

In contrast, thymus-independent antigens (Chapter 7) can provoke an antibody response in the absence of T cells. This category of antigens is small in comparison to the thymus-dependent group and includes mainly polysaccharide antigens with repeating subunits, such as those from pneumococcus. These antigens are comparatively weak and provoke only an IgM antibody response as opposed to thymus-dependent antigens that induce antibody formation in all of the different immunoglobulin classes. Thymus-independent antigens can apparently interact directly with immunoglobulin receptors present on B cells, triggering their differentiation into antibody-secreting plasma cells. The effectiveness of such antigens is thought to be related to their repeated polymeric structure, a common feature of such molecules, which allows for cross-linking between immunoglobulin receptors. This cross-linking event is considered necessary for B cell activation and differentiation. Most of the thymus-independent antigens also exert a mitogenic effect on B cells; it has been postulated that the proliferation and differentiation of B lymphocytes is triggered by the mitogenic activity of the antigen following attachment to the immunoglobulin receptors.

Most research on the regulation of antibody synthesis has concentrated on defining the sequence of steps that occur in the initiation of antibody synthesis to thymus-dependent antigens and the corresponding regulatory events. Such studies have utilized antigens with a restricted number of antigenic determinants in order to minimize the heterogeneity of the immune response. These studies have established that the initiation of antibody synthesis to a specific antigen depends on a critical interrelationship between an antigen-presenting cell, which appears to be the macrophage, and T lymphocytes; the key factors in this regulation are the products of the I region of the major histocompatibility gene complex.

GENETIC REGULATION OF MACROPHAGE–T CELL INTERACTIONS[3, 29, 33, 35, 40, 42, 43]

Cell culture systems have proved to be a useful tool for demonstrating the interaction of macrophages with lymphocytes in the in-

Table 9–2. *In Vitro* Induction of Antibody Synthesis to BSA as Determined by the Incorporation of Radioactive Thymidine

Lymphocyte Donor*	Antigen†	Counts per Minute‡
BSA-immune	none	2,300
Nonimmune	none	3,150
BSA-immune	BSA	75,000
Nonimmune	BSA	3,300
BSA-immune	Hemocyanin	2,500
Nonimmune	Hemocyanin	3,100

*Spleen cells from mice immunized with BSA or from nonimmune animals.

†Spleen cells exposed in cell culture to BSA or a nonrelated antigen (hemocyanin).

‡Cultures exposed 5 days to antigen and then labeled with radioactive thymidine. Counts incorporated above background (determined by incorporation in the absence of antigen) are indicators of immune response to specific antigen.

duction of antibody synthesis. Antibody synthesis is initiated when T cells proliferate in response to antigenic stimulation. Stimulation in this manner can be measured by incorporation of radioactive thymidine. That this is a specific response to the immunizing antigen is shown by the absence of proliferation when cells are exposed to unrelated antigens. Table 9–2 illustrates these responses.

It is possible, therefore, to examine the responses of different lymphoid cell preparations following depletion of specific cell types. For example, mononuclear cell populations can be depleted of macrophages by allowing the latter to adhere to glass surfaces. Alternatively, macrophages may be allowed to phagocytize iron particles, which then permits their removal by passage through a magnetic field. Depletion of macrophages from the mononuclear cell populations abolishes the ability of these cell preparations to respond to the immunizing antigen. The macrophage is, therefore, essential to the initiation of antigen-induced proliferation of T lymphocytes. Similar results are noted with cell transfer experiments into lethally irradiated animals. Antibody responses in such animals can only be

induced when macrophages are present in the transferred lymphoid population. The response of macrophage-depleted populations to antigen can be reconstituted by the addition of normal macrophages, demonstrating their important role in antibody synthesis. T lymphocytes are activated to initiate antibody synthesis in the absence of antigen, provided the macrophages have been exposed briefly to the antigen. This suggests that the macrophage functions as an antigen-presenting cell (APC). Further, the macrophage is probably essential in the role of an antigen-presenting cell for the initiation of antigen-induced T cell proliferation in cell cultures. This is shown schematically in Figure 9–4.

Two additional important features of macrophage–T lymphocyte interactions have been defined. The proliferating T cell and macrophage must express the same histocompatibility antigens and the macrophage must express the major I region–associated antigens (Ia antigens) of that species.

The requirements for histocompatibility between the interacting cell types was first noted by Rosenthal and Shevach in 1973. T lymphocyte cell cultures were derived from two guinea pig strains, 13 and 2, which differ only at the I region of the MHC. Macrophages from either strain were primed with antigen and added to the cell cultures that had been depleted of macrophages. Following this exposure, the cultures were examined for evidence of antigen-induced T cell proliferation. T cells from strain 2 guinea pigs responded to antigen-primed macrophages from strain 2 or from the F_1 hybrid (2×13), but did not respond to antigen presented by strain 13 macrophages, and vice versa (Table 9–3). In addition, antibodies prepared against the appropriate MHC gene products (anti-2 or anti-13) blocked the appropriate antigen-induced proliferation, *i.e.*, anti-2 blocked T cell proliferation induced by strain 2 macrophages but not by strain 13, and vice versa. Similar studies in mice have yielded the same results. In mice, the important cellular antigens in this macrophage–T cell interaction

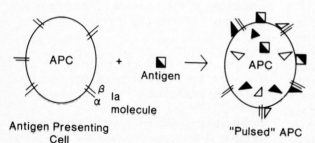

Figure 9–4. Schematic model showing the proposed uptake and processing of antigen by an antigen presenting cell *(APC)*, presumably the macrophage, in the initiation of antibody synthesis; α,β represent chains of Ia molecule. (Courtesy of Dr. David McKean, Department of Immunology, Mayo Foundation and Mayo Medical School, Rochester, Minn.)

Table 9–3. **Requirement for I Region Histocompatibility between T Cells and Macrophages in Antibody Synthesis**

T Cell Donor*	Macrophage Donor†	Immune Reaction
Strain 2	Strain 2	+
Strain 2	Strain 13	−
Strain 2	F₁ Hybrid(2 × 13)	+
Strain 13	Strain 2	−
Strain 13	Strain 13	+
Strain 13	F₁ Hybrid(2 × 13)	+

*Strain 2 and Strain 13 guinea pigs differ at I region only.

†Macrophages are exposed to antigen and then mixed with purified T cells and cultures monitored for antibody production.

map in the I–A subregion of the H-2 complex. Further, the activation of immune T cells by antigen-primed macrophages is dependent on the interaction of cell-surface structures encoded by genes in the I region of the MHC. Similar studies in humans have linked gene products of the DR region of the HLA complex with this function.

The activation and proliferation of T cells in this interaction requires the participation of soluble factors released by the respective cell types. One of these factors released by macrophages following stimulation by specific antigens, by different lectins, or by other stimulating agents, such as adjuvants, is the **lymphocyte-activating factor,** recently termed **interleukin 1.** This factor exerts its effects on the immune response by attaching to T lymphocytes through specific receptors, causing these cells to differentiate and produce a second factor—**T cell growth factor,** or **interleukin 2.** This latter factor stimulates proliferation of activated T helper cells (T_H cells) by binding to specific receptors and, in fact, is required for the continued proliferation of these cells *in vitro.* The production of these soluble factors

is essential for the initiation of the cellular events required for antibody synthesis.

In summary, experiments on macrophage–T cell cooperation in the initiation of antibody synthesis have provided evidence that (1) T_H cells require macrophages for proliferation in culture following antigen stimulation; (2) macrophages appear to be essential as antigen-presenting cells in the induction of antibody to T-dependent antigens (although there is still some controversy concerning this point); (3) the I region of the MHC regulates the interaction between T_H cells and macrophages; (4) macrophages must express in their cell membrane the gene product (Ia antigen) of the I region in order to interact with T_H cells; (5) T cells must possess two receptors for reacting with the macrophage-processed antigen, one for the antigenic determinant and a second receptor for the appropriate I gene product; and (6) soluble factors released by both macrophages and T lymphocytes participate in the initiation of antibody production to a specific antigen. A hypothetical scheme showing these interactions is shown in Figure 9–5.

INTERACTIONS BETWEEN B AND T CELLS[3, 12, 17, 28]

The I region of MHC also controls specific interactions between B and T cells. This has been determined by examining the antibody responses to haptens in irradiated animals reconstituted with antigen-activated T_H cells and antigen-primed splenic B cells. Following challenge of such animals with the appropriate antigen, antibody production to this antigen occurs only when the transferred T_H and B cells share the same histocompatibility antigens. No antibody is produced when the two cell populations are incompatible. Using appropriate congenic strains of mice, compatibil-

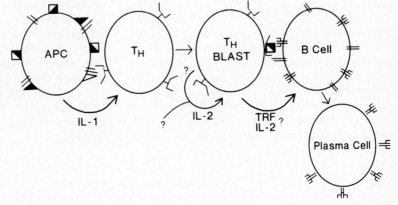

Figure 9–5. Schematic presentation of the cellular interactions that occur in the development of an immune response to an antigen. *APC,* antigen presenting cell; $T_H,$ helper T cell; *IL–1,* interleukin 1; *IL–2,* interleukin 2; *TRF,* T cell replacing factor. (Courtesy of Dr. David McKean, Department of Immunology, Mayo Foundation and Mayo Medical School, Rochester, Minn.)

ity at the I region has been found necessary for this T–B cell interaction. T_H clones, activated by the macrophage-processed antigen and which now possess the macrophage Ia antigen, can interact with B lymphocytes that bear the same Ia antigen, activating these lymphocytes into antibody-producing plasma cells (Fig. 9–5). It has been postulated that the processed antigen can recognize immunoglobulin receptors associated with the appropriate Ia antigen on B lymphocytes; antigen could then attach to the receptors, forming a bridge between the two cell types. However, current evidence suggests that the mechanism of B cell activation is probably more complex. It is also possible that soluble substances, carrying I-dependent antigen-specific factors, are released by activated T_H cells and promote B cell differentiation. One of these factors has been designated T cell replacing factor, since it can replace T_H cells in the activation of B lymphocytes. This is still an unsettled issue and the precise mechanism signaling the B lymphocyte to differentiate into an antibody-producing plasma cell still needs to be unraveled. It is apparent that simple binding of an antigen to the surface receptors of B lymphocytes is not an adequate stimulus to initiate B cell differentiation in most instances.

INDUCTION OF SUPPRESSOR T LYMPHOCYTES[10]

In addition to the activation of T_H cells by macrophage-processed antigen, a second population of T lymphocytes, called **suppressor T** (T_S) cells, defined in Chapter 7, can also be activated by antigen during the initiation of antibody synthesis. Such suppressor cells have an antigen-specific inhibitory effect on both T and B cell functions, and it is likely that several different classes of suppressor cells exist. Recognition of antigen by T_S cells seems not to be MHC-restricted, as is true for T_H cells, but this has not been completely resolved. Suppressor cells are considered to be important regulatory cells for controlling the initiation and levels of antibody synthesis. It is likely that these cells also participate in autoimmunity, in graft or tumor rejection, and in immunological tolerance, as discussed in the following two chapters. Genetic studies have shown that the production of suppressor cells is under the control

of the I–J region, located between I–B and I–C regions. These cells release a soluble factor capable of suppressing or controlling antibody synthesis, possibly by interfering with specific T_H cells; this factor is encoded by genes in the I–J region and has been partially purified. It has a molecular weight of approximately 70,000 daltons and is retained in columns coated with specific antigen, but not with immunoglobulin, suggesting that it is a protein with antigen-binding sites.

GENETIC CONTROL OF CYTOTOXIC LYMPHOCYTES[8, 45, 46]

The activity of cytotoxic T lymphocytes (T_C) or killer T (T_K) cells against virus-infected or tumor cells is also restricted by gene products of MHC. This was first described by Zinkernagel and Doherty as a result of studies of T cell immunity to mouse cells infected with lymphocytic choriomeningitis (LCM) virus. T_C lymphocytes isolated from immune animals lyse cells infected with LCM if the target cells express the same major histocompatibility antigens as the lymphocytes. Infected cells expressing unrelated MHC antigens are not lysed by these immune lymphocytes. This phenomenon occurs with a variety of viruses, such as the human herpesviruses, influenza virus, and measles virus. Tumor cells induced by different oncogenic viruses also show the same MHC restriction in regard to cytotoxic T lymphocytes. It is now generally accepted that this restriction is universal for virus-infected cells. Cytotoxic T lymphocytes must, therefore, recognize the foreign antigen plus a product of the MHC before exerting their cytotoxic effect. In contrast to the initiation of antibody responses against thymus-dependent antigens, genetic studies have established that the products of H-2K and H-2D in the mouse and of HLA–A and HLA–B in the human, are responsible for this MHC restriction. Presumably, virus-induced antigens inserted into the cell membrane form complexes with the products of these MHC loci, creating the structure recognized by the cytotoxic T lymphocytes. Whether these cytotoxic lymphocytes express one receptor site that recognizes the complex or two receptors, one for the new antigen and one for the MHC product, has not been resolved.

Clonal Selection and Other Theories for Antibody Production[6, 13, 16, 27, 32]

The mechanisms by which antibodies are generated still remains a largely unresolved question in immunology. Over the years a number of theories on antibody synthesis have been proposed, but none of them have provided completely for all known immunological phenomena, including specificity, diversity, and immunological memory. These theories have commonly been placed into two groups—**instructive** and **selective.**

The first modern theory on antibody production was proposed by Ehrlich in 1900 and essentially forms the basis for the current most popular theory of antibody production. Ehrlich proposed that circulating antibodies were identical to side chains (or receptors) bound to specific cells and that some of these receptors had structures which were complementary to specific antigens. Specific antigens could then attach to these receptors, causing the cells to produce more receptors of the same type, and these were then shed into the circulation. This theory proposed, therefore, a chemical basis for specific antigen-antibody reactions and suggested that antibody-producing precursor cells contained preformed surface receptors—now an accepted fact. This theory was threatened following Landsteiner's observation that antibodies could be produced against a variety of artificial antigens or haptens conjugated to carrier proteins. At that time, it was difficult to accept the idea that preformed receptors could exist against such a variety of antigens that included simple chemicals.

Ehrlich's theory was replaced by instructive (or template) theories for antibody production proposed by Breinl and Haurowitz and by Mudd and Alexander in 1930. These theories stated that antigen served as the template for the production of specific antibodies following contact with immunoglobulin molecules. According to the template hypothesis, contact with antigen modified the immunoglobulin molecule in such a way as to cause the formation of structures complementary to antigenic determinants. Thus, the antigen would instruct the immunoglobulin to form chemically specific structures that could then act as antibody binding sites for that antigen. This model was later amplified by Kerch, who proposed that antibodies consisted of reduced polypeptide chains that were secondarily folded in specific ways. In the presence of the antigen, this precursor molecule acquired a configuration complementary to the antigen and was stabilized in this configuration by disulfide bonds. Although this theory was satisfactory for explaining immunological specificity and diversity, it did not account for immune memory, characterized by rapid and increased antibody formation following second exposure to an antigen. Nor was it adequate to account for the fact, now established, that one cell produces antibodies with only one known specificity.

The first selective theory for antibody production was proposed by Jerne in 1955. He proposed that a multitude of antibody molecules were formed during embryonic life. Those antibodies with specificity against "self" were eliminated during fetal development by absorption into body tissues. Antigens then select from the remaining population of antibody molecules those antibodies with sites complementary to determinants on the antigen molecule and combine with such antibodies, forming antigen-antibody complexes. These complexes would then be taken up by phagocytic cells and provoke the cells to produce more antibodies of the same specificity. In this theory, then, the role of the antigen in triggering antibody synthesis is simply to select the preformed antibody with the right complementary structures.

In 1967, Burnet proposed the **clonal selection** theory, an extension of Jerne's theory. This theory ascribed to the cell what Jerne's theory attributed to circulating antibody. According to this theory, clones of cells have arisen through mutation or other inheritable changes, which contain receptors, now known to be immunoglobulins in nature, with specificity for a particular antigen. These clones developed from progenitor cells with surface receptors analogous to the antibody they would eventually produce following contact with the appropriate antigen. This theory has now proved to be generally correct. Particularly important supporting evidence has been reported by Wigzell and co-workers, who showed that passage of normal lymphoid cells through columns containing different antigens removes those cells capable of producing antibodies against each antigen. This type of experiment established the existence of precommitted clones possessing antigen-specific receptors. Further, antigen-binding is inhibited by antibodies to IgM or by anti-idiotypic anti-serums directed against the appropriate antibody specificity, providing further experimental proof for this conclusion. Other findings have established that each cell or clone of each cell is committed to the production of antibody with one specificity (one cell–one antibody), as predicted by the clonal selection theory.

According to this theory, therefore, induction of antibody synthesis to a specific antigen proceeds in two steps. In the first phase of clonal selection, pluripotential stem cells, originating in fetal liver, differentiate through a series of poorly defined steps into pre-B cells. These lymphocytes initially express IgM immunoglobulin molecules in their cytoplasm and, following subsequent maturation, express IgM on their cell surface as antigen receptors. At the end of this phase of clonal selection, each small lymphocyte is committed through all subsequent differentiation steps to express an antibody with a particular binding specificity. This specificity is determined when the differentiating lymphocyte is committed to express the specific light-chain and heavy-chain variable regions constituting the antibody combining site. This first phase of clonal selection occurs independently of antigen interactions with the differentiating cell.

The second phase of clonal selection occurs after the antigen is specifically bound to the cell surface immunoglobulin. This interaction stimulates the cell to divide and to differentiate into an antibody-producing plasma cell. This is, therefore, an antigen-dependent differentiation step. This clonal expansion increases the number of cells in the clone, and these undergo further differentiation into immunoglobulin-producing cells and memory cells. Daughter cells of a given clone can express different immunoglobulin classes (IgM, IgG, IgA, IgE) with the same antibody specificity, because a precommitted cell can express different heavy-chain constant regions (mu, gamma, alpha, epsilon) but maintains the same variable regions or idiotype, which constitutes the antibody combining site. For example, it is accepted that the first immunoglobulin generally produced in response to an antigen is IgM, with a later shift to IgG. This is known as **isotype switch** and usually occurs during the second phase of clonal selection. During this switch, it is believed that the $C\mu$ gene is repressed and the $C\gamma$ gene activated, resulting in an antibody with a new isotype but the same antigen specificity.

Genetic Basis for Antibody Diversity[14, 15, 27]

A very large repertoire of immunoglobulin molecules with different antigen-binding sites must exist in an individual to counter the large variety of antigens to which that individual is exposed in a lifetime. It has been conservatively estimated that this number is between 10^6 and 10^8. This immunoglobulin diversity is a feature of the primary structure of the antibody molecule (the variable regions of the H and L chains) and must reflect genetic rearrangements of the gene segments that encode for these variable regions. The actual mechanism by which this diversity is generated, however, is still largely speculative.

The genes that encode for the immunoglobulin polypeptides are arranged in chromosomal DNA in such a way as to maximize immunoglobulin diversity with a minimum of genetic material. In humans and mice, the genes coding for the synthesis of lambda L chains, kappa L chains, and the different H chains are located on different chromosomes. Within each of these families, each polypeptide is structurally different at its amino terminal half (variable region), but identical at the carboxy terminal half (constant region); for example, many different V regions are found in human kappa chains, yet all constant regions are identical except for a single amino acid substitution. Such a structural arrangement suggests that the synthesis of an antibody molecule does not follow the one gene–one polypeptide concept of genetics. In 1965, Dreyer and Bennett proposed a two gene–one polypeptide mechanism for the synthesis of immunoglobulin polypeptide chains in which the variable regions and the constant regions were encoded by two separate genes, joined through recombinational events during the first phase of clonal selection. This hypothesis is supported by recent evidence, reported by Hozumi and Tonegawa, generated through the use of DNA cloning techniques. Their results indicated that the two genes encoding for the kappa chain variable and constant regions are separated on the chromosome in embryonic cells, while in he fully differentiated plasma cell, the two genes are recombined to form a contiguous stretch of DNA. Several models have now been proposed and are currently being examined to explain a mechanism by which V and C regions are joined during B cell differentiation, an event that is likely to be more complex than suggested by this two gene–one polypeptide concept.

It is clear that the main source of antibody diversity lies in the V region genes, as indicated by studies of amino acids from different antibody molecules. Two general theories have been proposed to explain the origin of this genetic diversity in the V regions of antibody molecules. The **germline** or **phylogenetic** theory states that the genes responsible for coding for the large repertoire of antigen-binding sites (or V regions) are present in the germinal line of the organism and that diversity is generated by mutation and selection during evolutionary development. This could be accomplished by gene duplication and diversification. The V region genes are then passed to different cells during the somatic development of the organism without further generation of diversity. According to this theory, therefore, each V region would be encoded by a separate gene present in the germline of the organism. Although there is some evidence in support of this theory, the major objection is that it requires the presence of a large number of genes in the germline to account for the production of the vast array of antibody specificities.

An alternate proposal is presented in the **somatic diversification** and **ontogenetic** theories explaining the origin of antibody diversity. These theories differ from the germline hypothesis in that they postulate the existence of a limited number of V genes in the germinal line. Diversity in this situation is generated during somatic differentiation by a number of different mechanisms including (1) somatic point mutations, in which a small number of germline V genes become greatly diversified in somatic cells through successive point mutations and are subsequently selected by prevalent antigens; and (2) by recombination events through which germline V genes become greatly diversified during somatic cell differentiation, followed by selection by the prevalent antigens. Recent analysis of amino acid sequences of V_L and V_H regions, and from DNA sequence analysis, have provided evidence indicating that these theories may be partially correct.

In summary, the genetic basis of antibody diversity is a complex mechanism yet to be defined. Existing evidence indicates that there are probably a relatively large number of V region gene segments for both L and H chains present in embryonic DNA. These V region genes can probably be somatically modified during the lifetime of an individual, by somatic mutation or by recombination events, resulting in DNA rearrangement to generate antibody diversity.

References

1. Amos, D. 1969. Genetic and antigenic aspects of human histocompatibility systems. Adv. Immunol. **10**:251–297.
2. Baker, P. J. 1975. Homeostatic control of antibody responses. A model based on the recognition of cell-associated antibody by regulatory T cells. Transplant. Rev. **23**:3–20.
3. Benacerraf, B. 1978. A hypothesis to relate the specificity of T lymphocytes and the activity of I region-specific Ir genes in macrophages and B lymphocytes. J. Immunol. **120**:1809–1812.
4. Benacerraf, B., and R. W. Germain. 1978. The immune response genes of the major histocompatibility complex. Immunol. Rev. **38**:70–119.
5. Bevan, M. J. 1981. Thymic education. Immunol. Today **3**:216–219.
6. Burnet, F. M. 1957. A modification of Jerne's theory of antibody production using the concept of clonal selection. Australia J. Sci. **20**:67–69.
7. Cantor, H., and E. A. Boyse. 1975. Functional subclasses of T lymphocytes bearing different Ly antigens. I. The generation of functionally distinct T cell subclasses is a differentiation process independent of antigen. J. Exptl. Med. **141**:1376–1389.
8. Cantor, H., and E. A. Boyse. 1975. Functional subclasses of T lymphocytes bearing different Ly antigens. II. Cooperation between subclasses of Ly + cells in the generation of killer activity. J. Exptl. Med. **141**:1390–1399.
9. David, C. S. 1976. Serologic and genetic aspects of murine Ia antigens. Transplant. Rev. **30**:299–322.
10. Dutton, R. W. 1975. Suppressor T cells. Transplant. Rev. **26**:39–55.
11. Gershon, R. K. 1974. T cell control of antibody production. Contem. Topics Immunobiol. **3**:1–40.
12. Hämmerling, G. J., and H. O. McDevitt. 1975. Antigen-binding structures on the surface of T lymphocytes. Israel J. Med. Sci. **11**:1331–1356.
13. Haurowitz, F. 1965. Antibody formation and the coding problem. Nature **205**:847–851.
14. Hood, L. E. 1972. Two genes, one polypeptide chain—fact or fiction? Fed. Proc. **31**:177–187.
15. Hood, L. 1976. Antibody genes and other multigene families. Fed. Proc. **35**:2158–2167.
16. Jerne, N. K. 1960. Immunological speculations. Ann. Rev. Microbiol. **14**:341–358.
17. Katz, D. H., and B. J. Benacerraf. 1972. The regulatory influence of activated T cells on B cell responses to antigen. Adv. Immunol. **15**:1–94.
18. Klein, J. 1978. H-2 mutations: their genetics and effects on immune functions. Adv. Immunol. **26**:56–147.

19. Krco, C. J., and C. S. David. 1981. Genetics of immune response: a survey. CRC Crit. Rev. Immunol. **1**:211–257.

20. McDevitt, H. O. 1976. The evolution of genes in the major histocompatibility complex. Fedn. Proc. **35**:2168–2173.

21. McDevitt, H. O. 1980. Regulation of the immune response by the major histocompatibility system. New Engl. J. Med. **303**:1514–1517.

22. McDevitt, H. O., and B. Benacerraf. 1969. Genetic control of specific immune responses. Adv. Immunol. **11**:31–74.

23. McDevitt, H. O., and A. Chinitz. 1969. Genetic control of the antibody response: relationship between immune response and histocompatibility (H-2) type. Science **163**:1207–1209.

24. McDevitt, H. O., et al. 1972. Genetic control of the immune response. Mapping of the IR–I locus. J. Exptl. Med. **135**:1259–1278.

25. McDevitt, H. O. et al. 1976. Genetic and functional analysis of the Ia antigens: their possible role in regulating the immune response. Transplant. Rev. **30**:197–235.

26. Miller, J. F. A. P. 1975. T-cell regulation of immunoresponsiveness. Ann. N.Y. Acad. Sci. **249**:9–26.

27. Milstein, C., and A. J. Munro. 1970. Genetic basis of antibody specificity. Ann. Rev. Microbiol. **24**:335–358.

28. Mitchell, G. F., R. I. Mishell, and L. A. Herzenberg. 1971. Studies on the influence of T cells in antibody production. pp. 324–335. In B. Amos (Ed.): Progress in Immunology. Academic Press, New York.

29. Nagy, Z. A., et al. 1981. Ia antigens as restriction molecules in Ir-gene controlled T-cell proliferation. Immunol. Rev. **60**:59–80.

30. Neta, R., and S. B. Salvin. 1976. T and B lymphocytes in the regulation of delayed hypersensitivity. J. Immunol. **117**:2014–2020.

31. Paul, W. 1976. Genetic control of specific interactions of immunocompetent cells. Speculation on mechanisms and general biologic significance. Fedn. Proc. **35**:2044–2047.

32. Pauling, L. 1940. A theory of the structure and process of formation of antibodies. J. Amer. Chem. Soc. **62**:2643–2657.

33. Rosenthal, A. S., and E. M. Shevach, 1973. Function of macrophages in antigen recognition by guinea pig T lymphocytes. I. Requirement for histocompatible macrophages and lymphocytes. J. Exptl. Med. **138**:1194–1212.

34. Shreffler, D. C., T. Meo, and C. S. David. 1976. Genetic resolution of the products and functions of I and S region genes of the mouse H-2 complex. pp 3–29. In D. H. Katz and B. Benacerraf (Eds.): The Role of Products of the Histocompatibility Gene Complex in Immune Responses. Academic Press, New York.

35. Smith, K. A., and F. W. Ruscetti. 1981. T-cell growth factor and the culture of cloned functional T cells. Adv. Immunol. **31**:137–176.

36. Snell, G. D., M. Cherry, and P. Demant. 1973. H-2, its structure and similarity to HL–A. Transplant. Rev. **15**:3–25.

37. Strominger, J. L., et al. 1974. The immunoglobulin-like structure of human histocompatibility antigens. Transplant. Rev. **21**:126–143.

38. Talmage, D. W., J. Radovich, and H. Hemmingsen. 1970. Cell interaction in antibody synthesis. Adv. Immunol. **12**:271–282.

39. Tanigaki, N., and D. Pressman. 1974. The basic structure and the antigenic characteristics of HL–A antigens. Transplant. Rev. **21**:15–34.

40. Taussig, M. J., and A. J. Munro. 1976. Antigen-specific T-cell factor in cell cooperation and genetic control of the immune response. Fedn. Proc. **35**:2061–2066.

41. Thorsby, E. 1974. The human major histocompatibility system. Transplant. Rev. **18**:51–129.

42. Unanue, E. R. 1972. The regulatory role of macrophages in antigenic stimulation. Adv. Immunol. **15**:95–165.

43. Unanue, E. R. 1981. The regulatory role of macrophages in antigenic stimulation. II. Symbiotic relationship between lymphocytes and macrophages. Adv. Immunol. **31**:1–136.

44. Winchester, R. J., and H. G. Kunkel. 1979. The human Ia system. Adv. Immunol. **28**:222–292.

45. Zinkernagel, R. M., and P. C. Doherty. 1974. Immunological surveillance against altered self components by sensitized T lymphocytes in lymphocytic choriomeningitis. Nature **251**:547–548.

46. Zinkernagel, R. M., and P. C. Doherty. 1979. MHC restricted cytotoxic T cells: studies on the biological role of polymorphic major transplantation antigens determining T cell restriction. Specificity, functions and responsiveness. Adv. Immunol. **27**:52–178.

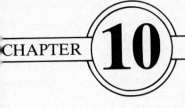

CHAPTER 10

Transplantation Immunology, Tumor Immunology, and Hypersensitivity

Gary R. Pearson, Ph.D.

The important role of cellular elements as effector components in the mediation of certain immunological phenomena has been established from studies involving the transplantation of organs or tissues between genetically dissimilar individuals (transplantation immunology); investigations on experimental tumors (tumor immunology); and the characterization of factors responsible for the induction of allergic states (hypersensitivity) to certain foreign substances. The rejection of tissue, organ, or tumor grafts has an immunological basis, as does the induction of hypersensitivity to soluble and cellular antigens. Lymphoid cells are the major effector components of these immunological reactions, although some hypersensitivity reactions are also mediated by certain classes of antibodies. Hypersensitivity reactions mediated by antibody are referred to as immediate, while those initiated by sensitized lymphoid cells and tending toward a slower time course are delayed hypersensitivity reactions.

Transplantation Immunology

The concept of transplantation immunology developed early in this century from studies on transplantable tumors. When transplanted among members of the same outbred species, tumors grew in some animals but not in others. The reasons for this variability remained unclear until the development of inbred strains of mice, when it became apparent that the growth of transplantable tumors depended on genetic identity between the tumor graft and the recipient mouse strains. Transplantable tumors from one inbred strain of mice grow in all members of that strain but not in other genetically dissimilar inbred strains (Table 10–1). These tumors will also grow in F_1 hybrid mice from a cross between the tumor donor

Table 10–1. **Influence of Histocompatibility Genes on the Acceptance or Rejection of Tumor Grafts**

Tumor Donor Strain	Recipient Strain	Graft Fate
A	A	Accepted
A	B	Rejected
A	$(A \times B)F_1$	Accepted
B	A	Rejected
B	B	Accepted
B	$(A \times B)F_1$	Accepted
$(A \times B)F_1$	A	Rejected
$(A \times B)F_1$	B	Rejected
$(A \times B)F_1$	$(A \times B)F_1$	Accepted

strain and another strain of mice, but tumors induced in the F_1 hybrid strains do not grow in the parental strains. Similar observations on skin grafts established the genetic control of tissue transplantation and the requirement for genetic identity between the donor and recipient before a graft is completely accepted. The cellular constituents responsible for determining whether a graft is accepted or rejected are the membrane-associated products of the major histocompatibility loci (H-2 in the mouse, HLA in humans) described in the preceding chapter. Rejection of genetically dissimilar grafts is mediated by an immune response of the recipient against the foreign, cell-surface antigens expressed on the donor tissue, the phenomenon of transplantation immunity.

Before discussing the various aspects of transplantation immunology, it is necessary to define the terminology used (Table 10–2). An **autograft** is a graft transplanted to another site on the same individual, *i.e.*, the graft donor also acts as the recipient. The donor is designated as **autologous** or **autochthonous.** Such grafts are readily recognized as "self" and, therefore, are not rejected. **Isograft** refers to a graft between genetically identical individuals, such as identical twins or members of the same inbred strain. The donor in this case is **isologous** or **syngeneic.** This type of graft is also recognized as "self" and is generally accepted. A graft between two genetically different individuals of the same species is designated as **allograft** or **homograft,** and the donor as **allogeneic** or **homologous.** These grafts are recognized as foreign by the recipient and are rejected. A **xenograft** is a graft between two individuals of different species and the donor of such grafts are **xenogeneic** or **heterologous** such grafts are normally rejected. A graft is called **histocompatible** if it is accepted by the recipient and **histoincompatible** if it is rejected because of the presence of foreign histocompatibility antigens.

THE IMMUNOLOGICAL BASIS OF GRAFT REJECTIONS[5, 7, 11, 12, 14, 35, 50, 51, 56]

It is well established that the rejection of grafts has an immunological basis. This has been determined primarily with allografts using a number of different criteria. First, the rejection of allografts shows an exquisite specificity similar to antigen-antibody reactions. Recipient individuals will only reject foreign or histoincompatible grafts. For example, if an autograft and allograft are placed next to each other on the same animal, only the allograft will be rejected. This was documented conclusively by eloquent experiments in inbred strains of guinea pigs. Pigmented A strain skin was grafted onto an unpigmented area of $(A \times B)$ F_1 hybrid guinea pigs. The grafts were accepted and with time the pigmented A cells migrated into the unpigmented area of the skin. Pieces of skin containing pigmented (A) and nonpigmented $(A \times B)$ regions were then grafted back onto unpigmented areas of A strain guinea pigs. Although the F_1 grafts were rejected because of the foreign antigens in the grafts provided by the B parent, the pigmented A cells were not rejected, as evidenced by the persistence of pigment in the graft area. Thus, the recipient A strain guinea pigs rejected the cells in the F_1 graft that expressed the antigens of the B parent, but not those pigmented cells that expressed antigens of the A parent only.

This specificity can also be shown by second-set rejection. When an animal is first exposed to an allograft, the graft usually becomes vascularized and remains healthy for approxi-

Table 10–2. **Description of Different Types of Tissue Grafts Employed in Transplantation Immunology**

Graft Designation	Other Names	Definitions
Autograft	Autologous, autochthonous	Graft to another site on same animal
Isograft	Isologous, syngeneic	Graft between genetically identical individuals
Allograft	Homograft, allogeneic, homologous	Graft between genetically dissimilar individuals of the same species
Xenograft	Xenogeneic, heterologous	Graft between members of different species

nately 10 days. However, from 10 to 14 days postgrafting, the graft is infiltrated by large numbers of mononuclear cells, the tissue is damaged, and it is then rejected. This is referred to as **first-set rejection.** If animals that have rejected a graft are now regrafted with tissue from the same donor as the first graft, the new graft will be rejected more rapidly, usually within 5 to 6 days. This is known as **second-set rejection.** The second-set response is specific for grafts containing the same major histocompatibility antigens as those expressed in the initial graft and is systemic, since it can be demonstrated with grafts placed at different sites on the body. This accelerated rejection noted with second-set grafts is due to the ability of the immunized animal to mount a memory, *i.e.,* secondary, or anamnestic, immune response against antigens expressed in the primary graft.

The immunological basis of allograft rejection has also been shown through the use of immunosuppressive measures. Suppression of the cellular immune response before grafting, using irradiation, cytotoxic drugs, or removal of the thymus, results in the prolongation of allografts and even xenografts. Such grafts will be rejected when the immunosuppressive measures are removed and the animal regains its ability to mount an immune response.

The mechanism of allograft rejection involves primarily immune lymphoid cells, although under certain circumstances, immunity to grafts can also be transferred by serum antibodies. Most of the work on the mechanisms of graft rejection has been done with allografts; transfer techniques and cell depletion has been used to identify the active immune effector cells. Transfer experiments test the ability of cells or serum from an immunized donor to transfer allograft immunity to a normal donor, as evidenced by the mediation of a second-set rejection. The transfer of cells is referred to as **adoptive transfer,** as opposed to **passive transfer,** involving the transfer of serum. Cells or serum from an immune animal are transferred to normal, nonimmune recipients, and these are then grafted with the same tissue used to sensitize the donor; the grafted animals are followed for evidence of second-set rejection. Generally, lymph nodes draining the graft area of the donor animal are used in adoptive immunity studies, although spleen and peripheral blood lymphocytes have also been successfully employed. The bulk of the evidence demonstrates that transplantation immunity is transferred by lymphoid cells, but not by antibody, and that the specificity of the adoptively transferred immunity is the same as that noted in regular tissue grafting. This has also been shown through the use of diffusion chambers containing the target tissue. When the chambers are implanted into the peritoneal cavity of mice, the target tissue is destroyed only if the pore size of the chambers allows the passage of sensitized cells into the chamber. The role of lymphoid cells in the rejection of allografts is further supported by the finding that mice thymectomized at birth or mice born lacking a thymus (athymic nude mice) are unable to reject allografts. T lymphocytes are implicated as the major mediator of allograft rejection. Administration of large quantities of immune serum is ineffective in mediating accelerated graft rejection, with some exceptions, as discussed below.

Depletion experiments have been valuable in identifying the specific subpopulation of lymphocytes responsible for mediating graft rejection. Several methods are used to eliminate one specific subpopulation from mixtures of lymphoid cells before employing them in transfer experiments. If T lymphocytes are killed with antibody and complement, the ability of the depleted lymphoid cell population to adoptively transfer allograft immunity is generally abolished, providing further evidence that the T lymphocyte is the major effector cell in transplantation immunity. The exact nature of the specific T cell subpopulation responsible for acute allograft rejection is still unknown, but depletion studies indicate that both cytotoxic T cells (Ly 1^-, 2, 3^+) and T lymphocytes that release lymphokines (Ly 1^+, 2, 3^-) participate in this immunological event. Macrophages possibly also interact with T lymphocytes in transplantation immunity, particularly at the recognition phase, although this requires further clarification.

Antibody, under certain circumstances, may also participate in graft rejection. The transfer of high-titered antiserum in dogs and goats causes the accelerated rejection of renal allografts; antibody may also function in the rejection of renal transplants in humans. Renal allograft rejection may be caused, at least in part, by the deposition of antigen-antibody complexes in the kidneys to result in infarction and later rejection. Similarly, antibody has been reported to be important in the rejection of skin allografts transplanted to hyperimmunized recipients; rejected grafts do not become vascularized following the grafting procedure and are referred to as **white grafts.** Passive transfer of high-titered antiserum reportedly produces this white graft reaction.

GRAFT VERSUS HOST DISEASE[12, 24]

In allograft reactions, the immune system of the recipient recognizes foreign antigens on the graft and rejects it. Under certain circumstances, the reverse can also happen and the graft reacts against host cell antigens. This is known as the **graft versus host** (GVH) reaction. GVH reactions occur when the graft contains significant numbers of T lymphocytes or their precursors; the recipient cells express antigens recognized as foreign by the donor cells; or the recipient is temporarily or permanently incapable of rejecting the graft. With inbred strains of mice, this third point can be genetically determined. Injection of parental strain lymphocytes into an F_1 hybrid allows the development of the GVH reaction because the parental donor cells will not be rejected in the F_1 host. On the other hand, the parental strain lymphocytes can respond to the other parental antigens expressed in the hybrid. As an example, GVH reactions may occur in $A \times B$ F_1 hybrid recipients following injection of cells from the A parent because the B antigens expressed in the F_1 recipients are recognized as foreign; GVH reactions occur, too, in immunologically immature animals or in animals that have been immunosuppressed with x-ray irradiation, cytotoxic drugs, anti-thymocyte serum, or other immunosuppressive measures, so that they can no longer reject foreign cells. GVH disease denotes the complex syndrome resulting from the effects of this immune reaction. Typical GVH lesions, consisting of necrotic nodules, occur in most organs but are most apparent in the spleen; a severe rash may also occur. Immature animals receiving an allograft of lymphoid cells from spleen, peripheral blood, or bone marrow do not develop normally but instead develop a fatal wasting syndrome called **runt disease.**

GVH disease is a significant clinical problem, particularly in patients receiving bone marrow transplants. Because the recipients cannot make their own bone marrow cells, they are immunodeficient and do not respond normally to foreign substances. The transplanted bone marrow cells can respond against the recipient's own antigens, however, if these antigens are dissimilar to those expressed on the grafted cells. Until recently, the incidence of acute GVH disease in bone marrow transplant recipients was 50 to 70 per cent, with about one-third of these patients eventually succumbing to the disease. Because of advances in tissue matching, diagnosis, and clinical management, the incidence of GVH disease in these patients has decreased 20 to 30 per cent.

As in allograft reactions, GVH reactions are principally cell-mediated, with antibody apparently playing an insignificant role in pathogenesis. Whether this immune reaction is mediated by one or more specific subpopulations of T lymphocytes is still not known, but there is suggestive evidence that more than one subpopulation participates in GVH reactions; this requires further exploration.

IMMUNOLOGICAL TOLERANCE[8, 16, 52]

Immunological tolerance is a state of immunological unresponsiveness to a specific antigen or foreign substance. The classic example of tolerance is the failure to mount an immune response to the individual's own tissue. In this case, the host recognizes its tissue antigens as self. When tolerance to self tissues breaks down for unknown reasons, the result often is the development of **autoimmune disease,** resulting from immune reactivity to the normal components of the individual's own body. In addition to natural tolerance, it is possible to induce a tolerance state to specific antigens under appropriate conditions. This is **acquired tolerance** and is the basis for studies directed at identifying the specific mechanisms regulating the development of the immune response to specific antigens.

The idea of tolerance stems from the observation by Owens in 1945 that the blood of most dizygotic cattle twins contained a mixture of erythrocytes. The chorioallantoic membranes of twin fetuses fuse early in development, resulting in a common blood supply. In this way, red blood cell **chimeras** are formed, in which a stable mixture of red blood cell serotypes is maintained throughout life. Later, skin grafts between cattle twins were found to be accepted even when the recipients were clearly nonidentical twins of different sexes. It was concluded that this was a consequence of the *in utero* exchange of antigenically different tissues between the twins. The formation of chimeras was experimentally duplicated in 1953 by Billingham, Burnet, and Fenner, who inoculated mice *in utero* with a mixture of cells from a genetically different strain of mice. After birth, these animals accepted skin grafts from the donors of the inoculated cells. This acquired tolerance was specific, because the mice rejected skin grafts from animals that differed genetically from the original donor strain.

In 1949, Burnet and Fenner proposed a theory of antibody formation to explain why animals did not produce antibodies to "self." They proposed that the critical phase, during which recognition of "self" took place, was during an early period of fetal development when the ability to respond to an antigen was absent or poorly developed. Any antigen, whether natural or acquired, present during this period before the maturation of the immunological system, would subsequently be accepted as "self" and would not thereafter provoke an immune response in the mature animal. This theory provided an explanation for the findings outlined above on the experimental induction of acquired tolerance.

Immunological tolerance was later demonstrated in a reverse manner, that is, by removal of a normal component of the body during fetal life and then re-exposing the adult animal to this same tissue. In these situations, the materials removed during fetal life, normally recognized as self, were immunogenic when reinoculated into the deficient host. In a classical study by Triplett in 1962, the buccal component of the pituitary gland in frog embryos was removed at birth and maintained in viable condition in the test tube. Following metamorphosis, reinoculation of the adult frogs with this tissue resulted in its rejection. Thus, these frogs rejected what was basically an autograft. These experiments established the existence of immunological tolerance to "self" antigens and further demonstrated that the induction of tolerance, either natural or acquired, required the presence of the antigen during the maturation of the immune system. The actual mechanism of tolerance induction was unknown but was thought to involve the elimination or inactivation of clones of antigen-reactive cells during this developmental period.

In 1956, Billingham and Brent demonstrated that tolerance could also be induced in newborn animals by the intravenous injection of foreign spleen cells. These animals did not later reject skin grafts from the spleen donor, although skin grafts from other genetically different strains were still rejected. Contrary to then prevalent opinion, induction of tolerance was not necessarily confined to the embryo. Nevertheless, large numbers of spleen cells had to be inoculated in order to induce tolerance in the newborn, while the injection of small numbers generally produced immunity; tolerance induction in the newborn was, therefore, dose dependent. Subsequent experiments in adult animals resulted in similar findings.

It is now apparent that tolerance to many different antigens can be induced if the antigen is presented to the animal when the immune system is not functioning, as occurs during fetal development; in the newborn, or in adult animals treated with immunosuppressive measures, such as x-ray irradiation, immunosuppressive drugs, or anti-lymphocyte serum. Tolerance to nonliving antigens, such as BSA, is dependent on the amount of antigen injected and the rate at which it is eliminated from the body. In many instances, the tolerant state can be maintained by continuous antigen injections. The presence of living, replicating antigens, as occurs with red blood cell chimeras or tissue grafts, permits the tolerance state to be maintained indefinitely.

The nature of the antigen also influences its capacity to induce a tolerant state. For example, heat-aggregated human gamma globulin is immunogenic in mice, but is tolerogenic when injected in the nonaggregated form. This difference between aggregated and nonaggregated gamma globulin appears to be at least partially related to macrophage functions. It has been postulated that aggregated antigens are more likely to be phagocytized by macrophages and, therefore, to be immunogenic. It has also been suggested that antigens are more likely to induce tolerance, rather than an immune response, if they interact directly with lymphocytes as opposed to presentation to lymphocytes by macrophages.

With protein antigens, tolerance can be induced in two different dose ranges. Mice can be made tolerant to BSA with both high and low concentrations, as illustrated in Figure 10–1. Mice preimmunized with repeated doses of approximately 1 μg. of BSA were tolerant

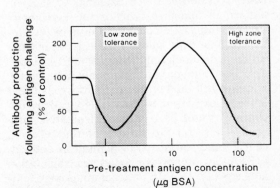

Figure 10–1. Illustration of low zone and high zone tolerance following immunization with different concentrations of BSA.

when subsequently challenged with BSA in adjuvant, as evidenced by the lack of antibody production. In contrast, mice preimmunized with doses of approximately 10 μg. of BSA responded like immune animals, while those preimmunized with doses of 100 μg. or higher were tolerant to BSA. This gave rise to the concepts of **low-zone** and **high-zone tolerance.** Later studies at the cellular level indicated that low-zone tolerance probably results from inactivation of helper T cells, while high-zone tolerance results from the induction of unresponsiveness in both T and B cell populations.

The exact mechanism of immunological tolerance is still not clear. Some consider the phenomenon of acquired tolerance as a specific, "central failure" of immunological responsiveness. In contrast, others suggest that acquired tolerance is, in fact, due to either the elimination or the inactivation of antigen-specific clones of lymphocytes. At this time, it is not possible to choose between these two alternatives. A third explanation for tolerance requires the involvement of suppressor T cells. There is some indication that tolerance cannot be induced in the absence of T cells. Moreover, it is well established that suppressor T cell populations can suppress antibody formation, lymphocyte blastogenesis, and cytotoxic T cell responses to specific antigens. Specific suppressor T cells are able to confer a tolerance-like state to different proteins and synthetic polymers of amino acids by adoptive transfer. These findings suggest that suppressor T cells possibly function in acquired tolerance by inactivating helper T cells. Whether these cells also function in the establishment of immunological tolerance to "self" or natural antigens remains to be resolved. If so, inactivation of a specific clone of suppressor T cells could result in the production of antibodies to "self" antigens, thereby providing a possible mechanism for the development of autoimmune disease.

Tumor Immunology[9, 13, 22, 43]

Tumor cells contain a variety of antigens that vary in specificity, location in the cell, and, most likely, biological importance. Antigens that are uniquely expressed on tumor cells and are not found in normal adult or embryonic cells are referred to as **tumor-specific** antigens. Sometimes, however, it is not possible to demonstrate convincingly this type of restriction. For example, some putative tumor-specific antigens are not found on corresponding normal adult cells, but can sometimes be detected on fetal or embryonic cells. Therefore, it has been common to refer to such antigens as **tumor-associated,** instead of tumor-specific, until the absolute tumor specificity is established. An example of such an antigen in human cancers is the **carcinoembryonic** antigen detected in tumors of the gastrointestinal tract and in fetal tissues, but not in the corresponding adult tissues. Tumor-associated antigens are commonly found in the nuclei of cells and on the cell surface. Nuclear antigens expressed in tumors induced by oncogenic viruses have been designated **T antigens.** Those on the surface of the cells are called **tumor-specific transplantation antigens** (TSTA) or **tumor-associated transplantation antigens** (TATA). In tumor immunology, particular attention has been directed toward the membrane-associated antigens, since these presumably serve as targets for a rejection-type immune response directed against the tumor. The definition of such antigens has required stringent controls to distinguish them from other types of antigens frequently expressed on the surface of tumor cells. These latter antigens include normal histocompatibility antigens, fetal antigens, organ- or tissue-specific antigens, and virus-specified antigens. Tumor-specific transplantation antigens may be identified by transplantation studies in appropriately immunized animals or by *in vitro* cytotoxic assays to demonstrate specific immune responses mediated by cellular or humoral immune mechanisms.

Interest in tumor-associated antigens can be traced back to the early 1900s. During this early period of tumor immunology, there were indications that tumors, particularly those experimentally induced in animals, might express new antigens as shown by immunization. In early studies, mice were immunized with mouse tumor A and then inoculated with viable cells of the same tumor. No tumors grew in mice immune to tumor A, while a high proportion of mice in the nonimmune group developed tumors. This was interpreted as being due to the existence of a tumor-specific immunity in the immunized mice, which resulted in tumor rejection in a manner similar to the rejection of a skin graft. Unfortunately, these early studies used outbred strains of animals. After identification of transplantation antigens, it became evident that histocompatibility antigens, and not tumor-specific antigens, were responsible for the apparent immunization against cancer cells. With the development of inbred strains of mice there was a new surge of interest in the existence of *bona fide* tumor-specific antigens.

Probably the first definitive evidence for the existence of TSTA was reported by Gross in 1943. He observed that tumors induced by methylcholanthrene could be transplanted among members of the same inbred strain by intradermal inoculation of viable cells. The transplanted tumor cells grew for a period of time at the inoculation site and then regressed. If these mice were reinoculated with the same tumor following this regression, no growth was observed, indicating that these mice were now resistant or refractory to the tumor. About 10 years later, Foley and co-workers injected mice with transplantable tumor cells induced by methylcholanthrene and then surgically removed the tumors after a period of growth. These mice were then reinoculated with cells from the same tumor. The incidence of tumor takes in this group of "immune" mice was significantly reduced in comparison to a control group of nonimmune mice. As an additional control, some mice were skin-grafted with grafts from other members of the mouse strain in which the tumor had been induced to determine whether resistance was associated with the presence of residual or minor histocompatibility antigens expressed on the tumor. Tumors failed to grow only in those mice previously exposed to or immunized with the same tumor, indicating that these tumors expressed an antigen not present in normal tissues and that immunity was not induced by normal cellular antigens. Final proof for the existence of new antigens in tumors induced by this chemical was reported by Klein and associates, who demonstrated that the autologous host was resistant to a second exposure of its own tumor, thereby eliminating any possible involvement of histocompatibility antigens in the development of resistance to tumor growth. It was later demonstrated that animals could be rendered resistant to the growth of tumors induced by chemicals, viruses, and physical agents, and even to some tumors that arose spontaneously, and that this resistance had an immunological basis. In addition, the specificity of tumor-specific antigens differed, depending largely on the agent responsible for tumor induction.

ANTIGENS IN TUMORS INDUCED BY CHEMICALS AND VIRUSES[22, 38, 39, 49]

Different tumors induced by the same chemical express individually distinct tumor-specific transplantation antigens. This specificity was shown initially by transplantation experiments, but has been confined by *in vitro* cell-mediated immunity studies. Table 10–3 illustrates the specificity of different tumor-specific antigens. If mice are immunized with tumor A induced by methylcholanthrene (MC–A) and then inoculated subcutaneously with graded doses of MC–A, tumors are not produced at the lower inoculum levels in immune mice, but are produced in some mice receiving large numbers of cells. In contrast, tumors are produced in most or all nonimmune control animals regardless of the initial inoculum level. If mice immune to MC–A are now challenged with a second methylcholanthrene tumor, MC–B or MC–C, this tumor grows as well in the immune mice as in the controls, *i.e.*, mice immunized with MC–A are not resistant to MC–B or MC–C. This type of experiment, performed with many different tumors induced by a variety of chemicals, illustrates two important points about immunity to chemically induced tumors. First, immunity is relatively weak in comparison to allograft immunity. A threshold number

Table 10–3. **Demonstration of TSTA in Chemically Induced Tumors***

| Cell Inoculum | Challenge Tumor | | | | | |
| | MC–A | | MC–B | | MC–C | |
	Control	Immune	Control	Immune	Control	Immune
10^5	5/5†	2/5	5/5	5/5	5/5	5/5
10^4	5/5	0/5	5/5	5/5	5/5	5/5
10^3	4/5	0/5	3/5	3/5	3/5	3/5
10^2	2/5	0/5	1/5	1/5	1/5	1/5
10^1	0/5	0/5	0/5	0/5	0/5	0/5

*Immunizing tumor = methylcholanthrene (MC)-induced tumor A; challenge tumor = MC-induced tumors A, B, and C.

†Number of animals developing tumors/number of animals inoculated with tumor cells.

Table 10–4. **Demonstration of TSTA in Virus-Induced Tumors***

Cell Inoculum	Challenge Tumor					
	Py-A		Py-B		SV-40	
	Control	Immune	Control	Immune	Control	Immune
10^5	5/5†	2/5	5/5	1/5	5/5	5/5
10^4	5/5	0/5	5/5	0/5	5/5	5/5
10^3	3/5	0/5	4/5	0/5	4/5	4/5
10^2	0/5	0/5	1/5	0/5	0/5	0/5

*Immunizing tumor = polyoma virus (Py)-induced tumor A; challenge tumor = Py virus tumors A and B; SV-40 virus-induced tumor.

†Number of animals developing tumors/number of animals inoculated with tumor cells.

of cells is required to demonstrate this immunity. When the cell inoculum is increased above the threshold level, the tumor cells grow as well in immune animals as in normal controls, masking the existence of tumor-specific immunity. Second, each chemically induced tumor expresses individually distinct tumor-specific antigens.

This specificity differs from that observed with virus-induced tumors, as illustrated in Table 10–4. Mice immunized with tumors induced by the oncogenic polyoma virus (PY), are resistant to the growth of the immunizing tumor (PY–A) when inoculated subcutaneously with threshold numbers of PY–A tumor cells. This resistance disappears as the inoculum is increased. However, animals immune to PY–A are also resistant to other tumors induced by the same virus (PY–B), but not to tumors induced by different oncogenic viruses (SV-40 virus) or to tumors induced by other agents. Thus, in this situation, all tumors induced by the same virus share the same TSTA.

This same type of specificity is also observed with *in vitro* cell-mediated immunity assays (Chapter 8). Lymphocytes from animals immunized with a specific chemically induced tumor are usually cytotoxic against that tumor, but are not active against other tumors induced by the same or different chemical or against tumors induced by viruses. In contrast, lymphocytes from animals immunized with tumors induced by a specific virus are cytotoxic against all tumors induced by this same virus, but not against tumors induced by other viruses or chemicals. Thus, chemically induced tumors express individually distinct TSTA, while tumors produced by a specific virus share a common TSTA.

In vitro assays for cell-mediated immunity also demonstrated the presence of other antigens on tumor cells that are normally not expressed in the corresponding adult tissues. The most common of these are embryonic antigens which become expressed in tumor cells, as discussed earlier. Whether these antigens function actively in immunity to cancer is still a controversial issue.

IMMUNOLOGICAL BASIS OF TUMOR RESISTANCE[10, 14, 26–30, 47, 48, 54]

Resistance to tumor growth has an immunological basis primarily involving the cellular immune system, as first demonstrated in immunosuppressed animals. Immunosuppression can be induced by thymectomy of animals at birth, whole body irradiation, immunosuppressive drugs, or anti-lymphocyte serum plus complement. Transplantable tumors grow more readily in such animals, and it is usually possible to induce tumors with small numbers of inoculated tumor cells. Immunization of these animals does not induce resistance to tumor growth. Further, virus-induced tumors that grow for a period of time and then regress in normal animals will grow progressively in immunosuppressed animals. These observations suggest that, in fact, resistance to tumor growth is mediated by immunological factors.

Support for this conclusion derives from adoptive transfer experiments. Specific tumor resistance is transferable to normal donors using lymphoid cells from immunized animals; the specificity of this adoptive immunity is identical to that observed in transplantation studies, *i.e.*, distinct antigen specificity for chemically induced tumors and common antigen specificity for virus-induced tumors. This can be demonstrated in two ways. In the Winn assay, lymphoid cells are mixed with the tumor cells before inoculation into normal animals; tumor growth does not occur when immune lymphoid cells are present in the mixture. Alternatively, lymphoid cells are inoculated into one site of the normal recipient and the tumor at a separate site; if the lymphoid cells are from an immune donor, tumor growth is suppressed. With a few exceptions, resistance cannot be consistently transferred with antiserum from resistant animals. To the contrary, the passive administration of serum to normal donors sometimes results in enhancement of tumor growth (see below).

Adoptive transfer experiments have established the importance of lymphoid cells in resistance to tumor growth; subsequent studies demonstrated the central role of T lymphocytes in this immunity. The important role of T lymphocytes is demonstrated by cytotoxicity and other *in vitro* cell-mediated immunity assays. T lymphocytes from animals immune to a specific tumor are usually capable of lysing such cells *in vitro* or inhibiting their growth. In order to demonstrate specific lymphocyte-mediated cytotoxicity of chemically or virus-induced tumor cells, the T lymphocytes and target cells must share some portion of the major histocompatibility locus (MHC), *i.e.,* lysis is MHC restricted. In mice this MHC restriction is associated with the K and/or D regions of the H-2 complex. Similar studies suggest that T cell–mediated cytotoxic resistance against some human tumors is also MHC restricted.

In addition to T lymphocytes, other elements in the immune system appear to function in tumor immunity. These include cytotoxic antibodies, natural killer (NK) cells, killer (K) cells, and macrophages.

Antibodies are effective in resistance to some types of tumors, particularly those of lymphoid nature. The mechanism of antibody-mediated tumor immunity probably involves complement-mediated lysis and, possibly, destruction of tumor cells by interaction with K cells in an antibody-dependent cellular cytotoxicity (ADCC) type of reaction.

The evidence implicating NK cells is still largely circumstantial and based mainly on indications that tumor resistance is greater in strains of mice selected for high NK activity. Nude (athymic) mice that lack T cells also appear to be relatively resistant to spontaneous tumor development. Nude mice usually exhibit high levels of NK activity, and it has been postulated that this cell is primarily responsible for the low incidence of spontaneous tumors in these animals. Of potential therapeutic importance is the observation that NK activity can be enhanced by interferon and interferon inducers and by nonspecific immune stimulators, such as avirulent tubercle bacilli (BCG). It is currently believed that the activation of NK cells may have beneficial effects against human cancers, at least partially accounting for the current interest in interferon therapy.

Macrophages and monocytes also play several important roles in tumor immunity. Be-sides being necessary in an auxiliary role for the generation of cytotoxic T lymphocytes, macrophages are activated to an increased cytotoxic potential by a variety of immunological stimulators. Activation of macrophages, resulting in the release of various lymphokines, is probably of importance in the enhanced resistance to tumor growth mediated by some immune stimulators, such as BCG.

The demonstration of tumor immunity mediated by T lymphocytes has provided support for the **immunosurveillance theory** first proposed by Burnet and modified by Thomas in 1959. As presented by Thomas, this theory states that "allograft rejection will turn out to represent a primary mechanism for natural defense against neoplasia," implying that the allograft reaction arose in evolution primarily as a defense against incipient neoplastic disease. This theory requires, therefore, the presence of unique antigens on tumors that the host sees as foreign. Indeed, there is substantial evidence in support of this theory, particularly in relation to virus-induced tumors. Possibly the strongest evidence against the generality of immunosurveillance is the presence of very weak TSTA, or their apparent absence, in most spontaneous tumors and the fact that the incidence of most tumors (except lymphomas) is not significantly increased in immunosuppressed individuals. It is, therefore, still too early to draw any general conclusions about this theory.

IMMUNOLOGICAL ENHANCEMENT OF TUMOR GROWTH[25, 36, 52]

Manipulation of the immune system sometimes results in the enhancement rather than resistance of tumor growth. This enhancement phenomenon has an immunological basis, although the exact mechanisms have not been clearly defined. Enhancement of tumor growth following immunization was noted as early as 1907, in Flexner's report that rats immunized with nonviable Jensen rat sarcoma and challenged with viable tumor cells exhibited tumor progression rather than regression. Casey, in 1932, demonstrated that this tumor-promoting factor was specific for each individual tumor and first labeled this phenomenon as **immunological enhancement.** In 1952, Kaliss ascribed enhancement to antibodies by showing that passive transfer of antibodies from immunized animals to normal animals, prior to tumor challenge, frequently resulted in en-

Table 10–5. **Enhancement of Tumor Growth with Serum from Animals with Progressively Growing Tumors***

Serum Donor	No. of Progressively Growing Tumors/No. of Animals Inoculated with Challenge Tumor	(%) Survivors
None	4/10	60
Immune	0/10	100
Tumor-bearing†	10/10	0

*Animals injected with serum from donor animals before being inoculated with an appropriate number of tumor cells.

†Serum donors bear progressively growing tumors of same type as challenge tumor.

hanced tumor growth. The Hellströms subsequently identified serum factors in mice bearing progressively growing, virus-induced tumors that blocked specific cell-mediated cytotoxicity *in vitro* against the appropriate tumor cell line. It was proposed that these blocking factors participated in immunological enhancement. Their findings suggested that blocking factors represented circulating antigen-antibody complexes, which blocked cell-mediated immunity, possibly by binding to specific receptors on sensitized lymphocytes.

Immunological enhancement can best be illustrated *in vivo* with the Moloney sarcoma virus (MSV). In mice, this virus induces sarcomas, most of which grow for a period of time and then regress; transplantable MSV-induced tumors behave similarly. If serum from animals with progressively growing tumors is used to pretreat normal mice before challenge with viable tumor cells, a high proportion of the challenged animals develop progressively growing tumors that eventually kill the host (Table 10–5). This enhancement effect is specific for the inducing tumor. Blocking of *in vitro* cell-mediated immunity assays and enhancement of tumor growth *in vivo* are apparently mediated by the same serum factor.

Exactly which phase of immune recognition is altered in immunological enhancement is unknown. Both afferent and efferent mechanisms have been proposed. According to the afferent proposed, enhancing factors block immune recognition of the tumor, allowing the tumor cells to grow unimpeded. Masking of tumor antigens by antibody to prevent recognition by the immune system is a possible explanation. According to the efferent proposal, immune cells are generated but are unable to attack tumor cells. Either some receptor on the lymphocyte required for im-

munological destruction of the tumor cell is blocked, possibly by antigen-antibody complexes, or the antigen on the target cell is masked by antibody, preventing immune recognition. Both mechanisms have evidential support, and it is likely that both function in tumor enhancement *in vivo*.

OTHER TUMOR ESCAPE MECHANISMS

Mechanisms other than enhancement may also function in allowing a tumor to grow in the face of an active immune response. Some of these are listed in Table 10–6. **Immunoselection** occurs if a population of tumor cells contains cells with varying antigenic expression. The most antigenic of such cells will be destroyed, resulting in selection of the less antigenic variants that can escape immune recognition. Supporting this possibility is the fact that metastatic cancer cells are frequently less antigenic than the primary tumor cells. **Antigenic modulation** by antibody can also result in changes in or complete disappearance of tumor antigens, allowing the tumor cell to grow in the presence of an active tumor-specific immune response. Recent evidence suggests that tumor cells, or factors released from tumors, can induce the appearance of specific suppressor T cells, which will suppress antitumor immunity. Finally, tumors induced by some agents induce a state of immunological tolerance, preventing the development of a specific anti-tumor response. This is particularly well documented for RNA-containing tumor viruses that are transmitted vertically through the germline from parent to offspring. Animals carrying such viruses are not capable of generating a detectable immune response to

Table 10–6. **Possible Mechanisms That Allow Tumors to Grow in the Presence of Specific Tumor Immunity**

1. *Enhancing or blocking factors:* Antibody or antigen complexes block some phase of immune recognition.

2. *Immunoselection:* Population of tumor cells contains variants with weak TSTAs which are resistant to tumor immunity.

3. *Antigen modulation:* Tumor antigens are altered or removed by, for example, antibody-induced capping.

4. *Tumor induction of suppressor cells:* Tumor acts to suppress cell-mediated immunity against tumor.

5. *Immunological tolerance*

the virus or its products. Therefore, tumors induced by such viruses will be recognized as self and will not be rejected. All of these mechanisms might function *in vivo*, enabling the tumor to circumvent immune surveillance mechanisms.

HUMAN TUMOR ANTIGENS[22, 23, 43, 49]

The demonstration of tumor-specific transplantation antigens on experimental tumors induced in animals has led to extensive examination of human cancers for similar antigens. In general, the results from such studies have been unrewarding. Antigens classified as tumor-associated have been detected in a few tumors, *e.g.*, bladder cancers, melanomas, and adenocarcinomas of the gastrointestinal tract (carcinoembryonic antigens), and in two tumors of apparent virus etiology—Burkitt's lymphoma and nasopharyngeal carcinoma. Examinations of other human cancers have been generally inconclusive or negative.

The search for tumor-specific antigens on human tumor cells have employed mainly cell-mediated immunity assays. Cell lines established from various types of cancers have served as targets, in cellular immunity assays, for lymphocytes from patients with the same or different cancers. The criteria for the existence of tumor antigens associated with a specific cancer have depended upon the demonstration of a specific cellular immune response with lymphocytes from patients with that specific cancer, but not with lymphocytes from normal individuals or patients with other malignancies. Although initial findings were promising, they have not been readily confirmed. Therefore, the question of the existence of tumor antigens associated with most human cancers remains largely unresolved.

The demonstration of tumor-specific antigens in animal systems has resulted in the development and evaluation of different ways to enhance this immunity for the treatment of antigenic cancers. This is known as **immunotherapy** and has been very successful in the treatment of animal cancers. Immunological approaches to the treatment of animal tumors have included nonspecific enhancement of the immune system, with substances such as BCG and *Corynebacterium parvum*; adoptive transfer of specific immunity with lymphocytes, or transfer factor prepared from such lymphocytes; immune serum; inducers of interferon production; and, recently, monoclonal antibodies directed against tumor-specific antigens in experimental tumors. All of these have been used successfully in the treatment of animal cancers, particularly as adjuncts to conventional therapy. These successes have generated optimism that they would also be successful against human neoplasms. Such optimism appears to be unfounded. Whether new advances, particularly the use of monoclonal antibodies directed against putative tumor-specific antigens, will yield effective therapies against human cancers remains to be determined.

Hypersensitivity

Besides having a protective nature, antibodies and immune cells can also have harmful effects by inducing damage to cells and tissues. These latter manifestations are referred to as **allergic** or **hypersensitivity** reactions and can be induced by a variety of substances, including environmental antigens, infectious agents, and simple chemicals. Hypersensitivity reactions are exemplified by the tuberculin skin reactions in individuals infected with *Mycobacterium tuberculosis*; food or drug allergies; hay fever; serum sickness; and, in some instances, autoimmune diseases. Antigens that induce a hypersensitive state are generally called **allergens.** Some allergens are complete antigens, capable of both inducing and eliciting a hypersensitivity reaction, while others act as haptens and must form complexes with a carrier molecule to induce this immunological state.

Hypersensitivity is categorized as **immediate** or **delayed,** depending on whether the reaction is mediated by serum or by sensitized lymphoid cells, and based on differences in the time interval required to elicit the hypersensitive state. Immediate reactions are mediated by antibody and are manifest within a few minutes to a few hours after exposure to antigen. Delayed hypersensitivity reactions, on the other hand, are mediated by sensitized lymphocytes and require a latent period of 48 to 72 hours before producing a visible reaction. Some examples of these hypersensitivity states

Table 10–7. **Examples of Immediate and Delayed Hypersensitivity Reactions**

Immediate Hypersensitivity
Anaphylaxis
Serum sickness
Drug allergies
Bronchial asthma
Allergies to ragweed (hay fever)
Hemolytic anemias
Transfusion reactions
Acute allograft rejection (white graft)

Delayed Hypersensitivity
Microbial antigens (tuberculin)
Contact dermatitis (simple chemicals, poison ivy)
Allograft rejections

are listed in Table 10–7. Based on the mechanisms by which antibodies and immune lymphoid cells produce these effects, hypersensitivity states have been classified by Gell and Coombs into four categories: anaphylactic reactions (type I); cytotoxic reactions (type II); immune complex reactions (type III); and delayed reactions (type IV). Distinguishing characteristics of these categories are listed in Table 10–8. Hypersensitivity reactions types I to III are mediated by antibody and are categorized as "immediate," while those of type IV are cell mediated and categorized as "delayed."

Type II cytotoxic reactions are those mediated by antibody to red blood cells or other tissue antigens. Antibodies are commonly produced following transfusions with unmatched blood or by Rh factor incompatibility, resulting in hemolytic anemia (Chapter 7). This type of reaction is also responsible for acute kidney rejection. These immune reactions are generally mediated by IgG or IgM antibodies and

complement, although complement-independent mechanisms, such as ADCC, might also function *in vivo*. Type III reactions are mediated by immune complexes and are discussed in more detail in the following chapter. This section will focus on the type I and type IV categories—the most common hypersensitivity reactions.

IMMEDIATE HYPERSENSITIVITY

ANAPHYLACTIC REACTIONS[1, 2, 17, 20, 40, 41, 45, 46, 53]

The term anaphylaxis was first used in 1902 to describe a fatal reaction in dogs that followed the second administration of a toxin obtained from sea anemones. Animals responded to the second sublethal inoculation of this toxin with symptoms suggestive of vasodilation followed by vascular collapse and death. This phenomenon was termed "anaphylaxis" to distinguish it from immunity—the "prophylactic state." Anaphylaxis now describes an acute, shock-like reaction that follows second exposure of a sensitized individual to an antigen. Systemic reactions are referred to as **generalized anaphylaxis. Local anaphylaxis** is demonstrated by injection of the appropriate antigen into the skin of a sensitized individual. The latter reaction is characterized by localized swelling, edema, and inflammation at the site of inoculation shortly following antigen injection. Both systemic and local anaphylactic reactions have now been demonstrated in most species, including humans.

Besides the anaphylactic syndromes described above, all allergic, or **atopic,** states

Table 10–8. **Categories of Hypersensitivity Reactions**

Type	Description
I. Anaphylactic (allergy or atopy)	Mediated by circulating or cell-bound antibody, predominantly IgE; immediate in onset; affects primarily smooth muscle components.
II. Cytotoxic reaction	Mediated by antibody and complement; antigen associated with cell membrane; immediate in onset.
III. Toxic complex reaction (immune complex or Arthus-type)	Mediated by soluble antigen-antibody complexes and complement; complexes deposited in blood vessels or in base membranes with resultant local inflammation; variable in onset.
IV. Delayed (cellular) reaction	Mediated by sensitized T lymphocytes following reaction with antigen; reaction sites in skin and parenchymatous organs; delayed in onset (24–72 hours).

such as food and drug allergies, hay fever, and asthma are also consequences of local anaphylactic reactions. This type of hypersensitivity is linked to antibodies in the IgE immunoglobulin class and to various mediators affecting smooth muscle that are released from mast cells and basophils.

The immunological basis of an anaphylaxis was established initially by the recognition of certain requirements similar to those necessary for the initiation of an immune response to an antigen: (1) prior exposure to the inciting substance is required to elicit the reaction, since anaphylaxis reactions rarely, if ever, occur following primary exposure to the agent; (2) an incubation or latent period, sufficient for the development of an antibody response, is required between the first and subsequent exposure to the agent; (3) the specificity of these reactions parallels that of antigen-antibody reactions; and (4) it is possible to transfer the hypersensitive state to normal hosts with specific antiserum from a sensitized host. In a classical study, Prausnitz and Küstner were able to transfer an allergic reaction against fish to a normal individual. The serum from an individual sensitive to a certain species of cooked fish was injected into the skin of a normal, nonsensitive individual. After 24 hours, this individual was injected subcutaneously with a small quantity of the fish allergen. Within a few hours, a local wheal and flare reaction occurred at the second site of inoculation. Now known as the **Prausnitz-Küstner** reaction, this simple test is widely used to identify immediate hypersensitivity to a variety of allergens.

Specific participants in anaphylaxis include a specific type of antibody capable of binding to certain cell types; cells that contain vasoactive amines; and the inducing antigen or allergen.

The basic mechanism of anaphylaxis involves the induction of special antibody (IgE) and its attachment to mast cells or basophils through specific cellular receptors. Subsequent reaction of antigen with the cell-bound antibody triggers the release of pharmacologically active substance from the cells; these exert their effects on the smooth muscle components of target tissues. These reactions are summarized in Figure 10–2.

The target tissue for anaphylaxis varies in different species, but in all cases it is the smooth muscle element of the organ or tissue that is affected. In the guinea pig, for example, anaphylaxis is characterized by suffocation brought about by contraction of the smooth

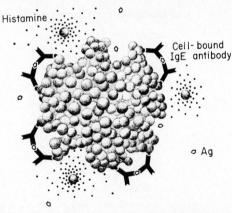

Figure 10–2. Diagram of the essential features of the immediate hypersensitivity reaction, which results in the release of histamine from mast cells. Note the requirement for attachment of antigen to two antibody molecules to initiate this reaction. (Courtesy of Dr. Gerald Gleich, Departments of Immunology and Internal Medicine, Mayo Foundation and Mayo Medical School, Rochester, Minn.)

muscles of the bronchi. In rabbits, the major target sites are pulmonary arteries, while in humans and dogs, smooth muscles in different areas of the vascular system are affected, ending in vascular collapse and death.

In addition to this immediate reaction, there is a late-phase hypersensitivity reaction, which is more intense and destructive to normal tissues. Both the immediate and late-phase reactions are mediated by IgE antibodies and are characterized by cutaneous erythema and edema. Late reactions, in which basophils appear to play a major role, are characterized by significant tissue damage leading to blood vessel necrosis and hemorrhage. Cells infiltrating the tissues in the late phase are predominantly mononuclear, but neutrophils, eosinophils, and basophils are also present. Eosinophils frequently infiltrate the sites of allergic reactions, and their presence is considered the hallmark of such reactions. Late hypersensitivity reactions mediated by IgE are often seen in the lungs of patients with bronchial asthma. A schematic diagram showing the immediate and late-phase reactions is presented in Figure 10–3.

Cytotropic Antibodies[3, 4, 32–34, 42, 46]

The nature of antibodies responsible for anaphylactic reactions has been of great interest over the past few years. It is now generally accepted that there are two categories of antibodies, originally referred to as **reagins,** mediating this reaction. IgE is the major class of antibody responsible in all species, possibly excepting guinea pigs. In addition, some subclasses of IgG can mediate the reaction in

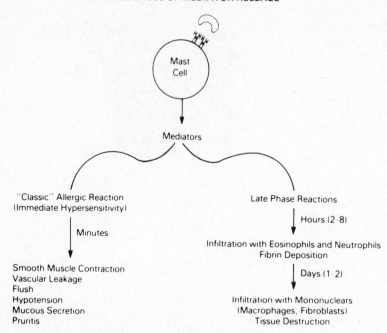

Figure 10–3. Schematic diagram showing the immediate and late phase of reactions of immediate hypersensitivity. (Oertel, H. L., and Kaliner, M., J. Immunol. **127**:1398–1402, 1981)

guinea pigs and mice. Interestingly, neither IgE nor the active IgG subclasses readily fix complement by the classical pathway; they both can, however, activate complement through the alternate pathway.

A fundamental characteristic of these antibodies is their ability to bind to receptors on mast cells or basophils. This binding takes place between the Fc portion of the antibody molecule and a specific receptor on the cell surface. Antibodies with this specialized ability to bind to certain cells are called **cytotropic antibodies.** Antibodies that bind to mast cells or basophils of their own or closely related animal species are referred to as **homocytotropic.** An example of this type of antibody is human IgE, which binds to human and monkey mast cells, but not to guinea pig cells. In contrast, some antibodies do not bind to cells of their own species, but do bind to those of a phylogenetically distant species. For example, human IgG binds to guinea pig cells, but not to human cells. These antibodies are designated **heterocytotropic antibodies.**

The necessity for cytotropic antibodies in the initiation of anaphylaxis is demonstrable by **passive cutaneous anaphylaxis** (PCA). Antibody is injected intradermally into a normal host and, after a suitable latent period, a mixture of Evan's blue and antigen is injected intravenously. Staining of the skin occurs at the site of the antigen-antibody reaction, due to increased capillary permeability, and its dimensions are a measure of the intensity of the antigen-antibody reaction. PCA reactions are readily demonstrated in the guinea pig and have, therefore, been studied most extensively in this animal. This is a very sensitive test and is capable of detecting as little as 0.1 μg. antibody. The important point about this assay is that a latent period is required for effective sensitization of the tissue. The latent period required between the time of IgG antibody administration and antigen challenge can be as short as 1 hour in the guinea pig, but is usually optimal after 4 hours and persists for less than 24 hours. In contrast, a latent period of 24 to 48 hours is required for PCA reactions with IgE antibodies. The latent period represents the time required for the antibody to react with and become fixed to receptor sites on mast cells and basophils. Noncytotropic antibodies are ineffective in the PCA reaction. The order of antigen and antibody injection can be reversed in this test if the antigen is a cytotropic immunoglobulin, such as IgG in the guinea pig. Anti-IgG can then be injected intravenously to demonstrate a cutaneous anaphylactic reaction. This is **reverse passive anaphylaxis,** and has been useful to demonstrate the importance of the cytotropic character of antibody in the mediation of anaphylaxis.

Anaphylaxis may also be demonstrated *in vitro*. The Schultz-Dale reaction has been particularly useful in establishing the role of cytotropic antibody in this phenomenon. Anaphylactic shock is manifest in isolated smooth muscle as a sharp and abrupt contraction. Uterine strips from sensitized animals are suspended in a bath of Ringer's solution with one end tied fast and the other attached to a kymograph. The addition of antibody to the bath causes measurable contraction of the sensitive muscle strip. All the essential features of anaphylaxis can be reproduced *in vitro* by this method, including passive sensitization, *i.e.*, normal uterine muscle can be first sensitized with antibody before adding antigen.

Mediators of Anaphylaxis[1, 31, 41, 44, 53]

Interaction of antigen with antibody bound to mast cells triggers release of vasoreactive amines of low molecular weight. Among these substances are histamine, serotonin, kinins, a substance called the slow reacting substance of anaphylaxis (SRS–A), platelet activating factor (PAF), eosinophil chemotactic factor of anaphylaxis (ECF–A), and neutrophil chemotactic factor (NCF). Some characteristics of these factors are shown in Table 10–9.

Release of these mediators from mast cells, a process called **degranulation**, requires crosslinking or bridging of the antibody molecules by a polyvalent antigen; univalent antigens are ineffective. The reason for this is unclear but is thought to involve a change in membrane structure necessary to activate the degranulation process. This is schematically illustrated in Figure 10–2. Histamine is the most important mediator of anaphylactic reactions in man. All of these factors, with the exception of SRS–A and PAF, exist preformed in granules within mast cells and basophils and are released by the antigen-antibody reaction at the cell surface. SRS–A and PAF are generated just before release from the cell. Release of histamine, serotonin, or kinins causes contraction of smooth muscle, increased vasodilation, and capillary permeability of vessels and is particularly active on human bronchiolar smooth muscle. The activity of histamine and serotonin can be countered with antihistamines and antiserotonin agents. **Anaphylatoxins,** high-molecular-weight substances formed during the activation of the complement system, also causes the release of histamine from mast cells (Chapter 7). These breakdown products of the C3 and C5 components of complement can be produced in the presence of IgE antibodies by activation of the alternate complement pathway and are designated C3a and C5a, respectively. Release of these substances is an active process requiring energy, an intact glycolytic pathway, and activation of serine esterase.

ATOPIC ALLERGIES[37, 53]

Atopic allergies are those human hypersensitivity states for which an inheritable basis is suspected. These include such disorders as hay fever, food allergies, and asthma. Allergies to food usually present as acute gastrointestinal distress with urticarial rashes, while local reactions, such as hay fever, usually affect the nasal mucosa and upper respiratory tract. Asthma results from constriction of the bronchi, hampering air flow into the lungs. These symptoms are all caused by localized anaphylactic events involving IgE antibodies to the inciting agents and the release of low-molecular-weight mediators, such as histamine and SRS–A, which affect the smooth muscle components of the surrounding tissues. The release of histamine from mast cells or basophils can

Table 10–9. **Chemical Mediators of Anaphylaxis**

Mediator	Manifestations
Histamine	Increased vascular permeability; enhancement of eosinophil migration; contraction of smooth muscle.
Serotonin	Contraction of smooth muscle.
Slow reacting substance of anaphylaxis (SRS–A)	Contraction of human bronchiole; increased vascular permeability.
Platelet activating factor (PAF)	Aggregation and lysis of platelets.
Eosinophil chemotactic factor of anaphylaxis (ECF–A)	Chemotactic attraction and inactivation of eosinophils.
Neutrophil chemotactic factor (NCF)	Chemotactic attraction and inactivation of neutrophils.

be demonstrated *in vitro* by exposing leucocytes from a sensitized or allergic individual to the appropriate allergen. Similarly, serum from allergic individuals can be used to sensitize cells from a normal individual, so that these cells will also release histamine following exposure to the allergen.

An atopic individual can be desensitized to a specific allergen by repeated injections with small doses of the antigen. The mechanism of this desensitization appears to involve the induction of noncytotropic IgG antibodies, which are capable of binding to the antigen, competitively inhibiting its reaction or combination with cytotropic IgE antibodies. Such desensitizing antibodies are commonly referred to as blocking antibodies. This has been a very effective means of preventing allergic reactions, particularly those of seasonal nature.

DRUG ALLERGIES[20, 53]

Drug allergies are also manifestations of anaphylactic responses mediated by IgE antibodies. These are generally not directed against the native substance but against metabolites or breakdown products of the natural substances produced by the action of microsomal enzymes of the liver. Therefore, it is frequently difficult to isolate the exact component responsible for eliciting the drug reaction for use in desensitization. It is believed that such allergens form complexes with the host cell proteins to constitute a complete antigen, since the drugs themselves are generally nonimmunogenic. They become immunogenic, however, after coupling to a carrier protein.

Allergy to penicillin is probably the most common drug allergy, affecting 1 to 5 per cent of the population. The allergic response appears to be directed against a metabolic product of penicillin, which becomes immunogenic following attachment to host cell proteins. Reactions to penicillin are of two kinds. Sudden reactions occur in individuals previously sensitized to this drug, and the symptoms resemble those of systemic anaphylaxis. This response occurs within seconds or up to a few hours following administration of penicillin. Late reactions occur in individuals with no history of prior exposure to penicillin. Symptoms generally appear 5 to 14 days following administration and are characterized by urticaria, polyadenopathy, joint swelling, and pain. Treatment of allergic reactions is by the use of catecholamines such as epinephrine to inhibit the effect of histamine on smooth muscles and vascular permeability, or by antihistamines to block histamine at its site of action.

DELAYED HYPERSENSITIVITY REACTIONS[6, 15, 18, 19, 21, 55]

Koch was the first to note that guinea pigs, recovered from previous infection with the tubercle bacillus and reinjected with the same organism, responded with an indurated non-necrotic lesion at the site of the second inoculation; the lesion reached a maximum size in 24 to 48 hours and then subsided. The microorganisms also did not spread systemically, as occurred following the first inoculation, but remained localized in enlarged regional lymph nodes. Thus, animals surviving primary exposure to the bacilli developed a resistance to systemic spread of the organism upon re-exposure. This phenomenon is recognized as an example of **delayed hypersensitivity** and has an immunological basis. It is distinguished from immediate hypersensitivity by the time elapsing between antigen re-exposure and appearance of symptoms, *e.g.,* 24 to 48 hours for delayed reactions as opposed to minutes to a few hours for immediate reactions. Delayed hypersensitivity is also fundamentally different, since it is mediated by immune lymphoid cells, in contrast to antibody mediation of immediate hypersensitivity. Delayed hypersensitivity is commonly observed following a second exposure to infectious agents, both bacterial and viral, and is also responsible for the clinical manifestations of **contact dermatitis** or **eczema,** which sometimes develops following skin contact with such substances as simple chemicals, synthetic resins, cosmetics, or locally applied drugs and ointments.

In humans, the prototype delayed-type hypersensitivity (DTH) reaction is characterized by erythema and induration. In other species, the appearance of erythema is variable, so that delayed hypersensitivity reactions are commonly detected by increases in skin thickness at the inoculation site 24 to 48 hours after exposure. For example, in mice these reactions are usually elicited in the footpad and are scored by increases in the thickness of the footpad at 24 to 48 hours. Histologically, delayed reactions are characterized by infiltrates of mononuclear cells and neutrophils that increase in numbers to reach a maximum between 24 and 48 hours following a second antigen exposure. The mononuclear infiltrate consists of monocytes and small to medium-sized lymphocytes, with the majority of cells having characteristics of activated macrophages. Only a small proportion of the cells in such lesions are T lymphocytes. This was first shown by McClusky and co-workers, who transferred radiolabeled lymphocytes from sensitized to nonsensitized guinea pigs, exposed these animals to the appropriate antigen, and examined the skin lesions after 48 hours for both radioactivity and specific cell types. Only 3 to 4 per cent of the cells in these lesions were derived from the donor lymphocytes, while the remainder of the cells, mainly macrophages, were derived from the host. The presence of macrophage infiltrates in these lesions is, therefore, considered to be the hallmark of delayed hypersensitivity reactions.

Although macrophages are the predominant cell in these lesions, delayed hypersensitivity reactions directed against infectious agents or chemicals are initiated by a subpopulation of T lymphocytes, and the immunological specificity is determined by this cell type. In classical experiments, Landsteiner and Chase established that delayed hypersensitivity could be transferred to a normal host with sensitized cells, but not with antibody. They successfully transferred tuberculin sensitivity to normal animals using peritoneal exudate, spleen, and lymph node cells from immune donors; successful transfers also required viable cells. The requirement for T lymphocyte participation is illustrated by the failure to elicit delayed hypersensitivity in animals lacking a thymus. This has also been shown by eliminating T cells in lymphocytic preparations before adoptive transfer by treatment with antithymocyte serum and complement. Elimination of macrophages does not, however, abolish the ability of these lymphoid preparations to transfer delayed hypersensitivity. B lymphocytes do not appear to participate directly in delayed hypersensitivity reactions, although they may be indirectly involved by producing various lymphokines that are important in the pathogenesis of these reactions (see below). With the recent demonstration of Ly cell surface markers that characterize different mouse T cell subpopulations, it has been noted that the T cell population active in delayed-type hypersensitivity reactions (T_{DTH}) expresses only the Ly-1 surface marker, a similarity shared with T_H cells that act as helpers for antibody production (Chapter 9).

Antigens capable of inducing delayed hypersensitivity must have a protein component; polysaccharide antigens will not generally induce a delayed state unless coupled to a protein. Similarly, small molecules such as dinitrofluorobenzene, picryl chloride, or compounds containing metallic groups will not induce delayed hypersensitivity by themselves, but are very effective inducers when coupled to a protein carrier. In the case of contact sensitivity, the chemical combines with protein in the epidermis to form the immunogen.

Interestingly, proteins by themselves, however, are not potent inducers of delayed hypersensitivity under most conditions. For example, hypersensitivity to the tubercle bacillus is effectively induced by viable microorganisms, and the sensitive state can be demonstrated by skin testing with the purified protein component, tuberculin. However, tuberculin itself is ineffective for inducing the hypersensitive state. The active component of the tubercle bacilli required for induction of hypersensitivity is the complex glycolipid called Wax D in the cell wall, while the specificity of the reaction is directed against the protein moiety. If purified tuberculin is mixed with Wax D, the mixture will now induce a hypersensitive state, whereas neither alone is effective. Similarly, many proteins are far more effective as sensitizing antigens when incorporated into complete Freund's adjuvant (containing mycobacteria). In the absence of adjuvant, sensitization to soluble proteins generally occurs only following immunization with small quantities. Larger amounts result in the induction of antibody formation. The reason for this is still not completely understood, but might be related to the necessity of inducing an inflammatory response, with infiltration by macrophages, before a delayed hypersensitivity state can be induced. The Wax D cell wall component appears to be necessary for inducing this inflammatory response.

The route of inoculation of the antigen is also critical to the induction of the delayed hypersensitivity state. Intradermal inoculation is by far the most effective route for sensitization. Intravenous inoculation is not effective, while subcutaneous and intramuscular injections will induce delayed hypersensitive responses if the antigen is administered in complete Freund's adjuvant. Contact sensitivity to simple chemicals is normally induced through the skin and requires the binding or coupling of the chemical to skin proteins to form an immunogen. This can be bypassed, however, if the chemical coupled to a carrier protein is inoculated in the presence of complete Freund's adjuvant.

Skin proteins participate in the specificity of

DTH reaction to chemicals or other antigens introduced by this route. Guinea pigs sensitized by painting the skin with picryl chloride will react strongly to this compound readministered through the skin or when coupled to skin proteins, but not when the chemical is coupled to other nonrelated proteins. Similarly, guinea pigs sensitized with picryl chloride coupled to a nonskin protein, even when given with complete Freund's adjuvant, will not produce a delayed hypersensitivity reaction to the chemical itself when readministered through the skin. These results indicate that in contact sensitization, the immune cells need to recognize the protein carrier as well as the chemical before initiating a delayed hypersensitivity reaction.

The antigen recognition phase of delayed hypersensitivity is similar to that described for the development of other types of immune responses, *i.e.*, a specific subpopulation of T lymphocytes is stimulated by antigen-presenting cells, presumably macrophages. As with other immune reactions, this phase requires identity at the MHC locus between the macrophage and T lymphocyte, as shown in adoptive transfer experiments. Successful transfer of delayed hypersensitivity only occurs when there is complete identity at the MHC between the recipient and donor. This restriction maps to the I–A region of the H-2 complex in mice. This MHC-restricted interaction results in the activation of T_{DTH} cells, which then recruit and activate other macrophages to the inoculation site during the second phase of the reaction. This is believed to take place by the release of soluble lymphokines from the activated T_{DTH} cells, to recruit, activate, and immobilize macrophages in the reaction area. Some of the factors secreted by T_{DTH} cells that appear to be important in the pathogenesis of delayed hypersensitivity reaction include **migration inhibitory factor** (MIF), described in Chapter 8, believed to immobilize macrophages at the site of reaction; **macrophage activating factor** (MAF), possibly responsible for the activation of macrophages; and **chemotactic factor**, thought to be reponsible for recruiting bone marrow–derived macrophages to the reaction site. All of these factors are present in cell-free supernatant fluids from cultures containing both sensitized lymphocytes and antigen, showing that the production of such factors is triggered by antigen stimulation. Injection of supernatant fluids containing these factors into the skin of normal animals elicits an inflammatory response with histological characteristics of delayed hypersensitivity.

This proposed mechanism for DTH would account for the predominance of macrophages in the reaction site and for the presence of only a small number of T lymphocytes. Macrophages, therefore, are important cells in both the sensitization phase and the second phase of the development of the DTH reaction, which results in the manifestations of this immune reaction.

TRANSFER FACTOR

It has been recognized for a number of years that delayed hypersensitivity in humans can be transferred with extracts prepared from sensitized lymphocytes. Individuals treated with such preparations become reactive to specific antigens within a week following administration, and sensitivity to the antigens persists indefinitely. The active substance in these preparations is termed transfer factor. The exact nature of this factor is still unknown after many years of study. It is dialyzable, with a molecular weight of less than 10,000; stable in solution and upon storage; sensitive to heating at 56°C. for 30 minutes; resistant to digestion by trypsin, RNAse, and DNAse; and nonantigenic. It has been postulated that transfer factor converts recipient lymphocytes into an antigen-sensitive state whereupon the cells can proliferate in the presence of a specific antigen. This is supported by the fact that cells can be sensitized *in vitro* to respond to a specific antigen, using transfer factor. For example, lymphocytes from a tuberculin-negative individual can be converted to a sensitive state by *in vitro* treatment with transfer factor from a tuberculin-positive individual. It is also possible to transfer specific cell-mediated immunity to skin grafts with transfer factor. More importantly, transfer factor might be of clinical value in the treatment of disseminated infections in immunodeficient individuals. For example, transfer factor is effective in the treatment of both disseminated vaccinia and *Candida* infections. There has also been a great deal of interest in the use of transfer factor for treatment of human cancers. Further clarification of the nature of transfer factor would be of great importance in developing a complete understanding of delayed hypersensitivity reactions and cellular immunity in general.

References

1. Austen, K. F., and R. P. Orange. 1975. Bronchial asthma: the possible role of the chemical mediators of immediate hypersensitivity in the pathogenesis of subacute chronic disease. Amer. Rev. Respir. Dis. **112**:423–436.
2. Becker, E. L. 1971. Nature and classification of immediate-type allergic reactions. Adv. Immunol. **13**:267–313.
3. Bennich, H., and S. G. O. Johansson. 1971. Structure and function of human IgE. Adv. Immunol. **13**:1–57.
4. Bloch, K. J. 1969. The antibody in anaphylaxis. pp. 1–12. *In* H. Z. Movat (Ed.): Cellular and Humoral Mechanisms in Anaphylaxis and Allergy. Karger, New York.
5. Bloom, B. R. 1971. In vitro approaches to the mechanism of cell-mediated immune reactions. Adv. Immunol. **13**:101–208.
6. Bloom, B. R., and B. Bennett. 1970. Relation of the migration inhibition factor (MIF) to delayed-type hypersensitivity reactions. Ann. N.Y. Acad. Sci. **169**:258–265.
7. Bloom, B. R., and R. David. 1976. In Vitro Methods in Cell-Mediated Immunity and Tumor Immunity. Academic Press, New York.
8. Brent, L., and I. V. Hutchison. 1981. The principles and practice of transplantation tolerance. pp. 33–60. *In* T. Hraba and M. Hašek (Eds.): Cellular and Molecular Mechanisms of Immunologic Tolerance. Immunology Series, Vol. 16. Marcel Dekker, Inc., New York.
9. Burnet, F. M. 1967. Immunological aspects of malignant disease. Lancet **1**:1171–1174.
10. Burnet, F. M. 1970. Immunological Surveillance. Pergamon Press, New York.
11. Carpenter, C. B., A. J. F. d'Apice, and A. K. Abbas. 1976. The role of antibodies in rejection and enhancement of organ allografts. Adv. Immunol. **22**:1–65.
12. Carpenter, C. B., and T. B. Strom. 1980. Transplantation immunology. pp. 376–444. *In* C. W. Parker (Ed.): Clinical Immunology. W. B. Saunders Co., Philadelphia.
13. Castro, J. E. (Ed.). 1977. Immunological Aspects of Cancer. University Park Press, Baltimore.
14. Cerottini, J. and K. T. Brunner. 1974. Cell-mediated cytotoxicity, allograft rejection, and tumor immunity. Adv. Immunol. **18**:67–132.
15. Chase, M. W. 1965. Delayed hypersensitivity. Med. Clin. North Amer. **49**:1613–1646.
16. Cinader, B. 1981. Tolerance as a facet of immune regulation—the trail from the past into the future. pp. 3–32. *In* T. Hraba and M. Hašek (Eds.): Cellular and Molecular Mechanisms of Immunologic Tolerance. Immunology Series, Vol. 16. Marcel Dekker, Inc., New York.
17. Coombs, R., R. A. Gell, and P. G. H. Gell. 1968. Classification of allergic reactions responsible for clinical hypersensitivity and disease. pp. 575–596. *In* P. G. H. Gell and R. R. A. Coombs (Eds.): Clinical Aspects of Immunology. F. A. Davis Co., Philadelphia.
18. Crowle, A. J. 1975. Delayed hypersensitivity in the mouse. Adv. Immunol. **20**:197–264.
19. David, J. R. 1968. Macrophage migration. In vitro correlates of delayed hypersensitivity. Fedn. Proc. **27**:6–12.
20. DeWeck, A. L. 1971. Immunochemical mechanisms of hypersensitivity to antibiotics. Solutions to the penicillin allergy problems. pp. 208–215. *In* U. Serafini *et al.* (Eds.): New Concepts in Allergy and Clinical Immunology. Excerpta Medica, London.
21. DeWeck, A. L. 1977. Immune responses to environmental antigens that act on the skin: the role of lymphokines in contact dermatitis. Fedn. Proc. **36**:1742–1747.
22. Fahey, J. L., and J. Zighelboim. 1980. Tumor immunology. pp 445–472. *In* C. W. Parker (Ed): Clinical Immunology. W. B. Saunders Co., Philadelphia.
23. Gold, P., and S. O. Freedman. 1965. Demonstration of tumor-specific antigens in human colonic carcinomata by immunologic tolerance and absorption techniques. J. Exptl. Med. **121**:439–462.
24. Grebe, S. C., and J. W. Streilein. 1976. Graft-versus-host reactions: a review. Adv. Immunol. **22**:120–221.
25. Hellström, K. E., and I. Hellström. 1970. Immunological enhancement as studied by cell culture techniques. Ann. Rev. Microbiol. **24**:373–398.
26. Hellström, K. E., and I. Hellström. 1976. Cell-mediated immunity to mouse tumors: some recent findings. Ann. N.Y. Acad. Sci. **276**:176–187.
27. Herberman, R. B. 1974. Cell-mediated immunity to tumor cells. Adv. Cancer Res. **19**:207–264.
28. Herberman, R. B., and H. T. Holden. 1978. Natural cell-mediated immunity. Adv. Cancer Res. **27**:305–355.
29. Herberman, R. B., and H. T. Holden. 1979. Natural killer cells as antitumor effector cells. J. Natl. Cancer Inst. **62**:441–445.
30. Herberman, R. B., *et al.* 1979. Natural killer cells: characteristics and regulation of activity. Immunol. Rev. **44**:43–70.
31. Hugli, T. E., and H. J. Müller-Eberhard. 1978. Anaphylatoxins: C3a and C5a. Adv. Immunol. **26**:1–55.
32. Ishizaka, K. 1969. Characterization of human reaginic antibodies and immunologloglobulin E. pp. 63–89. *In* H. Z. Movat (Ed.): Cellular and Humoral Mechanisms in Anaphylaxis and Allergy. S. Karger, New York.
33. Ishizaka, K., and T. Ishizaka. 1971. Immunoglobulin E and homocytotrophic properties. pp. 859–874. *In* B. Amos (Ed.): Progress in Immunology. Academic Press, New York.
34. Ishizaka, K. 1976. Cellular events in the IgE antibody response. Adv. Immunol. **23**:1–75.
35. Kahan, B. D., and R. A. Reisfeld. 1969. Transplantation antigens. Science **164**:514–521.
36. Kaliss, N. 1958. Immunological enhancement of tumor homografts in mice: a review. Cancer Res. **18**:992–1003.
37. King, T. P. 1976. Chemical and biological properties of some atopic allergens. Adv. Immunol. **23**:77–105.
38. Klein, G., and H. F. Oettgen. 1969. Immunologic factors involved in the growth of primary tumors in human or animal hosts. Cancer Res. **29**:1741–1746.
39. Law, L. W., M. J. Rogers, and E. Appella. 1980. Tumor antigens on neoplasms induced by chemical carcinogens and by DNA- and RNA-containing viruses: properties of the solubilized antigens. Adv. Cancer Res. **32**:201–237.
40. Lichtenstein, L. M. 1979. Anaphylactic reactions. pp. 13–28. *In* S. Cohen, P. A. Ward, and R. T. McCluskey (Eds.): Mechanisms of Immunopathology. John Wiley & Sons, New York.

41. Lichenstein, L., M., and A. G. Osler. 1964. Studies on the mechanisms of hypersensitivity phenomena. 9. Histamine release from human leucocytes by ragweed pollen antigens. J. Exptl. Med. **120**:507–530.

42. Metzger, H. 1978. The IgE-mast cell system as a paradigm for the study of antibody mechanisms. Immunol. Rev. **41**:186–199.

43. Oettgen, H. F., L. J. Old, and E. A. Boyse. 1971. Human tumor immunology. Med. Clin. North Amer. **55**:761–785.

44. Orange, R. P., and K. F. Austen. 1971. Chemical mediators of immediate hypersensitivity. pp. 115–125. *In* R. A. Good and D. W. Fisher (Eds.): Immunobiology. Sinauer Associates, Stamford, Conn.

45. Ovary, Z. 1964. Passive cutaneous anaphylaxis. pp. 259–275. *In* J. F. Ackroyd (Ed.): Immunological Methods. Blackwell, Oxford.

46. Ovary, Z., B. Benacerraf, K. J. Block. 1963. Properties of guinea pig 7S antibodies. 2: Identification of antibodies involved in passive cutaneous and systemic anaphylaxis. J. Exptl. Med. **117**:951–964.

47. Pearson, G. R. 1978. In vitro and in vivo investigations on antibody-dependent cellular cytotoxicity. Curr. Topics Microbiol. Immunol. **80**:65–96.

48. Perlmann, P., and G. Holm. 1969. Cytotoxic effects of lymphoid cells in vitro. Adv. Immunol. **11**:117–193.

49. Reisfeld, R. A. 1981. Tumor antigens. Fedn. Proc. **40**:228–230.

50. Roehm, N. W., B. K. Alter, and F. M. Bach. 1981. Lyt phenotype of alloreactive precursor and effector cytotoxic T lymphocytes. J. Immunol. **126**:353–359.

51. Strober, S. 1981. Regulation by T lymphocyte subsets. Fedn. Proc. **40**:1462.

52. Stuart, F. P., and F. W. Fitch. 1978. Immunological Tolerance and Enhancement. University Park Press, Baltimore.

53. Sullivan, T. J., and A. Kulczacki, Jr. 1980. Immediate hypersensitivity reactions. pp. 115–142. *In* C.W. Parker (Ed.): Clinical Immunology. W. B. Saunders Co., Philadelphia.

54. Takasugi, M., M. R. Mickey, and P. I. Terasaki. 1973. Reactivity of lymphocytes from normal persons on cultured tumor cells. Cancer Res. **33**:2898–2902.

55. Turk, J. L. 1975. Delayed Hypersensitivity. Frontiers of Biology, Vol. 4. American Elsevier, New York.

56. Wilson, D. B., and R. E. Billingham. 1967. Lymphocytes and transplantation immunity. Adv. Immunol. **7**:189–273.

CHAPTER 11

Immunity, Autoimmunity, and Immunopathology

Gary R. Pearson, Ph.D.

THE IMMUNE RESPONSE IN
  ACQUIRED IMMUNITY
KINETICS OF ANTIBODY
  PRODUCTION
MECHANISMS OF IMMUNITY
VACCINES

Inactivated Vaccines
Component Vaccines
Attenuated Vaccines
Passive Immunity
AUTOIMMUNITY
IMMUNE COMPLEX DISEASES

Immunity is generally discussed in the context of infectious diseases and refers to the resistance of an individual to second infections by the same or closely related infectious agent. This type of immunity is commonly known as **acquired immunity,** as opposed to natural immunity, discussed in Chapter 12. Since it develops following initial exposure to the inciting agent, it reflects the development of specific **immunological memory** to an antigen following the primary encounter. This memory phenomenon allows an individual to respond immunologically more quickly and more efficiently following any subsequent exposure to the same or closely related antigen. Such an individual is, therefore, considered "immune" to that antigen or, in the case of infectious agents, to the disease manifestations caused by a specific microorganism. Immunological memory forms the basis for the rational development of vaccines for the prevention of infectious diseases.

In addition to immunity, however, other manifestations of the immune response to a specific antigen can initiate disease processes. In one category of diseases with an immunological basis, the immune response is directed against self components, thereby disrupting the tolerance to "self" antigens that exists under normal conditions. Immune response to "self" components can cause tissue damage by a variety of mechanisms and result in disease symptoms characteristic of **autoimmune diseases.** Other immunologically induced disease manifestations can also be initiated following the *in vivo* interaction of antigen with antibody to form circulating immune complexes. These complexes can cause tissue damage when deposited in excess in a specific organ, such as the kidney, or when present in large quantities in the circulation. This chapter will focus on some of the different manifestations associated with the immune response.

The Immune Response in Acquired Immunity

KINETICS OF ANTIBODY PRODUCTION

There is a marked difference in the antibody response following the first or primary exposure to an antigen compared to that seen after secondary or subsequent exposure. These differences are reflected in both the time of

antibody appearance and the immunoglobulin class of the antibody formed. Following the initial encounter with a specific antigen, circulating antibody is usually detected after a latent period of 10 to 14 days, rises slowly to moderate levels, and then declines to low or undetectable levels. The factors influencing longevity of antibody in the peripheral circulation are the nature and concentration of the antigen and the serum half-life of the immunoglobulin molecule. With nonreplicating agents, antibody declines to undetectable levels in serum within 1 to 3 months following the initial encounter. In contrast, antibodies directed against a replicating antigen, such as an infectious agent, may persist for years. For example, herpesviruses establish a latent state following a primary infection and persist in the infected individual for life. Antibodies to these viruses, generally of the IgG class, also persist for life, at moderate levels. The presence of such antibodies in the serum is normally indicative of immunity to a superimposed infection with the same agent.

In contrast to the temporal pattern of antibody synthesis noted following primary antigenic exposure, a second exposure to the same antigen results in the appearance of antibody after a shorter latent period, generally within a few days, and usually reaching higher levels than noted following the primary response. In the case of nonreplicating antigens, antibodies persist in the peripheral circulation for a longer time. This secondary, or **anamnestic,** antibody response is attributed to immunological memory, which develops following the initial encounter with an antigen. Memory to a specific antigen persists for life, under most circumstances, and appears to be due to the persistence of memory cells in both B and T cell subpopulations.

The cellular immune response active in graft and tumor rejection and in the mediation of delayed hypersensitivity responses also shows a similar pattern following primary and secondary exposure to the appropriate antigen. This is most easily illustrated with skin grafts, as discussed in Chapter 10. Primary allogenetic skin grafts are generally rejected within 14 days. In contrast, secondary skin grafts are rejected in an accelerated fashion, reflecting the existence of T cell immunological memory.

The nature of the antibodies synthesized following primary exposure differs from the nature of those formed after secondary exposure to an antigen, as depicted in Figure 11–1. This difference can be of diagnostic importance, as will be discussed below. In most cases, the first antibody produced following the initial encounter with an antigen is of the IgM class. Except for thymus-independent antigens, such as pneumococcus polysaccharides that induce only IgM antibody formation, this IgM antibody response is transitory and is later replaced by a more sustained IgG antibody response persisting for a longer period of time.

In contrast, antibodies of the secondary, or anamnestic, response are predominantly of the IgG class. In some instances there may also be a transitory IgM antibody response following a second exposure to an antigen, but this is an inconsistent finding.

Following the secondary exposure to an antigen, there is usually a change in antibody affinity. Antibody produced during the secondary response is directed against a larger number of epitopes associated with the antigen and has a higher affinity. Consequently, this antibody will bind more firmly to its corresponding antigen. This change in antibody affinity reflects a continuing temporal change in the affinity constant of the binding site of the antibody population, probably as a result of clonal selection.

These important features that distinguish the primary antibody response from the secondary, or memory, response can be utilized to diagnose infectious diseases or to identify individuals immune to a particular microorganism. This is also depicted in Figure 11–1. Of major importance from the diagnostic point of view is the demonstration of specific IgM antibodies during the acute phase of an illness. Since IgM antibodies to an infecting agent are present in significant levels only during the acute phase of disease, the presence of such antibodies is often used as an indicator of a primary infection in the diagnosis of viral and bacterial diseases. For example, it is often difficult to diagnose primary herpesvirus infections, since IgG antibodies to these viruses persist for life following original infection. However, the presence of IgM antibodies to a particular herpesvirus can indicate recent primary infection by that virus. In addition, IgG

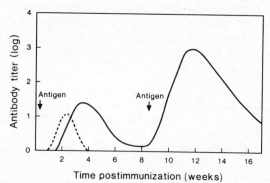

Figure 11–1. Antibody response patterns following a first (primary) and second (secondary) immunization with an antigen. (Dotted line = IgM antibody response; solid line = IgG antibody response). Note both the transient IgM antibody response following the primary immunization with an antigen and the higher IgG antibody peak titers following the second immunization.

antibody levels are generally higher during convalescence than during the acute phase of an infectious disease. Thus, a rise in specific serum antibody levels offers evidence of an active infection with a particular agent. When antibody titers in acute and convalescent serum samples are compared, an increase in titer of fourfold or greater in the convalescent serum is indicative of an active, specific infection. This has considerable diagnostic utility in many infections.

Besides being of diagnostic value, detection of antibodies to different antigens associated with an infectious process can also be used for prognostic purposes. For example, generally during an active viral infection, antibodies will be produced against a variety of viral proteins synthesized during the viral replication cycle. Such antibodies against the multitude of viral proteins will persist as long as the infection is active. However, when the infectious process subsides, antibodies to most of the viral antigens will decrease to low or undetectable levels. Continuous monitoring of antibody levels to different antigens associated with a suspected causative agent can, therefore, provide the clinician with important information in regard to the course of a disease.

MECHANISMS OF
IMMUNITY[4, 6, 11, 13, 14, 18, 21–23, 27–29, 32]

Antibodies and immune lymphoid cells participate in immunity to infectious agents through a variety of mechanisms. Some of these are listed in Table 11–1. As discussed in the preceding chapter, lymphoid cells generally function in immunity to foreign antigens through destruction of cells expressing the foreign antigens or through the release of lymphokines that serve to recruit cytotoxic cells to the site of antigen localization. Antibodies, on the other hand, mediate their protective effects through a variety of different mecha-

Table 11–1. **Major Mechanisms of Immunity**

Cellular
Cytotoxicity
Lymphokine production
Phagocytosis

Humoral
Neutralization
Aggregation
Lysis (complement-dependent, ADCC)
Opsonization
Immobilization

nisms. One major defense mechanism is the neutralization of toxic effects or infection mediated by the inciting agent. Neutralizing activity can be directed against the infecting agent or against toxic products released by it. For example, antibodies directed at specific sites on the surfaces of viruses will neutralize viral infections by blocking an essential step in the virus replication cycle. Antibodies directed against a specific component of a bacterial toxin will neutralize its toxic activity. In both examples, antibodies with neutralizing activity are directed against specific components, *i.e.,* not all antibodies against virus or toxin components have neutralizing capacity. With some viruses, complement also participates or enhances neutralization by antibody. This is particularly true for viruses with an outer envelope, such as members of the herpesvirus group. Complement presumably enhances antibody neutralizing activity by lysing the viral envelope, a component essential to initiation of the infectious process.

Antibodies can also mediate cytotoxic effects against cells expressing the appropriate antigens through complement-mediated lysis or by an antibody-dependent cellular cytotoxicity (ADCC) mechanism. It is known that both mammalian cells and many bacteria can be lysed *in vitro* in the presence of antibody and complement. Presumably such a lytic phenomenon is also active *in vivo*. This is supported by the fact that mice deficient in certain components of complement are more susceptible to certain bacterial infections, suggesting that complement-mediated antibody cytolysis is an important defense mechanism. In humans, it is also well documented that individuals lacking certain components of complement, particularly C3, are highly susceptible to recurrent infections. The role of ADCC as an active *in vivo* defense mechanism against infectious agents is less clear, but it is likely that this cytotoxic mechanism does function against certain virus infections. This is supported by *in vitro* observations showing that cells supporting the replication of certain viruses are very susceptible to ADCC. Indirect evidence supports the *in vivo* role of ADCC as an active defense mechanism against infectious diseases, including certain forms of virus-induced cancers.

A fourth mechanism of antibody-mediated immunity is the enhanced phagocytosis of antigens coated with antibody or complement or both, termed **opsonization** (Chapter 12). The serum factors responsible for this immune phenomenon are called **opsonins.** Phagocytes do not efficiently ingest particles suspended in physiological saline, but in the presence of normal or immune serum the number of particles or microorganisms ingested is greatly enhanced. This can be shown by direct counts of the number of bacteria ingested by phagocytes in the presence or absence of immune serum. Opsonization appears to involve the attachment of antigen-antibody complexes to the phagocyte through Fc receptors or receptors for C3b, present in the membranes of the phagocytic cells. Phagocytosis is enhanced under these conditions; antibody and C3b, therefore, function as opsonins. It should be pointed out, too, that C3 can be activated by various pathways, including the properdin (or alternate) pathway, and properdin can also be considered an opsonin. This opsonization process is an important defense mechanism against infectious agents (Chapter 12) and is also an active mechanism for the elimination of antigen-antibody complexes from the peripheral circulation.

It should be emphasized that antibodies are generally not directly effective in immunity against intracellular pathogens. As noted above, cells supporting the replication of some viruses might be eliminated through an ADCC mechanism, but antibody is not effective in neutralizing intracellular viruses. Once a pathogen enters a host cell, it is protected from the humoral immune environment, since antibody cannot penetrate intact host cells. In these cases, cellular factors (T cells, NK cells, phagocytes) appear to be the major defense elements. Besides viruses, intracellular pathogens include bacteria, such as *Brucella,* which reside in macrophages in the infected host. The important role of cells in immunity against these agents is exemplified by the fact that animals with impaired T cell or macrophage functions are highly susceptible to infections with intracellular pathogens. In fact, humans with defects in their T cell immunity frequently develop disseminated viral infections even in the presence of high levels of neutralizing antibodies.

Different immunoglobulins vary in their ability to mediate the various immunological activities that function in immunity to infectious agents. IgM antibodies fix complement more efficiently than those of other immunoglobulin classes and therefore are most active in complement-dependent immune defense mechanisms. IgG antibodies, on the other hand, are the principal mediators of ADCC; whether or not IgM antibodies can participate in ADCC reactions is not yet resolved. IgA antibodies and antibodies of the IgG4 subclass are very inefficient in complement-fixation reactions.

All three of these major immunoglobulin classes are capable of neutralizing infectious agents, although IgG antibodies appear to be the most active in systemic infections. Secretory IgA antibodies, however, play an important role in protecting against infections of the mucous membranes (local immunity). This is due to the fact that IgA is the major antibody-containing immunoglobulin class in external secretions and therefore plays an important role in mucosal defense. As noted earlier, most of the IgA in external secretions is produced locally by plasma cells residing in the submucosal tissues. An important defense activity associated with secretory IgA is the inhibition of bacterial adherence to epithelial cells of the mucosal surface. For example, secretory IgA from parotid fluid specifically inhibits the attachment of certain strains of streptococci to human buccal epithelial cells. Similarly, secretory IgA inhibits the adherence of *Neisseria gonorrhoeae* to human cervical epithelium, thereby preventing infection. Thus, secretory IgA appears to be the immunoglobulin of major importance in local immunity at mucosal surfaces. The relevance of this observation will be discussed further in the next section on vaccines.

Finally, IgG antibodies appear to be of major importance in conferring immunity to the newborn, since this is the only immunoglobulin class that will cross the placenta. Placental transfer of IgG antibodies from the maternal circulation to that of the fetus is a form of passive immunization, protecting the newborn from some infective agents.

VACCINES[2, 5, 12, 15, 16]

The identification of the immune factors that protect against different pathogenic microorganisms has led to the development of vaccines to prevent initial infections with these agents. The process of **vaccination** is, therefore, an attempt to induce immunity in the absence of disease. To accomplish this, vaccines are composed of those antigens that induce immune factors that can block, neutralize, or prevent the establishment of infectious processes. The immunity induced in this fashion is highly variable, depending largely on the method used to prepare the vaccine as well as the strength of the antigen. For example, the immunity produced to highly antigenic toxoids,

Table 11–2. **Different Types of Vaccines Used for Preventing Human Diseases**

Vaccine	Diseases
Inactivated	Diphtheria
	Tetanus
	Influenza
	Cholera
	Whooping cough
	Polio
	Rabies
	Typhoid fever
Attenuated	Smallpox
	Tuberculosis
	Polio
	Yellow fever
	Mumps
	Measles
	German measles
Component	Influenza
	Herpesvirus diseases*
	Hepatitis*

*Vaccine in preparation.

such as those of tetanus or diphtheria, persists for years without the need for re-exposure to the antigen in the form of booster injections. Similarly, immunity induced with attenuated viral vaccines, such as vaccinia, yellow fever, and polioviruses, also persists for years because of the prolonged persistence of the viruses in the tissues. In contrast, vaccines against typhoid fever are relatively ineffective and require multiple inoculations to maintain an effective level of immunity.

The kinds of vaccines that have been used to induce immunity against different diseases can be grouped into three different categories, as listed in Table 11–2. These include inactivated vaccines, living attenuated vaccines, and component vaccines. Most of the vaccines now employed for immunization against human diseases are of the inactivated or attenuated types.

Inactivated Vaccines

Inactivation involves various forms of treatment to render the agent noninfective or nonviable while retaining its immunogenicity. Inactivation is usually accomplished by heating or by treatment with an agent such as formalin. Parenteral administration of inactivated vaccines commonly induces both humoral and cellular systemic immunity. The duration of immunity varies, depending on the strength of the antigens in the preparations. Little local immunity, associated with secretory IgA, is induced by such preparations. Since these are nonreplicating antigens, periodic booster injections are required to maintain immunity against the appropriate infection.

Component Vaccines

The development of component vaccines is of great interest, particularly those directed against viral infections (Table 11–2). Component vaccines against hepatitis virus and members of the herpesvirus group induce essentially the same type of immunity as inactivated vaccines. Since component vaccines are composed only of those specific antigens that elicit selective immune responses, their main advantage is the absence of any genetic material (DNA or RNA) from the original virus or microorganism. The presence of genetic material in vaccine preparations is a major concern, for example, in vaccines against herpesviruses. Since many of these viruses contain a gene capable of changing a normal cell into a cancer cell, it is ill-advised to use a vaccine containing this genetic information, even in inactivated form, to immunize human populations. A more acceptable approach is to use a component vaccine free of the viral DNA. Such vaccines are now difficult and expensive to produce for widespread use. However, because of recent advances in genetic engineering, it should be possible to produce large quantities of inexpensive synthetic component vaccines in the relatively near future.

Attenuated Vaccines

Attenuation is currently the procedure of choice in preparing vaccines to produce a long-lasting immunity. The attenuation process basically selects an organism that has lost some element required for the production of disease but maintains its infectivity and immunogenicity. Attenuated vaccines are now available against diseases such as smallpox, polio, tuberculosis, yellow fever, mumps, measles, and rabies, to name a few; others are under development. Attenuated vaccines have the advantage over inactivated vaccines in that they provide for a continuous antigenic stimulation, thereby eliminating the need for additional booster injections. In addition, such vaccines generally induce a local or mucosal immunity characterized by the production of secretory IgA antibodies. This is thought to be of particular importance for effective immunity against virus infections. Of major concern in the use of such vaccines is that, through back mutational events, they have the potential to revert to a fully virulent state.

Passive Immunity

An alternative approach to prevention of disease is through **passively acquired immunity.** This entails the inoculation, into nonimmune individuals, of serum or serum components containing antibody against specific microorganisms. This has been found effective in preventing infection and disease over the short term, but passively transferred antibody is not long-lived in the host. To be effective, large quantities of antibody are usually required. Because such antibodies are often produced in a foreign animal species and are, therefore, immunogenic in humans, it is prudent to minimize reactivity to the foreign protein. To this end, the IgG fraction is usually isolated from the whole antiserum; antigenic determinants are sometimes further removed by treatment with enzymes. This approach toward prevention is routinely used in individuals bitten by animals suspected of being rabid or for treatment of those who have ingested food possibly containing botulinum toxin; it is otherwise of limited value.

Human gamma globulin preparations, isolated from the pooled serum from normal adult donors, have also been found to contain significant levels of antibody to a variety of infectious agents and have been used successfully for passive immunity. Human pooled gamma globulin usually contains antibody to such viruses as measles, varicella, herpes simplex, rubella, and hepatitis. It is frequently given as a preventive for hepatitis or to protect immunosuppressed individuals from infection with adventitious agents; more recently, it has been used to treat patients with chronic viral infections, such as chronic infectious mononucleosis. Gamma globulin is also routinely given to pregnant women who are not immune to rubella if they are exposed to this virus during the first trimester of their pregnancy, since infection during this period places the fetus at great risk of developing congenital abnormalities.

Autoimmunity[1, 3, 9, 10, 17, 19, 20, 24, 30, 31]

As discussed in Chapter 10, an individual does not normally produce antibodies to his own tissues. This is known as "tolerance to self." Under some circumstances, however, tolerance breaks down and self antigens become recognized as foreign. This results in the production of antibodies, called **autoantibodies,** to the individual's own tissues. This abnormal immune response is referred to as **autoimmunity** and sometimes, but not always, can lead to **autoimmune disease.**

The phenomenon of self-tolerance was originally described in the early 1900s by Paul Ehrlich as "horror autotoxicus." However, it was recognized even at that time that there were exceptions to the role of self-tolerance and that under some circumstances an individual did, in fact, produce antibodies against components of his own tissues. For example, after the introduction of Pasteur's rabies vaccine, prepared from spinal cords of rabbits infected with an attentuated strain of rabies virus, it was observed that an occasional individual who received the vaccine would develop an encephalomyelitis that could not be attributed to rabies virus infection. It was suspected that this occurrence was induced by immune response to rabbit brain tissue, resulting in antibodies cross-reactive with normal brain tissues of the immunized individual. This was subsequently proved to be the case in the middle 1900s.

A number of diseases are categorized as autoimmune because of the frequency of appearance of autoantibodies in the serum of patients with these different disease manifestations. Clinically, diseases considered to have an autoimmune pathogenesis can be grouped into two categories: (1) **organ-specific,** to identify those diseases that primarily affect a specific organ, and (2) **multisystemic,** for those diseases affecting several tissues and organs. This classification is not absolute, however, and a number of so-called autoimmune disorders overlap both categories. A list of some of the putative major autoimmune diseases is shown in Table 11–3. Diseases for which an organ-specific pathogenesis is suspected or proved include Graves' disease, Hashimoto's thyroiditis, juvenile diabetes mellitus, pernicious anemia, Addison's disease, myasthenia gravis, Goodpasture's syndrome, and glomerulonephritis, but only myasthenia gravis and Goodpasture's syndrome have a proven autoimmune pathogenesis. The best known autoimmune multisystem diseases are rheumatoid arthritis, systemic lupus erythematosus, and Sjögren's disease. All of these are char-

Table 11–3. **Diseases Suspected of Having an Autoimmune Basis**

Organ-Specific Diseases
Hashimoto's thyroiditis
Graves' disease
Addison's disease
Goodpasture's syndrome*
Myasthenia gravis*
Juvenile diabetes mellitus
Pernicious anemia
Glomerulonephritis

Systemic Diseases
Rheumatoid arthritis
Systemic lupus erythematosus (SLE)
Sjögren's disease
Scleroderma
Ulcerative colitis

*Proven autoimmune etiology.

acterized by the presence of serum autoantibodies to numerous cellular constituents. The disease symptoms produced in autoimmune multisystem diseases are attributed largely to the presence of circulating immune complexes that become deposited in various tissues and initiate the disease processes. These diseases will be considered in more detail in the next section (Immune Complex Diseases). This discussion focuses on the organ-specific diseases, initiated by immune responses against antigenic components of a specific tissue or organ.

The exact mechanisms by which organ-specific autoimmune diseases are induced are not fully understood, but in diseases proved to have an autoimmune basis, autoantibodies directed against cell membrane receptors or against endocrine hormones appear to be largely, if not exclusively, responsible for the disease symptoms. For example, in myasthenia gravis, one of the best understood autoimmune diseases, antibodies to acetylcholine receptors are responsible for the impaired neuromuscular transmission that characterizes this disease. These antibodies react with receptors located in the postsynaptic membrane and can block the acetylcholine binding site. Complement-mediated lysis of the postsynaptic membranes, initiated by the antibody-antigen reaction, is the major mechanism of receptor loss. This mechanism was proven by showing that serum containing antibodies to acetylcholine receptors can transmit this disease to experimental animals only in the presence of an intact complement system. Myasthenia gravis is also induced experimentally in rats by active immunization with purified acetylcholine receptors. Similarly, Graves' disease is mediated by antibodies directed against receptors for thyroid-stimulating hormone (TSH) on thyroid epithelial cells. Interaction of these antibodies with the TSH receptors induces an increased secretion of thyroid hormones, resulting in symptoms characteristic of this disease. Other autoimmune diseases associated with the presence of autoantibodies to antigens expressed on endocrine glands include juvenile diabetes mellitus, Hashimoto's thyroiditis, and Addison's disease. In early stages of juvenile diabetes mellitus, antibodies against pancreatic islet cells are transiently present at high frequency. In patients with an unusual form of juvenile diabetes associated with extreme insulin resistance, autoantibodies capable of blocking the binding of insulin to its receptors have been demonstrated. Individuals with Hashimoto's disease possess serum autoantibodies to thyroglobulin, while patients with Addison's disease generally possess serum antibodies to antigens on the surface of adrenal glands. In both diseases, the autoantibodies are thought to be the major factors in the production of specific disease manifestations.

In other autoimmune organ-specific diseases, autoantibodies are directly cytotoxic to the tissues in which they are deposited. This is most evident in the glomerulonephritis of Goodpasture's syndrome. In this disease, antibodies are produced that react directly with the glomerular basement membrane. The localization of these antibodies has been convincingly demonstrated by immunofluorescent staining of diseased kidneys. Following their binding to the basement membrane, these antibodies activate complement, resulting in the chemotactic attraction of polymorphonuclear leucocytes and subsequent destruction of the basement membrane. Similar lesions occur in the basement membrane of the lungs in Goodpasture's syndrome. Glomerulonephritis can be induced in experimental animals by immunization with basement membrane preparations or by passive transfer of serum containing high levels of antibodies to antigens of the glomerular basement membrane. These observations provide evidence for the participation of organ-specific antibodies in the pathogenesis of this disease.

Although the factors responsible for induction of autoimmunity are not clear, the underlying mechanism appears to be the breaking of tolerance to self-components. A number of theories have been advanced to explain the breaking of tolerance. One possible explanation is that tolerance to self is broken through the modification of an autoantigen, introducing foreign determinants acting as haptens. The altered antigen is no longer recognized as "self" and provokes an immune response. This response must be at least partially directed against carrier determinants, resulting in the production of autoantibodies. Autoantigens could be modified in this way by environmental agents, such as by-products of viral infection, or by chemicals. This proposal assumes that tolerance to self occurs at the helper T cell level. The modified autoantigen would, therefore, bypass the tolerant helper T cells to induce antibody synthesis in B lymphocytes.

A second popular theory is that autoimmunity results from the loss of suppressor T cell control of antibody synthesis; this theory has some experimental support. The NZB strain of mice develops a disease similar to systemic lupus erythematosus (SLE) late in life. These mice also show a loss of nonspecific suppressor T cell function with age that parallels the development of SLE-like disease. Transfer of thymus cells from young mice to older mice prevents both disease and formation of the antinuclear antibodies that is characteristic of

SLE. This observation has been interpreted to indicate that suppressor T cell functions are lost or become nonfunctional in older animals, resulting in the loss of tolerance and the development of autoimmunity. Although this theory is attractive, its relevance to human disease remains to be proved.

Other possible explanations for the induction of autoimmunity are (1) cross-reactivity between organ-specific antigens and those associated with certain microorganisms, (2) release of sequestered antigens not normally accessible to the immune system and for which self-tolerance does not exist, and (3) polyclonal activation of B lymphocytes by viruses, bacterial products, or other activators, resulting in the production of autoantibodies. It is clear from experimental studies that all of these mechanisms could be active in the induction of autoimmunity, depending on circumstances. It is, therefore, not necessary to suppose at this stage that the different types of autoimmune diseases will have a common mechanism for induction.

Immune Complex Diseases[7, 8, 25, 26]

Circulating immune complexes can induce disease manifestations when deposited in various tissues. Examples of such disorders include glomerulonephritis, since many complexes are deposited in the kidney; rheumatoid arthritis; and systemic lupus erythematosus (SLE). These types of disorders, which are characterized by inflammation, are categorized as **Type III hypersensitivity reactions** (Chapter 10) and are caused by deposition, in blood vessel walls or in basement membranes, of immune complexes containing complement. The resultant local inflammation is mediated largely through activation of the different components of complement.

The type III hypersensitivity reaction was originally reported by Arthus in 1903. He noted that repeated subcutaneous injection of horse serum into the skin of rabbits was followed by local inflammatory reactions at subsequent sites of injection of the same antigen. This was reproduced in other mammals, including humans. It was further observed that this type of hypersensitivity reaction was not confined to the skin but could also be induced in other tissues. For example, it is now known that inhalation of an antigen frequently induces congestion of the lung, with a histological

picture of pneumonia. This is caused by the formation of antigen-antibody complexes in the lungs, involving the inhaled antigen.

This immune complex reaction is now known as the **Arthus reaction** and requires the participation of large amounts of complement-fixing antibody and complement. The following sequence of events leads to the Arthus reaction: (1) antigen diffuses through the tissues, making contact with antibody to form antigen-antibody complexes that are then deposited in the walls of blood vessels; (2) these complexes activate the complement system, resulting in the formation of chemotactic factors (C3a, C5a, C6, C7) which attract neutrophils to the reaction site; (3) the neutrophils phagocytize the immune complexes, resulting in the release of lysosomal enzymes that mediate tissue damage. Damage to vessel walls allows for leakage of plasma and blood cells and necrosis of the surrounding tissue. The Arthus reaction can readily be transferred to normal animals with serum containing large quantities of precipitating antibodies.

The Arthus reaction differs from anaphylaxis in a number of ways. The most important differences are in the time course of events, the nature of the participating antibodies, and the requirement for complement. The Arthus reaction generally does not begin until 1 to 2 hours after the injection of antigen, peaks at about 4 hours, and then subsides after 8 to 12 hours. The length and intensity of the reaction is dependent on the concentrations of both antigen and antibody and on the quantities of immune complexes that are subsequently formed. In contrast, immediate anaphylactic reactions occur generally within minutes following antigen injection, peak within 30 minutes, and then subside quickly. As mentioned in Chapter 10, anaphylactic reactions are mediated by IgE antibodies that become fixed to mast cells via their Fc fragment. These antibodies are effective even in very small quantities. Arthus reactions, in contrast, are initiated by antibodies that do not fix to tissues (IgG or IgM), but are capable of activating complement. Complement is required for Arthus reactions, but not for anaphylactic reactions. Arthus reactions cannot be induced in complement-deficient animals, even in the presence of large quantities of antibodies.

The **serum sickness** syndrome frequently noted following injections of foreign serums, such as antitoxins against diphtheria and tetanus toxins prepared in horses, is mediated by an Arthus-like mechanism. Symptoms of serum sickness include localized urticarial rash at the site of antigen injection followed by generalized urticaria, enlargement of lymph nodes draining the site of injection, fever, edema, and joint pains. Symptoms generally appear 1 to 2 weeks following antigen injection. Laboratory studies have established that serum sickness occurs at a time when the immunized host starts to develop antibodies against the serum components and while these antigens still persist in the circulation. With continued antibody production, antigen is eliminated and free antibody starts to appear in the circulation. The clinical manifestations of serum sickness start to disappear at about this time.

Dixon and co-workers established that the symptoms of serum sickness coincided with the appearance of circulating immune complexes. Definitive proof of the role of immune complexes in the pathogenesis of serum sickness was provided by the demonstration that lesions similar to those of this syndrome could be induced with immune complexes preformed *in vitro*. Only those complexes formed in moderate antigen excess were active, while complexes formed at equivalence or in extreme antigen excess were inactive. This appears to be due to the fact that antigen-antibody complexes formed at equivalence, which tend to be particulate, or those with molecular sizes greater than 11S are readily removed from the circulation by phagocytic cells.

In addition to serum sickness, there are certain chronic multisystem human diseases that occur spontaneously and are considered to be immune complex diseases. Rheumatoid arthritis and SLE are the prototypes of these diseases. The clinical symptoms of both of these disease conditions are believed to be closely linked to the formation and persistence of circulating immune complexes. Rheumatoid arthritis, a chronic inflammatory disease primarily affecting the joints, also involves other tissue and organs. The histological picture of this disease includes the accumulation of lymphocytes and plasma cells at the site of inflammation. One of the major characteristic immunological findings for this disease is the presence of an autoantibody, designated as **rheumatoid factor,** in the serum and synovial fluid of these patients and directed against the Fc fragment of aggregated IgG. These antibodies can be of either the IgG or the IgM classes, although IgM rheumatoid factors are more common. These antibodies fix complement and can react with native IgG, but react more intensely with the aggregated form of this immunoglobulin molecule. Other immunological characteristics of this disease include low levels of complement in synovial fluids. Immune complexes, formed between rheumatoid factor and IgG and containing complement components, are routinely detected in the serum and synovial fluids of patients with rheumatoid arthritis; they are thought to be important factors in the pathogenesis of this disease. Activation of the complement system by immune complexes in the synovial fluid may produce the chronic inflammation of the joints noted in these patients. The mechanism is probably similar to that of the Arthus reaction, *i.e.*, formation of chemotactic agents, accumulation of neutrophils, and release of lysosomal enzymes. Why patients with rheumatoid arthritis produce antibodies to IgG is not yet known, but any or all of the proposed mechanisms for autoimmunity discussed above could be involved.

The serum of patients with SLE contains autoantibodies to a variety of normal cellular components. Most relevant to the pathogenesis of the disease are those antibodies directed against single- and double-stranded DNA and DNA-histone complexes. One other common characteristic is the presence of low levels of serum complement, a feature which correlates with the disease course. In addition, cytotoxic autoantibodies reactive with surface antigens on erythrocytes, platelets, and leucocytes are frequently detected in the serum of these patients. High levels of antibodies to double-stranded DNA are considered of diagnostic significance in this disease, since such antibodies are not frequently encountered in other disease conditions. The major symptoms of this disease include rash, polyarthritis, vasculitis, central nervous system abnormalities, and glomerulonephritis. Antigen-antibody complexes composed of double-stranded DNA, anti-DNA antibodies, and complement are frequently found in the kidneys of SLE patients who develop glomerulonephritis and are thought to be responsible for the development of this complication. These deposits are usually located between the endothelial cells and the basement membrane, as demonstrated by immunofluorescence. Antibodies eluted from the kidneys of such patients react specifically with double-stranded DNA. The sequence of events that leads to the development of these autoantibodies and the subsequent formation of immune complexes is not completely clear, but animal studies indicate that the production of the different antibodies characteristic of this disease might be the result of the loss of suppressor T cell control of antibody synthesis.

References

1. Briggs, W. A., *et al.* 1979. Antiglomerular basement membrane antibody-mediated glomerulonephritis and Goodpasture's syndrome. Medicine **58**:348–361.
2. Chanock, R. M. 1981. Strategy for development of respiratory and gastrointestinal tract viral vaccines in the 1980s. J. Infect. Dis. **143**:365–374.
3. Cochrane, C. G. 1968. Immunological tissue injury mediated by neutrophilic leukocytes. Adv. Immunol. **9**:97–162.
4. Collins, F. M. 1971. Mechanisms in anti-microbial immunity. J. Reticuloendothel. Soc.**10**:58–99.
5. Harrison, H. R., and V. A. Fulginiti. 1980. Bacterial immunizations. Amer. J. Dis. Child. **134**:184–193.
6. Humphrey, J. H., and R. R. Dourmashkin. 1969. Lesions in cell membranes caused by complement. Adv. Immunol. **11**:75–115.
7. Inman, R. D., and N. K. Day. 1981. Immunologic and clinical aspects of immune complex disease. Amer. J. Med. **70**:1097–1106.
8. Kunkel, H. G. 1980. The immunopathology of SLE. Hosp. Pract. **15**:47–56.
9. Lennon, V. 1979. Immunologic mechanisms in myasthenia gravis—a model of a receptor disease. pp. 259–289. *In* E. Franklin (Ed.): Clinical Immunology Update. Reviews for Physicians. Elsevier North Holland, New York.
10. Lindstrom, J. 1979. Autoimmune response to acetylcholine receptors in myasthenia gravis and its animal model. Adv. Immunol. **27**:1–51.
11. MacKaness, G. B. 1971. Resistance to intracellular infection. J. Infect. Dis. **123**:439–445.
12. Mestecky, J., *et al.* 1978. Selective induction of an immune response to human external secretions by ingestion of bacterial antigens. J. Clin. Invest. **61**:731–737.
13. Metzger, H. 1970. Structure and function of γM macroglobulins. Adv. Immunol. **12**:57–116.
14. Miller, I. 1970. Specific and non-specific opsonins. Curr. Top. Microbiol. Immunol. **51**:62–78.
15. Ogra, P. L., and D. T. Karzon. 1969. Poliovirus antibody response in serum and nasal secretions following intranasal inoculation with inactivated poliovaccine. J. Immunol. **102**:15–23.
16. Ogra, P. L., and D. T. Karzon. 1969. Distribution of poliovirus antibody in serum, nasopharynx and alimentary tract following segmental immunization of lower alimentary tract with poliovaccine. J. Immunol. **102**:1423–1430.
17. Osoba, D. 1972. Thymic function, immunologic deficiency and autoimmunity. Med. Clin. North Amer. **56**:319–335.
18. Pearson, G. R. 1978. *In vitro* and *in vivo* investigations on antibody-dependent cellular cytotoxicity. Curr. Top. Microbiol. Immunol. **80**:65–96.
19. Rose, N. R. 1981. Autoimmune diseases. Scient. Amer. **244**:80–84.
20. Shulman, S. 1971. Thyroid antigens and autoimmunity. Adv. Immunol. **14**:85–185.
21. Silverstein, S. 1970. Macrophages and viral immunity. Semin. Hematol. **7**:185–214.
22. Sissons, J. G. P., and M. B. A. Oldstone. 1980. The antibody-mediated destruction of virus-infected cells. Adv. Immunol. **29**:209–260.
23. Spiegelberg, H. L. 1974. Biological activities of immunoglobulins of different classes and subclasses. Adv. Immunol. **19**:259–294.
24. Talal, N. (Ed.). 1977. Autoimmunity: Genetic, Immunologic, Virological, and Clinical Aspects. Academic Press, New York.
25. Theofilopoulos, A. N., and F. J. Dixon. 1979. The biology and detection of immune complexes. Adv. Immunol. **28**:89–221.
26. Theofilopoulos, A. N., and F. J. Dixon. 1981. Etiopathogenesis of murine SLE. Immunol. Rev. **55**:179–216.
27. Tomasi, T. B. 1971. The gamma A globulins: first line of defense. pp. 76–83. *In* R. A. Good and D. W. Fisher (Eds.): Immunobiology. Sinauer Associates, Inc., Stamford, Conn.
28. Tomasi, T. B., and H. M. Grey. 1972. Structure and function of immunoglobulin A. Prog. Allergy **16**:81–213.
29. Tomasi, T. B., *et al.* 1980. Mucosal immunity: the origin and migration patterns of cells in the secretory system. J. Allergy Clin. Immunol. **65**:12–19.
30. Weigle, W. O. 1980. Analysis of autoimmunity through experimental models of thyroiditis and allergic encephalomyelitis. Adv. Immunol. **30**:159–274.
31. Wilson, C. B., and F. J. Dixon. 1979. Immunologic mechanisms in nephritogenesis. Hosp. Pract. **14**:57–69.
32. Youmans, G. P. 1971. The role of lymphocytes and other factors in antimicrobial cellular immunity. J. Reticuloendothel. Soc. **10**:100–119.

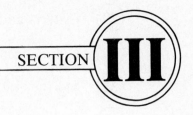

SECTION III

Medical Bacteriology

CHAPTER **12**

The Pathogenic Microorganisms and Disease

The Earth's biosphere contains untold numbers and kinds of microorganisms, most of which are unknown, even unsuspected, by man. Some we know by their activities in nature, such as the microorganisms of the nitrogen cycle that contribute to soil fertility and others that cause decay and mineralization of organic matter. Still others are nurtured for their beneficial properties in the production, preservation, and improvement of foods and beverages, such as cheese, wine, and beer; in the synthesis of organic solvents and antibiotics; and in the biological disposal and degradation of organic wastes.

Only a tiny portion of microorganisms are capable of entering into intimate, and usually innocuous, host-parasite relationships with man, colonizing on the skin and mucous membranes. Of these, only a few can cause disease in man and animals, usually after entering the tissues and injuring the host. Pathogenicity is, however, merely incidental and has significance to the parasite only as it relates to the establishment of an ecological niche and the survival of the pathogen.

The interaction between man and microorganisms is not static over time, but is frequently modified by many factors. Technological advances effect better control of some infectious agents, new chemotherapies are devised, and economic and social patterns of the population evolve; new diseases thereby emerge and the relative importance of older infectious agents is altered.

The Specific Microbial Etiology of Infectious Disease

From the time of van Leeuwenhoek, many suspected that microbes were involved in disease, but it was not until Koch published his classic paper on anthrax that these suspicions were subjected to rigid experimental analysis. Koch preferred a logical chain of evidence as unequivocal proof of the etiological connection between a specific bacterium, now called *Bacillus anthracis,* and the disease anthrax.

Koch's Postulates

The basic criteria necessary for such proof, known as Koch's postulates, have been universally applied in the intervening years, even though developing technology has required some expansion of the original tenets.

The First Postulate. The first criterion is that the microorganism must be observed in association with the disease. This is relatively simple when the agent occurs alone in otherwise germ-free tissues. When the causative agent is found mixed with other, often similar, forms, as in infections of the intestinal and respiratory tracts, it must be differentiated from them.

The requirement for this preliminary observation is self-evident. Yet, the first postulate must be emphasized for several reasons. First, closely similar, even indistinguishable, clinical syndromes may have quite different etiology. For instance, two similar diseases—cholera and bacillary dysentery—caused by different microorganisms often cannot be differentiated on clinical grounds alone. It is also true that a variety of different bacteria may be the cause of urinary tract disease, and the common cold is due to a wide variety of viruses that can give rise to substantially the same symptoms.

Second, the term "observation" must be broadly interpreted. In many bacterial diseases, there may be no morphological differences between the pathogen and related nonpathogens of the normal flora, *e.g.,* disease-causing enteric bacilli and nonpathogenic coliforms are morphologically indistinguishable. The first postulate then merges with the second, in that characterization and differentiation of the microorganism, in an isolated state, are required to establish its association with the disease.

Finally, the first postulate implies not only the presence of the microorganism in association with the disease, but also the corollary that it not be present in the absence of disease. Confusion then arises when the suspected pathogen is present in individuals with no symptoms of the disease, *viz.,* carriers and those with inapparent or asymptomatic infections.

In practice, it is necessary to qualify the dogmatic first postulate. For example, observation must be stretched to include cytopathology in tissue cultures inoculated with infectious material; association must be observed in at least a majority of cases of the disease; and a microorganism must be regarded as suspect even though it may be found in some healthy persons. Such association is by no means proof of an etiological relation, and further evidence is required.

The Second Postulate. The second postulate is that the microorganism must be isolated and grown in pure culture. This is clearly essential to effect a separation of the causative agent from other microorganisms when they are present and is often an integral part of the first postulate. Fortunately, most pathogenic bacteria can be isolated and grown in pure culture, although there are sometimes practical difficulties in devising appropriate culture mediums; a very few suspected pathogens cannot be grown in pure culture, however.

The leprosy bacillus, regularly found in enormous numbers in leprous lesions, is morphologically distinctive both in its acid-fast staining character and in the arrangement of the individual cells; it has not, however, been cultivated in the laboratory. The spirochete of syphilis also has not been cultivated, but its etiological relation to the disease is firmly established because supportive evidence is relatively strong. This includes a specific immune response to the spirochetal substance appearing during the course of the disease and reproduction of the disease by direct inoculation of infectious material containing only the spirochete. In some instances, then, the second postulate may be circumvented when there is a high degree of probability for the presumed etiological relation.

With the rickettsiae and viruses, isolation necessarily means growth in cell culture or in the embryonated hen's egg. It might be supposed that the purity of such cultures is questionable, but the occurrence of mixed viral infections in tissue culture is usually evident. Growth of these agents is often directly demonstrable by light or electron microscopy. Their presence may also be indicated by pathology of the tissue substrate, or by some unique feature, such as the development of hemagglutinin in the allantoic fluid of egg embryos infected with influenza viruses.

In some instances there may be no overt evidence of growth, and the agent may be carried by "blind passage" in a series of tissue or egg cultures. After several such transplants cytopathic effects often become apparent. The somewhat devious nature of such procedures does not invalidate them.

The Third Postulate. The third postulate requires that the disease be reproduced in a susceptible animal by inoculation with the microorganism grown in pure culture. This is sometimes difficult to accomplish for two reasons. First, the disease must be reproduced in a recognizable form and bear some similarity to the naturally occurring disease. Second, a susceptible animal may be difficult to find.

These are not matters of great importance in the diseases of domestic animals, for the natural host may be the experimental host also. For infectious diseases of man, however, a satisfactory animal must be found. The agents of human disease are often closely adapted parasites, so that they either fail to infect experimental animals or produce infections that are not recognizable as related to the naturally occurring human disease. Typhoid fever has not, for example, been reproduced in ordinary experimental animals.

In addition to variations in animal susceptibility, some infectious agents produce a delayed or seemingly indirect effect. The former include the "slow viruses," responsible for diseases such as scrapie in sheep, kuru in man, and mink encephalopathy. Scrapie, for example, may be reproduced in mice, but many weeks elapse before symptoms appear. Other viral infections, such as rubella, not only give rise to the known clinical picture of the disease, but also produce congenital defects when the infection occurs during pregnancy. To reproduce these teratogenic effects in experimental animals is frequently difficult.

The importance of reproducing infectious disease in an experimental animal cannot be overstated. Unless the disease can be studied under the controlled conditions of the laboratory, it must remain inadequately understood. It is equally obvious that unless this third postulate is fulfilled, it is not possible to establish fully the etiological relation of a given microorganism to a particular disease.

The Fourth Postulate. The microorganism must be found in the experimental infection produced in the susceptible animal and shown to be the same as that inoculated. If the first three postulates are met, the fourth ordinarily

follows without difficulty. It is nonetheless necessary to show that the animal was infected with the microorganism and that the disease or death so produced is specific, *e.g.,* a consequence of the inoculated agent rather than some intercurrent infection of the experimental animal.

Supporting Evidence. Less direct but supporting evidence for the etiology of a given disease assumes significance when the evidence provided by the four postulates is equivocal. In typhoid fever, for example, immunological evidence strongly supports the etiological relation of the microorganism to the disease. Typhoid fever can be prevented by immunization with vaccines prepared from cultures of the microorganism, and the naturally infected individual who recovers from the disease develops an immunity directed specifically toward the microorganism. Alternatively, the indirect supporting evidence may be epidemiological in nature, serving to associate a particular microorganism with a given disease, even though the disease cannot be reproduced experimentally.

Multiple Etiology[44]
Koch's postulates were intended, and are used, to describe the connection of a single microorganism to a particular disease. In certain naturally occurring diseases, however, several kinds of agents are sometimes involved. The etiological relationships are often complex, and three categories of such diseases are distinguished.

Secondary Infections. Secondary infection may occur when a primary invader reduces the resistance of the host so that a second kind of microorganism, of limited pathogenic powers and often a part of the normal microbial flora of the host, produces disease. Staphylococcal pneumonia, for instance, is rarely a primary disease but is most often seen as a secondary infection, commonly as a sequel to influenza. Predisposition to secondary infection is usually by alteration of cellular and humoral immunity, suppression of phagocytosis, or induction of anatomic changes in the host.

Mixed Infections. Other kinds of disease characteristically arise from mixed infections, in which more than one kind of agent is concerned from the outset. Thus, as many as eight different species of clostridia may cause gaseous gangrene; these occur in various combinations, but rarely is a single species responsible for the disease syndrome.

In both secondary and mixed infections the causative microorganisms are independently and individually capable of producing a disease condition, although often under severely restricted circumstances.

Dual Infections. The third kind of infection is that in which the etiology is a consequence of a synergistic relation between two microorganisms, the combination having pathogenic potential not possessed by the individual components.[61] Such dual etiologies become complex and are possibly more common than generally thought.

The classic example of dual etiology of disease is that of swine influenza, in which the two microorganisms are the porcine influenza bacillus, *Haemophilus suis,* and a variety of influenza virus. Swine influenza is not caused by either agent alone, but only by a combination of the two. Another, and potentially more significant, example is that of human diphtheria. For more than 70 years it was believed that the microbial etiology of this disease was fully and clearly established as due to a single kind of microorganism, *Corynebacterium diphtheriae.* In 1951, however, it was found that toxin formation by this bacterium, which accounts for its pathogenic potential, is due to lysogenic conversion by a specific bacterial virus or bacteriophage (Chapter 6). Thus, only the lysogenized bacterium, in effect a combination of two microorganisms, is capable of causing diphtheria.

It is not yet clear how common the phenomenon of true multiple etiology may be. There are indications that the etiology of many infections may not be as firmly established as has been thought. Infectious disease is a highly complex phenomenon, involving more than the nature and properties of the causative microorganism, and it is possible that observed discrepancies are due to an oversimplification of microbial etiology.

Microbial Pathogenicity and Virulence[66, 67, 73, 75]

Pathogenicity has been used above in its generally accepted sense as the ability of a microorganism to produce disease. Pathogenic potential varies widely, not only from one kind of microorganism to another, but also between strains of a single kind. The term virulence has often been used in a more or less synonymous fashion. The two terms will be used here in the sense suggested by Miles and now widely accepted. **Pathogenicity** refers to the potential capacity to cause disease and is applied to groups or species of microorganisms. Thus, for example, *Salmonella* are considered to be pathogens because they can produce disease in an animal host. **Virulence** refers to the degree of pathogenicity within a group or species and is generally measured by the number of microorganisms required to produce disease (see Measurement of Virulence). Thus, avirulent, virulent, or highly virulent strains may occur within a group of microorganisms that are said to be pathogenic.

Even though microorganisms may be introduced directly into the tissues of an animal host through cuts, burns, wounds, or inoculation by insect vectors, most infections begin when the agent penetrates the mucous membranes of the respiratory, gastrointestinal, or urogenital tract. Pathogenic bacteria possess qualities that set them apart from nonpathogens. With very few exceptions, pathogens must have the capacity to establish or colonize on the mucous membranes; in most cases they must penetrate the membranes and multiply in host tissues. Successful survival in the host is often further dependent on their capacity to avoid stimulating host defenses.

The first requirement of pathogenicity is, then, the ability to initiate infection, termed infectivity. Infection *per se* does not invariably lead to disease. To cause disease, the infecting agent must also meet a second requirement for pathogenicity, the ability to injure the host. In many instances, host damage is due to the production of toxic substances by the invading parasite.

The pathogenic potential of a given microorganism is determined by a multiplicity of factors, some of microbial and others of host origin. Knowledge of the microbial determinants of virulence is necessary for an understanding of disease mechanisms and often forms the scientific basis for control and management of disease.

It is self-evident that a complex interrelationship exists between a pathogen and its susceptible host and that microbial pathogenicity can be expressed only when disease is produced in the host. Conversely, host resistance to infectious disease is evident only as a response to the presence of the microorganism. Although resistance and disease are fundamentally inseparable, for convenience they will be considered individually.

INFECTION

Infection of the host is, in most circumstances, a necessary first step in production of microbial disease. The most notable exceptions are the food poisonings in which toxins, produced in foods as a consequence of microbial growth, are ingested and subsequently give rise to disease symptoms (Chapter 36). On the other hand, infection does not always cause disease. The colonization of a host animal by the normal microbial flora may be considered, in the broad sense, infection. These microbes are established on skin and mucous membranes soon after birth and persist in more or less stable form throughout the life of the host. Only rarely, as when host defenses are compromised, do they invade to cause disease. Indeed, they probably play an active role in host resistance by interfering with colonization by pathogens.

To initiate infection, most pathogenic agents must establish themselves on the mucous membranes and multiply. They must compete, in this process, with the indigenous microbial flora for attachment sites and for available nutrients. For some pathogenic microorganisms, no further penetration or invasion of tissues is necessary. As one illustration, the cholera vibrio does not invade the tissues of the intestine, but rather grows on the mucous membrane surface. Here it elaborates a toxin that is absorbed and attacks specific target cells, causing water and electrolyte loss to the intestinal lumen, which is the prominent character of this disease. In other instances, as exemplified in *Shigella* infections, the bacilli invade only to a minor degree; their penetration into the superficial layers of the intestinal epithelium is sufficient to injure these cells and to induce the bloody diarrhea that characterizes bacillary dysentery.

In most circumstances, however, pathogenic microorganisms penetrate a variety of host tissues, and their pathogenic potential is expressed by damage to tissues and organs apart from the mucosa at the invasion site. As a part of this invasion process, they must overcome host defenses and multiply within deeper host tissues. A number of microbial capabilities in this regard have been identified. Some microorganisms, by virtue of their surface capsules, are resistant to phagocytosis and thus escape destruction by this host defense mechanism; others may be phagocytized, but can survive and even multiply within phagocytic cells. Bacterial products that counteract host defenses are collectively termed aggressins and will be discussed later.

ADHERENCE[3, 4, 19]

Marine and aquatic microbiologists have long been aware that bacteria growing in nature are almost always adherent to solid surfaces, such as stones, pebbles, grains of sand, and other small particles. In this way they avoid being dispersed and swept away by water currents and take advantage of the concentration of nutrients at solid-liquid interfaces. Although there were isolated observations that bacteria could adhere to animal and plant cells, it is surprising that the ecological significance of cell-cell attachment so long escaped the attention of medical microbiologists.

Over the past two decades, it has been observed repeatedly that many bacteria have a propensity for association with the surface of a variety of animal host cells. This surface adherence can sometimes be demonstrated by agglutination of host cells, *e.g.*, erythrocytes, in which the adherent bacteria form bridges between cells. More often, the bacteria are seen to attach and colonize on the surface of cells or tissues, primarily the mucous membranes.

Mucous membranes are almost constantly exposed to bacteria from the environment— those found in food and water, inspired air and dust, and similar sources. Only bacteria with adherent capacity can establish and multiply at these sites. Many are removed mechanically before significant multiplication takes place through entrapment in and discharge with the mucus of the upper respiratory tract; lavage by urine, saliva, and tears; and entrapment and elimination with the intestinal contents. Bacteria that colonize these membranes share the ability to adhere closely and strongly to the membrane surfaces and, often, to multiply there.

A few bacteria adhere to seemingly inert surfaces. Attachment and colonization of the enamel surface of the teeth by *Streptococcus mutans* is an early event in the induction of dental caries. More widespread, however, is the attachment of bacteria to mucosal cells. Microorganisms entering such intimate associations include the indigenous microbial flora which do not cause disease, as well as pathogenic microorganisms that colonize and even invade from sites of original attachment.

Microbial adherence to eucaryotic cells is usually a specific process. Bacterial surface structures, called **adhesins,** react and combine with complementary receptors on the surface of eucaryotic cells. These specific interactions are generally thought to explain why individual bacterial strains show predilection for particular sites on body surfaces. Selective colonization of the teeth with *S. mutans* may be contrasted with the behavior of *Streptococcus salivarius*, the predominant streptococcus on the tongue, but a minor colonizer of tooth surfaces. Similarly, strains of *Streptococcus pyogenes* derived from pharyngeal infections adhere well to pharyngeal cells, whereas strains derived from pyoderma do not.

This adhesive property of pathogenic bacteria is recognized as an important determinant of virulence, and adhesion to mucosal surfaces is the first step in pathogenesis leading to infectious disease. A number of bacterial surface structures have been implicated in the attachment process, and current research seeks to determine the nature of the ligand-receptor interactions that result in adherence. Intervention in this important step in pathogenesis could aid in infectious disease control.

Mechanisms of Adherence[53]

Because the net surface charge for both eucaryotic and procaryotic cells is negative, repulsion would be expected to prevent adhesion between host and bacterial cells. The overall negative charge does not, however, preclude localized attractive zones on the cell surfaces that could arise from areas with higher density of hydrophobic molecules. These relatively weak, nonspecific attractive forces in localized areas can permit the approach of bacteria to the host cell surface; firm binding, however, depends upon interaction between **ligands** on the bacterial surface and complementary **receptors** on the host cell. The participation of large numbers of these specific attractive forces brings about a firm union between the cells.

Bacterial surface components that either contain or constitute the adherence ligand include fimbriae, fibrillae, surface polysaccharides, and specialized membrane locales, exemplified by the terminal structure on mycoplasma cells. These components of bacterial cells are collectively known as **adhesins.**

Fimbriae.[54] Many gram-negative bacteria possess surface fimbriae or pili, some of which function in adherence. Since most fimbriae are exclusively protein, they likely react with host cell receptors by virtue of a specific amino acid sequence or peptide configuration.

Efforts to define host cell receptors for fimbrial adhesins led to the observation that adherence by some fimbriated bacteria is blocked by the presence of D-mannose, suggesting that the host cell receptor for these bacteria contains mannose or mannose-like residues. Adhesins inhibited in this fashion are termed **mannose-sensitive,** and may be contrasted with **mannose-resistant** adhesins not so affected. Similar inhibition studies indicate that perti-

nent host cell receptors are probably membrane glycolipids or glycoproteins containing specific sugars, *e.g.,* mannose, fucose, sialic acid, or β-galactosyl residues.

Fimbriation is frequently correlated with other bacterial characters, such as colonial morphology, the tendency to form surface pellicles in liquid mediums, the ability to agglutinate certain erythrocytes, and adherence to a variety of other eucaryotic cells, and to other procaryotes, including those of plants and fungi.

Fibrillae. Fine, hair-like projections may be seen on the surface of gram-positive (and possibly some gram-negative) bacteria that are involved in adherence. These do not satisfy the morphological criteria for fimbriae and are termed fibrillae. In *Streptococcus pyogenes*, these fibrillae are composed of protein-lipoteichoic acid complexes. The lipid portion of lipoteichoic acid is thought to be the adhesive ligand that binds to protein or glycoprotein in the host cell membrane.

Surface Polysaccharides.[30] Certain oral bacteria, particularly *Streptococcus mutans*, adhere to the enamel surfaces of the teeth. In *S. mutans*, adherence is associated with production of an extracellular, water-insoluble glucan at the cell surface. The polymer, synthesized from sucrose by glucosyl transferase, is excreted from the cell and binds to the tooth. This polysaccharide matrix, with entrapped bacteria, becomes dental plaque and may ultimately lead to the production of caries. It is of interest that mature plaque also contains a variety of bacteria that coaggregate with one another in a specific manner, suggesting cell-cell adherence (Chapter 37).

Other Attachment Structures.[10] A few bacteria, notably *Mycoplasma* and certain filamentous bacteria, seem to attach by their ends to epithelial cells; specialized membrane zones at the tip of the cell probably constitute the attachment structure. Mycoplasmas, which have no cell wall, often exhibit a distinct terminal structure by which they attach to the membrane of host target cells (see Fig. 35–3, Chapter 35). The attachment ligand appears to be a surface protein of the bacterial membrane that reacts with a sialic acid–containing receptor in the host cell membrane.

Alterations in Adherence

Although adherence may be an important factor in colonization and infection, it can also adversely affect survival of the microorganism. Phagocytosis of fimbriated cells is, for example, more efficient than nonfimbriated cells, since attachment to phagocytes is the first step in phagocytosis and intracellular killing, as detailed in Phagocytic Defenses (p. 348). The successful pathogen must adapt to changes in the host environment; there is evidence that some bacteria do undergo alterations in their adherence potential after they enter the tissues. This is thought to have some survival advantage, since they might then avoid phagocytic killing. Similarly, many bacteria possess capsules that can either mask adhesins or alter the surface charge of the parent cell, thereby altering adherence.

Adherence may also be affected by intercurrent viral infections. Host cells infected by the influenza virus express new or additional receptors for staphylococci and certain other bacteria,[11] and oropharyngeal colonization by staphylococci is significantly increased during respiratory illness.[58]

Adherence may also be inhibited by the presence of specific antibodies to the adhesin. Attempted immunization against gonorrhea by use of fimbrial antigens is based upon this possible host defense mechanism.

Adherence and Virulence

It is already apparent that adherence is a factor in the capacity of a bacterium to infect a susceptible host and is often associated with virulence (Table 12–1). The association of adherence with virulence is not always evident, however. Many nonpathogens are able to adhere to eucaryotic cells and, even among pathogens, adherence is not always correlated with virulence. This should not be surprising, since virulence of a microorganism is multifactorial

and the host-parasite relationship is exceedingly complex, as will be evident in following sections.

PENETRATION AND MULTIPLICATION[73]

Although a few pathogenic bacteria—including *Vibrio cholerae*, some strains of enteropathic *Escherichia coli*, and *Bordetella pertussis*—can injure the host as a result of their proliferation on mucosal surfaces, most pathogens must penetrate into the tissues and multiply there before pathogenesis is evident. The mechanisms of penetration are not well understood and our knowledge is based largely on histological findings in animal models and in cell cultures. Microscopic studies on penetration of the mucosa of the small intestine by *Salmonella* have disclosed that when the microorganisms adhere closely to the brush border, the microvilli begin to degenerate. As the bacteria penetrate into the cell, further degeneration occurs and culminates in formation of a cytoplasmic vacuole, containing one or more bacteria. Subsequent regeneration of the microvilli ensues. The mechanism for further penetration into the lamina propria is not known. Mucosal penetration by *Neisseria gonorrhoeae* is somewhat different, at least in the early stages. Gonococci initially contact the microvilli of the columnar epithelium and are enveloped by them; they do not, however, cause host cell degeneration as seen with *Salmonella*. By a process analogous to phagocytosis, the gonococci then enter the epithelial cell enclosed in a membrane-bound vacuole. The bacteria subsequently multiply and spread, possibly by exocytosis from the originally infected cells.

The microbial virulence determinants associated with penetration and persistence in tissues are best exemplified in *Shigella*. Penetration of the intestinal mucosa by *Shigella* is largely dependent upon the presence of smooth lipopolysaccharide antigen on the bacterial cell surface and upon the chemical composition of the O-specific side chain, although other factors, as yet undefined, may also be involved.[29] Furthermore, the capability of multiplying in tissues is under separate genetic control from that of penetration.

The ability to grow *in vivo* constitutes, therefore, a virulence determinant for invasive microorganisms. It is likely that *in vivo* growth is frequently determined by the nutritional requirements of the microorganism and the adequacy of the host environment to provide

Table 12–1. Adherence Factors Associated with Virulence of Some Representative Bacteria

Bacteria	Adherence Factor
Escherichia coli	Fimbriae (MS*) Fimbriae (MR†)
Salmonella spp.	Fimbriae (MS)
Klebsiella spp.	Fimbriae (MS)
Neisseria gonorrhoeae	Fimbriae (MR)
Streptococcus pyogenes	Lipoteichoic acid
Streptococcus mutans	Glucan
Mycoplasma pneumoniae	Specialized terminal structure (protein)

*MS = mannose sensitive.
†MR = mannose resistant.

Table 12–2. **Siderophores in Pathogenic Bacteria***

Microorganism	Siderophore
Enteric bacteria	Enterobactin (enterochelins) Aerobactin
Mycobacterium spp.	Mycobactins
Neisseria spp.†	Gonobactins Meningobactins
Pseudomonas spp.	Pyochelins

*Neilands.[50]
†Yancey and Finkelstein.[79]

these nutrients. For example, the obligate intracellular parasite *Chlamydia psittaci* competes with its host cell for available isoleucine in the intracellular pool and does not grow when this amino acid is limiting.[31] Similarly, microorganisms require metallic ions for a variety of physiological reactions, and the requirement for iron is of particular importance in the host-parasite relationship.

Iron and Infection[8,51]

Iron in body fluids is not normally free, but is complexed by iron-binding host proteins, principally **transferrins.** These are reported to reduce available free iron to $10^{-8}M$, a level insufficient for bacterial growth. These chelators, collectively termed **siderophores,** are usually not iron saturated and are considered to play a role in host resistance to infection.

The mammalian iron-binding proteins have functional counterparts in many bacteria. Bacterial siderophores are low-molecular-weight molecules that scavenge iron and make it available to the bacterium for essential metabolism. Many pathogenic bacteria possess siderophores, permitting them to compete successfully for host iron during infection. Siderophores are, therefore, virulence determinants in such bacteria. Microbial siderophores are generally hydroxymates or phenolate-catechols and are found in both aerobic and facultatively anaerobic microorganisms. Some of the siderophores of pathogenic bacteria are listed in Table 12–2.

AGGRESSINS[66]

Once microbial invaders gain entry, the host responds in a variety of ways to eliminate the parasite, as described in the later section, Natural Resistance to Infection. Successful pathogenic bacteria must minimize the effectiveness of host defenses through mechanisms

such as the production of **aggressins,** nontoxic substances inhibiting the humoral and cellular elements of host defenses. Toxic bacterial products are discussed in a following section.

Microbial pathogens first contact the defenses of the host on the surfaces of the mucosal membranes, where they encounter elements of immune and natural resistance. Among the most effective immune defenses at these sites is a specialized form of immunoglobulin, **secretory immunoglobulin A** (sIgA). Although sIga does not activate complement or promote phagocytosis, it does inhibit bacterial adherence and plays a significant role in viral defenses; in addition, sIgA reacts with certain bacterial products to prevent their absorption through mucosal membranes. Many bacteria possess specific enzymes capable of cleaving and destroying human IgA, termed **IgA proteases.**[43] Such enzymes are aggressins in these bacteria, exemplified by a correlation between IgA protease production and virulence in certain *Neisseria*.

Aggressins Inhibiting Humoral Defenses[20]

Among the first barriers encountered by infecting bacteria are the several bactericidal factors found in blood and tissue fluids; these include β-lysins, complement, lysozyme, certain basic peptides, and the transferrins previously mentioned. Virulence, in a number of microorganisms, depends upon their ability to withstand these host microbicidal factors. For example, many strains of *Neisseria gonorrhoeae* causing uncomplicated gonorrhea are readily killed by normal serum, presumably because they become acutely deficient in iron in the presence of partially saturated transferrin. Other strains, causing disseminated infection, are serum resistant due to the synthesis of siderophores. Similarly, invasive strains of *E. coli* achieve serum resistance by the production of **enterobactin.** These siderophores are, therefore, aggressins.

Siderophore production is only one of several mechanisms for withstanding effects of serum, but the others have not been extensively studied. The ability of *E. coli* to repair damage to its membrane may determine resistance to antibody-complement lysis.[47] In other bacteria, serum resistance may depend upon surface components, including lipopolysaccharides and capsules.

Aggressins Inhibiting Cellular Defenses[12]

The cellular defenses of the normal mammalian host usually leading to phagocytosis and destruction of invading microorganisms include the relatively short-lived polymorphonuclear phagocytes and the more durable mononuclear cells. The former are most effective against extracellular pathogens, while the latter control infections due to the obligate and facultative intracellular parasites.

The mobilization and action of these phagocytic cells require several sequential steps, *viz.,* **chemotaxis,** or attraction of phagocytes to the site of microbial multiplication or tissue injury; **attachment** of the microorganisms to the phagocyte plasma membrane; **ingestion** into a phagosomal vacuole lying in the cytoplasm of the phagocyte; **degranulation** or fusion of lysosomes with the phagosome, to form the phagolysosome; and **destruction** of the parasite by a variety of microbicidal mechanisms in the phagolysosome. The details of phagocyte chemotaxis, phagocytosis, and intracellular destruction will be found in the following section on host resistance (p. 348).

It is evident that microbial virulence is enhanced by resistance to one or more of these phagocyte operations.

Inhibition of Chemotaxis. Phagocytes are often attracted to the site of injury and microbial proliferation as a part of the host inflammatory response; many microorganisms fail to elicit such responses. Some virulent strains of the gonococcus, for example, do not activate complement and thus do not stimulate chemotaxis. *Pseudomonas aeruginosa,* on the other hand, produces an extracellular protease which destroys complement components that initiate chemotaxis, acting as an aggressin.

Inhibition of Phagocytosis. Phagocytosis of invading microorganisms begins with their adherence to the phagocyte plasma membrane, a specific process involving cell-cell interactions analogous to epithelial cell colonization discussed earlier; adherence is usually followed by ingestion of the offending microorganism.

One of the classic observations relating to host-parasite relationships was the discovery that **capsules** on the surface of pneumococcal cells inhibit their phagocytosis. Since ingestion and subsequent destruction of the pneumococcus is the basis for host defense in this disease, the importance of this aggressin in virulence is unquestioned. Many other bacteria are also destroyed after ingestion by granulocytes; their capacity to avoid phagocytosis is, therefore, essential for persistence in the animal host. The aggressins responsible may be morphologically evident capsules, as in the pneumococcus, or other surface components (Table 12–3). Although attachment is usually followed by ingestion, this is not invariably the

Table 12–3. **Bacterial Surface Components (Aggressins) That Interfere with Phagocytosis**

Aggressin	Microorganism
Polysaccharide capsule	*Streptococcus pneumoniae* *Neisseria meningitidis* *Pseudomonas aeruginosa* *Klebsiella pneumoniae* *Haemophilus influenzae* *Staphylococcus aureus*
Protein A	*Staphylococcus aureus*
Polypeptide capsule	*Bacillus anthracis*
M protein, hyaluronic acid	*Streptococcus pyogenes*
Vi antigen	*Salmonella typhi*
K polysaccharide	*Escherichia coli*
Lipopolysaccharide	Enteric bacilli

case, as exemplified by certain virulent gonococci that attach to polymorphonuclear leucocytes but are not subsequently ingested. Such findings suggest that some virulence determinants are associated only with the ingestion step.

So far as known, antiphagocytic aggressins do not exhibit any common chemical characteristics, although many are polysaccharides. It is possible that physical characteristics are more important, since these seem to be surface structures of the cell. It has been suggested, for example, that capsules can mask or interfere with adhesins, thereby preventing attachment. It is also possible that surface aggressins may conceal bacterial components that would otherwise activate complement components to trigger chemotaxis and phagocytosis.[60]

It is usually possible to circumvent the action of antiphagocytic aggressins by reaction with specific antibody; antibody-treated bacteria are usually phagocytized without difficulty. Virulent encapsulated pneumococci, after reaction with anticapsular antibody, are rapidly ingested and killed, thereby furnishing the basis for effective immunity in pneumococcal pneumonia.

Resistance to Intracellular Destruction.[27, 70] After ingestion has occurred, resistance of the bacteria to intracellular destruction may take several forms: (1) inhibition of lysosome-phagosome fusion; (2) resistance to oxygen-dependent mechanisms of intraleucocytic killing, *e.g.,* myeloperoxidase and associated systems; or (3) resistance to lysosomal antimicrobial proteins, *e.g.,* lysozyme, lactoferrin, and cationic proteins.

Table 12–4. **Bacterial Aggressins and Resistance to Intracellular Destruction**

	Aggressins Interfering with		
Microorganism	Lysosome-Phagosome Fusion	Oxidative Attack	Lysosomal Antimicrobial Proteins
Salmonella typhimurium			Lipopolysaccharide
Escherichia coli		Superoxide dismutase (?)	Lipopolysaccharide
Staphylococcus aureus		Catalase	Coagulase (?)
Listeria monocytogenes		Catalase	
Mycobacterium	Elevated cAMP, sulfolipids	Catalase	Mycosides (?)
Streptococcus			C-polysaccharides, peptidoglycan
Brucella	Uknown aggressin	Catalase	Cell wall component
Chlamydia	Unknown aggressin		

Although a number of microorganisms have been shown to exhibit one or more of these, the microbial aggressins responsible are only now becoming known. Table 12–4 lists many of the known aggressins and their activity.

Not included are certain toxic substances produced by bacteria that are cytotoxic for phagocytes and other cells. These are discussed in the following section.

INJURY TO CELLS AND TISSUES[72]

The derangement of the normal physiological process that constitutes infectious disease is generally a consequence of the **toxicity** of proliferating microorganisms that have become established in the tissues. Toxic substances affecting tissues, cells, and possibly enzyme systems are formed by the microorganisms incidental to their metabolic activities. Some of these diffuse more or less freely from the microbial cells, and others are part of the cell soma. In addition, toxic effects may be produced indirectly, as by the activation of tissue enzymes by bacterial kinases, or by formation of inflammatory and similar toxic substances by the affected tissues, and by the development of hypersensitivity to the microbial cell substance (Chapter 10).

In many diseases, however, no toxins have yet been described that account for the disease symptoms. Indeed, even when toxic substances of microbial origin are known, their relevance to the disease process is not always clear. In only a few cases can pathogenesis be ascribed to a single toxic substance; these are exemplified in the intoxications attributable to the classic exotoxins.

The toxicities of microbial origin may be separated into three groups: the potent **exotoxins,** which are the classical bacterial toxins; the **endotoxins,** which occur as structural components of the bacterial cell wall; and a heterogeneous group of toxic substances, often enzymatic in function, which usually diffuse from the bacterial cell. Such separation is obviously artificial, and lines of demarcation between the groups are often indistinct, but it is useful for purposes of discussion.

EXOTOXINS[1, 24, 25, 33, 80]

The bacterial exotoxins are the most potent poisons known, and it has been calculated that as little as 7 ounces of crystalline botulinum type A toxin would suffice to kill the entire population of the world. These toxins have their counterparts in the less potent zootoxins, such as snake, spider, and scorpion venoms, and in the phytotoxins, such as ricin and abrin.

The nomenclature of microbial toxins, as with any arbitrary classification, is not entirely satisfactory. It is generally agreed that microbial toxins are antigenic poisons produced by bacteria. Those that are proteins of high toxicity and found in cell-free culture supernatants are considered to be classic **exotoxins.** Such arbitrary classification leaves uncertain the status of a number of less potent substances, such as hemolysins, some cytotoxins, and a variety

Table 12–5. **Bacterial Exotoxins with Predominant Roles in Disease**

Microorganism	Toxin	Disease	Effects of Toxin
Corynebacterium diphtheriae	Diphtheria toxin	Diphtheria	Damage to internal organs, *e.g.*, heart, lungs, liver, kidney, and nervous system; death is usually by cardiac arrest. Toxin inhibits cellular protein synthesis by inactivation of elongation factor 2 (EF-2).
Clostridium tetani	Tetanospasmin	Tetanus	Spastic paralysis of skeletal muscle. Toxin blocks synaptic release of certain neurotransmitters or interferes with their postsynaptic action.
Clostridium botulinum	Botulinum toxin	Botulism; botulinum food poisoning	Flaccid paralysis, breathing and swallowing difficulty, and double vision. Toxin prevents release of acetylcholine from cholinergic nerve endings of peripheral nervous system. There are 8 serotypes of toxin.
Vibrio cholerae	Cholera enterotoxin	Cholera	Diarrhea, with massive fluid and electrolyte loss leading to extreme dehydration. Adenylate cyclase is elevated, resulting in increased cAMP in ileal mucosal cells.
Escherichia coli	Heat-labile enterotoxin	*E. coli* enterocolitis	Diarrhea, with fluid and electrolyte loss. Toxin action is similar to that of cholera toxin.
Pseudomonas aeruginosa	Exotoxin A	Several opportunistic infections	Precise effect in humans not established; lethal for animals. Mode of action similar to diphtheria toxin.
Staphylococcus aureus	Enterotoxin	Staphylococcal food poisoning	Ingestion results in diarrhea and vomiting. Mode of action not established. Several serological types.
		Toxic shock syndrome	Fever, diarrhea, shock, and rash; putatively due to pyrogenic exotoxin.
	Exfoliatin	Scalded skin syndrome	Epidermal separation, resulting in blister-like lesions or bullae. Several serological types.
Clostridium perfringens	Enterotoxin	*C. perfringens* food poisoning	Diarrhea and vomiting.
Bacillus cereus	Enterotoxin	*B. cereus* food poisoning	Vomiting and diarrhea. Toxin(s) not well characterized.
Clostridium difficile	Enterotoxin	Antimicrobial enterocolitis	Disease usually follows antimicrobial therapy. Toxin is cytotoxic and causes colitis in animals and in man.

of necrotic and lethal microbial products. This latter group will, for convenience, be considered in the section on Other Bacterial Products. The classic exotoxins produced by *Clostridium botulinum, Clostridium tetani,* and *Corynebacterium diphtheriae;* the enterotoxins produced by a variety of microorganisms; and the exfoliating toxin of *Staphylococcus aureus* generally account for the specific pathology of the individual diseases. Table 12–5 summarizes the important characteristics of these and other bacterial exotoxins with predominant roles in disease production. The list is by no means exhaustive and does not include a number of exotoxins that are probably involved in virulence but do not play a major role in disease production.

Botulinum type A toxin is the most potent of the bacterial toxins. The minimum lethal dose (MLD) for the mouse is about 4×10^{-6} μg; that for the slightly less toxic type B toxin, about 8×10^{-6} μg. Tetanus toxin is somewhat less toxic. Highly purified diphtheria toxin is lethal for sensitive species (guinea pig, rabbit, man) at levels of 0.1 μg. per kilogram of body weight. These amounts are incredibly small, but many of the toxins are neurotoxins, and thus need react with only limited numbers of target cells in order to show effect. The lethal dose of botulinum in the mouse, for example, is about 20 million molecules, corresponding to about eight molecules per target nerve cell.

The potency of these exotoxins is, in general, paralleled by their efficiency as antigens. Antitoxic serums of high titer may be obtained against diphtheria toxin, such that 1 ml. of antitoxin will neutralize thousands of minimum lethal doses for the guinea pig.

The gross chemical composition of exotoxins is unremarkable. They are proteins with no unusual characteristics in their amino acid composition. Their structure may, however, be somewhat complex.

The larger toxins, *e.g.,* cholera, diphtheria, tetanus, and botulinum toxins and *E. coli* enterotoxin, range in molecular weight from about 62,000 to 150,000 daltons. In several cases they comprise subunits or fragments with differing functions. One subunit is usually responsible for binding of the toxin to susceptible cells, while the other possesses toxic activity. The smaller toxins, *e.g.,* exfoliatin and the enterotoxins of *S. aureus* and *C. perfringens,* have molecular weights of about 25,000 to 30,000 daltons and are not known to have subunit structure.

Most exotoxins are destroyed by proteolytic enzymes. Exceptions include botulinum toxin and the enterotoxins of staphylococci and *Bacillus cereus*. These are food poisoning toxins, as noted in Chapter 36, and their resistance to proteolytic enzymes is not surprising. Botulinum toxins are, however, partially degraded by gastrointestinal proteases, resulting in more readily absorbable active fragments of lower molecular weight. Thus, partial hydrolysis may contribute significantly to their toxicity by the oral route.

Following the experimental injection of exotoxins, a period of incubation elapses before symptoms of intoxication appear. This incubation period may be very short or may extend to 48 hours or longer. The usual incubation period for tetanus toxin is about 36 hours, but it may be reduced to an hour or less following injection of very large amounts—of the order of 500,000 MLD—of crystalline toxin.

The discovery that the toxic qualities of the soluble toxins are destroyed by treatment with formaldehyde—which, at the same time, leaves the antigenic and antitoxin-combining properties unimpaired—has been of the greatest practical importance in immunization procedures. Toxin so treated is called **toxoid.**

The details of biochemistry, mode of action, and pathogenetic role of exotoxins will be found in following chapters on relevant bacteria; those associated with food poisoning are discussed in Chapter 36.

ENDOTOXINS[7, 18, 40]

Gram-negative bacterial cells, whether living or dead, are toxic when injected into experimental animals. The toxic principle is a part of the outer membrane and has been called **endotoxin** to distinguish it from the exotoxins, which are easily released from cells without lysis. The term endotoxin is not an ideal one in light of present knowledge that the toxic substance can be found in small amounts in culture supernatants, but it remains in use as a descriptive term.

Endotoxin is, in general, synonymous with the **lipopolysaccharide** (LPS) of the outer membrane of gram-negative cells, as described in Chapter 2. Lipopolysaccharide is a structural component of the bacterial cell wall, represents the somatic O antigen, and is composed of a hydrophilic polysaccharide component linked to the hydrophobic **toxophore** group, lipid A. Endotoxins may be contrasted with exotoxins in the following particulars:

1. They are heat-stable, *i.e.,* resistant to boiling in neutral solutions.

2. They are not destroyed by proteolytic enzymes.

3. They are of relatively low toxicity, *e.g.,* the mouse LD_{50} is usually somewhat less than 0.1 mg.

4. Their toxicity is only partially neutralized by specific antiserum.

5. They are not convertible to toxoids.

The endotoxins can be derived from intact gram-negative bacterial cells by a variety of extraction procedures; the complexity of the preparations is greatly influenced by the method employed. Extraction with phenol-water mixtures yields the most homogeneous LPS, representing the endotoxic principle.

The chemical composition and toxic potency of endotoxin varies with the kind of cells extracted, the conditions of cultivation, and the purification methods applied. Most information on the composition and structure of endotoxic LPS is derived from studies on enteric bacteria, principally *Salmonella.* Lipopolysaccharide from these bacteria contains a polysaccharide component consisting of two regions—a **core region,** common to both smooth and rough forms, and a **specific region** made up of O-specific polysaccharide side chains that characterize the smooth form of these bacilli. The lipid component of LPS, the **lipid A region,** is attached to the core polysaccharide backbone structure (see diagram, page 35).

The central core polysaccharide is linked on the one hand to lipid A and on the other to the O-specific side chains. The core consists of a backbone structure made up of basal core sugars that are substituted with other sugars, ethanolamine, and phosphate. While a number of different sugars may be found in this region, 2-keto-3-deoxy-D-manno-octulosonic acid (KDO) is unique to LPS and is invariably present. The core polysaccharide in the LPS of enteric bacteria is group specific; for example, the core region is essentially identical in all species of *Salmonella,* but differs from that found in other genera of enteric bacilli.

As expected, based upon the great number of serotypes in smooth gram-negative bacilli, the O-specific side chain regions vary greatly in their chemical constitution. Although a great number of sugars may be encountered, those occurring with greatest frequency are mannose, fucose, rhamnose, and galactosamine. The chemical nature of the polysaccharides in the O-specific side chains determines the O antigen specificity of the bacterial strain.

Lipid A, the toxophore of LPS, consists of D-glucosamine, phosphorus, and, as major constituents, a variety of fatty acids. These include lauric, palmitic, myristic, and β-hydroxymyristic acids; with few exceptions, the latter seems to be a specific lipid A constituent.

Because of the lipid A component, isolated lipopolysaccharides are highly aggregated; apparent molecular weights range as high as 24×10^6 daltons. The tendency of endotoxin to form aggregates has greatly complicated purification and has compromised studies on the heterogeneity of the toxin and its biological activities.

Though it was long believed that endotoxin antigenicity, and its serological specificity, resided solely in the polysaccharide component, there is evidence that the lipid A component is also immunogenic and induces lipid A–specific antibodies. These cross-react with lipid A derived from a variety of other gram-negative cells and, under certain circumstances, protect against lipid A toxicity.[59]

Biological Effects[74, 76]

Despite chemical and physical differences, endotoxins have substantially similar activities regardless of their origin. A catalogue of the biological effects of endotoxin when administered to animals and humans is astounding in number and variety, and is probably unmatched for any other natural substance. The principal effects are listed in Table 12–6.

The underlying principles that may ultimately explain endotoxin action are beginning to emerge. The framework of endotoxic activity may be expressed diagramatically as follows:

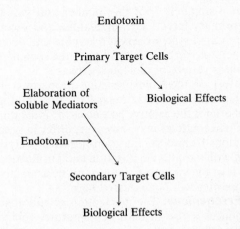

When introduced parenterally, endotoxin reacts with a variety of **primary target cells,** including macrophages, granulocytes, blood platelets, B lymphocytes, and fibroblasts. These cellular reactions are likely controlled

Table 12–6. **Principal Biological Effects Observed after Endotoxin Administration**

Pyrogenicity	Lymphocyte mitogenicity
Resistance to infection	Macrophage activation
Shock and lethality	Decreased phagocytosis
Diarrhea	Inflammation
Generalized Shwartzman	Leucopenia
Radiation protection	Leucocytosis
Tumor necrosis	Hematopoiesis
Adjuvancy	Endotoxin tolerance
Immunosuppression	Complement activation

by receptors on target cells, probably glycero-phosphatides, binding to the lipid A region. The direct action of endotoxin on the primary target system may elicit primary toxicity, apparent as metabolic perturbations of target cells, macrophage activation, lysosomal exocytosis, and the like.

More often, however, primary target cells are induced to release soluble **mediators or effectors** that excite or activate **secondary target systems**, yielding biological effects that, in summary, constitute endotoxicity. A variety of mediators have been described, including lymphocyte-activating factors, glucocorticoid-antagonizing factors, colony-stimulating factors, tumor-necrosis factors, prostaglandins, endogenous pyrogens, and vasoactive factors. It should be noted that several of these mediators may be similar or identical, since their description is based on the assay employed. It is also possible that some are potentiated by endotoxin reentering the system at the secondary target level.

It is apparent that the number and variety of primary target cells, mediators, and secondary target systems serve to amplify and diversify endotoxin actions, leading to the seemingly endless variety of biological effects.

Most of these host-reactive properties are induced by endotoxin regardless of its biological origin; the relative potencies for individual biological effects may, however, differ in preparations from different gram-negative bacteria and with variation in isolation and purification. A few of the more important host-reactive properties will be discussed here.

Pyrogenicity. The inoculation of endotoxin produces a rise in body temperature. Phagocytic cells absorb and often ingest the endotoxin, releasing fever-producing substances, called **endogenous pyrogens.** These are low-molecular-weight proteins that act on the hypothalamus. Released prostaglandins may also serve as mediators of the febrile response.

Blood Changes. Administration of endotoxin to animals first induces a transient leucopenia and later marked leucocytosis; thrombocytopenia is also produced. Secondary host effects derive from the production of mediators, such as **colony-stimulating factors** produced by lymphocytes and factors produced by platelets. Among the more significant blood changes is **disseminated intravascular coagulation,** a major complication in many gram-negative bacterial infections. Activation of the complement system produces secondary effects of vascular permeability, coagulation, and leucocyte chemotaxis. Increased capillary permeability, often observed in endotoxemia, may be severe, with the production of local hemorrhage.

Shock and Lethality. Among the more striking aspects of endotoxemia are the disturbances in capillary permeability and associated changes that affect circulation and blood pressure—the syndrome of **endotoxic shock.** Shock is the sum of endotoxin-induced reactions involving, but not limited to, effects on leucocytes and platelets, complement activation, release of vasoactive substances, and myocardial depression. High doses of endotoxin are fatal for experimental animals.

Tolerance. The repeated administration of endotoxin to animals produces a refractory state in which the host-reactive properties are progressively diminished; the effect is pronounced in the febrile response, but applies to most other reactive properties as well.

The foregoing has centered on the effects of endotoxin *per se,* but it is the role of toxin in infection that is of underlying importance to the student of pathogenesis. For example, irreversible endotoxin shock is seen in gram-negative sepsis, and the Shwartzman reaction (see below) may account for some, or even a major portion, of the toxicity seen in such infections. When a single dose of endotoxin is given, the effects, including fever and malaise, mimic those seen in gram-negative bacterial infections, but they are transient and do not always parallel those in naturally occurring diseases.

OTHER BACTERIAL PRODUCTS[5, 37, 46, 68]

A variety of other substances formed by microorganisms sometimes contribute to the disease process, either directly or by facilitating establishment of a focus of infection. Some of these products are **cytotoxic,** affecting red and white blood cells; others interfere with blood clotting mechanisms; and still others are enzymes catalyzing degradation of structural elements of the tissues. Currently, the fragmentary information does not permit unequivocal assessment of their individual roles in virulence, but it is apparent that a pathogenic bacterium may have at its disposal a unique series of mechanisms for successful invasion of the host tissues, with subsequent production of disease. The more important of these activities will be considered briefly.

Hemolysins

A variety of bacteria produce hemolysins, substances which bring about the dissolution, or lysis, of red blood cells in suspensions. With few exceptions, these hemolysins may be considered to be exotoxins, since most of them are heat-labile, immunogenic proteins that are convertible to toxoids, and are found in culture supernatants. They differ from the exotoxins discussed earlier, however, in that they are significantly less potent. Hemolytic activity may also be shown by cultivating bacteria on blood agar plates (see below). There is evidence that blood plate hemolysis will detect not only the soluble or filterable hemolysins but other hemolytic substances as well.

While bacterial hemolysins all show the common feature of red blood cell lysis, they vary in other characteristics such as immunological specificity; sensitivity to oxidation, heat, and acid; optimum temperature for hemolysis; and activity on erythrocytes of various animal species.

Although a great number of bacteria are known to produce filterable hemolysins or to exhibit blood plate hemolysis, those of the staphylococci, streptococci, and clostridia are best known. A single bacterial strain may produce more than one hemolysin. Certain staphylococci form at least two hemolysins. One, α-hemolysin, acts on both rabbit and sheep cells to bring about rapid lysis at 37° C.; the other, β-hemolysin, acts only on sheep cells, which are lysed after holding at a lower temperature for several hours—a phenomenon termed "**hot-cold**" lysis. The action of both may be shown on blood agar plates as illustrated in Figure 12–1.

Multiple hemolysin production is not limited to staphylococci. Many streptococci, for example, produce two hemolysins—oxygen-labile **streptolysin O**, and oxygen-insensitive **streptolysin S**. The occurrence of multiple hemolysins is especially marked among the clostridia; many strains of *Clostridium perfringens*, for example, produce two hemolysins, α- and θ-toxins.

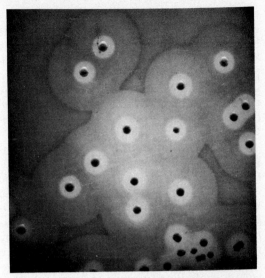

Figure 12–1. "Hot-cold" hemolysis by *Staphylococcus aureus* on sheep blood agar, produced by holding the plate alternately at incubator and refrigerator temperatures. The small clear zones are produced in the incubator by the α-hemolysis and the large zones in the refrigerator by the β-hemolysis.

Hemolytic toxins appear to bind and react with erythrocyte membranes; subsequent lysis is an all-or-none phenomenon in that a single cell is not partially lysed. Staphylococcal α-hemolysin initiates multiple blisters on rabbit erythrocyte membranes; as hemolysis occurs, the cell collapses, ghosts are formed, and large fragments separate from the red cell surface. Less sensitive cells, such as human erythrocytes, exhibit only finger-like protrusions from the surface.[42] Hemolysins may also affect cell membranes of other types of cells. Staphylococcal and streptococcal hemolysins have been found to lyse bacterial protoplasts and to bring about subtle changes in cytoplasmic membranes of cultured human cells.

Blood-Plate Hemolysis. Some bacterial colonies on blood agar produce visible changes in the surrounding medium attributable to hemolysis. Two types of changes are observed, one designated as α-**hemolysis,** in which there is a surrounding zone of greenish discoloration and the other, β-**hemolysis,** in which the zone is clear and uncolored, contrasting with the red opacity of the medium. Microscopic examination shows many discolored erythrocytes in α-hemolytic zones, but no cells are seen in β-hemolytic zones.

The relation between blood-plate hemolysis and the production of filterable hemolysins is sometimes uncertain, for microorganisms hemolytic on blood plates may not produce filterable hemolysin. It appears that the processes involved are different; filterable hemolysins alter red cell permeability and the hemoglobin simply escapes, while in blood-plate hemolysis the pigment is degraded to green or colorless states. Often, however, the two are congruent, as in the close association between β-hemolysis on blood plates by streptococci and the production of streptolysin O.

Hemolysins and Virulence. The relationship between hemolysin formation and virulence is not always apparent. It might be expected that infection with hemolytic bacteria would be accompanied by anemia and hemoglobinuria. Indeed, this is the case in *C. perfringens* infections that are characterized by gross blood destruction and consequent severe anemia due to α-toxin. The massive intravascular hemolysis and associated hemoglobinuria produced in direct hemolysis by scrub typhus rickettsia may be a significant part of pathogenesis in this disease. But in staphylococcal and streptococcal infections caused by hemolytic bacteria, no such major blood changes are evident. It should be noted, however, that hemolysis is only one of the toxic manifestations of these substances. Most also adversely affect leucocytes, macrophages, and blood platelets, even in sublethal concentrations. Several are cardiotoxic, while others disturb functions in the central nervous system; many are dermonecrotic. This range of effects possibly derives from perturbations of cellular and lysosomal membranes. Thus, hemolysins might be expected to contribute to host injury by mechanisms other than red blood cell lysis.

Leucocidin

A number of bacteria, notably staphylococci, streptococci, pneumococci, and *Pseudomonas,* form leucocidins—toxins that kill polymorphonuclear leucocytes. Often this is an accessory function of hemolysins, as noted above, but in others, the leucocidin is not related to red blood cell lysis. A case in point is the **staphylococcal leucocidin,** known to destroy human granulocytes and macrophages; no other cell types are susceptible to its action. Staphylococcal leucocidin is composed of two immunogenic protein subunits and is convertible to toxoid by formaldehyde. It increases cation permeability in susceptible cells.

The part played by leucocidins in virulence of the bacterium is not well established. Theoretically, the inhibition of host defenses by destruction of leucocytes should offer an advantage to the invading microorganism, but

these are complex relationships and have not been clarified.

The details of cytolysin action, including that of hemolysins and leucocidins, will be found in relevant chapters on individual microorganisms.

Coagulase

The formation of fibrin clots is accelerated by a bacterial product known as coagulase. Coagulase production is largely confined to the staphylococci and may be causally related to thrombus formation, common in infections with these organisms. Occasional strains of other bacteria may also exhibit coagulase activity.

Fibrin clot formation proceeds in two stages, *viz.,* interaction between the bacterial product and a plasma factor similar to prothrombin, yielding the clotting agent, coagulase. While the bacterial factor is, strictly speaking, procoagulase, it is commonly referred to as coagulase. It is a relatively heat-stable protein and, in staphylococci, appears in two forms, one free and the other cell-bound. Coagulase is immunogenic and comprises several serological types; more than one of these may be produced by a single strain. Other details of production and action will be found in Chapter 14.

Formation of coagulase in staphylococci is closely associated with virulence. The required plasma factor is not found in all animal species, and there is a correlation between its production and the susceptibility of the animal to staphylococcal infection. The virulence of coagulase-positive staphylococci is enhanced in plasma factor–deficient animals if the inoculated bacteria are suspended in coagulable plasma, *i.e.,* containing the plasma factor. Apparently, coating of bacteria with a fibrin network interferes mechanically with the phagocytic process. Furthermore, coagulase antagonizes the antibacterial action of normal serum; coagulase-positive bacteria grow in such serums while coagulase-negative bacteria do not.

Bacterial Kinases

Several kinds of bacteria, principally streptococci and staphylococci, are able to dissolve fibrin clots or to inhibit the clotting of plasma. The responsible substance is a bacterial kinase that acts indirectly to dissolve the clot. Bacterial kinase activates a plasma substance, plasminogen, to produce the active lytic agent, plasmin, which is responsible for fibrin dissolution. Therefore, the bacterial agent is not a fibrinolysin, as it was originally called, but is more properly referred to as a kinase. Those produced by streptococci are **streptokinases; staphylokinases** are formed by staphylococci.

The action of streptokinase is often antagonized by the presence in plasma of a substance, antiplasmin, which complexes with plasmin and renders it inactive.

A variety of other bacteria, including enteric bacilli and some clostridia, digest fibrin clots, but little is known about these activities; in some instances the digestion is due to proteolytic enzymes rather than kinases.

The streptokinases are immunogenic and those from different strains are immunologically similar. Antiserums specifically inhibit kinase activity and serum antikinase has been useful as an indicator of past infection with kinase-positive streptococci.

Streptokinase appears to be correlated with streptococcal virulence and invasiveness. One of the first host reactions to tissue destruction is the formation of fibrin clots, walling off and isolating the infected region; it is not surprising, therefore, that bacteria capable of lysing these clots would exhibit tendencies to extensive tissue invasion. Streptococci are demonstrably invasive, and this phase of their virulence may be partly attributable to streptokinase.

Hyaluronidase

Hyaluronic acid, a mucopolysaccharide consisting of acetylglucosamine and glucuronic acid, acts as a cementing substance in many mammalian tissues. When this substance is depolymerized by the enzyme hyaluronidase, the permeability of the tissues is remarkably increased. Hyaluronidase (Duran-Reynals factor, spreading factor, invasin) is present in certain tissues, notably testes, but it is also produced by a number of bacteria noted for their invasive properties, such as pneumococci and certain strains of staphylococci, streptococci, and clostridia. When injected along with hyaluronidase, bacteria, viruses, toxins, and India ink rapidly diffuse from the site of inoculation. Strains of staphylococci and streptococci that have no pronounced invasive powers may, in this way, be rendered highly invasive. Similarly, the invasiveness of strains of staphylococci is associated with the capacity to produce the enzyme; noninvasive strains produce little or no hyaluronidase.

Hyaluronidase decreases the viscosity of tissue hyaluronic acid by hydrolysis, facilitating tissue penetration by bacteria that produce it.

The effect is only temporary, however, and the dermal barrier is restored within 24 to 48 hours. The action of hyaluronidase in tissues is complex. Its action is antagonized by a plasma enzyme, anti-invasin I. This enzyme is destroyed by a bacterial enzyme, pro-invasin I, and it, in turn, is susceptible to another host enzyme, anti-invasin II. It is suggested that a balance among these determines whether or not invasion will occur. Furthermore, hyaluronidase is immunogenic and antibody is induced which neutralizes its activity; enzymes from different bacteria are, however, immunologically distinct and each would be neutralized only by homologous antibody.

It is of some interest that hyaluronic acid is found in the capsules of certain streptococci; not surprisingly, these strains do not produce hyaluronidase. When they are exposed to enzyme they are denuded of capsules and are more readily phagocytized. Thus, hyaluronic acid capsules, like many other bacterial capsules, act as aggressins.

TOXICITY OF HOST ORIGIN

In some diseases—tetanus, diphtheria, cholera, and a few others—pathogenesis is primarily attributable to the action of a single, highly toxic substance. In others, the etiologic agent is known to form one or more products that may cause host damage. Individually, these latter substances do not account for the total disease picture, yet acting in concert, they may be responsible for some or all of the observed effects in a particular disease.

It is not uncommon to observe signs of toxemia in infectious disease when the causative microorganism cannot be shown to form toxic substances *in vitro*. The classic example of this is the marked toxemia of acute pneumococcal infection, while the pneumococcal cell substance and metabolic products formed in culture are comparatively bland. Observations of this kind suggest either that the toxicity is of host origin, in that it is produced by the infected host tissues or cells, or that the microorganism forms toxic substances in the infected tissue environment but not in culture *in vitro*.

The formation of toxins by organisms in the unique environment of the host has been recognized. Both the cholera toxin and that of anthrax were first described as being formed by the bacteria within the host. They were later produced by *in vitro* culture, reflecting development of new techniques in laboratory manipulation.

Of primary concern here, however, is the possibility that host tissues and cells may, under the influence of invading bacteria, produce harmful substances. Some of these are linked to the immunological systems. **Hypersensitivity** reactions (Chapter 10), induced by relatively bland microbial antigens, sometimes lead to host damage. One such example is the **erythrogenic toxin** of *S. pyogenes* that induces the rash of scarlet fever by an immunologically mediated hypersensitivity reaction.

Emerging from recent research on the action of endotoxin is the clear indication that a significant portion of endotoxic reactions are due to mediators, induced by lipopolysaccharide, which have a "toxic" manifestation on secondary target cells. Endotoxin, for example, does not directly induce the febrile response, but rather causes the release of endogenous pyrogens from granulocytes; these **pyrogens** then act on the hypothalamus to affect temperature regulation. This and similar actions of endotoxin are discussed above.

Still another such phenomenon is the markedly increased sensitivity to histamine that develops in whooping cough and is perhaps attributable to an effect on the rate of histamine release from tissues. This sensitivity is possibly related to the pathogenesis of the disease in which the debilitating cough persists even after the bacilli are eliminated from the affected individual.

The Shwartzman Reaction[18]

The Shwartzman reaction may be regarded as a special case of a host reaction resulting in increased sensitivity to microbial substances, and is produced by two inoculations—a **"preparatory"** inoculation, followed a few hours (8 to 30) later by a **"provocative"** one. If the preparatory dose is given intradermally, and the provocative intravenously, the second inoculation is followed shortly by a local reaction inducing gross hemorrhage and necrosis at the site of the preparatory dose. A general reaction can be induced by giving both doses intravenously and is characterized by bilateral cortical necrosis of the kidneys. Although the Shwartzman reaction has no immunological basis, it overtly resembles the Arthus phenomenon (Chapter 11) and is intensified when the animal has received immunizing inoculations of the preparatory material.

Not all bacteria contain preparatory substances, but endotoxins are almost uniformly effective. It has been suggested that a part of the action of bacterial endotoxins may be a manifestation of the Shwartzman reaction.

This reaction may be enhanced by an immune response in which the preparatory dose is absorbed from the bowel as endotoxin from gram-negative members of the normal intestinal flora. There is a wider range of provocative than of preparatory substances; substances such as starch, agar, serum, or bacteria that have no preparatory effect may be provocative.

The participation of the host in this reaction is indicated in a number of ways. Following a preparatory intradermal inoculation, there is a local cellular reaction, with increased glycolysis associated with the influx of heterophils and a local accumulation of lactic acid. This response, and subsequent reaction to the provocative inoculation, is prevented by treatments that induce leucopenia. The significance of the cellular response is also indicated by the enhancement of the reaction when the macrophage system is blockaded and an increased sensitivity to endotoxin preparatory inoculation when the animal is treated with cortisone. In total, the evidence suggests that the preparatory inoculation interferes with a significant detoxifying mechanism.

Local infection with a variety of bacteria, such as tubercle, anthrax, and influenza bacilli, and streptococci, is preparatory even though the microorganisms themselves may not be preparatory. Thus, streptococci are not preparatory, though a local streptococcal infection may be, and preparatory activity may be demonstrated in extracts of the infected tissue. The extent to which the Shwartzman reaction contributes to the pathogenesis of infectious diseases is, however, not completely clear.

MEASUREMENT OF VIRULENCE

Virulence of a microorganism is rarely, if ever, attributable to a single characteristic. Rather, virulence represents a balance among a multiplicity of factors, some related to the microorganism and others related to host resistance. It is rarely possible to measure the contribution of a single determinant to the virulence of a microbial agent, although comparative virulence measurements of different strains are informative in this respect.

The measurement of virulence consists of testing for the ability to infect normal susceptible animals, such as a standard strain of mice, to produce observable consequences. The consequence is ordinarily an all-or-none phenomenon, such as death of the animal. On challenge inoculation of experimental animals with graded doses of the microorganism or substances such as bacterial toxins, it is apparent that virulence (or toxicity) is inversely related to the size of the effective dose, *i.e.*, the smaller the dose required to induce an observable effect, the greater the virulence. This is the basis of measurements of virulence (or toxicity) by determination of the **minimum lethal dose** (MLD), the smallest dose required to kill a standard experimental animal.

If each dose is given to groups of experimental animals, two additional points are apparent. First, the proportion of animals reacting in each group varies from none or practically none in the group of animals receiving the smallest dose, to all or practically all of the animals receiving the largest dose.

Second, when the groups of animals are sufficiently large and the doses graded appropriately, it is apparent also that the proportion of animals affected per unit increment of dose rises slowly at first, then rapidly, and finally slowly again as the proportion becomes large.

If the cumulative deaths or other effects are plotted against the logarithms of the dose, the points tend to fall on an S-shaped curve, which represents the integral of the frequency distribution of natural resistance in the experimental animals used. When the cumulative effect is plotted on probability paper, one scale representing the integral of the normal frequency distribution, against the logarithm of the dose, the points tend to fall on a straight line which may be fitted by inspection or by least squares.

The ED_{50}

The point on the dose scale at which this line intersects the 50 per cent point in the cumulative effect gives the interpolated dose which would produce the effect in half the animals inoculated, as shown in Figure 12–2. This is the 50 per cent effective dose, or ED_{50}. When death is the response measured, the dose is the 50 per cent lethal dose, or LD_{50}.

The ED_{50}, or LD_{50}, measure of virulence is subject to qualification in that virulence is also

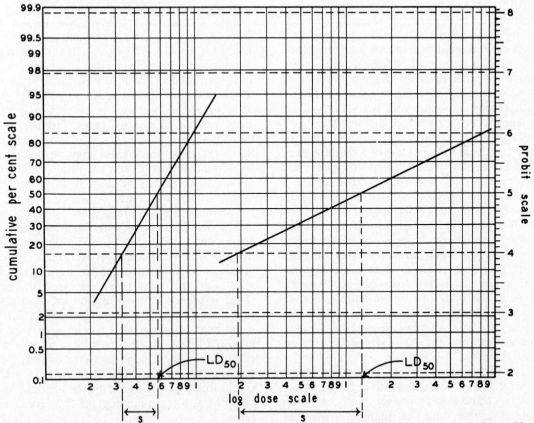

Figure 12–2. Graphical determination of the interpolated 50 per cent dose (LD_{50}, ED_{50}) and the standard error(s) on probability log paper. The vertical scale is the integral of the normal frequency distribution as per cent cumulative effect, and the horizontal scale is the dose. Two different types of dose response curves are shown.

The standard error is the standard deviate of the normal frequency distribution and is the distance on the dose scale from the center of distribution to the point of inflection on either side. The use of negative deviates is avoided by adding 5; the altered deviate is a probit (right scale in above figure).

indicated by the slope of the dose-response curve. Slopes may vary widely from one pathogenic microorganism to another. When a highly virulent strain of pneumococcus is titrated in the mouse, for example, the dose-response curve is steep and usually does not extend beyond a range of two logarithmic units on the dose scale. By contrast, when the virulence of *Salmonella* is titrated in the same animal, the dose-response curve is much less steep, extending over as much as six logarithmic units on the dose scale. Both types of dose-response curves are illustrated in Figure 12–2. The significance of slope is not clear, but it is obvious that the virulence of pneumococcus and that of *Salmonella* are not completely comparable using their respective LD_{50} values alone.

Protection Tests

The virulence titration is often used to assay the efficacy of some treatment, such as active or passive immunization or administration of drugs, by comparing directly or indirectly the LD_{50} of a given microorganism for normal animals and that for treated animals. From the analytical point of view, more reliable results may be obtained by using a standard challenge inoculum and varying the treatment. This preferred procedure is not always possible when the virulence of the challenge microorganism varies widely from one time to another. In such cases the protective material is given in constant dosage; the LD_{50} dose is titrated in both treated and control animals, and protection is measured by the ratio of the LD_{50} in treated animals to that in controls.

Natural Resistance to Infection[6, 16]

Although the ability to produce disease is conditioned by a series of mechanisms originating with the microorganism, pathogenicity must be evaluated in terms of host resistance. As a rule, a pathogenic microorganism is limited to a small number of hosts; microorganisms pathogenic for animals are not ordinarily pathogenic for plants; very few of the microorganisms that can infect mammals are also pathogenic for cold-blooded animals; some are even restricted to the tissues of a single species. **Resistance,** like virulence, depends upon many factors, some of which are known either in more or less specific form or in generalities that serve as a cloak for ignorance; others are, in all probability, as yet unsuspected. Resistance to infection is, in a sense, somewhat more complex than virulence. Not only are there specific barriers to infection which vary with species and even from one tissue to another in the body of a single animal, but the efficiency of these barriers is also a manifestation of general physiological well-being; hence, they are subject to extrinsic or environmental stress.

The factors operable in the host are of two general kinds: the **constitutive** group, which includes those host responses that occur in the normal animal; and the **adaptive** group, expressed only in the presence of the pathogenic microorganism. The latter are predominantly associated with the immune response and are considered elsewhere (Chapters 10 and 11).

Genetics and Host Resistance[38, 57]

Both animals and humans are known to differ greatly in their resistance to a given infectious disease. This knowledge is rooted in legend, folk medicine, clinical observation, and experimental findings. Resistance to infection is undoubtedly determined by the genetic makeup of the host and is evident as differences related to **species, races, families,** and **individuals.** In many cases resistance to infection is relative, for disease may be produced by administration of massive doses of microorganisms to a resistant animal, but in others it appears to be absolute.

The host-range of infectious agents is an indication of species resistance. Many viruses are highly species-specific, affecting a limited number of host species; for example, natural infection with hepatitis B virus occurs only in man. For the most part, this specific host-range is related to receptors on the host cells that interact with those on viruses. Similarly, it has been suggested that species resistance in bacterial infections may be related to adhesin-receptor specificities, as discussed earlier. Certainly the resistance of rats and mice to diphtheria toxin can be traced to the absence of a receptor for toxin-binding on their cell surfaces.

Other factors underlying differences in species resistance are not well understood, but in a few cases body temperature or anatomical differences account for the variation. Pasteur was able to infect the normally resistant hen with anthrax by lowering its body temperature; conversely, he produced anthrax in the resistant frog by raising its body temperature to 37° C. The insusceptibility of rabbits and guinea pigs to staphylococcal enterotoxin is attributed to their lack of a vomiting mechanism.

Resistance to a given infectious agent is not necessarily associated with phylogenetic relationship, and there is no pattern from which susceptibility or resistance of animal species can be predicted by logical processes; the tabulation of animals susceptible to a given disease represents information acquired by trial and error.

Even within a susceptible species, races, strains, and varieties may exhibit marked differences in susceptibility. The relative resistance of Algerian sheep to anthrax is well documented and inbred Berkshire swine are highly resistant to brucellosis. That these differences are genetic in origin is evident and has led to breeding of animals for disease resistance for both economic and scientific reasons.

It is not usually possible to associate resistance with any single character; rather, it appears to be dependent upon a complex interaction of different properties. Differences in susceptibility may, of course, be a reflection of alterations in immune responsiveness, or immunoregulation.

Resistance in Humans. The relative resistance of the human races to infection has been the subject of considerable interest and such investigation as has been possible. Under ordinary circumstances in the United States the nonwhite races are much more susceptible to infectious disease than are whites. There are, however, certain exceptions. The influenza epidemic of 1918 had a greater impact on the death rate for white youths than for nonwhites of similar age groups. A similar exception has been noted in diphtheria. Certain groups of black children showed a lower ratio of clinical diphtheria to immunizing infections than corresponding white children.

Special interest is attached to the white and nonwhite tuberculosis death rates, both crude and age-specific (Fig. 12–3). Whether the observed high mortality in nonwhites represents a racial susceptibility or is entirely a reflection of economic status is an unanswered question.

Although experimental studies in human disease resistance are not possible, genetic correlations in familial studies have provided useful information. Studies on monozygotic and dizygotic twins, particularly with respect to tuberculosis resistance, have indicated a hereditary element in susceptibility. The close relationship of resistance to elements of the immune system is indicated by an observed linkage between the genes of the human leucocyte antigen (HLA) and regulation of certain complement components. Gene defects leading to complement deficiency cause increased susceptibility to infection with pyogenic cocci and a variety of other agents.

One of the best established cases of heredi-

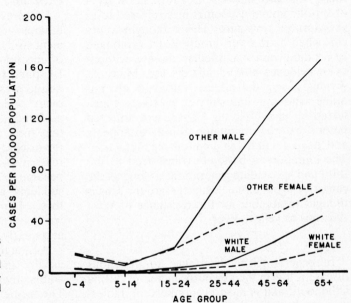

Figure 12–3. Reported cases of tuberculosis by race, age, and sex in the United States, 1978. (Centers for Disease Control, Annual summary 1978: reported morbidity and mortality in the United States. Morbidity and Mortality Weekly Report **27**[54], 1979.)

tary control of resistance to a specific infection is the resistance to malaria associated with **sickle cell anemia** and **thalassemia.** These diseases are almost invariably fatal in homozygous individuals, but those heterozygous for the appropriate gene are more resistant to malaria than those without the genes. In sickle cell anemia hemoglobin synthesis is directly affected to yield an abnormal hemoglobin (hemoglobin S). In thalassemia, excessive amounts of fetal hemoglobin (hemoglobin F) are produced. The presence of these in the red blood cell makes it less susceptible to infection with the malarial parasite. On the other hand, sickle cell disease decreases host resistance to bacterial infection, and deaths in children suffering from sickle cell disease are commonly due to infection.

Resistance may be expressed in several ways. A given disease may be mild in groups that have been in contact with it over a long period, but may assume a highly virulent form in other groups to which it is new. Measles, a mild disease in most developed countries, has been a scourge when introduced into certain primitive societies. Furthermore, diseases originally highly virulent have become less so with the passage of time; syphilis is considerably milder today than it was in the sixteenth century. Whether these changes represent increased racial immunity by selection of resistant individuals or changing virulence of the microorganism is unresolved; possibly both effects are operative.

In some circumstances what appears to be **racial resistance** may be, in reality, a low level of specific immunity, sometimes referred to as **pseudoracial resistance.** This is thought to occur when a race or group is in prolonged association with a particular disease without overt evidence of epidemic disease. Many individuals have the disease, survivors are immune, and this immunity is passively transferred to the offspring. These are infected before maternal immunity entirely disappears and have a mild, but immunizing, infection. The immunity is passively transferred to the third and succeeding generations as long as the causative agent circulates in the group. This is thought to account for the resistance of West Africans to yellow fever.

Age[23]

In general terms, resistance to infectious disease is low in the newborn, increases during childhood, and is most pronounced in adolescents and adults. With aging, resistance again declines, and the aged become increasingly susceptible to infections.

Embryonic and fetal tissues have little resistance to infections. The chick embryo, for instance, is exquisitely susceptible to infection, particularly with viruses and rickettsiae, to which the mature fowl is completely resistant. In humans and other mammals, resistance is afforded by the maternal environment as well as the natural and immune resistance of the mother. The innately low resistance of mammalian neonates is, however, illustrated by their susceptibility to exotic diseases in which there is no passive transfer of maternal antibodies to the offspring. Examples include the susceptibility of suckling mice to poliovirus infection and the enteric infection of suckling rabbits with the cholera vibrio.

One important factor in the susceptibility of the very young is the lack of an immune response. There is partial compensation by the presence of antibody of maternal origin, providing temporary protection during the first few months after birth, but this passive immunity is effective only for diseases in which humoral antibody is protective and for which the mother possesses circulating antibody. In humans, immunoglobulin M (IgM) is not placentally transferred; newborn children are, therefore, more susceptible to infections with gram-negative bacteria in which this Ig class is associated with resistance. By the age of about one year the immune mechanisms have matured sufficiently that children begin to develop acquired immunity to infectious agents in their environment (Fig. 12–4).

Diseases of childhood, such as measles, mumps, and chickenpox, are sufficiently prevalent in most populations that the probability of encountering them at an early age is great. By puberty, the average individual has acquired a variety of immunities with or without overt evidence of infection, described above as pseudoracial resistance. Isolation, as in certain rural areas, reduces this probability and the diseases tend to occur later in life. For this reason, so-called childhood diseases frequently become a problem when young adults are suddenly aggregated, as in military groups; these often include a proportion of individuals who have not contracted immunizing infections at an early age.

Although resistance to most infections is usually greatest in adolescents and young adults, there are some important exceptions. The incidence of tuberculosis is relatively low in young children, but there is a marked in-

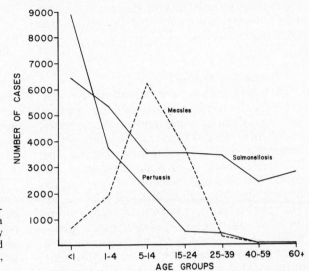

Figure 12–4. Reported cases of certain infectious diseases by age groups in the United States, 1980. (Data from Centers for Disease Control, Annual Summary 1980: reported morbidity and mortality in the United States. Morbidity and Mortality Weekly Report **29**[54], 1981.)

crease in infections at about the time of puberty; susceptibility continues to increase slowly until about age 65, when it begins a marked increase (see Fig. 12–3). The basis for the heightened susceptibility in young adults is not understood.

With the general aging of the population, the increased susceptibility of the elderly to infection has become of great importance. This generally lowered resistance is thought to be due to a combination of factors, *viz.*, environmental effects, physiological changes, alterations in the immunological mechanisms, and intercurrent or predisposing disease. An increase in incidence of infection occurs in such diverse diseases as tuberculosis, gram-negative bacterial infections, and a variety of urinary tract infections. Respiratory infections, both bacterial and viral, are markedly increased in the elderly; the greater susceptibility of the aged to pneumonia is well-known and generally regarded as an expression of accumulated degenerative changes and predisposing infections.

Degenerative changes are probably also related to increases in endocarditis, chronic skin ulcers associated with vascular obstruction, urinary tract infections in which local defenses are impaired, and respiratory infections arising from a decline in normal pulmonary function.

There is little evidence that aging induces changes in the cellular aspects of natural defenses, *e.g.*, phagocytic responses. Studies in both animals and humans, however, have revealed a decline in immunological responses with aging. Humoral responses are impaired,

but the most severe changes involve a broad loss of cell-mediated immune reactivity. These undoubtedly contribute to the greater incidence of infection in the aged.

Sex[41]

Knowledge of the relationship between sex and resistance to infection in humans is largely descriptive. Differences in incidence with respect to sex are exhibited in a few diseases and in almost all of these, infections are more common in males. Tuberculosis, in particular, exhibits a markedly greater incidence in males, as shown in Figure 12–3. On the other hand, toxic shock syndrome is almost exclusively a disease of menstruating women; only 1.5 per cent of cases in the United States in 1980 occurred in males.

Even in animals, the basis of infection resistance between sexes is not clear. Female chicks are more susceptible to the chicken malarial parasite, *Plasmodium gallinaceum*, than are males; this difference is unaffected by treatment with male or female hormones. Male mice are normally quite susceptible to streptococcal infection, but castration increases their resistance level to that of normally resistant females.

There appears to be no common mechanism explaining these observed differences, though some significance may be attached to the fact that the X-chromosome carries genes controlling immunoglobulin production. Immune responsiveness does differ between the sexes; for example, female mice are more responsive.[78] Any explanation of observed sex differences in resistance in humans must also take into consideration other factors such as occupation and risk.

Climate and Season[55]

That both climate and season of the year influence the incidence and mortality of many infectious diseases is well-known. Acute upper respiratory infections are more common in temperate than tropical zones, whereas the dysenteries more often occur as tropical diseases. The seasonal incidence of many infections is also common knowledge (Fig. 12–5). The upper respiratory infections, such as streptococcal pharyngitis, pneumococcal pneumonia, and meningococcal infections, are most often observed during the winter months. One of the most striking relationships between season and disease incidence is seen in cholera. The epidemic season coincides with hot weather and shows remarkable correlation with precipitation and relative humidity.

That climate has an effect on host resistance, rather than on the microorganism and its distribution, is suggested in the case of diphtheria. In the tropics, frank cases of diphtheria are rare, yet immunological studies indicate that inapparent, but immunizing infections are quite as common as in temperate zones.

In assessing the effect of climate and season on resistance, the influence of correlated factors must be considered. Transmission may, for example, be facilitated by seasonal and climatic factors, such as crowding and close association of individuals during colder months, or influenced by seasonal and geographic distribution of insect vectors. Seasonal variation in resistance may also be related to diet in some sociological groups or to summer activities such as swimming, which leads to increased incidence of otitis media in young children.

There is a great deal of experimental evidence substantiating the opinion that resistance varies with season, temperature, and related factors. For example, the brain reaction of mice inoculated with St. Louis encephalitis virus or guinea pigs inoculated with endemic typhus rickettsiae is more intense in summer than in winter. Mice, adapted to conditions of moist heat, are only one-fourth as resistant to infection with streptococci as those adapted to a cool environment. As a general rule, chilling reduces resistance to infection in experimental animals.[56]

Physiological State

Whatever disease resistance is conferred by genetic and other factors, resistance of the host is also profoundly influenced by its general physiological state. In general, resistance is at its height when an organism is functioning normally in every respect; it is reduced by factors that interfere with and alter its normal state. Altered physiological conditions and loss of resistance accompany many primary infections as noted earlier, leading to secondary invasion by less virulent organisms. In other instances, functional disorders such as diabetes bring about a reduced resistance to infection. More common, however, are the deleterious effects of inadequate diet and fatigue.

Nutrition.[9, 39] The relation between susceptibility to infection and faulty nutrition is of considerable interest in connection with deficiency diseases. It is indisputable that nutritional status is of significance to the incidence and mortality of infectious disease. In general, diets qualitatively and quantitatively inadequate predispose to bacterial infection, and this is most evident in gram-negative bacterial septicemia, tuberculosis, herpesvirus infections, measles, and candidiasis. Clinical studies on children in underdeveloped nations suggest that malnutrition and undernourishment lead to aberrations in the immune response, primarily reduced cell-mediated immunity and antibody responses to T lymphocyte–dependent antigens. There is generally, too, a marked

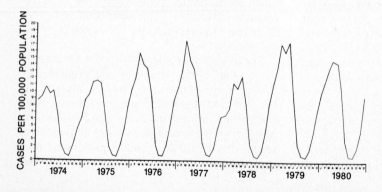

Figure 12–5. Seasonal incidence of chickenpox in the United States, 1974–80. Note that the seasonal pattern has remained constant. (Centers for Disease Control, Annual Summary 1980: reported morbidity and mortality in the United States. Morbidity and Mortality Weekly Report **29**[54], 1981.)

depression in the production of the C3 component of complement. Malnutrition also affects the nonspecific host responses; in particular, intracellular killing of bacteria is impaired.

It is obvious that clinical studies, while informative, are interpreted with difficulty. Controlled animal experiments generally support clinical studies in establishing that host resistance is markedly reduced by starvation or malnutrition. Both humoral and cell-mediated immunity is reduced, and cellular defenses, including phagocytosis, are impaired. The importance of adequate protein intake is emphasized; moderate depletion of protein reserves interferes markedly with antibody formation. Severe protein depletion interferes with normal functioning of cellular defenses.

The marked reduction in resistance associated with inadequate diets is not specific; rather, general resistance to infection is reduced. There appears to be no relation between lack of a single dietary factor and susceptibility to a particular infection, although vitamin A deficiency is almost universally inhibitory to general host resistance.

The unique aspects of **iron-deficiency** should be noted. As discussed earlier, microorganisms require iron for growth in the infected host; the requirement is met by synthesis of iron-binding siderophores that compete for transferrin- and lactoferrin-bound iron. It would be expected that iron deficiency in the host would deny this cation to the infecting bacterium. There is some indication that iron-deficiency does, in fact, increase host resistance; conversely, iron repletion decreases resistance to gram-negative sepsis, malaria, brucellosis, and tuberculosis.[2, 48]

Fatigue. It has long been known to the clinician that bodily rest is a valuable adjunct to the treatment of disease, and there is clinical evidence suggesting that resistance to the initial infection may be reduced by excessive fatigue. Experimental evidence on this point is scanty and to some degree conflicting, but it is probable that the unfavorable effect of fatigue on normal physiological well-being is reflected to some extent in an increase in susceptibility to infection. The normal white rat, for example, is highly resistant to anthrax, but when exhausted by work in a treadmill, becomes susceptible. Latent *Salmonella enteritidis* infections in the same experimental animal may be activated by fatigue to such a degree that the outcome is fatal. Exercise has been found to exacerbate tuberculous infection in the guinea pig by increasing dissemination

of the infection, but, curiously, stressed monkeys are more resistant to poliomyelitis.

Other mechanisms operative in the resistance associated with general physiological well-being are obscure. Studies on resistance to the common cold have strongly suggested that a constitutional factor, as yet undefined, is operative in the etiology of the clinical infection. There is evidence, too, that the capacity to maintain effective circulation and the ability to withstand the effects of sudden temperature changes are associated with resistance to experimental infections. The adverse effects of sudden changes in temperature and humidity on the organism, reflected in changes in the nasal mucosa, are perhaps a manifestation of temperature shock. Attempts to associate shock, fatigue, and other elements of nonspecific resistance with specific defense mechanisms, such as the capacity to form antibodies, have not been uniformly successful.

EXTERNAL DEFENSES OF THE HOST[49]

The cellular organization of the animal body is a closed system with respect to the outside environment, from which it is separated by the skin and mucous membranes. These structures, generally impermeable to particulate material of the size of bacteria, constitute the first line of defense against invading microorganisms and one that is, for the most part, highly effective. While mechanical obstruction contributes in no small part to the efficacy of these barriers, both skin and mucous membranes also play an active part in the protection of the organism against bacterial invasion.

Skin

As a rule, the unbroken skin presents an impassable barrier to microorganisms. Normally, bacteria are found on the skin between the superficial horny cells, but do not ordinarily penetrate into the underlying tissues in the absence of cutaneous injury. Although often claimed, it is improbable that pathogens can penetrate unbroken skin. More likely, bacteria such as leptospira and treponema gain entry through minute abrasions and fissures. Infection via sweat glands and hair follicles has been demonstrated experimentally in staphylococcal and streptococcal infections, resulting in acne, impetigo, boils, and similar affections.

The skin is not a completely inert surface on which bacteria die largely as a consequence of drying. On the contrary, healthy intact skin exerts demonstrable bactericidal activity on transient organisms as a consequence of the action of unsaturated fatty acids, especially oleic acid, present in sebaceous secretions. This bactericidal action is inhibited by serum albumin, which may be of significance in areas surrounding burns or other skin lesions producing a serous exudate. Possibly related is the fungistatic action of free saturated fatty acids in the sebaceous secretions of adults. Not all microorganisms are susceptible to these agents, however. Bacteria of the normal skin flora, such as *Staphylococcus epidermidis,* are not appreciably reduced in numbers after swabbing onto clean skin, a fact that probably accounts for their constant presence on the body.

Conjunctiva

Bacteria and dust particles settling in the eyes are removed relatively rapidly by the flushing action of tears. Lacrimal secretions are also bactericidal because of their lysozyme content; as described in Chapter 2, this enzyme breaks down the peptidoglycan of gram-positive bacteria, forming protoplasts. These are quite fragile, and the ultimate antibacterial effect of the enzyme is bacteriolysis.

Nose, Nasopharynx, and Respiratory Tract[52]

Bacteria and other particulate material in inspired air are rapidly removed as they travel through the tortuous nasal passages where they cling to the moist surfaces of the mucous membrane lining. In this way, air is largely freed of bacteria in the upper respiratory passages; those that pass the larynx are trapped in the bronchi and only a few reach the ultimate ramifications of the bronchioles. The process is so efficient that expired air contains almost no bacteria except those expelled in droplets by coughing and sneezing.

The mucosa of the nasal passages, sinuses, pharynx, and esophagus are covered with a continuous web or network of thin, but highly viscid, **mucus.** Bacteria removed from inspired air and those arriving via lacrimal secretions are trapped and embedded in this mucus web. The mucus film is in constant motion resulting from ciliary activity, which sweeps the mucus and its bacterial content toward the oropharynx, where it is swallowed. The exchange of mucus is rapid; that covering the posterior two-thirds of the nasal passages is replaced every 10 to 15 minutes, while that over the anterior third is removed every hour or two. Although mucus itself has no antibacterial ac-

tivity, it does inhibit adherence of bacteria to mucosal cells and the combination of mucus and ciliary activity is remarkably efficient in ridding the upper respiratory passages of bacteria. In rabbit models, particulates greater than 7 μm. in diameter, and about half of those between 3 and 7 μm., are retained in the upper respiratory passages. The remainder of these, plus practically all of those smaller than 1.5 μm. in diameter, penetrate into the lungs. The bacteria that reach the alveoli are phagocytized by macrophages.

Lysozyme is, of course, present in the nasal mucus and has a limited protective function. Normal serous secretions of the nose also contain a virus-inactivating agent, which is virucidal for influenza and certain other viruses. Its role in resistance, if any, is not clear.

Mouth, Stomach, and Intestinal Tract

The mouth contains a predominant normal bacterial flora and a minor transient flora. The normal flora consist of microorganisms that have established positions between the teeth, on dental plaques, and in the crevices between the teeth and gums; transient flora represents a constant contamination. Both are subject to continuous depletion because of the flushing action of the saliva. Saliva is mildly bactericidal, a part of the antibacterial mechanism being lysozyme, but the removal of bacteria appears to be largely a mechanical process. The microorganisms flushed to the back of the mouth meet with those from the nose and, with them, are swallowed.

Bacteria reaching the stomach are subject to the strongly acid environment of the normal gastric secretions, and there is no doubt that the great majority of them are destroyed there. This mechanism is, of course, inoperative in achlorhydric individuals. In the normal host, some viable microorganisms reach the intestinal tract, perhaps because they are embedded in solid particles of food and thus protected or because they are able to withstand a short exposure to the bactericidal action of the gastric secretions. Generally, very few viable bacteria are found in the stomach, but the numbers of microorganisms increase in the small intestine concomitantly with the rise in pH from the duodenum to the ileum. The large intestine contains great numbers of bacteria derived not only from the upper levels of the intestinal tract but also from the multiplication of bacteria present in the intestine as normal inhabitants. As in the respiratory passages, mucus plays an important part in the mechan-

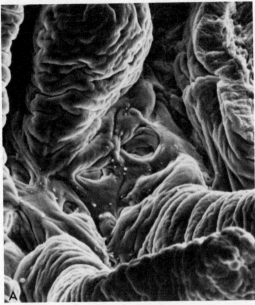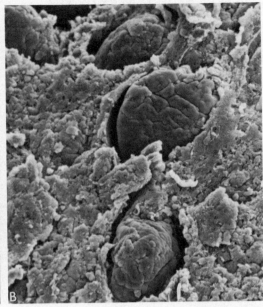

Figure 12–6. Scanning electron micrographs of the epithelial surface of mouse small intestine. *A*, Washed preparation showing the normal intestinal topography. Villi and crypts of Lieberkühn are visible. × 1000. *B*, Unwashed preparation showing mucus covering most of the epithelial surface. × 5000. Both fixed with osmium-glutaraldehyde. (Courtesy of Dr. Gordon D. Schrank.)

ical removal of bacteria. Here, however, the mucus does not form a uniform coating over the intestinal mucosa but is present as a meshwork. Villous movements help to trap bacteria and other particles in mucus, which is then rolled up into small masses, moved along the intestinal tract by peristalsis, and eventually eliminated with the feces.

Microorganisms present in the bowel, in-

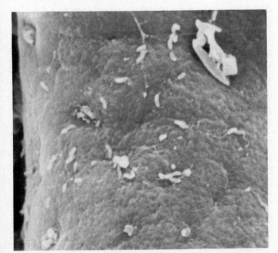

Figure 12–7. Scanning electron micrograph showing adherence of *Vibrio cholerae* to the microvillus surface of the mouse ileum. Note remnants of mucus covering. Washed preparation fixed with osmium-glutaraldehyde; × 5000. (Courtesy of Dr. Gordon D. Schrank.)

cluding those making up the normal intestinal flora, are, for all practical purposes, outside the tissues of the body. This flora contributes, in itself, a protective mechanism to the host. Invading pathogens must successfully compete with the normal flora in order to establish a focus of infection as described in the later section on normal flora (p. 350). Penetration of the tissues from the bowel, as in typhoid fever, is usually via Peyer's patches into the lymphatic system and the blood stream through the thoracic duct. Ordinarily this barrier is a highly effective one, but under certain circumstances, as in whole-body ionizing irradiation, the barrier is breached and treatment is followed by generalized invasion of the tissues by intestinal bacteria; the immediate cause of death in radiation sickness may be fulminating bacteremia.

The Genital Tract

The normal genital tract is remarkably free from bacteria. The urethra in both male and female is normally sterile, a consequence, perhaps, of the flushing action of the slightly acid urine. The few bacteria that may be present are confined to the region of the meatus. The normal vaginal secretion is acid in the postpubertal female, due to fermentation of glycogen by members of the normal flora, and is markedly bactericidal toward most pathogenic bacteria.

INTERNAL DEFENSES OF THE HOST

On gaining access to the tissues, a pathogenic microorganism must establish and maintain a focus of infection. A number of internal host factors may be distinguished that interfere with this microbial invasion. The more important of these include the relevant physiological responses subject to hormonal regulation and the antimicrobial activities demonstrable in tissues and organs.

Hormones

Hormonal imbalance and consequent disturbances of a wide variety of physiological functions are generally associated with increased susceptibility. Hormones do not act directly on the microorganisms, but affect host physiological responses to the stimuli provided by pathogenic microorganisms and their products.

The well-known predisposition of diabetics to infection, such as gangrenous diseases of the extremities, is probably associated with circulatory disturbance and illustrates the indirect relation between hormonal imbalance and host resistance. Of the hormones, those of the adrenocortical group have been of greatest interest because of the great depression in resistance that they induce. In essence, their action derives from depression of the inflammatory response and activity of the reticuloendothelial cell system, emphasizing the significance of these cells in natural resistance.

The administration of ACTH or corticosteroids to patients with acute febrile infections usually leads to a prompt defervescence, in proportion to the severity of symptoms. Nevertheless, the infecting microorganisms are not affected and the infection may spread. If secondary infections occur, they are often asymptomatic because of the effects of the hormone. Herpes simplex appears to be an important exception; topical application of corticosteroids to herpetic infections of the eye results in exacerbation of the disease, with spreading destructive involvement that can lead to perforation of the cornea.

When administered to normal animals, these hormones depress natural resistance to experimental infections and lead to activation of latent infections, if these are present. Immunological responses are also affected and antibody formation is depressed.

These hormones accentuate the activity of endotoxins, not by affecting the toxin directly, but by interfering with the cellular response mechanisms. Further, when given in combination with antibiotics, the efficacy of the chemotherapeutic agents is reduced, emphasizing the significant role of host resistance factors in successful chemotherapy.

Because of these effects, the appearance of infection is a major reason for discontinuing or altering therapy with ACTH or corticosteroids initiated for other reasons. It is also not surprising that impairment of resistance to infection is commonly seen in spontaneous hyperadrenalism and that the death rate in this disease was not appreciably altered with the introduction of antimicrobial therapy.

Fever[13, 62]

The possible beneficial effects of fever have been suspected for many years. Indeed, before antibiotics were known, there were several attempts to affect the outcome of infections by induction of fever. Induced hyperthermia was applied to syphilis and other infections, with some indication of benefits. In most clinical studies the results have not been definitive, although there has been a general impression of improved host defenses.

Increased interest in fever, or hyperthermia, related to infection resistance has, in recent years, led to more informative animal studies. The animal models employed have included artificially induced fever in homeothermic animals and environmentally induced hyperthermia in poikilothermic animals. With a few exceptions, such studies have indicated that fever is associated with increased resistance in infections, usually measured as increased survival time. Among the pathogens so affected are pneumococci, staphylococci, anthrax bacillus, pasteurellae, herpesviruses, polioviruses, and rabies viruses. Hyperthermia does not appear to have a direct effect on growth of the microorganisms, but is more likely related to host alterations. Although data are often conflicting, some investigators claim that there is evidence that cellular defenses are sometimes potentiated, resulting in leucocytosis, increased leucocyte motility, and improved phagocytosis and intracellular killing. There is also some indication that elevated temperatures improve the humoral antibody response. It has recently been reported that higher temperatures in the physiological range enhanced the antimicrobial activity of serum.[45]

Hyperthermia is not always beneficial. Fever potentiates the lethal action of endotoxin and latent herpesvirus infections may be reactivated by fever, with recurrence of cold sores, or fever blisters.

Serum Factors[14, 21]

The presence of antimicrobial factors in serum and tissue fluids has long been recognized, but their relation to host resistance has not always been clear. Individually, these factors are probably of minor influence in resistance, but, in concert with one another and with other defense mechanisms, contribute to the sum of host resistance.

A number of antimicrobial factors are found in tissue extracts and fluids, such as blood, tears, milk, and saliva. They exhibit antibacterial activity against a wide variety of microorganisms, including anthrax bacilli, streptococci, staphylococci, and tubercle bacilli. Two of these factors have been discussed earlier—lactoferrin in milk and transferrin in serum. These **iron-binding proteins** are bacteriostatic because they deny required iron to certain bacteria. Most of the other serum factors are bactericidal and are divided into two groups, viz., the heat-stable bactericidins comprising the β-lysins, and the heat-labile factors associated with the complement cascade. These are summarized in Table 12–7.

β-Lysins. The name β-lysin has been given to the heat-stable components of serum to distinguish them from heat-labile factors, including complement, that were originally called α-lysins. The β-lysins are listed in Table 12–7. Lysozyme, a heat-stable, basic protein, is the enzyme that catalyzes the breakdown of peptidoglycans and results in bacteriolysis of many gram-positive bacteria; it is found in serum, lacrimal secretions, and saliva. The other β-lysins are also cationic proteins of relatively low molecular weight found in serum, plasma, and, in lower concentrations, tears and saliva. They are bactericidal for many intact gram-positive organisms; streptococci are an important exception. The majority of β-lysin in serum appears to be derived from platelets, although some may be of nonplatelet origin. **Platelet β-lysins** are best known. They are immunogenic, and antibody neutralizes their activity; platelet β-lysins from several animal species are immunologically similar, but not identical. Platelet β-lysin is bactericidal for many gram-positive bacterial cells, with the exception of staphylococci; it acts against susceptible bacterial cells by nonenzymatic disturbance of cell membrane function. **Nonplatelet β-lysin** is distinguishable from platelet β-lysins, but, because of technical difficulties, is not well characterized; it is, for example, bactericidal for staphylococci and listeria.

The role of platelet β-lysin in host resistance is suggested by its release from platelets during processes associated with infection. Significant increases occur in serum during inflammation and bacteremia, and after endotoxin challenge in the generalized Shwartzman reaction, and accompany in vivo antigen-antibody reactions; as expected, blood coagulation results in increased serum levels of platelet β-lysin.

Alternative Complement System.[34] The importance of the complement system in bringing about the increased lysis of bacteria and erythrocytes has been known since the late nineteenth century. During those early days of microbiology it was also observed that normal serum contained heat-labile factors bactericidal for a number of gram-negative bacteria. The relationship between these lines of evidence began to emerge in the early 1950s, when Pillemer and his associates described the **properdin system**—normal serum components, including complement, that were bactericidal for gram-negative bacteria.

Subsequently, it has been shown that the properdin system consists of a series of proteins that are analogous to the proteins of the classical complement pathway. These are activated not by antibody, as in the classical

Table 12–7. **Normal Serum Components with Bactericidal or Opsonic Activity**

System	Components	Chemical Nature	Action
β-Lysins (heat-stable)	Lysozyme	Basic protein	Enzymatic lysis of gram-positive bacteria by hydrolysis of cell wall peptidoglycan.
	Platelet β-lysin	Basic protein	Nonenzymatic, nonlytic bacterial action on cell membrane of gram-positive bacteria.
	Nonplatelet β-lysin	Basic protein	Nonlytic bactericidal action on gram-positive bacteria, probably acting on cell membrane.
Alternative complement cascade (heat-labile)	Properdin and complement	Proteins	Cascading enzymatic reactions resulting from complement activation. Promote opsonization of both gram-positive and gram-negative bacteria and lysis of gram-negative bacteria.

pathway, but by surface components of bacterial cells, including lipoteichoic acids and lipopolysaccharides. The two pathways of complement activation then converge at the level of the C3 component of complement, as discussed in detail in Chapter 7.

The two pathways and biological activities may be summarized in the following simplified form:

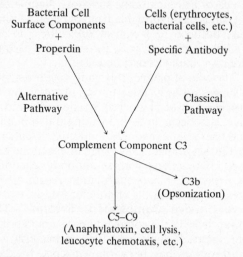

The alternative complement pathway, activated by bacterial surface components, can thus play a significant role early in the infection process. The C3b component can react with invading bacterial cells and promote their phagocytosis; opsonization in this way is considered to be the most important aspect of complement activation in host resistance, since it occurs with both gram-positive and gram-negative cells. Also, genetic deficiency of the C3 component is known to predispose to infection. Later events in the complement cascade may lead directly to bacterial cell lysis, but only gram-negative bacteria are susceptible.

As the infection progresses, specific antibody to the bacterial invader is produced by the host, thus activating the classical pathway. This immunological response is specifically directed toward the infectious agent and is more efficient than that accompanying alternative pathway activation.

In addition to the direct effects of **opsonization** and **bacteriolysis,** the complement cascade also has other important, but less direct effects, *viz.,* **anaphylatoxic** fragments induce local vasodilation that increases blood supply to the focus of infection, bringing fresh complement to the area, while **chemotactic** fragments help to mobilize and increase the number of leucocytes in the affected area.

Immunization or previous infection induces antibody specific to the infecting agent, and the protection of the host by these is often through activation of the classical pathway. Normal serum frequently contains factors that behave like antibodies in that such serums react with bacterial cells and activate complement. Although these have been referred to as natural antibodies, it seems likely that they represent specific antibodies induced by previous subclinical infection with the same, or antigenically related, bacteria. Alternatively, they may be induced in response to a variety of cross-reactive antigenic substances in the environment. These antigenic substances, possibly derived from plants, microorganisms, and the like, can be introduced into the host by the alimentary and respiratory routes.[64]

It must be noted that the bactericidal effects of the complement cascade may be amplified by β-lysins. Antibody-complement lysis of gram-negative cells is potentiated by lysozyme and by platelet β-lysins. Lysozyme may also act on the peptidoglycan of certain bacteria to yield products that are more effective in activation of the alternative pathway.[28]

Interferon[26, 35, 77]

Studies on the mechanisms of viral interference led to the finding that a host cell, normally susceptible to viral infection, may become resistant in consequence of exposure to certain viruses or viral components. This refractory state is associated with the synthesis, by the host cell, of a substance designated interferon.

The production of interferon by stimulated host cells may be demonstrated by viral challenge in animals as well as cell cultures. Since it is released from productive cells, it can be isolated and purified. When naive animals or cell cultures are treated with graded doses of interferon, their relative resistance to viral challenge becomes a measure of interferon activity.

In addition to viruses, a great many substances have been found to induce, or stimulate, host cells to interferon production. These vary widely in their induction capacity. Those most effective in inducing interferon production in both tissue culture and animals include viruses; double-stranded RNA (dsRNA) of normal cells; and synthetic dsRNA, composed of polyriboinosinate and polyribocytodilate (Poly rI:Poly rC). Those requiring higher doses for induction, and often failing to induce interferon in tissue cultures, include certain intracellular bacteria; protozoan parasites; bacterial products, *e.g.*, lipopolysaccharides; defined polymers; and a few low-molecular-weight substances.

Interferon is also produced by lymphocytes in response to mitogenic agents or by sensitized T lymphocytes in response to antigens. Their production is thus analogous to that of other lymphokines. This type of interferon is often referred to as immune interferon as opposed to the classical interferons induced by viruses and other substances listed above.

Interferon is not a single substance, but is a group of antiviral proteins, produced by several cell types and differing in physical, antiviral, and other properties. Three human interferons are recognized, *viz.*, leucocyte, fibroblast, and immune interferons; their properties are summarized in Table 12–8.

In addition to their antiviral properties, interferons produce a variety of other cellular effects, including growth inhibition and immunoregulation. Interferons have been found to exhibit antitumor effects which are believed to be due to activation of cellular elements in cell-mediated immunity.

In itself, interferon has no direct effects on viruses. Rather, its effect is on the host cell during viral replication. The initial steps in virus infection—adsorption, penetration, and uncoating—are not subject to the action of interferon. The principal action appears to be related to the inhibition of viral protein synthesis. In susceptible host cells, interferon affects the protein-synthesizing machinery by inducing two enzymes, a protein kinase and an oligonucleotide synthetase. These act in concert to inhibit mRNA translation—the ki-nase by interfering with initiation of mRNA translation, and the synthetase by promoting mRNA degradation.

The protective effect associated with interferon has a broad spectrum with respect to infecting viruses, but is narrowly specific with regard to host cells. Although the induction of interferon is effected by a wide variety of viruses and other inducers, the interferon produced may not exhibit antiviral activity in other species. As shown in Table 12–8, human interferons are antiviral in human cells, but human immune interferon is not active in cells of other species; human fibroblast interferon is active in only human, rabbit, and rat cells. Human leucocyte interferon has the broadest spectrum of activity.

Perhaps the most striking feature of the interferons is their potency. Purified human interferons, of either fibroblast or leucocyte origin, have been reported to be biologically active at levels as low as 10^{-9} mg. of protein. It has been suggested that because of their diverse biological activities and high potency interferons are remindful of hormones.

The antiviral protection afforded by interferon or its inducers is of limited duration, lasting only a few days, and is prophylactic rather than therapeutic. Extension of the prophylactic effect is difficult because of the refractoriness of cells to repeated induction. Narrow host cell specificity also effectively precludes the use of interferons of animal cell origin in human disease. The knowledge that interferon has antitumor effects has spurred efforts to develop effective chemotherapeutic modalities, employing either interferon induc-

Table 12–8. **Properties of Human Interferons***

| Property | Type I | | Type II |
	Produced by Leucocytes	Produced by Fibroblasts	
Protein	+	+	+
Stable at pH 2	+	+	−
Antiviral in:			
Human cells	+	+	+
Bovine cells	+	−	−
Rabbit cells	+	+	−
Rat cells	−	+	−
Neutralized by antiserum to:			
Type I—Leucocyte IF	+	−	−
Type I—Fibroblast IF	−	+	−
Molecular weight	15K; 21K	20K	30K; 70K†

*Adapted from Stewart.[71]
†Two components.

ers or exogenous interferon. The latter has been prepared by stimulation of human cell cultures or synthesis by bacterial or animal cells, using recombinant DNA technology. The practical and effective use of interferon as an antitumor or antiviral agent is not yet achieved, however.

PHAGOCYTIC DEFENSES[17, 22, 36, 63, 69]

When pathogenic microorganisms penetrate the mechanical barriers of the skin and membranes and establish a focus in the tissues, the host counters with inflammatory reactions that call forth a characteristic cellular response. The infection site is invaded by phagocytic cells, first by polymorphonuclear leucocytes (PMN), then by macrophages. This response, characterized by the appearance of host cells capable of phagocytizing and in many cases killing the invading microorganisms, is one of the most effective means of resistance to infection.

Leucocyte Chemotaxis

The cellular response to bacterial invasion is initiated when leucocytes are attracted to the invasion site. This attraction is mediated by a variety of chemoattractants produced in inflammation by kinin activation, complement activation, bacterial metabolism, or injuries to host tissues. The more important of these are listed in Table 12–9. The most potent bacterial chemotactic agents are the N-formylated peptides, a peptide configuration characteristically produced by procaryotes in protein synthesis. There is amplification when chemoattractants are produced by phagocytic cells during the ingestion process. Complement component C5a may arise from complement activation in either the alternate or classical pathway. Later, as immunological responses are stimulated, lymphokines are liberated and reinforce the normal resistance systems.

The chemoattractants are bound to specific

Table 12–9. **Chemoattractants for Leucocytes**

Complement component C5a
Lymphokines
Chemoattractants released from:
    Polymorphonuclear leucocytes
    Macrophages
    Mast cells
Metabolites of arachidonic acid:
    5-Hydroxyeicosatetranoic acid
    Leucotrienes
Bacterial products:
    N-formylated peptides

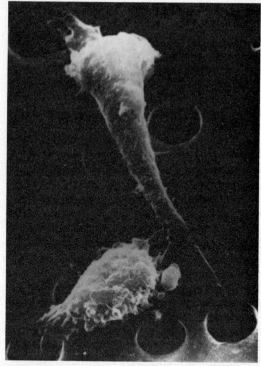

Figure 12–8. Scanning electron micrograph of monocytes migrating through pores of a polycarbonate filter in response to a chemotactic lymphokine. The cell at the top has emerged and has advanced across the filter surface. The bottom cell is just emerging from the pore. × 4000. (Snyderman and Goetzl.[69] Copyright 1982 by the American Association for the Advancement of Science.)

receptors on the leucocyte plasma membranes. In this manner leucocytes detect and move in the direction of increasing chemotactic gradients (Fig. 12–8). As noted in Chapter 2, bacteria sense chemotactic gradients in a temporal fashion and move by alternating tumbles and straight runs. Leucocytes are strikingly different, sensing gradients in a spatial fashion and moving continuously toward the attractant. This is so because they have a large number of specific receptor sites distributed along their surfaces and can sense spatial differences in concentrations of the chemoattractant.

Within a few minutes after sensing chemoattractants, leucocytes alter their morphology and orient toward the chemotactic gradient. They then move in a directed fashion toward the inflammatory site.

Ingestion and Degranulation

When leucocytes have been mobilized and attracted to the infection site, their role is to ingest and destroy the parasite; the cells most often involved are the neutrophils. When the mobilized leucocytes encounter the invading microorganism, the ingestion process is initiated by adherence of the bacteria to the leucocyte surface. This adherence is most often mediated by complement component C3b, generated by the complement cascade reactions described in the preceding section. Bacteria may also adhere to the leucocyte surface by adhesin-receptor reactions.

Following adherence, most bacteria are then engulfed by invagination of the leucocyte membrane through a complex sequence of reactions. After complete engulfment, the plasma membrane fuses and the ingested particles are internalized and enclosed in a vacuole surrounded by what was originally plasma membrane. The vacuole, with the enclosed particles, is the **phagosome.**

Granulocytes contain a number of intracytoplasmic granules, known as **lysosomes,** surrounded by a limiting membrane and containing a variety of enzymatic systems. Neutrophils have two types of lysosomal granules—**primary** and **specific granules.** Primary, or azurophilic, granules contain the important microbicidal enzyme, **myeloperoxidase,** along with acid hydrolases, neutral proteases, cationic proteins, and lysozyme. The specific, or secondary, granules possess a majority of the cellular lysozyme and lactoferrin. The role of these granules and their microbicidal systems are discussed below.

These lysosomal granules in the neutrophil cytoplasm contact the phagosomes formed during ingestion. Their membranes fuse, and the lysosomal contents are emptied into the phagosome, forming a **phagolysosome.** The process is called degranulation.

Degranulation of phagocyte lysosomes may also occur in other ways. Occasionally, microorganisms or other particles react with leucocyte plasma membrane receptors but phago-

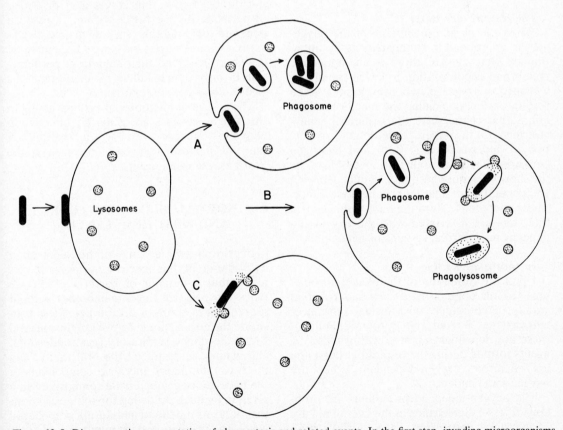

Figure 12–9. Diagrammatic representation of phagocytosis and related events. In the first step, invading microorganisms encounter leucocytes and adhere to their surface. The microorganism may be ingested and become enclosed in the phagosome *(A and B)*. Normally, lysosomes fuse with the phagosome to form the phagolysosome (pathway *B*). Intracellular degradation of the invader then follows, resulting in death of the microorganism. Occasionally, lysosomal fusion is inhibited and the microorganisms multiply in the phagosome (pathway *A*). With some microorganisms, phagocytosis does not take place, but lysosomes fuse with the plasma membrane and release their contents into the surrounding milieu (pathway *C*). The localized concentration of lysosomal contents is often sufficient to destroy the adherent microorganisms.

cytosis does not ensue, either because of the size of the particle or for other reasons. In response to these particles (or other stimuli), lysosomal granules may fuse to the plasma membrane and release their contents into the surrounding milieu. Certain fungi and metazoan parasites have been shown to be killed in this fashion, even though they are not phagocytized.

In other instances, notably in the case of certain obligate intracellular bacteria, phagocytosis is not followed by degranulation. The bacteria apparently inhibit lysosomal fusion with the phagosomal membrane, putatively by the production of cyclic adenosine monophosphate (cAMP). Such bacteria are, therefore, not subject to the microbicidal mechanisms described below. This may permit their survival and multiplication in the phagosome, although there is evidence that intracellular bacteria are able to multiply intracellularly even after lysosomal fusion has occurred.

The Respiratory Burst

When the plasma membrane of the phagocyte is appropriately stimulated, as by initiation of phagocytosis, there is an immediate membrane depolarization followed rapidly by a change in oxygen metabolism, known as the respiratory burst. Among the metabolic alterations that characterize the respiratory burst are: increase in oxygen consumption; production of superoxide ions (O_2^-) and hydrogen peroxide; increase in glucose metabolism *via* the hexose monophosphate shunt pathway; and generation of light, or chemiluminescence. These metabolic alterations are significant in that they are associated with the oxygen-dependent microbicidal systems of neutrophils.

Intracellular Killing

Upon the formation of the phagolysosome, ingested microorganisms are exposed to a great variety of potentially microbicidal substances and enzymes derived from lysosomes. Some of these are dependent upon powerful oxidizing agents formed during the respiratory burst and are, therefore, oxygen-dependent; others are oxygen-independent.

The oxygen-independent systems are probably of lesser significance in the overall picture of microbial destruction. These include lysozyme that acts upon some intact gram-positive bacteria. As noted earlier, however, lysozyme is of greater significance as an accessory factor in immune lysis. The specific granules also contain lactoferrin, which, as noted earlier, has high iron affinity and denies this required cation to many microorganisms.

Of greater interest and significance are the oxygen-dependent antimicrobial systems. One of these, the myeloperoxidase system (MPO), is generally thought to be the most active in microbial killing.

The **myeloperoxidase system** consists of a heme enzyme, found in primary granules, which acts on hydrogen peroxide in the presence of halides to form hypohalites. In most phagocytes, the halide is Cl^- and the antimicrobial effect is due to formation of hypochlorite, which probably halogenates proteins. The hydrogen peroxide in this system is derived from a single electron reduction of molecular oxygen (O_2) to superoxide O_2^- by action of a cellular oxidase; superoxide is then spontaneously dismutated to hydrogen peroxide, or this reaction may be enhanced by the enzyme superoxide dismutase.

Other products of oxygen reduction may also be effective, either directly or indirectly, in microbial killing. Superoxide is probably not directly active, but serves as a precursor of peroxide for the MPO system. It also can generate toxic radicals, such as hydroxyl radical (OH$^.$) and singlet oxygen ($^1O_2$), but these are short-lived and their significant participation in intracellular killing of microorganisms is still somewhat speculative.

These several microbicidal systems acting in the phagolysosomes are generally effective in eliminating phagocytized bacteria, thereby tipping the balance in favor of the host in the host-parasite relationship.

NORMAL MICROBIAL FLORA AND HOST RESISTANCE[32, 65]

In previous consideration of the colonization by bacteria of the mucosal surfaces, it was noted that a number of bacteria of diverse types can colonize these membranes without subsequent invasion or host injury; these constitute the normal flora. At each of the mucosal sites—the upper respiratory, gastrointestinal, and genitourinary tracts; the oral cavity; and the skin—the major microbial components of the flora are of characteristic composition in a given individual. Allowing for some variations that occur in childhood and during prepubertal years, the makeup in both numbers and types of the microbial flora at each mucosal site is remarkably constant through late adult years. Even when the composition is disturbed, as by antibiotics, it rapidly returns to the normal state when this stimulus is removed.

This remarkable constancy in composition of the normal flora implies resistance to the introduction and establishment of new members, including possibly pathogenic bacteria. Thus the normal flora is believed to aid in resistance to infection by regulating access to the tissues by pathogens. The composition of the normal flora and factors leading to its establishment are discussed in Chapter 37.

There is evidential support for several mechanisms whereby the normal microbial flora can influence host resistance to invading microorganisms. These may be divided into two categories—competition and antagonism.

Competition between resident flora and invading microorganisms may take two forms. One, already discussed, is the competition for available attachment sites on the mucosal cell surfaces. This can conceivably be specific, as two microorganisms competing for the same receptor, or it can be spatial, as when different receptors are in near proximity on the mucosal surface. For example, colonization of the umbilicus or nasopharynx of the newborn with staphylococci prevents subsequent colonization of these sites with other strains. This may be a mechanism for protection against virulent, invasive strains. Competition for growth-limiting nutrients has also been observed, such as the competition for carbon sources under the highly reducing conditions of the intestinal environment.

Another form of competition involves the production of antibiotic substances by microorganisms; this formed a part of the early history of microbiology. The possible regulation of ecological communities in natural environments by such antagonistic substances is intuitively obvious. In the intestinal and genitourinary tracts, the formation of volatile fatty acids by normal flora has an inhibitory effect on sensitive bacteria introduced into this environment. The complexity of these associations is suggested by the finding that *Shigella* in the mouse intestine is apparently inhibited by products formed by certain clostridia when stimulated by *Escherichia coli.*[15] Certain bacteria, especially gram-negative bacilli, produce substances called **bacteriocins** that are bactericidal for other microorganisms. It is suspected that these substances help regulate the flora of the intestinal tract.

REFERENCES

1. Arbuthnott, J. P. 1978. Role of exotoxins in bacterial pathogenicity. J. Appl. Bacteriol. **44**:329–345.
2. Barry, D. M. J., and A. W. Reeve. 1977. Increased incidence of gram-negative neonatal sepsis with intramuscular iron administration. Pediatrics **60**:908–912.
3. Beachey, E. H. (Ed.). 1980. Bacterial Adherence. Chapman and Hall, London.
4. Beachey, E. H. 1981. Bacterial adherence: adhesin-receptor interactions mediating the attachment of bacteria to mucosal surfaces. J. Infect. Dis. **143**:325–345.
5. Bernheimer, A. W. 1970. Cytolytic toxins of bacteria. pp. 183–212. *In* S. J. Ajl, S. Kadis, and T. C. Montie (Eds.): Microbial Toxins. Vol. I, Bacterial Protein Toxins. Academic Press, New York.
6. Björkstén, B. 1980. Unspecific host defence. Scand. J. Infect. Dis. Suppl. **24**:33–35.
7. Bradley, S. G. 1979. Cellular and molecular mechanisms of action of bacterial endotoxins. Ann. Rev. Microbiol. **33**:67–94.
8. Bullen, J. J. 1981. The significance of iron in infection. Rev. Infect. Dis. **3**:1127–1138.
9. Chandra, R. K., and P. M. Newberne. 1977. Nutrition, Immunity, and Infection. Mechanisms of Interactions. Plenum Press, New York.
10. Collier, A. M. 1980. Attachment of *Mycoplasma pneumoniae* to respiratory epithelium. pp. 159–183. *In* E. H. Beachey (Ed.): Bacterial Adherence. Chapman and Hall, London.
11. Davison, V. E., and B. A. Sanford. 1981. Adherence of *Staphylococcus aureus* to influenza A virus-infected Madin-Darby canine kidney cell cultures. Infect. Immun. **32**:118–126.
12. Densen, P., and G. L. Mandell. 1980. Phagocyte strategy vs. microbial tactics. Rev. Infect. Dis. **2**:817–838.
13. Dinarello, C. A., and S. M. Wolff. 1982. Molecular basis of fever. Amer. J. Med. **72**:799–819.
14. Donaldson, D. M., and J. G. Tew. 1977. Beta-lysin of platelet origin. Bacteriol. Rev. **41**:501–513.
15. Ducluzeau, R., *et al.* 1977. Antagonistic effect of extremely oxygen-sensitive clostridia from the microflora of conventional mice and of *Escherichia coli* against *Shigella flexneri* in the digestive tract of gnotobiotic mice. Infect. Immun. **17**:415–424.
16. Dunlop, R. H., and H. W. Moon (Eds.). 1970. Resistance to Infectious Disease. Saskatoon Modern Press, Saskatoon, Saskatchewan, Canada.
17. Edelson, P. J. 1982. Intracellular parasites and phagocytic cells: cell biology and pathophysiology. Rev. Infect. Dis. **4**:124–135.
18. Elin, R. J., and S. M. Wolff. 1976. Biology of endotoxin. Ann. Rev. Med. **27**:127–141.
19. Elliot, K., M. O'Conner, and J. Whelan (Eds.). 1981. Adhesion and microorganism pathogenicity. Ciba Foundation Symposium 80. Pittman Medical Ltd., London.
20. Elwell, L. P., and P. L. Shipley. 1980. Plasmid-mediated factors associated with virulence of bacteria to animals. Ann. Rev. Microbiol. **34**:465–496.
21. Frank, M. M. 1979. The complement system in host defense and inflammation. Rev. Infect. Dis. **1**:483–501.
22. Gabig, T. G., and B. M. Babior. 1981. The killing of pathogens by phagocytes. Ann. Rev. Med. **32**:313–326.
23. Gardner, I. D. 1980. The effect of aging on susceptibility to infection. Rev. Infect. Dis. **2**:801–810.
24. Giannella, R. A. 1981. Pathogenesis of acute bacterial diarrheal disorders. Ann. Rev. Med. **32**:341–357.
25. Gill, D. M. 1982. Bacterial toxins: a table of lethal amounts. Microbiol. Rev. **46**:86–94.
26. Gordon, J., and M. A. Minks. 1981. The interferon renaissance: molecular aspects of induction and action. Microbiol. Rev. **45**:244–266.
27. Goren, M. B. 1977. Phagocyte lysosomes: interactions with infectious agents, phagosomes, and experimen

tal perturbations in function. Ann. Rev. Microbiol. **31**:507–533.

28. Greenblatt, J., R. J. Boackle, and J. H. Schwab. 1978. Activation of the alternate complement pathway by peptidoglycan from streptococcal cell wall. Infect. Immun. **19**:296–303.

29. Hale, T. L., and P. F. Bonventre. 1979. Shigella infection of Henle intestinal epithelial cells: role of the bacterium. Infect. Immun. **24**:879–886.

30. Hamada, S., and H. D. Slade. 1980. Mechanisms of adherence of *Streptococcus mutans* to smooth surfaces *in vitro*. pp. 105–135. *In* E. H. Beachey (Ed.): Bacterial Adherence. Chapman and Hall, London.

31. Hatch, T. P. 1975. Competition between *Chlamydia psittaci* and L cells for host isoleucine pools: a limiting factor in chlamydial multiplication. Infect. Immun. **12**:211–220.

32. Hentges, D. J. 1975. Resistance of the indigenous intestinal flora to the establishmont of invading microbial populations. pp. 116–119. *In* D. Schlessinger (Ed.): Microbiology—1975. American Society for Microbiology, Washington, D.C.

33. van Heyningen, S. 1977. Cholera toxin. Biol. Rev. **52**:509–549.

34. Hirsch, R. L. 1982. The complement system: its importance in the host response to viral infection. Microbiol. Rev. **46**:71–85.

35. Ho, M., and J. A. Armstrong. 1975. Interferon. Ann. Rev. Microbiol. **29**:131–161.

36. Horwitz, M. A. 1982. Phagocytosis of microorganisms. Rev. Infect. Dis. **4**:104–123.

37. Jeljaszewicz, J., S. Szmigielski, and W. Hryniewicz. 1978. Biological effects of staphylococcal and streptococcal toxins. pp. 185–227. *In* J. Jeljaszewicz and T. Wadström (Eds.): Bacterial Toxins and Cell Membranes. Academic Press, London.

38. Jorgensen, G. 1981. Humangenetik und infektionskrankheiten. Münich. Med. Wochensch. **123**:1447–1452.

39. Jose, D. G., *et al.* 1975. Deficiency of immunological and phagocytic function in Aboriginal children with protein-calorie malnutrition. Med. J. Australia **2**:699–701, 703–705.

40. Kabir, S., D. L. Rosenstreich, and S. E. Mergenhagen. 1978. Bacterial endotoxins and cell membranes. pp. 59–87. *In* J. Jeljaszewicz and T. Wadström (Eds.): Bacterial Toxins and Cell Membranes. Academic Press, London.

41. Kernbaum, S., L. Tazi, and D. Champagne. 1976. Sexe et susceptibilité aux maladies infectieuses. Bull. Inst. Pasteur **74**:359–382.

42. Klainer, A. S., T.-W. Chang, and L. Weinstein. 1972. Effects of purified staphylococcal alpha toxin on the ultrastructure of human and rabbit erythrocytes. Infect. Immun. **5**:808–813.

43. Kornfeld, S. J., and A. G. Plaut. 1981. Secretory immunity and the bacterial IgA proteases. Rev. Infect. Dis. **3**:521–534.

44. Mackowiak, P. A. 1978. Microbial synergism in human infections. Parts 1 and 2. New Engl. J. Med. **298**:21–26, 83–87.

45. Mackowiak, P. A., and M. Marling-Cason. 1983. Hyperthermic enhancement of serum antimicrobial activity: mechanism by which fever might exert a beneficial effect on the outcome of gram-negative sepsis. Infect. Immun. **39**:38–42.

46. McCartney, A. C., and J. P. Arbuthnott. 1978. Mode of action of membrane-damaging toxins produced by staphylococci. pp. 89–127. *In* J. Jeljaszewicz and T. Wadström (Eds.): Bacterial Toxins and Cell Membranes. Academic Press, London.

47. Melching, L., and S. I. Vas. 1971. Effects of serum components on gram-negative bacteria during bactericidal reactions. Infect. Immun. **3**:107–115.

48. Murray, M. J., *et al.* 1978. The adverse effect of iron repletion on the course of certain infections. Brit. Med. J. **2**:1113–1115.

49. McNabb, P. C., and T. B. Tomasi. 1981. Host defense mechanisms at mucosal surfaces. Ann. Rev. Microbiol. **35**:477–496.

50. Neilands, J. B. 1981. Microbial iron compounds. Ann. Rev. Biochem. **50**:715–731.

51. Neilands, J. B. 1982. Microbial envelope proteins related to iron. Ann. Rev. Microbiol. **36**:285–309.

52. Newhouse, M., J. Sanchis, and J. Bienenstock. 1976. Lung defense mechanisms. Parts 1 and 2. New Engl. J. Med. **295**:990–998, 1045–1052.

53. Ofek, I., and E. H. Beachey. 1980. General concepts and principles of bacterial adherence in animals and man. pp. 1–29. *In* E. H. Beachey (Ed.): Bacterial Adherence. Chapman and Hall, London.

54. Pearce, W. A., and T. M. Buchanan. 1980. Structure and cell membrane-binding properties of bacterial fimbriae. pp. 289–344. *In* E. H. Beachey (Ed.): Bacterial Adherence. Chapman and Hall, London.

55. Piccardi, G. 1962. The Chemical Basis of Medical Climatology. Charles C Thomas, Springfield, Ill.

56. Previte, J. J., *et al.* 1970. Invasiveness of *Salmonella* administered orally to cold-exposed mice. Infect. Immun. **2**:274–278.

57. Quie, P. G., E. L. Mills, and W. Regelmann. 1979. Genetically determined abnormalities of host defense against bacterial diseases. pp. 246–248. *In* D. Schlessinger (Ed.): Microbiology—1979. American Society for Microbiology, Washington, D.C.

58. Ramírez-Ronda, C. H., Z. Fuxench-López, and M. Nevárez. 1981. Increased pharyngeal bacterial colonization during viral illness. Arch. Intern. Med. **141**:1599–1603.

59. Rietschel, E. T., C. Galanos, and O. Lüderitz. 1975. Structure, endotoxicity and immunogenicity of the lipid A component of bacterial lipopolysaccharides. pp. 307–314. *In* D. Schlessinger (Ed.): Microbiology—1975. American Society for Microbiology, Washington, D.C.

60. Robbins, J. B., *et al.* 1980. Virulence properties of bacterial capsular polysaccharides—unanswered questions. pp. 115–132. *In* H. Smith, J. J. Skehel, and M. J. Turner (Eds.): The Molecular Basis of Microbial Pathogenicity. Verlag Chemie, Weinheim, Germany.

61. Roberts, D. S. 1969. Synergic mechanisms in certain mixed infections. J. Infect. Dis. **120**:720–724.

62. Roberts, N. J., Jr. 1979. Temperature and host defense. Microbiol. Rev. **43**:241–259.

63. Root, R. K., and M. S. Cohen. 1981. The microbicidal mechanisms of human neutrophils and eosinophils. Rev. Infect. Dis. **3**:565–598.

64. Rozmiarek, H., R. W. Bolton, and F. W. Chorpenning. 1977. Environmental origin of natural antibodies to teichoic acid. Infect. Immun. **16**:505–509.

65. Savage, D. C., and J. S. McAllister. 1970. Microbial interactions at body surfaces and resistance to infectious diseases. pp. 113–127. *In* R. H. Dunlop and H. W. Moon (Eds.): Resistance to Infectious Disease. Saskatoon Modern Press, Saskatoon, Saskatchewan, Canada.

66. Smith, H. 1977. Microbial surfaces in relation to pathogenicity. Bacteriol. Rev. **41**:475–500.

67. Smith, H., J. J. Skehel, and M. J. Turner (Eds.). 1980. The Molecular Basis of Microbial Pathogenicity. Verlag Chemie, Weinheim, Germany.

68. Smyth, C. J., and J. L. Duncan. 1978. Thiol-activated (oxygen-labile) cytolysins. pp. 129–183. *In* J. Jeljaszewicz and T. Wadström (Eds.): Bacterial Toxins and Cell Membranes. Academic Press, London.

69. Snyderman, R., and E. J. Goetzl. 1981. Molecular and cellular mechanisms of leukocyte chemotaxis. Science **213**:830–837.

70. Spitznagle, J. K. 1979. Microbial cells as determinants of intraleukocytic degradation. pp. 100–104. *In* D. Schlessinger (Ed.): Microbiology—1979. American Society for Microbiology, Washington, D.C.

71. Stewart, W. E., II. 1980. Purification and properties of interferon proteins. pp. 208–210. *In* D. Schlessinger (Ed.): Microbiology—1980. American Society for Microbiology, Washington, D.C.

72. Stoner, H. B. 1972. Specific and non-specific effects of bacterial infection on the host. Symp. Soc. Gen. Microbiol. **22**:113–128.

73. Symposium. 1975. Pathogenic mechanisms in bacterial diseases. pp. 103–340. *In* D. Schlessinger (Ed.): Microbiology—1975. American Society for Microbiology, Washington, D.C.

74. Symposium. 1977. Bacterial antigens and host response. pp. 217–430. *In* D. Schlessinger (Ed.): Microbiology—1977. American Society for Microbiology, Washington, D. C.

75. Symposium. 1979. Mechanisms of microbial virulence. pp. 77–253. *In* D. Schlessinger (Ed.): Microbiology—1979. American Society for Microbiology, Washington, D.C.

76. Symposium. 1980. Endogenous mediators in host responses to bacterial endotoxin. pp. 1–167. *In* D. Schlessinger (Ed.): Microbiology—1980. American Society for Microbiology, Washington, D.C.

77. Symposium. 1980. Interferon: induction and action. pp. 197–216. *In* D. Schlessinger (Ed.): Microbiology—1980. American Society for Microbiology, Washington, D.C.

78. Terres, G., S. L. Morrison, and G. S. Habicht. 1968. A quantitative difference in the immune response between male and female mice. Proc. Soc. Exptl. Biol. Med. **127**:664–667.

79. Yancey, R. J., and R. Finkelstein. 1981. Siderophore production by pathogenic *Neisseria* spp. Infect. Immun. **32**:600–618.

80. Young, L. S. 1980. The role of exotoxins in the pathogenesis of *Pseudomonas aeruginosa* infections. J. Infect. Dis. **142**:626–630.

The Epidemiology of Infectious Diseases

Whatever the pathogenic powers of a microorganism and the efficiency of host defenses, an essential preliminary to the production of infectious disease is a meeting of the parasite and its prospective host. Saprophytic microorganisms usually enter the host by accident, as in tetanus, gas gangrene, and similar infections that follow traumatic introduction of the agent into host tissues. In most instances, however, microorganisms that produce disease are more or less adapted to a parasitic existence and pass from one animal host to another with only a relatively brief sojourn in the external world. Transmission of infection results from transfer of the causative microorganism, either directly or indirectly, from an infected to a healthy susceptible animal.

The elucidation of the mechanisms involved in this transfer is a matter of considerable importance. If the sequence of events that precedes infection is known, interruption of the process at its most vulnerable point can permit control of the spread of disease. Disease is not entirely a matter of host resistance and microbial virulence; it is, in a very real sense, the outcome of interaction between host and parasite populations. It is at this point that the study of infectious disease transcends the microbiology of clinical medicine, with its emphasis on the individual case, and assumes broad biological significance as a problem in interspecies competition.[3]

The equilibrium that tends to establish between host and parasite populations is an unstable one in that the factors which determine it—the character of the host and parasite populations and the environmental factors that bear upon their relationship—are constantly shifting, and the equilibrium ever has the tendency to establish at a new level. The shift may be sudden and dramatic, manifesting as an explosive outbreak of disease; less commonly, it may take the form of a gradual increase or decrease in the number of cases.

Factors associated with the maintenance or shift of this equilibrium are the subject matter of epidemiology. The term **epidemiology** is best regarded in this broad sense and therefore includes the study of factors influencing transmission of both endemic and epidemic disease. **Endemic** diseases are those which appear in a population at a relatively standard or expected frequency, while **epidemics** are characterized by an unusual accumulation or sudden upsurge in the number of cases. The term **pandemic** is usually applied to an epidemic of unusually great, often worldwide, proportions. These categories, although useful, are not mutually exclusive; a disease endemic in a community may, at times, attain the proportions of an epidemic and later subside again to the endemic level. A case in point is the experience with encephalitis in the United States, as shown in Figure 13–1.

Essential to the understanding of the epidemiology of disease are certain characteristics of the etiological agent and of the clinical infection that determine the possible channels of transmission. The more important of these are:

1. The route by which the infective agent enters the body

2. The route by which the infective agent leaves the body

3. The resistance of the microorganism to the deleterious effects of the environment outside of the host

4. Existence of an intermediate, or reservoir, host

5. The relation between clinically recognizable disease and the discharge of infectious microorganisms from the body

These are most readily and satisfactorily determined by direct study of the etiological agent under controlled conditions and by observations of the pathogenesis of the naturally occurring disease. Even when the causative agent is unknown, a first approximation of these properties may be inferred with surprising confidence from the observed epidemiological behavior of the disease. For example, in the famous Broad Street Pump epidemic, which occurred prior to discovery of the etiology of cholera, the indirect evidence plainly indicated to Snow that the infective agent left the body in feces and entered the gastrointestinal tract via contaminated well water.

Rates in Epidemiology

In epidemiological studies it is essential to measure the frequency of a disease or condition in a unit of population within some spec-

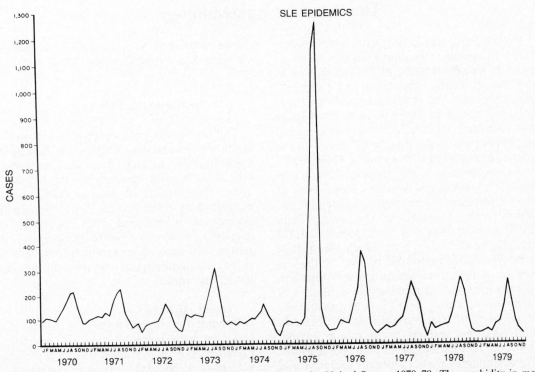

Figure 13–1. Reported cases of encephalitis by month of onset in the United States, 1970–79. The morbidity in most years was relatively constant, but in 1975 assumed epidemic proportions. (Centers for Disease Control, Annual summary 1980: reported morbidity and mortality in the United States. Morbidity and Mortality Weekly Report **29**[54], 1981.)

ified time frame. This measure is generally expressed as a fraction, or rate, in which the numerator is the number of afflicted and the denominator is the population at that time. Thus:

$$\text{Rate (in a time period)} = \frac{\text{Number of cases or deaths}}{\text{Population}}$$

When this rate is for cases of disease, it is the **morbidity (case** or **attack) rate**; rates of death are termed **mortality rates.**

Depending upon the requirements of an epidemiological study, the measures of morbidity may take one of two forms, incidence or prevalence rates. **Incidence rates** express the number of new cases of disease appearing in a population over an interval of time, usually one year, although any time period may be selected. Ideally, the population used in incidence rate calculations should be the population at risk, *e.g.,* should exclude those who are immune. In practice, this is difficult to determine and such corrections are not usually made.

Prevalence rates express the number of existing cases of disease in the total population at some specific point in time. Therefore, prevalence depends upon previous incidence as well as the duration of the illness. Most infectious diseases tend to be acute rather than chronic, so that incidence rates find greater application and are generally used to predict probability of illness in a given population.

Correction of morbidity and mortality rates are often a practical necessity. Such corrections take the form of **age-specific rates**—the proportion of cases or deaths in a specific age group—or **standardized (adjusted) rates,** which are not the observed rates, but rather what the rates would be if the age distribution of the population were that of a standard or reference population. In the United States, for example, the total population is usually taken as a standard and the population of states or other smaller groups is compared or adjusted to it. The age distribution is probably of greatest importance in infectious disease epidemiology, and most adjusted rates are so corrected; sex and racial distribution are of somewhat lesser practical significance, although some diseases are strikingly different in such groups and both sex- and race-specific rates are determined, as illustrated in Figure 12–3 (p. 337).

The Scope of Epidemiology[1, 5]

Epidemiological investigations are undertaken to establish the cause, modes of transmission, and distribution of disease, as well as the reasons for the appearance and disappearance of disease and environmental factors that act upon the population at risk. Knowledge and understanding of these features can lead to intervention in the disease process with the goal of terminating or preventing epidemics.

To accomplish these purposes, epidemiological investigations usually adopt one of three strategies: (1) descriptive epidemiology, which seeks to determine the amount and distribution of disease within a population; (2) analytic epidemiology, in which descriptive data are incorporated and related to the dynamics of infection, permitting identification of principles that determine the evolution of infectious processes; and (3) experimental epidemiology, wherein variables are deliberately controlled and studied, as in animal populations or vaccination of human populations. These strategies are not mutually exclusive and sometimes overlap; data accumulation that is a part of descriptive epidemiology is, for example, necessary to construct the mathematical models of analytic epidemiology.

DESCRIPTIVE EPIDEMIOLOGY

The most frequent method employed to study the occurrence of disease is descriptive epidemiology. In large measure it represents the accumulation and statistical analysis of data. The amount of disease that occurs is measured by rates and its distribution in the population is analyzed with respect to the variables of persons affected, geographic limitation, and time of occurrence; these are the classic epidemiological variables of **persons, place,** and **time.**

Persons Affected

Populations affected by disease may be characterized with respect to a large number of variables, but most studies specify three characteristics of persons—age, sex, and race.

Age. The age distribution of disease is often the most important of epidemiological variables. It is suggestive as a corollary to other epidemiological characteristics and often aids in their interpretation. Thus, a disease generally occurring in the early years of life, such as measles or diphtheria, often shows differences in age incidence between urban and rural populations; these differences are explained by the more frequent occurrence of immunizing infections, either apparent or subclinical, in the more crowded urban populations. Similar differentials are apparent in cerebrospinal meningitis; the age distribution of this disease, together with other of its epidemiological features, supports the view that it is prevalent as an inapparent infection.

Sex. Differentials of disease with respect to sex are expected in certain diseases, such as toxic shock syndrome, related to host anatomy and physiology (Chapter 14). In tuberculosis, on the other hand, the higher incidence and mortality rates in males is essentially unexplained, although it may be related to greater likelihood of exposure. Such is the case, too, in brucellosis; the higher incidence in males is probably due to occupational exposure to infected animals.

Race. Although epidemiological data classified by race is of considerable value, the distinction between true racial differences and differences associated with socioeconomic conditions are not easily discerned. Such data clearly identify high risk groups in diseases like tuberculosis (Fig. 12–3, p. 337).

Geographical Distribution

The area in which a disease occurs and the regularity of its geographic distribution are highly informative. The general occurrence of a disease indicates that environmental conditions peculiar to only parts of the area are not essential to its transmission. Similarly, restriction of a disease within geographic limits implies that special environmental conditions are necessary to its dissemination; these may include crowding, presence of an arthropod vector, water supplies, or animal reservoirs of infection. If the method of transmission is simple, as in measles, the disease is generally uniformly distributed, whereas irregular distribution, such as that of spotted fever, implies a more complex process dependent upon a source of infection or conditions necessary for transmission that are correspondingly irregularly distributed.

Seasonal Distribution

Seasonal distribution is also informative when considered together with other epidemiological features of a disease. Thus, occurrence of arthropod-transmitted infections is conditioned by season and effects of temperature. Others, particularly respiratory diseases, may be associated with the crowding and greater chances for transmission that occur during winter months. The seasonal variation that characterizes death from pneumonia-influenza is illustrated in Figure 13–2.

Levels of Disease

Levels or amounts of a disease in the population can suggest a source of infection. A high rate of incidence, as observed in measles outbreaks, indicates that observed cases are the most important, if not the only, source of

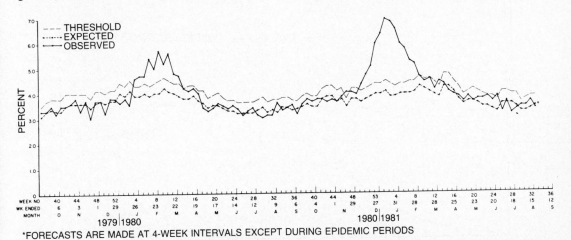

Figure 13–2. The effect of season on infectious disease as illustrated by the variations in death rate from pneumonia-influenza in 121 large cities in the United States. Deviations from the threshold are attributable to epidemics. (Centers for Disease Control, Annual summary 1980: reported morbidity and mortality in the United States. Morbidity and Mortality Weekly Report **29**[54], 1981.)

infection. Conversely, sporadic distribution of widely separated cases implies the existence of a concealed source of infection, such as a carrier or animal reservoir.

ANALYTIC EPIDEMIOLOGY[4]

Descriptive studies in epidemiology are useful in elucidating the occurrence of disease in both general and specific populations. Such studies do not, of course, answer the question of why a particular group is affected—an answer that is essential to the planning necessary for prevention and intervention. It is the province of analytic epidemiology to provide these answers, *i.e.,* identification of factors that establish causal relationships and the evolution of disease in a susceptible group.

Theoretical examination of the frequency of infectious disease consists of the formulation of hypotheses and the construction of epidemiological models that are often mathematical in nature. A number of variables and their interrelationships must be taken into account. These include the effective contact or dose required to produce overt disease; the degree of homogeneity of populations containing both infected and susceptible persons; the probability of spread from infected individuals in the incubation period, during the clinical stages,

or during the convalescent period; and the effectiveness of the immune response associated with recovery. The way in which relevant factors are presumptively defined prior to formulation in mathematical terms leads to two kinds of approaches, one deterministic and the other stochastic.

The **deterministic** approach is based upon the assumption that when the numbers of susceptible and infected persons are known, along with rates of attack, birth, death, and the like, any future state of the host population can be precisely defined.[2] From the **stochastic** point of view, the variables are regarded as probabilities and are so treated mathematically.

The deterministic theory of the epidemic process, developed by Kermack and McKendrick in 1927, established the general principle of the mechanism of epidemics by formulating the "threshold of density" of susceptible populations as the determining factor. Figure 13–3 illustrates this theory in diagrammatic terms; *i.e.,* when the number of susceptibles is above a mathematically determined threshold level, the number of cases will increase in an epidemic wave, whereas when the number of susceptibles falls below the threshold, the number of cases will decrease.

The rate at which the number of cases in-

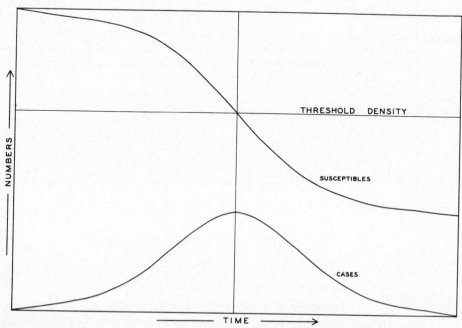

Figure 13–3. Diagrammatic representation of the course of an epidemic wave in terms of number of cases (lower curve) and number of susceptibles (upper curve). Note the coincidence of the peak of the epidemic wave with the threshold density of susceptibles. (After McKendrick.)

creases or decreases is a function of the **incubation period,** *e.g.,* the shorter the incubation period, the more explosive the character of the outbreak. **Generation time**—that elapsing between exposure of the susceptible individual to an effective dose and the point at which microorganisms are shed into the environment—is a more accurate measure than incubation time, because in many diseases, the individual is infectious before symptoms appear.

Each disease situation involves a series of unique combinations of assumptions to be reduced to mathematical form and is therefore not generalizable. The availability of computers has made possible the utilization of mathematical models of the spread of disease and their testing against its observed behavior. It follows that such methods may also be used to determine the theoretical effectiveness of control methods, singly and in combination; when extended to include costs, they permit cost-effectiveness and cost-benefit analysis of control measures.

EXPERIMENTAL EPIDEMIOLOGY

The information that can be derived from observation of naturally occurring disease—descriptive epidemiology—is limited, since the observer usually has no control over the process, the experiment being carried out for, rather than by, the observer.

In a few instances, "experiments" may be carried out in human populations, as in large-scale immunizations against naturally occurring disease, coupled with observations of its long-term effects. Thus, the effects of altering the levels of susceptibles in a population may be assessed.

Other epidemiological factors cannot be controlled in naturally occurring human disease. Experimental epidemics can be generated, however, in animal populations in which the conditions can be adjusted as desired. The experimental system, *i.e.,* agent and host population, are generally selected to mimic an epidemic situation in humans. For example, *Salmonella typhimurium* or *Pasteurella multocida* infections in mice are regarded as analogous to those human diseases, such as typhoid, in which there is imperfect immunity and a carrier state; mousepox (ectromelia) virus infections are similar to human diseases in which solid immunity is developed, such as diphtheria. The extent to which these analogies may be carried and to which the conclusions are applicable to complex populations is open to question; nevertheless, such studies have yielded valuable information.

Experimental animal epidemics are of two general types. A closed epidemic may be simulated by the simple introduction of infected animals into an animal colony. Alternatively, the experiment may be carried out in an infected animal population altered by the introduction of a new group of immigrant animals at regular intervals. Dispersal methods, simulating those sometimes employed in human disease, may be introduced by separation of groups from the original populations. The effects of immunization, either by immunizing infection and recovery or by artificial immunization, may also be assessed.

These kinds of experiments have yielded results that bear directly upon the interaction between host and parasite populations in nature. Perhaps the most important of these is the experimental demonstration of recurring epidemic waves resulting from continuous addition of new susceptibles to the infected population. Although such a sequence of events is predicted by theoretical epidemiology, the repeated flare-up of a disease of humans or domestic animals, thought to be stamped out in the interepidemic period, has been taken as evidence of reimportation of disease. The experimental demonstration of this phenomenon and the indicated futility of quarantine in the control of a disease that is widely disseminated are clearly of considerable significance.

The Natural History of Disease

An understanding of the disease process is a necessary antecedent to the prevention and control of that disease. The natural history of an infectious disease embodies the host-parasite interactions, as discussed in the previous chapter (Chapter 12). Taken from an epidemiological point of view, these involve relations between host and parasite populations, including influences of the environment. This ecological model—host, parasite, and environment—is often applied to the epidemiology of infectious diseases, implying that each component must be analyzed and interrelated in order to understand disease causation in populations. The infectious diseases of man, then, constitute a series of special cases of the host-parasite relationship, differing from one another with respect to the biology of the infectious agent, mode of transmission, incubation period, period of infectivity, immunity, case fatality, and the like.

The Carrier

In the early days of microbiology, it was assumed that the contact of host and parasite could have one or the other of two outcomes; either no infection occurred, owing presumably to high resistance on the part of the host, or clinically characteristic disease developed in the individual. Subsequently, it became clear that an intermediate state, a symptomless infection, can be established. Such an infection is, of course, inapparent and can be demonstrated only by isolation and identification of the infectious agent. An individual so infected is termed a carrier.

Two types of carriers are commonly differentiated: the **casual carrier** who harbors the microorganism only temporarily (a few days or weeks), and the **chronic carrier** who remains infected for a relatively long time, sometimes throughout life. These individuals serve to disseminate the infectious agent. Carriers of the diphtheria bacillus, meningococcus, pneumococcus, and streptococcus are, in the majority, casual carriers, whereas those carrying enteric bacilli, especially the typhoid bacillus, are most often chronic carriers. A third type of carrier is often specified, the **convalescent carrier,** who remains infected for varying periods after recovery from the disease, but these last do not fall into the category of inapparent infections. Sharp separation of these types is sometimes not possible, for the casual or chronic carrier may, in fact, be convalescent from the disease in a form either atypical or so mild as to be unrecognized.

While it is commonplace to recognize the existence of the carrier state, the implications of the general principle that infection can occur without overt disease are frequently neglected. If an important proportion of the infections are inapparent, the number of cases of disease cannot offer an accurate estimate of the incidence of infection. The implications of this are several. For example, sporadically occurring diseases, such as poliomyelitis, meningococcal infection, and pneumococcal infection, may be as widely disseminated and readily communi-cable as measles or the common cold, but the clinically distinctive disease is the exception rather than the rule. Furthermore, changes in morbidity, duration, or geographic distribution of an infectious disease may not reflect a corresponding variability in the occurrence of infection, but rather may be a consequence of variation in the case:carrier ratios. Similarly, carriers of virulent pneumococci do not occur predominantly in higher age groups, or diphtheria bacillus carriers in schoolchildren, where the morbidity of these diseases is highest; and diphtheria bacillus carriers are as common in the tropics as in temperate climates despite the relative rarity of clinical diphtheria in the warmer areas.

It is obvious that recognition of the carrier state and its implications is basic to sound epidemiological thinking and of primary importance in understanding the mechanisms of disease transmission.

Herd Immunity

As already noted, the probability of epidemic disease is directly related to the proportion of susceptibles in the population. The resistance of a population or group, herd immunity, is based upon the relative number of immunes, for the higher the proportion of immunes in a population, the smaller the probability of effective contact between infected persons and susceptibles. Under such circumstances, many of the contacts will be with immunes, and the population exhibits a group resistance which may be of such high order that an epidemic is no longer possible; consequently, the disease smolders in an endemic form. A susceptible member of such an immune population enjoys an immunity, not of his own making but arising from membership in the group.

It is evident that not all members of the group must be immune in order to prevent or abort an epidemic. The proportion of immunes required is variable, depending upon such factors as population density, the infectious dose, and the characteristics of the carrier state. In diphtheria, for example, immunization of 30 per cent of preschool children suffices to control epidemics in this group, whereas the proportion required is much higher in schoolchildren—70 per cent is the commonly accepted level—and if population density is great, even higher levels of herd immunity may be necessary. Since immunes are often casual carriers of the diphtheria organism, the potential sources of infection for susceptibles is increased, introducing a new variable in herd immunity. In other diseases, *viz.*, measles, immunization of 50 per cent of susceptible children has been shown to result in a 90 per cent reduction in cases.[8]

When the incidence of infection is high, a given individual will be subjected to a greater number of infectious particles per unit time; some, previously immune to smaller doses, will then become susceptibles, and the effective concentration of immunes declines with consequent effect on the herd immunity. This effect of dosage has been termed **infection pressure.** Successive epidemic waves then derive from increased infection pressure as well as from accumulation of new susceptibles.

THE MICROBIAL POPULATION

The well-known variation in the severity and "contagiousness" of infectious diseases is a consequence of corresponding variation from one species of pathogenic microorganisms to another in their ability to colonize the host, invade the tissues, and produce clinical disease (Chapter 12). As indicated in Chapter 6, a single species is potentially variable in these respects, for such variations can be induced by experimental manipulation. The possibility of such intraspecies variation in a bacterial population existing under natural conditions is one that has long intrigued students of infectious disease.

It is tempting to account for the genesis and rise of epidemic disease by postulating that the causative agent of endemic disease gains in virulence by successive passage from person to person until its virulence is so enhanced that an epidemic ensues. There is, however, no direct evidence that host-induced alterations in virulence play an important role in the evolution of single or secondary epidemic waves; in nature, microbial virulence, with few exceptions, appears to be a relatively stable character.

On the other hand, differences in the severity of a single disease from one epidemic to another are, in part, attributable to strains of the agent differing from one another in virulence, such differences possibly arising as a consequence of mutation. Smallpox is a case in point; before its eradication, it was seen in two forms—variola major and variola minor—differing only in severity of the disease.

It is possible that long-term changes in the morbidity and mortality of certain diseases may reflect alterations in virulence of the etiologic agent. Syphilis is no longer the scourge it was in the sixteenth century, and the decline in tuberculosis began before the institution of preventive and therapeutic measures. It has not yet been possible to assess these phenomena; possibly in some diseases there are long-term periodic fluctuations in microbial virulence, while in others an adaptive reduction in virulence or increase in host resistance (or combination of the two) may play a part. Perhaps the most elegant example of this phenomenon is illustrated by the attempt to control the rabbit population in Australia by introduction of myxomatosis virus. Initially, the rabbit population declined sharply, but with adaptation of the host and parasite, an equilibrium was established, with essentially complete defeat of the original objective.

In general, it may be said that the natural bacterial population, in the short term, is remarkably stable in its ability to produce disease in a host population. Although the severity of a disease may, and often does, vary from one epidemic to another, variation in virulence is not an important factor in the single epidemic wave. Over long periods, however, alterations in virulence may contribute to changes in morbidity and mortality.

THE HOST POPULATION

In contrast to the relative stability of the bacterial population, human populations are highly variable in their resistance to infection. These variations, attributable to both intrinsic and extrinsic factors, are frequently of such magnitude that the consequences are of great practical importance.

Since a population, human or infrahuman, is composed of individuals, it follows that its character is determined by the nature of the individuals and their relations to one another; reaction of the population to an external influence represents the aggregate of its members' reactions. The response of a human population to an infectious disease is measured as a composite of the responses of individuals, using statistical methods that involve rates, ratios, life tables, and similar numerical devices.

Intrinsic Factors

Of the intrinsic factors that determine the response of a human population to infectious disease, one of the most important is age distribution. The quantitative predominance of lower age groups, which characterizes an immature population, declines as the total population increases. With population growth, there is a corresponding increase in the older age groups. Consequently, the diseases of childhood and early adult life, including diphtheria, meningitis, and the like, are relatively more common in an immature population, but become progressively less so with time, while the diseases of old age increase in incidence with maturation of the population.

Extrinsic Factors

The extrinsic factors that alter host resistance to the spread of disease may exert their influence in either or both of two ways; first, by influencing the resistance of all or part of the individuals composing the population, and second, by influencing the relationships between individuals. Perhaps the most important factor in the first category is active immunity. If a sufficient portion of a population is immune to a disease as a result of artificial inoculation or recovery from an attack, the resistance of the entire group to epidemics of that disease is of high order—herd immunity. Other factors may reduce the resistance of the individual; in times of stress or calamity, for example, when relatively large groups are undernourished, fatigued, or exposed to inclement weather, epidemics may spread with great rapidity.

Equally important to the resistance of a population to epidemic disease are the factors that determine the interrelationships of its members. Crowding in large gatherings or the enforced close associations arising from inadequate housing obviously provide opportunities for the dissemination of respiratory and other diseases transmitted directly from person to person and for certain indirectly transmitted infections, such as louseborne typhus fever. Similarly, the spread of enteric infections is, to a large extent, dependent upon sanitary facilities and the solution to the twin problems of water supply and sewage disposal. Group living conditions that support a large rat population make bubonic plague a potential menace, and the presence of large numbers of mosquitoes of the appropriate species allows the dissemination of yellow fever and malaria. A vivid example of the effects of changing behavior patterns of a host population on the incidence of disease is that of kuru, a slow virus infection that occurs in the highlands of New Guinea (Chapter 42). First described in 1957, it then accounted for more than half of the postinfancy deaths. It is a progressive neurological disease occurring primarily in women and older children. It is transmitted by ritual cannibalistic practices in which dead tribesmen are consumed by their relatives; boys and men traditionally eat the flesh, while the brain and viscera are eaten by women and children. With a decline in this practice beginning in 1950, the death rate in women dropped sharply in the period 1960–65; while about the same number of persons born between 1945 and 1951 died each year of kuru, almost no children born after 1955 contracted the disease.

The epidemiological character of other diseases is altered by changing sociological patterns and individual life styles. The risk of infection with hepatitis B virus is, for example, increased in groups engaged in illicit drug use because of the parenteral mode of transmission of this disease. The incidence of gonorrhea exhibited an almost explosive increase after 1960 and ranks as the most widespread reportable communicable disease in the United States (Fig. 13–4); this increase must be partly attributable to changing social mores.

Such factors—political, sociological, or economic in nature—obviously exert a great influence on the resistance of a population to epidemic spread of a disease.

It is clear that the interaction between host and parasite populations is a highly complex phenomenon. Even assuming that the parasite population remains relatively constant in its ability to produce disease, the resistance of the host population is in a constant state of flux and the equilibrium between the two is rarely a steady state.

MECHANISMS OF TRANSMISSION

The epidemic character of infectious diseases is influenced in a significant way by the mechanisms of transmission, or the means of

Table 13–1. **Modes of Transmission of Infectious Diseases**

Direct Transmission	Indirect Transmission
Person-to-person contact	Airborne
	Droplet nuclei
Animal-to-person contact	Dust
	Vehicleborne
	Food
	Water
	Fomite
	Vectorborne

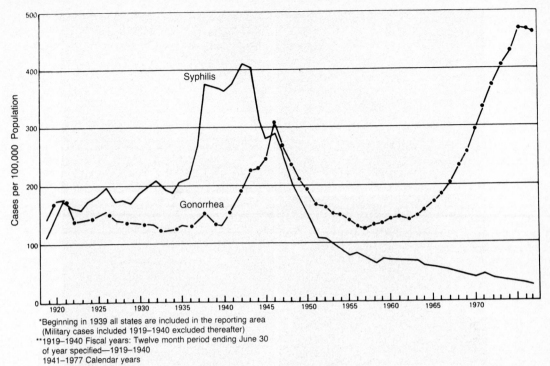

Figure 13–4. Reported cases of gonorrhea and syphilis per 100,000 population in the United States, 1919–1977. (Centers for Disease Control, Annual summary 1977: reported morbidity and mortality in the United States. Morbidity and Mortality Weekly Report **26**:[53], 1978.)

spread, from an infected person or animal to a susceptible human. As indicated in Table 13–1, mechanisms of transmission may be classified as direct or indirect.

DIRECT TRANSMISSION

The simplest form of transmission is that of direct contact between an infective source, or reservoir, and a susceptible host. Obvious examples of person-to-person transfer of the infective agent include kissing and sexual contact, routes of transmission that are typical of many respiratory and venereal diseases. Several animal diseases are also directly transmitted to man, *e.g.,* rabies, by the bite of an infected animal, and tularemia, contracted by hunters and others who handle infected flesh.

It is also common epidemiological practice to include among the direct contact diseases those transmitted by the inhalation of infective aerosol droplets expelled by coughing or sneezing, since there is essentially an immediate transfer of the agent, and the link between the source of infection and its recipient is not readily broken.

Aerosols

The processes of coughing, sneezing, and talking generate enormous numbers of tiny droplets in the environment, as illustrated in Figure 13–5. When these contain infective agents, as in many respiratory diseases, the aerosols may be inhaled directly by others in the vicinity. Inhalation infection has been studied extensively, particularly the effects of particle size on pulmonary penetration and mucosal deposition.

Infectious agents may be finely dispersed in air under laboratory conditions, and the aerosols so produced can be studied with respect to particle size, infectivity, and the like. Survival of bacteria in the ambient cloud is conditioned by relative humidity and the nature of the suspending menstruum.

The upper respiratory tract is remarkably efficient in the removal of particulate matter suspended in inhaled air by impingement of the particles on wet mucosal surfaces. In general, particles 10 μm. or greater in diameter are removed in the nasal passage, while those of 1 to 2 μm. penetrate to the alveoli and, by deposition, are retained there with great efficiency.

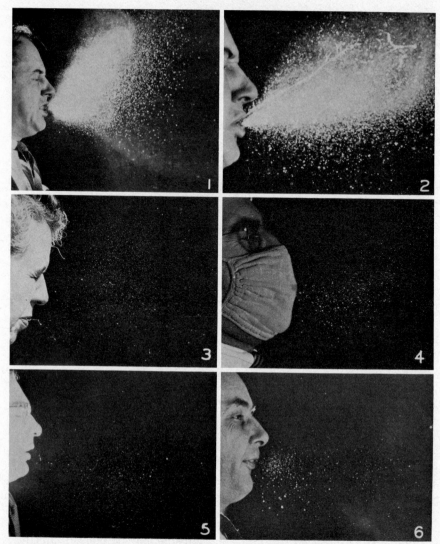

Figure 13–5. The atomization of mouth and nose secretions demonstrated by high-speed photography. *1,* A violent sneeze in a normal subject; note the close approximation of the teeth, resulting in effective atomization. *2,* Head cold sneeze; note the strings of mucus and the less effective atomization of the viscous secretions. *3,* A stifled sneeze. *4,* Sneeze through a dense face mask. *5,* Cough; note the smaller discharge than in the uninhibited sneeze. *6,* Enunciation of the letter "f". (Jennison, Amer. Assn. Adv. Sci., Publ. No. 17, 1942.)

Total body retention is, however, greater than indicated by examination of the respiratory tract alone. About 30 per cent of 1 μm. particles are retained in the respiratory tree, but there is essentially complete whole body retention; the remaining 70 per cent being retained predominantly in the gastrointestinal tract. The occurrence of inhaled material in this site is, of course, a consequence of the removal mechanism in which mucus of the upper respiratory tract, containing entrapped microorganisms, is swallowed.

INDIRECT TRANSMISSION

The indirect transmission of infectious diseases is more varied and complex than direct, and is generally classified as airborne, vehicleborne, or vectorborne.

Airborne Transmission

The indirect transmission by the airborne route involves two kinds of infectious particles, **dust** and **droplet nuclei.** The latter derive from aerosol particles, described above, which have lost water by evaporation. These particles are usually quite small and remain suspended for long periods of time. Their inhalation and deposition are subject to the same considerations as aerosol droplets.

Microorganisms in dust may have two origins: settling of bacteria-laden particles that are too large to remain suspended in air, and contamination of objects, especially textile products, with infectious secretions that become infectious dust after drying. The simple removal of clothing also disperses the bacteria colonized on the skin, contaminating the surrounding air.[11]

Inhalation of dustborne bacteria may be quantitatively more important than aerosol inhalation, *i.e.*, dust is probably a more prolific and constant source of air contamination.

Vehicleborne Transmission

The vehicles that can be involved in transmission are many and varied. Those of greatest importance include contaminated food and water as well as inanimate objects, or fomites, that may become contaminated and serve to transfer pathogenic microorganisms. Vehicles may serve as passive transfer agents, such as fomites, or they may support the growth of contaminating microorganisms, as in foods such as milk.

Water as a Vehicle. Some of the world's most devastating epidemics have been waterborne infections. The importance of water as a vehicle in such epidemics is attributable to two factors: first, water is subject to contamination with pathogens, particularly those of enteric disease, and second, it is universally consumed. The recreational use of water, especially swimming, also presents many opportunities for disease transmission.

Although natural waters contain bacteria derived principally from air and soil, contamination with pathogenic microorganisms usually originates from infected animals or humans. In a few instances, bacteria are dispersed in soil and water from the tissues of infected animals, as occurs in brucellosis, tularemia, and anthrax. Mostly, such pathogens do not survive for long periods under these conditions, but anthrax spores are an important exception (Chapter 27).

More frequently, infective organisms are shed from the diseased host in the urine, as in leptospirosis, or in excreta, as in the enteric diseases. In most cases, pathogenic bacteria do not multiply in soil and water, but they may survive for long periods, possibly for weeks or months. Some of the potential pathogens, *e.g.*, the bacilli of tetanus and gas gangrene, are not infective by the oral route, but the portal of entry for enteric organisms is the gastrointestinal tract, and these create a significant health problem, through contamination of soil and, ultimately, water.

The presence of excreta on watersheds can lead to contamination of both impounded and shallow ground waters. Water supplies may also be contaminated directly by the dumping of untreated or inadequately treated sewage into a community water supply. A variety of pathogenic microorganisms may be fecally shed and find their way into water supplies. Among the most commonly encountered are the enteric bacilli, such as *Salmonella* and *Shigella*; cholera vibrios; animal parasites, including *Ascaris, Entamoeba,* and *Giardia;* and enteroviruses, such as polioviruses, Coxsackie viruses, and echoviruses.

It is significant that modern sanitary practices, including bacteriological assessment of water quality, chlorination of potable water supplies, and adequate treatment and disposal of sewage, have virtually eliminated large-scale epidemics of enteric infections in developed nations. Waterborne epidemics that do occur are indicative not of a lack of knowledge, but of a failure to use that already existing.

Food as a Vehicle. Other than the ramifications of a common water supply, the most frequent vehicles for dissemination of microbial diseases are the wide variety of foods consumed by humans. Like water, food constitutes a link between the susceptible individual and the source of infection.

Historically, the food most often involved in disease transmission has been milk and its products. Unlike water, milk supports the active growth of many pathogens; moreover, it is the only major food of animal origin that is often consumed in a raw state. Since large quantities are consumed, its importance in disease transmission is evident. The diseases transmitted by milk fall into two categories. In the first group are the diseases of cattle that are transmissible to man, including bovine tuberculosis, brucellosis, and certain streptococcal infections. In the second group are the diseases of humans in which the milk serves as the link between individuals, principally the enteric infections. It must be borne in mind that milk in the udder is normally sterile; the presence of microorganisms is always a consequence of contamination either from tissue infection or from external sources, after it is drawn.

Disease transmission by milk and milk products is a specialized, but important case of a more general phenomenon of foodborne infection. As with milk, the contamination of foods may arise from an infection of the animal source, as in trichinellosis and other parasitic diseases, or it may result from contamination during handling or food preparation and storage. Like milk, many foodstuffs support the growth of bacteria under appropriate conditions of storage. In other instances their role is that of a passive vehicle for pathogenic microorganisms; a case in point is the contamination of vegetables with human excreta used as fertilizer, a common practice in rural areas of some underdeveloped nations.

Food may then serve simply as a vehicle for foodborne transmission of infectious diseases. In other instances, however, illness that is clinically and epidemiologically distinct may result from consumption of contaminated food, and is classified as bacterial food poisoning. These affections are described in Chapter 36.

Fomites as Vehicles. In many diseases, especially respiratory and enteric infections, microorganisms are shed in the secretions and excretions. When these contaminate inanimate objects, or fomites, the vehicle can then serve as the connection between cases or carriers and susceptibles. Common fomites are toys, books, clothing, bedding, towels, and medical instruments.

Vectorborne Transmission[16]

Several diseases of animals or humans are spread by means of an arthropod vector. The transmission can be strictly mechanical; in certain enteric infections, flies contaminate their legs or mouthparts in human wastes, *e.g.*, in open privies, and transfer pathogenic microorganisms to food or fomites, with subsequent ingestion by a susceptible person. In mechanical transmission the microorganisms do not multiply to any significant extent in the vector. In other cases, the microorganism may actually infect the arthropod vector, usually after feeding on blood or other body fluids, and undergo multiplication in the vector. The arthropod conveys the infection by subsequent feeding on a susceptible person. This kind of transmission is typical of bubonic plague (Chapter 23) and arbovirus infections (Chapter 42).

Occasionally, the infected arthropod passes the infection from one insect generation to the next through the egg—**transovarial infection**—thus maintaining a reservoir of infection in the vector population; transovarian passage is seen in certain tick infections by the rickettsiae of spotted fevers (Chapter 33). In malaria and some other infections by animal parasites, a more complex host-parasite relationship exists, in which the agent undergoes a part of its life cycle in the invertebrate host before further transmission.

Special Considerations

It is appropriate to consider here two unique kinds of disease transmission of special interest to microbiologists and infectious disease clinicians. These involve the laboratory and hospital as a setting for disease transmission.

Laboratory Associated Infections.[13] A wide variety of laboratory procedures—pipetting, decanting of culture supernatants, transferring freeze-dried and other cultures, and blender operation—generate infectious aerosols. The liquid-to-air dissemination of bacteria is especially hazardous because the number of bacteria in aerosol droplets may be concentrated up to 1000 times over that in the liquid medium. Infectious aerosols probably account for the majority of laboratory infections and are of serious concern, since medical laboratory workers exhibit a marked risk of acquiring many diseases.[6, 12] The control of laboratory infections is a matter of both proper equipment and appropriate technique.

Nosocomial Infections.[9] In the developed countries, there has emerged in the past few decades a changing pattern in the epidemiology of infectious diseases relating to the appearance of **hospital-associated** or **hospital-acquired** infections. There has been an upsurge of infections in hospitals that are caused by microorganisms normally considered to be noninvasive or invasive to only a low degree. These changing patterns reflect more effective control of highly virulent microorganisms, coupled with the use of medical procedures that alter the normal host defense mechanisms. For example, the normal microbial flora helps to hold in check many of the pathogens of low virulence (Chapter 12), but when this balance is perturbed by antimicrobial therapy, microorganisms considered to be nonpathogenic may cause disease. These "**opportunists**" include fungi and a number of gram-negative bacilli. Similarly, when host immunological defenses are compromised, as by the administration of cancer chemotherapeutic and immunosuppressive drugs, even "nonpathogens" may cause life-threatening diseases. Medical practices and procedures, including inhalation therapy and indwelling catheters and cannulas, as well as wound infections in surgical wards, tend to increase both the incidence and the severity of hospital-associated infections.

EPIDEMIC PATTERNS

It is obvious that the character of an epidemic will be determined by the origin, incubation period, and mode of spread of the agent within a population. In general, two principal patterns of epidemics are observed—common source and propagated. These can ordinarily be distinguished by the pattern of the epidemic curve, in which the case distribution is plotted against the time of onset (Fig. 13–6).

Common Source Epidemics
Outbreaks that occur in a single epidemic wave, with most cases appearing within approximately one incubation period, can usually be ascribed to a common event or source of infection. Such epidemics are common source, or **point source,** outbreaks. If the incubation period is fairly constant and the period of exposure is short, the epidemic curve will

exhibit a sharp increase and decline. A typical curve for a common source epidemic of hepatitis A is shown in Figure 13–6.

Propagated Epidemics
Propagated epidemics usually exhibit a more complex pattern than common source epidemics, and the epidemic extends over more than one incubation period. The epidemic progresses by the occurrence of secondary cases that serve as new sources of infection. As the number of cases rises early in the epidemic, the probability of contact between infected and susceptibles increases until the number of susceptibles falls below the critical threshold level (Fig. 13–4). The probability of contact then decreases and the number of new cases declines. Propagated epidemics, then, exhibit a longer course, usually with some variation in the rate of appearance of new cases. Figure 13–7 illustrates these features in an epidemic of chancroid.

THE CONTROL OF INFECTIOUS DISEASE

The control of infectious diseases in a population must depend upon an understanding of the contributions of the host, parasite, and

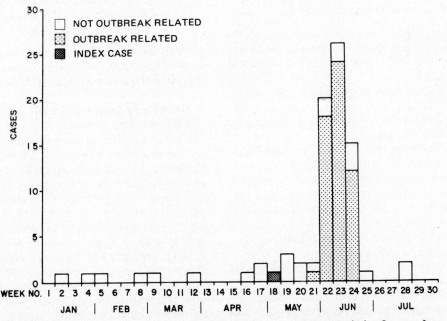

Figure 13–6. Hepatitis A cases, by week of onset, in Monmouth County, New Jersey, during January–June 1981. The usual incidence of hepatitis in this area averaged 3 to 4 cases per month. In June, a sharply increased incidence of infection was seen among patrons of a local restaurant. The index case, a food handler in the restaurant, was ill on May 9 and did not work thereafter. Outbreak-associated patients had eaten at the restaurant within the appropriate incubation period (1 to 6 weeks). (Centers for Disease Control, Morbidity and Mortality Weekly Report **31**[12]:150–152, 1982.)

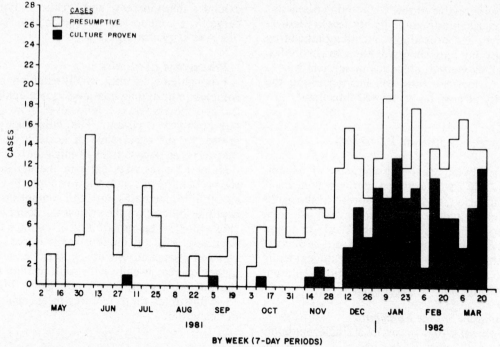

Figure 13–7. Cases of chancroid, by week of first clinic visit, in Orange County, California, during the period of May 1981 to March 1982. *Haemophilus ducreyii* was identified as the causative agent of the outbreak in late December 1981. (Centers for Disease Control, Morbidity and Mortality Weekly Report **31**[14]:173–175, 1982.)

mechanism of transmission, as just described. Thus, the control of a particular disease almost always constitutes a special case. In general, however, control measures are of three kinds:

1. Those directed toward reduction or elimination of the source of infection, such as:
   a. Quarantine and isolation of cases and carriers
   b. Destruction of an animal reservoir of infection
   c. Treatment of sewage to reduce water contamination
   d. Therapy that reduces or eliminates infectivity of the individual
2. Those designed to break the connection between the source of infection and susceptible persons, *i.e.,* general sanitation measures such as:
   a. Chlorination of water supplies
   b. Pasteurization of milk
   c. Supervision and inspection of foods and food handlers
   d. Destruction of arthropod vectors
3. Those that eliminate susceptibles and raise the general level of herd immunity by immunization, including:
   a. Passive immunization to give a temporary immunity following exposure

or when a disease threatens to take epidemic form
   b. Active immunization to protect the individual from disease and the host population from epidemic disease.

One or more of these control measures are applicable to most infectious diseases, depending upon the circumstances of transmission.

Diseases of Lower Animals Transmissible to Man[10]

Diseases in this group have in common an animal reservoir of infection. Direct control of the source of infection is, therefore, sometimes possible. When the transmission is direct, as in rabies, the reservoir of infection in the domestic dog may be controlled by immunization and quarantine of animals. The reservoir in wild animals, however, is not subject to such control, and complete elimination of the disease cannot be accomplished except locally under favorable circumstances. The animal reservoir of bovine tuberculosis is subject to direct control by testing and slaughter of infected animals; by these methods this reservoir has been virtually eliminated in the United States. Pasteurization of milk also provides protection to the human population.

Vectorborne Diseases

Control of these diseases is most readily accomplished by control of the vector. Malaria control, for example, depends upon elimination or reduction of the appropriate mosquito population, and louseborne typhus is controlled by measures directed against the human body louse, as well as by immunization of humans. In instances such as these the vector is closely tied to humans, but when a disease has a reservoir of infection in wild animals and is transmitted by a vector that bites both these animals and man, control is more difficult. Plague is an example of an intermediate disease in this respect. The rat reservoir of infection is closely associated with humans, and both the rat and flea populations are subject to an effective degree of control, but neither the wild rodent reservoir nor the insect vectors of sylvatic plague are subject to any appreciable degree of control. Similarly, tularemia and spotted fever, the latter having a reservoir in the tick, cannot be effectively controlled.

Diseases Transmitted from Man to Man[15]

When disease is transmitted from person to person indirectly, as by contaminated water, milk, or food, it is susceptible to control by interruption of the connecting link. Thus, the chlorination of water supplies and pasteurization of milk over many years in the United States have led to significant reduction in the incidence of water- and milkborne diseases, and epidemics seldom occur. Foodborne disease is more difficult to control in practice because of the element of human fallibility. Food poisoning of staphylococcal or *Clostridium perfringens* etiology (Chapter 36) results most often from contamination of human origin, and the source of infection in foodborne *Salmonella* infection is made possible by improper handling of food.

Airborne Infection. As yet it has not been possible to control airborne infection effectively by interference with transmission as, for example, by ultraviolet irradiation or by the production of microbicidal aerosols. Such infections are commonly respiratory, but at times other diseases may be so transmitted.

Quarantine. Probably the oldest method of control of the spread of infectious disease is the separation of the infected and susceptible persons by quarantine. With rare exceptions, notably the effective quarantine of cases of rabies in England, this is not as effective as might be supposed, largely because of the occurrence of inapparent cases and carriers. Although it has tended to fall into disuse in community outbreaks, quarantine continues to be applied on a global scale to international travel. Diseases to which international quarantine continues to be applied are plague, cholera, and yellow fever. The mobility of populations and the wide use of air travel between countries has introduced complications;[14] a case of cholera occurring in Australia, for example, was found to have been acquired in Bombay immediately preceding departure by air.

Immunization

The effectiveness of prophylactic immunization varies greatly from one disease to another. Mass immunization, when a solid and lasting immunity is produced, is a highly effective method of controlling epidemic disease through the mechanism of herd immunity, or even of practical eradication. For example, smallpox has been abolished by a combination of mass immunization and effective case location and quarantine. This eradication program was uniquely possible with smallpox because of the effectiveness of vaccination, the fact that there is no normal animal reservoir of infection, and the virtual absence of carriers and subclinical infections. It now appears that measles is similarly subject to eradication, and public health authorities now envision its eradication in the United States.

When immunity produced by prophylactic inoculation is only partial and of limited duration, as in diseases like typhoid fever and influenza, repeated immunization is required to maintain the partial degree of control attainable by this means. Since a solid and lasting immunity to infectious disease is the exception rather than the rule, and other control measures are imperfect to greater or lesser degree in practice, the eradication of the majority of the infectious diseases confined to humans appears to be improbable.[7]

REFERENCES

1. Anderson, R. M.; and R. M. May. 1979. Population biology of infectious diseases; Part I. Nature **280**:361–367. Part II. (May and Anderson). *Ibid.* **280**:455–461.
2. Black, M. L., and I. D. Gay. 1965. Some kinetic properties of a deterministic epidemic confirmed by computer simulation. Science **148**:981–985.
3. Burnet, Sir M., and D. O. White. 1972. Natural History of Infectious Disease. 4th ed. Cambridge University Press, London.

4. Cvjetanović, B., B. Grab, and K. Uemura. 1978. Dynamics of acute bacterial diseases. Epidemiological models and their application in public health. Bull. Wld Hlth Org. **56** (Supplement No. 1):1–143.

5. Doege, T. C., and H. M. Gelfand. 1978. A model for epidemiologic research. J. Amer. Med. Assn **239**:328–330.

6. Harrington, J. M., and H. S. Shannon. 1976. Incidence of tuberculosis, hepatitis, brucellosis, and shigellosis in British medical laboratory workers. Brit. Med. J. **1**:759–762.

7. Hinman, E. H. 1966. World Eradication of Infectious Diseases. Charles C Thomas, Springfield, Ill.

8. Levitt, L. P., et al. 1970. Determination of measles immunity after a mass immunization campaign. Publ. Hlth Rep. **85**:261–265.

9. Montgomerie, J. Z. 1979. Epidemiology of *Klebsiella* and hospital-associated infections. Rev. Infect. Dis. **1**:736–753.

10. Muul, I. 1970. Mammalian ecology and epidemiology of zoonoses. Science **170**:1275–1279.

11. Noble, W. C., et al. 1976. Quantitative studies on the dispersal of skin bacteria into the air. J. Med. Microbiol. **9**:53–61.

12. Pike, R. M. 1976. Laboratory-associated infections: summary and analysis of 3921 cases. Hlth Lab. Sci. **13**:105–114.

13. Pike, R. M. 1979. Laboratory-associated infections: incidence, fatalities, causes, and prevention. Ann. Rev. Microbiol. **33**:41–66.

14. Prothero, R. M. 1977. Disease and mobility: a neglected factor in epidemiology. Internat. J. Epidemiol. **6**:259–267.

15. Report. 1977. Social and health aspects of sexually transmitted diseases. Principles of control measures. Public Health Papers No. 65, World Health Organization, Geneva.

16. Sellers, R. F. 1980. Weather, host and vector—their interplay in the spread of insect-borne animal virus diseases. J. Hygiene **85**:65–102.

The Staphylococci

The staphylococci are among the earliest recognized of the pathogenic bacteria, having been first characterized in the early 1880s. They are widely distributed in nature, and are often seen as members of the normal bacterial flora of the skin, the nares, and the upper respiratory tract. Many of the species found in humans are commensals, but several have limited pathogenic potential. The species predominantly pathogenic for man, *Staphylococcus aureus*, is the most common cause of localized suppurative infections in humans.[8, 15]

The genus *Staphylococcus* is classified in the family Micrococcaceae, along with *Micrococcus* and *Planococcus*. Members of the latter two genera are not pathogenic for man, but *Micrococcus* assumes some importance to the medical microbiologist, since micrococci are similar to staphylococci and the two must frequently be differentiated. Table 14–1 displays the characters that may be used to differentiate *Micrococcus* and *Staphylococcus*.

For several decades the taxonomy of the genus *Staphylococcus* has been controversial, reflecting the divergent needs and aims of medical microbiologists on the one hand and bacterial systematists on the other. A toxonomic scheme is now emerging that, while complex, may bring useful order to the classification of the genus.[19] At least 13 species are recorded; their identification is based upon biochemical characters, cell wall composition, protein homology, DNA relatedness, and natural host range.

Description of the Genus

Staphylococci are gram-positive, spherical cells, ranging from about 0.5 to 1.5 μm. in diameter; they typically appear in irregular, grape-like clusters in stained smears. Growth is best under aerobic conditions, but they are facultatively anaerobic; the optimum temperature for growth is from 30° to 37° C. Staphylococci are nonmotile and do not form spores. Table 14–2 lists the medically important *Staphylococcus* species, *i.e.*, those known to be pathogenic for humans, with their important identifying characteristics. Other species— *Staphylococcus capitis*, *S. warneri*, *S. cohnii*, *S. xylosus*, and *S. sciuri*—are found as commensals in humans, but are rarely, if ever, responsible for disease. Remaining species are found only in animals.

Morphology and Staining

Staphylococci exhibit a remarkable constancy in size and shape; they are uniformly near 1 μm. in diameter and are more nearly perfect spheres than other cocci. Among the more obvious morphological characteristics is the marked tendency to appear as masses of cells in grape-like clusters, a cell grouping that arises from the geometry of cell division.[21, 43] Cells divide sequentially in three perpendicular planes; normally, this would result in regular packets (Chapter 2), but following division, daughter cells are translocated by action of separation enzymes to yield the typical irregular clusters. In the usual stained smear, cells

Table 14–1. **Distinguishing Characters of Micrococcus and Staphylococcus***

Character†	Micrococcus	Staphylococcus
G + C content (mole %)	66–73	30–38
Cell wall teichoic acid	–	+
Lysostaphin susceptibility‡	R	S
Lysozyme susceptibility‡	S	R
Anaerobic growth§	–	+
Growth at 45° C.	–	+
Acid from glycerol‖	–	+

*Data from K. H. Schleiffer and W. E. Kloos, Internat. J. Syst. Bacteriol. **25**:60, 1975.
†Predominant and typical reactions are shown; some strain variations may occur.
‡R = resistant; S = sensitive.
§In thioglycolate medium.
‖By aerobic plate culture.

Table 14–2. **The Medically Important Species of Staphylococcus***†

	S. aureus	S. epidermidis	S. saprophyticus	S. simulans	S. hominis	S. haemolyticus
Morphology						
Cells						
Size (mm)	0.8–1.0	0.5–1.5	0.8–1.2	0.8–1.5	1.0–1.5	0.8–1.3
Colonies						
Elevation‡	R	R	LC	R	C	LC
Light transmission§	T	T	O	T	O	O
Diameter (mm)	6–8	2–4	5–8	5–7	3–4	4–8
Pigment‖	(+)	(–)	V	–	V	–
Cell Wall Teichoic Acid**	R	G	R, G	G	G	G
Physiology						
Anaerobic growth	+	+	+	+	+	+
Growth in 10% NaCl	+	W	+	+	W	+
Growth at 45° C.	+	+	V	+	+	+
Biochemical Reactions						
Coagulase	+	–	–	–	–	–
Hemolysis	(+)	W; –	–	W; –	(W; –)	(+)
Acetylmethyl carbinol	+	+	(+)	W; –	V	+; W
Nitrate reduction	+	(+)	–	+	+	(+)
Phosphatase	+	+	(–)	(W)	(–)	(–)
Deoxyribonuclease	+	(W)	–	(W)	W; –	W; –
Acid from Carbohydrate††						
Sucrose	+	+	+	+	+	+
Trehalose	+	–	+	(+)	+	+
Turanose	(+)	V	+	+	+	+
Mannitol	+	–	+	–	(+)	V
Xylitol	–	–	(+; W)	–	–	V
Antibiotic Sensitivity						
Novobiocin	+	+	–	+	+	+
Penicillin G	V	V	+	V	V	V
Tetracycline	+	(+)	+	V	V	V
Erythromycin	+	+	(+)	(+)	+	+

*Data from W. E. Kloos and K. H. Schleiffer, Internat. J. Syst. Bacteriol. **25**:62–79, 1975.
†Symbols alone = frequency of 90%; parentheses indicate 70–89% frequency; + = positive; W = weakly positive; – = negative; V = variable.
‡R = raised; LC = low-convex; C = convex.
§T = translucent; O = opaque.
‖Pigmented colonies range from orange, to yellow-orange, to yellow, to gray or white with yellow tint.
**R = ribitol type; G = glycerol type.
††Aerobic acid production by plate culture.

are also found singly, in pairs, and in tetrads, as seen in Figure 14–1.

Staphylococci stain readily and deeply with basic dyes and are strongly gram-positive. Although the majority of strains are not encapsulated, a few strains of *S. aureus* form capsules; these may be morphologically evident or they can be detected by immunological methods.

Growth on agar mediums is abundant; colonies are translucent to opaque, with some variation in colony profile and margin (Fig. 14–2). Such variations are useful for differentiation. Some staphylococci form carotenoid pigments,[25] yielding colonies with a golden-yellow, lemon-yellow, or creamy color (Table 14–2). Pigmentation occurs most often in *S. aureus*, where it is more or less constant in primary isolates; pigments are less frequently observed in strains of *S. saprophyticus* and *S. hominis*.

When cultured on blood agar plates, most *S. aureus* and *S. haemolyticus* colonies are surrounded by a zone of β-hemolysis; other species are typically nonhemolytic. α-Hemolysis is not observed in staphylococci.

Physiology

Staphylococci are relatively more resistant to heat and certain disinfectants than the vegetative forms of most pathogenic bacteria. Whereas other bacteria are killed in 30 minutes at 60° C., staphylococci require higher temperatures and longer times, such as 80° C. for one

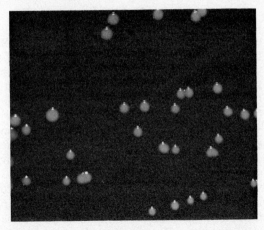

Figure 14–2. Colonies of *Staphylococcus aureus* on nutrient agar, 24–hour culture; × 3.

hour. Heat resistance is accompanied by higher maximum growth temperatures; staphylococci, unlike many bacteria, grow at 45° C. Resistance to drying is also marked, and staphylococci may remain infectious in the environment for extended periods.

The great majority of strains grow in the presence of 10 per cent sodium chloride, some even growing at concentrations as high as 15 per cent. This has some significance in salt preservation of foods, for staphylococci may grow and form enterotoxin in foods containing quantities of salt otherwise sufficient to act as a preservative. Salt tolerance frequently furnishes the basis for selective mediums used in isolation of these bacteria.

In common with other gram-positive organisms, these cocci are sensitive to the bacteriostatic action of triphenyl methane dyes and are characteristically susceptible to antibiotics effective against gram-positive bacteria, including penicillin and many of the broad-spectrum antibiotics. They are, however, especially prone to develop drug resistance, and generalizations on sensitivity may not be applicable to all current isolates.

Cultural Characteristics

Staphylococci are not highly fastidious in their nutritive requirements, growing readily on the usual meat extract–peptone mediums. Growth is most profuse on the blood agar commonly used for isolation and differentiation of the pathogenic forms. They may also be grown aerobically on synthetic mediums that contain amino acids and vitamins; anaerobic growth on these mediums requires the addition of uracil and a fermentable carbon source, such as pyruvate.[13]

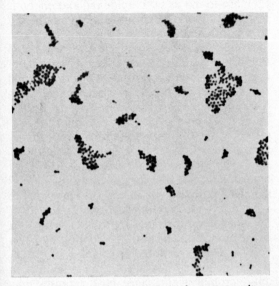

Figure 14–1. *Staphylococcus aureus* from pure culture. Note the characteristic clusters of the cocci. Fuchsin; × 1050.

A variety of carbohydrates are utilized aerobically with the production of acid; differences in carbohydrate utilization form one of the bases for species differentiation (Table 14–2). Glucose is fermented anaerobically, with lactic acid as the predominant end-product. Other biochemical characters are listed in Table 14–2.

The importance of **coagulase** production should be noted. *Staphylococcus aureus,* the predominant and most important pathogenic species for man, is the only *Staphylococcus* species that produces coagulase; its presence is also often correlated with hemolytic toxin formation, and these are considered to be virulence determinants. Coagulase production is, therefore, one of the characters of great utility in identification of pathogenic species.

Drug Resistance[22, 28]

Insusceptibility to the antimicrobial activity of antibiotics is of great practical importance among the staphylococci, since they exhibit such drug resistance more often than most other bacteria.

Staphylococcal strains become resistant to antibiotics by acquiring new genes that specify such resistance, usually by phage transduction, as described in Chapter 6. Resistance genes, or markers, are most often present on **plasmids** or extrachromosomal elements that replicate independently of the bacterial chromosome. Resistance to several drugs, or multiple resistance, is usually a consequence of the presence of several drug-resistance genes on a single plasmid. A bacterial cell may carry more than one plasmid, each with its own resistance markers. Resistance genes are also sometimes located on the bacterial chromosome. For example, the erythromycin resistance gene occurs occasionally on the penicillinase plasmid, but is more often located on the chromosome.

The emergence of drug-resistant strains almost inevitably follows the widespread therapeutic use of antibiotics, and the proportion of drug-resistant strains among the circulating staphylococci has steadily increased over several decades. For example, penicillin-resistant staphylococci appeared shortly after the introduction of this antibiotic in the 1940s. As new antibiotics came into use, staphylococci inexorably became resistant to each of them. Moreover, multiple drug resistance appeared, and strains resistant to several antibiotics are now the rule rather than the exception. The increasing prevalence of drug-resistant strains has prompted the search for more effective antimicrobial agents and has led to extensive sensitivity testing of isolates and careful selection of antibiotics used in therapy.

Many of the serious and life-threatening staphylococcal infections are now acquired in hospitals. Individuals in these settings are more susceptible to infection because of intercurrent disease and other predisposing factors. The staphylococcal carrier rate in both hospital patients and attendants is usually higher than in the general population; moreover, the proportion of drug-resistant strains in these carriers is also significantly higher. Thus, nosocomial infections with drug-resistant staphylococci, particularly in surgical wards and burn units, constitute a serious medical problem.[9]

It has been established in both natural and experimental circumstances that drug-resistant staphylococci tend to be replaced by drug-sensitive strains in cases and carriers, provided there is no pressure exerted by the use of the antibiotic in question. Therefore, careful control of the antibiotics used in therapy, based upon the frequency of isolation of resistant strains, can provide an effective approach to the problems posed by drug resistance.

Resistance to penicillin is of particular importance among the staphylococci. Penicillin resistance is usually associated with the production of penicillinase, an enzyme which degrades penicillin to an inactive compound, penicilloic acid. This resistance prompted the development of methicillin and related forms of penicillin that are not attacked by penicillinase. Unfortunately, staphylococci are now appearing that are resistant to methicillin, and they are found as both epidemic and endemic nosocomial pathogens in increasing numbers.[29]

A curious new type of penicillin resistance in *S. aureus* was reported in 1977. It was noted that some strains of *S. aureus,* although inhibited by penicillin concentrations in the normal range, were killed only by much higher concentrations; such strains were said to be **tolerant**.[32] Tolerance obviously cannot be detected by the ordinary disk diffusion sensitivity tests, since these measure only growth inhibition. The mechanism for tolerance is not yet determined, but such strains form less **autolysin** than normal cells in the presence of the antibiotic, inferring that normally sensitive, but not tolerant, strains are killed, partly as a consequence of cell wall degradation by autolytic enzymes. As noted in Chapter 12, bactericidal action is not always essential for an antimicrobial agent, since host defenses may effectively dispose of microorganisms whose multiplication is inhibited. Thus, it might be expected that tolerance would not present a problem in treatment, yet endocarditis caused by tolerant staphylococci is evidently an exception, requiring therapy with other antibiotics.[31]

Antigenic Structure[17]

The antigenic makeup of *Staphylococcus* is complex and heterogeneous. Many antigens are shared between the several species, and even with micrococci. Staphylococcal antigens include a variety of proteins, teichoic acids, and polysaccharides demonstrable by agglutination, precipitation, or passive hemagglutination. The human strains, particularly those of *S. aureus* and *S. epidermidis*, have been extensively studied and serotyping schemes have been proposed, but technical difficulties have largely precluded their practical use.

Aside from this, several of the staphylococcal antigens, particularly those of the cell surface, are of interest because of their possible interaction with host defenses in the host-parasite relationship. For example, **cell wall teichoic acid,** one of the major agglutinogens in staphylococci, enhances complement activation by these organisms,[47] and is also responsible for adherence of *S. aureus* to nasal epithelial cells.[2]

A cell wall protein, found in almost all strains of *S. aureus* and designated **protein A,** is thought to play a significant role in the host-parasite relationship. Protein A has the unusual capacity to bind to the Fc region of immunoglobulin G, a reaction that has many implications in relation to host defenses. Since antibody-mediated phagocytosis is Fc receptor–dependent, protein A is believed to interfere with opsonization. Additionally, protein A inhibits the activation of the alternative complement pathway, probably by covering the complement-activating sites of cell wall peptidoglycans; this results in decreased phagocytosis of protein A–rich staphylococci.[41]

A relatively few strains of *S. aureus* produce polysaccharide capsules. These are antigenic and are of several serological types; indeed, multiple antigens may occur in the capsule of a single strain. The capsule is sometimes microscopically visible, as shown in Figure 14–3; its presence may also be demonstrated by serological methods.

Encapsulated strains are poorly phagocytized and are, thereby, more virulent. The mechanisms of phagocytosis-inhibition have recently been set forth.[48] Both encapsulated and nonencapsulated strains activate complement by the cell wall peptidoglycan. The resulting C3 component associates with the cell wall, but is covered by the polysaccharide in encapsulated bacteria and is not available to leucocyte receptors (Chapter 12); these bacteria are not then efficiently phagocytized.

Phage Typing

The host specificity and lytic ability of bacterial viruses, or bacteriophages, provide an additional means of characterizing bacteria. This method, first applied to typhoid bacilli, permits the differentiation of strains not otherwise separable by biochemical and serological means. Bacteriophage, or phage, typing has been extremely useful for epidemiological purposes in tracing the origin of disease outbreaks.

Among the staphylococci, phage typing is most commonly applied to *S. aureus*, since this is the species most often encountered in human infections. Phage collections are available in several reference laboratories for typing of *S. epidermidis* under special circumstances.

Phage typing is based upon the lysis of a culture of *S. aureus* by a standard battery of phages, each with relatively narrow host specificity and arbitrarily designated by number.

The procedures used in phage typing require technical precision and standardization, and

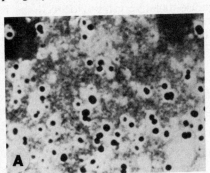
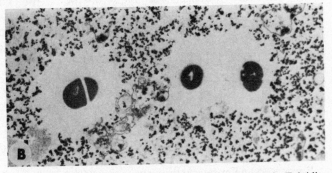

Figure 14–3. Capsules of *Staphylococcus aureus* prepared by India ink technique. *A*, Light photomicrograph. Toluidine blue; × 1500. *B*, Transmission electron micrograph. × 13,000. (Reprinted from J. Infect. Dis., **140**:605–609, 1979, by M. A. Melly, *et al.*, by permission of the University of Chicago Press. Copyright 1979 by the University of Chicago.)

Table 14–3. **Principal Virulence Determinants of** *Staphylococcus aureus*

| Adhesions | Aggressins Inhibiting: | | | | Toxins |
	Leucocyte Chemotaxis	Phagocytosis	Intracellular Killing		
Cell wall teichoic acid	Peptidoglycan	Protein A Capsules Coagulase (?)	Catalase		Hemolysins Leucocidins Enterotoxins Exfoliatin Pyrogenic exotoxins

such typing is usually performed only in larger clinical or reference laboratories. The principles are simple, however. A standardized suspension of each phage is dropped onto an agar plate seeded with the staphylococcus culture. After incubation, sensitivity to the phage is indicated by a clear zone of confluent lysis.

Individual cultures of *S. aureus* are often lysed by more than one of the phages employed, resulting in patterns of susceptibility. Because the number of patterns is impractically large, sets of phages are used and grouped as follows:

Group I: 29, 52, 52A, 79, 80
Group II: 3A, 3B, 3C, 55, 71
Group III: 6, 7, 42E, 47, 53, 54, 75, 77, 83A, 84, 85
Group IV: 42D
Miscellaneous: 81, 94, 95, 96

In this way a *Staphylococcus* strain may be characterized as belonging to one of these groups and phage types. Not all cultures are typable by this procedure and the susceptibility patterns of circulating strains vary in time and locality; the phages in the reference set thus require periodic revisions.

Virulence[44]

A number of staphylococcal properties, especially the production of **coagulase, hemolysins,** and **deoxyribonuclease,** correlate reasonably well with virulence, yet many of the determinants remain unknown, particularly among the coagulase-negative strains. Virulence undoubtedly is dependent upon a number of individual properties, each contributing in varying degrees. Determinants of virulence in *S. aureus* are best defined; the more important of these are listed in Table 14–3.

STAPHYLOCOCCAL TOXINS[17]

It was known very early that cell-free culture filtrates of staphylococci are toxic on parenteral inoculation and that the extracellular toxins are formed in considerable quantities. Such filtrates are necrotic and lethal when administered to experimental animals.

These ill-defined toxicities have yielded to searching investigation, and many of the toxic principles have been isolated and characterized to varying degrees. Among the more important of these are the **cytotoxins,** including hemolysins and leucocidins; the **enterotoxins;** the **exfoliatins;** the **pyrogenic exotoxins;** and the enzymatic activities exemplified by **coagulase, hyaluronidase,** and the **kinases.**

Hemolysins[30]

The coagulase-forming staphylococci are almost invariably hemolytic and upon primary isolation on blood agar they are surrounded by a clear zone of β-hemolysis. The hemolytic principle is soluble and is present in culture filtrates; it consists of several distinct protein hemolysins, or **staphylolysins.** The properties of these hemolytic toxins of *S. aureus* are summarized in Table 14–4.

The α-hemolysin (α-toxin, α-lysin) is produced by almost all strains of *S. aureus*; a vast majority also produce the β-hemolysin. Hemolysin production correlates well with the formation of coagulase, for only a few of the coagulase-negative strains are hemolytic (Table 14–2). When hemolysis does occur among the coagulase-negative staphylococci, it is thought to be attributable to α- or β-hemolysin, but there are claims that distinct and different hemolysins are formed by these strains.

Leucocidin

Although some of the staphylolysins possess leucocyte toxicity, only one staphylococcal toxin acts exclusively on leucocytes—the **Panton-Valentine (P–V) leucocidin.** By convention, this toxin is now the one referred to as leucocidin.

Leucocidin is cytotoxic for both human and

Table 14–4. **Hemolysins of *Staphylococcus aureus***

Property	α-Hemolysin	β-Hemolysin	γ-Hemolysin	δ-Hemolysin
Molecular weight	± 28,000	± 30,000	2 components (I = 29,000) (II = 26,000)	± 21,000
Distinct antigen	Yes	Yes	Yes	Probably
Erythrocytes	Rabbit	Sheep, ox	Rabbit, human, sheep	Human, sheep, rabbit, monkey
Cytotoxic for	Variety of cells, including leucocytes, platelets, and fibroblasts	Leucocytes, macrophages, fibroblasts	Human leucocytes and lymphoblasts	Lytic for bacterial protoplasts and spheroplasts, lysosomes, mitochondria
Other activities	Dermonecrotic, neurotoxic, and lethal	Weak lethality for rabbits	Lethal for guinea pigs	Inhibits water absorption in ileum of rabbits and guinea pigs
Mode of action	Controversial, possibly proteolytic; possibly surface active on membrane	Enzymatic, hydrolyzes sphingomyelin; requires Mg^{++}; hot-cold lysin	Unknown; probably not enzymatic; requires Na^+	Detergent-like action on membrane
Possible role in disease	Not well defined, but affects cardiovascular and central nervous systems in animals, probably by membrane damage	Not defined	Not defined, but lysosomal enzymes released may contribute	Suggested role in intestinal disturbances

rabbit leucocytes; it has no activity on other cell types, but is dermonecrotic in rabbits.[46] The toxin is antigenically distinct and is converted to toxoid by formaldehyde. Leucocidin comprises two components, designated F and S; these are separable by ion-exchange chromatography, with respective molecular weights of 32,000 and 38,000. Separately, the F and S components have no toxic activity.

Leucocidin-treated white cells are altered in cation permeability, which leads to a variety of secondary effects. The cell loses motility and swells to a spherical shape, with granules distributed around the cell periphery; eventually the cell is disrupted.

Administration of leucocidin to animals causes a transient leucocytopenia followed by extensive leucocytosis; the relationship of these effects to staphylococcal disease is, however, unclear. Antitoxin is produced in those with staphylococcal disease, and it has been suggested that such antibodies are essential for resistance to infection. Leucocidin may be a virulence determinant by destroying leucotyes, thus reducing phagocytosis of the microorganism in the host.

Enterotoxins[5]

The relation of staphylococci to the intoxication type of food poisoning described in Chapter 36 has been known since 1914. It was not until 1930 that Dack and his associates established that such illness could be produced by ingestion of culture filtrates of *S. aureus* strains that form enterotoxin.

Enterotoxins are relatively heat-stable proteins formed almost exclusively by coagulase-positive strains of *S. aureus,* but not by all such strains; it is estimated that the majority are capable of enterotoxin synthesis.

There are five well-characterized immunological types, designated A to E, which range in molecular weight from 28,000 to 35,000 daltons. Although each of these is immunologically distinct, there is some antigenic cross-relationship between several of them. A putative sixth type, designated enterotoxin F, has been described.[6] Although enterotoxic activity may be assayed in monkeys or chimpanzees, the method is expensive and unwieldy. Immunological methods are more specific and sufficiently sensitive that they can detect enterotoxin in culture filtrates and in extracts of foods containing enterotoxigenic *S. aureus.*[26]

Susceptibility to ingested enterotoxin is limited to man, certain apes, and monkeys. Ingestion by humans is followed within two to three hours by acute gastrointestinal distress characterized by projectile vomiting and diarrhea. Symptoms subside after a few hours with no aftereffects. The effective toxin dose for humans appears to be 1 to 4 μg.

Exfoliatins[30]

Although the association of staphylococcus with the dermatitis now known as **scalded skin syndrome** has been recognized since the turn of the century, the toxin responsible was not identified until 1971; it is now designated exfoliatin or exfoliative toxin. Within a short time after its discovery, the toxin had been purified and its fundamental properties described.

Exfoliatin is produced in broth cultures of *S. aureus* and may be recovered from cell-free supernatants. The toxin, or strains of staphylococci producing it, causes a generalized exfoliation of the epidermis when injected into neonatal mice, a technique employed for assay of biological activity. Exfoliatin is produced by *S. aureus* strains of phage Group II—in one study more than 85 per cent of the producing strains were in this group—although it has been encountered in a few strains of other phage groups.[3]

Two types of the toxin are known, exfoliatin A and exfoliatin B. Their important properties are summarized in Table 14–5.

Exfoliatin causes the scalded skin syndrome in humans, as described later in this chapter, by disturbing the adhesive forces between cells of the stratum granulosum to give rise to the characteristic bullae. It is a relatively potent exotoxin, 0.2 μg. of purified toxin causing skin separation in the neonatal mouse; somewhat higher doses are effective in adult humans.

The toxin is immunogenic and may be measured by bioassay or by serological tests, including gel diffusion, radial immunodiffusion, or radioimmunoassay.[49] Antitoxin neutralizes the effects of toxin and can be assayed in this way, but it may also be measured by passive hemagglutination.

Pyrogenic Exotoxins[33-36]

In 1979, Schlievert and his colleagues described a toxin isolated from *S. aureus* that is similar in many respects to the pyrogenic exotoxins of streptococci. This protein toxin is pyrogenic, is mitogenic for lymphocytes, and enhances susceptibility to certain effects of endotoxins—lethal shock and myocardial and liver damage. Subsequently, two additional pyrogenic toxins were described, and these are now designated pyrogenic exotoxins A, B, and C; their properties are described in Table 14–6. In common with streptococcal pyrogenic toxins, staphylococcal toxins produce a scarlatiniform rash by enhancing hypersensitivity; both streptococcal and staphylococcal pyrogenic toxins share a common core component which may induce delayed hypersensitivity. It has been suggested that the toxins may be associated with the scarlatiniform syndrome caused by staphylococci, with Kawasaki disease, and with the toxic shock syndrome.

Staphylococcal Enzymes[1,17]

Staphylococci synthesize a number of enzymatically active factors that act on host-associated substrates and often produce deleterious effects. The major factors are coagulases, hyaluronidase, and staphylokinases; these are generally thought to be related to virulence.

Coagulase.[42] The ability of some bacteria, staphylococci in particular, to clot plasma is described in Chapter 12. The staphylococcal coagulases exhibit a high degree of correlation

Table 14–5. **Exfoliative Toxins of *Staphylococcus aureus****

Property	Exfoliatin A	Exfoliatin B
Molecular weight	24,000	24,000
Cation requirement	Cu++	None
Stability at:		
100° C. for 20 min.	Stable	Inactivated
60° C. for 30 min.	Stable	Inactivated
−30° C.	Stable	Inactivated
	(>1 year)	(<1 year)
Toxoid formed†	+	+
Antigenicity	Specific	Specific
Gene location‡	Chromosomal	Plasmid

*Adapted from M. Rogolsky, Microbiol. Rev. **43**:320, 1979.
†After treatment with formaldehyde.
‡Applies to phage group II strains only; others not established.

Table 14–6. **Properties of Staphylococcal Pyrogenic Exotoxins***

Property	Pyrogenic Exotoxin Type		
	A	B	C
Molecular weight	12,000	18,000	22,000
Isoelectric point	5.3	8.5	7.2
Antigenicity	Specific	Specific	Specific
Pyrogenicity	+	+	+
Mitogenicity	+	+	+
Endotoxin shock enhancement	+	+	+

*Data from P. M. Schlievert, D. J. Schoettle, and D. W. Watson, Infect. Immun. **23**:609, 1979; P. M. Schlievert. Biochemistry **19**:6204, 1980; P. M. Schlievert. *et al.,* J. Infect. Dis. **143**:509, 1981.

with virulence; they aid in protection against intraleucocytic destruction by inhibiting phagocytosis and antagonize the bactericidal activity of normal serum, traits that plausibly relate to virulence.

Staphylococcal coagulase exists in two forms—one **free** and the other **cell-bound.** The two are immunologically dissimilar and have slightly different actions. Cell-free coagulase is protein in nature and four antigenic types have been identified.

In clotting plasma, coagulase reacts with a plasma factor similar to prothrombin to yield a complex composed of coagulase and a coagulase-reacting factor; the complex has thrombin-like enzymatic activity and cleaves fibrinogen, thus producing a fibrin clot.

Cell-bound coagulase, or **clumping factor,** is not released from the cell surface, so that when these cells are mixed with plasma they clump or agglutinate by virtue of fibrin precipitation on the cell surface, as shown in Figure 14–4. The substrate appears to be soluble fibrin monomers that cannot be clotted by thrombin and the mechanism is not, therefore, identical to that of free coagulase.

Coagulase activity may be assayed in two ways. One, measuring free coagulase, is a tube test in which bacterial cells induce a fibrin clot in the presence of human or rabbit plasma. In the second, bacteria are suspended in a drop of plasma on a slide; positive strains clump rapidly, giving the appearance of a bacterial slide agglutination test. Results of these tests are not always parallel. Coagulase formation is also demonstrable as a halo of opacity surrounding colonies of coagulase-positive staphylococci grown on agar mediums containing fibrinogen.

Coagulase is not highly toxic on parenteral inoculation, but in sufficient doses induces a rapid fall in fibrinogen and extensive intravascular coagulation, especially in the lungs, to produce rapid death in experimental animals.

Hyaluronidase. Hyaluronic acid, the ground substance of tissues, is depolymerized by hyaluronidase, an enzyme formed by the majority of *S. aureus* strains. Staphylococcal hyaluronidase is antigenically homogeneous, although multiple molecular forms (isoenzymes) are observed. Hyaluronidase enhances the invasiveness of staphylococci (Chapter 12).

Staphylokinase. A large number of staphylococci are able to dissolve fibrin clots by a bacterial kinase. The mechanism resembles that of streptokinase and is described in Chapter 12. Unlike streptokinase, the staphylococ-

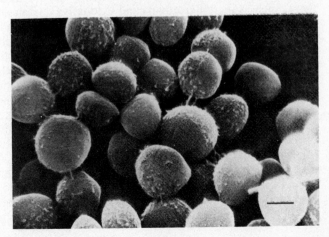

Figure 14–4. Scanning electron micrograph of *Staphylococcus aureus* (Cowan I strain) showing clumping in the presence of fibrinogen. Fibrinogen fibers are bound to clumping factor on the cell surface; some fibers form bridges between cells. Bar = 0.05 μm. (A. Umeda, T. Ikebuchi, and K. Amako, J. Bacteriol. **141**:838, 1980.)

cal kinase acts on the plasma of animals, including dogs, guinea pigs, and rabbits.

STAPHYLOCOCCAL DISEASE[17, 39]

The staphylococci are said to be ubiquitous, occurring as a part of the normal microbial flora of man and animals. In humans, the predominant staphylococci of the skin are the coagulase-negative strains, principally *S. epidermidis,* while coagulase-positive *S. aureus* is often found colonizing the nasopharynx. The presence of *S. aureus* on the skin is common, but these are thought to be contaminants derived from nasal secretions.

The staphylococci are considered to be **opportunistic** pathogens. They are involved in disease production when host resistance is compromised or when the particular microbial strain possesses a combination of virulence factors that permit invasion and host damage. The characteristic lesion caused by staphylococci is an **abscess**—a localized focus of purulent infection partially or completely walled off from surrounding tissues.

Although virulent staphylococci may penetrate the mucous membrane barrier to cause such infections as staphylococcal pneumonia, the most common type of infection is cutaneous, in which the microorganisms infect the hair follicles and sweat ducts or penetrate the skin barrier after trauma. The abscesses formed may be limited or the bacteria may spread via the blood stream to give rise to secondary foci of infection in multiple organs and tissues. Occasionally, a serious and fulminating bacteremia may result.[27]

It has already been noted that the staphylococci are extremely versatile in the number and kinds of metabolic products that contribute to their pathogenic potential. Some of these, such as the enterotoxins and exfoliative toxins, are demonstrably responsible for food poisoning and scalded skin syndrome. Other factors, such as protein A, coagulase, peptidoglycans, and leucocidin help to overcome or circumvent host defenses. The multifactorial nature of staphylococcal virulence has inhibited experimental assessment of the precise contribution of the dermonecrotic and lethal effects of the hemolytic toxins, as well as the roles of hyaluronidase and other staphylococcal enzymes. The combined effects of staphylococcal factors must, however, account for the pathogenic potential of these bacteria and for the observed character of the infections.

Carriers

Nasal and skin carriers are probably the most important reservoirs of staphylococcal infections in humans. Infants are colonized by these organisms within a few days after birth, probably from family members and hospital attendants. In the newborn, the umbilicus appears to be a preferred site of colonization for most staphylococci. The majority of humans continue to harbor these organisms, either intermittantly or continuously, throughout life.

The carrier rate is significantly greater in hospitals, in both patients and attendants. Many of the strains associated with hospitals are resistant to antibiotics, and serious staphylococcal infections occur in the hospital environment. The spread of infection, airborne or by contact, is of particular concern in nurseries, burn units, and surgical wards.[9]

Colonization with staphylococci, as in carriers, is not altogether lamentable. Since the early 1900s, it has been known that colonization with one strain of staphylococcus interferes with colonization by a second. Thus, if the original strain is of low virulence, the host may be protected from infection with more dangerous strains. This has practical application in nurseries; infants colonized with an avirulent *S. aureus* are resistant to colonization with virulent strains present in the hospital environment.[38]

There is some nonspecificity to this interference, since it occurs between strains of different taxonomic groups; colonization with *S. epidermidis* or gram-negative bacilli also protects against colonization by other staphylococci.[40] Interference is most likely associated with competition for receptor sites necessary for bacterial adherence.

Suppurative Infections

Infections by staphylococci are usually cutaneous. Since these organisms are commonly found on the skin, it is likely that most such infections follow a transitory decrease in host resistance, permitting local invasion of hair follicles and sweat glands to establish a focus of infection. Invasion may also accompany wounds or foreign body penetration.

The primary cutaneous infections may be relatively mild, as acne or simple boils, or may involve extensive carbuncles; these are possibly followed by metastatic abscesses or bacteremia that may result in acute disseminated disease, particularly in children.

The balance between the virulence of the microorganisms and host resistance determines whether the infection is initially established and also influences subsequent events of the disease process. In addition to the variety of cutaneous infections, staphylococci are responsible for the majority of cases of osteomyelitis, usually as a consequence of bacteremia following skin infections.

Bacteremia is a serious consequence of many localized infections, principally the more extensive skin infections, endocarditis, and osteomyelitis. Disseminated staphylococcal infection may involve bones and joints, lungs, central nervous system, kidneys, and heart. The staphylococci in bacteremia include both coagulase-positive and coagulase-negative strains, but the latter generally follow a more indolent course.

While urinary tract infections are most frequently due to gram-negative bacilli, principally *Escherichia coli,* an increasing number are now of staphylococcal etiology. In sexually active young women, the second most common cause of such infections is *S. saprophyticus.*[16, 45]

Staphylococcal Pneumonia

Pneumonia due to staphylococci is not common, except those occurring in influenza as secondary infections. Nevertheless, the case mortality rate is high, and it must be considered to be a serious disease requiring prompt and vigorous therapy.

Two general types of staphylococcal pneumonia are recognized. One is a primary infection of the lung and is predominantly seen in the very young or those with predisposing conditions, such as influenza. The other often follows bacteremia, as a secondary focus of infection.

The bacteria may be found, frequently in almost pure culture, in sputum, empyema fluid, or lung puncture specimens; and in blood culture when there is bacteremia. A gram stain of sputum can aid in differentiation from other pneumonia-causing bacteria and as a guide to initial therapy.

Scalded Skin Syndrome[10, 12, 30]

Staphylococci are associated with several kinds of dermatitis variously termed Ritter disease, toxic epidermal necrolysis, generalized exfoliative dermatitis, and bullous impetigo. Current usage favors the term scalded skin syndrome as descriptive of the dermatitis which is most often linked to the action of the exfoliative toxin produced by a few strains of *S. aureus.*

The generalized dermatitis usually begins with intense, tender erythema, often first localized about the face and trunk and later spreading to the extremities. The epidermis is loosened, with appearance of large flaccid bullae. The epidermal layers separate and large sheets of skin peel away, exposing the underlying, sensitive dermal surface. A secondary desquamation then ensues for several days, followed by healing, without scarring, within about two weeks of onset. In some patients, a scarlatiniform rash predominates, and in others localized bullae characterize the disease. The primary infection focus may be distant from the dermal lesions; the disease in male infants, for example, may be associated with primary infection of circumcision wounds.

Scalded skin syndrome is most often seen in infants and young children, although it has been observed in adults, most often in those with underlying disease. The epidermolytic reactions are undoubtedly due to the exfoliative toxin. However, the recent discovery of the staphylococcal pyrogenic exotoxin, which induces a scarlatiniform rash by hypersensitivity, suggests that cases exhibiting only the rash may be due to this toxin, rather than to exfoliatin.

The epidermolytic toxin apparently acts only on cells of the granular layer of the epidermis, where it disrupts desmosomes binding adjacent cells, resulting in cleavage of the layers.

The toxin is antigenic, and antibody is induced in humans following the disease. Antibody may be produced by rabbit immunization and the antitoxin passively protects neonatal mice against exfoliatin, but not against infection. Antitoxin has not yet been employed for therapy in human cases and pooled human serum globulin does not contain adequate amounts of antitoxin for protection.[18]

Toxic Shock Syndrome.[7, 11, 14, 37]

In 1978, Todd and associates described the toxic shock syndrome due to *S. aureus* infection. Subsequently, the disease has been found to occur predominantly in menstruating women, with significantly increased risk associated with tampon use. *Staphylococcus aureus* appears to be the etiologic agent, and vaginal infection the most common focus, although infections at other sites are sometimes seen; blood cultures are uniformly negative.

The disease is characterized by sudden onset with fever, diarrhea, shock, and a macular erythematous rash. The rash extends to a desquamation of the hands and feet after one or two weeks. Multiple organ systems may be involved.

The clinical and bacteriological findings in toxic shock syndrome suggest intoxication as the pathogenetic mechanism. Exfoliatins seem not to be the toxins involved, but the pyrogenic exotoxins, described earlier, appear to be a more likely cause. The production of pyrogenic exotoxin C, in particular, is significantly associated with *S. aureus* strains isolated from cases of toxic shock syndrome.[36] However, the possibility that several toxins are involved cannot presently be discounted.

As noted above, most of the recent cases of toxic shock syndrome have occurred in menstruating women using tampons. In 1980, more than 940 cases were reported in the United States; 99 per cent were in women and 98 per cent of these were associated with menstruation. The disease seems to be waning, probably due to public awareness of the role of tampons and changes in tampon-wearing habits.

Enterocolitis

Until recently, the pseudomembranous type of enterocolitis associated with oral administration of broad-spectrum antibiotics was thought to be due to staphylococci. Antibiotic-resistant staphylococci were believed to multiply in the bowel at the expense of the normal flora. While a few cases may be of staphylococcal etiology, the disease is primarily associated with intestinal overgrowth of *Clostridium difficile* following antibiotic administration (Chapter 28).

Bacteriological Diagnosis[20]

The isolation of staphylococci is usually not a difficult matter. Blood agar is the medium of choice for isolation and good growth obtains within 24 hours. The staphylococci grow in the presence of 7.5 per cent sodium chloride; selective mediums containing salt, mannitol, and sometimes antibiotics are employed for heavily contaminated specimens. These selective mediums are inhibitory for gram-negative bacteria but permit growth of staphylococci.

Examination of gram-stained smears from typical colonies will show characteristic morphology. The staphylococcal species most often encountered in human infections may be further differentiated by characters such as colony morphology, coagulase production, hemolysis, novobiocin resistance, phosphatase activity, and carbohydrate utilization, as listed in Table 14–2.

Immunity

Acquired immunity to infection with staphylococci is generally of low order and appears to be primarily cellular in nature, with phagocytosis as the most significant factor. A cell-mediated immune response has been documented, with release of lymphokines and activation of macrophages,[4, 23, 24] but these cells do not appear to have increased bactericidal capability.

Many of the toxins and enzymes produced by staphylococci serve as virulence determinants and are immunogenic. Nevertheless, antibody directed against them, with the possible exception of leucocidin, does not appear to play a significant role in effective immunity. Most immunity studies have failed to take into account the multiplicity of these factors, however, and their role in immunity is perhaps not yet resolved.

It must be noted that the nature of the infection process minimizes contact of the staphylococcal antigens with both antibody-forming cells and circulating antibody. Microorganisms present in abscesses find sanctuary from humoral elements. Even during hematogenous spread in bacteremia, they may be protected from antibody, since they are contained within leucocytes or masses of fibrin. Thus, active immunization against staphylococcal disease finds little support.

Chemotherapy

Sensitive strains of staphylococci are inhibited by sulfonamides, penicillins, tetracyclines, chloramphenicol, erythromycin, and other broad-spectrum antibiotics. Chemotherapy is, however, complicated by the prevalence of resistant strains and strains of multiple resistance. It is essential, therefore, that isolated strains be tested for sensitivity to a variety of potentially effective agents as a part of the laboratory procedure to provide a basis for rational and effective chemotherapy.

Cutaneous infections, if small, are effectively treated by drainage. If they are more extensive, antimicrobial drugs are generally employed; these include oral penicillin, erythromycin, or clindamycin. Bacteremia, endocarditis, osteomyelitis, and staphylococcal pneumonia require vigorous parenteral therapy with antimicrobials such as the penicillinase-resistant penicillins, cephalosporins, or gentamycin.

References

1. Abramson, C. 1972. Staphylococcal enzymes. pp. 187–248. *In* J. O. Cohen (Ed.): The Staphylococci. Wiley-Interscience, New York.
2. Aly, R., *et al.* 1980. Role of teichoic acid in the

binding of *Staphylococcus aureus* to nasal epithelial cells. J. Infect. Dis. **141**:463–465.

3. de Azavedo, J., and J. P. Arbuthnott. 1981. Prevalence of epidermolytic toxin in clinical isolates of *Staphylococcus aureus*. J. Med. Microbiol. **14**:341–344.

4. Baughn, R. E., and P. F. Bonventre. 1975. Cell-mediated immune phenomena induced by lymphokines from splenic lymphocytes of mice with chronic staphylococcal infection. Infect. Immun. **11**:313–319.

5. Bergdoll, M. S. 1972. The enterotoxins. pp. 301–331. *In* J. O. Cohen (Ed.): The Staphylococci. Wiley-Interscience, New York.

6. Bergdoll, M. S., *et al.* 1981. A new staphylococcal enterotoxin, enterotoxin F, associated with toxic-shock-syndrome Staphylococcus aureus isolates. Lancet **1**:1017–1021.

7. Chesney, P. J., *et al.* 1981. Clinical manifestations of toxic shock syndrome. J. Amer. Med. Assn **246**:741–748.

8. Cohen, J. O. (Ed.). 1972. The Staphylococci. Wiley-Interscience, New York.

9. Crossley, K., *et al.* 1979. An outbreak of infections caused by strains of *Staphylococcus aureus* resistant to methicillin and aminoglycosides. I. Clinical studies. II. Epidemiologic studies. J. Infect. Dis. **139**:273–279; 280–287.

10. Curran, J. P., and F. L. Al-Salihi. 1980. Neonatal staphylococcal scalded skin syndrome: massive outbreak due to an unusual phage type. Pediatrics **66**:285–290.

11. Davis, J. P., *et al.* 1980. Toxic-shock syndrome. Epidemiologic features, recurrence, risk factors, and prevention. New Engl. J. Med. **303**:1429–1435.

12. Elias, P. M., P. Fritsch, and E. H. Epstein, Jr. 1977. Staphylococcal scalded skin syndrome. Clinical features, pathogenesis, and recent microbiological and biochemical developments. Arch. Dermatol. **113**:207–219.

13. Evans, J. B. 1975. Uracil and pyruvate requirements for anaerobic growth of staphylococci. J. Clin. Microbiol. **2**:14–17.

14. Glasgow, L. A. 1980. Staphylococcal infection in the toxic-shock syndrome. New Engl. J. Med. **303**:1473–1475.

15. Jeljaszewicz, J. (Ed.). 1976. Staphylococci and staphylococcal diseases. Proceeding of III International Symposium on Staphylococci and Staphylococcal Infections. Zentbl. Bakt. I., Suppl. 5, pp. 1–1137.

16. Jordan, P. A., *et al.* 1980. Urinary tract infection caused by *Staphylococcus saprophyticus*. J. Infect. Dis. **142**:510–515.

17. Kaplan, M. H., and M. J. Tenenbaum. 1982. Staphylococcus aureus: cellular biology and clinical applications. Amer. J. Med. **72**:248–268.

18. Kapral, F. A. 1979. Levels of exfoliatin antitoxin in pooled human serum globulin. J. Infect. Dis. **139**:209–210.

19. Kloos, W. E. 1980. Natural populations of the genus *Staphylococcus*. Ann. Rev. Microbiol. **34**:559–592.

20. Kloos, W. E., and P. B. Smith. 1980. Staphylococci. pp. 83–87. *In* E. H. Lennette, *et al.* (Eds.): Manual of Clinical Microbiology. 3rd ed. American Society for Microbiology, Washington, D.C.

21. Koyama, T., M. Yamada, and M. Matsuhashi. 1977. Formation of regular packets of *Staphylococcus aureus* cells. J. Bacteriol. **129**:1518–1523.

22. Lacey, R. W. 1975. Antibiotic resistance plasmids of *Staphylococcus aureus* and their clinical importance. Bacteriol. Rev. **39**:1–32.

23. Lenhart, N., and S. Mudd. 1972. Staphylococcidal capability of rabbit peritoneal macrophages in relation to infection and elicitation: delayed-type hypersensitivity without increased resistance. Infect. Immun. **5**:757–762.

24. Lenhart, N., and S. Mudd. 1972. Staphylococcidal capability of rabbit peritoneal macrophages in relation to infection and elicitation: induction and elicitation of activated macrophages. Infect. Immun. **5**:763–768.

25. Marshall, J. H., and G. J. Wilmoth. 1981. Pigments of *Staphylococcus aureus*, a series of triterpenoid carotenoids. J. Bacteriol. **147**:900–913.

26. Miller, B. A., R. F. Reiser, and M. S. Bergdoll. 1978. Detection of staphylococcal enterotoxins A, B, C, D, and E in foods by radioimmunoassay, using staphylococcal cells containing protein A as an immunoadsorbent. Appl. Environ. Microbiol. **36**:421–426.

27. Nolan, C. M., and H. N. Beaty. 1976. *Staphylococcus aureus* bacteremia. Current clinical patterns. Amer. J. Med. **60**:495–500.

28. Plorde, J. J., and J. C. Sherris. 1974. Staphylococcal resistance to antibiotics: origin, measurement and epidemiology. Ann. N.Y. Acad. Sci. **236**:413–434.

29. Report. 1981. Methicillin-resistant *Staphylococcus aureus*–United States. Morbid. Mortal. Wkly. Rep. **30**:140–147.

30. Rogolsky, M. 1979. Nonenteric toxins of *Staphylococcus aureus*. Microbiol. Rev. **43**:320–360.

31. Sabath, L. D. 1979. Staphylococcal tolerance to penicillins and cephalosporins. pp. 299–303. *In* D. Schlessinger (Ed.): Microbiology—1979. American Society for Microbiology, Washington, D.C.

32. Sabath, L. D., *et al.* 1977. A new type of penicillin resistance of *Staphylococcus aureus*. Lancet **1**:443–447.

33. Schlievert, P. M. 1980. Purification and characterization of staphylococcal pyrogenic exotoxin type B. Biochemistry **19**:6204–6208.

34. Schlievert, P. M. 1981. Staphylococcal scarlet fever: role of pyrogenic exotoxins. Infect. Immun. **31**:732–736.

35. Schlievert, P. M., D. J. Schoettle, and D. W. Watson. 1979. Purification and physicochemical and biological characterization of a staphylococcal pyrogenic exotoxin. Infect. Immun. **23**:609–617.

36. Schlievert, P. M., *et al.* 1981. Identification and characterization of an exotoxin from *Staphylococcus aureus* associated with toxic-shock syndrome. J. Infect. Dis. **143**:509–516.

37. Shands, K. N., *et al.* 1980. Toxic-shock syndrome in menstruating women. Association with tampon use and *Staphylococcus aureus* and clinical features in 52 cases. New Engl. J. Med. **303**:1436–1442.

38. Shinefield, H. R., *et al.* 1972. Bacterial interference. pp. 503–515. *In* J. O. Cohen (Ed.): The Staphylococci. Wiley-Interscience, New York.

39. Shulman, J. A., and A. J. Nahmias. 1972. Staphylococcal infections. pp. 457–481. *In* J. O. Cohen (Ed.): The Staphylococci. Wiley-Interscience, New York.

40. Speck, W. T., *et al.* 1978. Effect of bacterial flora on staphylococcal colonisation of the newborn. J. Clin. Pathol. **31**:153–155.

41. Spika, J. S., H. A. Verbrugh, and J. Verhoef. 1981. Protein A effect on alternative pathway complement activation and opsonization of *Staphylococcus aureus*. Infect. Immun. **34**:455–460.

42. Switalski, L. M. 1976. Isolation and purification of staphylococcal clumping factor. Zentbl. Bakt. I., Suppl. 5, pp. 413–425.

43. Tzagoloff, H., and R. Novick. 1977. Geometry of cell division in *Staphylococcus aureus*. J. Bacteriol. **129**:343–350.

44. Verhoef, J., and H. A. Verbrugh. 1981. Host determinants in staphylococcal disease. Ann. Rev. Med. **32**:107–122.

45. Wallmark, G., I. Arremark, and B. Telander. 1978. *Staphylococcus saprophyticus:* a frequent cause of acute urinary tract infection among female outpatients. J. Infect. Dis. **138**:791–797.

46. Ward, P. D., and W. H. Turner. 1980. Identification of staphylococcal Panton-Valentine leukocidin as a potent dermonecrotic toxin. Infect. Immun. **27**:393–397.

47. Wilkinson, B. J., *et al.* 1978. Activation of complement by cell surface components of *Staphylococcus aureus*. Infect. Immun. **20**:388–392.

48. Wilkinson, B. J., *et al.* 1979. Localization of the third component of complement on the cell wall of encapsulated *Staphylococcus aureus* M: implications for the mechanism of resistance to phagocytosis. Infect. Immun. **26**:1159–1163.

49. Wuepper, K. D., D. H. Baker, and R. L. Dimond. 1976. Measurement of the staphylococcal epidermolytic toxin: a comparison of bioassay, radial immunodiffusion, and radioimmunoassay. J. Invest. Derm. **67**:526–531.

The Streptococci

The streptococci make up a relatively large, somewhat heterogeneous group of spherical forms that are characterized by arrangement of cells in chains. They are responsible for a variety of diseases in humans and certain diseases in lower animals. Many occur also as commensals in man and animals and some are saprophytes found in milk and milk products.

Of the five genera currently placed in the family Streptococcaceae, only *Streptococcus* and *Aerococcus* are associated with infections in man. *Aerococcus* is occasionally found in urinary tract infections and in endocarditis, but the members of greatest medical importance are found in *Streptococcus*. The genus comprises more than 20 species, many with varying pathogenic potential in man.

The present classification of *Streptococcus,* based primarily on physiological characters, is not entirely satisfactory from the viewpoint of the medical microbiologist. In 1933, Lancefield discovered that the pathogenic streptococci could be assigned to several serological groups on the basis of antigens of the cell wall; these groups were correlated, in a general way, with the epidemiology of the diseases concerned. It is now recognized that most pathogenic streptococci, with the exception of the pneumococci, possess these group antigens, and they can be at least partly classified on this basis. The Lancefield groups are of practical value to the systematist, and the serological groups correlate generally, though not invariably, with the taxonomy of streptococci based on other criteria.

As a matter of practical convenience and in keeping with usual conventions, *Streptococcus pneumoniae*—the pneumococcus—will be con-

385

sidered separately from other streptococci (p. 405). Pneumococci are differentiable from other streptococci, and the characteristics of

pneumococcal disease warrants separate discussion.

The Streptococci

Early in the history of bacteriology, streptococci were observed in the pus formed in suppurative inflammatory conditions; their frequent presence and pathological significance were first emphasized in the early 1880s. In addition to the more virulent pathogenic forms, relatively harmless parasitic streptococci are more or less constantly present in the human throat and in the intestinal tract; these assume a pathogenic role only under circumstances in which normal host resistance is markedly reduced, and they may be regarded, for all practical purposes, as a portion of the normal flora of the human body.

GENERAL FEATURES OF STREPTOCOCCI[6, 54]

Morphology and Staining

Except for the characteristic cell grouping, streptococci are similar in morphology and staining to *Staphylococcus*. They are gram-positive, spherical cells, 0.8 to 1.0 μm. in diameter. Some size variation results from cultural conditions, *e.g.*, cells are somewhat smaller when grown anaerobically. Smaller varieties, termed minute streptococci, are about one-half the size of typical cells.

Streptococci typically undergo binary fission in parallel planes; they usually remain united after division, developing characteristic chains of cells that account for the generic name (Fig. 15–1). Chain length is determined by the firmness of attachment of individual cells; some strains exhibit long chains, while others show only one or two pairs of diplococci. Typical chain formation is most regular in liquid growth mediums; stains prepared from cultures on agar, and to a lesser extent from exudates, reveal not only chains, but single cells, pairs, and sometimes aggregates resembling *Staphylococcus*.

Many of the streptococci form capsules; when present, the capsules of *Streptococcus pyogenes* and those of group C strains (Fig. 15–2) are composed of hyaluronic acid, while polysaccharide capsules are encountered in members of groups B and D. Hyaluronic acid

capsules are not, of course, found in strains that produce hyaluronidase (see below). Unlike the polysaccharide capsules of many other bacteria, the hyaluronic acid capsules of streptococci are not immunogenic. Additional surface antigens appear in *Streptococcus* that are not associated with the presence of true capsules. These are a part of the cell wall structure and are sometimes referred to as envelope antigens. For the most part, these antigens impart group- and type-specific characters to streptococci and are therefore of significance in classification and antigenic structure of these bacteria.

Streptococci do not form spores and they are nonmotile, with the exception of a few strains of group D.

Colonies of *Streptococcus* growing on solid mediums are usually quite small, about 0.5 mm. in diameter, with entire margins; translucent; and slightly granular (Fig. 15–3). Pigmentation is rare, and is confined to group B and D strains in which red and yellow pigments are sometimes observed. Encapsulated varieties may grow as mucoid colonies, but the

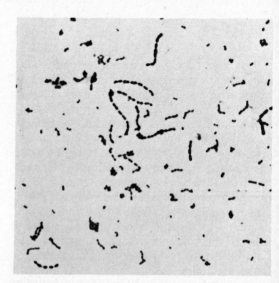

Figure 15–1. *Streptococcus pyogenes.* The tendency to remain attached is more pronounced between daughter cells after the first cell division, resulting in the diplococcus arrangement in the chains, as seen in this photomicrograph. Fuchsin; × 1500.

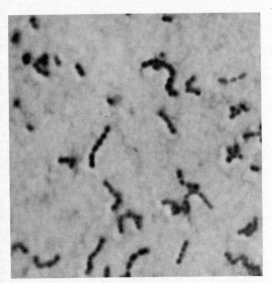

Figure 15–2. Group C streptococci stained with methylene blue to show capsules. Smear from serum broth. × 2400.

usual colonial form is smooth and glistening. Most of the human and animal strains of *Streptococcus* are hemolytic on blood agar mediums, exhibiting either β- or α-hemolysis, and this property is an important character for differentiation (see below).

Physiology

As noted above, streptococci are morphologically similar to *Staphylococcus* and other Micrococcaceae, but they may be separated from these by their failure to produce catalase. Streptococci are aerobic and facultatively an-

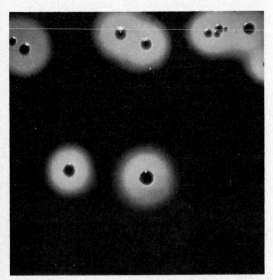

Figure 15–3. *Streptococcus pyogenes.* Pure culture on blood agar showing β-hemolysis. ×5.

aerobic. The growth of several varieties is markedly stimulated by increased CO_2 tension of about 10 per cent. As a group, these microorganisms grow over a wide temperature range from about 10° C. to as high as 50° C., and growth at temperature extremes is an important differential character among streptococci, as shown in Table 15–1.

These microorganisms are among the most exacting bacteria with respect to nutritive requirements. Growth is ordinarily poor, even on fresh meat infusion mediums, but these are improved by the inclusion of phosphate buffer and glucose. The most satisfactory are infusion mediums supplemented with fresh blood. Routine culture of the pathogenic forms is usually on sheep blood agar.

Although streptococci exhibit wide variation in nutritive requirements, the pathogenic species are the most exacting and are relatively fastidious. Most require glutamine, vitamins, and a variety of amino acids; group A strains must also be furnished with nucleic acid derivatives and their growth is stimulated by peptides. Only a relatively few strains can be cultivated on semisynthetic or synthetic mediums.

The biochemical activities of streptococci are diverse and constitute an important part of physiological classification schemes. All members of *Streptococcus* are **homofermentative,** *i.e.,* they produce dextrorotary lactic acid as the chief product of glucose fermentation by the hexose diphosphate pathway. A wide variety of other sugars are fermented and a number of polysaccharides hydrolyzed. Sodium hippurate, arginine, and polymers such as inulin, starch, and dextrin may be hydrolyzed and these have some differential significance, as can be seen in Table 15–1.

Classification[6]

Classification of species within *Streptococcus* has been of both theoretical and practical importance because of their etiological relationship to a number of widespread diseases of man and animals. This has been particularly difficult, since neither the physiological nor immunological methods of differentiation have been completely satisfactory.

Three general criteria have been used, *viz.,* hemolysis by cultures on blood agar, biochemical properties, and immunological reactions. Those concerned with the pathogenic streptococci make a preliminary separation on the basis of hemolysis, and define groups and types on an immunological basis. Workers with more

Table 15–1. **Some Differential Characters of the Principal Species of** *Streptococcus*

Streptococcus Species	Hemolysis	Growth at 10° C.	Growth at 45° C.	Growth 6.5% NaCl	Hydrolysis of Hippurate	Hydrolysis of Arginine	Hydrolysis of Bile-Esculin	Lancefield Group Antigen
S. pyogenes*	β	–	–	–	–	+	–	A
S. agalactiae†	β‡	–	–	–	+	+	–	B
S. equisimilis	β	–	–	–	–	+	–	C
S. zooepidemicus	β	–	–	–	–	+	–	C
S. equi	β	–	–	–	–	+	–	C
S. dysgalactiae	α	–	–	–	V§	+	–	C
S. faecalis	α; β; NH§	+	+	+	+	+	+	D
S. faecium	α; NH	+	+	+	V	+	+	D
S. durans	α; β; NH	+	+	+	V	+	+	D
S. avium	α; NH	–	+	+	–	–	+	D
S. bovis	NH	–	+	–	V	–	+	D
S. equinus	α	–	+	–	–	–	+	D
S. sanguis	α	–	–	–	–	+	–	H
S. anginosus	α	–	–	–	–	+	–	F; G
S. salivarius	NH	–	+	–	–	–	–	K; None
S. mitis (mitior)	α	–	+	–	–	V	–	O; None
S. mutans	α; NH	–	–	–	–	–	–	None
S. milleri	α; NH	–	–	–	–	+	–	Varies
S. pneumoniae‖	α	–	–	–	–	+	–	None
S. lactis	α; NH	+	–	–	V	+	–	N

*Susceptible to bacitracin.
†Produces CAMP factor.
‡Usually.
§V = variable; NH = nonhemolytic.
‖Bile soluble; optochin sensitive.

general interests rely primarily on physiological characters, such as those used in the Bergey classification.

Hemolysis. The use of blood plate hemolysis is especially convenient, since blood agar is the medium of choice in primary isolation. Hemolytic reactions on blood agar distinguish three kinds of streptococci:

1. The β-hemolytic streptococci, which produce a clear zone of hemolysis in the red opaque medium immediately surrounding the colony (see Fig. 15–3).

2. The α-hemolytic or green streptococci, which produce a zone of green discoloration with partial hemolysis about the colony on blood agar; the zone is usually considerably smaller than that seen in β-hemolysis.

3. The nonhemolytic, gamma, or indifferent streptococci, which produce no change in the medium.

These distinctions have some validity in that the highly virulent streptococci isolated from pathological conditions are almost invariably β-hemolytic varieties. Some heterogeneity is indicated, however, by the fact that a few nonpathogenic forms are also β-hemolytic.

The α-hemolytic streptococci embraces such seemingly diverse forms as fecal streptococci, or enterococci; the oral streptococci; certain animal forms; and the nonpathogenic varieties. The pneumococci, discussed in a later section, are also α-hemolytic. Some of the α-hemolytic streptococci, especially those found in the oral cavity, throat, and intestine, have only limited pathogenic potential. They sometimes produce localized infection in the gingival crevices of the teeth, on the heart valves in bacterial endocarditis, and in other locations, particularly if host resistance is impaired. They differ rather sharply, however, from the β-hemolytic streptococci in virulence.

The nonhemolytic streptococci are almost all saprophytic forms, most often found in milk and dairy products. They are only rarely encountered in human cases of subacute bacterial endocarditis.

Hemolytic capacity is, therefore, of great utility in preliminary differentiation, but taken alone is not sufficient to ascribe pathogenic potential to a given strain.

Immunological Differentiation. Through the pioneering efforts of Lancefield and her co-workers, the patterns of antigenic structure became the basis for the present understanding of the pathogenic streptococci. By extraction of soluble antigens and application of the precipitin test, Lancefield demonstrated the presence of both group- and type-specific antigens in the streptococci. Each of the **Lancefield groups** is characterized by a group-specific antigen (called the C-substance) shared by all of its members. These antigens are commonly polysaccharide in nature; in two groups, however, it is known to be teichoic acid. The group antigen is not capsular, but is a part of the cell wall, although it may be cryptic and demonstrable only by extraction of the cells. In most instances, the group antigen is nontoxic. Rhamnose appears to be a common constituent of those polysaccharide group antigens that have been studied; only the antigen of group O is known to be free of rhamnose.[33] The immunological specificity, however, usually resides in other residues. In the polysaccharide antigen of group A, for example, the specificity is due to N-acetyl glucosamine, which is linked to the cell wall peptidoglycan through rhamnose residues. The polysaccharide moieties of group antigens are haptens and they are immunogenic only when they are a part of the cell wall.

Based on the immunological specificity of group antigens, five streptococcal groups were originally described and were designated group A, B, and so on. Additional groups have since been found, up to and including group T. Not all of these have taxonomic standing, however, and many have not been given species rank. Some groups, too, comprise several species, separated on physiological grounds; group C, for example, is divided into four recognized species. The divergence between immunological and physiological methods for speciation is exemplified in *S. milleri*, strains of which may display one of several group antigens. In a few streptococci, no group antigens have been identified.

Most of the streptococcal groups may be further subdivided into serological types on the basis of other cell surface antigens. These are outlined in the following sections on individual groups of streptococci.

The biological significance of the Lancefield groups is indicated in Table 15–2, which shows the pathogenic species; their Lancefield groups, where applicable; and the principal human infections attributable to each.

Physiological Differentiation.[6, 15] Although it is not uniform, there is often some correlation between immunological groups of hemolytic streptococci and their physiological characteristics, as shown in Table 15–1.

Table 15–2. **The Principal Streptococci Responsible for Human Infections**

Lancefield Group		Streptococcus Species	Principal Human Infection
Designation	Antigen		
A	Rhamnose-N-acetyl glucosamine polysaccharide	*S. pyogenes*	Pharyngitis; pyoderma; erysipelas; wound infections
B	Rhamnose-glucosamine polysaccharide	*S. agalactiae*	Neonatal septicemia and meningitis
C	Rhamnose-N-acetyl galactosamine polysaccharide	*S. equisimilis* *S. zooepidemicus* *S. equi*	Pharyngitis; pyoderma; endocarditis
D	Glycerol teichoic acid with D-alanine and glucose	*S. faecalis** *S. faecium** *S. durans** *S. avium** *S. bovis* *S. equinus*	Endocarditis; urinary tract infections; neonatal septicemia and meningitis
H	Rhamnose polysaccharide	*S. sanguis*†	Endocarditis, gingival abscesses
K	Rhamnose polysaccharide	*S. salivarius*†	Endocarditis
NG‡	Not defined	*S. mutans*† *S. milleri*† *S. mitis (mitior)*†	Gingival abscesses; endocarditis; some are responsible for dental caries

*Enterococci.
†Viridans streptococci.
‡NG = not grouped.

A single species, *S. pyogenes,* is recognized in group A; as expected, this species shows a reasonable degree of homogeneity. *Streptococcus pyogenes* is differentiated from other β-hemolytic streptococci by susceptibility to the growth-inhibiting effect of bacitracin.

Group B, too, comprises only one species, *S. agalactiae,* and these are more or less homogeneous. *Streptococcus agalactiae* strains are usually, but not always, β-hemolytic, and they are differentiated from other species by the production of a factor that enhances β-hemolysis by *Staphylococcus aureus*—the CAMP test—as illustrated in Figure 15–4.

The streptococci of group C are somewhat more diverse, but they resemble group A in most physiological reactions. They are separable from group A, and from one another, by a variety of fermentative reactions.

Group D streptococci are considerably more heterogeneous, and the species casually grouped as enterococci—*S. faecalis, S. faecium, S. durans,* and *S. avium*—are characterized by greater temperature tolerance, growth in the presence of higher concentrations of sodium chloride, and the hydrolysis of bile-esculin.

Variation[9]

Alterations in the morphology of individual streptococci are frequently observed in old cultures, with cells swollen to several times normal size. Such aberrant morphology in aging cultures reflects the presence of involution forms that are degenerative in nature.

Streptococci may occur as L forms, *i.e.,* cells with little or no cell wall material. These can be induced by a variety of means, including the action of autolytic enzymes, such as lysozyme acting on peptidoglycan,[23] and by residence in human diploid cells.[45]

Changes in colonial morphology are well known and are often associated with the presence of **capsules.** The nonencapsulated varieties form smooth, glossy colonies, while those producing capsules grow as mucoid colony types. Immunological changes, not correlated with colonial morphology, have been noted, including loss of group-specific antigens as well as some irregularity in type-specific antigens (see below).

Variation in hemolysis is commonly reported in which β-hemolytic strains give rise to nonhemolytic or even α-hemolytic variants. This alteration is to some degree environmental, in that nonhemolytic variants may be hemolytic under anaerobic conditions, suggesting oxygen-inactivation of streptolysin O (see below). Similarly, some α-hemolytic varieties may be β-hemolytic in the presence of catalase.

Drug Resistance. The β-hemolytic streptococci initially were relatively uniform in their susceptibility to sulfonamides, penicillin, and tetracycline. Development of resistance to sulfonamides has been appreciable, possibly in consequence of their use in mass prophylaxis against other agents, primarily meningococcus. Tetracycline resistance appeared very soon after introduction of these antibiotics, and a majority of isolates are now resistant. Although strains resistant to penicillin are occasionally encountered, most β-hemolytic streptococci have remained sensitive to this antibiotic, and it remains as the most useful chemotherapeutic agent in most streptococcal infections.

The α-hemolytic streptococci vary widely in their sensitivity to chemotherapeutic drugs; such variations, however, do not appear to be due to acquired resistance factors.

Extracellular Products[13, 49]

The hemolytic streptococci produce a number of toxic substances. Certain of these are intracellular and are found in cell lysates, while others diffuse from the cell. In the former group, an intracellular hemolysin is formed, demonstrable in cell lysates, that is distinct from the extracellular streptolysins and is lethal for mice.

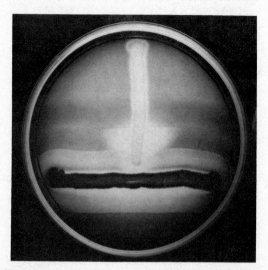

Figure 15–4. The CAMP test for group B streptococci. Note the arrow-shaped zone of accentuated β-hemolysis. The group B streptococci (vertical streak) produce CAMP factor that accentuates the normal zone of β-hemolysis produced by *Staphylococcus* (horizontal streak).

The extracellular products include the streptolysins, or hemolysins; streptokinase; streptodornase; hyaluronidase; and the pyrogenic exotoxins. The properties of these are summarized in Table 15–3.

Streptolysin S and **streptolysin O** are produced by group A, C, and G streptococci. Similar but distinct hemolysins are produced by the β-hemolytic group B streptococci. Streptolysin S is the principal hemolysin detected by aerobic blood plate cultures, while streptolysin O activity is expressed in anaerobic cultures.

Of these hemolysins, streptolysin O is the more important to the virulence of the hemolytic streptococci, since it is toxic for a wide variety of cells and is specifically cardiotoxic. Streptolysin O is antigenic, and toxins from group A strains are immunologically and functionally alike. Antibody to this lysin is formed in streptococcal infection and is used as an indicator of previous streptococcal infection (see Rheumatic Fever, p. 400); both the titer and the prevalence of antistreptolysin O (ASO) in human populations increase with age, indicating prior infection. The cytotoxicity and cardiotoxicity are thought to play a part in the sequelae following acute infections.

Erythrogenic Toxins.[56] The erythrogenic toxins are responsible for the rash of scarlet fever, a syndrome that sometimes accompanies acute infections with group A streptococci. These are also sometimes known as scarlatinal or Dick toxins. These toxins give rise to a marked erythema upon intradermal inoculation in humans (the Dick test), and in larger amounts they produce a generalized, erythematous rash.

For many years, it was believed that the scarlatinal rash represented the primary reaction to the toxin. It is now generally accepted, however, that the erythrogenic activity is expressed only as enhancement of hypersensitivity to other streptococcal products,[42] and that the primary toxicity of these substances is manifest as pyrogenicity, through hypothalmic stimulation; enhanced susceptibility to endotoxin shock; lymphocyte mitogenesis; and suppression of antibody response by alteration of the activity of T lymphocytes.[10, 43, 44] Thus, they are now more appropriately known as **streptococcal pyrogenic exotoxins.**

Three distinct immunological types (A, B, and C) of these toxins have been described, although they share some cross-reactive immunological determinants with one another. They are proteins of low molecular weight (less than 17,500 daltons) and stimulate antibodies that neutralize the primary toxic effects.

Only group A streptococci are known to

Table 15–3. **Biologically Active Products of *Streptococcus***

Product	Action	Properties
Streptolysin S	Hemolysis	Nonimmunogenic, low-molecular-weight hemolysin; not oxygen-sensitive; labile at 37° C.; produced in serum-containing mediums by groups A, C, and G; toxic for leucocytes and cells with sterol-containing membranes; inactivated by fixation to cell membranes; lethal for animals; inhibited by phospholipids.
Streptolysin O	Hemolysis	Immunogenic hemolysin produced by groups A, C, and G; oxygen-sensitive; activated by reducing conditions; labile at 37° C.; cardiotoxic; lethal for animals; neutralized by specific antibody.
Streptokinase	Fibrinolysis	Immunogenic plasmin activator, initiating dissolution of fibrin clots (Chapter 12); produced by groups A, C, and G; several immunogenic types.
Streptodornase	DNA hydrolysis	Immunogenic deoxyribonuclease; several immunogenic types.
Hyaluronidase	Hyaluronic acid hydrolysis	Immunogenic; promotes breakdown of hyaluronic acid of tissues to increase tissue permeability; not found in strains producing hyaluronic acid capsules.
Erythrogenic toxin	Induction of fever and rash	Pyrogenic exotoxins produced by some group A strains; three immunogenic types (A, B, and C); cytotoxic; mitogenic; enhances susceptibility to endotoxins; induces rash in hypersensitive individuals; lethal for animals; neutralized by antibodies.

form pyrogenic exotoxins, but not all strains are producers. The capacity for toxin production is apparently due to lysogenic conversion by bacteriophage. Nontoxigenic strains can be converted to toxin producers by lysogenization with appropriate phage.[21, 32]

Pathogenicity for Man[51, 54, 57]

The streptococci are responsible for a wide variety of human diseases, exhibiting a greater spectrum of disease production than most other kinds of bacteria. In addition to being a primary cause of disease, they have a marked tendency to appear in mixed and secondary infections with other pathogenic bacteria, especially staphylococci.[16] In general, streptococcal infections are characterized by suppurative lesions and very often by manifestations suggesting toxemia; the latter often take the form of nonsuppurative complications such as fever, arthritis, carditis, and nephritis.

Streptococcal infections exhibit considerable variation in extent and kind. These range from local infections, such as abscesses of the mucous membranes, joints, and serous membranes; infection of muscle, or cellulitis, which simulates gaseous gangrene; suppurative processes in all kinds of wounds; to those as generalized as pyemia or septicemia. Many streptococcal infections have no distinctive clinical manifestations, e.g., abscesses due to streptococci are not distinguishable from those of staphylococcal etiology. Others, however, such as erysipelas, have a more distinctive clinical character.

There are appreciable differences in the character of streptococcal infections as they appear in children and in adults, and lower age groups are relatively more susceptible. In infants, infections tend to be prolonged and low grade, with frequent suppurative complications, but rheumatic fever and nephritis seldom follow. In older children and adults, the infection tends to be more acute and self-limited, with nonsuppurative complications.

The β-hemolytic streptococci of Lancefield groups A, B, and C are the most virulent, with the greatest number of human infections due to group A. The very small proportion of infections with group C streptococci are not distinguishable from those of group A, except by isolation and immunological typing of the etiological agent. A significant and increasing number of human infections are attributable to group B streptococci. In adults, these are usually genital infections of a benign nature, but in very young children serious neonatal septicemia and meningitis are the usual manifestations.

While knowledge of the mechanisms of the pathogenic action of the β-hemolytic streptococci is far from complete, there is a considerable body of evidence indicating that the production of disease is at least partly due to streptococcal products, principally toxins. Strains of streptococci differ with respect to the kinds and amounts of such substances they produce, and this variability partially accounts for the differences in diseases they produce. Thus, strains that produce the pyrogenic exotoxins may have increased virulence over nontoxigenic strains, and scarlet fever may occur in certain individuals who are hypersensitive to streptococcal products. The route of infection and the immune status of the host are significant factors as well.

The α-hemolytic and nonhemolytic streptococci are much less virulent. The α-hemolytic forms constitute a portion of the normal bacterial flora of the mouth, upper respiratory tract, and intestine. It is probable that they seldom initiate primary infection of healthy tissues, but when host resistance is impaired they may initiate low-grade, essentially localized infections such as focal abscesses in the oral cavity. They are also the most common agents in subacute bacterial endocarditis, but while serious, the infection has little or no tendency to spread to other tissues despite the showering of streptococci into the blood. Pneu-

Table 15–4. **Lancefield Groups of Streptococci Isolated from Major Clinical Sources***

| Source | Streptococcal Groups | | | | | | | | | |
| | A | | B | | C | | G | | NG† | |
	No.	%	No.	%	No.	%	No.	%	No.	%
Upper respiratory	916	51.7	153	8.6	363	20.4	134	7.6	207	12.8
Lower Respiratory	143	18.8	222	29.3	95	12.5	94	12.5	203	22.8
Genitourinary	29	4.3	479	71.2	55	8.2	39	5.8	71	11.5
Wounds and exudates	1188	79.1	65	4.3	60	4.0	110	7.3	79	5.9
Total	2276	48.4	919	19.9	573	12.2	377	8.0	560	11.5

*Modified from H. M. Pollock, and B. J. Dahlgren, Appl. Microbiol. **27**:141–143, 1974.
†Not groupable.

monia due to α-hemolytic streptococci occurs from time to time, and tends to assume a chronic relapsing form. Meningitis due to these bacteria has also been reported, but is rare.

Epidemiology[37, 53, 57]

The primary sources of pathogenic streptococci are the individuals who carry these bacteria in the upper respiratory tract or, in the case of group B streptococci, in the genitourinary tract. The carrier state may represent subclinical infection, convalescent carriers, or true long-term carriers in the absence of disease. High carrier rates, up to 75 to 90 per cent, have been reported in schoolchildren. It is estimated that overt streptococcal infections occur in most individuals from time to time, but the incidence of subclinical infections is not known, other than in restricted groups. Those with overt symptoms of upper respiratory disease, such as tonsillitis, sinusitis, and pharyngitis, are prolific sources of infection. Streptococci are disseminated from the upper respiratory tract by sneezing, coughing, and contamination of hands and skin by nasal secretions. In most instances, group B streptococci are present in genitourinary discharges of adult carriers and are sexually transmitted; serious infections are then transmitted to the newborn *in utero* or during birth.

Skin infections, particularly streptococcal pyoderma, are also relatively common in both tropical and temperate zones and are circulated by direct contact.

Transmission from the infected person to a susceptible individual is by direct contact or by contamination of the environment. Direct contact infection is by inhalation of infected droplets or bodily contact such as hand-to-hand transmission. Most upper respiratory infection is airborne.

Bacteriological Diagnosis[15]

Isolation of streptococci from specimens of pathological material is ordinarily not difficult. Swabs from the throat, the nasopharynx, or skin lesions may be enriched in a variety of infusion mediums or they may be inoculated directly onto blood agar plates; other body fluids are usually inoculated directly. The medium of choice for isolation is sheep blood agar that is free of glucose; both α-and β-hemolysis are readily seen on such mediums. Incubation of the culture under anaerobic conditions results in improved detection of β-hemolytic streptococci, particularly those producing only streptolysin O.

Culture on selective mediums may be employed if the specimen is expected to contain large numbers of contaminants, *e.g.,* vaginal or rectal swabs. Selective agents employed include gentamycin, neomycin, nalidixic acid, polymixin, crystal violet, and sodium azide. The choice of such agents depends upon the origin of the specimen and the experience of the particular clinical laboratory.

The identification of streptococci on blood agar plates depends upon colonial morphology, hemolysis, and cellular morphology and arrangement as seen in Gram-stained smears.

Further identification of isolates depends upon the selective use of immunological and physiological tests. Immunological procedures are designed to establish the presence of relevant group antigens. If the isolate is β-hemolytic, the group antigen is extracted and reacted against antiserums to groups A, B, C, F, and G. If the strain is not β-hemolytic, extracts are tested with group B and D antiserums.

Streptococci that can be grouped by these procedures usually require no further differentiation, except for those of group D. The enterococci of group D are identified by growth in the present of 6.5 per cent sodium chloride. Physiological tests (Table 15–1) may be employed for other strains and species that cannot be grouped by these methods.

Although immunological methods are most accurate for identification of groupable streptococci, several physiological tests may yield presumptive group identification. For example, group A strains are β-hemolytic and are susceptible to bacitracin; group B strains exhibit a positive CAMP reaction and hydrolyze sodium hippurate; and group D isolates hydrolyze bile-esculin. Pneumococci are similar to viridans streptococci, but are differentiated by their solubility in bile, or sodium deoxycholate, and inhibition by optochin.

Immunofluorescence microscopy has some utility in the rapid identification of groups A and B streptococci. Enrichment broth cultures of throat or nasal swabs are usually employed, but direct smears have only limited value.

GROUP A STREPTOCOCCI[39, 53]

The streptococci that possess the Lancefield group A antigen are recognized as belonging to a single species, *Streptococcus pyogenes.* They are generally considered to be the most important streptococcus in cutaneous and up-

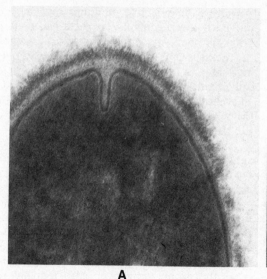
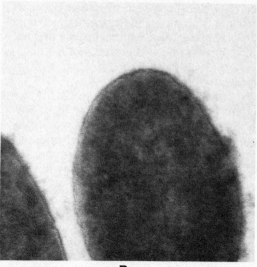

A   **B**

Figure 15–5. *A, Streptococcus pyogenes* containing the M antigen. Note the hairlike surface projections of M protein. *B, Streptococcus pyogenes* without M protein. × 82,500. (Courtesy of Dr. Edwin Beachey.)

per respiratory infections, not only because of their prevalence, but because such infections often are followed by serious sequelae, *e.g.,* rheumatic fever or glomerulonephritis.

Streptococcus pyogenes is similar to other streptococci in morphology and staining as previously described. Most strains possess a nonimmunogenic hyaluronic acid capsule that, when present, lends a mucoid appearance to colonies; capsules are not visible, however, in ordinary electron micrographs. These bacteria are β-hemolytic on sheep blood agar and are distinguished from other streptococci by the presence of the group A antigen, by their susceptibility to bacitracin, and by the physiological characters outlined in Table 15–1.

Antigenic Structure

Cells of *S. pyogenes* exhibit the fundamental structure common to other gram-positive cells, but are unique in composition. The relatively

thick cell wall contains peptidoglycan, the group A carbohydrate antigen, teichoic acid, and a variety of proteins. When observed by electron microscopy, virulent strains possess surface fibrillae that contain the M protein antigen, as shown in Figure 15–5. The other antigenic components are believed to occur in a mosaic pattern in the cell wall matrix. Table 15–5 lists the principal antigens that occur in *S. pyogenes*.

Group A streptococci are divided into many serological types, determined by two kinds of type-specific antigens. The most prevalent of these are the **M protein antigens**, located on the cell surface as a part of the hair-like fibrillae. It is likely that most strains of *S. pyogenes* contain M protein, but many of these are only weakly immunogenic, and antiserums are not available for all antigens in this series. Therefore, a portion of isolates cannot be typed on this basis. Nevertheless, more than

Table 15–5. **Antigens of *Streptococcus pyogenes****

Antigen	Serological Activity	Chemistry	
		Nature	**Properties**
C	Group-specific	Polysaccharide	Polymer of *N*-acetylglucosamine and rhamnose; occurs in cell wall.
M	Type-specific	Protein	Alcohol-soluble; resistant to heating in dilute acid; destroyed by proteolytic enzymes; related to virulence, and antibody is protective.
T	Occurs in several types but may be type-specific	Protein	Resistant to proteolytic enzymes; unstable to heat in dilute acid, but resistant in slightly alkaline solution.
R	Occurs in type 2, 3, 28, and 48 and in strains of Groups B, C, and G	Protein	Destroyed by peptic but not tryptic digestion; unstable to heat in dilute acid, but stable to heat in dilute alkali.

*Modified from R. C. Lancefield: Streptococcal Infections. Columbia University Press, 1954, pp. 3–18.

70 M-types of group A streptococci have been recorded. With only rare exceptions, each strain contains only one M antigen; however, some M proteins are similar, and presumably share antigenic determinants, so that there is occasional cross-reaction between M types.[59] The importance of the M antigen in the host-parasite relationship is emphasized by the fact that antibodies directed against the M antigen are protective in homologous type infections.

The other principal type-specific antigen is designated the **T antigen.** The T antigens are not so prevalent as the M antigens and they do not have the same theoretical importance, since antibodies against them are not protective. Thus, types 10 and 12 contain the same M antigens but different T antigens, while types 15, 17, 19, 23, and 30 contain similar T antigens but distinct M antigens. Some strains contain one, but not both antigens.

The typing of *S. pyogenes* has been rather generally applied, principally because of its utility in epidemiological investigations, as discussed later with streptococcal diseases. Serological typing is not, however, a part of routine identification of streptococci in clinical laboratories.

Virulence

The virulence determinants in *S. pyogenes* are many and varied, leading to an extremely complex host-parasite relationship, and one that is still incompletely understood.

Host-parasite interactions begin with the deposition of *S. pyogenes* on the mucosal surfaces (Chapter 12). Largely through the studies of Beachey and his colleagues,[3] the factors mediating attachment to these surfaces have been elucidated. **Lipoteichoic acid** (LTA) from the streptococcal cell membrane associates with the M protein, and possibly the T protein, to form a complex that is anchored to the cell surface; the fatty acid portion of LTA is then free to bind to receptors, such as fibronectin, on the host cell membrane, resulting in adherence.[48] This adherence and colonization must, of course, take place in competition with normal flora. The normal flora of the pharynx interferes with colonization by *S. pyogenes* and evolves slowly with age, perhaps explaining the greater resistance of adults to streptococcal infection.[41]

After infection is established, the streptococci produce an array of biologically active, often toxic, substances; acting in concert these probably account for pathogenesis by these microorganisms. Table 15–6 lists these prod-ucts along with their biological activities that relate to virulence and disease production.

One of the most important factors associated with disease production by streptococci is the development of a hypersensitivity to the cell substance of these bacteria, probably enhanced by action of the pyrogenic exotoxins. Subsequent infection, then, results in allergic phenomena that may be of considerable importance in pathogenesis. It seems probable that hypersensitivity plays a part in rheumatoid disease and arthritis of streptococcal etiology (see below).

Immunity[37]

Infection with group A streptococci is accompanied by humoral response to both cellular antigens and immunogenic extracellular products. The cellular antigens include the protein antigens—M, T, and R—and the group A carbohydrate substance, while the soluble antigens include streptolysin O, hyaluronidase, deoxyribonucleases, streptokinase, and the pyrogenic exotoxins.

Antibody formation has no diagnostic utility in acute streptococcal infections because there is not sufficient time for antibody response during the course of the disease. Antibody titration is useful, however, for retrospective diagnosis, *i.e.*, in associating antecedent streptococcal infection with sequelae such as rheumatic fever, arthritis, and glomerulonephritis. For example, patient's serum is often titrated for the presence of antistreptolysin O, or ASO, as an indicator of recent streptococcal infection. About 80 per cent of individuals with streptococcal respiratory infections exhibit ASO titers within three weeks of onset. If a broader antibody response is measured, as in the streptozyme test, about 95 per cent show antibody response. In this test, sheep erythrocytes are coated with a mixture of soluble streptococcal products; agglutination of these cells with patient's serum constitutes a measure of antibody response against the variety of soluble streptococcal antigens.

Antibody response to the cellular antigens is not generally employed for retrospective diagnosis. Antibodies to the group A carbohydrate appear at about the same time as antibodies to streptolysin O, but these are less sensitive indicators than ASO titers. Antibody response to M antigen is greatly delayed, since these proteins are poorly immunogenic in man, and a large number of individuals fail to develop antibody titers. Moreover, these are type-specific and their detection is complex.

Table 15–6. **Effects of Group A Streptococcal Products on Cells and Tissues***

Streptococcal Product	*In Vitro* Effects	*In Vivo* Effects
Streptolysin S	Lyses erythrocytes, leucocytes, tumor cells, mesenchymal cells, and platelets by altering membrane permeability; kills leucocytes; releases enzymes from lysosomes; inhibits phagocytosis.	Intravascular hemolysis; necrosis of parenchymatous organs; induces arthritis and renal tubule necrosis.
Streptolysin O	Lyses erythrocytes, leucocytes, tumor cells, mesenchymal cells, and platelets by altering membrane permeability; causes systolic contraction of perfused heart; constricts coronary arteries in perfused heart; releases lysosome enzymes.	Lethal to mice and rabbits; myocardial necrosis; intravascular hemolysis; cardiotoxicity; provokes Shwartzman reaction; releases acetylcholine.
Streptokinase	Activates plasminogen to plasmin, which hydrolyzes various proteins; liberates chondroitin sulfate from collagen; activates complement components and generates permeability and chemotactic factors.	Enhances spread of infection.
Hyaluronidase	Hydrolyzes hyaluronic acid.	Acts as spreading factor and may enhance spread of infection; localizes in RES, kidney, and endocardium but does not cause lesions.
Deoxyribonuclease	Cleaves DNA.	May enhance multiplication of virulent streptococci.
Erythrogenic toxin	Cytotoxic in tissue culture; mitogenic.	Induces skin rash, probably by delayed hypersensitivity; pyrogenic; lethal to rabbits; causes myocardial necrosis; suppresses RES function; inhibits antibody formation; inhibits phagocytosis; increases host response to streptolysin O and endotoxin; causes carditis.
Hyaluronic acid	Antiphagocytic.	Enhances invasiveness of streptococci, inhibits attachment to peritoneal macrophages.
M antigen	Toxic to leucocytes and platelets; antiphagocytic.	Enchances invasiveness of streptococci; protective antigen of streptococci; may cause glomerulonephritis in rats by immune-complex formation; inhibits activation of the alternate complement pathway.
C-polysaccharide	Group antigen.	Causes granulomas when injected; with edestin, causes necrotic lesions of myocardium; cross-reacts with mammalian connective tissue antigens; in immune complex, causes toxic manifestations in animals.
Peptidoglycan†	Cell wall polymer.	Toxic manifestions in rabbits, including fever and necrosis; activates alternative complement pathway.
Lipoteichoic acid‡	Mediates attachment to epithelial cells.	Adhesin for attachment to mucosal surfaces; activates alternative complement pathway.

*Modified, in part, from I. Ginsburg, J. Infect. Dis. **126**:419–456, 1972.
†J. Greenblatt, R. J. Boackle, and J. H. Schwab, Infect. Immun. **19**:296. 1978.
‡E. H. Beachey, J. Infect. Dis. **143**:325, 1981; B. A. Fiedel and R. W. Jackson, Infect. Immun. **22**:286, 1978.

Antibodies to the M protein are, however, protective and persist for many years; their titer is increased by anamnestic response to the homologous M protein.

Differentiation must be made between immune response, in the sense of antibody formation, and effective immunity that prevents and/or modifies the infection or disease. In general, immunity to streptococcal infections is of low order, although some degree of immunity is indicated by recovery from and elimination of the infective agent in naturally occurring disease.

Unfortunately, such immunity as exists is type-specific, since it is associated with antibody to M antigen. The effective immune response is opsonic, and studies utilizing the phagocytic index and similar criteria show correlation between effective immunity and this humoral antibody. Effective immunity to streptococcus is, then, theoretically obtainable and has been reported following immunization with M protein vaccine,[11] but the multiplicity of M-types, coupled with the toxicity of native M proteins, presents many obstacles in practical and widespread prophylaxis.

INFECTIONS OF THE SKIN AND SUBCUTANEOUS TISSUES

Streptococcal infections of the skin are of two general types. Those which are superficial in nature, frequently with secondary staphylococcal infection, are termed streptococcal pyoderma, while the more deeply seated infections include erysipelas and wound infections. These two types are distinguished by their characteristic lesions and by their epidemiology.

Streptococcal Pyoderma[29, 35, 37]
This disease, also known as impetigo contagiosa, is a skin infection resembling chickenpox. It begins with a vesicular rash that rapidly becomes pustular. In the later stages, the lesions are covered over with a thick crust, and streptococci, often in pure culture, may be found in the fluid beneath the crust. As the lesion ages staphylococci appear as secondary invaders, but seem to contribute little to pathogenesis. The disease is endemic in the southern United States and in most tropical areas. Usually, the etiologic agent is a strain of β-hemolytic, group A streptococcus. A number of M-types seem to be associated with the disease, often those of higher number, e.g.,

M49 and M52 to M61. These are frequently referred to as pyoderma strains, since they seldom are encountered in streptococcal pharyngitis (see below). Many strains cannot be typed by known M antiserums and are generally identified by their T antigen pattern. Occasional outbreaks are caused by other streptococci, including groups G and C.

The disease is normally spread by close, direct contact between individuals; thus, several cases may appear in family groups or others living under crowded and unsanitary conditions. The microorganisms colonize the skin, usually in minute breaks or in skin lesions from other causes, such as scabies infestation and insect bites. Children are most often affected, with much higher incidence in the summer months.

Pyoderma usually results in an increase of type-specific antibodies to the causal strain; there is evidence, too, that pharyngeal carriage of pyoderma-causing strains may also induce a type-specific antibody response, and this may be a mechanism of acquired immunity. Pyoderma is accompanied by the appearance of antibodies to other streptococcal antigens. The antibody response to streptolysin O is not great, however, so that the ASO titration does not have the clinical significance in pyoderma that it has in pharyngeal infections. Serum antibody titers to DNAse B and hyaluronidase are, however, useful in retrospective diagnosis of pyoderma antecedant to acute glomerulonephritis.

The most serious complication of streptococcal pyoderma is acute glomerulonephritis, which sometimes follows the skin infection after two to three weeks. Acute glomerulonephritis as a poststreptococcal sequel is discussed later in this chapter. Rarely, if ever, does acute rheumatic fever follow skin infection with streptococci.

Erysipelas
The second kind of skin disease caused by S. pyogenes, erysipelas, is an inflammatory disease of skin and adjacent tissues that spreads in the subepidermal tissues, usually of the face and head, but occasionally in other areas of the body. It is somewhat more serious than streptococcal pyoderma, but is seen much less frequently. The etiological relationship of S. pyogenes to the disease is indicated by its presence, frequently in enormous numbers, in the lesions. There is some evidence that an attack of the disease is preceded by streptococcal infection of the throat or elsewhere in

the upper respiratory tract, and it has been found that some individuals have the same immunological type of streptococcus in the throat as in the skin lesions. It is possible that hypersensitivity may contribute to the pathogenesis of the disease.

Streptococci are not present in the central portion of the inflamed area, but are found on its periphery, and can be isolated most readily by excision of portions of the tissue, other methods rarely succeeding. In the skin they occur chiefly in the lymph spaces, which are often packed with them, and may be recovered by skin puncture as far as 3 cm. beyond the advancing edge of the lesion, where there is no gross evidence of inflammation. The hypothesis that the inflammatory reaction is due in part at least to erythrogenic toxins has been an attractive one, but it seems definitely established that there is no relation; immunization against erythrogenic toxin, for instance, in no way prevents or reduces the inflammatory reaction in erysipelas.

Wound Infection

Streptococcus pyogenes is occasionally the cause of suppurative infections of the skin following trauma. This organism is not normally present on the skin, and, in fact, normal skin has a bactericidal effect upon it, probably as a consequence of skin lipids such as oleic acid.[50] The relative rarity of infection of wounds by these bacteria is consistent with this, and streptococcal infection in most instances is a result of subsequent contamination by direct contact rather than of a primary infection. *Streptococcus pyogenes* may occur alone or in mixed infections with other pyogenic bacteria, such as *Staphylococcus*.

Cellulitis. Traumatic invasion of the skin and subcutaneous tissues may develop into an acute, spreading infection of the subcutaneous tissue with invasion of the muscle, giving rise to gangrenous myositis. The infection of the subcutaneous tissues may show little or no evidence of localization and is characterized by the formation of a seropurulent exudate. It tends to spread rapidly via the lymphatic tissues and generalize into septicemia. This kind of streptococcal infection has been termed cellulitis, and may result from *S. pyogenes* alone or, in the development of the gangrenous process, more often in mixed infection with anaerobic streptococci.

Chemotherapy

Although streptococcal skin infections are occasionally self-limited, their chronicity and the possibility of extension and secondary foci warrant antibacterial therapy. There are public health advantages, too, in reducing the infective reservoirs.

Topical treatment has included débridement, the use of antibacterial soaps, and topical antibiotic ointments. These are not particularly effective, however, and systemic antimicrobial therapy is much more efficacious in eliminating streptococci from the lesions. Parenteral benzathine penicillin is most effective, and oral penicillin or erythromycin somewhat less so. While these can effect clinical and bacteriological response, there is little evidence that they prevent poststreptococcal glomerulonephritis; they may, however, help to prevent spread of nephritogenic strains during epidemics.

INFECTIONS OF THE UPPER RESPIRATORY TRACT[37, 51]

As indicated earlier, the β-hemolytic streptococci occur most commonly as parasites and pathogens of the upper respiratory tract. By far the largest proportion of human disease caused by *S. pyogenes* results from infection of the upper respiratory tract and adjacent areas, symptoms arising not only from the acute infectious process, but also in connection with its complications and sequelae. The clinical character of the disease is determined by the relative prominence of the various results of the infection and, while seemingly different, is fundamentally the same. Thus, streptococcal pharyngitis or septic sore throat can become scarlet fever when the infecting strain of *S. pyogenes* produces erythrogenic toxin. Pharyngitis commonly extends into the tonsils or may be localized primarily there to give clinical tonsillitis; it may extend into the sinuses or middle ear to produce streptococcal sinusitis and otitis media, respectively; and by extension into the lungs results in bronchopneumonia of streptococcal etiology. Furthermore, late nonsuppurative complications of streptococcal infection include carditis, nephritis, and arthritis. While separation of β-hemolytic streptococcal infection into various clinical entities has some practical value, the basic infectious process is essentially the same.

Pharyngeal Infection

The β-hemolytic streptococci are responsible for an acute infection of the throat commonly known as **septic** or **streptococcal sore throat.** Epidemics of this disease appeared in the

United States and in England during the first decade of the present century. The immediate symptoms in these and subsequent epidemics have been strikingly similar and include an intense local hyperemia, with or without a grayish exudate, enlargement of the cervical lymph nodes, and usually fever. Rarely, extension of the infection into the lungs may occur, with resulting streptococcal pneumonia that may terminate in fatal septicemia. The disease, usually in a relatively mild form, is a common one, with the result that streptococci are now the most frequent bacterial agent causing primary sore throat.

The sequelae of streptococcal sore throat include those resulting from the extension of the infection into adjacent areas such as the sinuses and middle ear, and purulent, semichronic infections often develop. Streptococci also frequently persist in tonsillar crypts in a chronic type of infection that may flare up periodically in an acute form. Streptococcal tonsillitis, sinusitis, and otitis media are, then, a part of the pathology of hemolytic streptococcal infection of the throat. In addition to such extensions, secondary effects on other parts of the body are evident as carditis, nephritis, and arthritic involvement of the joints. The character of an epidemic is often recorded as percentage incidence of these various sequelae.

Streptococcal pharyngitis is most frequent in the 5 to 15 year age group. This group also shows high carrier rates, *i.e.,* the presence of β-hemolytic streptococci in the nasopharynx in the absence of overt disease. The highest incidence of infection occurs in the winter months, from December to May. Climatic conditions in the winter months frequently lead to crowded indoor living conditions, resulting in an increased number of close contacts that promote streptococcal spread.

Strains of *S. pyogenes* are for the most part responsible for the disease, although a small portion of the cases result from infection with streptococci of group C. There is reason to believe that so-called "epidemic strains" of high virulence and infectivity are often associated with epidemic disease.

It is probable that the infection is largely droplet- and airborne, but there is no doubt that in many instances direct contact is of considerable significance. It may also be transmitted occasionally through food and milk.

Scarlet Fever
Scarlet fever is a clinical entity because of the rash resulting from the action of the eryth-

rogenic toxin; otherwise it does not differ significantly from other streptococcal infections of the upper respiratory tract, and its sequelae are essentially the same.

While scarlet fever has declined in prevalence and severity since the turn of the century, it has behaved differently in different parts of the world. It increased in continental Europe after World War II and remained at high prevalence; in England and Wales it continued at a fairly constant level, but declined sharply in the same period in the United States and Canada.

The relationship of β-hemolytic streptococci to the disease was demonstrated by the reproduction of typical scarlet fever in human volunteers by inoculation of pure cultures, and by the demonstration of the existence of erythrogenic toxin. A conclusive demonstration of the etiological relation was required because of the contrast between the relatively lasting immunity to scarlet fever following recovery from an attack of the disease and the seemingly transient immunity to other streptococcal infections.

It is now established that immunity to infection by group A streptococci is type-specific and is associated with antibody to the M antigen. Immunity to the erythrogenic effects of the scarlatinal toxin is not associated with M-type and thus does not reflect resistance to infection *per se.* While the streptococci responsible for clinical scarlet fever are all members of group A, the ability to form erythrogenic toxin is not confined to any particular type within this group, although some types occur more frequently than others.

Immunity to erythrogenic toxin may be demonstrated by the **Dick test,** a skin test analogous to the Schick test in diphtheria; *i.e.,* the local erythema is due to the action of the toxin and is absent in the presence of circulating antitoxin. In this connection it is of interest that Schultz and Charlton earlier observed that when a scarlet fever patient with a bright red rash is injected with convalescent serum, the rash begins to fade after about six hours and soon disappears completely. The significance of this phenomenon, the Schultz-Charlton blanching phenomenon, was not recognized until the discovery of the erythrogenic toxin.

Chemotherapy
Streptococcal pharyngitis is essentially a self-limiting disease, subsiding within about five days. Rationale for chemotherapy is, therefore, related to the prevention of complications and sequelae, both suppurative and nonsup-

purative, rather than symptomatic treatment of the pharyngitis.

Penicillin is the antibiotic of choice to eliminate infecting streptococci. Penicillin-resistant strains are rare, and the microorganisms remain remarkably sensitive. Penicillin therapy, either oral or parenteral, administered for a period of 10 days eradicates the infection in 90 per cent or more of the cases, and is effective in preventing rheumatic fever. Orally administered erythromycin or clindamycin is also effective and may substitute for penicillin in allergic individuals. Other chemotherapeutic agents are seldom employed.

NONSUPPURATIVE SEQUELAE TO STREPTOCOCCAL INFECTION[39]

Rheumatic Fever [24, 31, 51]

As indicated earlier, some of the sequelae to β-hemolytic streptococcal infection are carditis and arthritic involvement of the joints. These are emphasized and assume a major role in the symptomology and pathology of the poststreptococcal, nonsuppurative inflammatory disease known as rheumatic fever or rheumatic heart disease. These sequelae follow streptococcal infection in about 3 per cent of cases in closed populations, but at a lower rate in the general population.

The most common manifestation of rheumatic fever is arthritis, which is of greater frequency in older age groups. The most significant lesion is carditis, which includes the connective tissue degeneration characteristic of the damaged heart valves and specific inflammatory myocardial lesions characterized histologically by nodular collections of cells known as Aschoff nodules. Carditis is more frequent in younger age groups.

The epidemiological association between streptococcal pharyngitis and rheumatic fever has long been recognized. The relationship is now regarded as etiological, a view that is reinforced by evidence of immunological response to streptococcal infection that accompanies rheumatic fever. Rheumatic fever does not occur, for example, in the absence of significant antibody response as measured by rising antibody titers to streptolysin O, DNAse, or hyaluronidase.

The streptococcal infection antecedant to rheumatic fever is almost always streptococcal pharyngitis; seldom, if ever, does rheumatic fever follow streptococcal pyoderma. The onset of rheumatic fever does not necessarily coincide with acute streptococcal disease. Three stages are recognized; first, an acute streptococcal infection of the nasopharynx; second, a latent or quiescent period during which streptococci may remain in the throat; and third, the stage in which electrocardiographic changes appear and symptoms of acute rheumatic fever are observed. The average time between the pharyngeal infection and onset of rheumatic fever is 18 to 19 days, with a range from one to five weeks. Throat cultures are often negative by the time the third stage is reached. It was the temporal lag between the first and third stages, along with the fact that the primary infection is sometimes asymptomatic, that delayed recognition of the etiological association of streptococci with rheumatic fever.

Subsequent attacks of the disease may result from reinfection with streptococci and, occasionally, follow nonspecific febrile events.

Since it is not always possible to find streptococci in the throat of rheumatic fever patients, and earlier streptococcal infection is sometimes uncertain, the clinician must rely heavily upon immunological procedures such as antistreptolysin O, anti-DNAse B, antifibrinolysin, and antihyaluronidase titers as diagnostic aids.

Since clinical rheumatic fever occurs some time after infection, antibiotic therapy is without effect in modifying the attack. Most authorities, however, recommend the use of penicillin at this time to eradicate any residual streptococci. Control of subsequent or secondary episodes of rheumatic fever is effected by chemoprophylaxis. Penicillin, in the repository form, is the drug of choice; sulfonamides and oral penicillin are less effective. The time over which prophylaxis must be continued is uncertain, but most agree that five years after the last episode is minimal, and consideration should be given to environmental and other variables.

The mechanism whereby streptococci induce rheumatic fever is not at all clear. The possibility that one or more of the toxins discussed earlier could be responsible has always had a degree of plausibility, but precise causal relationships have not been established. Indeed, antibodies are induced to many of these substances, such as streptolysin O, erythrogenic toxins, and hyaluronidase, but are apparently without protective effect in the disease. Theories of immunological damage are now more popular. There is considerable evidence that streptococci and their products induce a hypersensitive state; for instance, joint pains are often produced in rheumatic patients by inoculation of sterile streptococcal filtrates and have followed immunization with purified M protein antigen. The possibility that autoimmunity may be involved in the pathogenesis of rheumatic fever is increasingly evident. Observed antigenic similarities between streptococci and host tissue components could result in production of antistreptococcal antibodies that lead to autoimmune damage to the heart. Streptococci are known to possess at least four such cross-reactive antigens that are components of streptococcal cell walls and cell membranes; circulating antibodies to these antigens are encountered in rheumatic fever patients. The precise role of autoimmune mechanisms in the pathogenesis of rheumatic fever is not yet resolved, but the plausibility is obvious.

Acute Glomerulonephritis[12, 36]

The association of acute glomerulonephritis with streptococcal infection has been known for many years; it was first associated with scarlet fever in 1836.

Like rheumatic fever, it is a nonsuppurative sequel to streptococcal infection, usually pyoderma, and generally follows this infection within 10 days to two weeks. It is characterized by hematuria, fluid retention and edema, and hypertension. The latter may give rise to secondary effects of headaches and nausea, as well as circulatory congestion.

The poststreptococcal attack rate, in contrast to that of rheumatic fever, is highly variable and extremes of 0.03 and 18 per cent have been reported. The disease may occur in epidemic form, especially in children, suggesting variable temporal and geographic distribution of nephritogenic strains of S. pyogenes.

The group A streptococci that are associated with glomerulonephritis, the **nephritogenic strains,** are those generally causing pyoderma and are usually the higher numbered M serotypes. Some of these are of greater importance in both prevalence and geographic distribution. Thus, types 2, 49, 57, 59, and 60 are the principal M serotypes causing pyoderma-nephritis. In a few instances, pharyngeal strains are nephritogenic, particularly types 1 and 12. Glomerulonephritis is not, however, an invariable sequel to infection with nephritogenic strains; it is estimated that the attack rate usually ranges from 1 to 10 per cent of infections. Other than association with serotype, nephritogenic strains of S. pyogenes cannot be differentiated from those which are not associated with kidney disease.

As in rheumatic fever, immunological response to the originating infection is of clinical importance in patients with suspected glomerulonephritis. Antistreptolysin O titers are generally low or absent following pyoderma, however, and significance is most often attached to increases in anti-DNAse B and antihyaluronidase titers.

The pathogenesis of poststreptococcal glomerulonephritis is generally thought to be immunologically mediated by the deposition of immune complexes in the glomeruli. The nature of the streptococcal antigens involved is controversial, but in some cases appears to be M protein or M-associated proteins. There is no evidence that these deposits result from immunological cross-reactions between tissue and streptococcal antigens. Since complement is activated by the immune complexes, damage to the glomeruli probably results from complement-mediated lysosomal exocytosis by polymorphonuclear phagocytes.

GROUP B STREPTOCOCCI[20, 27, 57]

The streptococci that possess the Lancefield group B antigen are placed in a single species, *Streptococcus agalactiae.* These bacteria are important animal pathogens, causing bovine mastitis; in veterinary microbiology they occupy a position analogous to the group A streptococci in human infections. Although occasional human infections with S. agalactiae were encountered earlier, it was not until the late 1960s that their importance in human disease became evident.

It is now clear that S. agalactiae is a part of the indigenous microbial flora of humans, appearing in the vagina, urethra, and gastrointestinal and upper respiratory tracts of healthy adults; in these populations it is probably circulated by sexual intercourse. In adults, these bacteria may, on rare occasions, be responsible for upper respiratory infections, meningitis, bacteremia, endocarditis, and a variety of other infections. Their pathogenicity is, however, more evident in neonates, in whom they are often responsible for meningitis and undifferentiated septicemia.

Differentiation

As noted earlier, the group B streptococci are morphologically indistinguishable from other members of the genus. Colonies may be somewhat larger than those of S. pyogenes, however, and sometimes display an orange or red-brown pigmentation, particularly under anaerobic conditions. Most, but not all, strains are β-hemolytic on sheep blood agar, but the hemolysin is different from streptolysins S and O; hemolysis zones are usually smaller and slightly different from those of group A strains.

Apart from immunological differences, the group B streptococci may be separated from other human strains of streptococci by the **CAMP test.** In this reaction, group B strains produce an extracellular protein factor[4] that sensitizes red cells to the action of staphylococcal β-hemolysin (Fig. 15–4); other physiological reactions are listed in Table 15–1.

Antigenic Structure

In addition to the group B carbohydrate, *S. agalactiae* strains are separated into serotypes on the basis of capsular polysaccharide antigens. These were originally designated types I, II, and III. Type I is now further divided into Ia, Ib, and Ic, whose specificity is attributable to both polysaccharide and protein capsular antigens. Thus the principal group B serotypes are now Ia, Ib, Ic, II, and III, and about 95 per cent of the group B strains are typable by these antigens. Some strains, particularly from cattle, possess additional protein antigens, designated R and X, but these are not a part of the typing scheme.

It is clear that the serotyping scheme, with only five serotypes, is not as discriminating as the M-typing used with *S. pyogenes*. A phage typing system has been proposed that should offer improved discrimination for epidemiological investigations.[52]

Antibodies to the type-specific antigens are protective, probably acting as opsonins, through complement activation by the classical pathway.[47]

Extracellular Products

Like group A streptococci, the group B strains produce several biologically active extracellular products. These include hemolysins, CAMP factor, deoxyribonuclease, hyaluronidase, protease, and neuraminidase. Erythrogenic toxins do not appear to be produced by these bacteria.

It has already been noted that the group B hemolysins are different from those produced by group A strains. Similarly, deoxyribonucleases and hyaluronidase are serologically different in *S. agalactiae*.

Virulence[14]

The virulence factors operative in *S. agalactiae* infections are even more obscure than those in group A infections. Adherence of group B streptococci to epithelial cells is known, but the nature of the adherence factors is not yet established, and the influence of extracellular products on pathogenesis is still speculative. Only the type-specific antigens are known to affect virulence. They are capsular antigens inhibiting phagocytosis and antibodies are protective against the homologous type, probably by opsonic action.

Epidemiology

Group B streptococci are a part of the indigenous microbial flora of many adult humans, yet overt disease is a rare occurrence in these populations. The common sites of colonization in adults are the vagina, particularly in pregnant females; the urethra of both sexes; and the rectum; they are less often found in the pharynx. The prevalence of colonization varies widely, but most studies indicate vaginal colonization in nonpregnant women is usually under 10 per cent, while as many as one-quarter of pregnant females harbor the organism. One-fourth to one-half of the male partners of carrier women also exhibit urethral colonization. Thus, the adult infection appears to be sexually transmitted.

The greatest importance of group B streptococcal disease is in the newborn. Infants are infected by direct maternal transmission *in utero,* during birth, or soon thereafter by nosocomial transmission. The great majority of infants born of culture-positive mothers become colonized; a significant number of infants from culture-negative mothers also become colonized in the nursery or at home soon after birth. About one per cent of infants that are colonized develop disease. Currently, the serotypes involved in these infections seem to be about equally distributed.

Since these organisms are frequently the etiological agents for mastitis in cattle, there arises the possibility of transmission from animals to man.[5] This remains unresolved, but there is yet no convincing evidence that such transmission is epidemiologically significant.

Perinatal Infections

Group B streptococcal disease of the newborn is categorized as either early- or late-onset disease. The **early-onset** type is thought to be due to infection *in utero* or during vaginal passage and is ordinarily a critical illness. The disease appears within 24 hours of birth, but can be delayed up to a week. The primary infection site is the lungs, presumably infected by aspiration of infected maternal secretions. The respiratory infection is often followed by septicemia and meningitis.

Late-onset disease is probably most often acquired in the nursery or home and, therefore, appears late, usually 7 to 10 days after birth, but sometimes much later. It is not so severe as early-onset disease, and is more varied in clinical appearance. Although the fatality rate is lower than that of early-onset disease, there is a high incidence of residual effects, often of a neurological nature.

The mortality in these infections is usually extremely high, about 50 per cent. Even with early penicillin therapy, the more severe type may have a 30 per cent fatality rate. This has led to proposals to reduce the incidence by immunization, administration of antibiotics to culture-positive mothers during labor, and immediate antibiotic prophylaxis to children born of colonized mothers. Whether these will prove effective, or even feasible, remains to be determined.

OTHER STREPTOCOCCAL GROUPS

The majority of human infections with β-hemolytic streptococci are caused by group A and B streptococci, but group C is sometimes involved. The α-hemolytic, nongroupable streptococci, casually referred to as viridans streptococci, have limited pathogenic potential for humans, and they are often involved in wound infections, endocarditis, and abscess formation; certain species are related to dental caries formation.

Group C Streptococci

The streptococci of group C include several species that are primarily animal pathogens, viz., *Streptococcus equi, S. equisimilis, S. dysgalactiae,* and *S. zooepidemicus.* These may be responsible for rare human infections similar to those caused by *S. pyogenes,* but there is no evidence that they are responsible for rheumatic fever or glomerulonephritis.

Group D Streptococci

The streptococci that possess the Lancefield group D antigen are more heterogeneous than those discussed previously. The group D species normally grow at higher temperatures (45°C.) and hydrolyze bile-esculin. Those that occur as normal inhabitants in the intestinal tract of man, known as enterococci, includes *S. faecalis, S. faecium, S. durans,* and *S. avium;* these are distinguished by higher salt-tolerance (Table 15–1). There is considerable deviation, too, in hemolysis. Many strains are nonhemolytic; hemolytic strains usually exhibit α-hemolysis; but some strains of *S. faecalis* and *S. durans* are β-hemolytic.

Group D streptococci may be regarded as opportunistic pathogens. They are often found in causal relationship to subacute bacterial endocarditis (see below) and in urinary tract infections. They do not cause pharyngeal infections, though they are sometimes found in the respiratory tract. Interestingly, it has been suggested that an association exists between *S. bovis* endocarditis, or colonization, and adenocarcinoma of the colon.[26]

The separation and identification of the enterococci has some significance in that they are resistant to penicillin; thus, infections by these must be treated with other antibiotics, such as vancomycin or streptomycin-penicillin combinations.

Oral Streptococci[17]

The α-hemolytic and nonhemolytic streptococci of the normal oral flora do not fall within any single Lancefield group; indeed, several do not possess a defined group carbohydrate, whereas strains of some species may exhibit one of several group antigens. As expected, they are quite heterogeneous and their common characteristic is occurrence in the normal oral microflora; even in this ecological niche, however, they tend to colonize different tissues and the ecosystem is very complex. *Streptococcus salivarius,* for example, colonizes the dorsum of the tongue and is found in saliva; *S. mutans* and *S. milleri* are found in gingival crevices and in dental plaque; the remaining species, *S. sanguis* and *S. mitis (mitior),* are found in varying numbers in dental plaque, saliva, and gingival crevices and on the surface of the tongue. Their colonization sites are probably determined by specific adhesin-receptor interactions as described in Chapter 12. The physiological characters of these bacteria are listed in Table 15–1.

Current interest in the oral streptococci centers largely upon their role in the oral ecosystem and the association between *S. mutans* and dental caries. These ecological relationships are more fully discussed in Chapter 37. In the present context, it is the systemic infective capacity of oral streptococci that is of interest. Several of the oral streptococci, principally *S. mutans, S. sanguis,* and *S. milleri,* have been found, apparently in causal relationship, in gingival abscesses. Of even greater significance is the association of several species, especially *S. mutans* and *S. sanguis,* with subacute bacterial endocarditis; *S. milleri* may also be associated with suppurative infections, including abscesses and peritonitis.[34]

These and the other so-called viridans streptococci are not highly invasive, and the infections that lead to subacute infective endocarditis (see below) usually result from entry of the organism into the circulatory system, followed by colonization on damaged cusps of the heart valves. The oral streptococci probably enter the bloodstream following periodontal infections, tooth extractions or other dental treatment, brushing, or even vigorous chewing. These organisms probably do not effectively colonize healthy heart valves, but can establish an infective focus if the valves are damaged. It has been suggested that heart valve adherence is mediated by glucans on the bacterial surface, exopolysaccharides which are produced in considerable quantities by both *S. mutans* and *S. sanguis.* In this connection, it is interesting that *S. bovis,* a group D streptococcus, is also frequently a causal agent in endocarditis and that it, too, produces glucans.

SUBACUTE BACTERIAL ENDOCARDITIS[40]

Infections of the heart valves leading to subacute bacterial endocarditis may occur with many kinds of bacteria. By far the most common are the α-hemolytic, or viridans, streptococci. Staphylococci, $gb-hemolytic streptococci, gonococci, meningococci, *Haemophilus, Brucella,* and *Salmonella* are found in similar infections, but with these more highly virulent bacteria, the infection is generally acute, rather than subacute. Table 15–7 shows the agents found to be responsible for infective endocarditis in one study.

The infection of the heart valves may be primary or secondary to an infection focus elsewhere in the body. It is generally accepted that healthy heart valves are not usually colonized, but bacterial colonization and lesions develop when there is predisposition by congenital abnormality or prior valvular damage, as by rheumatic fever. The source of infection is usually the tonsils or other pharyngeal infection, periapical infection of the teeth, or low-grade infection of the gingiva or other sites.

Table 15–7. **Agents of Infective Endocarditis***

Microorganism		% of Total
Streptococci		
Viridans streptococci		50
Streptococcus mitis (mitior)	36%†	
Streptococcus sanguis	25	
Streptococcus mutans	7	
Streptococcus milleri	4	
Streptococcus salivarius	1	
Streptococcus bovis	27	
Unclassified	1	
Streptococcus faecalis		7
β-Hemolytic streptococci		1
Streptococcus pneumoniae		1
Total streptococci		58
Staphylococci		
Staphylococcus aureus		15
Staphylococcus epidermidis		11
Total staphylococci		26
Other (diphtheroids; gram-negative bacilli; fungi; etc.)		13
Culture-negative		3

*Isolated from 243 patients with infectious endocarditis at the New York Hospital (New York, N.Y.) during the period 1970–1978. Data from R. B. Roberts, *et al.,* Rev. Infect. Dis. **1**:955, 1979.

†Percentage of patients with viridans streptococcal endocarditis from whom indicated species was isolated.

There seems to be an occasional leakage of streptococci from these foci, and disturbance of an infected area, as by tooth extraction, tonsillectomy, or manipulation of an infected cervix, results in transient bacteremia. Although the bacteria are rapidly removed from the bloodstream by phagocytic cells, some may escape this defense and become adherent to abnormal or damaged heart valves.

The bacteria may establish in small platelet thrombi on the valvular surface and convert this initial lesion into the vegetation that characterizes bacterial endocarditis. They are, under these circumstances, sheltered from phagocytic destruction by deposits of platelets and thrombi. The lesion continues to develop, with progressive damage leading to valvular perforation or destruction. In the absence of appropriate antimicrobial therapy, the disease is almost always fatal.

Despite the sanctuary afforded by the structure of the vegetation, bacteria are more or less constantly shed from the lesion, resulting in continuous bacteremia. It is probably an indication of their low virulence that they are unable to establish secondary foci at other sites in spite of their continuous shedding into the bloodstream.

The Pneumococci[38]

The bacterium most commonly found in pneumonia in humans is a small lanceolate diplococcus, casually known as pneumococcus. The formal name assigned to this microorganism is *Streptococcus pneumoniae*, recognizing its close relationship to the streptococci discussed above. The characteristics of pneumococcal disease, as noted earlier, warrant separate discussion from other streptococcal diseases.

Of the generally recognized anatomical types of pneumonia, that classified as lobar pneumonia is nearly always due to the pneumococcus, although other bacteria are occasionally involved. The pneumococcus is by far the most prevalent single bacterial agent in pneumonia and in otitis media in children.

Morphology and Staining[6]

The pneumococcus is typically a small, slightly elongated coccus, one end of which is pointed or lance-shaped. They usually appear as pairs, or diplococci, but variation in size, form, and cellular arrangement are frequently observed. Chain formation is common, especially in laboratory cultures, although the chains are usually shorter than those of *S. pyogenes*. Pneumococcus is nonmotile and asporogenous. In exudates, a well-defined capsule appears to envelop the diplococci, but is less readily demonstrable in cultured strains, unless they are grown in mediums containing blood or serum.

These microorganisms are readily stained by aniline dyes and are typically gram-positive. There is, however, a tendency to become gram-negative in older cultures, since the integrity of the cell wall is lost by autolysis (see below). In stained preparations, particularly from exudates, the capsule is seen as an unstained halo surrounding the cells, as demonstrated in Figure 15–6. Alternatively, the capsule itself may be stained by special methods.

Colonies of pneumococcus on infusion or blood agar are typically small, moist, translucent, and granular, with well-defined margins. On some mediums, large amounts of capsular polysaccharide give the colonies a mucoid appearance. On blood agar, they are typically α-hemolytic, yielding colonies that are indistinguishable from those of the α-hemolytic streptococci described earlier; a few strains exhibit β-hemolysis when grown under anaerobic conditions. Cellular and colonial morphology are illustrated in Figure 15–7.

Physiology

The nutritional requirements for growth of pneumococci are complex. Some strains may grow sparsely on ordinary nutrient agar, although most do not. Infusion mediums, particularly when supplemented with blood, support good growth. A number of semisynthetic mediums have been developed that contain protein hydrolysates supplemented with additional amino acids, vitamins, and growth factors such as choline, purines, and pyrimidines. Nutritional studies utilizing these mediums have revealed widely different requirements among strains.

Pneumococci grow over a relatively narrow temperature range, 25°C. to 42°C., with an optimum of 37°C. They are sensitive to variations in pH from the optimum of 7.8, with pH limits of 6.5 to 8.3. Like other streptococci, they are aerobic and facultatively anaerobic.

In general, a variety of sugars are fermented, with production of large amounts of lactic acid;

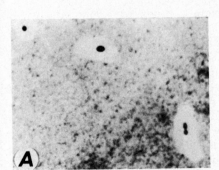
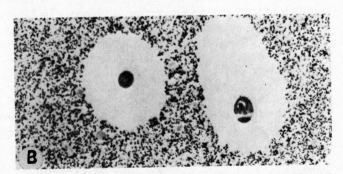

Figure 15–6. Capsules of *Streptococcus pneumoniae* prepared by the India ink technique. *A,* Light photomicrograph (toluidine blue; × 1500); *B,* transmission electron photomicrograph (× 9000). The capsule is seen as a halo surrounding the cell. (Reprinted from J. Infect. Dis. **140**:605–609, 1979, by M. A. Melly, *et al.,* by permission of the University of Chicago Press. Copyright 1979 by the University of Chicago.)

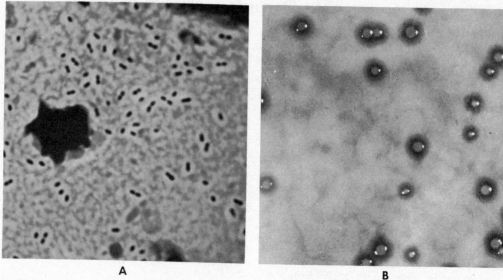

Figure 15–7. *A,* Pneumococcus in the peritoneal fluid of a mouse. Note the capsules. Fuchsin; × 2200. *B,* Colonies of the pneumococcus on blood agar. The areas of green hemolysis have been accentuated in the photograph. × 3.

they are therefore homofermentative. Fermentations are not, however, of great utility for differentiation.

Pneumococci are structurally delicate organisms and autolyze much more readily than most kinds of bacteria. **Autolysis** results from the activity of autolysin, *N*-acetylmuramyl-L-alanine amidase. This enzyme, produced by the bacteria, solubilizes the peptidoglycan of the cell wall.[19] Associated with the autolytic process is the lysis of pneumococci by bile and bile salts, in which the autolysin is activated by these substances; heat-killed cells, for example, are not lysed by bile salts. Sodium lauryl sulfate and other detergents also cause dissolution of pneumococcal cells.

Bile solubility is sufficiently constant in pneumococci that it can be used to separate them from other α-hemolytic streptococci. Other differential characteristics include inhibition by optochin and their greater virulence for mice.

Peroxide is produced by pneumococci in culture and accumulates after prolonged incubation because of the lack of catalase in these bacteria. This, coupled with their sensitivity to peroxide, results in autosterilization of cultures kept in the incubator for several days. They may be preserved, however, by storage in the refrigerator or by lyophilization.

Pneumococci are more sensitive to the usual antiseptics and disinfectants than are many other bacteria. Soaps, such as sodium ricinoleate and sodium oleate, are bactericidal in concentrations as low as 0.004 per cent; disinfectants such as phenol and mercuric chloride are also highly effective in destroying these bacteria.

Toxins

The severe intoxication observed in human pneumococcal infections suggests toxin formation by these bacteria. Despite countless searches, however, no toxin has yet been described that explains this syndrome.

Nevertheless, some products formed by these microorganisms exhibit toxic activity. A filterable hemolysin, called **pneumolysin**, accounts for the α-hemolytic activity on blood agar. Pneumolysin is lytic for sheep, guinea pig, and human erythrocytes, and reportedly has lethal and dermonecrotic properties in animals. It has been purified and the kinetics of hemolysis determined.

Leucocidin is produced, along with a necrotizing substance, similar to that formed by some staphylococci. Many strains produce hyaluronidase, especially when cultured in the presence of hyaluronic acid. A purpura-producing substance, described by a number of workers, has recently been purified and characterized. Upon injection into albino mice the substance induces purpura, with discoloration of the skin of the feet, tail, ears, and nose. The purpura-producing principle is probably a high-molecular-weight, nonimmunogenic cleavage product of cell wall peptidoglycan formed by action of the pneumococcal autolysin.[7, 8]

Antigenic Structure

Although *S. pneumoniae* is not accorded group status in the Lancefield scheme, they share a common somatic antigen, a choline phosphate–containing teichoic acid of the cell wall, which is immunologically identical in all strains. It is frequently referred to as C-substance.

Pneumococcus Types. Unlike *S. pyogenes,* wherein types are differentiated on the basis of the M protein surface antigens, pneumococcal types are distinguished by their immunologically specific capsular carbohydrates, sometimes called **soluble specific substance,** or **SSS.** Eighty-three types of pneumococcus are now recognized, and the biochemical nature of several of the type-specific polysaccharides has been established. They also contain envelope proteins, similar to M antigens of *S. pyogenes,* but these are not used for typing. The presence of capsules usually masks agglutination by antibody to cell wall and protein antigens, so that antiserums to the capsular carbohydrate are sharply type-specific.

There are two different nomenclatures for pneumococcal types. That used in the United States assigns consecutive numbers to the types in the order of discovery; in the Danish system, serologically related types are grouped together as subtypes. For example, U.S. types 6 and 26 are equivalent to Danish types 6A and 6B, respectively, and are serologically related, but not identical.

The serological typing of pneumococcus may be carried out in several ways. Typing is not a routine diagnostic procedure, but has great utility in epidemiological studies. The typing methods are of three kinds: (1) agglutination of encapsulated cells with type-specific antiserum, (2) precipitin reaction of capsular polysaccharide with type-specific antiserums, and (3) the **Quellung reaction.** In the last method, encapsulated bacteria are mixed with antiserum and a small amount of methylene blue. Microscopic observation reveals an apparent marked swelling of the capsule in the presence of its homologous antiserum, but not with heterologous antiserums.

Virulence and Host Defenses[18, 22, 58]

The early steps in infection and pathogenesis by *S. pneumoniae* are topics of current research interest. Colonization of the mucous membranes of the upper respiratory tract is well known, and is undoubtedly related to the high carriage rate in healthy individuals, as discussed below. Adherence of *S. pneumoniae* to pharyngeal cells has been reported; adherence capacity is greatest in strains associated with otitis media and those from healthy carriers.[1] Their capacity to maintain association with mucous membranes may also be related to the production, by virulent *S. pneumoniae,* of an immunoglobulin A1 protease that cleaves IgA.[30]

Penetration of tissues from colonization sites on mucous membranes undoubtedly takes place, but by mechanisms yet obscure. In spite of this, the interplay of bacterial virulence factors and host defenses is beginning to emerge. The several toxic factors produced by *S. pneumoniae* may contribute to virulence, since preparations containing these factors reportedly increase the invasive capacity of relatively avirulent pneumococcal strains when injected simultaneously with the bacteria. Yet, virulence of pneumococci is directly dependent not upon toxic factors, but upon the polysaccharide capsule that interferes with phagocytosis; it is the capsule that is the primary aggressin in these bacteria. Loss of the capsule renders pneumococci susceptible to phagocytosis and, thus, avirulent.

Host resistance to infection depends upon the rapid clearance of the invading microorganism by phagocytic cells, since *S. pneumoniae* are rapidly killed after ingestion. Host resistance is, therefore, dependent upon activation of the complement system, which in turn promotes phagocytosis (see Chapter 12).

In the nonimmune host, the alternative complement pathway is activated by the teichoic acids of the pneumococcal cell wall; the pneumococcal polysaccharides probably are not able to activate this pathway. In immune hosts, pneumococci activate the classical pathway when they are sensitized by antibody directed against their capsular substance. Since activation of the classical pathway requires capsular-specific antibody, it occurs either late in the disease after antibody synthesis has begun or upon subsequent infection with the same capsular type.

In either activation pathway, complement component C3b is the active factor in promoting phagocytosis, but its effectiveness in this regard is dependent upon several variables. The most important of these is the location of C3b on the bacterial surface. When C3b is activated by the alternative pathway, it apparently is fixed to the subcapsular surface of the bacterial cell. In this location, the capsule acts as a physical barrier to the recognition of C3b by phagocytes, and the opsonizing effect of

C3b is diminished or lost. Classical pathway activation, on the other hand, results in the generation of C3b that associates with antibody at the capsular surface, where it is recognized by phagocytes and ingestion ensues. Therefore, activation of the classical pathway by specific capsular antibody is much more effective in promoting opsonization and serves as the theoretical basis for immunization, discussed below. Alternative pathway activation is less effective in this regard, but may promote phagocytosis if large amounts of C3b are formed; different pneumococcal strains differ in this respect, and those which activate large amounts of C3 are more effectively opsonized and are, thereby, less virulent.

It is appropriate to note the possible effects of these host responses in the pathogenesis of pneumococcal infection. As mentioned above, such infections are characterized by an apparent toxemic reaction. It seems likely, but it has not yet been proved, that activation of complement and action of phagocytic cells may give rise to inflammatory tissue injury. For example, the activation of C3a and C5a complement components stimulates the release of histamine and serotonin. C5a is also chemotactic and stimulates the release of enzymes and toxic oxygen metabolites from neutrophils; these substances are also released during the ingestion of bacterial cells. There is, then, potential for tissue injury during those processes that accompany the defensive host responses to pneumococcal infections.

Variation

The **smooth** and **rough variants** that are found in a number of bacteria are also observed in S. pneumoniae. As in other cases, there are various intermediate colonial types between the two extremes, and the pneumococcus is virulent in the smooth form and almost completely avirulent in the rough form. The change from smooth to rough is reflected in the microscopic morphology of the cells as a loss of capsule, emphasizing its importance as an aggressin.

Since type specificity is determined by the capsular polysaccharide, the loss of capsule is accompanied by a complete loss of type specificity; the somatic antigen then predominates and, irrespective of original type, the pneumococci become immunologically identical. The dissociative change may be reversed, although with difficulty, by animal passage or by cultivation of the rough strains in anti-R immune serum. The R form may also be converted to a smooth form by cultivation in the presence of heat-killed cells from a smooth culture. This conversion is an example of **transformation**, first accomplished with pneumococci, and one of the most important early findings in microbial genetics, as discussed in Chapter 6.

Drug Resistance.[55] Since it was first used in 1940, penicillin has served as an effective chemotherapeutic agent in pneumococcal infections. Until 1967, almost all strains were sensitive to less than 0.05 μg./ml. of penicillin; subsequently, moderate levels of penicillin resistance began to appear in a few strains, first in Australia, then in other parts of the world. These strains were sensitive to about 1.0 μg./ml. or less of penicillin, and most infections could still be treated with penicillin, albeit with larger doses. Resistance to tetracycline and a few other antibiotics had been noted earlier, but multiple antibiotic resistance was rare. In 1977, S. pneumoniae strains appeared in South Africa that were resistant to high levels of penicillin (2 to 10 μg./ml.). These also had similar levels of resistance to other β-lactam antibiotics, and some showed multiple antibiotic resistance. Interestingly, resistance to β-lactam antibiotics was not due to β-lactamases.

Although strains with high resistance to penicillin are rare, and largely confined to Africa, there is evidence of spread to other parts of the world, including the United States.

Pathogenicity for Man[25]

Pneumococcal infections are among the leading cause of deaths throughout the world; particular vulnerability attaches to the very young and the elderly. The clinical syndromes associated with S. pneumoniae infections are many and varied, but pneumonia, otitis media, meningitis, and septicemia are the most prominent, as illustrated in Table 15–8.

Carriers. Pneumococci are strict parasites and are not found in the environment. They are found, however, in the upper respiratory tract of a significant number of healthy carriers. Transmission of disease is favored by high carriage rates in the population and by such environmental factors as crowding and the prevalence of other respiratory diseases, including viral infections.

Carriage rates are highest in the very young, and many infants are colonized within hours of birth. Numerous studies indicate that about one-third of preschool children are colonized by S. pneumoniae, with somewhat lower carriage rates in children from 6 to 12 years of

Table 15–8. **Estimated Occurrence of Serious Pneumococcal Disease in the United States***

Pneumococcal Disease	Estimated Cases (thousands/yr)	Estimated Incidence†	Case/Fatality Ratio (%)
Pneumonia	150–570	68–260	5–7
Meningitis	2.6–6.2	1.2–2.8	32
Bacteremia	16–55	7–25	20

*Morbidity Mortality Weekly Report **30**:411, 1981.
†Per 10^5 population/year.

age. Adolescent children and adults exhibit still lower rates of colonization, usually less than 10 per cent. The carrier state is not permanent, but is rather sporadic and intermittent; many persons may carry the bacteria for a short time, particularly during episodes of other upper respiratory infections. There is some seasonal fluctuation, with lower rates during the summer months.

Colonization is not, then, a predictor of overt disease, yet the reasons why some individuals are colonized while others develop disease are unknown. Susceptibility to overt infection may be related to the virulence of the colonizing strain but is more often due to an array of predisposing factors that include viral infections of the upper respiratory tract, other systemic disease, severe or sudden exposure to cold, fatigue, splenic disfunction, alcohol consumption, inadequate nutrition, or advanced age. Children with sickle cell disease are particularly susceptible to infection with pneumococci. Conversely, resistance is to be associated with a state of physiological well-being.

Pneumonia. The precise incidence of pneumococcal pneumonia in the United States is not known, but it is estimated that about one-half million cases occur annually, with an overall mortality rate of 5 to 10 per cent. The elderly are especially susceptible, particularly those with intercurrent infection or with pre-disposing factors noted above; the part played by pneumococcal pneumonia in the fatal termination of many diseases is, for example, well known.

Pneumococci are also a leading cause of pneumonia in children, most frequently during the second year of life. Bacteria are not confined to the lung, for they may be distributed hematogenously to other foci. Bacteremia is common and the microorganisms may be recovered by blood culture, even when the clinical signs of pneumonia are equivocal. The prognostic value of blood cultures is recognized, and in most instances both the case fatality rate and the incidence of complications are considerably higher when bacteremia is present.

The case fatality rate in untreated pneumococcal pneumonia is relatively high, indicating the pathogenic potential of these bacteria once they are established in the tissues. There is, however, some variation in the invasive capacity of the serotypes. For example, types 6 and 14 are often present in childhood bacteremia and meningitis.

Meningitis. Pneumococcal meningitis is not so prevalent in the United States as that caused by *Haemophilus influenzae* and meningococci, but manifests a higher mortality rate, up to 40 per cent, even when appropriately treated with antibiotics (Table 15–9). Survivors display a high incidence of neurological sequelae, in-

Table 15–9. **Agents of Bacterial Meningitis***

Bacterial Agent	Number of Cases	Incidence†	Case/Fatality Ratio (%)
Haemophilus influenzae	1885	1.24	7.1
Neisseria meningitidis	1095	0.72	13.5
Streptococcus pneumoniae	456	0.30	28.2
Streptococcus agalactiae (Group B)	130	0.09	22.4
Listeria monocytogenes	68	0.04	29.5
Other	235	0.15	36.6
Unknown	212	0.14	16.7
Total	4081	2.69	13.6

*Reported to the Centers for Disease Control from 38 states in 1978. Morbidity Mortality Weekly Report **28**:277, 1979.
†Cases per 10^5 population.

cluding deafness, convulsions, and retardation. The disease most often affects children under one year of age, with peak incidence during the third to fifth month. Meningitis may represent a primary infection, or develops secondarily by hematogenous spread from a pulmonary focus. Although the predominant serotypes vary with time, types 6, 14, 18, 19, and 23 have been the most frequent recent isolates from childhood meningitis and bacteremia in the United States.

Otitis Media. Acute otitis media is one of the most widespread childhood infections; it is estimated that more than 70 per cent of children will suffer at least one episode by the age of three. The most frequent causative agent is *S. pneumoniae,* found in about one-third of the cases cultured. Peak incidence is in children six months to one year of age. Type 19 is the principal serotype responsible for otitis media in the United States, but types 3, 6, 14, and 23 are also prevalent.

It is likely that primary otitis media is derived from microorganisms present in the nasopharynx, which pass through the eustachian tube to the middle ear; alternatively, the infection can be secondary to other foci.

Bacteriological Diagnosis[15]

Streptococcus pneumoniae is usually isolated by culture or animal inoculation from clinical specimens such as sputum, pleural exudate, blood, spinal fluid, or pus. Primary culture is normally on blood agar plates, although some specimens, such as blood, may require enrichment in infusion broth. Blood agar is the preferred medium for preliminary identification, since colonies develop within 24 hours and α-hemolysis is easily seen. The techniques for isolation and identification are essentially those employed for streptococci. Differentiation from viridans streptococci is not possible by colonial and microscopic morphology, but pneumococci are distinguished by bile solubility and optochin sensitivity, as well as by immunological means. The physiological reactions of *S. pneumoniae* are shown in Table 15–1. Virulence may be determined by intraperitoneal inoculation into mice; with virulent strains, the animal shows signs of illness in 5 to 8 hours, and microscopy of peritoneal exudate reveals large numbers of encapsulated diplococci.

Although complete serotyping of pneumococcal isolates is not routinely performed, commercial typing serums are available for epidemiological studies, if required. More often, isolates are tested, usually by the Quellung test, with polyvalent pooled antiserums to establish identification as *S. pneumoniae.*

The isolation and identification of *S. pneumoniae* as an aid in diagnosis of pneumococcal infection is necessarily slow. To overcome this deficiency, serological methods have been proposed to permit the rapid and accurate detection of pneumococcal polysaccharides in sputum, serum, and urine as an indicator of infection.[28]

Chemotherapy[55]

Until recently, *S. pneumoniae* had been uniformly and markedly sensitive to penicillin. In the mid-1960s, a few strains were recovered that exhibited moderate levels of resistance (see above, Drug Resistance). Nevertheless, most infections by these still responded to penicillin therapy. The appearance of highly resistant forms in South Africa aroused concern about the future usefulness of penicillin in these infections. Fortunately, the vast majority of isolates have remained fully sensitive; moderately resistant strains represent a small portion of circulating *S. pneumoniae,* averaging fewer than 5 per cent in most areas.

Antibiotic sensitivity testing of isolates has not, therefore, been routine, but the possibility of highly resistant strains has prompted recommendations for such testing in serious infections, or those not responding to therapy. It should be noted that penicillin susceptibility, as measured by zone size in the Kirby-Bauer technique, is not appropriate for pneumococci, although methacillin or oxacillin disks can be used for screening purposes. Accurate penicillin susceptibility testing requires the more cumbersome tube dilution methods to establish minimum inhibitory concentrations.

Pneumococci are often encountered that are resistant to other antibiotics, tetracycline in particular, but this has not yet been of great clinical importance. There is concern, however, regarding the occasional appearance of multiple resistance patterns, including strains resistant to (1) penicillin and tetracycline, (2) penicillin, tetracycline, and chloramphenicol, and (3) penicillin, tetracycline, chloramphenicol, erythromycin, and clindamycin (and sometimes rifampicin). Thus far, isolates with greatest resistance have been those found in Africa.

Bacteremic infections due to moderately penicillin-resistant pneumococci may be successfully treated by high-dose parenteral therapy, since achievable blood levels of antibiotic exceed the resistance levels of these strains.

Therapy of meningitis caused by these is less successful, however, reflecting the difficulty of achieving inhibitory antibiotic levels in spinal fluid. Therapy with alternative antibiotics, selected on the basis of resistance patterns, is required in such infections or in those due to highly resistant strains.

Immunity[2, 46]

Immunity to pneumococcal infection is associated with antibody against the capsular polysaccharide and, as indicated previously, involves complement activation and subsequent opsonization of the bacterial cells. The hallmark of immunity is, therefore, antibody with type-specificity to the polysaccharide antigen.

Active immunization of humans to pneumococcal infection has been of interest since mass inoculation studies in 1918–1919 suggested its usefulness. The multiplicity of capsular types and effective chemotherapy, however, inhibited the development of prophylactic vaccines. Therapeutic use of specific antiserums, however, found widespread application between the two world wars; serum therapy, based on serological typing of the infecting strain, was of great practical importance until the introduction of effective chemotherapeutic agents in the early 1940s. Nevertheless, passive immunotherapy established the protective capacity of type-specific capsular antibody.

Continued high incidence of pneumococcal disease in both children and the elderly, coupled with the appearance of drug-resistant strains, led to the development of a new polyvalent pneumococcal vaccine in the late 1970s. Based upon the serotypes most frequently found in adult infections, a pneumococcal vaccine was licensed in the United States in 1977, which contains purified capsular polysaccharides from the 14 most prevalent pneumococcus types (Table 15–10). The types represented in the vaccine are responsible for about 70 per cent of pneumococcal infections in the United States. In immunized populations the vaccine is said to protect against 70 to 90 per cent of disease due to these types. Although not yet resolved, there is the possibility that protection may extend to serologically related types that are not present in the vaccine.

Immunization with the vaccine is believed to enhance the resistance to serious disease by humoral antibody response. It does not, however, effectively reduce the nasopharyngeal

Table 15–10. **Pneumococcal Types Represented in the Current Polysaccharide Vaccine**

American Nomenclature	Danish Nomenclature
1	1
2	2
3	3
4	4
6	6A
8	8
9	9N
12	12F
14	14
19	19F
23	23F
25	25
51	7F
56	18C

colonization rate by the pneumococcal types represented in the vaccine. This probably denotes a less effective mucosal antibody response. Although the vaccine induces a significant antibody response in most individuals, the levels of antibody are sometimes transient, particularly against certain serotypes. Moreover, reimmunization is not to be recommended, since antibody levels are not significantly boosted and adverse reactions are commonplace.

Although the view is sometimes challenged, it is generally believed that the vaccine offers protection against the severe effects of pneumococcal disease in certain high risk groups, *e.g.,* the elderly, particularly in closed populations such as nursing homes, and those predisposed by chronic disease, impaired splenic function, chronic alcoholism, sickle cell disease, and leukemia. The vaccine is not recommended, however, for children under two years of age. Thus, immunoprophylaxis is not yet achieved for the group at greatest risk.

REFERENCES

1. Andersson, B., *et al.* 1981. Adhesion of *Streptococcus pneumoniae* to human pharyngeal epithelial cells in vitro: differences in adhesive capacity among strains isolated from subjects with otitis media, septicemia, or meningitis or from healthy carriers. Infect. Immun. **32**:311–317.
2. Austrian, R. 1977. Prevention of pneumococcal infection by immunization with capsular polysaccharides of *Streptococcus pneumoniae:* current status of polyvalent vaccines. J. Infect. Dis. **136**(Suppl):S38–S42.
3. Beachey, E. H. 1981. Bacterial adherence: adhesin-receptor interactions mediating the attachment to mucosal surfaces. J. Infect. Dis. **143**:325–345.

4. Bernheimer, A. W., R. Linder, and L. S. Avigad. 1979. Nature and mechanism of action of the CAMP protein of group B streptococci. Infect. Immun. **23**:838–844.

5. Brglez, I. 1981. A contribution to the research of infection of cows and humans with *Streptococcus agalactiae.* Zentbl. Bakt. I **172B**:434–439.

6. Buchanan, R. E., and N. E. Gibbons (Eds.). 1974. Bergey's Manual of Determinative Bacteriology. 8th ed. Williams & Wilkins Co., Baltimore.

7. Chetty, C., and A. Kreger. 1980. Characterization of pneumococcal purpura-producing principle. Infect. Immun. **29**:158–164.

8. Chetty, C., and A. Kreger. 1981. Role of autolysin in generating the pneumococcal purpura-producing principle. Infect. Immun. **31**:339–344.

9. Clewell, D. B. 1981. Plasmids, drug resistance, and gene transfer in the genus *Streptococcus.* Microbiol. Rev. **45**:409–436.

10. Cunningham, C. M., and D. W. Watson. 1978. Suppression of antibody response by group A streptococcal pyrogenic exotoxin and characterization of the cells involved. Infect. Immun. **19**:470–476.

11. D'Alessandri, R., et al. 1978. Protective studies with group A streptococcal M protein vaccine. III. Challenge of volunteers after systemic or intranasal immunization with type 3 or type 12 group A *Streptococcus.* J. Infect. Dis. **138**:712–718.

12. Dillon, H. C., Jr. 1979. Post-streptococcal glomerulonephritis following pyoderma. Rev. Infect. Dis. **1**:935–943.

13. Duncan, J. L. 1975. Streptococcal toxins. pp. 257–262. *In* D. Schlessinger (Ed.): Microbiology—1975. American Society for Microbiology, Washington, D.C.

14. Durham, D. L., et al. 1981. Correlations between the production of extracellular substances by type III group B streptococcal strains and virulence in a mouse model. Infect. Immun. **34**:448–454.

15. Facklam, R. R. 1980. Streptococci and aerococci. pp. 88–110. *In* E. H. Lennette, et al. (Eds.): Manual of Clinical Microbiology. 3rd ed. American Society for Microbiology, Washington, D.C.

16. Freeman, R. 1971. Streptococcal infection in a large general hospital. J. Clin. Pathol. **24**:300–313.

17. Hamada, S., and H. D. Slade. 1980. Biology, immunology, and cariogenicity of *Streptococcus mutans.* Microbiol. Rev. **44**:331–384.

18. Horwitz, M. A. 1982. Phagocytosis of microorganisms. Rev. Infect. Dis. **4**:104–123.

19. Howard, L. V., and H. Gooder. 1974. Specificity of the autolysin of *Streptococcus (Diplococcus) pneumoniae.* J. Bacteriol. **117**:796–804.

20. Jelínková, J. 1977. Group B streptococci in the human population. Curr. Topics Microbiol. Immunol. **76**:127–165.

21. Johnson, L. P., P. M. Schlievert, and D. W. Watson. 1980. Transfer of group A streptococcal pyrogenic exotoxin production to nontoxigenic strains by lysogenic conversion. Infect. Immun. **28**:254–257.

22. Johnson, R. B., Jr. 1981. The host response to invasion by *Streptococcus pneumoniae:* protection and the pathogenesis of tissue damage. Rev. Infect. Dis. **3**:282–288.

23. Joseph, R., and G. D. Shockman. 1976. Autolytic formation of protoplasts (autoplasts) of *Streptococcus faecalis:* location of active and latent autolysin. J. Bacteriol. **127**:1482–1493.

24. Kaplan, M. H. 1979. Rheumatic fever, rheumatic heart disease, and the streptococcal connection: the role of streptococcal antigens cross-reactive with heart tissue. Rev. Infect. Dis. **1**:988–996.

25. Klein, J. O. 1981. The epidemiology of pneumococcal disease in infants and children. Rev. Infect. Dis. **3**:246–253.

26. Klein, R. S., et al. 1977. Association of *Streptococcus bovis* with carcinoma of the colon. New Engl. J. Med. **297**:800–802.

27. Knox, J. M. 1979. Group B streptococcal infection. A review and update. Brit. J. Vener. Dis. **55**:118–120.

28. Leach, R. P., and J. D. Coonrod. 1977. Detection of pneumococcal antigens in the sputum in pneumococcal pneumonia. Amer. Rev. Resp. Dis. **116**:847–851.

29. Leyden, J. J., R. Stewart, and A. M. Kligman. 1980. Experimental infections with group A streptococci in humans. J. Invest. Dermatol. **75**:196–201.

30. Male, C. 1979. Immunoglobulin A1 protease production by *Haemophilus influenzae* and *Streptococcus pneumoniae.* Infect. Immun. **26**:254–261.

31. McCarty, M. 1981. An adventure in the pathogenic maze of rheumatic fever. J. Infect. Dis. **143**:375–385.

32. McKane, L., and J. J. Ferretti. 1981. Phage-host interactions and the production of type A streptococcal exotoxin in group A streptococci. Infect. Immun. **34**:915–919.

33. Mukasa, H., and H. D. Slade. 1972. Chemical composition and immunological specificity of the streptococcal group O cell wall polysaccharide antigen. Infect. Immun. **5**:707–714.

34. Murray, H. W., et al. 1978. Serious infections caused by Streptococcus milleri. Amer. J. Med. **64**:759–764.

35. Nelson, K. E., et al. 1976. The epidemiology and natural history of streptococcal pyoderma: an endemic disease of the rural southern United States. Amer. J. Epidemiol. **103**:270–283.

36. Nissenson, A. R., et al. 1979. Poststreptococcal acute glomerulonephritis: fact and controversy. Ann. Intern. Med. **91**:76–86.

37. Peter, G., and A. L. Smith. 1977. Group A streptococcal infections of the skin and pharynx. Parts 1 and 2. New Engl. J. Med. **297**:311–317; 365–370.

38. Quie, P. G., G. S. Giebink, and J. A. Winkelstein (Eds.). 1981. The pneumococcus. A symposium held at the Kroc Foundation Headquarters, Santa Ynez Valley, California, February 25–29, 1980. Rev. Infect. Dis. **3**:183–371.

39. Read, S. E., and J. B. Zabriskie (Eds.). 1980. Streptococcal Diseases and the Immune Response. Academic Press, London.

40. Roberts, R. B., et al. 1979. Viridans streptococcal endocarditis: the role of various species, including pyridoxal-dependent streptococci. Rev. Infect. Dis. **1**:955–966.

41. Sanders, C. C., G. E. Nelson, and W. E. Sanders, Jr. 1977. Bacterial interference. IV. Epidemiological determinants of the antagonistic activity of the normal throat flora against group A streptococci. Infect. Immun. **16**:599–603.

42. Schlievert, P. M., K. M. Bettin, and D. W. Watson. 1979. Reinterpretation of the Dick test: role of group A streptococcal pyrogenic exotoxin. Infect. Immun. **26**:467–472.

43. Schlievert, P. M., D. J. Schoettle, and D. W. Watson. 1980. Ganglioside and monosaccharide inhibition of nonspecific lymphocyte mitogenicity by group A streptococcal pyrogenic exotoxins. Infect. Immun. **27**:276–279.

44. Schlievert, P. M., and D. W. Watson. 1978. Group A streptococcal pyrogenic exotoxin: pyrogenicity, alteration of blood-brain barrier, and separation of sites for pyrogenicity and enhancement of lethal endotoxin shock. Infect. Immun. **21**:753–763.

45. Schmitt-Slomska, J., A. Boúe, and R. Caravano. 1972. Induction of L-variants in human diploid cells infected by group A streptococci. Infect. Immun. **5**:389–399.

46. Schwartz, J. S. 1982. Pneumococcal vaccine: clinical efficacy and effectiveness. Ann. Intern. Med. **96**:208–220.

47. Shigeoka, A. O., et al. 1978. Role of antibody and complement in opsonization of group B streptococci. Infect. Immun. **21**:34–40.

48. Simpson, W. A., and E. H. Beachey. 1983. Adherence of group A streptococci to fibronectin on oral epithelial cells. Infect. Immun. **39**:275–279.

49. Smyth, C. J., and J. L. Duncan. 1978. Thiol-activated (oxygen-labile) cytolysins. pp. 129–183. In J. Jeljaszewicz and T. Wadström (Eds.): Bacterial Toxins and Cell Membranes. Academic Press, London.

50. Speert, D. P., et al. 1979. Bactericidal effect of oleic acid on group A streptococci: mechanism of action. Infect. Immun. **26**:1202–1210.

51. Stollerman, G. H. 1975. Rheumatic Fever and Streptococcal Infection. Grune & Stratton, New York.

52. Stringer, J. 1980. The development of a phage-typing system for group-B streptococci. J. Med. Microbiol. **13**:133–144.

53. Wannamaker, L. W. 1979. Changes and changing concepts in the biology of group A streptococci and the epidemiology of streptococcal infections. Rev. Infect. Dis. **1**:967–975.

54. Wannamaker, L. W., and J. M. Matsen (Eds.). 1972. Streptococci and Streptococcal Diseases. Academic Press, New York.

55. Ward, J. 1981. Antibiotic-resistant Streptococcus pneumoniae: clinical and epidemiological aspects. Rev. Infect. Dis. **3**:254–266.

56. Watson, D. W., and Y. B. Kim. 1970. Erythrogenic toxins. pp. 173–187. In T. C. Montie, S. Kadis, and S. J. Ajl (Eds.): Microbial Toxins. Vol. III, Bacterial Protein Toxins. Academic Press, New York.

57. Wilkinson, H. W. 1978. Group B streptococcal infection in humans. Ann. Rev. Microbiol. **32**:41–58.

58. Winkelstein, J. A. 1981. The role of complement in the host's defense against Streptococcus pneumoniae. Rev. Infect. Dis. **3**:289–298.

59. Wittner, M. K. 1976. Antigenicity of the M proteins of group A hemolytic streptococci: further evidence for shared determinants among serotypes. Infect. Immun. **13**:634–642.

CHAPTER 16

Neisseria:
The Gram-Negative Cocci

The gonococcus and the meningococcus are the chief representatives of a small group of gram-negative diplococci classified in the genus *Neisseria*. Other members are usually nonpathogenic, but all typically colonize the mucous membranes of the mouth, upper respiratory tract, or genitourinary tract of man. In addition to *Neisseria*, the family Neisseriaceae comprises the genera *Branhamella, Moraxella,* and *Acinetobacter.* Both *Moraxella* and *Acinetobacter* sometimes inhabit the mucous membranes of humans, but they are not considered to be primary pathogens. They are usually distinguished from *Neisseria* by their coccobacillary morphology.

Branhamella rarely cause disease, but are opportunistic pathogens often found as commensals of the upper respiratory tract and are morphologically similar to *Neisseria*. These related microorganisms are briefly discussed later in this chapter.

As a practical matter, the pathogenic species, *Neisseria gonorrhoeae,* the gonococcus, and *N. meningitidis,* the meningococcus, must be differentiated from the nonpathogenic *Neisseria* and *Branhamella,* which similarly colonize mucous membranes. Differential characteristics of greatest utility are shown in Table 16–1.

The Gonococcus[30, 33]

Neisser in 1879 first called attention to the constant presence of a peculiar coccus in gonorrheal exudates. In cases of gonorrhea of recent origin this was the sole organism found; it occurred in urethral and vaginal discharges of ordinary gonorrhea and also in the exudate of conjunctivitis due to gonorrheal infection. Pure cultures of this organism were first isolated in 1885 and its etiological relation to gonorrhea demonstrated by inoculation of hu-

Table 16–1. **Differentiation of the Aerobic Gram-Negative Diplococci**

Species	Growth on MTM*	Acid from					Reduction of	
		Glucose	Maltose	Fructose	Sucrose	H₂S	NO₃	NO₂
Neisseria gonorrhoeae	+	+	–	–	–	–	–	–
Neisseria meningitidis	+	+	+	–	–	–	–	V†
Neisseria sicca	–	+	+	+	+	+	–	+
Neisseria subflava	–	+	+	V	V	+	–	+
Neisseria flavescens	–	–	–	–	–	+	–	+
Neisseria mucosa	–	+	+	+	+	+	+	+
Neisseria lactamica	+	+	+	–	–		–	+
Branhamella catarrhalis	V	–	–	–	–	–	+	+

*Modified Thayer-Martin medium.
†V = variable.

man volunteers. This bacterium, known generally as the gonococcus, is formally designated *Neisseria gonorrhoeae.*

Morphology and Staining

In stained preparations of gonorrheal exudates, gonococci usually appear within polymorphonuclear leucocytes as shown in Figure 16–1. Their typical appearance is that of coffee bean–shaped cells occurring in pairs with the flattened sides in juxtaposition. In stains prepared from pure cultures (Fig. 16–2), the cocci usually appear as oval or spherical cells occurring singly or sometimes aggregated in irregular masses, without the typical diplococcal arrangement. Transient tetrad arrangements sometimes appear in young cultures.

The gonococcus and other *Neisseria* are **gram-negative**, a staining characteristic that sets them apart from other pyogenic cocci and is of considerable differential value. Gonococci from young cultures stain evenly, while older cultures contain larger swollen forms that stain poorly. The latter forms are associated with loss of cell wall integrity brought about by the action of autolytic enzymes. L-forms are occasionally seen as either large, vacuolated round bodies or as smaller granular bodies.

The architecture of the gonococcal cell is similar to that of other gram-negative bacteria as detailed in Chapter 2. A thin peptidoglycan layer is found in the periplasmic space between the cytoplasmic and outer membranes; the outer membrane contains a number of anti-

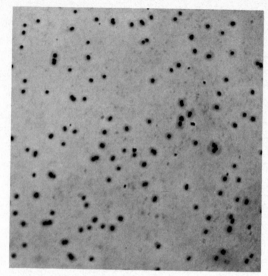

Figure 16–2. The gonococcus from pure culture. Fuchsin; × 1050.

genic proteins as well as lipopolysaccharides. Freshly isolated strains possess pili, or fimbriae, on their cell surface; pili are related to virulence and may also be responsible for a peculiar twitching motility that is sometimes observed. Newly isolated strains also exhibit a carbohydrate capsule that can be demonstrated by special techniques (Fig. 16–3); it is rapidly lost during *in vitro* cultivation unless special precautions are taken for its preservation.

Colonial Morphology. Colonies of *N. gonorrhoeae,* when viewed by ordinary transmitted light are small, translucent to grayish white, raised, and glistening (Fig. 16–4). Colonial appearance is, however, subject to variation, which depends upon virulence and the possession of surface pili and certain outer membrane proteins.

Differences in the colonial appearance of gonococci have been observed since the turn of the century, but these differences were not associated with virulence until the mid-1960s. Five distinct colonial types are recognized and designated types 1 through 5. Upon isolation from pathological processes, gonococci are almost always either type 1 or type 2. When observed by obliquely transmitted light, type 1 colonies are small, irregular, flattened, translucent, and golden; type 2 colonies are somewhat smaller, round, opaque, and raised with a slightly convex and uneven surface. Both have proved to be virulent when inoculated into human volunteers. Colony types 3, 4, and 5 usually arise after laboratory cultivation. They are distinguished by larger, flattened,

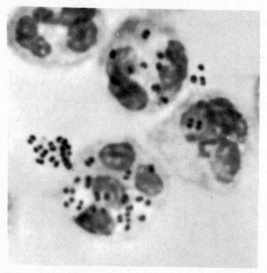

Figure 16–1. Urethral smear from gonorrhea patient. Note the intracellular and extracellular positions of the gonococci and their typical coffee-bean shape and arrangement in pairs. Gram stain; × 2400.

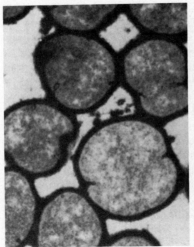
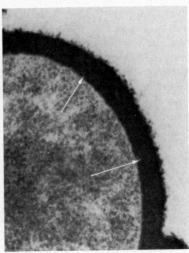

Figure 16–3. Electron photomicrographs of *Neisseria gonorrhoeae* showing thin capsules, demonstrated by staining *in situ* with alcian blue. *Left,* Most cells possess capsular material. × 27,000. *Right,* The capsular material is seen external to the outer membrane (arrows). × 81,600. (Reprinted from J. Infect Dis. **143**:796–802, 1981, by J. O. Hendley *et al.,* by permission of the University of Chicago Press. Copyright 1981 by the University of Chicago.)

and less colored colonies; they are generally considered to be avirulent for man, although type 5 has some virulence, as assayed in chick embryos.[18] Virulence and colonial type are also correlated with the presence of **pili.** Virulent types 1 and 2 are piliated, but these organelles are lacking in the avirulent varieties. Although their presence is correlated with colonial morphology, pili are not believed to be directly responsible for the colonial appearance. Their role in virulence is discussed below (see Virulence, p. 419).

A second type of colony variation, not related to possession of pili, is detected by differences in color and opacity of the colonies. Colonies that are dark colored and opaque by transmitted light are characterized by a high degree of cellular aggregation within the colony and by the possession of a unique, heat-modifiable protein in their outer membrane, termed the **colony opacity-associated** protein, or hmP$_{OP}$. Lighter colored and translucent colonial variants exhibit lesser cellular aggregation and lack the opacity-associated protein in the outer membrane.[43] It has been suggested that piliated translucent variants are more virulent than piliated opaque forms.[38]

As noted earlier, gonococci are occasionally seen as L-forms. Under appropriate conditions of osmotic stabilization, such cell wall–defective bacteria are isolated from infections, and grow as typical L-phase colonies. The significance of spontaneous or antibiotic-induced L-forms in the etiology of gonorrheal infections is uncertain.

Physiology

Gonococci are among the most nutritionally fastidious bacteria, particularly upon primary isolation. Complex and rich mediums are employed for isolation and cultivation, including chocolate (heated blood) agar or some variation containing additional enrichment as described later in the section on bacteriological diagnosis.

Despite their complexity in growth requirements, some strains may be subcultured on tryptic digest–glucose agar containing added cystine, since cysteine or cystine is required by all *N. gonorrhoeae;* relatively complex synthetic mediums have also been devised. Stock strains are commonly less exacting than those recently isolated.

Strains of *N. gonorrhoeae* may be typed by

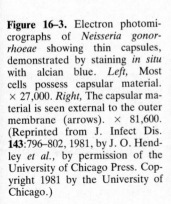

Figure 16–4. Colonies of the gonococcus on blood agar. × 6.

evaluating their nutritional requirements, a procedure that is called **auxotyping.**[7] Growth patterns of individual strains are observed on a series of synthetic mediums with addition or deletion of nutrients, such as amino acids and vitamins. Auxotypes so identified are more constant than serotypes and have proved to be useful markers in epidemiological studies.

Physical conditions for growth of the gonococcus are of considerable importance. A sufficient supply of moisture is essential, and the incubation atmosphere must be kept saturated with water. Gonococci also require increased CO_2 tension for initiation of growth, although this requirement usually diminishes upon continued subculture in the laboratory. Carbon dioxide tension of 3 to 10 per cent is generally supplied for primary isolation; the requirement for both moisture and CO_2 may be satisfied by incubation in candle extinction jars. In certain mediums, the gaseous CO_2 requirement can be replaced by incorporating sodium bicarbonate into the medium. Although gonococci grow scantily under anaerobic conditions, they are essentially aerobic in character. The optimum growth temperature for these bacteria is around 37° C., with some strain variation. The minimum temperature for growth is near 25° C. and the maximum is 41° C.

Even under laboratory conditions, gonococci are difficult to preserve, tending to autolyze readily in older cultures held at 37° C. and less readily at room temperature; they are best preserved by storage in the cold.

The gonococcus is a delicate microorganism. It is readily killed by moderate temperatures and by dilute disinfectants; 1 per cent phenol, for example, kills in 1 to 3 minutes. It is remarkably sensitive to certain flavin dyes and is rapidly destroyed by silver salts.

The microorganism is sensitive to drying, and under ordinary conditions survives exposure in the environment for only a few hours; this may be extended somewhat under humid conditions. In dried urethral exudates, gonococci may survive for a day or so, but rarely longer. It is clear, therefore, that gonococci do not long remain viable and infective when free in the environment, a characteristic of considerable importance in the epidemiology of the disease.

The gonococcus is not very active biochemically. Glucose is fermented, principally to lactic acid, but most other sugars are not attacked. Glucose fermentation, and the failure to ferment maltose, distinguish it from other *Neisseria* (Table 16–1). The fermentative reactions are generally reliable, provided the basal medium used supports growth of the microorganism. Cystine-tryptic digest agar is the usual choice for this purpose.

In common with other neisseriae, gonococci produce both catalase and indophenol oxidase; the latter characteristic has been turned to practical differential use as the **oxidase test.** Colonies of bacteria forming indophenol oxidase turn a bright purple color when sprayed with a 1 per cent solution of tetramethyl-*p*-phenylenediamine, as demonstrated in Figure 16–5. Other *Neisseria* and a few gram-negative bacilli also yield positive oxidase reactions, but only the latter will grow on the selective me-

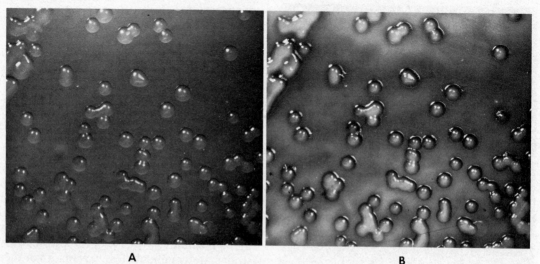

A   B

Figure 16–5. The oxidase test for the identification of gonococcus colonies. Pure culture on blood agar. *A,* Gonococcus colonies before the application of tetramethyl-*p*-phenylenediamine solution. *B,* The same colonies after the application of the reagent. Note the greater intensity of color about the edges of the colonies immediately after application and the discoloration of the medium. × 5.

diums employed for primary isolation of gonococci. Therefore, a positive oxidase reaction, coupled with examination of smears of typical colonies for gram-negative diplococci, offers presumptive evidence for *N. gonorrhoeae.*

Toxins

Other than a weak hemolysin, gonococci apparently form no extracellular toxic substance, but the cell substance is toxic to experimental animals on parenteral inoculation and has been reported to produce suppuration when instilled into the human urethra.

This toxicity is likely due to the presence of endotoxin, or lipopolysaccharide (LPS), present in the outer membrane of *N. gonorrhoeae.* It is similar to the LPS present in other gram-negative bacteria (see Chapter 12), and its pharmacological activity is overtly like that of other endotoxins, with lipid A being responsible for the toxicity. Although the role of LPS in the pathogenesis of gonococcal disease is uncertain, it has recently been shown to be responsible for fallopian tube mucosal damage in an organ culture system.[17]

Drug Resistance

Resistance of gonococci to chemotherapeutic agents is readily acquired under experimental conditions, and resistant strains have appeared in nature coincident with the general application of these drugs. When sulfonamides were introduced, 80 to 90 per cent of infections could be cured by them. Just over a decade later, as few as 15 per cent responded to sulfonamide therapy.

Meanwhile, penicillin therapy became available in the early 1940s and has since become the most widely used antibiotic in gonorrhea. Resistant strains did not appear until about 10 years after its introduction, but by the late 1950s, 20 per cent or more of strains in some areas were resistant to concentrations as much as 20 times those originally effective. The proportion of resistant strains continued to increase throughout most of the world until the late 1970s, when it apparently reached a plateau, and even declined, in the Scandinavian countries and other parts of Europe, the United Kingdom, and the United States. In other parts of the world, particularly Southeast Asia and the Western Pacific, the proportion of resistant strains continued to increase and has reached 100 per cent in some areas.

During these years, it was evident that penicillin resistance was not due to production of β-lactamase by the microorganism, and resistance levels could be overcome by the expedient of larger therapeutic doses.

In 1976, however, an alarming note was raised when strains of *N. gonorrhoeae* appeared that were resistant to penicillin by the mechanism of plasmid-mediated penicillinase production. A primary focus appeared to be East Asia, but by 1981 resistant strains were being isolated in most parts of the world; in some areas up to 19 per cent of isolates produce β-lactamase. In the United States, such strains are still rare—fewer than 1 per cent— and alternative treatment with spectinomycin has been effective in controlling these infections. It should be noted that penicillinase-producing strains that are also resistant to spectinomycin have been reported.[34]

Penicillinase production in resistant strains is specified by R plasmids that occur in one of two sizes (4.5 and 3.2×10^6 daltons). A large transfer plasmid (24.5×10^6 daltons), which occurs in the majority of strains harboring the larger R plasmid,[10] has been shown to transfer penicillin resistance at a frequency of 10^{-2} to 10^{-4} per recipient cell, indicating a possibility of natural transfer of resistance among gonococci by this mechanism.[36]

Resistance to other antibiotics has also been observed following their introduction. Resistance to streptomycin, tetracycline, and erythromycin has often paralleled that of penicillin, including the decline in resistance noted in some parts of the world in recent years.

Therapeutic failures with penicillin and other antibiotics are not always a consequence of antibiotic resistance of the infecting strain. Some cases may be refractory because of failure of the antibiotics to affect intracellular gonococci, which can be shown experimentally to survive concentrations of penicillin that are normally effective. Also, strains of moderate penicillin resistance bind considerably less drug than highly sensitive strains, thus requiring higher concentrations of penicillin for therapeutic efficacy. Certain treatment failures in urethritis may also be related to the occurrence of nongonococcal urethritis caused by organisms, such as *Chlamydia,* that are unaffected by the chemotherapeutic agent used.

Pathogenesis and Virulence [21, 43-46]

The highly infectious nature of gonococcal disease is unquestioned. More than one million cases are reported each year in the United States, transmitted primarily by sexual means. The virulence of gonococci is also demonstrated by the low dose required for infection;

only 1000 organisms instilled into the urethra is sufficient to lead to urethritis.

In the pathogenesis of gonorrheal disease, gonococci must first adhere to the mucosal surface, a process mediated either by pili, outer membrane proteins, or both. This attachment permits the gonococci to resist removal by shearing forces of urine and mucus flow. At this site, gonococci are also subject to the inhibitory effects of the normal bacterial flora. It has been found, for example, that growth of N. gonorrhoeae is inhibited by many of the bacterial species that constitute the normal flora of the human urogenital tract, including a number of anaerobes, streptococci, staphylococci, and lactobacilli.[29, 37] The presence of gonococcal capsules could also be expected to inhibit attachment, especially that mediated by outer membrane proteins, since they are masked by the overlying capsule. Pili, on the other hand, might penetrate the capsule to a degree sufficient to permit them to react with host cell receptors.

The initial interaction of adherent gonococci is with the microvilli of the columnar epithelium; they become enfolded in the villous processes and are brought into direct contact with the host cell surface (Fig. 16–6). Ciliated epithelium does not offer appropriate attachment sites, and stratified squamous epithelium is more resistant to penetration than columnar epithelium. Once bound to the epithelial surface, they are internalized by phagocytic processes and lie within the cytoplasm, enclosed in membrane-bound vesicles. Gonococci adherent to the mucosal surface elaborate toxic substances, probably lipopolysaccharides, that cause sloughing of adjacent cells, particularly nonciliated mucosal cells, which are not themselves infected.[17, 27]

Following ingestion by epithelial cells, the microorganisms reach subepithelial connective tissues, possibly through intracellular spaces, from which they spread by local extension or by transport in lymphatic or blood vessels. The characteristic tissue reaction is an intense inflammation with infiltration of polymorphonuclear leucocytes, plasma cells, and mast cells. Eventually these are replaced by fibrous tissue, and this fibrotic healing process is of considerable significance, particularly in urethral stricture.

Once within the tissues, the gonococci are subject to several of the host defenses, including normal serum bactericidal factors and phagocytes. Iron is essential for the growth of gonococci, and they must successfully compete

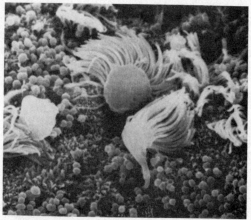

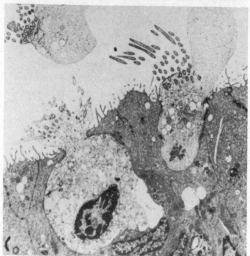

Figure 16–6. Human fallopian tube organ culture infected with *Neisseria gonorrhoeae* colony type 1 (piliated) cells. *Top,* Scanning electron micrograph showing gonococci attached almost exclusively to microvilli of nonciliated cells; mucosal damage is exemplified by two sloughing ciliated cells (center); intact ciliated cells are also shown (far right and top). × 3,126. *Bottom,* Transmission electron micrograph showing sloughing of ciliated cells from the mucosa or free in the lumen; no gonococci are attached to ciliated cells. × 3,600. (Reprinted from J. Infect. Dis. **143**:413–422, 1981, by Z. A. McGee, *et al.,* by permission of the University of Chicago Press. Copyright 1981 by the University of Chicago.)

for available iron in the host tissues. It is of some significance that strains causing disseminated gonococcal infection, as described in a later section, are considered to be more virulent, are usually serum-resistant, and have enhanced capacity to compete for iron.

Many gonococcal factors are probably active in the host-parasite interactions that result from gonococcal exposure, infection, and subsequent disease. The principal ones are listed in Table 16–2, although not all of these can be categorized as virulence determinants.

Table 16–2. **Gonococcal Mediators in Host-Parasite Interactions**

Mediator	Action
Capsule	Surface polysaccharide that inhibits phagocytosis; may interfere with pilus- or outer membrane–mediated adherence.
Pili	Gonococcal surface structures that mediate adherence to a variety of human cells; antiphagocytic; may promote penetration into epithelial cells; found in virulent colonial types 1 and 2; several serological types.
Protein I	Principal outer membrane protein; found in all gonococci; not trypsin sensitive; heat-modifiable; several serological types and are the major determinant of serological specificity; induce specifically protective and bactericidal antibodies; determinant of sensitivity or resistance to normal serum bactericidal activity.
Protein II (heat-modifiable protein, hmP)	Family of minor proteins of the outer membrane; trypsin sensitive; colony opacity proteins (hmP_{OP}) are responsible for cellular aggregation and optical appearance of gonococcal colonies and for sensitivity to normal serum bactericidins; leucocyte-association proteins (hmP_{LA}) promote gonococcal adherence to leucocytes and subsequent ingestion; some species enhance gonococcal adherence to certain epithelial cells.
Lipopolysaccharides	Outer membrane components that have endotoxin properties; probably responsible for some mucous membrane damage in infection; induce bactericidal antibodies.
Gonobactin	Hydroxymate siderophore that permits iron acquisition and assimilation by gonococci in host tissues.
IgA_1 Protease	Gonococcal enzyme that destroys certain IgA molecules and possibly interferes with antibody defenses at the mucosal surface.

The association of colonial morphology with the virulence of *N. gonorrhoeae* was mentioned earlier. Only colonial types 1 and 2 are found in disease and these are the virulent varieties that possess pili. The remaining colonial types result from variation in culture and are both nonpiliated and avirulent.

Because of high correlation with virulence, gonococcal pili have received most attention as the prime virulence determinant, being largely responsible for the binding or adherence of gonococci to mucosal and other eucaryotic cells. Pili, which appear in varying numbers on the cell surface, are 0.5 to 4 μm. in length and are 800 to 850 nm. in diameter. Figure 16–7 demonstrates the appearance of piliated and nonpiliated cells by electron microscopy. In some strains, two types of pili have been detected, designated α and β. The pilus protein in each is slightly different in molecular weight (19,000 and 20,500 daltons, respectively) and they have differing cohesive properties; α-pili bind to sialic acid-containing receptors on human cells and appear to confer greater virulence than β-pili.

Pilus-mediated binding is the principal mode of attachment of gonococci to a variety of cells and tissues, including erythrocytes, urethral and vaginal mucosal cells, fallopian tube organ cultures, buccal epithelial cells, and human sperm, as shown in Figure 16–8. The possibility that sperm can carry gonococci into the upper female genital tract is an intriguing aspect of their mode of spread.

For several years it has been the central dogma of gonococcal pathogenesis that their adherence to mucosal surfaces prevents mechanical removal of the bacteria from the epithelial cells and facilitates their later penetration, a function that is clearly associated with bacterial pili. In addition, piliated strains are more resistant to phagocytosis and are less likely to be destroyed after phagocytosis than are the nonpiliated, avirulent forms.

Yet the pathogenesis of gonococcal infection is obviously complex, and pilus-mediated adhesion must be only one of the host-parasite interactions that lead to disease. In this regard, a number of the outer membrane proteins may play a role in host-parasite interactions, as outlined in Table 16–2. Some of these may promote attachment to mucosa; others may render the gonococcus resistant to the bactericidal action of normal serum components; and others, as yet unidentified, are believed to mediate penetration into host cells. It is of

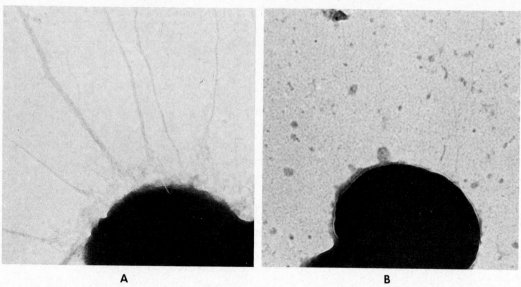

Figure 16–7. Pili of *Neisseria gonorrhoeae. A,* Type 1 gonococcus with pili. *B,* Type 4 gonococcus without pili. × 37,000. (Courtesy of Dr. Edwin Beachey.)

some interest that strains possessing the heat-modifiable protein responsible for aggregation and colony opacity (hmP$_{OP}$) are less virulent than those producing transparent colonies. Other possible virulence determinants include capsules, which inhibit phagocytosis; gonococcal siderophores, or gonobactin, which promotes iron utilization;[12] and IgA protease which cleaves IgA$_1$ and thereby interferes with this local defense mechanism at the mucosal surface.[2]

Some of these factors are not invariably correlated with virulence, *e.g.,* capsules are found in avirulent strains and pili are encountered in saprophytic neisseriae. This is not surprising, since virulence is multifaceted and is expressed only when all necessary factors are present and acting in concert.

Antigenic Structure[8]

The gonococci are of uncertain antigenic composition when assayed by conventional methods of antigenic analysis, such as agglutination and complement-fixation. It is apparent that they are antigenically heterogeneous and that they share antigenic determinants with certain other *Neisseria.*

Several of the antigenic components have been characterized and an antigenic mosaic has begun to emerge. The principal immunological components of the bacterial surface include pili and the proteins and lipopolysaccharides of the outer membrane. Many of these surface antigens participate in host interactions, as detailed in Table 16–2, and interest has centered on their roles in virulence and protective immunity, as well as the delineation of immunotypes that may aid in epidemiological investigations.

Because of their relationship to virulence, the pilus antigens of the gonococci have been of great interest. Pili from colonial types 1 and 2 are antigenically similar, but there is some antigenic heterogeneity among gonococcal strains. On the basis of these antigens, strains may be differentiated by hemagglutination inhibition reactions; these are sufficiently sensitive that shared antigenicity between strains is also apparent.[6] Indeed, gonococcal strains may be readily differentiated into pilus serotypes,

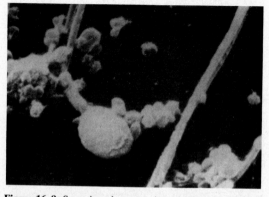

Figure 16–8. Scanning electron micrograph showing pilus-mediated attachment of *Neisseria gonorrhoeae* to human sperm head and tail. × 5800. (C. I. Gomez, *et al.,* Brit. J. Vener. Dis. **55**:245, 1979.)

using enzyme-linked immunosorbent assays (ELISA).[3] Purified gonococcal pili are immunogenic in humans, and antibody prevents adherence of homologous strains to human buccal epithelial cells.[26]

Aside from pilus antigens, the majority of the important antigens are located in the outer membrane of gonococcal cells. These have been extensively studied in recent years, and the antigenicity and function of these surface antigens are beginning to be understood. In common with other gram-negative bacteria, the gonococci possess lipopolysaccharides (LPS) in the outer membrane, as well as a variety of proteins.

The LPS of *N. gonorrhoeae* has not been so extensively studied as that of the Enterobacteriaceae, and some of the available information is contradictory. Nevertheless, it appears that LPS from gonococci contains both O-antigen polysaccharides and a core oligosaccharide region linked to lipid A. Studies on polysaccharides derived from gonococcal LPS indicate at least six serogroup-specific determinants, along with other determinants, some of which are common to all serogroups.[1] Antibody directed against LPS is bactericidal for gonococci.

Outer Membrane Proteins.[31, 44] The protein composition of the gonococcal outer membrane is relatively simple. Three classes of proteins, designated proteins I, II, and III, account for most of the total protein of the outer membrane, although a few other proteins have been reported; proteins I and II are best known. The significance of outer membrane components is emphasized by the observation that, in animal models, antibodies to outer membranes are protective against infection by homologous strains.

Protein I is the major outer membrane protein and accounts for most of the total protein of the membrane; it apparently occurs in all gonococcal strains. Protein I is the major determinant of serological reactivity in gonococci, and probably contributes strain-specific antigenic determinants; protein III may contribute cross-reactive determinants.[22] At least nine different serotypes of protein I have been recognized, with molecular weights of 36,000 to 39,000 daltons, and constitute the basis for one gonococcal serotyping scheme, employing the ELISA procedure.[5]

Protein II, comprising a family of minor outer membrane proteins, differs from protein I antigenically and in physicochemical properties and function, as shown in Table 16–2.

Although protein II varies in occurrence among different gonococcal strains, it undoubtedly contributes to the antigenic mosaic of these organisms.

In spite of recent progress, it is evident that much remains to be learned concerning gonococcal antigenic structure, including further knowledge of the immunoprotective antigens as well as a simplified and generally acceptable immunotyping scheme.

GONORRHEA

Gonorrhea is typically an infection of the mucous membranes of the genitourinary tract, although an accompanying anorectal infection is common in females. With few exceptions, the infection is spread by sexual contact and is therefore most commonly seen in sexually active young adults. Among these, groups at particularly high risk include prostitutes and homosexual males.

Gonorrhea in Males

Following an incubation period of 2 to 8 days, acute gonorrhea in males is characterized by urethritis accompanied by a profuse purulent discharge. Gonococci are present in these exudates in great number, usually within polymorphonuclear leucocytes. In the absence of complications, acute urethritis usually subsides within a few weeks; the individual remains infectious, however, and continues to shed gonococci, probably from infection of the prostate. Complications of gonorrheal infection in males includes epididymitis, chronic urethritis, prostatitis, and urethral stricture; infertility may result from epididymitis.

Most infections in males are symptomatic, *i.e.*, with urethritis and obvious urethral discharge. It is increasingly evident, however, that some portion of gonorrheal infections are mild or asymptomatic; the figure most often given is about 10 per cent, but in some populations, as many as 60 per cent of infections were without symptoms.[32] Such individuals may still transmit the disease, however, and they constitute a serious, but hidden, reservoir of infection.

In heterosexual males, gonorrhea is almost always an infection of the genitourinary tract; other sites are seldom invaded. Genitourinary disease is common in homosexual males, but extragenital infections are also manifest. The extragenital sites infected are most often the oropharynx and rectum.

Oropharyngeal infections are almost always asymptomatic, but may present as tonsillitis or pharyngitis resembling mild streptococcal pharyngitis in clinical appearance. The asymptomatic infections usually are self-limited and resolve without treatment. Oropharyngeal mucosa does not offer a particularly suitable site for colonization and these infections are not common, usually less than 10 per cent.

Rectal infections are more frequent, representing up to 50 per cent of the infections in homosexual males. About half of these are asymptomatic, the remainder presenting as proctitis, with varying degrees of severity.

Gonorrhea in Females

Gonococcal infection in women is more cryptic than in men. Following the incubation period there may be a mild and transient urethritis; infection of the cervix may give rise to a mucopurulent discharge that varies from mild to profuse. Anorectal infection in females often results from contiguous spread from the urogenital site of infection and occasionally produces proctitis. Pharyngeal infection can result from orogenital sexual practices, but is rare.

The primary infection in a large number of cases is asymptomatic and this is more common than in males. Such individuals are, however, carriers and can transmit the disease.

The most important complication of gonorrheal infection in women is acute pelvic inflammatory disease, with involvement of fallopian tubes, ovaries, and peritoneum. Gonococcal salpingitis is thought to result from ascending infection rather than from hematogenous spread; sterility can result from occlusion of the fallopian tubes.

Other Gonococcal Infections

When the gonococcus invades the blood stream from local lesions and is carried to various parts of the body, it gives rise to **disseminated infections** with a variety of extragenital lesions.[20] Disseminated infections, which include bacteremia, endocarditis, and arthritis, are more likely to appear after untreated primary infections and are more frequent in women, possibly because of the high incidence of asymptomatic, and therefore untreated, infections.

Gonococci seem to have special predilection for synovial membranes of the joints, where they cause gonococcal arthritis, often accompanied by skin lesions.

Since gonococci that cause disseminated infection must be hematogenously transported to extragenital sites, it is considered significant that strains responsible for such infections are usually resistant to the bactericidal action of normal serum, in contrast to those causing uncomplicated infections, which are usually serum-sensitive.

In infants, **conjunctivitis** is the most common manifestation. Gonococcal ophthalmia of the newborn is acquired from the infected mother; the infection may arise *in utero,* during birth, or by intimate contact after birth. Arthritis has also been observed in infants, the infection having been acquired *in utero* or during birth.[25] In preadolescent girls, vulvovaginitis is sometimes seen. It is most often contracted by close contact with infected mothers, by contaminated fomites, and by precocious sexual contact.

Epidemiology

Few diseases are so widely disseminated through all classes of society as gonorrhea. In the United States gonorrhea is now the most common, by a wide margin, of all reportable diseases, with more than 440 cases per 100,000 population, as shown in Figure 16–9; more than one million cases have been reported each year since 1976. However, these figures must be regarded as minimums, since most asymptomatic infections are not included and a high proportion of cases are probably not reported. The incidence of gonorrhea is even more striking in certain age groups. In 1980, the case rate reached more than 2100 per 100,000 in males between the ages of 20 to 24 years. Gonorrhea has assumed epidemic proportions in Europe, as well as in the United States, and effective control has proved to be an elusive goal.

Neisseria gonorrhoeae is a strict human parasite and infected humans constitute the sole reservoir. Adult infections are almost invariably the result of direct contact, usually sexual. Once infected, an individual may remain infective for long periods. Gonococci can persist in genitourinary secretions for years after apparently complete recovery and such persistent infections can be transmitted. Asymptomatic infection in both males and females constitute a particularly critical source of infection.

Gonorrheal vulvovaginitis sometimes occurs in epidemic form in little girls, with transmission effected by bedclothes, towels, and other fomites. Such epidemics are frequently exceedingly difficult to control and can pose a serious problem in institutions, such as children's wards in hospitals.

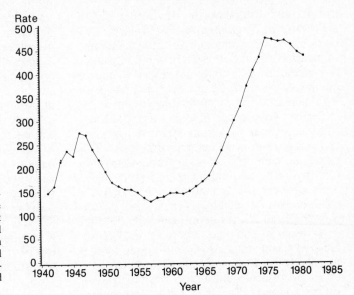

Rate

Figure 16–9. Reported case rates of gonor-rhea, United States, 1941–1980. Note the sharp increase after 1960 and the apparent leveling off of case rates after 1975, believed to be due to control programs initiated in 1973. (Centers for Disease Control, Annual summary 1981: reported morbidity and mortality in the United States. Morbidity and Mortality Weekly Report, **30**[54], 1982.)

Gonorrheal ophthalmia of the newborn is a well-known consequence of maternal infection and has been a significant cause of blindness in children. Infection is prevented by the pro-phylactic instillation of silver salts or antimi-crobial drugs into the eyes of the newborn.

Bacteriological Diagnosis[28]

A diagnosis of gonorrhea is established with certainty only by isolation and identification of *N. gonorrhoeae.* This assumes significance in view of the fact that a high proportion of cultures may show *Neisseria* other than gono-cocci. Also, nongonococcal urethritis may be more prevalent in certain groups than gonor-rhea, the condition being associated with other microorganisms, including *Chlamydia* and, possibly, mycoplasmas.

Specimens for culture are collected on cal-cium alginate swabs or, in the case of urethral specimens, by bacteriological loops. These may be cultured directly or if direct plating is not possible, they may be placed in appropriate transport mediums designed to protect these delicate microorganisms, since they rapidly lose viability under adverse environmental conditions.

Direct microscopic examination of exudates is often appropriate and informative. The dem-onstration of intracellular, gram-negative di-plococci in urethral smears from symptomatic males constitutes presumptive diagnosis. Di-agnosis on the basis of stained cervical smears in females is much less reliable, because of the presence of microorganisms easily confused with gonococci. Furthermore, gonococci may be few in number and not detectable by micro-

scopic examination in a substantial portion of infected females. Gram stains should also be performed on conjunctival exudates and joint fluids.

In pharyngeal infections, Gram stains are of little value, due to the frequent presence of commensal neisseriae that are morphologically indistinguishable from gonococci. Anorectal smears are difficult to interpret and are inform-ative only in homosexual males exhibiting mu-copurulent proctitis.

In culturing *N. gonorrhoeae,* the selection of appropriate mediums is exceedingly impor-tant. Specimens that are not expected to con-tain large numbers of contaminating microor-ganisms, including joint fluids or conjunctival swabs, may be inoculated onto a nonselective medium such as infusion chocolate agar. Ure-thral specimens or anorectal swabs are usually heavily contaminated, requiring the use of selective mediums.

Several excellent mediums are available that contain antibiotics to inhibit most contami-nants, including commensal neisseriae. Per-haps the most widely used is modified Thayer-Martin agar, consisting of an infusion choco-late agar base with nutritive supplement, and the antibiotics vancomycin, colistin, nystatin, and trimethoprim lactate. The medium devel-oped in the New York City Department of Health, NYC agar, also is an excellent medium with some added advantages, *viz.,* it is trans-parent and permits the growth of certain my-coplasmas that also can cause urethritis. The medium contains complex peptones, starch, yeast dialysate, hemoglobin, horse plasma, and the antibiotics vancomycin, colistin, amphotericin B, and trimethoprim. Unfortunately, a few strains of *N. gonorrhoeae* are inhibited by the vancomycin contained in these mediums. In practice, then, both selective and nonselective mediums are usually inoculated. Cultures are incubated at 37° C. in a humid atmosphere with increased CO_2, usually 3 to 10 per cent.

Typical gonococcal colonies are presumptively identified by Gram stain and oxidase test. Oxidase-positive colonies may be subcultured and identified by sugar fermentations in carbohydrate-containing cystine-tryptic digest agars or by rapid fermentation kits that are commercially available. Typical *N. gonorrhoeae* produce acid from glucose, but not from fructose, maltose, sucrose, or lactose. Isolated strains may also be confirmed by serological tests, as with specific fluorescent antibody or by coagglutination with *Staphylococcus aureus*. In the latter procedure, antigonococcal antibody is bound, by its Fc region, to protein A on *S. aureus* cells; when gonococci are mixed with these coated staphylococci, they react with the specific region of antibody to form mixed aggregates of cells.

Chemotherapy

A wide variety of chemotherapeutic agents are available for treatment of gonococcal infections. Except for infections due to penicillinase-producing *N. gonorrhoeae*, uncomplicated gonorrhea usually responds to single-dose therapy with aqueous procaine penicillin G combined with probenecid. Alternatively, multiple-dose therapy with tetracycline is usually successful. Other antibiotics that have been found effective include ampicillin, amoxicillin, erythromycin, and spectinomycin. Complicated gonococcal infections may require extended and more vigorous therapy; cases due to penicillinase-producing strains are usually treated with spectinomycin or cefoxitin.

Animal Models

Under natural conditions, the gonococcus is a strict human parasite, although some other primates may be experimentally infected. Clinical gonorrhea has been produced in chimpanzees by urethral inoculation of virulent gonococci from human exudates and may be successfully passed from infected to noninfected animals by artificial inoculation and by sexual transmission.

The gonococcus does not produce infection in common laboratory animals when given by ordinary routes, but a mouse model has been proposed in which animals are inoculated intravaginally. Although the infective dose required is large, histological changes in the uterus are similar to those found in human disease.[24] A guinea pig model, in which gonococci are grown in chambers implanted subcutaneously, has been extensively used, particularly in virulence and immunization studies; it is not suited, however, to studies of interactions between host cells and gonococci.

The chick embryo is also susceptible to infection with *N. gonorrhoeae* and has found wide application in studies on virulence. The virulence of colonial types in this model appears to parallel that observed in humans.

Each of these models has deficiencies, and it is apparent that knowledge of the pathogenesis of gonococcal disease suffers from the lack of a suitable animal model.

Immunity

The observation that repeated gonococcal infections may occur in the same individual and that acute infections may be superimposed upon old chronic infections suggests that little immunity is acquired as a result of infection. Failures in effective immune response are, however, thought to be at least partially related to antigenic differences between gonococcal strains. As discussed previously, there is antigenic heterogeneity in pilus proteins and in the outer membrane proteins. The importance of these antigenic differences in immunity have been established in experimental systems. For example, immunization of chimpanzees with *N. gonorrhoeae* results in strain-related protection against experimentally induced urethritis. Similarly, outer membrane preparations from different gonococcal strains are markedly protective against homologous strain challenge in guinea pigs, but yield only low levels of protection against a heterologous strain.[4] Immunization with purified pilus vaccines in human volunteers induces specific local genital antibody that blocks attachment of gonococci to human epithelial cells. The antibody response is largely strain specific, but there is evidence of cross-reaction with heterologous strains.[26]

It is plausible that a vaccine against gonococci, or some subunit of the cells, could offer protective immunity. Nevertheless, the antigenic heterogeneity of the protective antigens presents practical problems unless some protective antigen common to all or most strains is defined.

Some degree of immunological response during infection is evident. Genital secretions of infected individuals often possess antigono-coccal antibody, most often in the IgA and IgG classes. Based upon the mode of pathogenesis, it seems probable that a secretory IgA response could play a role in effective immunity at the mucosal surface by inhibiting gonococcal adherence.

Systemic antibody response is also evident in infected individuals, with IgA, IgG, and IgM responses documented. Humoral immunity is likely related to opsonic and bactericidal activity, and may be strain related. Serum antibody response in infection may also be measured by complement fixation, ELISA, or fluorescent antibody techniques, but these have not been of great utility as diagnostic aids.

The Meningococcus[9]

Inflammation of the meninges or investing membranes of the brain and spinal cord can be provoked by a variety of microorganisms and may occur either as a primary affection or secondarily in the train of an infection originating elsewhere. One form of meningitis, characterized especially by epidemic spread and usually designated as **epidemic cerebrospinal meningitis** is caused by a specific microorganism commonly known as the meningococcus, or more formally as *Neisseria meningitidis*.

This bacterium was described in meningeal exudates as early as 1884, but was first isolated in pure culture and described in detail by Weichselbaum in 1887, who found it in cases of acute cerebrospinal meningitis.

Morphology and Staining
In stained films of meningeal exudates (Fig. 16–10) the meningococcus is very like the gonococcus and occurs in pairs and tetrads, both within leucocytes and free; the diplococci are flattened along their adjacent sides like gonococci. There is considerable variability in the size of different cells in the same smear. In stains from pure cultures, size variation is also apparent; average cells are a little less than 1 μm. in diameter and, as a rule, appear in pairs; short chains are seen more rarely (Fig. 16–11). Involution forms are commonly observed in older cultures.

The fine structure of meningococcus is similar to that of the gonococcus. The cell wall is typical of gram-negative forms, with a thin peptidoglycan layer located in the periplasmic space between the cytoplasmic and the outer membranes. The outer membrane is characterized by several protein constituents, as well as rough-type lipopolysaccharide, *i.e.*, without the O-specific side chains. Although capsules are not readily apparent by ordinary staining, in the presence of specific immune serum they become swollen and are easily observed—the

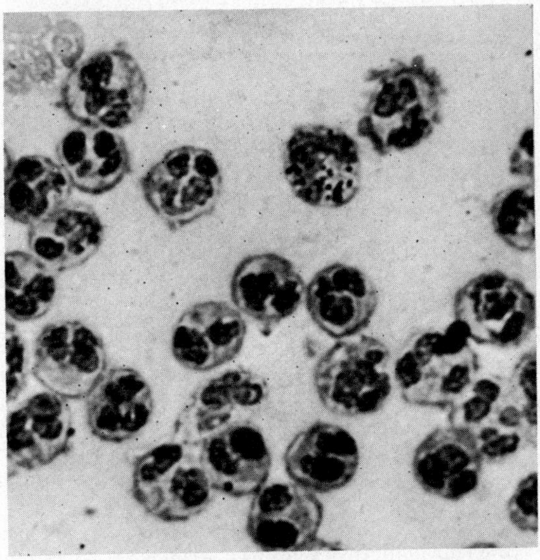

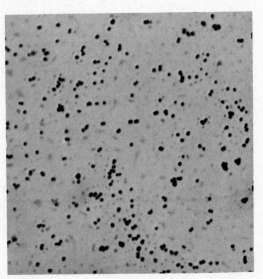

Figure 16–10. Meningococci in spinal fluid, showing phagocytosis of the microorganisms. Gram stain; × 1050.

Figure 16–11. Meningococcus, pure culture. Note the typical diplococcus arrangement. Fuchsin; × 1050.

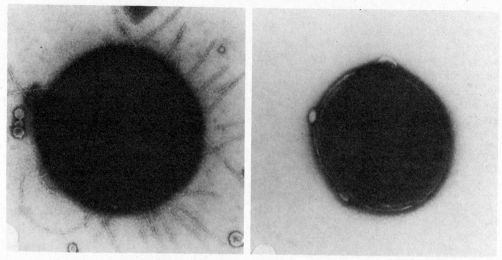

Figure 16–12. Electron photomicrographs of *Neisseria meningitidis*. *Left,* Cultured on medium which preserves pili. *Right,* Cultured on medium that results in loss of pili. × 41,560. Z. A. McGee, *et al.,* Infect. Immun. **24**:194, 1979.)

Quellung reaction. Like gonococci, meningococci usually possess surface pili when freshly isolated from the infected host. Piliated meningococci attach more readily to human nasopharyngeal cells than do nonpiliated variants, suggesting a relationship to virulence as in gonococci. Piliation is, however, not constant in cultivated strains and is, to a considerable degree, dependent upon cultural conditions, as seen in Figure 16–12.

On blood agar, colonies of meningococcus are moist, elevated, and smooth and have a bluish-gray tinge (Fig. 16–13). Neither α- nor β-hemolysis is produced, thus permitting their differentiation from hemolytic and viridans streptococci and pneumococcus. The colonies are not so white and opaque as those of staphylococci. Strains producing large amounts of capsular material sometimes form mucoid colonies, but colonial form is not related to piliation as in the gonococcus.

Meningococci stain readily with the usual dyes and are gram-negative. No sure distinction between the meningococcus and other

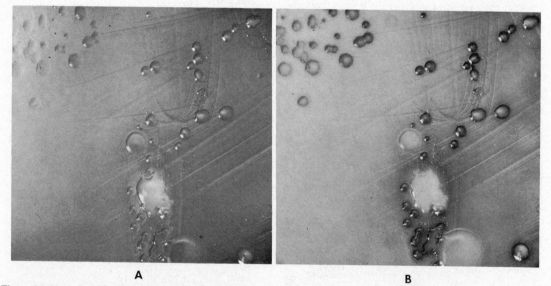

Figure 16–13. The oxidase test for the identification of meningococcus colonies. Mixed culture on blood agar. *A,* Colonies of meningococci and contaminants before the application of tetramethyl-*p*-phenylenediamine solution. *B,* The same colonies after the application of the reagent. Note that the meningococcus colonies show the development of color first about the edges and there is slight discoloration of the medium. × 5.

neisseriae, including the gonococcus, can be made on morphological grounds. Since both meningococci and gonococci may be found at the same infection sites, *viz.*, pharynx and anogenital region, isolation and identification is required for differentiation.

Physiology

Strains of meningococci vary considerably in the ease with which they may be cultivated. Although some strains will grow sparsely on nutrient and infusion mediums, more complex mediums are generally employed, *viz.*, chocolate infusion and blood agar. Nutritive requirements of meningococci are similar to those of gonococci, but most strains grow in the absence of cysteine or cystine, thus providing differentiation from gonococci. Stock strains have been grown on synthetic mediums containing glutamic acid and lactate or glucose, but the growth of freshly isolated strains is usually not supported on these mediums. Since there is little variation in nutritional requirements between strains, auxotyping has not been applied to *N. meningitidis.*

Growth of meningococcus is favored, especially upon primary isolation, by incubation in an atmosphere containing 3 to 10 per cent carbon dioxide. These bacteria will grow over a temperature range of 25° C. to 42° C., with an optimum at 37° C. Although some growth will occur under anaerobic conditions, the meningococcus is, for all practical purposes, aerobic.

Continued laboratory cultivation usually results in more luxuriant growth, but meningococcal cultures are difficult to maintain, tending to die out as a consequence of autolysis. They may be maintained by frequent transfer or preserved by stab cultures in starch agar kept at 37° C. Their limited viability when not transferred, as well as the relatively early appearance of involution forms, is attributable to the formation of an autolysin. Autolysis occurs in a short time in saline at 37° C.; since the autolysin is heat-labile, suspensions prepared for agglutination should be inactivated at 65° C. for 30 minutes.

The meningococcus, like the gonococcus, is a delicate microorganism. It is killed in a short time by drying or exposure to dilute disinfectants. It is particularly sensitive to heat and cold and, unlike most bacteria, rapidly loses viability at refrigerator temperatures.

The meningococcus exhibits little biochemical activity. Only glucose and maltose are fermented with formation of considerable quantities of acid. Maltose fermentation serves to distinguish the meningococcus from the gonococcus.

Toxin

Meningococcal infection in humans and in experimental animals is usually accompanied by symptoms of extreme toxemia. No soluble toxins have been found, but the cell substance is toxic, a consequence of endotoxic lipopolysaccharides (LPS) present in the outer membrane. These lipopolysaccharides are structurally similar to the R-type LPS of enteric bacilli, *i.e.*, they contain a core polysaccharide and covalently bound lipid A, which is responsible for endotoxicity; strains that have been studied do not, however, appear to possess the O-specific side chains characteristic of complete LPS.

It is probable that the LPS of meningococci is responsible for the endotoxemia that characterizes disseminated infections, such as meningococcemia. The toxic reaction appears to be more severe than that observed in infections with other gram-negative bacteria.

Antigenic Structure and Classification

The meningococci are closely related to the gonococci, not only morphologically, but immunologically as well, and antigenic cross-reactions between the two are common. They also share antigenic determinants with certain enteric bacteria. It is likely that many of these cross-reactions are due to similarities in the lipopolysaccharides.

Meningococci contain a genus-specific, carbohydrate-containing antigen that is detectable by a variety of serological tests. The antigen probably represents common polysaccharide determinants of the lipopolysaccharides. Within the species, serological groups are distinguished on the basis of serological reactivity of capsular polysaccharides on the bacterial surface. Nine of these serogroups are now recognized, *viz.*, A, B, C, D, X, Y, Z, W135, and 29E. The serogroup of *N. meningitidis* isolates is determined by agglutination or capsular swelling by Quellung reaction, using group-specific antiserums; a few strains are not groupable by these techniques, either because they are autoagglutinable, because they are not encapsulated, or because they contain none of the known group polysaccharides.

In most of the serogroups, additional serotypes can be distinguished, based on proteins and lipopolysaccharides located in the outer membrane. These serotype antigens are distinct and independent of the serogroup antigens. Thus, the protein type 2 antigen is found in strains of serogroups B and C; other serotype antigens are restricted to a single serogroup, *e.g.*, LPS serotype antigens L10 and L11 are found only in group A strains.[47] In many cases, a single strain may contain multiple serotype antigens, including both proteins and lipopolysaccharides. Not surprisingly, many strains are not typable, suggesting that not all serotype antigens are yet recognized.

Clinical isolates of meningococci may be serogrouped by agglutination, using commercially available grouping serums. Serotyping is, however, quite complex and is not routinely performed. Both serogrouping and serotyping have considerable utility in epidemiological studies on the distribution of strains which occur in carriers or cases of the disease and in connection with efforts to develop effective immunizing vaccines. For example, antibody to the capsular polysaccharides of groups A, C, Y, and W135 are bactericidal and thus are protective against infection with the homologous meningococcal group. On the other hand, the capsular polysaccharide of group B is poorly immunogenic in humans and protection is possibly associated with serotype antigens (see Immunity, p. 434).

Virulence

The characteristics of meningococcal disease in humans, including the frequency of an asymptomatic carrier state and the profound toxemia, suggest an exceedingly complex host-parasite relationship.

Virulence determinants of meningococci, as they are presently known (Table 16–3), appear to operate at two levels in the process of pathogenesis. Meningococci first colonize the mucous membranes, usually in the oropharynx or nasopharynx. If the infection does not progress beyond this point, pharyngeal carriage results and is usually short-lived. Depending upon the relative virulence of the microorganism and the effectiveness of host defenses, meningococci may penetrate the mucous membranes and gain entry to the tissues; they may then cause meningococcemia or they may be transported to the central nervous system, where they cause inflammation of the meninges and the symptoms of meningitis.

The attachment and colonization of meningococci on the pharyngeal surfaces appears to be mediated by pili, since piliated strains exhibit greater adherence than nonpiliated strains.[39, 42] Furthermore, piliated meningococci demonstrate greatest adherence to na-

Table 16–3. Possible Virulence Determinants in Meningococcus

Bacterial Factor	Action
Pili	Adhesion for colonization of mucous membranes of the pharynx; may inibit phagocytosis.
Capsule	Inhibits phagocytosis; decreases adherence by pili.
Iron Acquisition System	Promotes the acquisition of iron from transferrin and other iron chelators in the host during systemic infection.
IgA Protease	Cleaves certain subclasses (1 and 2) of IgA at mucosal surfaces, presumably interfering with this host defense; within the host, may promote defenses by inactivating IgA that interferes with bactericidal antibody systems.
Serotype Antigens	Certain serotypes (2 and 15) are more often associated with epidemic disease.
Endotoxin	Probably accounts for toxemia in meningococcal disease.

sopharyngeal cells, the cell type most often colonized by these bacteria. Progressively poorer adherence occurs with buccal, urethral, and bladder mucosal cells and there is almost no adherence to anterior nasal epithelial cells. These observations are interpreted as reflecting decreasing numbers of specific host cell receptors for the bacterial adhesion.

Adherence is also modified by the presence of capsules on the bacterial cells. In general, encapsulated cells are considered to be more virulent in that they are most often associated with invasive disease; yet, encapsulated cells are generally less adherent *in vitro,* the capsule presumably interfering with pilus-mediated attachment. It has been suggested that virulent encapsulated cells may have a compensatory increase in piliation or have pili of different composition from avirulent or lowly virulent strains.

Colonization may also be affected by the capacity of virulent cells to overcome specific host defenses at the mucosal surface. Meningococci secrete proteases that cleave human IgA; since it is believed that IgA inhibits pilus-mediated attachment, the destruction of IgA could interfere with specific immunity associated with IgA at the mucosal surface.

Bacterial factors that might influence penetration are not known. However, several microbial virulence determinants are known to influence the host-parasite interactions after tissue invasion has occurred. The best known of these is the capacity of meningococci to acquire iron, which is necessary for their growth. As noted in Chapter 12, meningococci produce an iron siderophore, meningobactin, which can chelate iron and make it available for meningococcal growth. Virulent meningococci, but not commensal neisseriae, can also acquire iron from transferrin. Transferrin in body fluids is recognized by an iron sequestering system of the meningococcal cell surface. Iron is then removed from transferrin and made available to the bacterial cell. This high-affinity iron acquisition system requires a functional respiratory chain and is enhanced, as is virulence, in cells grown under conditions of iron starvation. It is specific for transferrin and is trypsin-sensitive; thus, it differs from meningobactin and may be associated with increased synthesis of certain outer membrane proteins.

As noted above, meningococci secrete IgA protease that enhances their capacity to colonize mucous membranes. Within host tissues, the protease may have an entirely different effect. During meningococcal carriage or infection, bactericidal antibodies of the IgM and IgG classes are produced. At the same time, IgA may be induced, which is not bactericidal, but does block the bactericidal effect of the other antibody classes. IgA protease, produced by meningococci, could then inactivate IgA and, thereby, increase the effectiveness of the bactericidal antibodies in eliminating the bacteria. Thus, within host tissues, meningococcal IgA protease would be an antagonist to bacterial virulence.

Most invasive strains of meningococci are encapsulated and piliated, but the role of these structures in promoting virulence within the tissues is somewhat uncertain. As in other pathogens, meningococcal capsules inhibit phagocytosis, but phagocytosis and intracellular killing do not seem to have a pivotal role in defense. It has been suggested that meningococcal pili may be antiphagocytic, as they are in gonococci, but such a role is not yet established.

Certain of the serotype antigens have also been proposed as markers of virulence. In a number of outbreaks, epidemic meningococcal infections have been due to serotype 2 and, to a lesser degree, serotype 15. The reason for this seemingly enhanced virulence of certain serotypes is unknown. Endemic and sporadic meningococcal infections, however, do not appear to be consistently associated with any specific serotypes.

The profound toxemia that marks meningococcal disease is believed to be associated with the endotoxin of these microorganisms and the toxemia is more severe in meningococcal infections than those caused by other gram-negative bacteria. This enhanced toxicity may be due either to increased production of endotoxin or to the absence of long O-specific side chains, presumably permitting more effective binding of the endotoxin to susceptible cell membranes.

It is evident that, in most cases, *N. meningitidis* is able to colonize membranes but unable to gain entry to tissues, indicating either a lack of virulence factors or effective host defenses. Some are capable of invasive disease, however, and the normal host defenses seem not to be effective in containing such infections. Thus, resistance to systemic infections depends primarily upon a specific, bactericidal antibody response (see Immunity, p. 434).

MENINGOCOCCAL DISEASE[13-15, 40]

Like gonococci, meningococci are exclusively parasites of man, natural infections not occurring in animals. *Neisseria meningitidis* is best regarded as a commensal parasite in man, causing disease only when there is a failure of host resistance or when a particularly virulent strain colonizes the mucous membranes.

The commensal relationship is exemplified by the high rates of meningococcal carriage— 25 to 40 per cent in some populations of young adults—without symptomatic disease; this rate can increase to 100 per cent in case contacts during epidemics. The host contributes to the commensal relationship by restricting colonization to the upper respiratory tract, inhibiting penetration and disseminated infection by the production of complement-dependent bactericidal antibodies. The susceptibles in the community include noncarriers and others who may not have antibodies to circulating strains, or those with reduced capacity to respond immunologically to meningococcal antigens. Predisposing factors, such as intercurrent viral infections, also increase susceptibility.

Meningococcal disease begins with colonization of the mucosa of the upper respiratory tract. In healthy carriers the infection remains confined to the pharynx and in this case is short-lived there, producing few or no symptoms. In susceptible individuals, disseminated disease usually begins with pharyngitis that is often mild. If the microorganism gains access to the circulatory system, **meningococcemia** is produced; the infection can then metastasize to the skin, joints, eyes, heart, adrenals, or meninges. In about 90 per cent of cases, **purulent leptomeningitis** follows the bacteremia, and about half of these also exhibit small skin hemorrhages (petechiae) or larger hemorrhagic lesions (purpura) after 12 to 36 hours. Similar hemorrhagic lesions are also found on mucosal or serosal surfaces in a variety of organs. Vascular damage includes injury to the endothelium, inflammation of the vessel walls, necrosis, and intravascular coagulation. Other symptoms include sudden onset, chills, fever, and meningeal symptoms, such as headache and drowsiness. Pain in the arms and legs is common.

Meningococci can be recovered from the nasopharynx or oropharynx in early stages, from the later dermal lesions, from the blood in meningococcemia, from synovial fluid in septic arthritis, or from cerebrospinal fluid in meningitis.

Invasion of the blood stream may, in rare cases, take the form of a highly fatal, fulminating meningococcemia of sudden onset and short course (**Waterhouse-Friderichsen syndrome**), accompanied by rapid development of massive petechial or purpuric lesions, often within a few hours. The most common systemic manifestation of this syndrome is myocarditis, often with congestive heart failure. Bilateral hemorrhagic destruction of the adrenals occurs in a small number of cases. The disease picture is that of an acute, generalized endotoxemia and shock.

In rare instances, the bacteremia may take a more chronic form with intermittent fever, chills, and arthralgia. The skin manifestations are not so common in this chronic form as in acute infections.

Upon reaching the central nervous system, the meningococcus sets up a suppurative lesion of the meninges with inflammation involving the spinal cord together with the base and cortex of the brain. In fulminant cases there is severe cerebral hyperemia and tissue swelling along with petechial hemorrhage. Meningococci are present in the spinal fluid, and are often found in great numbers, both free and within the leucocytes. Purulent meningococcal meningitis is almost invariably fatal in the absence of vigorous antimicrobial therapy.

Chemotherapy has markedly reduced the mortality rate, but long-term sequelae include deafness, blindness, and mental deficiency; these are rare and most often follow delays in initiating therapy.

In addition to the classical forms of meningococcal disease just described, *N. meningitidis* is also a rare cause of sexually transmitted infections of the anogenital region. The microorganism has been found in rectal infections, primarily in male homosexuals, where it may be responsible for proctitis, but is more often asymptomatic. It has also been responsible for urethritis, in both heterosexual and homosexual populations, presumably initiated by orogenital contact. Sexually transmitted infections probably do not give rise to bacteremia or meningitis but remain localized to the anogenital region.

Epidemiology

Like most respiratory infections, meningococcal disease is usually spread by direct contact and droplet infection through the secretions of the upper respiratory tract. Infection is spread by patients and convalescents to a limited extent, but healthy **carriers** are of primary importance. Most persons are temporary carriers, while a few are chronic carriers, discharging meningococci more or less continuously or in a sporadic fashion. During epidemics, the contacts of cases tend to carry the epidemic strains, and the carriage rate is very much higher in close contacts, such as families or barracks groups. In the absence of epidemics, the serogroups and serotypes encountered are usually varied.

Resistance to symptomatic infections in these carriers is associated with circulating bactericidal antibodies, engendered by serogroup and/or serotypic antigens of colonizing meningococcal strains or by exposure to antigens from other bacteria that cross-react with meningococci. Thus, resistance arises from and is reinforced by pharyngeal carriage of meningococci, and by colonization with other antigenically similar bacteria.

Susceptibility to meningococcal infection is biphasic. It is greatest in children between the ages of three months and five years; a second peak of susceptibility appears in adolescents and young adults. It is thought that the resistance of infants derives from maternal antibody; resistance in older children follows the acquisition of carrier strains that have immunizing potential.

Epidemics of meningococcal meningitis occur with some frequency in military popula-

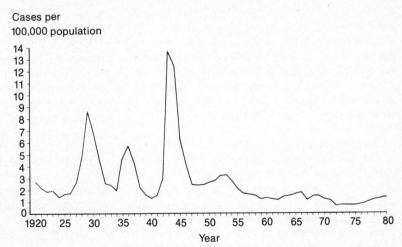

Figure 16–14. The reported case rates of meningococcal infection in the United States, 1920–1980. Note the epidemic periodicity prior to the 1950s. (Centers for Disease Control, Annual summary 1980: reported morbidity and mortality in the United States. Morbidity and Mortality Weekly Report, **29**[54], 1981.)

tions. It has long been thought that such outbreaks occur when susceptibles encounter new meningococcal strains by close contact with colonized, but essentially immune carriers. Griffiss has, however, proposed an intriguing model to explain these and similar epidemics in adolescents and young adults.[15] It is suggested that susceptibility arises not from the absence of bactericidal antibody, but from the presence of serum IgA which, as noted earlier, blocks the bactericidal action of specific IgM and IgG. Such individuals would then appear to lose their effective immune state, concomitantly with the production of specific IgA. The blocking IgA is thought to arise not from meningococcal immune stimulus, but from antigens present on other microorganisms, primarily enteric bacteria colonizing the intestinal tract, that induce IgA antibodies which cross-react with surface meningococcal antigens.

Throughout the world, serogroups A, B, and C account for about 90 per cent of meningococcal infections. Those of serogroup A are responsible for most of the large epidemics, while serogroups B, C, and Y are more often responsible for sporadic cases.

In the United States, serogroup B strains are the most prevalent in meningococcal disease, followed by group C. The latter has, however, shown a decrease following the introduction of vaccines against serogroup C. Serogroups Y and W135 have increased in prevalence in recent years, primarily in young adults and older individuals, but the number of cases remains well below that of the more commonly encountered strains. Infections due to serogroup A represent a small minority of cases, and other groups are rarely encountered.

Whether occurring in civilian or military populations, epidemics of meningococcal meningitis have a number of distinctive characteristics. The carrier rate is relatively high, while the morbidity rate is low. Thus, there is a high degree of resistance to disease. On the other hand, the high case fatality rate indicates that, once established in the host, the course of the disease is a serious one. The relative resistance of the general population results in disease spread that is spotty in nature. Direct transmission from case to case is rare; usually carriers constitute the link between cases. Further, epidemics frequently consist of a series of recurring outbreaks rather than the well-marked single epidemic wave often observed in other diseases. Prior to 1953, epidemics of meningococcal infections in this country occurred at 6- to 12-year intervals and lasted from 3 to 5 years, but since that time the case rate has varied only slightly from year to year, as shown in Figure 16–14. *Neisseria meningitidis* is the second leading cause of meningitis in the United States, after *Haemophilus influenzae*.

The seasonal incidence is marked in temperate climates, with peak incidence in the winter months in the United States. Males are more frequently attacked than females, although this may be an expression of risk. Attack rates are somewhat higher in blacks, American Indians, and Alaskan natives.

Chemotherapy

Of the antimicrobial agents available, the sulfonamides, especially sulfadiazine, were the drugs of choice for many years. Later, sulfonamide resistance increased markedly, probably reflecting widespread use of these drugs to eliminate the carrier state. Penicillin is now the preferred chemotherapeutic agent, but should be given in large doses in order to assure adequate penetration of the drug into the cerebrospinal fluid. For prophylaxis in case contacts, rifampin has proved to be effective, as are sulfonamides when the·strain is known to be sensitive to these agents.

Bacteriological Diagnosis[28]

The meningococcus is usually present in the spinal fluid in meningitis, and provisional diagnosis is established by the finding of characteristic gram-negative diplococci in stained smears of the sediment from centrifuged spinal fluid. Gram stains of joint fluid and petechial aspirates are also informative, but stains from sputum and nasopharyngeal swabs are of little value, owing to the frequent presence of morphologically indistinguishable saprophytic neisseriae.

Specimens for culture should be collected before initiating chemotherapy; these include blood and spinal fluid, aspirates of joint fluid or petechiae, sputum, and nasopharyngeal swabs. Specimens expected to be contaminated, such as sputum or nasopharyngeal swabs, may be cultured on modified Thayer-Martin or NYC agar, under conditions as used for gonococci. Cerebrospinal fluid or petechial or joint aspirates may be inoculated to blood or chocolate agar and incubated under increased carbon dioxide and humidity. Blood culture may be carried out under standard conditions. In all cases, specimens should be protected from drying and extreme changes in temperature; in no case should they be refrigerated before culture.

Cultures should be examined for oxidase-positive, gram-negative diplococci exhibiting the typical colonial morphology of N. meningitidis. The isolated meningococci may be identified by fermentation tests (Table 16–1) and agglutination by polyvalent antiserum or by fluorescent antibody techniques, using specific meningococcal antiserum. If required, they may be grouped by high-titer specific antiserum using agglutination or capsular swelling.

A valuable adjunct to bacteriological culture is the detection of meningococcal polysaccharide antigen in the spinal fluid of patients with meningitis, using countercurrent immunoelectrophoresis and high-titered group-specific antiserum. This method is most successful in infections due to serogroup A or C.

Animal Models

Although natural infections with meningococci occur only in humans, several animal models have been developed. Rhesus monkeys have been infected by intraspinal inoculation of large numbers of meningococci, with development of an acute disease. Meningitis has been reproduced in rabbits and guinea pigs by intracisternal infection of virulent meningococci. As in humans, the experimental disease is both a purulent meningitis and general toxemia. Similarly, fatal meningoencephalitis is produced in mice by intracerebral inoculation.

Usually, mice are not susceptible to infection with these microorganisms when given by ordinary routes. Lethal doses approach 10^8 living cells, which is only slightly less than the lethal dose using killed cells. These findings suggest that lethality is due primarily to endotoxin, and not infection in the usual sense. However, if the inoculum is suspended in mucin, mice become very sensitive to infection, developing fatal septicemia within a few days after intraperitoneal injection. The infection-promoting effect of mucin is due to its high iron content. Other iron-containing substances, such as iron dextran, will achieve the same effect; most studies with the mouse model now involve pretreatment of the animals with iron dextran. This model has been employed for virulence determination of meningococcal strains and to study the effects of iron on infection. The mouse LD_{50} of highly virulent strains may be as low as 1 to 10 cells. The developing chick embryo has also been employed as an animal model; 12-day embryos develop septicemia and hemorrhagic lesions simulating fulminating meningococcemia in man.

Animal models have not been particularly successful in immunization studies. Many antigens that induce bactericidal antibodies in animals do not do so in man. Therefore, the effectiveness of vaccines can only be assessed after field trials in humans.

Immunity[35]

In the preantibiotic era, epidemics of meningococcal disease occurred with some regularity. Since the mid-1940s, large epidemics have been rare; the disease is, however, still endemic in most parts of the world, including the United States. Small epidemics have occurred in military recruits, giving impetus to vaccine development. In civilian populations in this country, disease appears as sporadic cases with occasional small outbreaks; secondary cases are common in family members and other close contacts.

Effective immunity, whether engendered by artificial immunization, subclinical infection, or nasopharyngeal carriage, is correlated with the presence of **complement-dependent bac-**

tericidal antibodies. The importance of complement is emphasized by the marked susceptibility of individuals who are deficient in the higher complement components—C5 to C8—which are required for immune bacteriolysis.

In many of the meningococcal serogroups, including groups A, C, Y, and W135, bactericidal antibody is induced in humans by immunization with purified, serogroup-specific, capsular polysaccharides. These antigen preparations are essentially nontoxic and elicit both bactericidal and opsonizing antibodies; protection is achieved within a week of immunization, thus permitting their use in control of outbreaks. It has also been established that, with groups A and C at least, antibodies also participate in antibody-dependent cell-mediated antibacterial activity.[41]

Vaccines that contain polysaccharides of groups A and C are licensed for use in the United States, as well as several other countries, and have proved to be efficacious against infections in older children and adults caused by these serogroups. The group A vaccine is effective in controlling outbreaks when given to children beyond their first year; indeed, there is evidence that it is protective when administered as early as three months. The group C vaccine, while effective in children over two years of age, is poorly immunogenic and apparently not protective in younger children; unfortunately, about 30 per cent of group C cases are in children less than 2 years of age.

Preliminary trials in military recruits, testing serogroup Y and W135 vaccines, indicate that these will be protective, since they induce significant bactericidal antibody response.[16]

It is evident that serogroup B remains as the group causing significant human disease and for which there is no satisfactory vaccine. It has been repeatedly demonstrated that the group B polysaccharide is essentially nonimmunogenic in humans. There is, of course, the possibility that serotypic antigens can induce protective immunity. However, attempts to demonstrate bactericidal antibodies in humans inoculated with purified outer membrane proteins have not been successful, although animals may be protected by such preparations. The diversity of serotype antigens in group B strains will further complicate efforts at serotype immunization, although serotypes 2 and 15 are likely candidates, since they are found most often as the responsible agent in many epidemic infections.

Other Neisseria, Branhamella, Moraxella, and Acinetobacter[19]

Other Neisseria

In addition to the primary pathogenic species, *N. gonorrhoeae* and *N. meningitidis*, several other *Neisseria* are recognized. These are considered to be commensal forms that often inhabit the mucous membranes of the upper respiratory and genitourinary tracts. The principal species and some of their differential characteristics are listed in Table 16–1. Two species, *N. flavescens* and *N. subflava,* are pigmented and easily distinguished from the pathogenic members. The remainder are not pigmented and may be confused with the more virulent species, since their morphology is similar and they are normally oxidase-positive.

Neisseria lactamica is a normal inhabitant of the nasopharynx, primarily in infants and young children. It closely resembles *N. meningitidis* in cultural characteristics, including growth on modified Thayer-Martin and NYC mediums, and is serologically related. *Neisseria lactamica*, however, degrades lactose and is differentiated from the meningococcus on this basis.

Except for *N. gonorrhoeae* and *N. meningitidis*, *Neisseria* appear to be opportunists with only low virulence. On rare occasions, they have been isolated from normally sterile tissues under conditions implicating them as disease agents, as in meningitis, bacteremia, endocarditis, and pneumonia.

Branhamella catarrhalis[11]

This nonpigmented, oxidase-positive diplococcus, formerly known as *Neisseria catarrhalis,* is found commonly in the nasopharynx of healthy individuals and in persons suffering from colds and other respiratory infections. As a rule, *B. catarrhalis* is somewhat smaller than meningococcus and is less exacting in its nutritive requirements, growing readily on nutrient agar at 37° C. and on enriched mediums at 22° C.; no carbohydrates are fermented (Table 16–1). Although most strains fail to grow on modified Thayer-Martin medium, occasional strains are sufficiently resistant to the antibiotics in the medium that growth occurs.

While *B. catarrhalis* has long been consid-

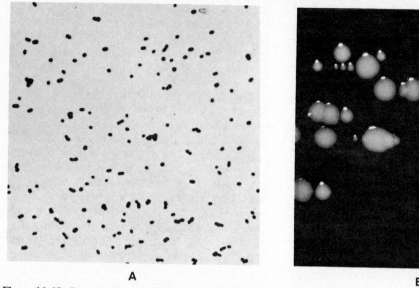

A

B

Figure 16–15. *Branhamella catarrhalis. A,* Smear from a pure culture. Note the diplococci and elongated forms which have not yet divided. Fuchsin; × 1050. *B,* 24-hour culture on blood agar. × 5.

ered to be an innocuous inhabitant of the upper respiratory tract, its pathogenic role is becoming evident. In children, it is known to cause otitis media and may be responsible for persistent coughs and bronchitis. In compromised adults, it has been found as the apparent etiologic agent of serious lower respiratory infection and bacteremia; it may also be the causative agent in some cases of laryngitis. Since many strains produce β-lactamase, the choice of antibiotics used to treat proven infections should be based on appropriate sensitivity testing.

Moraxella

The members of the genus *Moraxella* are short, plump, gram-negative diplobacilli, which sometimes give the appearance of diplococci; in other respects they closely resemble *Branhamella.* One species, *Moraxella lacunata,* was first described in 1896 and is the etiologic agent of a rare form of conjunctivitis in man.

The short rods, 1 μm. by 2 to 3 μm., frequently appear end to end in pairs or in short chains, as seen in Figure 16–16. *Moraxella lacunata* does not grow on ordinary nutrient mediums, but requires more complex mediums, such as blood or chocolate agar; colonies on blood agar are small, flat, and translucent.

As far as known, this bacterium is pathogenic only in humans, since inoculation of experimental animals is without effect. Instillation of the bacilli into the conjunctival sac of humans has resulted in blepharoconjunctivitis,

in either acute or chronic form, usually with severe inflammation of the cornea. Treatment with zinc sulfate solution produces a rapid cure, while silver salts are without effect. Both chlortetracycline and streptomycin, used topically, are reportedly also effective. Although rare, the disease is widely distributed and has been reported in Europe, Africa, and North America.

Other *Moraxella* may occasionally be found in the respiratory or genitourinary tract of humans, but they appear to be essentially nonpathogenic. *Moraxella bovis* has been associated with many outbreaks of keratoconjunctivitis in cattle.

Acinetobacter [23]

Like *Moraxella, Acinetobacter* are short, gram-negative rods related to other Neisseriaceae; they are, however, oxidase-negative. *Acinetobacter calcoaceticus* produces coccoid

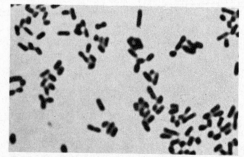

Figure 16–16. *Moraxella lacunata* (Morax-Axenfeld bacillus); pure culture. Gram stain; × 2400.

cells that occur in pairs and are easily confused with *Neisseria*. Their nutritional requirements are not complex, and they grow on ordinary nutrient mediums as domed, mucoid colonies; they are strict aerobes. They are biochemically active and exhibit great strain variation in this respect.

Typically, *A. calcoaceticus* is a common inhabitant of soil, water, and sewage; thus, these microorganisms are frequently found as contaminants in cultures from humans. There is, however, considerable evidence that they can be opportunistic pathogens for man, causing meningitis and septic infections, primarily in compromised hosts.

REFERENCES

1. Apicella, M. A., and N. C. Gagliardi. 1979. Antigenic heterogeneity of the non-serogroup antigen structure of *Neisseria gonorrhoeae* lipopolysaccharides. Infect. Immun. **26**:870–874.
2. Blake, M., K. K. Holmes, and J. Swanson. 1979. Studies on gonococcus infection. XVII. IgA₁-cleaving protease in vaginal washings from women with gonorrhea. J. Infect. Dis. **139**:89–92.
3. Buchanan, T. M. 1978. Antigen-specific serotyping of *Neisseria gonorrhoeae*. I. Use of an enzyme-linked immunosorbent assay to quantitate pilus antigens on gonococci. J. Infect. Dis. **138**:319–325.
4. Buchanan, T. M., and R. J. Arko. 1977. Immunity to gonococcal infection induced by vaccination with isolated outer membranes of *Neisseria gonorrhoeae* in guinea pigs. J. Infect. Dis. **135**:879–887.
5. Buchanan, T. M., and J. F. Hildebrandt. 1981. Antigen-specific serotyping of *Neisseria gonorrhoeae*: characterization based upon principal outer membrane protein. Infect. Immun. **32**:985–994.
6. Buchanan, T. M., and W. A. Pearce. 1976. Pili as a mediator of the attachment of gonococci to human erythrocytes. Infect. Immun. **13**:1483–1489.
7. Catlin, B. W. 1978. Characteristics and auxotyping of *Neisseria gonorrhoeae*. pp. 345–380. *In* T. Bergan and J. R. Norris (Eds.): Methods in Microbiology, Vol. 10. Academic Press, London.
8. Danielsson, D., and J. Maeland. 1978. Serotyping and antigenic studies of *Neisseria gonorrhoeae*. pp. 315–344. *In* T. Bergan and J. R. Norris (Eds.): Methods in Microbiology, Vol. 10. Academic Press, London.
9. DeVoe, I. W. 1982. The meningococcus and mechanisms of pathogenicity. Microbiol. Rev. **46**:162–190.
10. Dillon, J.-A. R., M. Pauzé, and A. G. Jessamine. 1981. Penicillinase-producing *Neisseria gonorrhoeae* in Canada. Can. Med. Assn J. **125**:851–855.
11. Doern, G. V., and S. A. Morse. 1980. *Branhamella (Neisseria) catarrhalis*: criteria for laboratory identification. J. Clin. Microbiol. **11**:193–195.
12. Finkelstein, R. A., and R. J. Yancey. 1981. Effect of siderophores on virulence of Neisseria gonorrhoeae. Infect. Immun. **32**:609–613.
13. Galazka, A. 1982. Meningococcal disease and its control with meningococcal polysaccharide vaccines. Bull. Wld Hlth Org. **60**:1–7.
14. Geiseler, P. J., *et al*. 1980. Community-acquired purulent meningitis: a review of 1,316 cases during the antibiotic era, 1954–1976. Rev. Infect. Dis. **2**:725–745.

15. Griffiss, J. McL. 1982. Epidemic meningococcal disease: synthesis of a hypothetical immunoepidemiologic model. Rev. Infect. Dis. **4**:159–172.
16. Griffiss, J. McL., B. L. Brandt, and D. D. Broud. 1982. Human immune response to various doses of group Y and W135 meningococcal polysaccharide vaccine. Infect. Immun. **37**:205–208.
17. Gregg, C. R., *et al*. 1981. Toxic activity of purified lipopolysaccharide of *Neisseria gonorrhoeae* for human fallopian tube mucosa. J. Infect. Dis. **143**:432–439.
18. Hafiz, S., *et al*. 1978. *N. gonorrohoeae:* pathogenicity of colonial type 5. J. Clin. Pathol. **31**:437–438.
19. Henriksen, S. D. 1976. Moraxella, Neisseria, Branhamella and Acinetobacter. Ann. Rev. Microbiol. **30**:63–83.
20. Holmes, K. K., G. W. Counts, and H. N. Beaty. 1971. Disseminated gonococcal infection. Ann. Intern. Med. **74**:979–993.
21. James, J. F., *et al*. 1982. Relation of protein I and colony opacity to serum killing of *Neisseria gonorrhoeae*. J. Infect. Dis. **145**:37–44.
22. Judd, R. C. 1982. Surface peptide mapping of protein I and protein III of four strains of *Neisseria gonorrhoeae*. Infect. Immun. **37**:632–641.
23. Juni, E. 1978. Genetics and physiology of *Acinetobacter*. Ann. Rev. Microbiol. **32**:349–371.
24. Kita, E., H. Matsuura, and S. Kashiba. 1981. A mouse model for the study of gonococcal genital infection. J. Infect. Dis. **143**:67–70.
25. Kohen, D. P. 1974. Neonatal gonococcal arthritis: three cases and review of the literature. Pediatrics **53**:436–440.
26. McChesney, D., *et al*. 1982. Genital antibody response to a parenteral gonococcal pilus vaccine. Infect. Immun. **36**:1006–1012.
27. McGee, Z. A., A. P. Johnson, and D. Taylor-Robinson. 1981. Pathogenic mechanisms of Neisseria gonorrhoeae: observations on damage to human fallopian tubes in organ culture by gonococci of colony type 1 or type 4. J. Infect. Dis. **143**:413–422.
28. Morello, J. A., and M. Bohnhoff. 1980. *Neisseria* and *Branhamella*. pp. 111–130. *In* E. H. Lennette, *et al*. (Eds.): Manual of Clinical Microbiology. 3rd ed. American Society for Microbiology, Washington, D.C.
29. Morin, A., *et al*. 1980. In vitro inhibition of *Neisseria gonorrhoeae* growth by strict anaerobes. Infect. Immun. **28**:766–770.
30. Morse, S. A., A. F. Cacciapuoti, and P. G. Lysko. 1979. Physiology of *Neisseria gonorrhoeae*. Adv. Microbial Physiol. **20**:251–320.
31. Newhall, W. J., *et al*. 1980. High molecular weight antigenic protein complex in the outer membrane of *Neisseria gonorrhoeae*. Infect. Immun. **27**:475–482.
32. Potterat, J. J., and R. D. King. 1981. A new approach to gonorrhea control. The asymptomatic man and incidence reduction. J. Amer. Med. Assn **245**:578–580.
33. Report. 1978. Neisseria gonorrhoeae and gonococcal infections. Wld Hlth Org. Technical Report Series 916. World Health Organization, Geneva.
34. Report. 1981. Spectinomycin-resistant penicillinase-producing *Neisseria gonorrhoeae*—California. Morbid. Mortal. Wkly Rep. **30**:221–222.
35. Robbins, J. B. 1978. Vaccines for the prevention of encapsulated bacterial diseases: current status, problems and prospects for the future. Immunochemistry **15**:839–854.
36. Roberts, M., and S. Falkow. 1979. In vivo conjugal

transfer of R plasmids in *Neisseria gonorrhoeae*. Infect. Immun. **24**:982–984.

37. Saigh, J. H., C. C. Sanders, and W. E. Sanders, Jr. 1978. Inhibition of *Neisseria gonorrhoeae* by aerobic and facultatively anaerobic components of the endocervical flora: evidence for a protective effect against infection. Infect. Immun. **19**:704–710.

38. Salit, I. E., and E. C. Gotschlich. 1978. Gonococcal color and opacity variants: virulence for chicken embryos. Infect. Immun. **22**:359–364.

39. Salit, I. E., and G. Morton. 1981. Adherence of *Neisseria meningitidis* to human epithelial cells. Infect. Immun. **31**:430–435.

40. Shaad, U. B. 1980. Arthritis in disease due to *Neisseria meningitidis*. Rev. Infect. Dis. **2**:880–888.

41. Smith, L. F., and G. H. Lowell. 1980. Antibody-dependent cell-mediated antibacterial activity of human mononuclear cells. II. Immune specificity of antimeningococcal activity. J. Infect. Dis. **141**:748–751.

42. Stephens, D. S., and Z. A. McGee. 1981. Attachment of *Neisseria meningitidis* to human mucosal surfaces: influence of pili and type of receptor cell. J. Infect. Dis. **143**:525–532.

43. Swanson, J. 1980. ^{125}I-labeled peptide mapping of some heat-modifiable proteins of the gonococcal outer membrane. Infect. Immun. **28**:54–64.

44. Swanson, J. 1981. Surface exposed protein antigens of the gonococcal outer membrane. Infect. Immun. **34**:804–816.

45. Virji, M., and J. S. Everson. 1981. Comparative virulence of opacity variants of *Neisseria gonorrhoeae* strain P9. Infect. Immun. **31**:965–970.

46. Watt, P. J., and M. E. Ward. 1980. Adherence of *Neisseria gonorrhoeae* and other *Neisseria* species to mammalian cells. pp. 251–288. *In* E. H. Beachey (Ed.): Bacterial Adherence. Chapman and Hall, London.

47. Zollinger, W. D., and R. E. Mandrell. 1980. Type-specific antigens of group A *Neisseria meningitidis*: lipopolysaccharide and heat-modifiable outer membrane proteins. Infect. Immun. **28**:451–458.

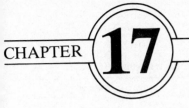
The Enteric Bacilli: Classification and Properties of Enterobacteriaceae

CLASSIFICATION AND NOMENCLATURE OF ENTEROBACTERIACEAE
PROPERTIES OF ENTEROBACTERIACEAE
Morphology
Biochemical Reactions
Antigenic Structure

Toxins
Genetic Variation
ISOLATION AND IDENTIFICATION OF ENTEROBACTERIACEAE
Specimen Collection
Isolation
Biochemical Screening

The gram-negative, nonspore-forming bacilli make up a large group of bacteria that includes intestinal commensals, such as *Escherichia* and *Proteus;* enteric pathogens, such as *Salmonella, Shigella,* and some strains of *Escherichia; Klebsiella* as respiratory and urinary tract pathogens; *Yersinia,* including the plague bacillus; and a variety of saprophytes and plant pathogens. Distant relatives of these are the generally more virulent *Haemophilus, Bordetella, Pasteurella,* and *Brucella.*

The **facultative anaerobic** forms constitute the largest segment of these gram-negative rods. Two families make up this group: Enterobacteriaceae and Vibrionaceae. The Vibrionaceae are rigid, curved bacilli and are usually motile by polar flagella. The more important members of this family, *Vibrio,* are discussed in Chapter 21. The subject of this and the following three chapters are the Enterobacteriaceae, or enteric bacilli, distinguished by the usual presence of peritrichous flagella, as well as certain physiological traits.

For the most part, these bacteria are found in the intestine of humans and other animals, where they behave as commensals of limited pathogenic potential, sometimes causing diarrheal disease or, much less commonly, infections of the tissues. Some are free-living saprophytes of soil and water, while still others are pathogenic for plants.

Classification and Nomenclature of Enterobacteriaceae[2, 14]

The differentiation and characterization of the Enterobacteriaceae are based upon a variety of biochemical and cultural reactions and differences in antigenic structure; these bacteria are better known by these conventional criteria than are any other group of microorganisms. When the more important of them—*Salmonella, Shigella,* and *Escherichia*—were first described and studied, it was not difficult to characterize them with reasonable precision, and they appeared to fall within well-defined genera and species.

With increasing knowledge, it has become obvious that enteric bacilli make up a more or less continuous series of forms, showing almost every conceivable combination of differential characteristics. Combinations which have not been found in nature can be created in the laboratory by recombination and transduction, with demonstrable fertility groups crossing accepted taxonomic lines. Sharp distinction between species is often not possible, therefore, and intermediate strains are sometimes difficult to categorize.

439

Table 17–1. **Taxonomic Relationships of the Enterobacteriaceae***

Tribe	Genus	Species
Escherichieae...............	Escherichia..................	E. coli
	Shigella.....................	S. dysenteriae S. flexneri S. boydii S. sonnei
Edwardsielleae...............	Edwardsiella.................	E. tarda
Salmonelleae.................	Salmonella...................	S. cholerasuis S. typhi S. enteritidis
	Arizona......................	A. hinshawii
	Citrobacter..................	C. freundii C. diversus C. amalonaticus
Klebsielleae.................	Klebsiella...................	K. pneumoniae K. ozaenae K. rhinoscleromatis K. oxytoca
	Enterobacter.................	E. aerogenes E. cloacae E. agglomerans E. sakasakii E. gergoviae
	Hafnia.......................	H. alvei
	Serratia.....................	S. marcescens S. liquifaciens S. rubidaea
Proteeae.....................	Proteus......................	P. mirabilis P. vulgaris
	Providentia..................	P. rettgeri P. stuartii P. alcaliquifaciens
	Morganella...................	M. morganii
Yersinieae...................	Yersinia.....................	Y. pestis Y. pseudotuberculosis Y. enterocolitica Y. intermedia Y. frederiksenii Y. ruckeri
Erwinieae....................	Erwinia Pectinobacterium	

*Adapted from the proposals in Brenner, et al.[1]

The inadequacy of the usual differential criteria as a basis for formal classification, as distinct from a differential key, is clearly evident in this family. It is now generally recognized that subdivision of Enterobacteriaceae into conventional tribes, genera, and species must ultimately be based upon genetic relatedness, especially interspecies integration of chromosomal genes; similarity of gene order in the chromosome; comparative chemistry of the genome; and structural homology of specific proteins.

Genetic relatedness is not, however, routinely applicable and, as a matter of practical expendiency, the separation of enteric bacilli into genera, species, and varieties is accomplished by application of biochemical and immunological methods. Quite apart from the requirements of a soundly based taxonomic system, a workable system of nomenclature is essential and should be based upon general usage and familiarity. Accordingly, the nomenclature used here for the enteric bacilli will be based on current usage in the United States as proposed by the Centers for Disease Control.[1]

The taxonomic relationships of the Enterobacteriaceae are displayed in Table 17–1 and are based upon a variety of biochemical reactions, antibiotic sensitivity, bacteriophage sensitivity, and DNA hybridization. The designation of tribal subdivisions has, at this time, no formal standing, but serves to illuminate the relationships among genera. Detailed consideration of several of the medically important members will be found in succeeding chapters: *Escherichia* and *Shigella* in Chapter 18; *Salmonella* in Chapter 19; *Klebsiella, Proteus,* and related forms in Chapter 20; and *Yersinia* in Chapter 23. *Erwinia* and *Pectobacterium,* although important as plant pathogens, will not be considered in detail here.

Properties of Enterobacteriaceae

Since the enteric bacilli are closely related in morphology, structure, biochemistry, and antigenic makeup, we shall first examine some of their common properties.

Morphology

Enteric bacteria are aerobic, facultatively anaerobic, gram-negative, nonsporulating bacilli. Capsules are formed by a few, principally *Klebsiella,* as well as some strains of *Enterobacter* and *Serratia;* loose slime is frequently produced by *Erwinia.* Most of the enteric bacteria are motile and, when motility occurs, it is by means of peritrichous flagella; *Shigella, Klebsiella,* and *Yersinia* are typically nonmotile. Individual cells vary somewhat in size, but typically they are in the range of 1.0 to 1.5 × 2.0 to 6.0 μm.; they occur singly and in pairs. Some variation in size and morphology is encountered, even within a species. In some groups, *e.g., Proteus,* there is evidence of filaments, spheroplasts, and other aberrant forms. *Yersinia* tend to be somewhat coccoid or oval in shape and are smaller than other members. Fimbriae are produced by many enterobacteria, being found principally in *Escherichia, Klebsiella, Proteus, Salmonella,* and *Shigella*

In colonial morphology, the enteric bacteria are all very much alike, and it is not possible to make valid distinctions by these characters. On ordinary bacteriological mediums, they tend to be smooth, convex with entire margins, moist, and shiny and are usually gray in color. Rough colonial forms are frequently seen. These are often dry, friable, and not easily emulsifiable in saline. The presence of capsules or loose slime is usually reflected in dome-shaped colonies of mucoid and viscous consistency. Some strains, particularly of *Escherichia* and *Proteus,* are hemolytic on blood agar. Although pigment production is rarely seen in most genera, *Serratia* produce a red pigment under certain growth conditions, while many *Erwinia* colonies are cream to yellow in color.

Biochemical Reactions[11]

The Enterobacteriaceae are differentiated from other gram-negative bacteria by several biochemical characters. All are aerobic and facultatively anaerobic; oxidase-negative; and ferment glucose, although gas is not always produced in this fermentation. With very few exceptions, nitrates are reduced to nitrites, but nitrites are not reduced.

Within the family, further differentiation to tribes, genera, and, often, species, is by biochemical reactions as well. The biochemical reactions that characterize the tribes of Enterobacteriaceae are summarized in Table 17–2.

A useful primary differentiation of genera can be made on the basis of **lactose fermentation.** In general, *Escherichia, Klebsiella,* and *Enterobacter* ferment lactose rapidly, as do

Table 17–2. Biochemical Reactions of the Tribes of Enterobacteriaceae*

Test	Tribe					
	Escherichieae	*Edwardsielleae*	*Salmonelleae*	*Klebsielleae*	*Proteeae*	*Yersinieae*
H_2S production	−	+	+	−	+	−
Urease	−	−	−	−	+	+
Indole production†	+	+	−	−	+	−
Methyl red‡	+	+	+	−	+	+
Voges-Proskauer§	−	−	−	+	−	−
Citrate utilization	−	−	+	+	V	−
Phenylalanine deaminase	−	−	−	−	+	−

*Adapted from Martin and Washington.[11] Symbols: +, most strains positive; −, most strains negative; V, variable.
†From tryptophane.
‡A determination of final pH of a glucose broth culture after 2 to 4 days. The test is positive when the indicator turns red, signifying accumulated organic acids.
§A test for the presence of acetylmethylcarbinol, a late end-product of glucose fermentation.

some strains of *Citrobacter* and *Arizona*. A few, including *Shigella sonnei,* are slow lactose fermenters. The production of gas from the fermentation of glucose is also of utility in primary differentiation of genera, as discussed below.

Although without formal taxonomic standing, the lactose-fermenting Enterobacteriaceae have been casually grouped together as **coliform** bacilli since the first description by Escherich of *Bacterium coli* (now *Escherichia coli*). Coliform bacilli usually encompass the lactose-fermenting *Escherichia, Citrobacter, Klebsiella,* and *Enterobacter,* and include, on other biochemical grounds, the nonlactose-fermenting *Edwardsiella* and *Serratia*.

The bacilli occurring in specimens from pathological processes in humans are separable by systematic application of their biochemical characteristics. The enterobacteria are generally isolated on mediums made selective by inclusion of dyes, bile salts, or other inhibitors and often made differential by the inclusion of sugars along with acid-base indicators, as noted in the following section.

Antigenic Structure

Among the Enterobacteriaceae the designation of genus and, in many cases, species, is based primarily on biochemical parameters. Further differentiation, to specific rank in some instances and to serogroups, serotypes, and varieties, is dependent upon serological reactions that detect surface antigens. These antigens fall into three major classes: **somatic O antigens; flagellar H antigens;** and **capsular** or **envelope K antigens**.

O Antigens. The somatic O antigens are the heat-stable lipopolysaccharides common to all smooth, gram-negative bacteria. They are present in the outer membrane (Chapter 2) and are responsible for the endotoxic activity allied with gram-negative bacteria (Chapter 12). The antigenic specificity of these O antigens resides in the **O-specific side chains** of the lipopolysaccharide and is dependent upon the kinds of sugar residues and their arrangement in the side chain. Occasional O antigen cross-reactions are observed between different enteric bacteria, and these are due to similarities in the polysaccharide composition of the O-specific side chains. Reactions of surface O antigens with homologous antibody result in agglutination of the bacterial cells, yielding closely adherent cellular aggregates, appearing macroscopically as fine granules which rapidly settle from suspension. These cellular aggregates are not easily dispersed by shaking.

Variation from the **smooth** to **rough** colonial form (S–R variation) is accompanied by a progressive loss of the smooth O antigen and, ultimately, results in a rough (R) bacterial strain whose lipopolysaccharide lacks the O-specific side chains, retaining only the basal core structure. Rough strains do not, therefore, react with O-specific antibody.

H Antigens. The flagella of motile bacteria contain serologically specific proteins (flagellins) which, unlike the O antigens, are heat-labile and are destroyed by ethanol. When these motile bacteria are reacted with specific antiflagellar antibodies, microscopic observation reveals a loose association of many cells with tangling and intertwining of their flagella. Macroscopically, this type of agglutination is seen as fluffy or flocculent masses that settle from suspension. Vigorous shaking disperses the floccules, but they re-form upon further incubation. The terminology of the H and O antigens arises from the fact that motile bacteria frequently grow as a thin film on moist mediums. This film was termed *Hauch* (puff, or film) by German workers; motile strains, and their flagellar antigens, were then designated H. Strains which grow as discrete colonies on moist mediums (*Ohne Hauch,* without cloud or film) are nonmotile and are designated O.

Motile bacteria may lose their capacity to produce flagella, yet still retain their O antigen specificity. This is known as the HO–O variation.

K Antigens. A third class of antigens, the K antigens, appear in Enterobacteriaceae as **capsules,** or as **envelope antigens,** which overlie the surface O antigens. Because of this, the K antigens block agglutination by O-specific antibody. Antigens of this class are generally polysaccharides and their reactivity is usually altered by heating, so that treatment in this way yields strains agglutinable with O antiserums. *Klebsiella,* as well as some strains of other genera, produce microscopically visible capsules. In other species, however, the K antigens on the cell surface are serologically reactive but not otherwise demonstrable; in these strains, therefore, they are envelope antigens. The K antigen terminology varies somewhat in different genera. In the few *Salmonella* that possess K antigen, it is designated the Vi antigen. K antigens of *Escherichia* are generally polysaccharide, but in a few cases, they are composed of protein and occur as fimbriae on the cell surface.

Enterobacterial Common Antigen.[8, 9, 13] In 1962, Kunin and his colleagues described a haptenic substance of wide distribution among enterobacteria that is now called the enterobacterial common antigen (ECA) or Kunin antigen. The hapten occurs in two aggregative forms in the outer membrane. In a few bacteria, the hapten is linked to the lipopolysaccharide (LPS) and is immunogenic; in the majority of enteric bacteria, however, it is in a free form and is not capable of eliciting antibody response. The LPS-linked ECA is relatively rare, but is found in some R mutants of *Escherichia coli* and *Shigella*. By appropriate methods, the ECA can be separated from the bacterial cell and, when attached to the surface of erythrocytes, sensitizes these cells to agglutination by ECA-specific antibody. Chemical analysis of ECA has revealed that it is a low-molecular-weight (ca. 2700 daltons) linear polymer predominantly composed of alternating units of *N*-acetyl-D-glucosamine and *N*-acetyl-D-mannosaminouronic acid, partly esterified by palmitic acid; it is also thought to contain an unknown lipid component. Although antibodies to ECA may be detected in human serum, particularly in severe or chronic enterobacterial infections, the role of this substance in virulence and pathogenesis has not been established.

Fimbrial Antigens. Most members of the Enterobacteriaceae produce fimbriae, or pili. The "common" pili are usually numerous on the bacterial surface, whereas the F, or sex, pili are limited in number—1 to 4 per cell— and differ morphologically from common pili. Common pili possess strong adhesive properties; thus, piliation of bacteria is often demonstrated by their capacity to bring about agglutination of red blood cells. Bacteria with these surface appendages are also readily agglutinated in pilus-specific antibody, a reaction that resembles flagellar agglutination. Richly fimbriated cells are not readily agglutinated, however, by antiserum to their O antigens, *i.e.*, the fimbriae interfere with O agglutination. Boiling destroys these fimbriae, and cells so treated become O-agglutinable.

Protein Antigens. In common with other gram-negative bacteria, the Enterobacteriaceae contain several major proteins in the outer membrane (Chapter 2). These are antigenic and contribute to the antigenic mosaic of enterobacteria. There is considerable serological cross-reactivity between major outer membrane proteins from related strains, *e.g.*, *Escherichia,* and at least one of these may be common to all Enterobacteriaceae.[6]

In addition to the major outer membrane proteins, Enterobacteriaceae appear to possess a common lipoprotein antigen.[5] This lipoprotein occurs in the inner leaflet of the outer membrane, linked to the peptidoglycan of the cell wall, and probably plays a role in the structure and organization of the cell wall. Antibody to the lipoprotein is produced in a significant number of individuals suffering systemic enterobacterial infections.

Toxins

In addition to the endotoxic activity associated with the lipopolysaccharide of the outer membrane, and common to all wild strains of enterobacteria, several other toxins may be produced.

Those enterobacteria that exhibit hemolytic activity, *i.e.*, enteropathic strains of *E. coli* and some *Proteus*, usually produce extracellular hemolytic toxins that may have other cytotoxic properties as well. Of considerably greater significance is the **diarrheagenic enterotoxin,** produced by some strains of *E. coli,* and responsible for the secretion of fluids and electrolytes into the lumen of the small intestine (Chapter 18). It resembles the enterotoxin of *Vibrio cholerae* (Chapter 21) in both mode of action and constitution. Several shigellae, especially *Shigella dysenteriae* type 1, produce substances with cytotoxic and enterotoxic activity, probably acting to inhibit protein synthesis (Chapter 18). Enterotoxins are also occasionally encountered in certain *Salmonella*.

Genetic Variation

The enterobacteria, by virtue of the close physical and ecological associations in their natural habitat, exhibit considerable genetic variation. The conditions of enterobacterial ecology may promote the exchange of genetic information, largely through transduction and conjugation, thereby probably accounting for common physiological reactions, shared antigenic constituents, and multiple drug resistance.[7, 12] Gene transfer in microorganisms is discussed fully in Chapter 6. Of particular importance in the Enterobacteriaceae is the conjugative transfer of **R plasmids** to recipient strains, because these plasmids carry genes specifying **drug resistance.** Resistance genes for several antibiotics are often present on a single plasmid.[3] The biochemical mechanisms for resistance vary with the antibiotic in question. Resistance to penicillin usually depends upon the synthesis of penicillinase; tetracycline resistance appears when cells fail to concentrate the antibiotic intracellularly; and in chloramphenicol resistance, an enzyme is formed which inactivates the antibiotic.

Although resistant enteric bacteria have been encountered in geographic areas where the antibiotic had not been previously used, the incidence of drug resistant strains markedly increases where antibiotics are widely employed in treatment or prophylaxis. The addition of antibiotics to animal feeds, in order to promote weight gain and improve disease resistance, has been particularly troubling, since the practice leads to increased incidence of multiple drug resistance of enteric bacteria in these animals; it is believed that the resistance plasmids are passed from animal to human strains.[10]

Isolation and Identification of Enterobacteriaceae[4, 11]

The isolation and identification of the enteric bacilli is a relatively complex process and is best undertaken by clinical laboratories with trained and experienced personnel. Nevertheless, the general principles of specimen collection and transport, isolation, and screening of isolates will be discussed here. More detailed differentiation of genera and species will be found in succeeding chapters.

Specimen Collection

Depending upon the site of infection, enteric bacilli may be found in stools, urine, abscesses, blood, wounds, sputum, and body fluids of infected individuals. Specimens should be carefully collected to avoid exogenous contamination. They should be rapidly transported and cultured to prevent overgrowth of contaminating microorganisms and to preserve the viability of the suspected pathogen. Specimens may be refrigerated for short periods, but if delay in culturing is anticipated, they should be placed in appropriate transport solutions, *e.g.*, buffered glycerol-saline.

Isolation

A variety of mediums have been devised for the primary isolation of enterobacteria. The selection of an appropriate isolation medium depends upon the number and kind of enteric bacilli expected to be present as well as the degree and type of contamination. Stool cultures, for example, contain large numbers of contaminating microorganisms and require selective mediums. If the relative number of pathogenic forms is low, preliminary enrichment culture may be necessary to increase their numbers and to improve chances for their isolation. Several of the recommended plating and enrichment mediums are listed in Table 17–3.

Biochemical Screening

A preliminary differentiation of isolates may be accomplished by a combination of biochemical tests, as illustrated in Tables 17–2 and 17–4. Further differentiation among genera and species requires multiple biochemical and

Table 17–3. **Mediums for Enrichment and Isolation of Enterobacteriaceae**

Plating Mediums	Enrichment Mediums
Nonselective	
Nutrient or infusion agars	GN (gram-negative) broth
Blood agar	Tetrathionate broth
	Tetrathionate–brilliant green broth
Nonselective, differential	Selenite F broth
Indicator-lactose agars	
Lowly selective, differential	
Eosin–methylene blue agar	
MacConkey's agar	
Deoxycholate agar	
Moderately selective, differential	
Salmonella-Shigella agar	
Deoxycholate-citrate agar	
Hektoen-enteric agar	
Xylose-lysine-deoxycholate agar	
Highly selective	
Bismuth sulfite agar	
Brilliant green agar	

Table 17–4. **Reactions of Enterobacteriaceae in Triple Sugar-Iron Agar***

Genus	Slant	Butt	Gas	H₂S
Escherichia	A	A	+	−
Shigella	K	A	−	−
Salmonella	K	A	+ or −	+
Arizona	K	A	+	+
Citrobacter	K	A	+	+
Edwardsiella	K	A	+	+
Klebsiella	A	A	+	−
Enterobacter	A	A	+	−
Hafnia	K	A	+	−
Serratia	A or K	A	−	−
Proteus	A or K	A	+	+
Morganella	K	A	−	−
Providentia	K	A	+ or −	−
Yersinia	A or K	A	−	−

*Adapted from Martin and Washington.[11] Symbols: A, acid; K, alkaline. An acid slant indicates the fermentation of sucrose and/or lactose, whereas an acid butt indicates glucose fermentation, with or without gas production. Usual reactions are shown, but a few strains may differ in some reactions.

sometimes serological testing. These more definitive reactions are treated in immediately following chapters.

REFERENCES

1. Brenner, D. J., *et al.* 1977. Taxonomic and nomenclature changes in *Enterobacteriaceae*. Centers for Disease Control, Atlanta, Ga.
2. Buchanan, R. E., and N. E. Gibbons (Eds.). 1974. Bergey's Manual of Determinative Bacteriology. 8th ed. Williams & Wilkins Co., Baltimore.
3. Davies, J. E., and R. Rownd. 1972. Transmissible multiple drug resistance in Enterobacteriaceae. Science **176**:758–768.
4. Edwards, P. R., and W. H. Ewing. 1972. Identification of Enterobacteriaceae. 3rd ed. Burgess, Minneapolis, Minn.
5. Griffiths, E. K., S. Yoonessi, and E. Neter. 1977. Antibody response to enterobacterial lipoprotein of patients with varied infections due to *Enterobacteriaceae*. Proc. Soc. Exptl Biol. Med. **154**:246–249.
6. Hofstra, H., and J. Dankert. 1979. Antigenic cross-reactivity of major outer membrane proteins in Enterobacteriaceae species. J. Gen. Microbiol. **111**:293–302.
7. Jones, R. T., and R. Curtiss, III. 1970. Genetic exchange between *Escherichia coli* strains in the mouse intestine. J. Bacteriol. **103**:71–80.
8. Mäkelä, P. H., and H. Mayer. 1976. Enterobacterial common antigen. Bacteriol. Rev. **40**:591–632.
9. Männel, D., and H. Mayer. 1978. Isolation and chemical characterization of the enterobacterial common antigen. European J. Biochem. **86**:361–370.
10. Marsik, F. J., J. T. Parisi, and D. C. Blenden. 1975. Transmissible drug resistance of *Escherichia coli* and *Salmonella* from humans, animals and rural environments. J. Infect. Dis. **132**:296–302.
11. Martin, W. J., and J. A. Washington, II. 1980. *Enterobacteriaceae*. pp. 195–219. *In* E. H. Lennette, *et al.* (Eds.): Manual of Clinical Microbiology. 3rd ed. American Society for Microbiology, Washington, D.C.
12. Neu, H. C., P. J. Huber, and E. B. Winshell. 1973. Interbacterial transfer of R factor in humans. Antimicrob. Agents Chemother. **3**:542–544.
13. Rinno, J., J. R. Golecki, and H. Mayer. 1980. Localization of enterobacterial common antigen: immunogenic and nonimmunogenic enterobacterial common antigen–containing *Escherichia coli*. J. Bacteriol. **141**:814–821.
14. Sanderson, K. E. 1976. Genetic relatedness in the family Enterobacteriaceae. Ann. Rev. Microbiol. **30**:327–340.

CHAPTER 18

The Enteric Bacilli: Escherichia and Shigella

Escherichia coli, one of the first of the enteric bacilli to be described and cultured, is a normal inhabitant of the intestinal tract of man and animals. At this site of colonization, *E. coli* is a rare agent of gastroenteritis, but is a significant cause of urinary tract infections and of neonatal septicemia and meningitis. *Shigella* are the agents of bacillary dysentery, a gastroenteritis uniquely affecting humans, first described by Shiga in Japan in 1898. *Escherichia* and *Shigella* are closely similar, both bacteriologically and in the types of infection they cause. In the classification scheme used here, they are placed together in the tribe Escherichieae of the family Enterobacteriaceae. Table 18–1 illustrates some of the biochemical tests that may be used to differentiate between these two genera.

Escherichia[12]

Since their discovery by Escherich in 1886, the lactose-fermenting *Escherichia coli* have fascinated and intrigued microbiologists. They are widely distributed, being universally found in the intestinal tract of man and both warm- and cold-blooded animals. For this reason, they are often employed as indicators of fecal pollution of water supplies. As is evident in earlier chapters, *E. coli* has been one of the most important tools of the microbial geneticist and microbial physiologist. Long considered to be nonpathogenic commensals, their role in both opportunistic and frank infections is now universally recognized.

Morphology
These gram-negative bacilli conform to the general description given earlier for Enterobacteriaceae, although they exhibit some variation in size. Many strains are encapsulated and most are motile by peritrichous flagella. Cellular architecture generally conforms to that given in Chapter 2 for gram-negative bacteria. *Escherichia* are generally fimbriate,

Table 18–1. **Differential Reactions of *Escherichia*
and *Shigella****

Test	Escherichia	Shigella
Gas from glucose	+	−
Lactose fermentation	+	−
Motility	+	−
Lysine decarboxylase	+	−
Mucate utilization	+	−

*Adapted from Martin and Washington.[30] Symbols: +,
most strains positive; −, most strains negative.

possessing both **sex pili** and **adhesive fimbriae.**
Figure 18–1 illustrates the morphology of *E.
coli* and that of the type 1 adhesive fimbriae.

Colonies, especially on nutrient gelatin, are
opaque to partially translucent, smooth, and
homogeneous in consistency and exhibit the
maple-leaf colonial appearance common to
many enterobacteria. When grown on certain
mediums, particularly eosin–methylene blue
agar, the colonies take on a curious metallic
sheen. Some varieties are β-hemolytic on
blood agar; hemolytic strains are more frequent in pathological processes than in the
intestine.

Physiology

These bacteria grow luxuriantly on ordinary
nutrient mediums and may be cultivated in the
simplest of synthetic mediums, *i.e.,* those with
an inorganic nitrogen source and glucose.
Growth occurs over a temperature range of
10° to 46°C.; optimum growth temperature is
37°C.

Various sugars, including lactose, are rapidly
fermented, producing acid and gas. The principal acid formed is lactic acid; smaller quantities of formic and acetic acids are produced,
together with ethyl alcohol.

Most strains are killed by exposure to 60° C.
for 30 minutes, but occasionally more resistant
varieties are encountered. In common with
other gram-negative bacteria, they are more
resistant to the bacteriostatic action of dyes
than are gram-positive bacteria. Thus, selective mediums containing dyes are commonly
used in primary isolation of these and other
enteric bacteria. Their ability to grow in the
presence of bile salts is likewise marked and
these are often incorporated into selective mediums.

Biotypes. Strains of *Escherichia* frequently
exhibit differences in biochemical reactions,
e.g., carbohydrate fermentation, decarboxylation of lysine and ornithine, and hydrolysis of
esculin. It has often been proposed that biotypes differentiated in this way should prove
useful for epidemiological purposes; biotyping
has gained only limited acceptance, however,
and epidemiological typing is usually by serological means.

Antigenic Structure[35]

The antigenic structure of *Escherichia* has
been elucidated in great detail, and serotypes
may be identified with a high degree of precision. Serotyping is based on the distribution
of O, K, and H antigens (Chapter 17).

The O antigens represent the specific polysaccharide side chains that are a part of the
cell wall lipopolysaccharides of smooth cells.

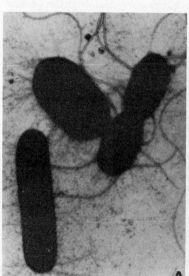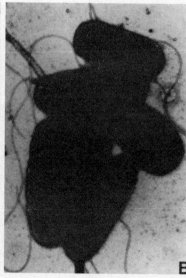

Figure 18–1. Electron micrograph
of *Escherichia coli*. *A,* Fimbriate
strain possessing both flagella and
type 1 fimbriae. *B,* Nonfimbriate
strain, possessing only flagella.
× 20,400. (B. I. Eisenstein, Science **214**:337, 1981. Copyright
1981 by the American Association
for the Advancement of Science.)

Their presence is detected by bacterial agglutination in O-specific antiserums. With respect to the heat-stable O antigen constitution of *E. coli,* serological O groups, rather than types, are designated, since several of the O groups contain related, but immunologically specific, antigens called O factors. Group O1, for example, is made up of factors O1a and O1b. About 160 O groups are recognized.

There is some cross-reactivity between *E. coli* O groups and similar antigens in other enterobacteria. These cross-reactions are frequently noted with shigellae and, to a lesser extent, with other genera, emphasizing the close relationships between *Escherichia* and *Shigella.*

Many *Escherichia* possess polysaccharide capsules that overlie the O antigen structures of the outer membrane. These interfere with agglutination by O-specific antiserums and such cells are said to be O-inagglutinable. Agglutination by O antiserums may be restored by heating, which destroys the capsular antigens. These antigens are designated as K antigens (from the German, *Kapsel*) and are numbered in sequence, K1, K2, etc., more or less in order of discovery. More than 100 K antigens are designated.

Although most K antigens are acidic polysaccharides, the terminology has been extended to include several surface antigens that are protein in nature. These appear on the cell surface as fimbrial structures. The fimbrial antigens designated as K antigens (K88 and K99) are found in strains that are associated with diarrheal disease in animals. They differ from other fimbrial antigens of *E. coli* in that their hemagglutinating activity is not inhibited by D-mannose.

Not all *Escherichia* contain K antigens; when they are present, only one serological type is found in a given strain. Strains containing these antigens are generally more resistant to phagocytosis and to the bactericidal action of antibody and complement. Certain K antigens appear to correlate with other virulence properties. Strains carrying the K1 antigen, for example, have been repeatedly incriminated in neonatal meningitis outbreaks.

The synthesis of capsular polysaccharides is controlled by chromosomal genes of *E. coli,* while the fimbrial K antigens are transferable and directed by plasmids.

The flagellar, or H, antigens of *Escherichia* are sometimes poorly developed, at least on primary isolation, but their use completes the serotyping of this group. More than 50 H antigens are known.

Colicins [23]

A number of bacteria, both gram-positive and gram-negative, produce protein substances that are bactericidal for other microorganisms, usually those closely related to the producing strains. The generic term for these antibiotic principles is **bacteriocins,** but they are often given more specific names to indicate the producer; those produced by *E. coli,* for example, are called colicins. Colicins are proteins, ranging in molecular weight from about 20,000 to 90,000 daltons, whose synthesis is governed by plasmids. They act against other, sensitive strains of *Escherichia,* as well as some closely related enterobacteria. Colicins bind to specific receptors on the outer membrane of susceptible cells; following this they penetrate the cytoplasmic membrane. Some act by forming ion-permeable channels in the membrane that results in collapse of the membrane proton motive force. Others enter the cytoplasm and interrupt protein synthesis, in some cases by ribonuclease activity and in others by action as DNA endonuclease.

It is often assumed that colicin production confers selective advantage, particularly in the competitive environment of the intestinal tract. Although colicin producers tend to predominate at this location, there is no direct evidence of enhanced survival attributable to colicin production.

Toxins [39]

In addition to the classical endotoxin commonly produced by gram-negative bacteria, *Escherichia* produce several extracellular toxins.

Enterotoxin. The great majority of enteropathic strains of *E. coli, i.e.,* those associated with diarrheal disease, produce one or more enterotoxins. These toxins mediate the movement of water and ions from tissues into the bowel lumen to give a net secretion that manifests as diarrhea. Two different kinds of enterotoxins can be distinguished; one is a **heat-stable toxin (ST),** the other is **heat-labile (LT).** The properties of each are listed in Table 18–2. Both kinds of toxin cause fluid accumulation in ligated ileal loops of rabbits and may be assayed in this way, or by biological responses in a variety of *in vitro* cell systems.

The heat-labile toxin is best known and its mode of action is well understood. The toxin first binds to the G_{M1}-ganglioside receptor on susceptible cells through the **binding (B) subunit.** The **active (A) subunit** then activates cellular adenyl cyclase to increase the levels of cyclic adenosine-5'-monophosphate (cAMP),

Table 18–2. *Escherichia coli* Enterotoxins

Property	Heat-Labile Toxin	Heat-Stable Toxin
Molecular weight*		
Whole toxin	72,000–91,400	2500–5100
A subunit	25,500–28,000	none
B subunit	11,500–12,700	none
Heat sensitive	+	–
Acid sensitive	+	–
Trypsin sensitive	+	–
Immunogenic	+	weak
Neutralized by antitoxin	+	+
Subtypes	several	several
Principal receptor	G_{M1}-ganglioside	unknown
Plasmid coded	+	+

*From published data.[1, 4, 11, 13, 18, 29]

which, in turn, brings about water and electrolyte loss. This mode of action is quite similar to that of cholera toxin (Chapter 21). Curiously, the two toxins are similar structurally and immunologically as well.

In contrast, the ST toxin activates guanyl cyclase and elevates tissue cyclic guanosine-5′-monophosphate (cGMP) to induce water and electrolyte secretion in the intestine.[20]

Hemolysins. A number of *E. coli* strains are hemolytic and this property is often associated with those responsible for disease production. Two kinds of hemolysins are produced. One, designated α-hemolysin (not to be confused with α-hemolysis by streptococci) is a soluble hemolysin released from the cell; its synthesis is controlled by transmissible plasmids.[50] The synthesis of hemolysin is correlated with virulence; it is cytotoxic for leucocytes,[9] and, at sublethal levels, inhibits phagocytosis and chemotaxis.[10] Hemolytic activity is neutralized by homologous antibody. The other, β-hemolysin, is a cell-bound hemolysin.

Virulence

The virulence factors of *E. coli* are unusually complex and the contribution of individual determinants cannot be considered in isolation. Indeed, the relevant determinants may vary with the locus and nature of the infection.

Table 18–3 displays the determinants that appear to be directly related to virulence. In addition to these, several factors are known to correlate with virulence. The production of hemolysin appears to correlate with certain O groups and with serum resistance. Another correlate is the frequent association of certain serotypes with enteropathogenesis (see below).

Virulence in microorganisms is associated with the capacity to attach and colonize at the site of infection, with subsequent damage to the host, usually by production of toxins. Virulence is promoted by aggressins that interfere with host defenses. All of these are observed in pathogenic *E. coli*.

Colonization.[14] Adherence of *E. coli* to epithelial cells is mediated by one or more of the **adhesins** listed in Table 18–3. For the most part, these are fimbrial in nature. Present evidence indicates that these react with specific receptors on the eucaryotic cells; the distribution of the receptors on host cells determines their susceptibility to colonization by particular strains of *E. coli*. For example, *E. coli* adherence to phagocytes is mediated by mannose-sensitive pili or by cell wall adhesins, but not by mannose-resistant pili.[6] Porcine enteropathic strains usually adhere to the intestinal mucosa by virtue of their mannose-resistant, fimbrial K antigens (K88). The bacilli are not found in the crypts, but adhere to the sides and tips of the villi. Human strains of enteropathic *E. coli* do not possess fimbrial K antigens but do attach and colonize intestinal epithelium. Their adherence is often mediated by plasmid-directed, heat-labile, mannose-resistant fimbriae functioning as colonization factors. Two of these colonization factor antigens are recognized, **CFA/I** and **CFA/II,** which differ from one another, and from other fimbrial adhesins, in serological reactivity and receptor specificity.[16] Antibody to fimbrial adhesins specifically protects against colonization. Other fimbrial antigens, both mannose-resistant and mannose-sensitive, are usually responsible for adherence at sites such as the urinary tract epithelium. In a few instances, surface antigens

Table 18–3. **Virulence Determinants in *Escherichia coli***

Adhesins	Toxins	Aggressins
Fimbrial K antigens	Heat-stable enterotoxins	Capsular K antigens
Colonization factor antigens (CFA/I and CFA/II)	Heat-labile enterotoxins	Iron siderophores and transport systems
Fimbriae, mannose-resistant		Serum resistance factors
Fimbriae, mannose-sensitive		Antibody-complement resistance factors
Nonfimbrial, surface adhesions		

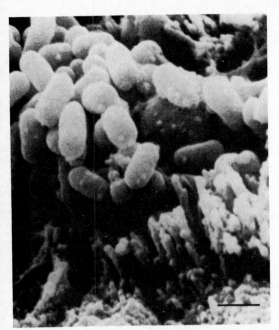

Figure 18–2. Scanning electron micrograph of *Escherichia coli* adherent to the mucosal surface of the rabbit cecum. Bar = 1 μm. (A. Takeuchi, *et al., Infect. Immun.* **19**:686, 1978.)

other than fimbriae are associated with adherence, but these are not well defined. Figures 18–2 and 18–3 illustrate the adherence of *E. coli* to intestinal epithelium.

While colonization is probably a requisite first step in pathogenesis, enteropathic *E. coli* subsequently cause diarrheal disease by one of two distinct mechanisms. Some are able to invade the intestinal epithelium in a manner

analogous to the *Shigella;* pathogenesis by this mode does not appear to involve enterotoxin production. As in the *Shigella,* invasiveness often correlates with the possession of plasmids.[24] Others are not invasive, however, but produce diarrhea by production of enterotoxin, which is absorbed from the site of villus colonization. Occasionally, infant diarrhea is caused by *E. coli* strains that are neither enterotoxic nor enteroinvasive; the mechanism of pathogenesis by these remains unknown.

Aggressins. When *E. coli* invade the tissues, as in neonatal meningitis and pyelonephritis, other virulence factors become important. These include resistance to phagocytosis and to the bactericidal action of serum, as well as the ability to capture utilizable iron in tissue.

Encapsulated strains of *E. coli, i.e.,* those containing polysaccharide K antigens, are resistant to phagocytosis, and their survival in tissues is enhanced. The capsular layer inhibits complement activation and opsonization, as described in Chapter 12. Similarly, encapsulated strains are generally resistant to the bactericidal action of normal serum, indicating diminished capacity to activate complement. Serum resistance may also be determined by the structural components of the outer membrane, resistance being conferred not by interference with complement activation but by resistance to the action of terminal (C6–C9) complement components.[5]

In order to grow within the tissues, *E. coli* must be able to sequester iron that is bound to tissue siderophores (Chapter 12). Many strains form **enterochelin** to satisfy this require-

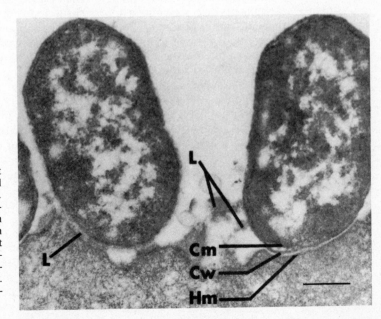

Figure 18–3. *Escherichia coli* adherent to the invaginated host epithelial cell membrane *(Hm)* of the rabbit cecum. Note that remnants of the lanthanum-stained glycocalyx are still present on the host cell surface *(L)* and between the bacterial cell wall *(Cw)* and host membrane. *Cm,* bacterial cell membrane. Alcian blue-lanthanum treatment, lead citrate–uranyl acetate stain. Bar = 0.2 μm. (A. Takeuchi, *et al., Infect. Immun.* **19**:686, 1978.)

ment, but other mechanisms may also be operative. Several systems for iron uptake have been detected, including a cytoplasmic membrane transport system for uptake of hydroxamate siderophores.[25] One of the colicin plasmids, *colV*, codes for an iron-uptake system in invasive strains of *E. coli* that includes an extracellular iron-chelator, aerobactin, and a cell-membrane iron-transport component.[53]

ESCHERICHIA COLI INFECTIONS[21]

Escherichia are a part of the normal intestinal flora in humans and are the predominant members of the aerobic bacteria of the bowel. Except for the relatively few enteropathogenic strains, they are commensals at this site, but they are potentially pathogenic elsewhere in the body. Several kinds of *E. coli* infections can be distinguished—urinary tract infections; septicemic infections, sometimes with meningitis; and diarrheal disease.

Urinary Tract Infections[22]
Among the most frequent bacterial infections in humans are those of the urinary tract, and *E. coli* predominates as the causative agent. Fortunately, the greatest proportion of these infections are asymptomatic and manifest only as bacteriuria with significant numbers of bacteria in the urine ($\geq 10^5$ per ml.). Others—pyelonephritis and acute cystitis—are more serious. Complications may lead to renal insufficiency and hypertension. In young children, both sexes are susceptible, but in adults the frequency is greatest in women. Several of the virulence determinants discussed above are found in uropathogenic strains of *E. coli*. Polysaccharide K antigens appear to be significant, with the K1 antigen most often associated with virulent strains. Adherence to uroepithelium is characteristic of uropathogenic strains, and the principal adhesins are the mannose-resistant fimbriae; nonfimbrial surface adhesins may also be involved. Strains responsible for acute pyelonephritis exhibit a greater resistance to the bactericidal action of normal serum.

Neonatal Meningitis[52]
Escherichia coli is a leading cause of neonatal septicemia and meningitis. Infection characteristically occurs in the first 30 days of life, with premature infants at more than four times greater risk than full-term infants. The mortality of meningeal infections in the newborn is remarkably high, 40 to 80 per cent,

and even when appropriately treated a majority of the survivors exhibit severe neurological sequelae.

The elevated susceptibility of neonates is likely due to deficiencies in host defense systems. Antibodies against the somatic O antigen of enteric bacilli are those of the IgM class; newborn infants are deficient in these, since neither IgA nor IgM is placentally transferred from the mother. Further, IgM is the antibody class most efficient in opsonization and complement-mediated bacterial killing. Infants are deficient, too, in complement components of both the classical and alternate pathways. Infants that are not breast-fed may also be deprived of the protection afforded by lactoferrin and IgA, which are contained in mother's milk.

Escherichia coli strains with the greatest virulence in neonatal meningitis are those that possess the K1 polysaccharide antigen. Antibody to the K1 antigen is passively protective, at least in animal models. It is of considerable theoretical interest that the K1 antigen of *E. coli* is immunologically identical to the polysaccharide antigen of group B meningococci, also a significant cause of meningitis. The importance of iron in the virulence of *E. coli* is emphasized by the finding that Polynesian infants receiving iron dextran to correct iron deficiencies exhibited a marked susceptibility to neonatal sepsis by this microorganism.[3]

Diarrhea[19, 38, 41]
The association between *E. coli* and animal diarrheas has been known for over 80 years, but an established relationship to human diarrhea came much later. Even though Escherich suspected that the colon bacillus was responsible for infant diarrhea, the presence of *E. coli* in the intestinal tract of normal individuals promoted the assumption by most workers that these were commensal microorganisms. Nevertheless, by the early 1950s, a number of studies had established the etiological role of certain antigenically distinct strains of *E. coli* in human diarrheal disease, particularly in infants.

The *E. coli* that cause diarrheal disease are conveniently grouped into three categories, based on mechanisms of pathogenesis, and differing in serology and epidemiology: (1) **enterotoxigenic**, (2) **enteropathic**, and (3) **enteroinvasive**.

In the pathogenesis of *E. coli* diarrhea, there is a complex interrelationship between host defense factors and bacterial virulence factors. Among the more important of the host defenses are the bactericidal action of gastric acid; the mucosal immune defenses, including IgA; intestinal motility, which helps to remove ingested bacteria; and the normal bacterial flora of the bowel inhibiting colonization by pathogens. Virulence determinants vary in each of the *E. coli* pathogenic types and are discussed below.

Enterotoxigenic Escherichia. Enterotoxigenic *E. coli* produce one or both of the enterotoxins—ST or LT—discussed earlier. These induce the net secretion of fluid and electrolytes into the lumen of the small intestine, thereby generating the characteristic diarrhea. Adherence and colonization of the intestinal mucosa is a necessary antecedent to toxin production and is mediated by *E. coli* adhesins, particularly colonization factors CFA/I and CFA/II.

Diarrheal disease caused by enterotoxigenic *E. coli* ranges from a mild illness to severe, cholera-like disease, and can occur in either children or adults. In children under two years of age, these strains are a major cause of the sporadic and epidemic diarrheas that occur in underdeveloped countries, but are uncommon in industrialized nations. In adults, they are the leading agent of traveler's diarrhea, acquired by tourists visiting in developing countries. Although infant diarrhea of this type is infrequent in the United States and England, a few outbreaks in nurseries have been documented. A few large outbreaks have occurred among adults in this country, spread by contaminated water or foods; it appears that case-to-case spread is an exception.

The O serogroups associated with enterotoxigenic *E. coli* are shown in Table 18–4 and are compared to the serogroups usually found in other types. Although a high proportion of the enterotoxigenic strains possess one of the serogroup antigens shown, the agreement is not perfect. Not all members of the particular serogroup produce toxin, and enterotoxigenic strains sometimes are found in other serogroups. Similar admonitions apply to serogroups associated with enteropathogenic and invasive *E. coli*.

Enteropathogenic Escherichia. The *E. coli* strains of this type are not known to produce enterotoxins, and their mode of pathogenesis is not clear. They do, however, possess adhesins and colonize the small bowel as a part of pathogenesis. It is possible that they produce toxins yet to be recognized; if they form enterotoxins, these are not detectable by the usual tests.

Enteropathogenic *E. coli* have been responsible for frequent epidemic episodes of infantile diarrhea, although these largely disappeared from the United States and England after about 1971. Sporadic cases still occur, however, usually in the summer months. Occasional waterborne and foodborne outbreaks occur in adults in developed countries.

Enteroinvasive Escherichia. A third group of *E. coli* cause diarrheal disease distinguished by invasion of the intestinal mucosa. These strains are designated enteroinvasive; they do not produce enterotoxins and their mode of pathogenesis is similar to that of *Shigella*. Indeed, they resemble *Shigella* in other respects as well. Lactose may be fermented late, or not at all, and gas may not be formed; they are frequently nonmotile. Furthermore, many of the invasive strains share major antigens with certain of the *Shigella*. The O124 serogroup antigen, for example, is identical to the major somatic antigen of *Shigella dysenteriae* type 3. As with *Shigella*, their invasive capacity is established by the production of keratoconjunctivitis when instilled into the guinea pig eye (the Serény test).

As expected, the clinical manifestation of enteroinvasive *E. coli* disease is usually indistinguishable from bacillary dysentery caused by *Shigella*. The disease is normally seen in older children, either as sporadic cases or in institutional outbreaks. Adult disorders often appear as water- or foodborne episodes, with worldwide distribution.

Nosocomial Infection.[2, 49] *Escherichia coli* is the leading cause of hospital-acquired, or nosocomial, infections; hospital-based studies in the United States reveal that almost 20 per cent of all such infections are due to *E. coli*. In a few instances, it is responsible for epidemics of gastroenteritis, but more often, the infections are endemic in nature.

Of the latter, the urinary tract is the most

Table 18–4. **Serogroups of *Escherichia coli* Associated with Diarrheal Disease***

Type	O Serogroup†
Enterotoxigenic *E. coli*	8, 25, 78, 115, 128
Enteropathic *E. coli*	18, 20, 25, *26*, 28, 44, **55**, 86, **111**, 112, 114, **119**, 125, 126, **127, 128**, 142
Enteroinvasive *E. coli*	28ac, 112ac, 124, 136, 143, 144, 152, 164

*Data from Report, Bull. Wld Hlth Org **58**:23, 1980.
†The O serogroups in boldface are particularly common.

common site of infection; about 40 per cent of all nosocomial infections involve the urinary tract, and *E. coli* is the etiological agent in approximately 50 per cent of these. In large measure, nosocomial bacteriuria follows catheterization or other urological manipulations; greatest risk attaches to the use of indwelling catheters with open drainage.

Immunity

Despite the apparent parallels between the serogroup and pathogenic potential of *E. coli,* there is no convincing evidence that protection against infection is afforded by antibody response to O antigens. Rather, it is more likely that immune protection is induced by the recognized virulence factors acting as antigens.

The epidemiology of *E. coli* diarrhea suggests a naturally acquired immunity, at least to those strains circulating in the population. Young children in endemic areas are at risk, but older children and adults seem to acquire some level of immunity, presumably by continued exposure. Adults entering the endemic area, without previous exposure to the circulating strains, develop traveler's diarrhea. The basis for acquired immunity is uncertain. It may arise from antitoxic immunity to the enterotoxins; from antibody to the adhesins, resulting in decreased colonization; or from antibody against other surface antigens leading to opsonization and intracellular destruction of the bacteria.

In one study of Swedish soldiers in Cyprus, diarrheal episodes were followed by the appearance of serum antibodies against the LT enterotoxin. Even those who did not develop diarrhea often exhibited antitoxin titers after residence in the endemic area. A high proportion of the area residents also had significant levels of serum antibodies.[45]

A number of studies in animals have indicated that immunization with enterotoxin protects against challenge with either enterotoxigenic *E. coli* or toxin alone. Immunization and challenge of human volunteers, on the other hand, suggest that antitoxin is not the protective mechanism;[28] more likely, immune protection arises from antibody to other surface antigens, probably colonization factor antigens or other adhesins.

Based upon numerous veterinary studies disclosing protection of animals by anti-pilus antibody, it can be speculated that human protection is engendered in the same fashion. Mucosal IgA directed against colonization factor antigens would be expected to interfere with colonization by *E. coli* in the intestinal tract; fimbriae and polysaccharide K antigens in uropathogenic strains might render similar protection.

Chemotherapy and Drug Resistance

Escherichia coli is normally susceptible to a variety of chemotherapeutic agents, including tetracycline, ampicillin, erythromycin, neomycin, streptomycin, trimethoprim, and sulfonamides. Drug-resistant strains are increasingly prevalent, however, and a major portion of these carry R plasmids directing resistance to one or more drugs. Indeed, a single R plasmid in enterobacteria has been shown to determine resistance to nine antibiotics.[46]

Uncomplicated urinary tract infections in women usually respond successfully to therapy with amoxicillin, sulfisoxazole, or trimethoprim-sulfomethoxazole.[44] In infant diarrhea, trimethoprim-sulfomethoxazole or mecillinam has yielded clinical cure in 73 to 79 per cent of those treated.[47] Both doxycycline and erythromycin have been successfully used as prophylactic agents against traveler's diarrhea in visitors to endemic areas.

Laboratory Diagnosis

The laboratory diagnosis of disease caused by *E. coli* has been systematized and is discussed in Chapter 17. Although detailed serotyping of isolates may have epidemiological significance, it is complex and time-consuming, and is not generally performed in clinical laboratories. The value of serogrouping by clinical laboratories is controversial, since there has been variation in the serogroups associated with *E. coli* diarrheal disease over periods of time. Tests for enterotoxin production by isolated strains are possible, but are not routinely performed.

Animal Models[38]

Naturally occurring *E. coli* diarrheal disease of neonatal animals is relatively common. The diarrhea of young calves, known as scours, is due to *Escherichia,* as is a similar, sometimes epidemic, disease of piglets.

Enterotoxic colibacillosis is the name most often applied to these infections that affect very young swine, calves, and lambs, since the responsible strains of *E. coli* form enterotoxins of both ST and LT types. Strains of *E. coli* responsible for these infections are uniquely pathogenic for animals, owing to the specificity of their adherence factors. Several adhesins are recognized, including two protein K antigens, K88 and K99, along with a fimbrial antigen designated 987P. Strains affecting swine may possess any one of these adhesins, while the K99 antigen is usually found in those strains colonizing calves and lambs; these particular adhesins have not been identified in human strains.

Enterotoxins synthesized by animal strains are similar, but not identical, to those of human strains. Studies in animal models have contributed to an understanding of the pathogenesis of *E. coli* disease, particularly in adherence and immune intervention against colonization and infection. Animal models for the assay and study of enterotoxins have developed from those used originally to study cholera toxin (Chapter 21). These include infection of a ligated ileal segment of the rabbit intestine (ileal loop) described by De, which detects both enterotoxin types. This is an unwieldy method and has largely been supplanted by *in vitro* models using tissue cultured cells to detect activation of adenyl and guanyl cyclase.

Shigella: The Dysentery Bacilli

Dysentery is a clinical rather than an etiological entity, and its characteristic symptoms—diarrhea, abdominal pain, and bloody stools—may occur either alone or as a part of the syndrome of a number of diseases. In the former instance, dysentery may be of protozoan, viral, or bacterial etiology. A dysentery-like infection is produced by some *Salmonella* and by enteroinvasive *Escherichia coli*, but in most cases of bacterial dysentery, *Shigella* is the agent responsible.

Shigella are gram-negative, nonspore-forming rods related to the other enteric bacteria (Fig. 18–4). Some of them resemble anaerogenic *Escherichia* and the typhoid bacillus in that they ferment carbohydrates with the production of acid but without gas. None of the dysentery bacilli are motile; hence, they do not contain flagellar antigens. As a group they differ from one another biochemically and immunologically. They are presently classified with *Escherichia* in the tribe Escherichieae.

Shigella are aerobic and facultatively anaerobic, and their optimum temperature for growth is 37°C. Their nutritive requirements are not complex, since they will grow upon ordinary nutrient mediums containing peptones and beef extract. They ferment glucose without gas, producing the same end products as the other enteric forms—lactic acid together with smaller amounts of formic and acetic acids and ethyl alcohol. Like the other gram-negative bacilli, they are relatively resistant to the bacteriostatic action of dyes, and these substances may be incorporated in differential mediums for their isolation, as described in Chapter 17.

Classification[8, 15]

In the present classification of the genus *Shigella*, four species are recognized, separated primarily on the basis of biochemical reactions. The more important and informative of these are shown in Table 18–5. There is some variation in biochemical characters and in several of the species biotypes are identified by differences in biochemical tests.

Mannitol fermentation is one of the more useful characters; all species excepts *S. dysenteriae* typically ferment mannitol. *Shigella sonnei* differs from the other mannitol-fermenting species by the slow (four to seven days) fermentation of lactose. Fermentations by *Shigella* are anaerogenic, *i.e.*, without gas formation.

Some workers prefer to designate the species as groups, as shown in Table 18–5; within each of these species or groups, one or more serotypes are distinguished.

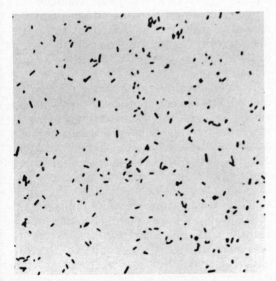

Figure 18–4. *Shigella flexneri*. Smear from a pure culture. Fuchsin; × 1050.

Table 18–5. **Selected Biochemical Reactions of** *Shigella**

Test	*Shigella dysenteriae* (Group A)	*Shigella flexneri* (Group B)	*Shigella boydii* (Group C)	*Shigella sonnei* (Group D)
Mannitol fermentation	–	A	A	A
Lactose fermentation	–	–	–	A†
Ornithine decarboxylase	–	–	–	+
Tartrate utilization	+	–	–	+

*The reactions shown are those exhibited by most strains. A number of biotypes can be separated by use of these and additional biochemical tests. Symbols: +, most strains positive; –, most strains negative; A, acid only.
†Delayed fermentation, 3 days or longer.

Antigenic Structure[43]

As noted above, *Shigella* are not motile and do not, therefore, possess H antigens. The differentiation of serotypes is based on their smooth lipopolysaccharide O antigens.

Members of each of the species are characterized by both cultural and antigenic similarities, and individual serotypes are separated on the basis of O-specific, somatic antigens. Many *Shigella* also produce heat-labile K antigens, which are of interest because they interfere with O-agglutination, but they have not been employed for serotyping as in *Escherichia*.

Identification[30]

As a practical matter, each of the species of *Shigella* is identified by a combination of biochemical and serological reactions. Isolates are differentiated from similar enteric bacilli and identified as *Shigella* by biochemical and cultural reactions; species separation is accomplished by fermentations and other tests (Table 18–5) and by serology. Polyvalent antiserums are available for each of the *Shigella* groups, and their use confirms the species identification. It is important to note that the O antigens of *Shigella* are frequently similar or identical to those of other enteric bacilli, especially *Escherichia*. They must, therefore, be identified as *Shigella* before agglutination in polyvalent antiserums has meaning.

Serotyping is more complex and requires a large battery of highly specific serological reagents; consequently, serotyping is usually available only in reference laboratories. Knowledge of serotype is not required for management of bacillary dysentery cases, but has great utility in epidemiological studies.

SHIGELLA DYSENTERIAE (GROUP A)

The dysentery bacilli making up this group are set apart by their inability to ferment mannitol. *Shigella dysenteriae* is an immuno-logically heterogeneous species, made up of 10 sharply separable serotypes arbitrarily designated by numbers. The serotypes are antigenically unrelated except for unilateral cross-reactions between some strains of types 2 and 10. These two serotypes are also serologically related to *Shigella boydii* type 1 (see below).

Shigella dysenteriae Type 1

This was the first of the dysentery bacilli to be described, found by the Japanese bacteriologist Shiga to be the etiological agent of epidemic dysentery in Japan in 1898. It is often referred to as the **Shiga bacillus.**

Toxins.[7, 33] Like other enteric bacteria, the Shiga bacillus produces an endotoxic lipopolysaccharide which is also responsible for the O antigenicity of the bacillus; the chemical and serological differences between O antigens determine the serotypes of *S. dysenteriae*. The Shiga bacillus is considered to be unique, however, in that it also produces one or more **exotoxins.** As known for many decades, the bacillus produces a **neurotoxic exotoxin** that affects the central nervous system of experimental animals to induce paralysis and subsequent death. This trait is generally thought to explain the usually more severe dysentery caused by this serotype.

Recently there has been renewed interest in Shiga toxins. Highly purified toxin exhibits a variety of biological activities. In addition to the neurotoxic and lethal properties originally described, the toxin is also cytotoxic for HeLa cells and behaves as an enterotoxin in a manner similar to the *E. coli* and cholera enterotoxins. Current evidence suggests that these activities reside in a single toxic entity.

Knowledge of the mode of action of the Shiga toxin has come from studies on the cytotoxic activity.[34, 37] In common with many other bacterial protein exotoxins, the cytotoxin consists of subunits, including one **heavy (A) chain** and 6 to 7 **light (B) chains.** The A chain is the active subunit, inhibiting protein synthesis in susceptible cells, while the B chains are thought to serve as binding units by reacting with receptors on cell surfaces. Protein synthesis is interrupted when the A subunits inactivate 60 S ribosomes in eucaryotic cells.

Shiga bacillus infections have been observed most frequently in India, Japan, China, and other parts of Asia and have occurred in explosive epidemic form in Central America; the infection has been imported by tourists to the United States, where otherwise it is relatively rare.

Shigella dysenteriae Type 2

This serotype was described by Schmitz in 1917 as a cause of dysentery in prisoners of war. The serotype is immunologically homogeneous, and is serologically related to *E. coli* O112 and to *S. boydii* types 1 and 15. *Shigella dysenteriae* type 2 has been found most often in Europe, India, and the Sudan. It is not as common as some of the other *Shigella,* but is encountered occasionally in institutional and other outbreaks of dysentery.

Other serotypes of *S. dysenteriae* are sometimes isolated, but they are not significant agents of disease in most geographical areas.

SHIGELLA FLEXNERI (GROUP B)

Soon after Shiga's discovery, Flexner discovered dysentery bacilli in the Philippines that differed from *S. dysenteriae,* both serologically and in the fermentation of mannitol. These were subsequently named *S. flexneri.*

Shigella flexneri is made up of a group of immunological types that are distinct and yet related to one another. The commonly accepted serological types of *S. flexneri* are shown in Table 18–6. Six serotypes are recognized and each of these possesses a single major somatic antigen, designated in the antigenic formula by Roman numerals. Subserotypes are identified within several of these, based upon minor antigens.

Attempts to subdivide the bacilli of the Flexner group by biochemical methods have not been particularly successful. Serotypes 1 through 5 are relatively homogeneous in cultural and biochemical characters; those of type 6 frequently show delayed fermentation of dulcitol.

Phage typing, useful with staphylococci and *Salmonella,* has not generated great interest, although it has been reported that phage sensitivity correlates closely with serological groups.

Colonial morphology, as accentuated by

Table 18–6. **Serotypes of *Shigella flexneri***

Serotypes	Subserotypes	Antigenic Formula*
1	1a	I:3,4,(7,8)
	1b	I:(3,4),6
2	2a	II:3,4
	2b	II:7,8
3	3a	III:6,7,8
	3b	III:(3,4),6,7,8
	3c	III:(3,4),6
4	4a	IV:3,4
	4b	IV:(3,4),6
5		V:7
6		VI:(3,4)

*Major antigens are shown in Roman numerals; minor antigens are designated by Arabic numerals. Minor antigens in parentheses may be absent from some strains.

oblique transmitted light, appears to be associated with both virulence and antigenic content. Highly virulent colonial types contain a full complement of antigens, while morphologically distinct avirulent forms do not contain specific, or type, antigen, and are apparently transitional in the change from smooth to rough.

Shigella flexneri is worldwide in distribution and has been the most commonly found of the dysentery bacilli, making up more than half of the isolates. Within the past two decades, *S. sonnei* has tended to replace it in the United States, Europe, and the Far East. In the United States, for example, *S. flexneri* represented about 62 per cent of all isolates in 1964; by 1970 it was reduced to about 27 per cent and remained at this level in 1980.

Toxins

The cell substance of *S. flexneri,* like that of all Enterobacteriaceae, is toxic, due to the endotoxic activity of the lipopolysaccharides that make up the somatic antigens (Chapter 2). The O antigens have been studied in some detail,[43] and their structure found to resemble that of other enteric bacilli. The basal core structure of the lipopolysaccharide is similar, if not identical, in all *S. flexneri* serotypes; each serotype differs in the constitution of the O-specific side chains of the smooth antigen.

Shigella flexneri type 2a, and possibly other serotypes, produces a toxin with properties similar to that of *S. dysenteriae* type 1; indeed, the two are serologically related.[32]

SHIGELLA BOYDII (GROUP C)

Shigella boydii represents a group of mannitol-fermenting dysentery bacilli closely similar to *S. flexneri* in biochemical characteristics, but unrelated serologically to the Flexner group. Although there is no common group antigen in *S. boydii* and most members are antigenically distinct, some are related to *Escherichia* as well as to certain of the other Boyd types; specifically, types 10 and 11 share antigens with *E. coli* O105 and with *S. boydii* type 4.

The pathogenicity of these forms appears to be closely similar to that of *S. flexneri,* and their distribution seems to be ubiquitous. They have not, however, been studied in the same detail as the Flexner bacilli with respect to chemical characterization of the somatic antigens and effective immunity.

SHIGELLA SONNEI (GROUP D)

In contrast to the other mannitol-fermenting *Shigella* just described, those designated as *Shigella sonnei* are set apart by the fermentation of lactose. **Lactose fermentation** is slow and may be delayed for a week or 10 days; strains of this kind were doubtlessly confused with Flexner bacilli by earlier workers.

Shigella sonnei is serologically distinct and homogeneous. Although there is only one serotype, it may appear in one of two forms, designated I and II. The antigen that characterizes form I is plasmid directed, and spontaneous loss of the plasmid results in failure to synthesize the form I antigen.[27] The **form I antigen** is one of several factors required for invasion by *S. sonnei* and form I strains tend to predominate in acute disease. Form II strains occur for the most part in carriers and are not virulent.

Shigella sonnei has become the most common species responsible for shigellosis in the United States. In 1980 it was isolated from about 70 per cent of cases, as compared to only 37 per cent in 1964.

Bacteriocin Typing.[31] Serotyping of *S. sonnei* does not yield a number of differentiable types that would be useful in epidemiological studies. For this reason, strain differentiation by bacteriocin production has been of interest. At least 16 types may be distinguished on the basis of the bacteriocins produced by *S. sonnei* and their activity against a series of indicator strains of known susceptibility. Although quite useful, bacteriocin typing is subject to greater variation than serotyping.

BACILLARY DYSENTERY

Bacillary dysentery is a relatively common disease of man, more so in warmer climates, and tends to be associated with crowding under conditions favoring spread of the infection from the human reservoir. It is more prevalent in underdeveloped countries, especially in the tropics and subtropics. It has been a perennial problem in military operations; for example, more men died of diarrheal disease during the Civil War in this country than were killed in battle. As a serious epidemic disease, it continued to be a problem in the two World Wars and in subsequent situations such as the landing of American troops in Lebanon in the late 1950s. While the proportion of Shiga bacillus infections has sharply declined, with consequent reduction in mortality, bacillary dysentery remains an important incapacitating disease.

Human Disease

The infecting dose of *S. flexneri* has been found, in studies on human volunteers, to be of the order of 10^4 to 10^8 microorganisms, and that of other species is probably similar. The incubation period is generally short, about 48 hours, and the disease may be acute or chronic. Symptoms of shigellosis range from simple diarrhea to true dysentery. The latter is characterized by fever; diarrhea; bloody, mucous stools; tenesmus; and abdominal pain. Apart from occasional inflammatory lesions in the intestine (ulcerative colitis), the anatomical picture of dysentery presents little that is characteristic. Dysentery bacilli are sometimes found in immense numbers in the dejecta, often in almost pure culture. They may be found at autopsy in the mesenteric glands, but, as a rule, not in the spleen or other internal organs, nor do they commonly occur in the blood or urine. The pathogenesis of the disease in experimental animals (see below) simulates that in man, *viz.*, an initial penetration of the epithelial cells and the development of infection foci in the lamina propria. Bacillary dysentery is, therefore, localized in the alimentary tract. Recurrent diarrheal disease may be caused by dysentery bacilli, indicating that the bacilli may persist in the superficial layers of the intestinal epithelium for long periods.

In the United States, children under about 10 years of age are most susceptible to *Shigella* infection, with greatest incidence in those around 2 years old. Mortality, even in untreated cases, is usually quite low. The Shiga dysentery of the tropics is considerably more severe and more often fatal; complications, such as arthritis, are more frequent in these infections.

Carriers. It is probable that *Shigella* infection is very common, many infections going

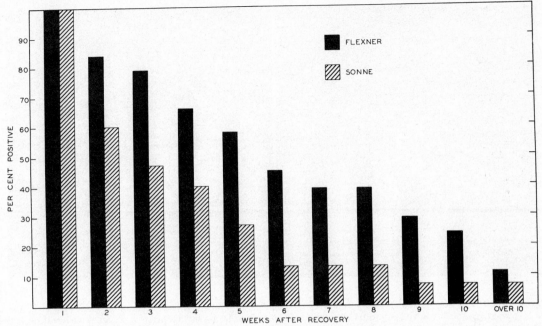

Figure 18–5. The persistence of dysentery bacilli in the feces of convalescents. (Prepared from data of Watt, Hardy, and De Capito.[51])

unrecognized because of the mildness of the symptoms. Persons with such infections are, of course, convalescent carriers who continue to discharge the bacilli for several weeks (Fig. 18–5). It is the casual carrier and changing groups of casual carriers or ambulatory cases that are of primary importance in the maintenance and spread of the infection, and the disease persists in smoldering, endemic form.

Animal Models

Although primates, *e.g.*, chimpanzees, may become infected with *Shigella*, the disease is essentially one of humans. A number of experimental infections have been described which vary in the degree to which they approximate the human disease. The fatal fulminating bacteremia produced in various experimental animals, such as the mouse, on intraperitoneal inoculation is at best only distantly related to the human disease. An infection of the urinary bladder of the guinea pig may be produced by direct instillation of dysentery and certain other enteric bacilli, but it does not remain localized. The inoculation of a ligated loop of the small bowel of the rabbit or guinea pig, extensively used as an experimental model of cholera (Chapter 21), gives positive reactions, *e.g.*, intraluminal fluid accumulation and bacterial multiplication, with virulent dysentery bacilli but not with avirulent strains. A keratoconjunctivitis may be produced in the guinea pig eye by instillation of

the bacilli—the Serény test for invasiveness—and in this infection the histopathology closely resembles that found in experimental enteric infections.

Although enteric infections can be produced in mice and guinea pigs by oral administration of dysentery bacilli, these require extensive pretreatment of the animals to increase susceptibility, and their relationship to natural disease is suspect. The experimental enteric infection produced in monkeys closely simulates the human disease and does not depend upon pretreatment to break down resistance.

Pathogenesis[48]

The pathogenesis of *Shigella* infections derives from several virulence features of the microorganism, *viz.*, adherence to the mucosal epithelium of the bowel; penetration of epithelial cells and into the lamina propria; and multiplication in the lamina propria as a focus of infection (Fig. 18–6). The bacilli do not generally penetrate further into the tissues, but induce an inflammatory response that results in local tissue degeneration and ulceration to engender the clinical picture described earlier.

The **adhesive factors** in *Shigella* are not as well understood as those of *E. coli*. Only *S. flexneri* is known to produce pili and these are of the mannose-sensitive type; they do not appear to correlate with virulence. Adherence may be more dependent upon physical forces,

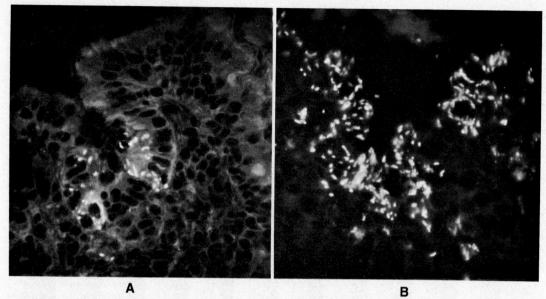

A   **B**

Figure 18–6. The pathogenesis of bacillary dysentery. *A,* Penetration of the ileal epithelium in the guinea pig at 12 hours by *S. flexneri* 2a; bacilli can be seen in the epithelial cells and some in the lamina propria. *B,* Small micro-ulcer in the colonic epithelium in the monkey 24 hours after infection; bacilli are present in the epithelial cells and in the lamina propria of the tubular glands of the colon. (LaBrec.) (*B* courtesy of Journal of Bacteriology.)

including surface hydrophobicity and charge, than on specific receptor-ligand interactions.

The ability of *Shigella* to invade epithelial cells and multiply in the mucosal lining has been intensively studied using the techniques of microbial genetics. It is established that invasion and multiplication are required for virulence and are under polygenic control; a mutation in any one of the genes results in loss of virulence. Several regions of the bacterial chromosome are involved in virulence and the locus controlling invasiveness is separate from that involved in multiplication in tissues. Recently, the importance of plasmid control of virulence has been emphasized. The production of form I surface antigen, one of several requirements for invasion by *S. sonnei,* is mediated by a large plasmid;[27] similarly, a large plasmid in *S. flexneri* affects some function required for penetration of epithelial cells.[42]

The ability of virulent *Shigella* to invade epithelial cells may be demonstrated in tissue culture by use of HeLa cells; the process consists of attachment of the bacilli to the cell membrane, with subsequent engulfment by pinocytosis. Attachment may be prevented by specific secretory immunoglobulin A, but not by immunoglobulins G or M.[36] It has been noted that the dysentery caused by the Shiga bacillus is usually more severe than that caused by other *Shigella,* presumably because of the action of the Shiga toxin. Since other species

also produce similar toxins, it becomes more logical to assume a role for the toxin in pathogenesis. The precise role, however, must await more definitive evidence.

Bacteriological Diagnosis[30]

Since, as indicated earlier, dysentery is a clinical rather than an etiological entity, the causative microorganism must be isolated and identified to allow a diagnosis of bacillary dysentery. The bacilli may be found in fecal specimens, and rectal swabs are cultured for the detection of carriers. The methods of enrichment culture and direct plating are described in Chapter 17. Deoxycholate-citrate and Salmonella-Shigella (SS) agar are the most useful of the agar mediums; bismuth-sulfite is not suitable because species other than *S. flexneri* are inhibited. Colonies are subcultured and identified by biochemical reactions and slide agglutination. For tentative serological indentification, polyvalent antiserums for each species may be used. For precise identification, monospecific antiserums are required; this kind of serotyping is best performed by reference laboratories.

Chemotherapy

The sulfonamides are highly effective chemotherapeutic agents in bacillary dysentery and have been widely used for both therapy and prophylaxis. Streptomycin and the broad spectrum antibiotics—tetracycline, ampicillin, and chloramphenicol—are also effective, and all have been of interest as chemoprophylactic agents.

With the general use of sulfonamides, sulfonamide-resistant strains of dysentery bacilli became more and more common. This led to increased usage of the other antimicrobial agents, with the consequence that strains with **multiple antibiotic resistance** are encountered with increasing frequency. In 1960 it was found in Japan that the multiple resistance (simultaneous resistance to sulfonamide, streptomycin, tetracycline, and chloramphenicol) acquired by sensitive strains of *Shigella,* as well as other enteric bacilli, is plasmid-mediated (Chapter 6). This kind of acquired drug resistance has worldwide occurrence and continues to increase.

Although resistance may be encountered to many of the usual antimicrobial agents, *Shigella* are most often sensitive to ampicillin, rifampicin, co-trimoxazole, aminoglycosides, chloramphenicol, and nalidixic acid. While not all cases of bacillary dysentery require antimicrobial therapy, the unpredictable nature of resistance argues for sensitivity testing of *Shigella* isolates as a guide to therapy.

Epidemiology

Infections caused by dysentery bacilli are probably far more common than is generally recognized. Attacks of severe illness grade off into mild and almost trivial attacks of simple diarrhea. In a number of localities where careful bacteriological studies have been made, dysentery bacilli have been found widely distributed both in patients with gastrointestinal derangements and in the general population. Probably the most important single reservoir of infection is the human carrier, either convalescent or with inapparent infection.

Dysenteric infections seem to be most common in tropical countries and in the summer months in temperate climates, although they can occur at any season of the year. The acute diarrheal disease, appearing routinely in tropical countries and known locally as "Gyppy tummy," "Delhi belly," and the like, is frequently bacillary dysentery, usually of *S. flexneri* and *S. boydii* etiology.

The spread of the disease is due to the more or less direct transfer of the specific bacillus from infected intestinal discharges to the alimentary tract of another individual. The manner of this transfer varies with geography and socioeconomic conditions within the population. In developed countries of temperate climates, the majority of cases involve person-

to-person spread. Conditions for this type of contact include crowding and lapses in personal hygiene, as occurs in some family groups and in institutions, such as mental hospitals. The case rate in mental institutions in the United States is abnormally high. In 1967 it was 1350 cases per 10^5 patients compared to 5.9 per 10^5 in the general population. Wherever it gains a foothold in these institutions it seems to be kept alive by chronic carriers and constitutes an obstinate problem.

Outside of such institutions, shigellosis also appears in large epidemics and these are usually water- or foodborne. Waterborne epidemics result from fecal pollution of water supplies, often those of semipublic nature, when there is inadequate chlorination. Disease may also be contracted by swimming in contaminated water.[40]

Foodborne outbreaks of shigellosis can almost always be traced to contamination by infected food handlers. The foods involved are often salads or other uncooked foods subject to handling; the circumstances of contamination usually include poor habits of personal hygiene by the infected carriers.

In underdeveloped countries, many of these same modes of spread may be operative, but the opportunities for transmission are expanded by generally lower sanitary standards and inadequate treatment of both sewage and water supplies. Improper disposal of human wastes may be commonplace, permitting dissemination by flies in the classic chain of feces→flies→food.

In the United States, bacillary dysentery tends to be prevalent among Indians on reservations; in 1970 a case rate of 170 per 10^5 population in reservations contrasted with a rate of 5.4 per 10^5 persons for the entire country. Shigellosis has emerged, too, as a venereal contact disease among homosexuals, the transmission link being sexual practices in this group. Epidemic bacillary dysentery is also a disease of armies in the field, where opportunities for the dissemination of infection are frequently very great, and extensive outbreaks are common.

In the United States, shigellosis exhibits seasonal variation, with rises in late summer and fall. The most common type is now *S. sonnei;* about 70 per cent of isolates in 1980 were this species. Except for *S. flexneri,* the remaining species are now only rarely isolated in this country.

Immunity

The development of some degree of effective immunity is indicated by the relative resis-

462 o Medical Bacteriology

tance of the resident population of an endemic area to the acute disease which affects recent arrivals, *e.g.,* "acclimatization diarrhea." This phenomenon is well known to residents of temperate climates visiting tropical and subtropical areas.

Infection with dysentery bacilli results in the formation of antibodies, predominantly agglutinins to the O antigens, usually appearing after the sixth day. The titer is relatively low as a rule. The diagnostic significance of agglutinins is somewhat uncertain largely because "normal" agglutinins are common, ranging in titers from 1:20 to 1:150.

There appears to be no significant relationship between serum antibody as such and effective immunity to the naturally acquired disease. This is perhaps to be expected, since the infection remains localized in the bowel, and a local immunity may be independent of serum antibody response. *Shigella* infection results in the appearance of 11S immunoglobulin A in diarrheal stools. Immunoglobulin A, by interfering with bacterial attachment to mucosal cells, can lead to localized intestinal immunity. Infections with *S. dysenteriae, S. flexneri,* and *S. sonnei* result in the production of antibodies that neutralize the Shiga toxin;[26] whether *S. boydii* infection also engenders such antibodies is not known. These results suggest a role for the toxin in pathogenesis and raise the possibility of antitoxic immunity.

Immunization[48]

An artificially induced effective prophylactic immunity would be a valuable adjunct in the control of bacillary dysentery, not only because of multiple drug resistance of the microorganisms, but also because it could be applied in situations where the disease is difficult to control, *viz.,* mental institutions, Indian reservations, and military personnel in the field. Such a possibility has been of continued interest and encouraging results have been obtained.

Parenterally administered vaccines consisting of suspensions of killed bacilli are relatively toxic and have not yielded significant immunity. More recently, interest has centered on induction of local immunity in the bowel by administration of **oral vaccines.** Killed vaccines given by mouth have yielded only equivocal results, but living attenuated bacilli, particularly those able to colonize the intestine, appear to be more promising.

Several kinds of attenuated *Shigella* strains have been constructed for use as oral vaccines. Some of these have proven successful in both laboratory and field studies. Nevertheless, they have not been widely applied because of diffi-

culties in obtaining safe, genetically stable strains that proliferate sufficiently to induce significant protection. As our understanding of virulence determinants improves, it should be possible to create effective and safe vaccine strains. For example, the genes controlling form I antigen of *S. sonnei* can be transferred to a strain of *Salmonella typhi* that has already been shown to be a safe and effective oral vaccine for typhoid.[17] Whether this hybrid strain can also offer protection against intestinal *S. sonnei* infection awaits confirmation.

The type-specificity of the immunity produced by such vaccines would appear to limit their utilization in view of the multiplicity of dysentery bacilli. Almost invariably, however, bacillary dysentery in a given area is caused by two or three kinds of bacilli; in the United States in 1980, for example, *S. sonnei* and *S. flexneri* types 2a and 3a represented more than 80 per cent of *Shigella* isolates. In practice, therefore, immunization against a few kinds of dysentery bacilli should suffice to control a very large portion of naturally acquired infections.

REFERENCES

1. Alderette, J. F., and D. C. Robertson. 1978. Purification and chemical characterization of the heat-stable enterotoxin produced by porcine strains of enterotoxigenic *Escherichia coli*. Infect. Immun. **19**:1021–1030.
2. Allen, J. R., *et al.* 1981. Secular trends in nosocomial infections: 1970–1979. Amer. J. Med. **70**:389–392.
3. Barry, D. M. J., and A. W. Reeve. 1977. Increased incidence of gram-negative neonatal sepsis with intramuscular iron administration. Pediatrics **60**:908–912.
4. Bergan, T., and Ø. Olsvik. 1980. Produktion und Reinigung des thermolabilen *Escherichia coli*-enterotoxins. Infection **8** (Suppl. **3**): S226–233.
5. Binns, M. W., J. Maydon, and R. P. Levine. 1982. Further characterization of complement resistance conferred on *Escherichia coli* by the plasmid genes *traT* of R100 and *iss* of ColV, I–K94. Infect. Immun. **35**:654–659.
6. Blumenstock, E., and K. Jann. 1982. Adhesion of piliated *Escherichia coli* strains to phagocytes: differences between bacteria with mannose-sensitive pili and those with mannose-resistant pili. Infect. Immun. **35**:264–269.
7. Brown, J. E., *et al.* 1982. Purification and biological characterization of Shiga toxin from *Shigella dysenteriae* 1. Infect. Immun. **36**:996–1005.
8. Buchanan, R. E., and N. E. Gibbons (Eds.). 1974. Bergey's Manual of Determinative Bacteriology. 8th ed. Williams & Wilkins Co., Baltimore.
9. Cavalieri, S. J., and I. S. Snyder. 1982. Effect of *Escherichia coli* alpha-hemolysin on human peripheral leukocyte viability in vitro. Infect. Immun. **36**:455–461.
10. Cavalieri, S. J., and I. S. Snyder. 1982. Effect of *Escherichia coli* alpha-hemolysin on human peripheral leukocyte function in vitro. Infect. Immun. **37**:966–974.

11. Clements, J. D., R. J. Yancey, and R. A. Finkelstein. 1980. Properties of homogeneous heat-labile enterotoxin from *Escherichia coli*. Infect. Immun. **29**:91–97.

12. Cooke, E. M. 1974. *Escherichia coli* and Man. Churchill Livingston, Edinburgh.

13. Dallas, W. S., D. M. Gill, and S. Falkow. 1979. Cistrons encoding *Escherichia coli* heat-labile toxin. J. Bacteriol. **139**:850–858.

14. Duguid, J. P., and D. C. Old. 1980. Adhesive properties of Enterobacteriaceae. pp. 184–217. *In* E. H. Beachey (Ed.): Bacterial Adherence. Chapman and Hall, London.

15. Edwards, P. R., and W. H. Ewing. 1972. Identification of Enterobacteriaceae. 3rd ed. Burgess, Minneapolis, Minn.

16. Evans, D. G., and D. J. Evans, Jr. 1978. New surface-associated heat-labile colonization factor antigen (CFA/II) produced by enterotoxigenic *Escherichia coli* of serogroups 06 and 08. Infect. Immun. **21**:638–647.

17. Formal, S. B., *et al.* 1981. Construction of a potential bivalent vaccine strain: introduction of *Shigella sonnei* form I antigen genes into the *galE Salmonella typhi* Ty21a typhoid vaccine strain. Infect. Immun. **34**:746–750.

18. Geary, S. J., B. A. Marchlewicz, and R. A. Finkelstein. 1982. Comparison of heat-labile enterotoxins from porcine and human strains of *Escherichia coli*. Infect. Immun. **36**:215–220.

19. Gianella, R. A. 1981. Pathogenesis of acute bacterial diarrheal disorders. Ann. Rev. Med. **32**:341–357.

20. Guerrant, R. L., *et al.* 1980. Activation of intestinal guanylate cyclase by heat-stable enterotoxin of *Escherichia coli*: studies of tissue specificity, potential receptors, and intermediates. J. Infect. Dis. **142**:220–228.

21. Hanson, L. Å. 1976. *Esch. coli* infections in childhood. Significance of bacterial virulence and immune defence. Arch. Dis. Childh. **51**:737–743.

22. Hanson, L. Å., *et al.* 1981. Biology and pathology of urinary tract infections. J. Clin. Pathol. **34**:695–700.

23. Hardy, K. G. 1975. Colicinogeny and related phenomena. Bacteriol. Rev. **39**:464–515.

24. Harris, J. R., *et al.* 1982. High-molecular-weight plasmid correlates with *Escherichia coli* enteroinvasiveness. Infect. Immun. **37**:1295–1298.

25. Kadner, R. J., *et al.* 1980. Genetic control of hydroxamate-mediated iron uptake in *Escherichia coli*. J. Bacteriol. **143**:256–264.

26. Keusch, G. T., and M. Jacewicz. 1977. The pathogenesis of Shigella diarrhea. VI. Toxin and antitoxin in *Shigella flexneri* and *Shigella sonnei* infection in humans. J. Infect. Dis. **135**:552–556.

27. Kopecko, D. J., O. Washington, and S. B. Formal. 1980. Genetic and physical evidence for plasmid control of *Shigella sonnei* form I cell surface antigen. Infect. Immun. **29**:207–214.

28. Levine, M. M., *et al.* 1979. Immunity to enterotoxigenic *Escherichia coli*. Infect. Immun. **23**:729–736.

29. Madsen, G. L., and F. C. Knoop. 1980. Physiochemical properties of a heat-stable enterotoxin produced by *Escherichia coli* of human origin. Infect. Immun. **28**:1051–1053.

30. Martin, W. J., and J. A. Washington, II. 1980. Enterobacteriaceae. pp. 195–219. *In* E. H. Lennette, *et al.* (Eds.): Manual of Clinical Microbiology. 3rd ed. American Society for Microbiology, Washington, D. C.

31. Morris, G. K., and J. G. Wells. 1974. Colicin typing of *Shigella sonnei*. Appl. Microbiol. **27**:312–316.

32. O'Brien, A. D., *et al.* 1977. Biological properties of *Shigella flexneri* 2A toxin and its serological relationship to *Shigella dysenteriae* 1 toxin. Infect. Immun. **15**:796–798.

33. Okamoto, K., Y. Takeda, and T. Miwatani. 1982. Purification of a lethal toxin produced by *Shigella dysenteriae*. Toxicon **20**:451–456.

34. Olsnes, S., R. Reisbig, and K. Eiklid. 1981. Subunit structure of *Shigella* cytotoxin. J. Biol. Chem. **256**:8732–8738.

35. Ørskov, I., *et al.* 1977. Serology, chemistry, and genetics of O and K antigens of *Escherichia coli*. Bacteriol. Rev. **41**:667–710.

36. Reed, W. P., and A. H. Cushing. 1975. Role of immunoglobulins in protection against Shigella-induced keratoconjunctivitis. Infect. Immun. **11**:1265–1268.

37. Reisbig, R., S. Olsnes, and K. Eiklid. 1981. The cytotoxic activity of *Shigella* toxin. Evidence for catalytic inactivation of the 50S ribosomal subunit. J. Biol. Chem. **256**:8739–8744.

38. Report. 1980. *Escherichia coli* diarrhoea. Bull. W.H.O. **58**:23–36.

39. Richards, K. L., and S. D. Douglas. 1978. Pathophysiological effects of *Vibrio cholerae* and enterotoxigenic *Escherichia coli* and their exotoxins on eucaryotic cells. Microbiol. Rev. **42**:592–613.

40. Rosenberg, M. L., *et al.* 1976. Shigellosis from swimming. J. Amer. Med. Assn **236**:1849–1852.

41. Sack, R. B. 1975. Human diarrheal disease caused by enterotoxigenic *Escherichia coli*. Ann. Rev. Microbiol. **29**:333–353.

42. Sansonetti, P. J., D. J. Kopecko, and S. B. Formal. 1982. Involvement of a plasmid in the invasive ability of *Shigella flexneri*. Infect. Immun. **35**:852–860.

43. Simmons, D. A. R. 1971. Immunochemistry of *Shigella flexneri* O-antigens: a study of structural and genetic aspects of the biosynthesis of cell-surface antigens. Bacteriol. Rev. **35**:117–148.

44. Souney, P., and B. F. Polk. 1982. Single-dose antimicrobial therapy for urinary tract infections in women. Rev. Infect. Dis. **4**:29–34.

45. Svennerholm, A.-M., E. Bäck, and J. Holmgren. 1977. Enterotoxin antibodies in relation to diarrhoea in Swedish soldiers in Cyprus. Bull. W.H.O. **55**:663–668.

46. Tantulavanich, S., *et al.* 1981. An R plasmid of broad host-range, coding for resistance to nine antimicrobial agents endemic in gram-negative nosocomial isolates. J. Med. Microbiol. **14**:371–380.

47. Thorén, A., *et al.* 1980. Antibiotics in the treatment of gastroenteritis caused by enteropathogenic *Escherichia coli*. J. Infect. Dis. **141**:27–31.

48. Thorne, G. M., and S. L. Gorbach. 1977. Shigella vaccines, Shigella pathogens—Dr. Jekyll and Mr. Hyde. J. Infect. Dis. **136**:601–604.

49. Turck, M., and W. Stamm. 1981. Nosocomial infection of the urinary tract. Amer. J. Med. **70**:651–654.

50. Waalwijk, C., *et al.* 1982. Hemolysin plasmid coding for the virulence of a nephropathogenic *Escherichia coli* strain. Infect. Immun. **35**:32–37.

51. Watt, J., A. V. Hardy, and T. M. De Capito. 1942. Studies of the acute diarrheal diseases. VII. Carriers of *Shigella dysenteriae*. Publ. Hlth. Rep. **57**:524–529.

52. Wilfert, C. M. 1978. *E. coli* meningitis: K1 antigen and virulence. Ann. Rev. Med. **29**:129–136.

53. Williams, P. H., and P. J. Warner. 1980. ColV plasmid-mediated, colicin V-independent iron uptake system of invasive strains of *Escherichia coli*. Infect. Immun. **29**:411–416.

CHAPTER 19

The Enteric Bacilli: Salmonella, Arizona, and Citrobacter

The enteric bacilli constituting the large *Salmonella* group are all pathogenic for humans to a greater or lesser degree. They include the typhoid bacillus and a wide variety of forms whose natural hosts are usually animals, especially rodents and birds.

Long before the typhoid bacillus was discovered, the infectious nature of typhoid fever was apparent; in 1856, on the basis of epidemiological evidence, William Budd suggested that the disease was spread by sewage-contaminated water and that the source of the infection was human feces. The typhoid bacillus was found by Eberth in 1880 in the spleen and mesenteric nodes of persons dying from typhoid fever, and was cultured in 1884 by Gaffky.

For a good many years, the kinds of microorganisms making up the "typhoid-paratyphoid" group were few in number and were differentiable by cultural and biochemical reactions. With the development of the techniques of antigenic analysis and their application to these microorganisms in the 1920s, very many serologically differentiable types were described, so that the *Salmonella* group is now made up of many hundreds of serotypes.

Over a long period, each new serotypic isolate has been given a specific epithet, thus implying species status for each serotype. The taxonomy of *Salmonella* was, thereby, complex and somewhat at variance from that used for most other microorganisms. Since the needs of the clinical microbiologist are not those of the taxonomist, the classification system used here will be that advocated and presently used by the Centers for Disease Control.

In this system of taxonomy and nomenclature, the tribe Salmonelleae comprises three genera, *Salmonella*, *Arizona*, and *Citrobacter*. These may be differentiated from one another by cultural and biochemical reactions, as indicated in Table 19–1. *Salmonella* are important human pathogens, colonizing the intestinal tract of humans and a number of animal species. *Arizona* are characteristically found in the enteric contents of reptiles, but they are pathogenic for man in a fashion similar to that of *Salmonella*. *Citrobacter* are rarely the primary agent of disease in humans, but they are widely distributed in nature, occurring as normal intestinal inhabitants; they must, therefore, be differentiated from the pathogenic enterobacteria.

Table 19–1. **Biochemical Differentiation of Genera Within the Tribe Salmonelleae***

Test	Salmonella	Arizona	Citrobacter
Urease production	−	−	+
Lysine decarboxylase	+	+	−
Lactose fermentation	−	(+)	V
Tartrate utilization	+	−	+
β-Galactosidase	−	+	+

*Symbols: +, most strains positive; (+), most strains positive after 3 days or more; −, most strains negative; V, variable reactions.

Salmonella

In the classification scheme used here, three species of *Salmonella* are distinguished. These are differentiated on the basis of biochemical reactions, as indicated in Table 19–2. *Salmonella enteritidis* is separated into several hundred serotypes, each assigned a serotype name replacing the binomial designation used in the older literature. For example, *S. pullorum* has become *S. enteritidis* serotype *pullorum*.

Morphology and Staining

The *Salmonella* are gram-negative bacilli whose cellular morphology closely resembles and is indistinguishable from the other enterobacteria. They stain readily with the usual dyes, with no particular arrangement of the cells apparent on microscopic examination (Fig. 19–1). All members except *S. enteritidis* serotypes *pullorum* and *gallinarum* are actively motile by peritrichous flagella. No capsules are distinguishable by light microscopy, although a polysaccharide surface antigen, designated Vi, occurs in most *S. typhi* and a few other *Salmonella*. Of the *Salmonella* that have been studied, most possess adhesive fimbriae, usually of the mannose-sensitive type.

The colonial form of representative *Salmonella* is illustrated in Figures 19–2 and 19–3. Colonial variation, from smooth to rough (S–R), occurs in cultures of these bacilli, as in many other bacteria. The change from smooth to rough is manifest not only as an alteration in colonial morphology but in loss of virulence as well. The change is reflected immunologically as a loss of the O-specific side chains of the smooth lipopolysaccharide, leaving the basal R core and lipid A; flagellar antigens are unchanged in this variation.

Physiology

The bacteria of this group have simple nutritional requirements, growing readily on the usual nutrient mediums. Adequate growth obtains in synthetic mediums containing ammonium salt as a nitrogen source and simple carbon sources such as glucose, pyruvate, or lactate. The great majority of strains do not require vitamins or amino acids; some strains of *S. typhi* require added tryptophan. The optimum growth temperature is 37° C., but good growth is observed at room temperature. They are facultative anaerobes, growing equally well under either aerobic or anaerobic conditions.

The significant biochemical reactions of the three species of *Salmonella* are displayed in Table 19–2. The list is by no means exhaustive; these and other tests may be employed to identify biotypes of the individual species, but have limited utility in this regard.

Toxins[5, 16]

All *Salmonella* form endotoxin, the lipopolysaccharide of the outer membrane (Chapter 12). The O-specific side chains of the lipo-

Table 19–2. **Biochemical Differentiation of *Salmonella****

Test	Salmonella cholera-suis	Salmonella typhi	Salmonella enteritidis
Gas from glucose	+	−	+
Trehalose	−	+	+
Arabinose	−	−	+
Rhamnose	+	−	+
Ornithine decarboxylase	+	−	+
Citrate utilization	(+)	−	+

*Symbols: +, most strains positive; (+), most strains positive after 3 days or more; −, most strains negative.

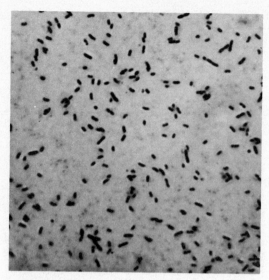

Figure 19–1. *Salmonella typhi.* Smear from a pure culture, Sommersby strain. Note the variation in size from coccoid to bacillary forms. Fuchsin; × 1050.

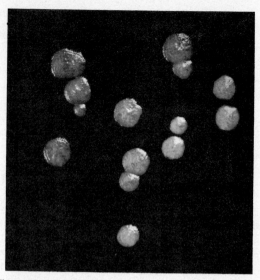

Figure 19–3. Colonies of typhoid bacillus on nutrient agar. Note the characteristic "maple leaf" irregular margin and slightly roughened glistening surface. × 6.

polysaccharide constitute the smooth O antigens of these bacteria, as discussed below.

The clinical manifestation of *Salmonella* gastroenteritis suggests the involvement of an entertoxin analogous to that of *Escherichia coli* and *Vibrio cholerae.* Production of an enterotoxin by *Salmonella* was first reported in 1975, and subsequent studies have established its close relationship to the *E. coli* and cholera toxins. The toxin is a heat-labile protein, with molecular weight greater than 110,000 daltons. It induces fluid accumulation in the rabbit ileal

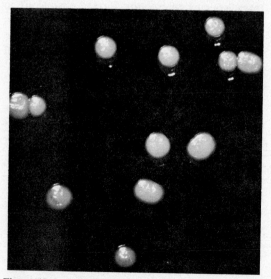

Figure 19–2. Colonies of *Salmonella enteritidis* serotype *typhimurium* on nutrient agar, 24-hour culture. × 3.

loop and stimulates adenyl cyclase. Antigenic similarity to the cholera toxin is indicated, since it is neutralized by antiserum to either whole cholera toxin or the B subunits. Toxin appears to be produced by a significant number of *S. enteritidis* serotypes, the salmonellae most often associated with gastroenteritis.

Pathogenesis and Virulence

With respect to the underlying pathogenesis, *Salmonella* infections are of two kinds, **enteric fevers** and **gastroenteritis.** In both kinds of infection, the bacteria are ingested in food or drink, and initiate the infection by adherence and colonization in the intestinal tract. In the enteric fevers the bacteria first invade the intestinal epithelium and subsequently multiply in the intestinal lymph follicles and draining mesenteric lymph nodes, reaching the blood stream via the thoracic lymph. The *Salmonella* responsible for these generalized infections are most often *S. typhi*, causing typhoid fever, and the paratyphoid bacilli.

Salmonella gastroenteritis differs in that the invasion is essentially superficial and is limited to the intestinal epithelium. Multiplication at this location is presumably accompanied by the production of enterotoxins, which in turn give rise to the symptoms of gastroenteritis. Such infections are often known as *Salmonella* food poisoning and are caused by serotypes of *S. enteritidis.*

The microbial factors that contribute to the virulence of *Salmonella* are not yet known with certainty. As with other enteric bacilli, *Salmonella* possess **fimbriae**, a fact that raises the question of their potential role as adherence factors in intestinal infection. The presence of fimbriae does, in fact, correlate with virulence; fimbriated strains of *S. enteritidis* serotype *typhimurium* are significantly more virulent by the oral route than nonfimbriate strains.[11] Adherence is only one possible factor, however, and is probably not sufficient for virulence. Although the ability to **penetrate** intestinal mucosa may be important, microbial factors mediating penetration have not been established. **Enterotoxin** production, by strains causing gastroenteritis, is likely a significant virulence factor.

Invasive strains of *Salmonella* must possess virulence factors that permit them to overcome tissue defenses. Unfortunately, little information is available on human invasive strains, but a similar disease in animals, mouse typhoid caused by *S. enteritidis* serotype *typhimurium*, has provided understanding of these factors.

The fact that the S–R mutation is accompanied by loss of virulence in mouse infection models has focused attention upon the virulence role of the **somatic O antigens** and the changes in the lipopolysaccharide that accompany such mutations. Not only is the smooth antigen required for mouse virulence, but certain O antigens are more effective than others in this regard.[33] The presence of **enterobacterial common antigen** seems to increase virulence,[34] probably by inhibition of phagocytosis, thus reducing intraphagocytic killing, and reduction of susceptibility to the bactericidal action of serum. The lipopolysaccharide content of the bacteria also determines their resistance to oxygen-independent bactericidal activity of neutrophils.[25]

One of the significant host defenses against systemic *Salmonella* infection is the entrapment and killing of bacteria by hepatic clearance mechanisms. When *Salmonella* are perfused through normal liver, those that possess type 1 pili are more effectively cleared than nonpiliated bacteria, presumably because they adhere to liver cells.[20] Thus, pilus-mediated adherence to mucosal epithelial cells increases virulence by permitting colonization; yet, *in vivo*, the survival of piliated cells is diminished. A similar phenomenon has been extensively studied in *Proteus* infections, with evidence that virulent piliated *Proteus* undergo a change to the nonpiliated state *in vivo*. Whether such changes occur during *Salmonella* infection is not known.

Finally, the ability to capture **iron** is necessary for *in vivo* survival and virulence of *Salmonella*. Mice that are nutritionally deficient in iron are more resistant to infection than normal animals,[27] and the injection of iron into *Salmonella*-infected mice induces an overwhelming and rapidly fatal infection.[19] The microbial virulence factor is a siderophore, **enterochelin,** that promotes iron-acquisition by the bacteria.[39]

Antigenic Structure

The antigenic structure of *Salmonella* is basically similar to that of other Enterobacteriaceae (Chapter 17), with two major kinds of antigens present—somatic O antigens and flagellar H antigens. A third kind is found in a few strains, occurring as a surface antigen, and is functionally analogous to the K antigens in other genera. Because it was originally thought to be associated with virulence, this antigen was designated the **Vi antigen.**

The O antigens are the lipopolysaccharides (LPS) of the outer membrane. These heat-stable antigens owe their antigenic specificity to the O-specific polysaccharides of the smooth LPS. Many different O antigens, designated by Arabic numerals, are found among the *Salmonella*. A single bacterial strain may contain more than one O antigen and they tend to appear in recurring combinations.

The flagellar antigens are the proteins that make up the peritrichous flagella of these bacteria. In contrast to the O antigens, the H antigens are labile to heat and to treatment with ethanol or acid.

The flagellar antigens may appear in two, usually reversible, phases. The **phase 1 antigens**, also called the specific phase, are individualistic and contribute to the immunological identity of a serotype. **Phase 2 flagellar antigens** are limited in number and tend to be shared by various serotypes. Individual bacterial cells do not contain antigens of both phases, but generally about half of the bacterial population will be in one phase and half in the other. Subculture of a bacterial clone from one phase will result in appearance of progeny representing both phases. The variation is not a mutational event, but is due to genetic regulation, as discussed in Chapter 6

Phase 1 flagellar antigens are arbitrarily designated by lower-case letters (an unfortunate choice, since the more recently discovered antigens are designated z_1, z_2, etc.) and those of phase 2 by Arabic numerals. Strains containing both kinds of flagellar antigens are

diphasic, while those with only a single kind are **monophasic** and may be either phase 1 or 2.

Both H and O antigens may be demonstrated by agglutination reactions, as described in Chapter 8. By appropriate techniques of antigenic analysis, *i.e.,* by reciprocal agglutinin adsorption, the components of both somatic and flagellar antigenic mosaics may be determined. Each of the serological types of *Salmonella* may be defined in immunological terms by **antigenic formulas** (see Serological Differentiation).

A heat-labile surface polysaccharide antigen, designated Vi, is found in *S. typhi* and a few strains of *S. enteritidis*. The Vi antigen is presumably superficial to the O antigen, since it blocks agglutination by O antiserums; agglutinability in O antiserum may be restored when this Vi antigen is destroyed by heating. The Vi antigen is present in practically all strains of *S. typhi* on primary isolation, but in only a few strains of the paratyphoid bacilli. The Vi antigen content may be progressively diminished upon continued laboratory cultivation, a dissociation known as **VW variation.**

Classification

The *Salmonella* group is relatively homogeneous in that these bacteria resemble one another more closely than other enteric bacilli. Their close relationship is indicated by similarities in biochemical reactions, antigenic structure, and polynucleotide sequences of their DNA.[10]

Nomenclature within the genus has long been complex. Certain well-established species, such as *S. typhi*, can be differentiated by physiological methods. Others, although similar in physiology, differ from one another in antigenic makeup. As new and different serological types were discovered, it was customary to assign names, usually the place of first isolation, that implied species status, *viz., S. newport, S. panama,* and the like. Hundreds of such "species" have now been described.

There now seems to be acceptance, at least in the United States, of a modified taxonomic scheme that preserves three species of *Salmonella*—*S. typhi, S. cholera-suis,* and *S. enteritidis*—each differentiated by biochemical patterns, as described above.[22] In this system, the familiar serotypes are placed within the species *S. enteritidis, e.g., S. enteritidis* serotype *newport.* Obviously, numbered serotypes would be less cumbersome, but some of the flavor of *Salmonella* bacteriology would be lost.

Serological Differentiation

By application of the techniques of **antigenic analysis,** the antigenic mosaic of isolated strains of *Salmonella* may be defined by an antigenic formula that describes the individual principal antigens, *viz.,* the formula 6,7:c:1,5 represents the major O antigens (6 and 7), the phase 1 flagellar antigen (c), and the phase 2 flagellar antigens (1 and 5). The classification of serotypes in this fashion is known as the **Kauffmann-White scheme.**

Salmonella Typing. Partial or complete identification of serotypes is carried out by the use of appropriate antiserums; monospecific antiserums may be prepared, by appropriate adsorption, to contain antibody to a single antigenic component. The serological identification of strains in this way is known as *Salmonella* typing.

The somatic antigens provide the basis for primary separation into serogroups, as shown in Table 19–3. There are more than 60 O antigen groups, each possessing a unique somatic antigen or combination of these, but about 98 per cent of *Salmonella* isolates fall into groups A through E.

It is, then, a relatively simple matter to assign a strain to one or another of these groups by the use of grouping antiserums, and identification may be carried considerably further with relatively few additional antiserums to H antigens. While the assignment of an isolate to a serotype is a complex matter, to be undertaken in only a few reference laboratories, these may be extremely useful in tracing epidemics; serotyping is not required in management of illness. Table 19–4 displays the O group and antigenic formulae of a few of the more important serotypes of *Salmonella.*

Table 19–3. **Principal O Antigen Groups of *Salmonella***

Group	Major O Antigens
A	1, 2, 12
B	4, 5, 12
C_1	6, 7
C_2	6, 8
D_1	9, 12
D_2	9, 46
E	3
F	11
G_1	13, 22
G_2	13, 23
H	6, 14

Table 19–4. **Important Serotypes of _Salmonella_**

Serotype	O Group	Antigenic Formula*
typhi	D	9, 12 [Vi]: d: —
paratyphi A	A	1, 2, 12: a: —
paratyphi B	B	1, 4, [5], 12: b: 1, 2
paratyphi C	C₁	6, 7, [Vi]: c: 1, 5
cholera-suis	C₁	6, 7: [c]: 1, 5
typhimurium	B	1, 4, [5], 12: i: 1, 2
enteritidis	D	1, 9, 12: g, m: —
heidelberg	B	1, 4, [5], 12: r: 1, 2
newport	C₂	6, 8: e, h: 1, 2
agona	B	1, 4, 12: f, g, s: —
saint-paul	B	1, 4, [5], 12: e, h: 1, 2
oranienburg	C₁	6, 7: m, t: —

*Symbols: [ ], may be lacking.

Phage Typing

Salmonella strains of the same serotype, indistinguishable by biochemical tests, may be subdivided into phage types (phagovars) on the basis of their susceptibility to lysis by different races of bacteriophage. Such differentiation is extremely useful for epidemiological purposes, particularly when the primary source of infection is a human carrier.

Phase typing of Vi-containing strains of _S. typhi_ is applied on an international scale; the paratyphoid bacilli are also typed, but to a lesser extent. There is considerable variation in the geographic distribution of _S. typhi_ phagovars throughout the world, but type E_1 is the most common all over the world, including the United States, with type A a close second.

Since the most frequently isolated _Salmonella_ serotype is _typhimurium_, a phage typing system has also been devised for these strains. At least 207 phage types are known, designated by Arabic numerals. A similar system, with 19 numbered types, is available for the _enteritidis_ serotype.

Ecology

All _Salmonella_ are obligate parasites and are found in a number of animal hosts, including man. Certain of these are restricted to man— _S. typhi_ and _S. enteritidis_ serotype _paratyphi A_—in whom they cause disease or persist in the carrier state. The remainder of the _Salmonella_ are parasites of lower animals, especially rodents and birds, although some are frequently found in reptiles and other poikilothermic animals. The natural host of _S. enteriditis_ serotype _enteritidis_, for example, is the rat, while the _typhimurium_ serotype is a natural pathogen of mice, causing mouse typhoid. Fowl are commonly infected, notably chickens, turkeys, and ducks. Among other domestic animals, pigs are sometimes infected, usually with _S. cholera-suis_.

A wide variety of _Salmonella_ serotypes are isolated from cases of human salmonellosis in the United States. The most frequently isolated serotype is _typhimurium_, as it is in most developed countries of the world. There is some variation in the predominant serotypes in different geographical areas; the figures for the United States in 1980 are shown in Table 19–5.

Salmonellosis in Animals

Salmonella infect a wide variety of animals, and their importance as animal reservoirs of human infection is well known. Food-producing animals, including swine, cattle, and fowl, may be naturally infected; man contracts salmonellosis by consumption of infected flesh of such animals. _Salmonella_ infection is also widespread in rodents; when the bacteria are excreted in the feces, contamination of food and water permits transmission of the infection to humans.

The _Salmonella_ responsible for animal infections include _S. cholera-suis_, most often found in swine, and serotypes of _S. enteritidis_, which infect many animals species. _Salmonella typhi_, in contrast to most other _Salmonella_, is almost completely nonpathogenic for lower animals, but a disease closely resembling typhoid fever is produced in chimpanzees by oral inoculation. There is no animal reservoir for _S. typhi_, since naturally occurring infections appear only in humans.

Salmonella enteritidis is generally responsible for infection in rats and mice, and these animals become healthy carriers of the bacilli,

Table 19–5. **The 10 Serotypes of _Salmonella_ Most Frequently Isolated in the United States During 1980***

Serotype†	Number	Percentage	Median Age (years)
typhimurium	10,443	34.8	9
heidelberg	1,975	6.6	3
enteritidis	1,904	6.3	18
newport	1,651	5.5	14
infantis	1,428	4.8	4
agona	1,402	4.7	7
saint-paul	757	2.5	20
montevideo	665	2.2	17
typhi	605	2.0	24
oranienburg	503	1.7	14

*Adapted from Morbid. Mortal. Weekly Rep. **30**:377, 1981.

†These serotypes accounted for 71.1 per cent of all _Salmonella_ isolated.

a point of importance in connection with outbreaks of gastroenteritis. Infection with the *typhimurium* serotype is by far the most prevalent in the United States.

Birds are quite commonly infected with salmonellae. Epidemics due to serotype *typhimurium* cause great destruction among canaries and other songbirds. Infections in turkeys occur and may be of such magnitude as to assume both economic and public health importance. Two barnyard diseases of great importance are due to specific types: the bacillary white diarrhea of chicks is caused by serotype *pullorum* and fowl typhoid is caused by *gallinarum*. The former may survive in ovaries of fowl that recover from infection; diseased chicks then develop from infected ova and communicate the disease to other members of the flock. Occasional human infections are due to the *pullorum* type, usually associated with consumption of infected eggs.

Other domestic animals contract salmonellosis. Infectious abortion of mares is usually due to the *abortus-equi* type of *S. enteriditis,* while a similar disease of sheep is caused by the *abortus-ovis* serotype. Most animal infections are, however, caused by serotype *typhimurium*.

It is well known that cold-blooded animals may be infected with *Salmonella*. Ordinarily such reservoirs of infection do not relate to human disease, but a number of human infections have been acquired from turtles and other aquarium pets.[7] As a part of this problem, freshwater aquarium snails may also harbor the microorganism,[2] along with other potentially pathogenic, gram-negative bacilli. It is estimated that 280,000 cases of human salmonellosis in the United States in 1970 were derived from pet turtles. Legal restrictions on the sale of these animals have effectively reduced this source of infection.[9]

Insects, especially flies and cockroaches, are potential vectors of salmonellae and thus are of some importance as reservoir hosts. Cockroaches fed *Salmonella* can harbor the bacteria for long periods, with fecal excretion up to 21 days after infection.[18] In some instances, the bacilli may multiply in this vector.

As noted earlier, experimental infections, produced by intragastric inoculation with *S. enteritidis* serotypes, may closely resemble the naturally occurring disease, with enteritis, invasion of the blood stream, and production of metastatic foci of infection.

Bacteriological Diagnosis[15]

The principles of isolation and identification of *Salmonella* do not differ from those used for other enteric bacilli and are summarized in Chapter 17. The identification of serotypes has been previously described.

SALMONELLA INFECTIONS OF MAN

Salmonellosis in humans is almost always acquired by ingestion of the microorganisms, usually in contaminated food, milk, or water. There are two kinds of salmonellosis, one an **acute gastroenteritis** characterized by vomiting and diarrhea in which a small proportion of patients, usually young children, become septicemic. The other is **typhoid**, also called enteric fever, a disease in which bacteremia and tissue invasion is noted in the initial stages and symptoms are more general in nature. In most cases of the latter disease the etiological agent is *S. typhi*, or the *paratyphi B* type of *S. enteritidis*. Occasionally, *paratyphi A* or *paratyphi C* is responsible and, in rare instances, other *Salmonella*. Acute salmonella gastroenteritidis, on the other hand, is practically never caused by *S. typhi* or the paratyphoid bacilli. Most infections of this type are due to the *typhimurium* serotype, but almost any of the myriad *Salmonella* serotypes are potential etiological agents.

In addition to these syndromes, other diseases are occasionally associated with *Salmonella* infection. These microorganisms appear to have a predilection for the bone marrow or joints, appearing occasionally as osteomyelitis or septic arthritis; there is a frequent association between acute osteomyelitis and sickle-cell anemia.[26] Other localized infections include those of the central nervous system, usually in children less than one year of age; *typhimurium* is the most common single serotype isolated from cerebrospinal fluid in such infections, as it is from stools in enteric infections.[37]

A **carrier state** often follows *Salmonella* infections, with discharge of the microorganisms in the feces. The carrier state may be chronic after *S. typhi* infections but is usually transitory with other serotypes. Carriers may spread the disease and should not, for example, be food handlers. With the exception of the enteric fevers, *Salmonella* infections are derived directly, or indirectly through index cases, from lower animals. The transmission from animals usually results from contamination of food with rodent feces, contamination of bulk and dried eggs by infected fowl, or contamination of animal carcasses or products during slaughter and processing.

SALMONELLA GASTROENTERITIS[3, 8]

Gastroenteritis of *Salmonella* etiology is characterized by a short incubation period, as little as 8 to 12 hours in some cases; acute vomiting and diarrhea; slight rise in temperature; and rapid recovery, usually within a few days. The disease is most often acquired by ingestion of contaminated food; it is, therefore, often called *Salmonella* food poisoning. A more complete description of the epidemiology and clinical aspects of this disease will be found in Chapter 36, including a comparison with other food poisoning syndromes.

The salmonellae responsible for this syndrome are generally serotypes of *S. enteritidis;* the types most often responsible for disease in the United States are listed in Table 19–5. With some exceptions, these are the serotypes that generally circulate in animal populations and animal reservoirs are, in large measure, the source of human infection. Outbreaks of salmonellosis are generally traced to contamination of foods by *Salmonella* of animal origin. The predominant vehicles include poultry, meat, eggs, and dairy products, but transmission from infected pets, particularly aquarium animals, has been significant; person to person transmission has also been noted.

Most outbreaks of salmonellosis in humans follow the consumption of food subjected to poor handling practices, usually inadequate refrigeration, that permit growth of the contaminating bacteria. The result is a large infecting dose, leading to disease in the majority of those exposed. Early studies indicated that infection by the oral route required about 10^6 bacteria. It is now evident that much lower doses can be infective. The size of the infectious dose depends upon the relative virulence of the bacterial strain, the protection from gastric acidity afforded by the vehicle, and the relative susceptibility of the host.

In the latter instance, epidemiological data indicate that host susceptibility is greatest among the very young, the elderly, and those with predisposing conditions, such as gastrectomy, sickle-cell disease, malignancies, and underlying infections.

It is popularly supposed that this kind of *Salmonella* infection is peculiar to underdeveloped nations. Yet it is estimated that as many as 2 million cases occur in the United States each year, with highest incidence in the summer months. The disease is primarily one of children under 5 years of age, with a significantly higher morbidity rate in neonates (Fig. 19–4). Death from the disease is rare in uncomplicated infections, but mortality is greatest in infants, the elderly, and those with intercurrent disease.

Complications
Most cases of *Salmonella* gastroenteritis are self-limiting, with little or no tissue invasion, and range from asymptomatic carriage to severe diarrhea. There may be a transient bacteremia, generally of a benign nature. Occasionally, however, septicemia results from infection, with the usual symptoms of an invasive disease, including chills and fever. Most infections of this nature occur in the elderly and in those with underlying disease, especially malignancies; the mortality rate may be high in septicemic infections.

Therapy
Uncomplicated cases of *Salmonella* gastroenteritis do not require antibiotic therapy. Indeed, there is evidence that it may be deleterious, prolonging the carrier state and exacerbating symptoms. It is likely that antibiotics interfere with the protective effects of normal intestinal flora. Fluid and electrolyte replacement may be indicated in cases with severe dehydration. Antidiarrheal agents, such as Lomotil, are not to be recommended, since they may facilitate adherence and invasion, thereby increasing severity and length of illness.

Disseminated infections, on the other hand, require vigorous therapy. The chemotherapeutic agents of choice are chloramphenicol, ampicillin, or trimethoprim-sulfamethoxazole. In all cases, the antibiotic sensitivity of the causative strains should be determined, since a large proportion of *Salmonella* strains are resistant to one or more antibiotics. *In vitro* sensitivity testing against other antibiotics is not warranted, since sensitivity frequently is not correlated with clinical effectiveness.

THE ENTERIC FEVERS: TYPHOID AND PARATYPHOID[28, 30]

Salmonella infection that results in a continued febrile disease with tissue invasion is characteristically typhoid fever, caused by *Salmonella typhi*. A similar disease, somewhat milder in form, may be due to other *Salmonella*, usually *S. enteritidis* serotypes *paratyphi A, B, or C*—the paratyphoid bacilli. Typhoid and paratyphoid fevers are indistinguishable except by isolation and identification of the etiologic agent.

Typhoid fever was long one of the most widespread and important of all bacterial dis-

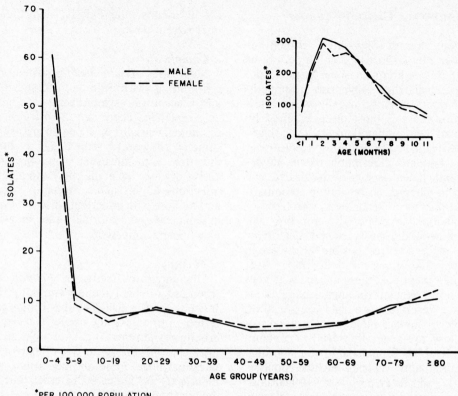

Figure 19–4. Reported isolations of *Salmonella* from humans, by age, United States, 1980. (Centers for Disease Control, Annual summary 1980: reported morbidity and mortality in the United States. Morbidity Mortality Weekly Report, **29**, 1981.)

eases. In the United States in 1900, there were about 350,000 cases of typhoid with more than 35,000 deaths reported. The incidence has markedly decreased with improvement of sanitary conditions and personal hygiene. Typhoid still persists, however, as large epidemic foci in underdeveloped countries, and as sporadic cases and small outbreaks in the United States and similar developed nations.

Sometimes considered primarily an intestinal infection, typhoid fever in fact represents a generalized invasion of the body, particularly of the lymphatic system. The gastrointestinal tract is first colonized, followed by invasion of the intestinal epithelium and later multiplication in the mesenteric lymph nodes.[13] The bacteria reach the blood stream via the thoracic lymph, and the characteristic lesions of typhoid fever are in the lymphoid tissue of the intestinal wall and mesenteric lymph nodes. It has long been assumed that the general symptoms of the disease are attributable to the endotoxic activity of bacterial lipopolysaccharide, but the central role of endotoxin in pathogenesis has been challenged.[14] Typhoid fever may also be accompanied by disseminated in-

travascular coagulation[32] and intestinal hemorrhage.

In the majority of cases, typhoid bacilli are found in the blood during the first 10 days of the disease. This is thought to represent a bacteremia rather than septicemia, since little or no multiplication takes place. At this time, too, bacilli may be present in the bone marrow. During and after the second week, *S. typhi* is excreted in the stools and the proportion of positive blood cultures decreases (Fig. 19–5). The bacilli are also excreted in the urine in about 25 per cent of the cases.

A variety of complications may occur. The gall bladder is often infected, and cystitis is sometimes observed. Suppurative and inflammatory processes may appear in other parts of the body, including laryngeal ulcer and lesions of the bones and joints. Osteomyelitis may develop as long as 6 or 7 years after apparent recovery from typhoid fever, indicating long term latent infections.

Carriers

In studies carried out in the preantibiotic era, about one-third of patients still discharged

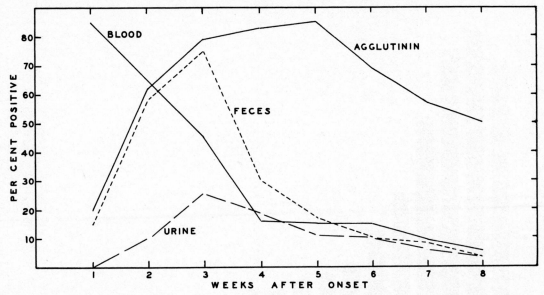

Figure 19–5. The approximate incidence of positive culture of blood, feces, and urine and the agglutinin response in typhoid fever.

bacilli 4 weeks after onset of typhoid fever; fecal discharge continued in about 10 per cent for 8 to 10 weeks. These represent convalescent carriers. A small proportion become long-term carriers and continue to excrete *S. typhi* for 6 months or more, sometimes for many years (Fig. 19–6).

The fecal carrier state is usually a consequence of persistent infection in the gallbladder. Persistence of the infection in the urinary bladder results in urinary carriers but is much less common than fecal carriage. In any case, the carrier state may be intermittent and weeks may elapse with negative cultures before the bacteria reappear; the necessity for repeated examination is obvious.

Attempts to cure typhoid carriers by non-surgical means, such as chemotherapy or vaccine use, have not been generally successful and are not advocated at present. Removal of the gallbladder has eliminated the fecal carrier state in about 70 per cent of cases.

The carrier rate in the United States is not known, but the low incidence of typhoid fever indicates that it is very low. Limited studies on the infrequent outbreaks of typhoid fever in this country have usually identified carriers as the source, and about one-fourth of the sporadic cases can be traced to carriers.[30]

Chemotherapy[6]
The typhoid bacillus is generally sensitive to many of the broad-spectrum antibiotics, but chloramphenicol is the most effective *in vivo* and has for many years been the drug of choice. Prior to 1972, only a few antibiotic resistant strains of *S. typhi* were reported. In that year, an epidemic of more than 10,000 cases of typhoid fever in Mexico was due to *S. typhi* resistant to both chloramphenicol and ampicillin by R plasmid acquisition. More than 60 cases due to this resistant strain were imported to the United States. Fortunately this epidemic subsided and the number of resistant strains has markedly diminished. Strains of *S. typhi* resistant to multiple antibiotics, including both chloramphenicol and ampicillin, continue to be reported from all parts of the world, but their number and significance remain low. In most instances, then, chloramphenicol is still the drug of choice, followed by ampicillin and trimethoprim-sulfamethoxazole. Nevertheless, drug sensitivity testing of isolates is recommended.

Epidemiology
The typhoid bacillus is an **obligate human parasite,** and probably does not multiply in nature outside of the human host. The organism is excreted from cases or carriers in the feces or urine and enters a susceptible host by ingestion. The epidemiology of typhoid fever is then predicated upon the connection between contamination of food, water, or fomites and ingestion by susceptibles. The extent of spread of the disease is dependent upon the nature of the connecting link, giving rise to two epidemiological types of disease—epidemic and endemic typhoid.

Epidemic Typhoid Fever. Extensive out-

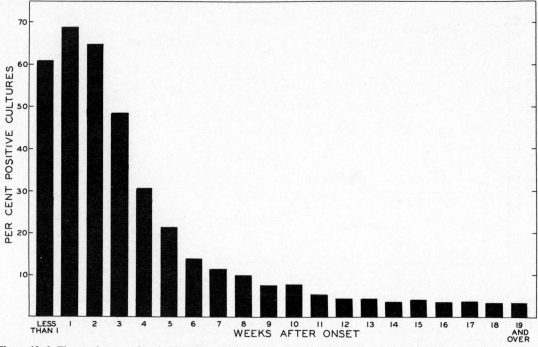

Figure 19–6. The persistence of typhoid bacillus infection as indicated by percentage of positive fecal cultures by weeks after onset. (Data from 374 cases in New York State, exclusive of New York City, by Ames and Robins.[1])

breaks of typhoid necessarily involve a connecting link common to a great many people; the most important vehicle of this kind is water. Once common throughout the world, waterborne typhoid fever is rare in most communities in the industrialized countries, illustrating the significance of water purification and treatment and the proper disposal of sewage. Thus, waterborne epidemics are readily preventable. When such epidemics do occur, the disease incidence is unaffected by age, sex, and economic status. Waterborne epidemics are seen occasionally in the United States and Europe, as in Florida in 1973, Heidelberg in 1974, and on a cruise ship in 1970. Milkborne typhoid fever, once second in importance only to waterborne typhoid, has been practically eliminated in most nations by the pasteurization of milk.

Foodborne typhoid fever may take on epidemic proportions in certain instances. An epidemic due to contaminated corned beef, for example, appeared in Aberdeen, Scotland, in 1964. The very serious epidemic in Mexico in 1972 was probably food- and milkborne.

Endemic Typhoid Fever. Although epidemic typhoid fever is largely eliminated by effective sanitary control of water and milk,

an endemic form remains which is manifest as occasional cases or small clusters of cases of sporadic appearance. In the United States, about half of the cases are acquired during foreign travel. In the remainder, the infection source is most often a chronic carrier. Carriers are particularly important in that they constitute a semipermanent focus of infection. Transmission from carriers or cases may be by direct contact or by vehicles such as food. The most notorious instance of the latter kind was that of Mary Mallon, "Typhoid Mary," who was unknowingly the source of 26 cases of typhoid fever in seven different families. Recently, it has become apparent that typhoid fever may be contracted in the microbiology laboratory, emphasizing the need for adequate laboratory safety procedures in handling of bacterial pathogens.[4]

Endemic typhoid is much more difficult to control than the epidemic form. The detection and supervision of carriers is a practical impossibility, and even if identified, elimination of the carrier state by chemotherapy is not yet a certainty. Yet, effective control of the epidemic form may result in reduced incidence of endemic cases and number of carriers. Certainly, the reduction in cases of typhoid fever

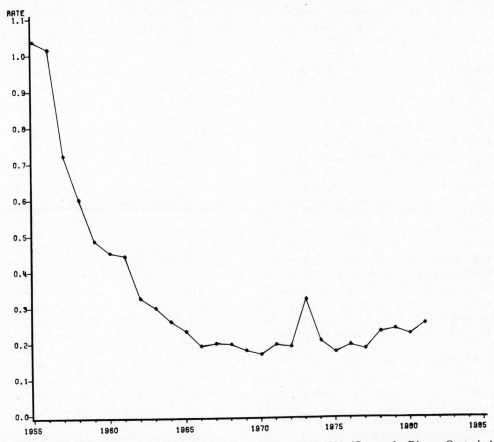

Figure 19–7. Reported case rates of typhoid fever in the United States, 1955–1981. (Centers for Disease Control. Annual summary 1981: reported morbidity and mortality in the United States. Morbidity and Mortality Weekly Report, **30**, 1982.)

in the United States has been marked since the early 1940s, and has remained at a relatively low level since 1970 (Fig. 19–7).

Immunity[36]

While it is widely believed that an attack of typhoid fever confers a degree of immunity to subsequent infection, instances of two and even more attacks in the same individual have been noted. Indeed, in controlled human experiments, infection with *S. typhi* did not significantly protect against subsequent challenge with the same strain.[12] In the Aberdeen epidemic, on the other hand, prior immunization modified the disease; immunized individuals more often exhibited mild disease than did nonimmunized persons.[29] It is clear that immunity to typhoid fever following either infection or immunization is not absolute. The immune state may be effective against exposure to low numbers of bacteria, but not against very high numbers. Further, the im-

mune state may not protect against infection, but may only modify severity of disease.

Exposure to the antigens of typhoid bacilli induces a substantial **humoral response,** with production of agglutinins, precipitins, and complement-dependent bactericidal antibodies. During the course of typhoid fever in humans, serum agglutinins appear, sometimes as early as the fifth day; by 4 weeks they are present in 90 per cent of cases. This agglutinin response is of some diagnostic value and may be measured by the **Widal test,** a macroscopic tube agglutination test using dilutions of the patient's serum and known *S. typhi* cell suspensions. In general, O or H agglutinin titers of 1:200 or greater offer presumptive evidence of infection, particularly if increases are noted with time. Interpretation is more difficult in patients previously immunized with typhoid vaccine or in adults in endemic areas, since low titers may be present in these individuals. Furthermore, other febrile conditions, such as typhus, may induce an anamnestic response to *S. typhi* antigens. Recently, a hemagglutination test for Vi antibodies has been introduced, using highly purified Vi antigen to sensitize red blood cells. It is reported to detect carriers of *S. typhi* as effectively as stool culture.[24]

While humoral response may be useful in laboratory diagnosis of typhoid fever, the presence of serum antibodies does not appear to correlate with effective immunity. On the other hand, experience with other enteric pathogens has supported the hypothesis that **intestinal antibodies,** such as IgA, may be protective by preventing bacterial adherence and colonization. This is the theoretical basis for oral immunization, as discussed in the following section. It has long been assumed that systemic immunity is associated with a cell-mediated immune response, but substantial proof has been elusive. The development of a cell-mediated immune response in typhoid fever has recently been shown to correlate with uncomplicated recovery from the disease.[31]

Prophylactic Immunization[36]

Vaccination against typhoid fever has been practiced since the turn of the century, particularly in military populations, since these were often devastated by the disease. These attempts at immunoprophylaxis were largely empirical, and it was not until the early 1960s that well-controlled field trials were carried out. Nevertheless, immunization was accompanied by lowered incidence of disease in army personnel and the character of epidemics was altered. Since immunization of United States Army personnel became compulsory in 1911, typhoid has practically disappeared in this population. Absolute protection is unlikely, and cases, while rare, have appeared from time to time. Moreover, the role of improved sanitary measures during this period cannot be assessed but is undoubtedly significant.

Parenteral Vaccines.[38] The most widely used prophylactic vaccines are suspensions of killed typhoid bacilli, administered parenterally. In practice, such vaccines also contain paratyphoid bacilli A and B as well. The bacilli may be killed with heat and preserved with phenol, or inactivated with acetone.

Prospective field trials with these vaccines since the 1960s have indicated that both types provide significant immunity, although the acetone-inactivated type is more successful.

Depending upon the geographical area of the trial, the number of vaccine doses administered, and the follow-up period, protection by the acetone-inactivated vaccine ranged from 50 to 94 per cent. Results in field trials are paralleled by vaccination and challenge in human volunteers. Volunteer studies have also demonstrated that immunity can be overwhelmed by large infective doses, but that good protection is offered against exposure to relatively low numbers of *S. typhi*.

Oral Immunization. With a new understanding of the mechanisms of pathogenesis in intestinal infection, *e.g.*, the role of adherence and colonization, attention has focused on the role of local immunity. Oral vaccines can be expected to stimulate the production of IgA in the intestinal tract that might, in turn, inhibit adherence and invasion by the bacilli. Both killed and live oral vaccines have been devised. Field trials in India, using high doses of killed vaccine, demonstrated no beneficial effect. Results with live oral vaccines are, however, more promising. In 1975, an attenuated mutant of *S. typhi* was described which lacked galactose epimerase. This strain, designated Ty21a, is unable to cause disease because of growth inhibition and cell lysis that follows uptake of galactose. This attenuated *S. typhi* strain has been tested as an oral vaccine in volunteers and in a field trial in Egypt. In immunized volunteers challenged with virulent *S. typhi*, an 87 per cent efficacy was attained with no side effects. In the field trial in children, the protection was 100 per cent, although the incidence in the control population was low.[35] If future trials are in general agreement with these findings, the vaccine may prove the best yet devised.

Paratyphoid Fever[23]

Paratyphoid fever was differentiated in 1896, when a microorganism similar to, but not identical with, the typhoid bacillus was isolated from typhoid-like disease.

Many cases of paratyphoid infection tend to run a relatively mild course and are marked by sudden onset with chills. Otherwise, they are clinically similar to infections with typhoid bacilli, presenting with fever, diarrhea, nausea, and vomiting; neurological complaints include headache and stiff neck. A certain proportion of apparent typhoid fever cases with negative Widal tests may, in fact, be paratyphoid fever. The only method to distinguish typhoid from paratyphoid fever is by isolation and identification of the causal microorganism.

Both scattered cases and limited epidemics of paratyphoid fever have been reported. Infection is probably most often acquired from human carriers. The bacilli may be excreted for some weeks by convalescents; undiagnosed subclinical cases are a similar source of infection. In general, the mode of dissemination of paratyphoid fever is practically identical with that of typhoid fever.

The frequency of paratyphoid infection varies in different localities. Paratyphoid bacilli are rarely isolated in the United States, although they are encountered in other parts of the world, including Asia, Africa, and southeastern Europe.

The causal agent is most often one of the *paratyphi* serotypes (*A, B,* or *C*) of *S. enteritidis,* although other serotypes have been found to cause enteric fevers of this nature. Pathogenesis is identical to that of typhoid fever.

Arizona[17]

A single species of *Arizona* is recognized, *A. hinshawii.* These organisms closely resemble *Salmonella;* indeed, in the 1974 Bergey classification they are included as serotypes of *Salmonella.* They may be biochemically separated from the salmonellae, however, by the reactions listed in Table 19–1. It can be seen that most strains ferment lactose, although the fermentation is frequently delayed.

These microorganisms appear to be normal intestinal parasites in **reptiles** and many strains have been isolated from such animals. Their antigenic structure is similar to that of *Salmonella,* being made up of somatic (O) antigens and flagellar (H) antigens of both phase 1 and 2. Indeed, the antigenic formulae for *Arizona* adopts the same designations as *Salmonella,* including the same O groups. There is, then, considerable sharing of antigens with *Salmonella.* The serotype designation is by complete antigenic formula, rather than specific epithets as used for *Salmonella.*

Strains of *Arizona* cause a spectrum of human disease indistinguishable from that of *S. enteritidis.* Occasional cases of gastroenteritis are usually associated with aquarium pets, such as turtles. Although rare, several cases of systemic infection have been documented, the organism being isolated from blood cultures. There is evidence that systemic infections occur principally in individuals with severe underlying disease.

Citrobacter[21]

The genus *Citrobacter* comprises three species—*C. freundii, C. amalonaticus,* and *C. diversus.* Their significant biochemical reactions are listed in Table 19–6.

Citrobacter is commonly found in soil and water and in the intestinal contents of humans and animals, in which they behave as commensals. These bacteria are rarely the primary etiological agents in human infections but may be pathogenic in elderly or debilitated patients. The predominant type of infection is that of the urinary tract, especially in individuals with abnormalities or with indwelling catheters. They have also been incriminated in pulmonary infections, wounds, osteomyelitis, peritonitis, and endocarditis, although such infections seem to be rare. *Citrobacter* is sometimes the cause of neonatal meningitis, representing a small portion of the gram-negative meningitides, but with high mortality rates and significant neurological sequelae in survivors.

Table 19–6. **Biochemical Reactions of *Citrobacter****

Test	C. freundii		C. amalonaticus	C. diversus
	Biotype A	Biotype B		
H₂S production	+	−	−	−
Indole production	−	−	+	+
Malonate utilization	−	−	−	+
Potassium cyanide inhibition	+	+	+	−

*Adapted from Lipsky, *et al.*[21]

REFERENCES

1. Ames, W. R., and M. Robins. 1943. Age and sex as factors in the development of the typhoid carrier state, and a method for estimating carrier prevalence. Amer. J. Publ. Hlth **33**:221–230.
2. Bartlett, K. H., and T. J. Trust. 1976. Isolation of Salmonella and other potential pathogens from the freshwater aquarium snail *Ampullaria*. Appl. Environ. Microbiol. **31**:635–639.
3. Blaser, M. J., and L. S. Newman. 1982. A review of human salmonellosis. I. Infective dose. Rev. Infect. Dis. **4**:1096–1106.
4. Blaser, M. J., et al. 1980. *Salmonella typhi*: the laboratory as a reservoir of infection. J. Infect. Dis. **142**:934–938.
5. Capioli, A., et al. 1982. Isolation of *Salmonella wein* heat-labile enterotoxin. Toxicon **20**:254.
6. Cherubin, C. E. 1981. Antibiotic resistance of *Salmonella* in Europe and the United States. Rev. Infect. Dis. **3**:1105–1126.
7. Chiodini, R. H., and J. P. Sundberg. 1981. Salmonellosis in reptiles: a review. Amer. J. Epidemiol. **113**:494–499.
8. Cohen, M. L., and E. J. Gangarosa. 1978. Nontyphoid salmonellosis. Southern Med. J. **71**:1540–1545.
9. Cohen, M. L., et al. 1980. Turtle-associated salmonellosis in the United States. Effect of public health action, 1970 to 1976. J. Amer. Med. Assn **243**:1247–1249.
10. Crosa, J. H., et al. 1973. Molecular relationships among the salmonellae. J. Bacteriol. **115**:307–315.
11. Duguid, J. P., M. R. Darekar, and D. W. F. Wheater. 1976. Fimbriae and infectivity in *Salmonella typhimurium*. J. Med. Microbiol. **9**:459–473.
12. DuPont, H. L., et al. 1971. Studies of immunity in typhoid fever. Protection induced by killed oral antigens or by primary infection. Bull. Wld Hlth Org. **44**:667–672.
13. Gaines, S., et al. 1968. Studies on infection and immunity in experimental typhoid fever. VII. The distribution of *Salmonella typhi* in chimpanzee tissue following oral challenge, and the relationship between the numbers of bacilli and morphologic lesions. J. Infect. Dis. **118**:293–306.
14. Greisman, S. E., et al. 1969. The role of endotoxin during typhoid fever and tularemia in man. IV. The integrity of the endotoxin tolerance mechanisms during infection. J. Clin. Invest. **48**:613–629.
15. Harvey, R. W. S., and T. H. Price. 1979. A review. Principles of salmonella isolation. J. Appl. Bacteriol. **46**:27–56.
16. Houston, C. W., F. C. W. Koo, and J. W. Peterson. 1981. Characterization of *Salmonella* toxin released by mitomycin C-treated cells. Infect. Immun. **32**:916–926.
17. Johnson, R. H., et al. 1976. *Arizona hinshawii* infections. New cases, antimicrobial sensitivities, and literature review. Ann. Intern. Med. **85**:587–592.
18. Klowden, M. J., and B. Greenberg. 1976. *Salmonella* in the American cockroach: evaluation of vector potential through dosed feeding experiments. J. Hygiene **77**:105–111.
19. Kochan, I., J. Wasynczuk, and M. A. McCabe. 1978. Effects of injected iron and siderophores on infections in normal and immune mice. Infect. Immun. **22**:560–567.
20. Leunk, R. D., and R. J. Moon. 1982. Association of type 1 pili with the ability of livers to clear *Salmonella typhimurium*. Infect. Immun. **36**:1168–1174.
21. Lipsky, B. A., et al. 1980. Citrobacter infections in humans: experience at the Seattle Veterans Administration Medical Center and a review of the literature. Rev. Infect. Dis. **2**:746–760.
22. Martin, W. J., and J. A. Washington, II. 1980. *Enterobacteriaceae*. pp. 195–219. *In* E. H. Lennette, et al. (Eds.): Manual of Clinical Microbiology. 3rd ed. American Society for Microbiology, Washington, D.C.
23. Meals, R. A. 1976. Paratyphoid fever. A report of 62 cases with several unusual findings and a review of the literature. Arch. Intern. Med. **136**:1422–1428.
24. Nolan, C. M., et al. 1981. Vi serology in the detection of typhoid carriers. Lancet **1**:583–585.
25. Okamura, N., and J. K. Spitznagel. 1982. Outer membrane mutants of *Salmonella typhimurium* LT2 have lipopolysaccharide-dependent resistance to the bactericidal activity of anaerobic human neutrophils. Infect. Immun. **36**:1086–1095.
26. Ortiz-Neu, C., et al. 1978. Bone and joint infections due to *Salmonella*. J. Infect. Dis. **138**:820–828.
27. Puschmann, M., and A. M. Ganzoni. 1977. Increased resistance of iron-deficient mice to Salmonella infection. Infect. Immun. **17**:663–664.
28. Rodriguez-Leiva, M. 1979. Typhoid fever 1979—a new perspective on an old disease. J. Infect. Dis. **140**:268–270.
29. Russell, E. M., A. Sutherland, and W. Walker. 1968. The ·Aberdeen typhoid epidemic. Lancet **1**:423–424.
30. Ryder, R. W., and P. A. Blake. 1979. Typhoid fever in the United States, 1975 and 1976. J. Infect. Dis. **139**:124–126.
31. Sarma, V. N. B., et al. 1977. Development of immune response during typhoid fever in man. Clin. Exptl Immunol. **28**:35–39.
32. Setiadharma, S., and L. K. Kho. 1973. Disseminated intravascular coagulation in typhoid fever in childhood. S. E. Asian J. Trop. Med. Publ. Hlth **4**:461–467.
33. Valtonen, M. V. 1977. Role of phagocytosis in mouse virulence of *Salmonella typhimurium* recombinants with O antigen 6,7 or 4,12. Infect. Immun. **18**:574–582.
34. Valtonen, M. V., et al. 1976. Effect of enterobacterial common antigen on mouse virulence of *Salmonella typhimurium*. Infect. Immun. **13**:1601–1605.
35. Wahdan, M. H., et al. 1980. A controlled field trial of live oral typhoid vaccine Ty21a. Bull. Wld Hlth Org. **58**:469–474.
36. Warren, J. W., and R. B. Hornick. 1979. Immunization against typhoid fever. Ann. Rev. Med. **30**:457–472.
37. Wilson, R., and R. A. Feldman. 1981. Reported isolates of *Salmonella* from cerebrospinal fluid in the United States, 1968–1979. J. Infect. Dis. **143**:504–506.
38. Woodward, W. E. 1980. Volunteer studies of typhoid fever and vaccines. Trans. Roy. Soc. Trop. Med. Hygiene **74**:553–556.
39. Yancey, R. J., S. A. L. Breeding, and C. E. Lankford. 1979. Enterochelin (Enterobactin): virulence factor for *Salmonella typhimurium*. Infect. Immun. **24**:174–180.

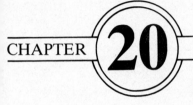

CHAPTER 20

The Enteric Bacilli: Klebsiella, Enterobacter, Serratia, Proteus, Providentia, and Morganella

KLEBSIELLA
   Immunological Types
   Virulence
   Pathogenicity
ENTEROBACTER AND SERRATIA

PROTEUS, PROVIDENTIA, AND MORGANELLA
   Morphology and Staining
   Physiology
   Antigenic Structure
   Pathogenicity

Klebsiella, Proteus, and related forms are generally regarded as enteric bacilli because they are frequently present in the enteric tract, but their pathogenic potential is usually expressed at other locations in the body. In general, when these bacteria are present in the intestine they behave as commensals. Nevertheless, their colonization at this site provides a source or reservoir for infection and disease production at other locations, including pulmonary and urinary tract infections.

Klebsiella, Enterobacter, and *Serratia* are members of the tribe Klebsielleae of the family Enterobacteriaceae. *Proteus, Providentia,* and *Morganella* are all quite similar bacilli classified in the tribe Proteeae. Characterization of these tribes and their differentiation from other Enterobacteriaceae is discussed in Chapter 17.

Klebsiella[10]

The taxonomy of *Klebsiella* is not altogether satisfactory, and there is some divergence between the systems employed by American and British workers.[1] In the United States, three species are generally recognized: *K. pneumoniae, K. ozaenae,* and *K. rhinoscleromatis.* The significant biochemical reactions of these species are found in Table 20–1. Occasionally, a fourth species is delineated, *K. oxytoca,* which is similar to *K. pneumoniae,* except that indole is produced from tryptophan.

The frankly pathogenic forms of *Klebsiella* are usually *K. pneumoniae* strains, and these are casually known as Friedländer's bacillus.

Table 20–1. **Biochemical Reactions of *Klebsiella* Species***

Test	*Klebsiella pneumoniae*	*Klebsiella ozaenae*	*Klebsiella rhinoscleromatis*
Urease	+	−	−
Methyl red	−	+	+
Voges-Proskauer	+	−	−
Citrate utilization	+	V	−
Lysine decarboxylase	+	V	−
Malonate	+	−	V

*Adapted from Martin and Washington.[10] Symbols: +, most strains positive; −, most strains negative; V, variable reactions.

Other strains of *K. pneumoniae* are widely distributed in nature, being found in soil and water as free-living forms. They are also normally found in the intestinal tract of man and animals as commensals. *Klebsiella ozaenae* is infrequently associated with chronic upper respiratory infection; *K. rhinoscleromatis* may be responsible for rhinoscleroma but such infections are quite rare.

Friedländer's bacillus was first described by him as an etiological agent of pneumonia. Strains of *K. pneumoniae* found in the upper respiratory tract are usually heavily encapsulated (Fig. 20–1). *Klebsiella* are typically nonmotile, encapsulated, gram-negative rods, often somewhat thicker than other enteric bacilli. Many strains of *K. pneumoniae* possess fimbriae; these act as adhesins and are therefore virulence factors for these strains, as noted below. Colonies on blood agar are usually large, with mucoid and viscous consistency (Fig. 20–2), reflecting the large amounts of polysaccharide capsular material.

There is considerable variability among *Klebsiella* in many of the biochemical reactions. In *K. pneumoniae,* biotypes have been designated on this basis but these have not found great practical use in clinical laboratories.

Immunological Types

Klebsiella contain both O and K antigens, the latter as morphologically evident capsules. At least 11 serogroups are differentiated on the basis of their O antigens, but routine grouping is not practiced, since the heat-stable capsules block O agglutination. Typing of *Klebsiella* is based on capsular K antigens; at least 80 capsular types have been described. The capsular substance is polysaccharide, usually comprising hexoses and uronic acid. Although reaction with anticapsular antiserum does not induce apparent swelling of the capsule as seen in the typical Quellung reaction, immune precipitation takes place at the periphery of the capsule, making the margin highly refractile; typing may be accomplished by this procedure. Virulence does not seem to be associated with capsular type, although the lower-numbered serotypes tend to predominate in human infections.

For epidemiological purposes, other typing methods have been explored. **Bacteriocin typing,** in which *Klebsiella* strains are subjected to a battery of known bacteriocins, has been the basis for several such schemes, but these are often not completely reproducible and

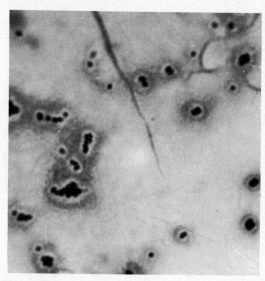

Figure 20–1. *Klebsiella pneumoniae* (Friedländer's bacillus) in pure culture on blood agar, showing capsules. Crystal violet; × 1200.

have not gained wide acceptance. A recently proposed system may overcome these technical difficulties.[2]

Virulence

The wide distribution of Klebsiellae and the epidemiology of infections indicate that virulence varies widely between strains. Some possess limited pathogenic potential, occurring as opportunistic pathogens after colonization at a variety of sites, while a few behave as primary invaders, presumably possessing higher viru-

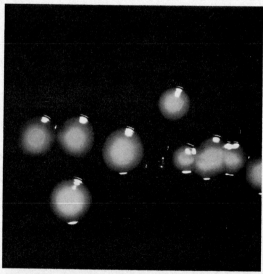

Figure 20–1. Colonies of *Klebsiella pneumoniae* on blood agar. Note the large size and mucoid appearance. × 3.

lence. The virulence determinants are not completely understood, although several factors are putatively involved. Current evidence indicates that mannose-sensitive pili are virulence factors, serving as **adhesins** that permit colonization of mucosal surfaces. Their role is best established in urinary tract infections as studied in animal models.[5] These pili are also capable of inhibiting phagocytosis and intracellular killing of *Klebsiella.*[12] Certain physiological states and intercurrent disease predispose to *Klebsiella* infections. It appears that these disease states somehow increase the number of **receptor sites** on epithelial cells for adherence of *Klebsiella.*[8] **Capsules** are also probably involved in virulence, inhibiting phagocytosis and impairing intraphagocytic killing. Some *K. pneumoniae* strains are known to produce a low-molecular-weight, heat-stable enterotoxin similar to that of *E. coli,* but its relationship to pathogenesis is unknown at present. Similarly, some strains produce **siderophores** that may behave as aggressins by competition for available iron in the host.

Pathogenicity[6, 11]

As noted above, *Klebsiella* are often a part of the normal flora of humans. Perhaps a third or more of human subjects harbor the microorganism in the bowel without evidence of pathogenesis. The degree of colonization is often increased in hospitalized patients. The normal intestinal flora are known to interfere with colonization by *Klebsiella;* antibiotic administration perturbs the sensitive normal microflora, permitting colonization by the more resistant *Klebsiella.* Other sites, such as the upper respiratory and urinary tracts, are sometimes colonized, and this colonization is believed to be fostered by extensive antibiotic usage, predisposing disease, surgery, alcohol-

ism, or the use of instruments such as indwelling urethral catheters.

Thus, *Klebsiella* infections are most often **hospital-associated** and are ultimately derived from the fecal flora of colonized individuals. In the hospital environment, patient-to-patient transfer is probably by hand contamination of hospital personnel.

The spectrum of serious *Klebsiella* disease is broad and includes bacteremia; pneumonia, often with necrosis; and urinary tract infections. In hospitals, serious epidemics have occurred among newborns, and endemic infections are seen in urological wards.

Pneumonia due to *Klebsiella* makes up a small proportion of all cases of pneumonia, but the case-fatality rate is high, 90 per cent or more in untreated cases. The microorganism has a greater tendency to produce necrosis than pneumococcus. Although similar to pneumococcal pneumonia in the early stages, progression of *Klebsiella* infection leads to disintegration of the alveolar wall and necrosis of the lung parenchyma. The bacilli may be isolated by blood agar culture of sputum, and the demonstration of typical colonial forms along with observation of thick, ovoid, gram-negative rods is presumptive evidence for *Klebsiella.*

Klebsiella infections do not respond to penicillin therapy but have in the past yielded to many of the sulfonamides and broad-spectrum antibiotics. Plasmid-mediated antibiotic resistance has, however, become prominent and most strains are now resistant to several antibiotics. In one study, more than 90 per cent of strains were resistant to at least 10 commonly used antibiotics.[3] Gentamicin has been widely and successfully applied, but increasing numbers of *Klebsiella* are now resistant.

Enterobacter[9] and Serratia[7, 15]

The *Enterobacter* and *Serratia* are closely related to *Klebsiella,* so that differentiation from *Klebsiella* and from one another is often difficult; several species of *Enterobacter* are now recognized. These species are morphologically indistinguishable from other Enterobacteriaceae. Unlike *Klebsiella,* capsules are not evident in these bacilli. The important species and their biochemical reactions are shown in Table 20–2.

Enterobacter are found as commensals in the intestine and are frequently isolated from soil and water. They are only rarely encountered as infectious agents in the community but may be responsible for a variety of hospital-associated or nosocomial infections. The predominant species responsible are *E. cloacae* and *E. aerogenes. Enterobacter* is responsible for about 4 to 12 per cent of gram-negative bacteremias, many of these arising in burn pa-

Table 20–2. **Biochemical Reactions of** *Enterobacter**

Test	Enterobacter cloacae	Enterobacter aerogenes	Enterobacter sakazakii	Enterobacter gergoviae	Enterobacter agglomerans	Enterobacter hafniae†
Urease	+	−	−	+	V	−
Citrate utilization	+	+	+	+	+	(+)
Sorbitol	+	+	−	−	−	−
Lysine decarboxylase	−	+	−	(+)	−	+
Arginine dehydrolase	+	−	+	−	−	−
Ornithine decarboxylase	+	+	+	+	−	+

*Adapted from Martin and Washington.[10] Symbols: +, most strains positive; (+), positive reactions may be delayed 3 days or more; −, most strains negative; V, variable reactions.
†Now *Hafnia alvei*.

tients. Hospital-acquired infections have also been traced to contaminated intravenous infusion fluids.

The taxonomy of the genus *Serratia* has been fluid for some years. In conformance with the classification used by the Centers for Disease Control, three species are recognized here. These are listed in Table 20–3, along with the more important biochemical reactions of each.

Serratia are, for the most part, free-living saprophytes. For many years they were considered nonpathogenic, but they are indeed capable of causing serious infections under some circumstances and are regarded as opportunistic pathogens. They have been implicated in infections of the respiratory tract, urinary tract, meninges, and endocardium. They are often the cause of bacteremia in hospitalized patients, particularly those with underlying disease or with preceding surgical intervention. *Serratia* endocarditis is often associated with intravenous drug abuse, and pneumonia has resulted from contaminated inhalation equipment. As in the genus *Klebsiella*, *Serratia* are frequently resistant to multiple antibiotics, thus complicating the management of clinical infections.

The most familiar of the *Serratia* are the red pigmented varieties of *S. marcescens*. Growth of these varieties on food has been mistaken for drops of blood and was accorded great religious significance in ancient writings. The pigment is not apparent in cultures incubated at 37°C., but the colonies are a bright pink-red at lower temperatures; the majority of strains are not pigmented, however.

Proteus, Providentia, and Morganella[10]

The tribe Proteeae is made up of three genera: *Proteus*, *Providentia*, and *Morganella*. These were, until recently, all classified as *Proteus* and are thus related to one another as well as to other enteric bacilli. Except for some of the *Providentia*, these microorganisms are found with some frequency in the intestinal tract of normal humans. They are common inhabitants in soil and water that contain decaying organic matter of animal origin and are usually found in sewage.

These microorganisms are regarded as opportunistic pathogens, and most infections are hospital-associated. Urinary tract infections are the predominant type and these are most often due to *Proteus mirabilis*.

Table 20–3. **Biochemical Reactions of** *Serratia**

Test	Serratia marcescens	Serratia liquefaciens	Serratia rubidaea
Sorbitol	+	+	−
Arabinose	−	+	+
Raffinose	−	+	+
Malonate	−	−	+
Ornithine decarboxylase	+	+	−

*Adapted from Martin and Washington.[10] Symbols: +, most strains positive; −, most strains negative.

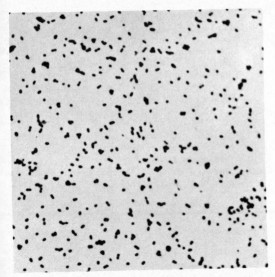

Figure 20–3. *Proteus vulgaris.* Smear from a pure culture. Note the coccobacillary form. The occasional occurrence of paired cells is a result of active multiplication. Fuchsin; × 1050.

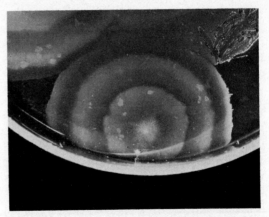

Figure 20–4. *Proteus vulgaris* colony on blood agar. Note the swarming, exhibited as successive waves of growth. (Dack.)

Morphology and Staining

They are similar in morphology to other gram-negative enteric bacilli (Chapter 17). Ovoid forms (Fig. 20–3) are common, however, and long, curved, filamentous cells predominate in swarming cultures. Proteeae are actively motile by peritrichous flagella; fimbriae are commonly found and, in *Proteus,* constitute the attachment structure for adherence to epithelial cells. Capsules are not formed.

The phenomenon of swarming[14] is typical of *Proteus* and is a consequence of the production of elongated cells with excessive numbers of flagella. On agar mediums the colonies do not remain compact and discrete, but spread rapidly, and in successive waves, over the agar surface as a thin, scarcely visible film (Fig. 20–4). This property is a source of considerable inconvenience in the isolation of other bacteria from mixed cultures containing *Proteus.*

Physiology

These microorganisms have simple nutritive requirements and are readily cultivated on ordinary nutrient mediums. Although they are facultative anaerobes, anaerobic growth is generally poor. Genera and species are separated on a biochemical basis by the reactions shown in Table 20–4.

Antigenic Structure

Like other motile enteric bacilli, these microorganisms possess both H and O antigens. Although typing schemes have been proposed, based upon specific O antigens, routine typing is not practiced.

Certain *Proteus* strains are agglutinated by serum of patients having typhus fever (Chapter 33). These so-called X-strains contain O antigens that share determinants with antigens of certain rickettsiae. Thus, patients infected with

Table 20–4. **Biochemical Reactions of *Proteus, Providentia,* and *Morganella***

Test	Proteus mirabilis	Proteus vulgaris	Providentia alcalifaciens	Providentia stuartii	Providentia rettgeri	Morganella morgani
Indole	−	+	+	+	+	+
Urease	+	+	−	−	+	+
H₂S production	+	+	−	−	−	−
Ornithine decarboxylase	+	−	−	−	−	+
Acid from:						
Mannitol	−	−	−	−	+	−
Maltose	−	+	−	−	−	−
Xylose	+	+	−	−	−	−

*Adapted from Martin and Washington.[10] Symbols: +, most strains positive; −, most strains negative.

these rickettsiae develop serum antibodies that agglutinate the X-strains of *Proteus*. An agglutination test employing *Proteus* cells (the Weil-Felix reaction) has been used in the diagnosis of typhus fever.

Pathogenicity[4, 13]

Members of the tribe Proteeae have been found in association with a variety of pathological conditions. Infections of the eye and ear, peritonitis, and suppurative abscesses at various sites are among the infectious processes in which an etiological role is probable. Many infections with these bacilli are hospital-associated and the strains responsible tend to show multiple drug resistance. Cystitis and pyelonephritis due to *Proteus* are frequent nosocomial infections, and their prevalence is exceeded only by *Escherichia coli* and, perhaps, by *Klebsiella*. There is evidence that ureases produced by *Proteus* are nephrotoxic, favoring the intracellular infection of the tubular epithelium and creating an alkalinity in the kidney that may lead to necrosis of renal epithelium and the formation of calculi.

In certain affections of the digestive tract, *Proteus* has been held to be the responsible agent. In diarrheic stools, especially those of infants, it has been found in large numbers and many regard it as a cause of infant diarrhea; the true relationship to intestinal disease is, however, still obscure.

REFERENCES

1. Barr, J. G. 1977. Klebsiella: taxonomy, nomenclature, and communication. J. Clin. Pathol. **30**:943–944.
2. Bauernfeind, A., C. Petermüller, and R. Schneider. 1981. Bacteriocins as tools in analysis of nosocomial *Klebsiella pneumoniae* infections. J. Clin. Microbiol. **14**:15–19.
3. Casewell, M. W., and I. Phillips. 1981. Aspects of the plasmid-mediated antibiotic resistance and epidemiology of Klebsiella species. Amer. J. Med. **70**:459–462.
4. Chow, A. W., *et al.* 1979. A nosocomial outbreak of infections due to multiply resistant *Proteus mirabilis*: role of intestinal colonization as a major reservoir. J. Infect. Dis. **139**:621–627.
5. Fader, R. C., and C. P. Davis. 1980. Effect of piliation on *Klebsiella pneumoniae* infection in rat bladders. Infect. Immun. **30**:554–561.
6. Goldmann, D. A. 1981. Bacterial colonization and infection in the neonate. Amer. J. Med. **70**:417–422.
7. Grimont, P. A. D., and F. Grimont. 1978. The genus *Serratia*. Ann. Rev. Microbiol. **32**:221–248.
8. Johanson, W. G., Jr., D. E. Woods, and T. Chaudhuri. 1979. Association of respiratory tract colonization with adherence of gram-negative bacilli to epithelial cells. J. Infect. Dis. **139**:667–673.
9. John, J. F., Jr., R. J. Sharbaugh, and E. R. Bannister. 1982. *Enterobacter cloacae*: bacteremia, epidemiology, and antibiotic resistance. Rev. Infect. Dis. **4**:13–28.
10. Martin, W. J., and J. A. Washington, II. 1980. *Enterobacteriaceae*. pp. 195–219. *In* E. H. Lennette, *et al.* (Eds.): Manual of Clinical Microbiology. 3rd ed. American Society for Microbiology, Washington, D. C.
11. Montgomerie, J. Z. 1979. Epidemiology of *Klebsiella* and hospital-associated infection. Rev. Infect. Dis **1**:736–753.
12. Pruzzo, C., E. Debhia, and G. Satta. 1982. Mannose-inhibitable adhesins and T3–T7 receptors of *Klebsiella pneumoniae* inhibit phagocytosis and intracellular killing by human polymorphonuclear leukocytes. Infect. Immun. **36**:949–957.
13. Turck, M., and W. Stamm. 1981. Nosocomial infection of the urinary tract. Amer. J. Med. **70**:651–654.
14. Williams, F. D., and R. H. Schwarzhoff. 1978. Nature of the swarming phenomenon in *Proteus*. Ann. Rev. Microbiol. **32**:101–122.
15. Yu, V. L. 1979. *Serratia marcescens*. Historical perspective and clinical review. New Engl. J. Med. **300**:887–893.

Vibrio and Campylobacter

The slightly curved, gram-negative bacilli casually known as vibrios were first described as the causative agent of Asiatic cholera by Robert Koch in 1883 during the fifth great pandemic of that disease. The recognition of water as a transmission vehicle for cholera led to the discovery of similar microorganisms in water and in the intestinal contents of man and animals. Several different *Vibrio* species were described, but they were considered to be nonpathogenic and for many years were studied only in relation to the pathogenic cholera vibrios. The unique pathogenicity of the cholera vibrio was unchallenged until the early 1950s, when a marine vibrio was reported in Japan as the cause of a new type of food poisoning. This microorganism, *V. parahaemolyticus*, was the first halophilic bacterium found to cause human disease.

The subsequent appearance of the seventh pandemic of cholera in the 1960s prompted renewed interest in vibrios as etiological agents of human illness. The present detailed knowledge of these microorganisms is a direct outgrowth of these events.

As knowledge of vibrios increased, their taxonomy has predictably become more complex. Their relationship to the enteric bacilli described in the preceding chapters has been clarified, and the gram-negative, facultatively anaerobic bacilli are now divided into two families: Enterobacteriaceae and Vibrionaceae. The latter contains the cholera and other vibrios of similar ecology. Vibrionaceae are distinguished from Enterobacteriaceae by their polar flagellation and, usually, by positive oxidase reaction.

The family Vibrionaceae is made up of five genera, but only three of these are of importance to the medical microbiologist: *Vibrio, Aeromonas,* and *Plesiomonas*. These may be separated on the basis of biochemical and physiological reactions as shown in Table 21–1.

Members of the genus *Vibrio* are found in fresh and salt water and in the intestine of animals and humans. Some are pathogenic for man, generally causing diarrheal illness that ranges from mild to severe. The best known is the agent of Asiatic cholera, *Vibrio cholerae*.

The natural habitat of *Aeromonas* is also fresh and salt water; they are morphologically and physiologically similar to *Vibrio*. *Aeromonas* commonly cause infections in certain cold-blooded vertebrates, such as frogs, but are only feebly pathogenic for man. Although they sometimes inhabit the intestinal tract without pathogenesis, in debilitated individuals rare infections take the form of diarrhea, septicemia, or wound infections.

Plesiomonas have been isolated from fresh water and from the intestinal discharges of animals. Rare human infections are usually associated with diarrheal disease.

Certain vibrio-like microorganisms have

Table 21–1. **Biochemical Characteristics of** *Vibrio,* *Aeromonas,* *Plesiomonas,* **and** *Campylobacter**

Test	Vibrio	Aeromonas	Plesiomonas	Campylobacter
Oxidase	+	+	+	+
Catalase	+	+	+	V
Lysine decarboxylase	+	−	+	
Glucose (acid)	+	+	+	−
Mannose (acid)	+	+	−	−
Indole	+	+	+	−
Growth in:				
0% NaCl	V	+	+	+
6% NaCl	V	−	−	−
Motility	+	+	+	+
Gelatinase	+	+	−	−
Aerobic growth	+	+	+	−

*Symbols: +, most strains positive; −, most strains negative; V, variable reactions.

long been recognized as causative agents of animal diseases, often causing abortion. Once classified as *Vibrio,* their physiological characters set them apart and they are now classified as *Campylobacter* in the family Spirillaceae *Campylobacter* do not ferment or oxidize carbohydrates, they are microaerophilic to anaerobic, and they differ from *Vibrio* in guanine plus cytosine content of their DNA. In addition to their role in animal diseases, *Campylobacter* are a significant cause of enteritis and other infections in humans, rivaling *Salmonella* and *Shigella* in prevalence.

Vibrio cholerae[2, 38, 50]

Although cholera has doubtless smoldered endemically in India for many centuries, the year 1817 marked its first considerable extension beyond the borders of that country. Europe was first invaded in 1831, and since that date, a series of great epidemics has carried the disease over a large part of the world. The disease entered the United States during the pandemic of 1832–33, resulting in thousands of deaths. During the 1846–62 pandemic, cholera appeared in New Orleans in 1848 and spread up the Mississippi Valley. The fourth pandemic, that of 1864–75, affected Asia, Africa, Europe, and the United States. The fifth pandemic covered the period 1881–96 and the sixth 1898–1923. Subsequently a few small outbreaks occurred in various parts of the world, such as the Egyptian epidemic in 1947. The current, seventh, pandemic began in 1960–61 in Macao and has gripped much of Asia and Africa. Fortunately, Europe and the Western Hemisphere have largely escaped the ravages of the current pandemic, suffering only a few small outbreaks.

Morphology and Staining
The etiological agent of Asiatic cholera, *V. cholerae,* is a short, slightly curved and twisted gram-negative rod, 1.5 to 3 μm. in length and about 0.5 μm. in breadth (Figs. 21–1 and 21–

2). It generally occurs singly, but short chains may give the appearance of a loosely wound spiral. The vibrios are actively motile by a single polar flagellum (Fig. 21–1).

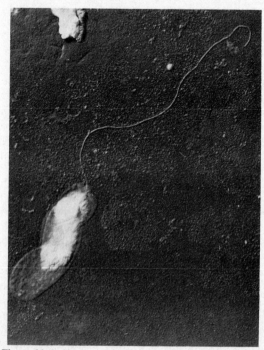

Figure 21–1. Shadow-cast electron micrograph of *V. cholerae,* Inaba 569B. × 12,800. (Felsenfeld.)

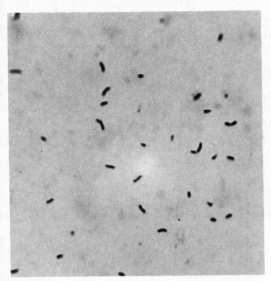

Figure 21–2. *Vibrio cholerae;* pure culture in peptone water. Gram stain; × 1200.

Colonies resemble those of other enteric bacilli, but can be distinguished by their thin opalescent appearance at 24 hours (Fig. 21–3). Upon continued incubation they become larger and more granular (Fig. 21–4). Vibrio colonies are 1 to 2 mm. in diameter, low, convex, finely granular, and grayish yellow in color. Some strains are hemolytic on blood agar.

Physiology
The cholera vibrio is **strongly aerobic,** growing only sparsely under anaerobic conditions.

The optimum temperature for growth is 37°C., but growth obtains over the range of 16° to 42°C. Although the bacteria may be cultivated over a pH range of 6.4 to 9.6, growth is markedly favored by alkaline reactions, pH 7.8 to 8.0. **Alkali tolerance** is somewhat unusual among bacteria, and selective mediums for the cholera vibrio are usually adjusted to this range. They are not nutritionally fastidious, growing well in simple peptone-water mediums. The relative resistance of the cholera vibrio to inhibitory substances such as bile salt, bismuth sulfite, and tellurite is used to advantage in a variety of selective mediums.

The biochemical reactions that have proven valuable for characterization of cholera vibrios and differentiation of *Vibrio* species are found in Table 21–2.

The cholera vibrio is sensitive to many physical and chemical agents. It is killed by moderately high temperatures (10 minutes at 55°C.) and is destroyed quickly by disinfectants. It is particularly sensitive to drying; if a drop of broth culture is dried on a slide, the vibrios are dead in about two hours. The transmission of cholera is usually by fecally contaminated food and water. Thus, cholera vibrios must survive and even multiply in the environment. In general, the atypical cholera vibrios seem to be more durable in this respect than typical strains, as discussed in a later section (see below, Epidemiology).

Biotypes of Vibrio cholerae. At the time of their original isolation by Koch and for many decades thereafter, the vibrios isolated

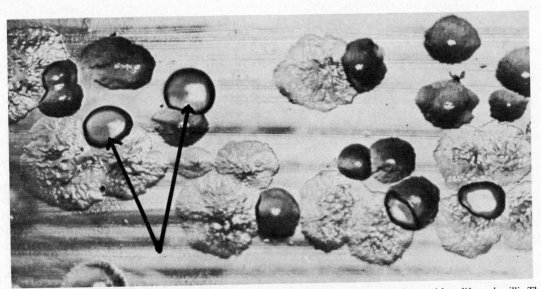

Figure 21–3. The colonial morphology of *Vibrio cholerae* on bile salt agar in mixed culture with coliform bacilli. The minute, translucent, raised colonies of the cholera vibrio contrast with the roughened appearance of coliform bacillus colonies in the presence of taurocholate. × 10.

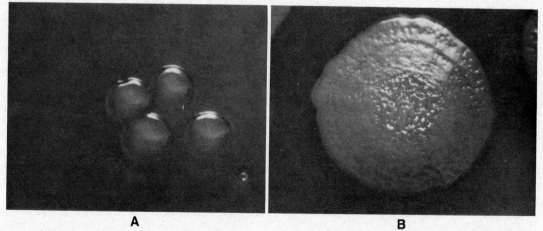

Figure 21–4. Colonial morphology of *V. cholerae* grown on alkaline peptone agar. *A,* after 24 hours' incubation; *B,* after seven days' incubation. × 5. (Felsenfeld.)

from cases of cholera were relatively homogeneous in physiological and antigenic properties and easily differentiated from nonpathogenic and saprophytic vibrios. Yet it has become clear with detailed study that while the general character of cholera vibrios holds true, causative vibrios occur as a number of differentiable biotypes.

At the turn of the century, vibrios were isolated from pilgrims passing through the quarantine station at El Tûr (Tor) on the Gulf of Suez. Some of these were immunologically indistinguishable from *V. cholerae,* but differed in that a soluble **hemolysin** was produced. The extracellular hemolysin is demonstrated by mixture of a broth culture with sheep red blood cells (the Grieg test), but not reliably by hemolysis on blood agar plates.

Vibrios producing hemolysins were designated **El Tor vibrios** and were considered to be nonpathogenic. The question of pathogenicity arose again with the occurrence of epidemic cholera in Sulawesi (Celebes) during 1937–38, caused by the hemolytic vibrios. After spreading through the southwest Pacific, these El Tor vibrios gave rise to a severe epidemic in Macao and Hong Kong in 1960–61 and subsequently have been responsible for the seventh pandemic of cholera.

In view of their now undoubted pathogenicity, these hemolytic vibrios are considered to be a biotype of *V. cholerae* and the classic cholera vibrio is, from this point of view, also a biotype. A number of tests are employed to separate the **classical** and **El Tor biotypes**; the usual reactions are displayed in Table 21–3. As might be anticipated with the application of several differential tests, intermediate forms

have been found. The hemolytic property is somewhat unstable and the production of soluble hemolysin has tended to disappear with pandemic spread of infection; most isolates are now "nonhemolytic" El Tor.

Toxins

As in other gram-negative microorganisms, cholera vibrios contain lipopolysaccharides in the cell wall which have endotoxic activity (Chapter 12). The polysaccharide portion determines the O antigenic specificity (see below, Antigenic Structure) and is responsible for the agglutination of vibrios in specific antiserum.

Enterotoxin.[13, 22, 23] The cholera vibrio was the first enteric pathogen shown to form an extracellular, heat-labile enterotoxin. The toxin, produced by vibrios colonizing the small intestine, mediates the movement of water and ions from the tissues into the bowel lumen to give a net secretion and produce the purging diarrhea characteristic of the disease.

The structure and pathophysiology of the toxin has been established in rich detail. Enterotoxin is a protein exotoxin of about 84,000 molecular weight. The holotoxin comprises two immunologically distinct regions, designated A and B. The **A (active) region** has a molecular weight of about 28,000 daltons and is made up of two subunits—A_1 (about 24,000 daltons) and A_2 (about 5000 daltons)—joined by disulfide linkages. The **B (binding) region** consists of five identical peptides, each of about 11,500 daltons.

The mechanism of cholera enterotoxin action has captured the attention of many investigators, not only those concerned with the pathogenesis of cholera but also those inter-

Table 21-2. **Representative Biochemical Reactions of *Vibrio* Species***

Test	V. cholerae	V. parahaemolyticus	V. alginolyticus	V. anguillarium	V. metschnikovi	Group F Vibrio	V. vulnificus
Arginine dihydrolase	−	−	−	+	+	+	−
Lysine decarboxylase	+	+	+	−	V	−	+
Ornithine decarboxylase	+	+	+	−	−	−	V
Acid from:							
Lactose	(+)	−	−	+	V	−	+
Sucrose	+	−	+	V	+	+	−
Arabinose	−	V	−	+	−	+	−
Voges-Proskauer	V	−	+	+	+	−	−
Growth in:							
0% NaCl	+	−	−	−	−	V	−
3% NaCl	+	+	+	+	+	+	+
6% NaCl	V	+	+	V	+	+	+
10% NaCl	−	−	+	−	−	−	−

*Adapted from several authors.[38,50] Symbols: +, most strains positive; (+), most strains positive after 3 days; −, most strains negative; V, variable reactions.

Table 21–3. **Differentiation Between *Vibrio cholerae* Biotypes**

Biotype	Soluble Hemolysin	Phage IV Sensitivity	Chicken Red Cell Agglutination	Polymyxin Sensitivity	Voges-Proskauer
V. cholerae biotype cholerae	–	+	–	+	–
V. cholerae biotype eltor	+	–	+	–	+

ested in membrane and cellular physiology. The holotoxin binds to eucaryotic cells by interaction of the B region with host cell membrane receptors. The **natural biological receptor** is G_{M1} ganglioside (galactosyl-*N*-acetyl-galactosaminyl-[sialyl]-galactosyl-glucosylceramide) which forms a very tight bond with the B region of toxin. This receptor is present in the cell membrane of a wide variety of eucaryotic cells, including those of the intestinal epithelium. Initial binding, which takes place very rapidly, is followed by a slow conformational change in the toxin molecule, leading to internalization of the A_1 subunit into the host cell. The A_1 subunit then interacts with the adenyl cyclase system of the cell, located on the inner surface of the cell membrane, in a series of events that involve nicotinamide adenine dinucleotide (NAD), adenosine triphosphate (ATP), and an acceptor protein in the cellular cytosol. The A_1 subunit has adenosine 5′-diphosphate (ADP)-ribosyl transferase activity, catalyzing the cleavage of NAD and transfer of (ADP)-ribose to a guanosyl triphosphate (GTP)-binding protein of the adenylate cyclase system. The GTP-binding protein normally has GTPase activity, inactivating the GTP-bound, active form of adenylate cyclase; ADP-ribosylation of this protein inhibits its GTPase activity, thereby inhibiting the normal "turn-off" reaction of adenylate cyclase and maintaining the enzyme in its activated state. These events then lead to an increase in intracellular cyclic 3′, 5′-adenosine monophosphate (cAMP), which mediates the intestinal secretion of water and electrolytes.

It is noteworthy that the action of cholera toxin resembles that of diphtheria toxin, which also requires ADP-ribosylation of a specific protein, elongation factor 2 (Chapter 30).

Cholera toxin activates adenylate cyclase in a variety of eucaryotic cell systems. The susceptibility of these cells is dependent upon the presence of the receptor, G_{M1} ganglioside, on the cell membrane. Since this receptor is widely distributed, a number of these cell systems can be employed for assay of cholera enterotoxin. For example, cholera toxin induces morphological alterations in Chinese hamster ovary or Y-1 mouse adrenal tumor cells in culture. Such assay systems have largely supplanted the animal models that measured diarrhea in infant rabbits or the accumulation of fluids in ligated ileal loops of rabbits and guinea pigs (see below, Animal Models).

Like other exotoxins, cholera enterotoxin is an effective immunogen, inducing antibodies with toxin-neutralizing activity. For purposes of immunization, toxoids may be formed from the enterotoxin by treatment with glutaraldehyde, heat, or formaldehyde.[19, 37] Antitoxic immunity is protective and primarily directed against the B region of the toxin molecule. Indeed, a naturally occurring toxoid, composed of the B region of the molecule, has been found in broth cultures of *V. cholerae*.

Hemolysin.[24] Hemolysins are produced by some *V. cholerae*, particularly biotype *eltor*, and are found in liquid culture supernatants. The hemolysin is thermolabile and of relatively low molecular weight (ca. 20,000 daltons). Relevance to cholera pathogenesis is probably remote, but the hemolysin does possess cytotoxic, cardiotoxic, and lethal activity.

Mucinase. The cholera vibrio and related forms produce mucinase that desquamates the intestinal epithelium of guinea pigs. More than one serological type of enzyme is produced by *V. cholerae*, and potent mucinases are produced by other vibrios. The relationship of this activity to cholera pathogenesis is doubtful.

Antigenic Structure

The vibrios contain both somatic, heat-stable O antigens (lipopolysaccharides) and flagellar, heat-labile, H antigens. Many serological groups have been established, based on the O antigenic makeup. The epidemic strains of *V. cholerae* fall into the serogroup designated **O group 1**, or *V. cholerae* O1. Little detailed knowledge is available on the antigens of other O groups.

For a number of years, vibrios were isolated from water, and from cases of diarrhea, that were biochemically indistinguishable from *V. cholerae* yet did not agglutinate in O group 1 antiserum. These strains were usually referred to as nonagglutinating, or NAG, vibrios. They

Table 21–4. **Serological Types of O Group 1 Cholera Vibrios**

Name	O-Antigen Factors
Inaba	AC
Ogawa	AB
Hikojima	ABC

were, however, readily agglutinated by homologous antiserum, leading to some confusion in the terminology. Such strains are now termed **non-O group 1**, or non-O1, *V. cholerae;* these strains are associated with sporadic cases and small outbreaks of diarrheal illness but are not considered to cause epidemics of cholera. Thus, the present nomenclature is both unfortunate and confusing. There seems little logic in designating strains that do not cause cholera as *V. cholerae*. Several investigative groups are now engaged in studies to establish serological relationships in these non-O1 vibrios.

Among the **epidemic strains,** or *V. cholerae* O1, individual serotypes may be further differentiated by specific factors that are a part of the O antigen complex. The predominant serotypes are listed in Table 21–4, along with the O antigen factors that are believed to determine the serotype. The A factor is common to all types and is, therefore, the group antigen; B and C are type-specific antigens. Most epidemic strains are either **Ogawa** or **Inaba** type; the **Hikojima** type is rare and appears to occur primarily in China, along with Ogawa and Inaba types. Vibrios containing only the group antigen (A) have been found and thus constitute a new type, having no formal name. Flagellar, or H, antigens are designated, but they are widely shared with other O group vibrios and are not used in typing schemes.

Cholera vibrios are serologically related to certain other bacteria, and cross-agglutination reactions are sometimes observed with enteric bacilli and *Brucella.*

Serotype Variation. While a single serotype of the vibrio is commonly observed in a given epidemic of cholera, multiple types are occasionally found, sometimes in the same individual. These could arise either from a mixed infection or instability of serotype. The latter is the most likely explanation. Serotype sometimes changes in culture, usually from Ogawa to Inaba, and both serotypic alteration and changes from smooth to rough colonial morphology have been shown in gnotobiotic mice. In an accidental laboratory infection with an Ogawa strain, the Inaba type was later iso-

lated, obviating the possibility of mixed infection. Vibrio phages have also been shown to convert serotype Ogawa to the Hikojima type in culture.[35]

Virulence[15, 17, 26, 43]

The virulence of cholera vibrio is believed to be dependent upon their ability to adhere to mucosal surfaces (as shown in Fig. 21–5); to multiply at this site; and to secrete the enterotoxin. Invasion of the intestinal mucosa does not occur. Cholera toxin is absorbed from the intestine and induces the water and electrolyte loss that is the hallmark of the disease.

Adherence of vibrios to the mucosal surface of the small bowel is a necessary step in pathogenesis. The mechanism of adherence is, however, not completely clear. Convincing evidence of adherence organelles, such as pili, is not available, although *Vibrio cholerae* produces several hemagglutinins, some of which may act as adhesins. Adherence may be in some way associated with motility, since nonmotile strains do not adhere well and are less virulent than motile strains. The adhesive factor is probably not flagella, *per se,* but may be associated with the flagella. It is also possible that flagella promote colonization by other means. For example, many *V. cholerae* respond to chemotactic stimuli, moving by flagellar activity. It has been proposed that chemotaxis plays a role by promoting penetration

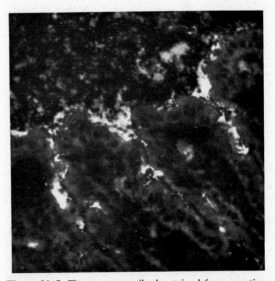

Figure 21–5. Fluorescent antibody–stained frozen section of the small bowel of a guinea pig infected with cholera. The vibrios are apparent in the lumen, sticking to the epithelial cells at the villus tips, extending into the crypt areas, and filling indentations of the epithelium. Failure to penetrate the epithelium is evident. (LaBrec.)

of the mucus gel under the influence of chemotactic stimuli.

Whatever the adherence mechanism, *Vibrio* colonize the mucosal surface and produce the enterotoxin that is directly responsible for diarrhea. The production of enterotoxin, as shown by onset of fluid and electrolyte loss in the intestinal lumen of infected rabbits, occurs concomitantly with colonization of the villi and crypts with vibrios.[41] The presence of other intestinal organisms predictably interferes with attachment and colonization by vibrios.[42]

Virulent strains of *V. cholerae* are, therefore, toxigenic, adherent, and motile, and respond to chemotactic stimuli.

CHOLERA

The causal connection between cholera and the microorganisms discovered by Koch has been repeatedly established both by accidental infections and by human feeding experiments in volunteers.

The **incubation period** in cholera is short, usually 3 to 5 days, although it may occasionally be as short as 24 hours, depending on the number of vibrios ingested. The infection begins when the ingested vibrios pass the barrier of gastric acidity in sufficient numbers to set up a focus of infection in the small bowel. As the microorganisms multiply on the epithelial surface, toxin is elaborated, and fluid and electrolytes are rapidly lost in the resulting purging diarrhea. There is no inflammation or apparent mucosal damage. The "rice water" stool, innocuous in odor and appearance, consists of plasma minus protein and contains flakes of mucus, shed epithelial cells, and enormous numbers of vibrios; leucocytes are usually absent. With continued loss of water and electrolytes, **marked dehydration** and **metabolic acidosis** become prominant features. This stage of disease is characterized by circulatory failure, subnormal temperature, and anuria.

Susceptibility to cholera infection appears to vary considerably in different individuals. Although the factors that contribute to this variation are not completely understood, gastric acidity is thought to be of great importance, since cholera vibrios are sensitive to low pH. The infectious dose may be as low as 10^2 to 10^3 vibrios in hypochlorhydric individuals or when administered with bicarbonate. Vibrios contained in food are also protected from gastric acidity.

Etiologic Agent

True cholera, with the clinical picture just described, is almost invariably due to the epidemic strains, *i.e., V. cholerae* O1, that produce enterotoxin. Substantially identical clinical disease is produced by the different biotypes *(classic* or *eltor)* and serotypes (Ogawa, Inaba, or Hikojima) of *V. cholerae* O1.

Atypical Vibrio cholerae O1. The worldwide spread of cholera during the present pandemic has led to increased surveillance for cholera vibrios, particularly in the environment. These studies have revealed the presence of certain vibrios in sewage and surface waters, which are similar to the epidemic strains but apparently not capable of causing cholera. These strains usually agglutinate in O group 1 antiserum and, in biochemical tests, often behave much like the epidemic strains. They differ, however, in that they apparently do not produce enterotoxin and are not susceptible to the classical or El Tor phages. They are usually designated as **atypical** *V. cholerae* O1. Although not responsible for cholera, these vibrios have been found in rare extraintestinal illness such as wound infections. For the most part, atypical *V. cholerae* O1 are encountered in the environment, where they are believed to be free-living.

Epidemiology

As in other enteric infections, the ultimate source of cholera infection is the **fecal excretions** from cases, carriers, or those with inapparent infections. In consequence, the disease is frequently **waterborne,** particularly in large epidemics, or **foodborne** when such foodstuffs are subject to fecal contamination. In the United States, for example, where water supplies and sewage disposal are hygienically controlled, cholera was absent for more than 70 years. A few cases appeared in coastal areas of Louisiana in 1978 that were traced to consumption of inadequately cooked, contaminated saltwater crabs.[5] Cholera may also be transmitted by contact with infected persons, but the qualitative importance of this mode is not yet clear and is somewhat controversial.[11] Cholera differs from other enteric diseases in the highly explosive character of the outbreak, attributable to the short incubation period; the high case-fatality rates; and rapid disappearance when the outbreak has subsided.

As a major waterborne disease, cholera should be subject to control by the application of modern methods of sewage treatment and disposal, and provision of clean water supplies. Yet the geographic foci of *V. cholerae* infections are in areas that are generally poor and where modern technologies are difficult to apply. Therefore, global control of cholera is not yet achieved.

Carriers and Inapparent Infections.[11] The epidemiological control of cholera is complicated by the human reservoirs of infection in the form of carriers and individuals with inapparent infections. The convalescent carrier state is of limited duration, and excretion of vibrios in detectable numbers usually ceases by the end of one week; in some few cases excretion may continue for additional weeks or months. A true long-term or chronic carrier state is extremely rare.

Asymptomatic or inapparent infections, in which cholera vibrios are excreted, are found with some frequency in endemic areas. The reported point prevalence of excretion among apparently healthy individuals is somewhat variable, but is less than 1 per cent. In children, the prevalence appears to be higher; up to 20 per cent has been reported in some studies. The family contacts of index cases appear to be at higher risk of infection than the general population in endemic areas. About one-fourth of family contacts develop clinical illness and another one-fourth become asymptomatic excretors of cholera vibrios. Generally, asymptomatically infected individuals excrete 10^2 to 10^3 vibrios per gram of feces in contrast to the 10^8 vibrios per gram usually found in the rice water stool of active cases. Nevertheless, convalescent carriers and asymptomatic infection are believed to aid in perpetuating the infection during interepidemic periods.

Endemic Foci. Cholera persists in interepidemic periods in foci of endemic infections. Endemic areas are generally low-lying, adjacent to rivers, and densely populated. In such areas ponds and other stored water often contain cholera and related vibrios. The infection persists in carriers and as a small number of active human cases, which occur continuously between epidemics.

The classic focus of endemic infection is in Bengal, in the deltas of the Ganges and Brahmaputra rivers. There is also a major focus of infection in Burma, in the Irrawady and Salween deltas. Cholera has occurred in Nepal for many years, and this area is suspected of being an endemic focus. Following the epidemic spread during the current pandemic, infection has persisted in endemic form in the invaded areas of Southeast Asia, the Philippines, Africa, and the Middle East; it remains to be seen whether these will become permanent endemic foci.

Epidemic Spread. Each year epidemics of cholera arise in endemic areas such as Bengal. The factors that determine the timing of the "cholera season" are not yet understood. Indeed, there have been rapid changes during the past two decades. In Calcutta, cholera was once most prevalent in the early summer, but has now shifted to the late fall.

The extension of cholera beyond the Indian subcontinent and Southeast Asia into Europe and the Western Hemisphere has occurred as a series of **pandemics,** as described at the beginning of this chapter. The quarantine stations at Tur and Basra functioned to prevent spread into the Middle East, although a cholera epidemic appeared in Egypt in 1947, coincident with the British evacuation of India. The traditional route of spread to the Middle East and eastern Europe was through Afghanistan. These historic corridors have lessened in importance, with worldwide distribution facilitated by modern transportation.

The Seventh Pandemic.[28] From 1883, when Koch discovered the cholera vibrio, until 1937, all known epidemics had been due to the classic biotype. The El Tor biotype appeared for the first time in virulent form in Indonesia in 1937–38. The disease remained relatively quiescent, with small localized outbreaks, until it assumed epidemic form in Hong Kong in 1960 and originated the seventh pandemic. It spread through the Southwest Pacific and north to Korea in 1963. From there it followed the classic routes of previous pandemics, reaching into the Middle East, to Russia, and into Africa by 1971. The extension of the pandemic during the first 10 years is seen in Figure 21–6. The current pandemic has seen an increase in the number of countries reporting cholera—from 10 in 1968 to 36 in 1970, diminishing slightly to 34 in 1981. Despite this geographic spread, the number of cases notified has decreased in the past few years. More than 110,000 cases were reported in 1971, but this had diminished to slightly less than 37,000 in 1981. South America has not reported cases during the present pandemic, and Oceania, the United States, and Europe are now cholera-free except for rare cases. Most cases are now found in Asia and Africa. Many of the countries newly invaded during the current pandemic are now becoming endemic for cholera, and epidemics may be expected in these countries when sanitary precautions are relaxed.

In the seventh pandemic, the El Tor biotype

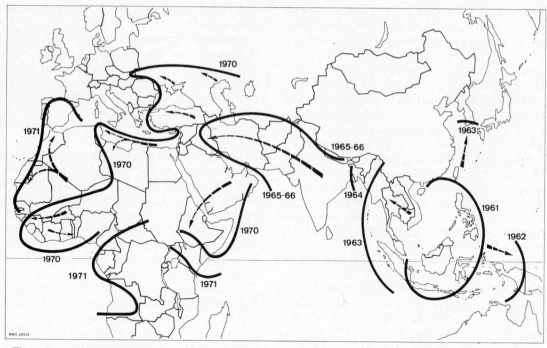

Figure 21–6. The global spread of cholera during the seventh pandemic, 1961–1971. (World Health Organization.)

has rapidly displaced the classic biotype, even in geographic areas where the latter was endemic, although rare cases of infection by the classic biotype still arise. Clinically, the disease caused by the two biotypes is identical, but some epidemiological differences are apparent. In El Tor epidemics the proportion of severe cases is smaller, while mild cases and asymptomatic infections are more frequent. The El Tor biotype also seems to be more resistant and to survive longer in the environment. It is of some interest that even the El Tor biotype has exhibited some changes since the beginning of the pandemic. Early in the pandemic, most strains were hemolytic, but the proportion of such strains has gradually decreased while other biotype characteristics have remained essentially unchanged.

Control of Epidemic Cholera.[10] In the absence of the hygienic control of food, water supplies, and sewage disposal—measures associated with relatively high living standards—the control of cholera is exceedingly difficult. International quarantine has not been successful, probably because air travel has led to rapid extension of the infection that is difficult to control. For example, an American tourist acquired an infection in Bombay and became ill upon arrival in Australia.[34] As noted below, mass immunization is expensive and of doubtful value. The relative inefficacy of present

vaccines has led to relaxation of immunization requirements for international travelers.

Bacteriological Diagnosis[1, 50]

Laboratory diagnosis of cholera is essential to establish the identity of the disease, particularly in sporadic cases and in early stages of an epidemic, because acute diarrheal disease of other etiology is common in most areas where cholera occurs.

Vibrios are present in very large numbers in the rice water stool and are apparent in gram-stained smears. They can be demonstrated by fluorescent antibody staining or by immobilization in the presence of specific antiserum observed by darkfield microscopy, but such observations are only provisional in the identification of cholera vibrios.

Stool specimens are cultured immediately or transported in buffered salts medium, in alkaline peptone water, or on blotter strips kept moist by sealing in plastic. Laboratory culture and isolation generally employs one or more of the several differential or selective mediums. The most widely used are MacConkey agar, taurocholate-gelatin agar (often also containing tellurite), and thiosulfate-citrate-bromthymol blue-sucrose (TCBS) agar. The selection of typical colonies is facilitated by use of oblique transmitted light in low-power stereomicroscopy.

Isolated colonies are subcultured on Kligler iron agar (KIA) and are used for slide agglutination with O group 1 antiserum. A typical reaction on KIA—red slant, yellow butt, no gas, and absence of H_2S—and a second slide agglutination test confirms the presence of O group 1 vibrios. *Vibrio* are differentiated from similar genera by the reactions listed in Table 21–1; species identification is by the reactions listed in Table 21–2. Biotype and serotype determinations may be carried out for epidemiological purposes, but these are generally performed in reference laboratories. Toxigenicity tests are difficult and expensive; they are only performed in reference laboratories when circumstances warrant.

Therapy[21]

Treatment of cholera is symptomatic and consists of the replacement of fluid and electrolytes. Usually there is acidosis, and patients literally minutes away from death can be saved by rapid intravenous administration of isotonic bicarbonate solution. Intravenous rehydration is usually followed by oral rehydration using glucose-electrolyte solution until diarrhea ceases and renal function is restored.

Chemotherapy occupies an anomalous position in that, when effective, it markedly reduces rehydration fluid requirements by shortening the period of diarrhea and vibrio excretion but does not seem to affect the case-fatality rate. Tetracyclines are the most effective antibiotics, but doxycycline and furazolidone are of comparable efficacy.

Chemoprophylaxis has been applied to contain epidemic spread in both case contacts and broader populations. There seems to be some benefit in this regard, but prophylaxis is generally discouraged owing to the appearance of strains with multiple antibiotic resistance following antibiotic use; such resistance is usually encoded by R plasmids.

The case-fatality rate in untreated cases has been as high as 50 to 60 per cent but can be reduced to 1 per cent or less under ideal conditions of therapy and management.

Immunity[9, 12, 14, 16, 51]

Recovery from an attack of cholera confers some immunity to subsequent infection. The duration appears to be limited, but protection for as long as three years has been documented.[31] Nevertheless, reinfections in the same individual have been noted.

With respect to the target immunogen, the antibody response is of two kinds—**antibacterial** and **antitoxic.** Antibacterial immunity is

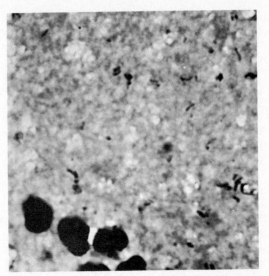

Figure 21–7. *Vibrio cholerae* in peritoneal exudate of a guinea pig. Note the swollen and aberrant forms. Gram stain; × 1250.

directed against the vibrios or their components and is manifest as agglutinating and vibriocidal (vibriolytic) antibodies (Fig. 21–7).

Since cholera vibrios do not invade tissues, antibacterial antibodies must act against vibrios in the intestine, presumably by vibriocidal action or by inhibiting adherence to mucosal surfaces. Parenteral immunization with killed vaccines primarily engenders a serum antibody response and, to a lesser extent, intestinally secreted antibodies. Oral immunization, on the other hand, is followed by earlier and higher intestinal antibody titers. Vibriocidal antibodies are directed against bacterial surface antigens, including the lipopolysaccharide O antigen and cell wall proteins, while agglutinating antibodies are induced by both O and H antigens. There is some indication that flagellar antigens may be protective, since rabbits immunized with flagella preparations and challenged with virulent vibrios do not exhibit intestinal fluid response and the vibrios fail to associate with intestinal mucosa.[52]

Cholera enterotoxin is immunogenic and antitoxin is usually induced in the cholera patient; in animal models, antitoxin has proved to be protective. Neutralizing antibodies are induced by both parenteral and oral immunization with either enterotoxin or toxoid. In experimental cholera, oral immunization with toxin induces intestinal immunoglobulin A (IgA) that correlates with protection.[47] Antitoxic antibodies are directed primarily against the binding, or B, region of the enterotoxin; in experimental cholera, colonization of animals with mutant strains that produce only the B region of the enterotoxin molecule yields protection against challenge with virulent strains.[8]

Vaccines.[27] The vaccines currently used for prophylactic immunization consist of saline suspensions of killed vibrios and are usually bivalent, consisting of equal numbers of Ogawa and Inaba serotypes. Immunization is by the subcutaneous route and booster inoculations are required at 6-month intervals.

Field tests indicate that fewer than 50 per cent of individuals are immune following one dose of vaccine. The proportion is increased to about 80 per cent after booster immunization, and protection is more long-lived in these individuals. Greatest immunization benefit is noted in children, the group at highest risk.[36] Mass immunization against cholera is expensive, however, and it is generally believed that treatment of active cholera cases is more cost-effective than large-scale immunization with the available vaccines.

Recent interest has focused on immunization measures designed to engender antitoxic immunity. Toxoid induces antitoxin in animals, but has not yet been evaluated in humans. The mutant strain described above, which produces only the B region of enterotoxin and is able to colonize the intestinal tract of animals, offers promise as a live oral vaccine to induce antitoxic and, perhaps, antibacterial immunity. Such vaccines could induce a more lasting immunity, comparable to that of natural infections.

Animal Models

The cholera vibrio is exclusively a parasite of man and naturally occurring infections of lower animals have not been described. Experimental infections can be induced by inoculation of mice and guinea pigs, usually facilitated by inclusion of mucin, but the bacteremia produced does not mimic the human infection.

Animal infections, simulating those of humans, have been devised. They have been utilized to assay immunogenic potency of vaccines and were pivotal in the very extensive studies that led to the discovery of enterotoxin and its mode of action.

Infant Rabbit. The infant rabbit model has been widely used in enterotoxin studies. Vibrios, or cell-free material, are administered orally, intragastrically, or directly into the lumen of the small bowel, to bring about diarrhea. Although degrees of reaction have been described, this animal model is essentially qualitative and has the disadvantage that it is not applicable to investigations on active immunity.

Ligated Intestinal Loop. In the late 1950s, De and his colleagues in Calcutta showed that a ligated section (loop) of the small bowel of adult rabbits can be infected with vibrios by intraluminal inoculation. Multiplication of the vibrios results in marked accumulation of fluid. Essentially the same reaction is produced by cell-free, enterotoxin-containing materials. The degree of fluid accumulation is a function of dose and becomes a quantitative assay for toxin. The model also may be used to measure antibody, using a standard amount of toxin. The reaction is not limited to rabbits, and similar assays have been performed in a variety of experimental animals.

Canine Model. Cholera infection of the dog has similarly been employed to study the pathophysiology of cholera and the action of enterotoxin. The model is used in two ways, one an infection or intoxication of the intact animal, either *per os* or by intraluminal inoculation of the small bowel, and the other making use of Thiry-Vella fistulae, prepared by transection of the jejunum.

NON–O GROUP 1 VIBRIO CHOLERAE[3, 25, 33]

For several decades, vibrios were isolated from the intestinal tract of man and from the environment that were biochemically similar to the epidemic strains of *Vibrio cholerae* but did not agglutinate in O group 1 antiserum. These were usually designated as nonagglutinating (NAG) vibrios or as noncholera vibrios because they were believed not to cause disease. On biochemical grounds they are now considered to be *Vibrio cholerae,* and are differentiated from epidemic strains by their somatic antigen makeup. Such strains now bear the cumbersome name, non–O group 1 *Vibrio cholerae* or *Vibrio cholerae* non-O1. More than 60 serotypes of these vibrios have been differentiated and a portion of isolates are not yet typable.

These vibrios have been isolated from the intestinal tract of humans, sometimes associated with gastrointestinal disease. They are widely encountered in the environment, most often in sewage, fecally-contaminated water, estuarine water, and seafood. They have also been found in the intestinal contents of animals. The most prolific source of environmental contamination appears to be the intestinal discharges of man and animals. These vibrios undoubtedly are also capable of free-living existence, and estuarine waters, in particular, harbor vibrios in the absence of fecal contamination. In many instances, human infections are associated with consumption of raw seafood, especially oysters; the latter presumably concentrate vibrios by filtration of contaminated water.

Pathogenicity

Although their pathogenic potential varies considerably, some *V. cholerae* non-O1 strains are capable of causing disease in humans. Most recognized infections are gastrointestinal and are manifest as small outbreaks and sporadic cases. The clinical syndrome is characterized by diarrhea and abdominal pain, often with vomiting and sometimes fever. Bloody diarrhea has been reported in some patients.

A few strains of *V. cholerae* non-O1 associated with intestinal disease produce an enterotoxin similar to that produced by epidemic strains, but most are not toxigenic by the usual laboratory tests; they appear to cause pathogenesis by other, ill-defined, mechanisms. In the United States, there has been a strong correlation between intestinal infection and consumption of raw oysters. Others appear to have been acquired during recent foreign travel; it is possible that these arise from consumption of contaminated food, including seafoods.

Non-O1 vibrios are also rarely associated with nonintestinal illnesses. Systemic infection in immunosuppressed or debilitated patients, including wound infections, otitis media, septicemia, and pneumonia, have been ascribed to these microorganisms. There appears to be some association with occupational or recreational exposure to salt water.

Halophilic Vibrios[3, 50]

In addition to *V. cholerae*, the genus *Vibrio* contains several species whose natural habitat appears to be marine environments and brackish water. Some of these are natural pathogens for saltwater fish, while others are free-living marine forms. A few are potential pathogens for humans, especially when large numbers are consumed in seafoods or when wounds are infected by exposure to contaminated sea water.

Vibrio parahaemolyticus[48]

A form of foodborne infection, prevalent in summer months and associated with the consumption of uncooked fish and shellfish, was reported in Japan in 1950. This gastroenteritis was found to be attributable to a halophilic vibrio, *Vibrio parahaemolyticus*.

The vibrios responsible are free-living, salt-loving forms and are most often found in marine environments. They have been isolated from bays, estuaries, and sediments in almost all parts of the world. In the colder months they are found only in sediment, but as temperatures rise their numbers increase in water and they may be isolated from finfish, shellfish, crustaceans, and plankton.

These aspects of the ecology of *V. parahaemolyticus* account for the seasonal incidence of the gastroenteritis and the association of most infections with consumption of raw, inadequately cooked, or improperly handled seafood. This gastroenteritis and other bacterial food poisoning syndromes are discussed in Chapter 36.

Vibrio parahaemolyticus may be distinguished from other halophilic vibrios by the biochemical reactions listed in Table 21–2. It requires 6 to 8 per cent sodium chloride in the medium, but fails to grow in 10 per cent NaCl. In this respect, as well as in other physiological characteristics, it may be separated from *Vibrio alginolyticus*, a similar vibrio that also grows in marine environments.

The vibrios contain O, K, and H antigens. The flagella of these vibrios are unusual. A single polar flagellum is present in all or most cells. The H antigen of this structure is common to all strains. During cultivation on agar, many cells develop lateral flagella that are not so thick or long as the polar flagellum. These lateral flagella are antigenically heterogeneous and are associated with increased motility and swarming. Figure 21–8 shows these two flagellar forms. Flagellar antigens, because of their heterogeneity and erratic presence, are not used in typing schemes. Rather, serotyping of *V. parahaemolyticus* is by O and K antigens. Twelve O antigenic groups are recognized, and these may be further typed by their K antigens; 59 K antigens are now designated. There is considerable sharing of antigens with *V. alginolyticus*, so that isolates for typing must first be established as *V. parahaemolyticus* by biochemical means.

Not all *V. parahaemolyticus* are clearly en-

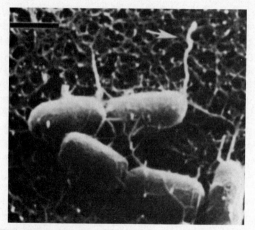

Figure 21–8. Scanning electron micrograph of *Vibrio para-haemolyticus* showing polar flagella (arrow) and thinner lateral flagella between cells. Bar = 1 μm. (M. R. Belas, and Colwell, R. R., J. Bacteriol. **150**:956, 1982.)

teropathogenic for man. Those isolated from intestinal contents of individuals with gastroenteritis are almost always hemolytic on the special, high-salt, Wagatsuma blood agar. Hemolysis in this medium is known as the **Kanagawa phenomenon** and such strains are said to be Kanagawa-positive. Most marine strains are not hemolytic on this medium and are, therefore, Kanagawa-negative. The soluble hemolysin responsible for the Kanagawa reaction is a 44,000 dalton, heat-stable protein[39] that is cytotoxic and lethal for mice.

Virulence of *V. parahaemolyticus* is correlated with the production of hemolysin, since Kanagawa-negative strains fail to produce disease when fed to volunteers. Kanagawa-positive strains also exhibit greater adherence to intestinal cells than Kanagawa-negative strains.[20] The mode of enteropathogenesis is not yet defined. Live vibrios cause mucosal destruction in the intestine, but there is no fluid accumulation in the ileal loop model, suggesting that enterotoxin is not produced.

One of the unexplained peculiarities of the epidemiology of *V. parahaemolyticus* gastroenteritis is the observation that only rarely are Kanagawa-positive strains encountered in seafoods, even those known to be responsible for outbreaks. It appears likely that the enteropathogenic strains occur in such low numbers, as compared to the nonhemolytic strains, that they may be missed in routine cultures of incriminated seafoods.

Although the most common *V. parahaemolyticus* infections are gastrointestinal in nature, other sites are occasionally invaded. These include wound and ear infections, usually with

sea water as the suspected transmission vehicle.

Vibrio alginolyticus

The halophilic *V. alginolyticus* is a marine vibrio of apparent worldwide distribution. Like *V. parahaemolyticus,* it is rarely found in sea water and seafoods during the colder months but its numbers increase as water temperature rises in the summer. As noted earlier, it is similar to *V. parahaemolyticus* in many ways but is distinguished by a higher salt tolerance and by the fermentation of sucrose (Table 21–2).

These vibrios apparently do not cause gastroenteritis in humans. Only a few infections have been recorded, principally wound and ear infections. Most of these have been noted in summer months and have been associated with exposure to sea water.

Vibrio vulnificus[4]

Although not as well known as the other halophilic vibrios just described, *V. vulnificus* is also a marine organism of apparent wide distribution. These vibrios are distinguished by their capacity to ferment lactose, and are casually known as **lactose-fermenting vibrios.** Their ecology is quite similar to that of other halophilic species.

Since the early 1960s, *V. vulnificus* has been occasionally incriminated in human infections. Less than half of the infections presented as infections of preexisting wounds or ulcers. The remainder began as primary septicemia. The latter were serious infections with high rates of mortality. In almost all cases there were predisposing factors that included diabetes, alcoholism, and hepatic disease. Thus, the microorganism may be regarded as an opportunistic pathogen.

Wound infections have often been associated with sea water exposure. In many cases, primary septicemia patients had consumed raw oysters shortly before onset.

Group F Vibrios

Vibrio-like organisms have been isolated from marine and estuarine environments around Britain and have been found associated with a cholera-like illness in several countries. Thought to be a new *Vibrio* species, they are informally known as Group F vibrios by British workers and as EF-6 in the United States. Although isolated from numerous cases of diarrheal disease, particularly in Bangladesh, their etiological relationship to these infections is equivocal.

Campylobacter[29, 40, 46]

The microorganisms now classified as *Campylobacter* have been recognized for over 70 years as the etiological agents of several diseases of domestic animals. Only in the last decade have certain members been established as important pathogens for man, causing outbreaks of enteritis as well as a variety of systemic infections.

Classification

Although once considered to be species of *Vibrio*, *Campylobacter* are now known to be quite different in physiology. They are more closely related to certain spiral organisms and are placed in the family Spirillaceae. The genus comprises four species: *C. fetus*, *C. jejunum*, *C. coli*, and *C. sputorum*. The distinctive biochemical features of these species are shown in Table 21–5.

The classification is somewhat confused; the currently approved classification, that of Véron and Chatelain,[49] will be used here. Nevertheless, other systems are often employed, particularly by many American workers. The taxonomy is considered fluid, therefore, with many questions remaining unanswered.

Campylobacter fetus is pathogenic for both man and animals. Cattle and sheep are infected to produce abortion in pregnant females. In bulls, campylobacteriosis is essentially asymptomatic, but is venereally transmitted to cows, leading to infertility and often resulting in abortion. In sheep it is not transmitted from rams, but by ingestion of fecally contaminated material. Ewes are not rendered infertile but may abort as a consequence of infection.

Human infections sometimes are seen, caused by *C. fetus* subspecies *fetus*. These are primarily systemic infections in debilitated or immunodeficient patients.

Campylobacter jejuni is a member of the normal intestinal flora of many animal species, particularly birds and domestic animals. It is apparently not a normal inhabitant of humans and, when present, is associated with an enteritis characterized by fever, bloody diarrhea, and abdominal pain. *Campylobacter coli* is bacteriologically a very similar microorganism, related to *C. jejuni* in both pathogenesis and ecology. Indeed, many workers prefer to designate these two species as the *C. jejuni/coli* group.

Campylobacter sputorum is divided into two subspecies. *Campylobacter sputorum* ss *sputorum* is a common inhabitant of the gingival crevice in humans; *C. sputorum* ss *bubulus* is a part of the normal genital and intestinal flora of sheep and cattle. Human disease by *C. sputorum* has not been described.

A fifth species, *C. fecalis*, is sometimes designated and members are a part of the normal flora of cattle and sheep.

The following discussion of *Campylobacter* focuses on those forms incriminated in human infections, *i.e.*, *C. fetus* ss *fetus* and the *C. jejuni/coli* group.

Morphology and Staining[44]

Campylobacter are curved or spiral-shaped, motile, gram-negative rods. Cell size ranges from 0.2 to 0.8 μm. in diameter and 0.5 to 5 μm. or greater in length. The shorter forms may appear as comma-shaped cells; cells of intermediate length may be S-shaped and longer forms are often spiral-shaped. Spiral forms vary from tightly coiled to open and undulating.

Motility is by polar flagella, located at one or both ends of the cell. In general, *C. jejuni/coli* are smaller and tightly coiled, and amphitrichous in flagellation. *Campylobacter fetus* ss *fetus* is longer in wavelength and is monotrichous. The morphology of *C. jejuni* is illustrated in Figure 21–9.

The colonial form of *Campylobacter* is somewhat variable, but colonies generally are small, round, and flat to convex, and range in color from gray to tan or brown. Colonies of the *C. jejuni/coli* group growing on mediums with low agar concentration exhibit swarming, producing a thin, translucent veil of growth on the agar surface.

Physiology

Campylobacter are microaerophilic forms that are inhibited by atmospheric concentrations of oxygen, but will grow at reduced oxygen tension in the presence of carbon dioxide (3 to 10 per cent). The physiological and biochemical features used in differentiating *Campylobacter* are shown in Table 21–5.

The human pathogenic strains grow at 37°C., but those of the *C. jejuni/coli* group are thermophilic, and grow best at temperatures of 42° to 45°C. The thermophilic nature of the latter is a differential character, used to advantage in their isolation from stools.

Campylobacter grow well on blood agar, and somewhat less luxuriantly on MacConkey agar. Growth in thioglycolate broth characteristically appears in a narrow zone a few millimeters beneath the surface of the medium. *Cam-*

Table 21–5. Nomenclature and Physiological Characters of *Campylobacter**

Approved Name†	Synonym‡	Oxidase	Catalase	Growth			1% Glycine	Nalidixic Acid	TTC§
				25°C.	37°C.	43°C.			
C. fetus									
ss fetus	C. fetus ss intestinalis	+	+	+	+	−	+	R	S
ss venerealis	C. fetus ss fetus	+	+	+	+	−	−	R	S
C. jejuni	C. fetus ss jejuni	+	+	−	+	+	+	S	S
C. coli	C. fetus ss jejuni	+	+	−	+	+	+	S	R
C. sputorum		+	−	+	+	−	+		

*Data from several authors.[30,44] Symbols: +, most strains positive; −, most strains negative; R, resistant; S, sensitive.
†Classification of Véron and Chatelain.[49]
‡From Smibert.[45]
§2,3,5-Triphenyltetrazolium chloride.

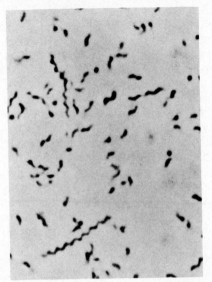

Figure 21–9. *Campylobacter jejuni/coli.* Phase-contrast photomicrograph of cells from 18-hour culture; × 2000. M. A. Karmali, and Fleming, P. C. Originally published in the Canadian Medical Association Journal, Vol. 120, June 23, 1979, p. 1525.)

pylobacter do not ferment or oxidize carbohydrates, rather tricarboxylic acid cycle intermediates are the primary energy sources. Chemically defined mediums, containing a variety of amino acids and vitamins, will support growth of many strains.

Campylobacter are sensitive to low pH, and die rapidly in acid environments; they are, therefore, rapidly killed in the stomach unless protected from acids by food or other means. At low temperatures, they survive in fecal material, milk, and water for several weeks, but for shorter periods at 25°C.[7]

Antigenic Structure

The antigenic makeup of *Campylobacter* has not been extensively studied, but two kinds of antigens are present. The flagellar, or H, antigens are heat-labile and seem to be heterogeneous. Heat-stable O antigens are lipopolysaccharide in nature and also are heterogeneous. Several serotyping schemes have been devised, but are not yet available for routine use.

Ecology of Campylobacter

The ecological distribution of campylobacters is shown in Table 21–6. The human diseases, especially enteritis caused by the *C. jejuni/coli* group, is thought to derive from animal reservoirs, as discussed in the following section.

ENTERITIS[6, 30, 39, 40]

Campylobacter of the *jejuni/coli* group are probably the most common bacterial agents causing human diarrheal disease. Intestinal infection with these bacilli is characterized by fever, bloody diarrhea, and abdominal pain that mimics appendicitis. Mucosal damage and inflammation is observed in the jejunum, ileum, and large bowel. Although these symptoms suggest an enterotoxemia, no enterotoxin has been detected. The mechanism of pathogenesis is presently unknown.

Infections usually occur in previously healthy individuals and follow ingestion of food or water containing campylobacters, or by occupational exposure to infected animals. The incubation period is variable and depends upon the number of microorganisms ingested;

Table 21–6. **Ecology of Campylobacter**

Species	Animals Colonized	Disease or Infection
C. fetus ss fetus	Humans	Systemic disease, including bacteremia, meningitis, and septic thrombophlebitis, in debilitated or immunodeficient patients.
	Cattle; sheep	Abortion in cattle and sheep; transmitted by fecal-oral route.
ss venerealis	Cattle	Abortion and infertility in cattle; venereal transmission.
C. jejuni/coli	Humans	Enteritis.
	Birds; domestic animals	Normal intestinal flora.
C. sputorum ss sputorum ss bubulus	Humans Sheep; goats	Normal flora of the gingival crevice. Normal genital flora.

most illnesses occur one to seven days after exposure. A proportion of exposed individuals develop asymptomatic infections, up to 25 per cent in one outbreak. Convalescent carriage may extend from several months, although most patients excrete the microorganisms for only two to three weeks.

The clinical features are not so distinct as to permit diagnosis on these grounds. The characteristic feature is a mild to moderate diarrhea, usually with blood, that lasts from one day to a week or more. Severe cases may require rehydration and chemotherapy. The etiological agent is susceptible *in vitro* to a variety of antimicrobial agents, including erythromycin, tetracycline, aminoglycosides, chloramphenicol, and furizolidone. Erythromycin is the preferred drug in severe cases, since it has been shown to eliminate intestinal campylobacters. In controlled trials, however, the course of the disease is not markedly altered by antimicrobial treatment.

Bacteriological Diagnosis

The laboratory aids to diagnosis of campylobacter enteritis include direct microscopic examination of diarrheal stools and the isolation and identification of the causative agent. *Campylobacter* exhibit a characteristic darting motion when observed in wet mounts by darkfield or phase-contrast microscopy. Thus, the presence of such microorganisms in diarrheal stools provides a rapid, but presumptive, diagnosis.

The isolation and identification of *Campylobacter* from cases of enteritis is relatively simple with current methods. Stools or rectal swabs are inoculated onto suitable selective mediums, usually containing blood and several antimicrobial agents to suppress normal fecal microorganisms. Cultures are incubated at 42° to 43°C. in an atmosphere of 5 to 10 per cent oxygen and 3 to 10 per cent carbon dioxide. After 24 to 48 hours, typical colonies are selected for confirmation by Gram stain, motility, and biochemical tests.

Epidemiology

As noted earlier, the *jejuni/coli* group of *Campylobacter* are found as normal intestinal flora of birds, both domestic and wild, and in a number of mammalian hosts. The latter include most domestic animals, such as swine, cattle, sheep, goats, and horses. A diarrheal disease may be produced in calves and lambs as well as dogs and cats. Man is infected by the fecal-oral route, so that there is ample opportunity for infection by contact with animals and by contamination of water and food supplies. Animal carcasses and milk frequently contain *C. jejuni* and outbreaks have been traced to these sources; raw milk and improperly cooked foods are the vehicles most often incriminated.

Cases of campylobacter enteritis also provide the source for spread by person-to-person contact. Young children with enteritis often proliferate the infection in day-care nurseries and in families; symptomatic patients excrete tremendous numbers of *C. jejuni* in stools, ranging up to 10^9 per gram. Those with asymptomatic infections excrete much lower numbers, but are potential infection sources. A chronic carrier state apparently does not occur.

Diarrheal illness due to *Campylobacter* is of worldwide distribution, presumably because of the variety and extent of infected animal reservoirs. Incidence of the disease appears to be greater in developing countries, but outbreaks and sporadic cases appear in industrialized nations as well. In temperate climates, incidence is greater in the warmer months and, in tropical areas, during the rainy season.

Campylobacter enteritis affects all age groups, but the greatest number of cases appears in children under five years of age. In developing countries, the infection is seen very early in life, often in those under one year of age. Most food and waterborne outbreaks, on the other hand, do not exhibit age-specific incidence.

Control. The control of *C. jejuni/coli* infections is based upon interruption of transmission, either from animal reservoirs to man or spread from person-to-person. Foods of animal origin should be properly cooked and stored, milk should be pasteurized, and water supplies should be chlorinated. Human cases of campylobacter enteritis must be recognized as infection sources and sanitary disposal of excreta and contaminated articles should be emphasized. Such individuals should not, for example, be permitted to work as food handlers until free of diarrheal symptoms.

SYSTEMIC INFECTIONS[40]

Although *C. jejuni* may occasionally be responsible for septicemia as a sequel to enteritis, most human systemic infections with *Campylobacter* are caused by *C. fetus* ss *fetus*. Although only relatively few cases have been documented, they tend to be serious, with high mortality.

The most common of the systemic infections

are manifest as bacteremia without localization. These have exhibited several clinical patterns, ranging from asymptomatic bacteremia to fulminant, fatal sepsis. Bacterial endocarditis, meningitis, and thrombophlebitis have also been noted in a portion of cases. In almost all instances, there is a history of underlying illness or predisposing medical condition. These have included alcoholism, diabetes mellitus, heart disease, lymphoproliferative disease, and immunodeficiency.

As noted above, *C. fetus* is an animal pathogen, causing abortion in cattle and sheep and often found in the intestinal tract of infected animals; in these animals it is transmitted by the fecal-oral route. Presumably, human infections can be derived from contamination of food or water by these animal campylobacters. Yet animal or environmental sources of infection are not evident in the majority of human cases. The mode of transmission is, therefore, not completely established.

Although definitive information on chemotherapy is lacking, it appears that chloramphenicol, aminoglycosides, and tetracycline are effective in treatment of these infections.

REFERENCES

1. Barua, D. 1974. Laboratory diagnosis of cholera. pp. 85–126. *In* D. Barua and W. Burrows (Eds.): Cholera. W. B. Saunders Co., Philadelphia.
2. Barua, D., and W. Burrows (Eds.). 1974. Cholera. W. B. Saunders Co., Philadelphia.
3. Blake, P. A., R. E. Weaver, and D. G. Hollis. 1980. Diseases of humans (other than cholera) caused by vibrios. Ann. Rev. Microbiol. **34**:341–367.
4. Blake, P. A., *et al.* 1979. Disease caused by a marine vibrio. Clinical characteristics and epidemiology. New Engl. J. Med. **300**:1–5.
5. Blake, P. A., *et al.* 1980. Cholera—a possible endemic focus in the United States. New Engl. J. Med. **302**:305–309.
6. Blaser, M. J., and L. B. Reller. 1981. Campylobacter enteritis. New Engl. J. Med. **305**:1444–1452.
7. Blaser, M. J., *et al.* 1980. Survival of *Campylobacter fetus* subsp. *jejuni* in biological milieus. J. Clin. Microbiol. **11**:309–313.
8. Boesman-Finkelstein, M., and R. A. Finkelstein. 1982. Protection in rabbits induced by the Texas Star-SR attenuated A⁻B⁺ mutant candidate live oral cholera vaccine. Infect. Immun. **36**:221–226.
9. Burrows, W., and J. Kaur. 1975. Current concepts of immunity to cholera. Bull. Haff. Inst. **3**:1–19.
10. Dorolle, P. 1974. International surveillance of cholera. pp. 427–433. *In* D. Barua and W. Burrows (Eds.): Cholera. W. B. Saunders Co., Philadelphia.
11. Feacham, R. G. 1982. Environmental aspects of cholera epidemiology. III. Transmission and control. Trop. Dis. Bull. **79**:1–47.
12. Feeley, J. C. 1974. Antitoxic immunity in cholera. pp. 307–314. *In* D. Barua and W. Burrows (Eds.): Cholera. W. B. Saunders Co., Philadelphia.
13. Field, M. 1979. Modes of action of enterotoxins from *Vibrio cholerae* and *Escherichia coli*. Rev. Infect. Dis **1**:918–925.
14. Finkelstein, R. A. 1975. Immunology of cholera. Curr. Topics Microbiol. Immunol. **69**:137–196.
15. Finkelstein, R. A., and L. F. Hanne. 1982. Hemagglutinins (colonization factors?) produced by *Vibrio cholerae*. pp. 324–326. *In* D. Schlessinger (Ed.): Microbiology—1982. American Society for Microbiology, Washington, D.C.
16. Freter, R. 1974. Gut-associated immunity to cholera. pp. 315–331. *In* D. Barua and W. Burrows (Eds.): Cholera. W. B. Saunders Co., Philadelphia.
17. Freter, R., and G. W. Jones. 1976. Adhesive properties of *Vibrio cholerae*: nature of the interaction with intact mucosal surfaces. Infect. Immun. **14**:246–256.
18. Freter, R., *et al.* 1981. Role of chemotaxis in the association of motile bacteria with intestinal mucosa: in vitro studies. Infect. Immun. **34**:241–249.
19. Germanier, R., *et al.* 1976. Preparation of a purified antigenic cholera toxoid. Infect. Immun. **13**:1692–1698.
20. Hackney, C. R., *et al.* 1980. Adherence as a method for differentiating virulent and avirulent strains of *Vibrio parahaemolyticus*. Appl. Environ. Microbiol. **40**:652–658.
21. Hirschhorn, N., *et al.* 1974. The treatment of cholera. pp. 235–252. *In* D. Barua and W. Burrows (Eds.): Cholera. W. B. Saunders Co., Philadelphia.
22. Holmgren, J. 1980. Cellular action and pathophysiological effects of cholera toxin. pp. 269–284. *In* H. Smith, J. J. Skehel, and M. J. Turner (Eds.): The Molecular Basis of Microbial Pathogenicity. Verlag Chemie, Weinheim.
23. Holmgren, J. 1981. Actions of cholera toxin and the prevention and treatment of cholera. Nature **292**:413–417.
24. Honda, T., and R. A. Finkelstein. 1979. Purification and characterization of a hemolysin produced by *Vibrio cholerae* biotype El Tor: another toxic substance produced by cholera vibrios. Infect. Immun. **26**:1020–1027.
25. Hughes, J. M., *et al.* 1978. Non-cholera vibrio infections in the United States. Clinical, epidemiologic, and laboratory features. Ann. Intern. Med. **88**:602–606.
26. Jones, G. W., and R. Freter. 1976. Adhesive properties of *Vibrio cholerae*: nature of the interaction with isolated rabbit brush border membranes and human erythrocytes. Infect. Immun. **14**:240–245.
27. Joo, I. 1974. Cholera vaccines. pp. 333–355. *In* D. Barua and W. Burrows (Eds.): Cholera. W. B. Saunders Co., Philadelphia.
28. Kamal, A. M. 1974. The seventh pandemic of cholera. pp. 1–14. *In* D. Barua and W. Burrows (Eds.): Cholera. W. B. Saunders Co., Philadelphia.
29. Kaplan, R. L. 1980. *Campylobacter*. pp. 235–241. *In* E. H. Lennette, *et al.* (Eds.): Manual of Clinical Microbiology. 3rd ed. American Society for Microbiology, Washington, D.C.
30. Karmali, M. A., and P. C. Fleming. 1979. Campylobacter enteritis. Can. Med. Assn J. **120**:1525–1532.
31. Levine, M. M. *et al.* 1981. Duration of infection-derived immunity to cholera. J. Infec. Dis. **143**:818–820.
32. Miyamoto, Y., *et al.* 1980. Simplified purification and biophysicochemical characteristics of Kanagawa phenomenon-associated hemolysin of *Vibrio parahaemolyticus*. Infect. Immun. **28**:567–576.
33. Morris, J. G., *et al.* 1981. Non-O group 1 *Vibrio cholerae* gastroenteritis in the United States. Clini-

cal, epidemiologic, and laboratory characteristics of sporadic cases. Ann. Intern. Med. **94**:656–658.

34. Newton-John, H. F., *et al.* 1971. Cholera: an imported case in Australia, 1969. Med. J. Australia **1**:135–138.
35. Ogg, J. E., M. B. Shrestha, and L. Poudayl. 1978. Phage-induced changes in *Vibrio cholerae:* serotype and biotype conversions. Infect. Immun. **19**:231–238.
36. Pal, S. C., *et al.* 1980. A controlled field trial of an aluminium phosphate-adsorbed cholera vaccine in Calcutta. Bull. Wld Hlth Org. **58**:741–745.
37. Rappaport, R. S. 1974. Development of a purified cholera toxoid. II. Preparation of a stable, antigenic toxoid by reaction of purified toxin with glutaral-dehyde. Infect. Immun. **9**:304–317.
38. Report. 1980. Cholera and other vibrio-associated diarrheas. Bull. Wld Hlth Org. **58**:353–374.
39. Report. 1980. Enteric infections due to *Campylobacter, Yersinia, Salmonella,* and *Shigella.* Bull. Wld Hlth Org. **58**:519–537.
40. Rettig, P. J. 1979. *Campylobacter* infections in human beings. J. Pediat. **94**:855–864.
41. Schrank, G. D., and W. F. Verwey. 1976. Distribution of cholera organisms in experimental *Vibrio cholerae* infections: proposed mechanisms of pathogenesis and antibacterial immunity. Infect. Immun. **13**:195–203.
42. Shedlofsky, S., and R. Freter. 1974. Synergism between ecologic and immunologic control mechanisms of intestinal flora. J. Infect. Dis. **129**:296–303.
43. Shrivastava, R., V. B. Sinha, and B. S. Shrivastava. 1980. Events in the pathogenesis of experimental cholera: role of bacterial adherence and multiplication. J. Med. Microbiol. **13**:1–9.

44. Skirrow, M. B., and J. Benjamin. 1980. "1001" Campylobacters: cultural characteristics of intestinal campylobacters from man and animals. J. Hygiene **85**:427–442.
45. Smibert, R. M. 1974. Campylobacter. pp. 207–212. *In* R. E. Buchanan and N. E. Gibbons (Eds.): Bergey's Manual of Determinative Bacteriology. 8th ed. Williams & Wilkins Co., Baltimore.
46. Smibert, R. M. 1978. The genus *Campylobacter.* Ann. Rev. Microbiol. **32**:673–709.
47. Svennerholm, A.-M., S. Lange, and J. Holmgren. 1978. Correlation between intestinal synthesis of specific immunoglobulin A and protection against experimental cholera in mice. Infect. Immun. **21**:1–6.
48. Symposium. 1975. Vibrio parahaemolyticus: occurrence, identification and clinical significance. pp. 229–262. *In* D. Schlessinger (Ed.): Microbiology—1974. American Society for Microbiology, Washington, D.C.
49. Véron, M., and R. Chatelain. 1973. Taxonomic study of the genus *Campylobacter* Sebald and Véron and designation of the neotype strain for the type species, *Campylobacter fetus* (Smith and Taylor) Sebald and Véron. Internat. J. Syst. Bacteriol. **23**:122–134.
50. Wachsmuth, I. K., G. K. Morris, and J. C. Feeley. 1980. *Vibrio.* pp. 226–234. *In* E. H. Lennette, *et al.* (Eds.): Manual of Clinical Microbiology. 3rd ed. American Society for Microbiology, Washington, D.C.
51. Watanabe, Y. 1974. Antibacterial immunity in cholera. pp. 283–306. *In* D. Barua and W. Burrows (Eds.): Cholera. W. B. Saunders Co., Philadelphia.
52. Yancey, R. J., D. L. Willis, and L. J. Berry. 1979. Flagella-induced immunity against experimental cholera in adult rabbits. Infect. Immun. **25**:220–228.

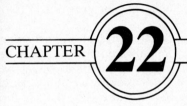

CHAPTER 22

Brucella: Undulant Fever; Contagious Abortion of Cattle

Morphology and Staining
Physiology
Antigenic Structure
Toxicity and Virulence
Variation
Pathogenicity for Lower
  Animals

Brucellosis in Humans
  Epidemiology
  Bacteriological Diagnosis
  Chemotherapy
  Immunity

While investigating the human disease known as Malta fever, in 1887 Bruce discovered a microorganism in the spleen in fatal cases of the disease which he called *Micrococcus melitensis.* A disease of goats transmissible to man, the affliction is common on the island of Malta, on neighboring islands, and in the Mediterranean littoral. It has since been reported from many other parts of the world, including the United States, and is variously known as Malta fever, Mediterranean fever, or undulant fever. Ten years later, Bang isolated a microorganism in Denmark, which he named *Bacillus abortus,* that was responsible for contagious abortion in cattle, a condition now known as Bang's disease.

These two diseases, one primarily of goats and secondarily of man, and the other one of cattle, were long studied quite independently. No connection between the two was recognized until 1918, when Evans demonstrated their remarkably close morphological, cultural, and serological relationships.

The microorganisms described by Bruce and Bang are now included in the genus *Brucella* and designated *Brucella melitensis* and *Brucella abortus,* respectively. A third species, *Brucella suis,* was discovered by Traum in 1914 in the aborted fetuses of infected swine. These three species are the principal causes of brucellosis in man. Although three additional species are

recognized—*B. neotomae, B. ovis,* and *B. canis*—these are animal pathogens and, except for *B. canis,* do not infect humans.

Morphology and Staining

The *Brucella* are small coccoid or short bacillary forms, 0.4 to 1.5 μm. in length and 0.4 to 0.8 μm. in breadth. Some variability is noted; both coccoid and bacillary forms may appear intermingled in stained smears, as shown in Figure 22–1. The bacilli usually occur singly or in pairs, but short chains are sometimes seen. *Brucella* are gram-negative; they are not encapsulated, do not form spores, and are nonmotile.

Colonies on agar mediums are small, circular, convex, amorphous, smooth, glistening, and translucent (Fig. 22–2). No pigment is formed, although colonies of *B. melitensis* and some strains of *B. abortus* become brown in older cultures.

Physiology

The nutritional requirements of *Brucella* are somewhat complex, at least upon primary isolation or when small inoculums are used. Best growth is obtained on enriched mediums containing meat infusion or on mediums with complex peptones, such as tryptose. Growth is usually slow and may require several days to develop. Many strains of *Brucella* can be

505

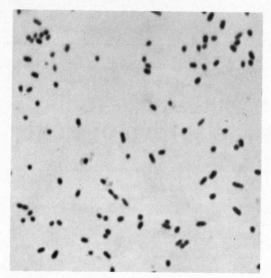

Figure 22–1. *Brucella melitensis* in pure culture. Note the coccobacillary morphology. Fuchsin; × 1050.

cultivated on chemically defined mediums containing amino acids and glucose, along with several vitamins—nicotinic acid, thiamin, pantothenic acid, and biotin. The temperature for growth ranges from 20° to 40° C., with an optimum at 37°C. These bacteria are somewhat unusual in that neither acid nor gas is produced from carbohydrates in peptone-containing mediums. Several carbohydrates and amino acids are, however, oxidatively metabolized. Catalase is formed, to a variable extent, and is reportedly associated with virulence of the

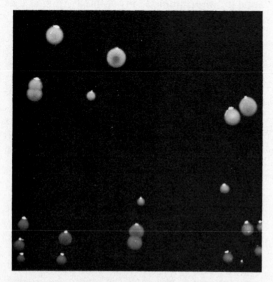

Figure 22–2. Colonial morphology of *Brucella melitensis* on liver infusion agar. The slight granularity is accentuated here, and the colonies are smooth, flattened, and slightly brownish in color. × 4.

strain. The optimum pH for growth is 7.0 to 7.2.

Brucella are strictly aerobic; *B. melitensis* and *B. suis* may be grown on primary isolation under the usual aerobic conditions but most strains of *B. abortus* require an atmosphere containing 5 to 10 per cent carbon dioxide for primary isolation. Upon subsequent transfers, *B. abortus* cultures gradually adapt to ordinary aerobic growth.

Biotypes. The several species of *Brucella* are differentiated by physiological and biochemical reactions (Table 22–1). Each of the three principal species are separated into biotypes, based on oxidative metabolism of several amino acids and carbohydrates; growth in the presence of dyes (basic fuchsin and thionin); requirement for increased carbon dioxide; and production of hydrogen sulfide.[4] A bacteriophage, isolated by Russian workers and designated Tb, lyses *B. abortus*, but not the other species. Biotypes have some epidemiological importance, since serotypes are not distinguished. Biotyping is not routinely carried out in clinical laboratories, however, since such knowledge is not required for management of the disease.

Brucella do not show unusual resistance to heat and disinfectants. Since they are found in the milk of infected cows, the rapid death of these bacteria at pasteurizing temperatures is of some practical importance; most are killed in three minutes at 143° to 145°F. They persist in soil, water, and dust for one to two months, but disappear within 10 days in milk. It is of interest that they survive two hours or more in milk mixed with gastric juice, and may survive for many weeks in certain cheeses.

Antigenic Structure

The smooth colonial form of each of the three classic species of *Brucella* possesses two heat-stable, surface O antigens, designated A and M: these lipopolysaccharide antigens are responsible for agglutination reactions. *Brucella melitensis* contains a relatively large amount of M and a small amount of A, while both *B. abortus* and *B. suis* contain large amounts of A and small amounts of M. The ratio of A to M antigens is said to be about 20:1 in *B. abortus* and *B. suis,* and about 1:20 in *B. melitensis*. It is possible, then, to differentiate *B. melitensis* from the other species by serological methods, but *B. abortus, B. suis,* and *B. neotomae* cannot be serologically distinguished from one another. In practice, monospecific antiserums, *i.e.,* those absorbed to remove antibodies to either A or M antigen,

Table 22–1. **Principal Differential Reactions of the *Brucella***

| | | | Growth in Presence of | | | |
| | | | Basic Fuchsin | Thionine | | |
Species	CO_2 Required	H_2S Produced	0.002%	0.004%	0.002%	Lysis by Phage Tb
B. melitensis (Biotype 1)	–	–	+	–	+	–
B. abortus (Biotype 1)	+*	+	+	–	–	+
B. suis (Biotype 1)	–	+	–	+	+	–
B. neotomae	–	+	–	–	+	–
B. ovis	+	–	+	+	+	–
B. canis	–	–	–	+	+	–

*Upon primary isolation.

are used. *Brucella ovis* and *B. canis* are rough colonial forms and do not contain the smooth somatic antigen. They are, however, agglutinated by antiserum directed against the rough, or core, lipopolysaccharide. Although detailed antigenic analysis reveals several other antigens, no serotypes are distinguished. The *Brucella* also share an O antigen with *Vibrio cholerae* and show cross reactions with some strains of *Yersinia enterocolitica*.[11]

Toxicity and Virulence

These bacteria are not known to form exotoxins, but the cell substance of *Brucella* is toxic by virtue of the lipopolysaccharide contained in the cell envelope. The biological activity of lipopolysaccharide from smooth virulent strains appears to be equivalent to that derived from rough strains.[7] Endotoxin is thought to contribute to the pathogenesis of disease, and is thus a component of virulence. Virulent smooth strains, unlike avirulent rough strains, appear to be able to multiply intracellularly. This capacity for **intracellular** growth appears to be associated with the O-specific components of the smooth lipopolysaccharide.[8] There is evidence, too, that phagocytes which have ingested *Brucella* do not undergo degranulation; thus the intracellular bacteria are not subject to intraphagocytic destruction.[9]

Variation

Smooth *Brucella* readily dissociate to give rise to the rough form. The smooth to rough (S–R) variation is characterized by a change to a rough colonial type; a loss of virulence; and alteration in immunological specificity, *i.e.*, loss of the O-specific side chains of the lipopolysaccharide.

The physiological conditions that determine the population change from smooth to rough are related to alanine metabolism. Alanine, produced by the S form, accumulates in the culture to toxic concentrations, and the S form

is then replaced by overgrowth of the alanine-resistant R form. Other environmental factors, including oxygen tension, also contribute. The antigenic alteration begins to take place before morphological changes are apparent and has been a source of considerable difficulty in the serological identification of these bacteria. It is, therefore, essential to use only smooth cultures for serological purposes.

A number of tests have been devised for the detection of antigenic variants. The rough forms are, of course, spontaneously agglutinated in saline. Slightly rough strains, but not smooth strains, are agglutinated by acriflavine. Colonies on glucose-glycerol agar may be differentiated morphologically by flooding the plate with aqueous crystal violet solution and examination by oblique, transmitted light. Smooth colonies are a light blue-green, while the nonsmooth vary from red to blue-red or violet-red.

Pathogenicity for Lower Animals[19]

Brucellosis is primarily a disease of domestic animals and is only secondarily communicated to man; the chief animal reservoirs are goats, cattle, and swine. The specific epithets of these bacteria reflect their host specialization.

Goats.[21] Goats can be artificially infected with *B. melitensis* by almost any route, and it is probable that under natural conditions the presence of bacilli in vaginal discharge at the time of abortion and shortly thereafter plays an important part in the dissemination of the infection. Bacilli are shed in the milk as well as in the urine of infected animals. Pregnant goats are highly susceptible to infection with *Brucella*. Bacteremia is initiated about 10 days after infection and persists for perhaps one month. This acute generalized infection becomes localized in the udder and uterus, where the microorganisms persist for months to several years.

The most obvious clinical symptom of infection is abortion, but it does not occur consistently. Pyrexia is apparent within 48 hours of the generalized infection, and there is slight diarrhea. The placenta is not often retained, but a copious vaginal discharge is frequently observed for two or three weeks after kidding. In lactating goats the milk may be physically altered and in extreme cases may appear as a clear fluid containing suspended clots.

Immature goats are highly resistant to infection. Kids born of infected dams may not be infected at birth and commonly do not become so in spite of the ingestion of enormous numbers of *Brucella* in the milk. Nonpregnant mature goats are also resistant to infection and respond to artificial inoculation with only a low and transient serum agglutinin titer.

Although more resistant than goats, sheep may be infected with *Brucella*, particularly with *B. ovis*. Infection results in epididymitis in rams, and, uncommonly, abortion in ewes.

Cattle. Brucellosis in cattle, sometimes termed Bang's disease or contagious abortion, is most commonly an infection with *B. abortus,* although both *B. melitensis* and *B. suis* have also been found. The microorganisms gain entrance by a variety of routes, including direct inoculation into the vagina, by way of the conjunctiva, or via the alimentary tract. The primary symptom of the disease is abortion of the fetus by pregnant cattle. The time elapsing between initial infection and abortion varies from three weeks to four months, and the period of gestation at which abortion may take place varies from two to nine months. Cattle do not abort, however, unless infected during pregnancy; even then no more than 30 per cent abort, but sterility sometimes results from infection. Subsequent pregnancies may proceed normally in spite of persistence of the infection; second abortions are not common; and third abortions are rare. As in the case of young goats, calves are relatively resistant to infection.

The bacilli are found in the blood in perhaps 10 per cent of infected animals and are very likely consistently present during the acute stages. Early in the disease, bacteria appear in the lymph nodes of the head and mesentery. By the end of the first month they are found throughout the body, and after the third month they are localized in the mammary glands, and found only in the udder. Chronic infection of the udder can persist indefinitely without significant differences in the quality of the milk. Bacilli may be excreted in the milk over a long period, perhaps for life. The uterus, on the other hand, becomes free of the bacteria rel-atively soon, and the vaginal discharges do not contain the bacilli for an extended period.

Animals infected during pregnancy develop serum agglutinins, but titers fall slowly over a period of six months or so. Cattle that continue to excrete bacilli in the milk generally show persistent agglutinin titers. Agglutinins are also present in milk and may be demonstrated in the whey after clotting with rennin.

Swine. Brucellosis of swine is almost always an infection with *B. suis*, though these animals may be artificially infected with *B. abortus*. Abortion sometimes occurs in infected sows, but is less frequent than in cows. The clinical symptoms may be mild or lacking and in a number of instances there is no outward evidence of disease in an infected herd. Under natural conditions infection may take place via the alimentary tract. Infected boars, in which a testicular localization occurs, are undoubtedly a significant element in dissemination of the infection by the genital route. Bacilli are eliminated with aborted fetuses and in vaginal discharges, urine, semen, and milk.

Dogs. It has long been recognized that dogs, particularly those in contact with infected cattle and swine, may become naturally infected with any of the three classic species of *Brucella*. In most cases, such infections are without overt clinical signs, although the animals develop *Brucella* agglutinins in their serums.

In 1968, a series of infectious canine abortions was noted in colonies of beagles and was found to be due to an organism designated *B. canis*.[5] The disease was subsequently found to be widespread in other dogs as well. Serological surveys have indicated that about 9 per cent of stray dogs show reactivity against *B. canis,* a rate much higher than observed in pets and confined animals.[3, 10] The disease is characterized by a generalized lymphadenitis and splenitis; in many females, early fetal deaths or abortions occur at about the 50th day of gestation, with subsequent prolonged vaginal discharge. Epididymitis, scrotal dermatitis, and testicular atrophy are prominent features in infected males. Although a persistent bacteremia occurs, there are few other clinical signs in most infected animals. Human infections due to this organism are infrequent. Some have resembled upper respiratory viral infections, but most infections are similar to classic brucellosis in symptomology.

The etiological agent, *B. canis*, is of rough colonial morphology and agglutinates in antiserum to rough, but not smooth, *Brucella*. The organisms have been found to have the same characteristics that define and identify *B.*

suis and are sometimes designated *B. suis* biotype 5.

Other Animals. Several other animals are naturally infected with *Brucella*. In Alaska, reindeer may serve as a reservoir host for the human disease. Man apparently becomes infected by consumption of caribou meat. Natural infection of rabbits with *B. melitensis* has been reported, as has *B. suis* infection of fowl. *Brucella neotomae* is a natural pathogen of wood rats, and wild rats may be artificially infected with other *Brucella*. Of the usual laboratory animals, guinea pigs are readily infected and are most often used for experimental purposes.

BRUCELLOSIS IN HUMANS[6, 13, 19, 20]

Humans are susceptible to infection with the three principal species of *Brucella*; infections with *B. melitensis* and *B. suis* are frequently more severe than those with *B. abortus*. *Brucella* are highly virulent microorganisms and the infective dose for man is relatively small; infection is usually acquired by the mucocutaneous route.

The epidemiology of brucellosis varies with geography and socioeconomic conditions. In developing countries and those with largely agricultural economies, transmission is usually by ingestion of unpasteurized milk and dairy products or by consumption of inadequately cooked flesh of diseased animals. In industrialized nations, where milk is pasteurized and animal disease control programs have been initiated, as they have in the United States, most cases are by occupational exposure to infected animal reservoirs. Agricultural and slaughterhouse workers acquire the infection from infected livestock or contaminated byproducts in the meat-processing industry. The microorganisms enter the body through cuts or skin abrasions, by inhalation of infected aerosols, or by contamination of the conjunctiva. A small, but significant, number of infections arise from laboratory accidents, and even the most skilled workers have acquired infection in this manner.

Following penetration of the skin or mucous membranes, the bacilli are first found in the lymphatic system and later in the bloodstream. They localize in a number of organs, including the spleen, liver, and bone marrow, where granulomas are the characteristic local lesion. *Brucella* are typically **intracellular parasites**, and the infection persists in infected macrophages and other cells of the reticuloendothelial system. The incubation period in man is highly variable and relatively long, ranging from one week to several months.

The human infection may have varied clinical manifestations. Undoubtedly many infections are effectively subclinical, as indicated by the isolation of *Brucella* from apparently healthy persons and the presence of specific agglutinins in the serum of individuals with no history of clinical disease. Clinically apparent brucellosis may be **acute** or **chronic**, with symptoms that are mild to severe; the prominent clinical features are listed in Table 22–2. The febrile response is generally intermittent, usually near normal in the morning but rising to 101° to 104° C. in the afternoon and evening. In typical undulant fever, there may be a stepwise, day-to-day increase in temperature to a maximum, followed by gradual decrease; successive repetitions of this sequence sometimes occur. In general, untreated brucellosis is a disease of long duration—one to four months—and relapses during convalescence are frequent. The case-fatality rate in untreated cases is relatively low—2 to 3 per cent. In chronic form, brucellosis is manifest as muscular stiffness, intermittent low fever, and emotional disturbance. Humans become sensitized to the cellular antigens of *Brucella*, a hypersensitivity that is sometimes manifest as skin eruptions, which may be macular or resemble the rose spots of typhoid fever. Endotoxin appears to contribute in large measure to the pathogenesis of the disease, through direct toxic effects and by elicitation of a hypersensitive state. Although abortions have been associated with brucellosis in pregnant females, such occurrences are extremely rare.

The clinical features of brucellosis, especially in the chronic form, are not particularly distinctive, so that physical findings and history of possible exposure establish suspicion, to be confirmed by laboratory tests. The bacilli are usually found in the blood, particularly during

Table 22–2. **Clinical Features of Brucellosis***

Symptom	% Reporting
Fever	89
Chills	69
Weakness and malaise	64
Body aches and sweating	61
Headache	51
Weight loss	41
Anorexia	39

*In 1288 cases reported in the United States between 1967 and 1974. Data from Fox and Kaufman.[6]

febrile episodes, and diagnosis is solidly established by their isolation and identification. The development of serum agglutinins is a significant diagnostic aid.

Epidemiology[17]

Brucellosis in man is probably always acquired from infected animals; man-to-man transmission is a possibility but rarely, if ever, occurs. As noted above, brucellosis is a foodborne infection in many parts of the world. Since *Brucella* are shed in great numbers in the milk of infected goats and cattle, milk and dairy products are common vehicles of transmission; pasteurization provides adequate protection from this mode of transmission. In the United States, milkborne transmission declined in importance following the initiation, in 1934, of elaborate programs to control bovine brucellosis. By the late 1950s, brucellosis in this country had become largely an occupational disease of farmers, livestock handlers, veterinarians, butchers, and slaughterhouse workers. Individuals become infected by the handling of the tissues of diseased animals or by close contact with other infected materials, such as aborted fetuses. The dramatic association of human cases with occupations involving the slaughter of animals is illustrated in Figure 22–3.

The epidemiology of brucellosis differs somewhat from one locality to another and is

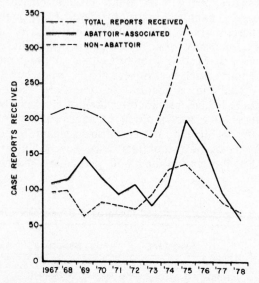

Figure 22–3. Cases of brucellosis reported in the United States during the period 1967–78, emphasizing the association of the disease with occupation. The proportion of infections found in abattoir workers includes packing-house employees, government meat inspectors, and rendering plant workers. (Morbidity and Mortality Weekly Report **28**:437–439, 1979.)

dependent upon the incidence and type of animal infections. During the period from 1959 to 1974, swine were the most common source of human brucellosis in the United States and the incidence was greatest in the midwestern states, where a significant number of these animals are infected with *B. suis*. In 1975, bovine brucellosis increased sharply, particularly in the southern states, and was followed by a concomitant increase in human cases. Cattle have now replaced swine as the predominant source of human infections. The reported incidence of human brucellosis in the United States from 1945 to 1981 is charted in Figure 22–4.

The prevalence of human brucellosis in the United States is not known with any degree of precision. The reported incidence reached a peak in 1947 with 6321 cases, declined to 262 in 1965 and has remained fairly constant since, although a slight increase occurred during the period from 1974 to 1977. The number of apparent cases of brucellosis tends to reflect either general interest or laxity in reporting. It is likely, too, that many infections go unrecognized. Although difficult to establish with certainty, the reporting rate is probably 10 per cent or less.

Although eradication of brucellosis has not been realized in the United States, efforts have been more successful in other countries. The Scandinavian countries are, for example, free of the disease. In others, brucellosis is still a serious public health problem. In the past decade, the disease has been epidemic in some Spanish provinces, where an estimated 80,000 cases occurred in 1974.[1] The case rate of 22.7 per 10,000 population was almost 2000-fold greater than in the United States for the same period.

Bacteriological Diagnosis[2, 16]

The laboratory diagnosis of brucellosis is best accomplished by the isolation and identification of the causative microorganism. Somewhat less definitive is the demonstration of specific agglutinating antibodies in the patient's serum; their presence indicates only an immune response to what may have been a past rather than present infection.

Brucella appear in the blood of infected individuals, particularly in the pyrexial period, but cannot always be isolated. Multiple blood cultures are, therefore, recommended in suspected cases. Blood or infected tissues are inoculated into tryptose broth or commercial blood culture bottles and incubated in an atmosphere of 5 to 10 per cent CO_2. These

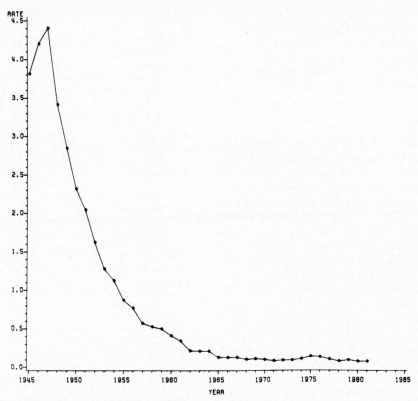

Figure 22–4. Cases of brucellosis per 100,000 population reported in the United States from 1945 to 1981. (Centers for Disease Control. Annual Summary 1981: reported morbidity and mortality in the United States. Morbidity and Mortality Weekly Report **30**(54), 1982.)

enrichment cultures should be subcultured on tryptose agar at four-day intervals and, if subcultures are negative, carried for a period of three weeks. Alternatively, Castañeda bottles may be used. These special bottles combine solid and liquid phases in the same bottle, thus facilitating regular subculture from the enrichment broth phase. They have an added advantage of increased safety for laboratory personnel.

The isolated bacteria may be identified as *Brucella* by agglutination with specific antiserum or by fluorescent antibody staining. Although not required for clinical management of disease, species may be identified by biochemical reactions (Table 22–1). Serological techniques, using monospecific A or M antiserum, can only distinguish between *B. melitensis* and *B. abortus/B. suis*. Biotype determinations are useful for epidemiological work, but are best carried out in specialized laboratories.

A presumptive diagnosis made on clinical grounds may be partially, but by no means absolutely, confirmed by an agglutinin titer of 1:320 or higher or by a rising antibody titer during the course of the disease. Unfortunately, agglutinin titers differ somewhat from one laboratory to another.

Interpretation of the agglutinin response is also complicated by cross-reactions with other microorganisms. Individuals immunized with cholera vaccine, for example, may exhibit serum agglutinins for *Brucella* because of the antigens shared by the two microorganisms.

Chemotherapy
Chemotherapy of brucellosis has not been uniformly successful, since the disease responds irregularly and temporarily to ordinary regimens of antibiotics. Therapeutic failures are probably due in part to the intracellular nature of the infection, since intracellular bacteria are not readily destroyed by antibiotics. Tetracyclines are considered the antibiotics of choice and usually terminate acute clinical episodes. Their use should be continued for a minimum of 21 days and may be repeated,

sometimes in combination with streptomycin, in severe or stubborn cases; nevertheless, relapses sometimes occur. It has also been observed that vigorous antibiotic treatment can induce endotoxin shock, which may be potentiated in hypersensitive individuals.

Immunity[12]

The resistance of calves and nonpregnant cows to clinically apparent brucellosis is clearly an expression of natural immunity, though the older animals respond to the microorganism with the production of antibodies and development of increased resistance to subsequent infection. Man likewise appears to have a high degree of natural resistance to the disease, and it is probable that there are many more infections than clinical cases of brucellosis.

An immune response is evident in humans by the appearance of agglutinins, opsonins, bactericidal antibodies, and hypersensitivity to preparations of the cell substance of the bacteria (brucellergin). It is not clear, however, that this response is associated with increased resistance, *i.e.,* effective immunity, to the infection. It is probable that effective acquired immunity is primarily cellular in nature. Since *Brucella* infection induces delayed hypersensitivity, the immunity may be analogous, in part, to that observed in tuberculosis, with activation of macrophages to restrict the intracellular multiplication of the brucellae;[14, 15] this restriction of growth is potentiated by immune serum. Consistent with this, the therapeutic use of antiserums in human brucellosis has given disappointing results, presumably because macrophages are not activated.

Vaccines.[18] The possibility of producing an effective prophylactic immunity, not only in man but also in animals, is of continued interest. Vaccines consisting of killed suspensions of the bacteria induce a serum antibody response, demonstrable as agglutinins, etc., but do not consistently produce immunity to the disease.

A live avirulent variant of *B. abortus,* strain BA 19, has been used extensively as an immunizing agent in cattle and sheep. Used in calves, it does not prevent infection but modifies the disease, as indicated by sharply reduced rate of abortion and shedding of the virulent bacteria. This strain is not completely avirulent for man, and a number of accidental infections have been reported. No effective vaccine is currently available for human immunization.

REFERENCES

1. Aller, B. 1975. Brucellosis in Spain. Internat. J. Zoonoses **2**:10–15.
2. Alton, G. G., L. M. Jones, and D. E. Pietz. 1975. Laboratory Techniques in Brucellosis. 2nd ed. Wld Hlth Org. Monogr. Ser., No. 55. Geneva.
3. Brown, J., *et al.* 1976. *Brucella canis* infectivity rates in stray and pet dog populations. Amer. J. Publ. Hlth **66**:889–891.
4. Buchanan, R. E., and N. E. Gibbons (Eds.). 1974. Bergey's Manual of Determinative Bacteriology. 8th ed. The Williams & Wilkins Co., Baltimore.
5. Carmichael, L. E., and D. W. Bruner. 1968. Characteristics of a newly recognized species of Brucella responsible for infectious canine abortions. Cornell Vet. **58**:579–592.
6. Fox, M. D., and A. F. Kaufman. 1977. Brucellosis in the United States, 1965–1974. J. Infect. Dis. **136**:312–316.
7. Jones, L. M., R. Diaz, and D. T. Berman. 1976. Endotoxic activity of rough organisms of *Brucella* species. Infect. Immun. **13**:1638–1641.
8. Kreutzer, D. L., and D. C. Robertson. 1979. Surface macromolecules and virulence in intracellular parasitism: comparison of cell envelope components of smooth and rough strains of *Brucella abortus*. Infect. Immun. **23**:819–828.
9. Kreutzer, D. L., L. A. Dreyfus, and D. C. Robertson. 1979. Interaction of polymorphonuclear leukocytes with smooth and rough strains of *Brucella abortus*. Infect. Immun. **23**:737–742.
10. Lovejoy, G. S., *et al.* 1976. Serosurvey of dogs for *Brucella canis* infection in Memphis, Tennessee. Am. J. Publ. Hlth **66**:175–176.
11. Marx, A., *et al.* 1975. Biochemical basis of the serological cross-reactions between *Brucella abortus* and *Yersinia enterocolitica* serotype O:9. Ann. Microbiol. (Inst. Pasteur) **126B**:435–445.
12. McCullough, N. B. 1970. Microbial and host factors in the pathogenesis of brucellosis. pp. 324–345. *In* S. Mudd (Ed.): Infectious Agents and Host Reactions. W. B. Saunders Co., Philadelphia.
13. McDevitt, D. G. 1973. Symptomatology of chronic brucellosis. Brit. J. Ind. Med. **30**:385–389.
14. McGhee, J. R., and B. A. Freeman. 1970. Osmotically sensitive *Brucella* in infected normal and immune macrophages. Infect. Immun. **1**:146–150.
15. Ralston, D. J., and S. S. Elberg. 1971. Sensitization and recall of anti-*Brucella* immunity in guinea pig macrophages by attenuated and virulent *Brucella*. Infect. Immun. **3**:200–208.
16. Renner, E. D., and W. J. Hausler, Jr. 1980. *Brucella*. pp. 325–329. *In* E. H. Lennette, *et al.* (Eds.): Manual of Clinical Microbiology. 3rd ed. American Society for Microbiology, Washington, D. C.
17. Report. 1979. Brucellosis—United States, 1978. Morbid. Mortal. Wkly Rep. **28**:437–439.
18. Roux, J. 1972. Les vaccinations dans les brucelloses humaines et animales. Bull. Inst. Pasteur **70**:145–202.
19. Roux, J. 1979. Epidémiologie et prévention de la brucellose. Bull. Wld Hlth Org. **57**:179–194.
20. Wise, R. I. 1980. Brucellosis in the United States: past, present, and future. J. Amer. Med. Assn **244**:2318–2322.
21. Zapatel, J., and H. Málaga. 1971. Epidemiologiá de la brucelosis caprina en el Perú. Bol. Of. Sanit. Panam. **71**:121–131.

CHAPTER 23

Yersinia; Pasteurella; Francisella; Actinobacillus

The small, gram-negative bacilli now distributed among the genera *Yersinia, Pasteurella,* and *Francisella* were, at one time, placed in the genus *Pasteurella.* While they are not as closely related taxonomically as the earlier classification would indicate, they are all primarily pathogens of lower animals and share some common characteristics in this regard.

The *Yersinia* and *Pasteurella* are the most closely related and exhibit some homogeneity in physiological and biochemical characters, as shown in Table 23–1; the *Francisella* are set apart by their fastidious nutritive requirements. The present taxonomic position of these groups is outlined in Chapter 2.

Yersinia

Yersinia was only recently adopted as a genus in the family Enterobacteriaceae, to include the plague bacillus, *Yersinia pestis*; the pseudotubercle bacillus, *Yersinia pseudotuberculosis;* and a relatively new bacillus, earlier known casually as *Pasteurella* X, and now designated *Yersinia enterocolitica.* The rela-

tionship between the plague and pseudotubercle bacilli is well established. They share many antigens and exhibit similar bacteriophage sensitivity and closely homologous DNA. Some of their biochemical and physiological characters are displayed in Table 23–1. The plague bacillus was discovered almost simultaneously by Yersin and Kitasato in 1894; the pseudotubercle bacillus was first described somewhat earlier, in 1893.

Recently, three new species of *Yersinia* have been described—*Y. frederikensii, Y. kristensenii,* and *Y. intermedia*—that were previously grouped together as *Y. enterocolitica*-like, or atypical yersiniae. They appear not to have great medical importance and are not otherwise included here.

YERSINIA PESTIS—THE PLAGUE BACILLUS[41, 42]

Plague is an ancient disease, probably originating in Central Asia. It is possible that the Biblical plague of the Philistines in 1320 B.C. was plague of specific etiology, and the great pandemic during the reign of the Emperor Justinian, A.D. 542, was certainly plague.

Plague prevailed extensively throughout Europe during the Middle Ages. It has been estimated that 25 million persons—one-quarter of all the inhabitants of Europe—perished in the "great mortality" or "Black Death" of the fourteenth century (1348–1349). Few diseases have left so deep a mark on general literature. Boccaccio's *Decameron* contains one of the most vivid descriptions of the plague ever written, and Defoe's fictitious *Journal of the Plague Year* provides a realistic picture of the devastation of London in 1665 by an outbreak of Black Death in which 70,000 persons perished.

For reasons that may only be conjectured, plague has had irregular periods of quiescence and recrudescence. Western Europe has been practically free from the plague since the middle of the eighteenth century, and the disease began its first great extension in modern times when it appeared in 1893 in Hong Kong and in 1896 in Bombay. Plague caused great loss of life in British India; official statistics show that in the period from 1896 to 1918 more than 10 million deaths were due to this disease. In October 1899, a case was recorded at Santos, Brazil; this is thought to be the first occurrence of plague in the Western Hemisphere. Plague first appeared in the United States in San Francisco in 1900; it is assumed that it was introduced by infected rats from the Orient. The infection apparently spread to ground squirrels and other wild rodents in the western part of the country, where it remains today as sylvatic plague.

The abatement of plague continues, but it is considered to represent only an extension of its decline from the most recent epidemics, rather than a prelude to its extinction. In fact, the infection is firmly established in endemic foci, and it may be a disease of the future.

Morphology and Staining
The plague bacillus is a short, plump, ovoid rod 0.5 to 1.0 μm. in breadth by 1 to 2 μm. in length; its morphology is illustrated in Figure 23–1. In the body fluids the bacilli may occur in pairs; long chains are rare and, in general, there is no characteristic arrangement (Fig. 23–2). The bacilli are nonmotile, and a surface slime layer is present (Fig. 23–3). The presence of this material, as an envelope or capsule,[14] is associated with resistance of the bacilli to phagocytosis. Involution forms are common, especially in older cultures, and coccus shapes, large rods, and giant swollen forms

Table 23–1. **Principal Reactions of *Yersinia* and *Pasteurella* Species**

Species	Motility		Indol	H₂S Production	Urease	Ornithine Decarboxylase
	22° C.	37° C.				
Yersinia pestis	−	−	−	+	−	−
Yersinia pseudotuberculosis	+	−	−	−	+	−
Yersinia enterocolitica	+	−	v*	−	+	+
Pasteurella multocida	−	−	+	+	−	+
Pasteurella haemolytica	−	−	−	v	−	v
Pasteurella pneumotropica	−	−	+	+	+	v
Pasteurella ureae	−	−	−	−	+	−

*v = most strains negative.

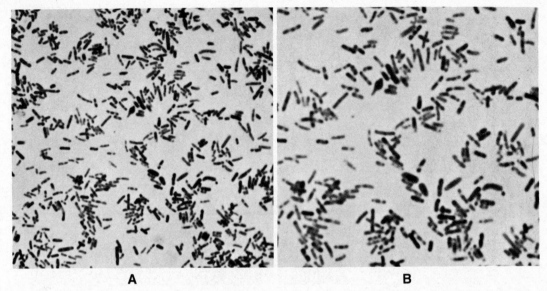

A   **B**

Figure 23–1. The plague bacillus. Smear from pure culture; fixed in methyl alcohol and stained methylene blue to show bipolar staining. Note the involution forms present even at 24 hours' incubation. *A*, × 1050; *B*, × 2100.

may be observed. The tendency of the plague bacillus to aberrant morphology is accentuated by cultivation on mediums containing 3 to 4 per cent sodium chloride.

Colonies on nutrient agar or gelatin have a delicate, drop-like appearance, with a round, granular center and a thin, granular, uneven margin. On blood or other hemin-containing mediums the colonies are dark brown in color,

the pigmentation being derived from absorption of hemin from the substrate.

The plague bacillus is uniformly gram-negative. It shows a marked tendency toward polar staining, *i.e.*, there are heavily stained areas at the ends of the cell separated by a lightly stained area in the center, when stained with methylene blue. The plague bacillus is best demonstrated in tissue sections by polychrome stains.

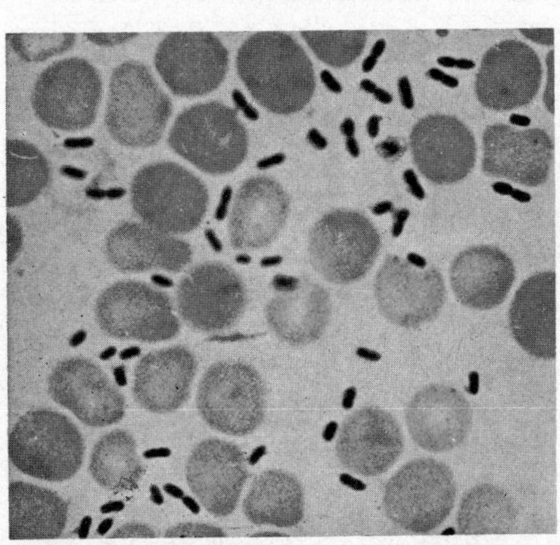

Physiology

Yersinia pestis is not nutritionally fastidious; growth occurs on the ordinary culture mediums provided the inoculum is heavy. Amino acids are required as nitrogen sources, but vitamins are not essential. Calcium is required for initiation of cell division at 37°C., but not at 26°C.[20] Casein hydrolysate furnishes adequate nutrients for growth in liquid culture, and has been used for vaccine and toxin production, but when prepared as a solid medium, supplementation with blood, heme, or reducing agents is required. Freshly isolated strains grow more slowly than adapted laboratory strains. Unlike most bacteria pathogenic for man, plague bacilli grow best at 25°C. to 30°C., with limiting temperatures of −2°C. and 45°C. In any case, the colonies on solid mediums grow slowly and never attain a large size. The

Figure 23–2. The plague bacillus in the blood of an infected mouse. × 2000. (J. R. Douglas, and C. M. Wheeler, J. Infect. Dis. **72**:18, 1943.)

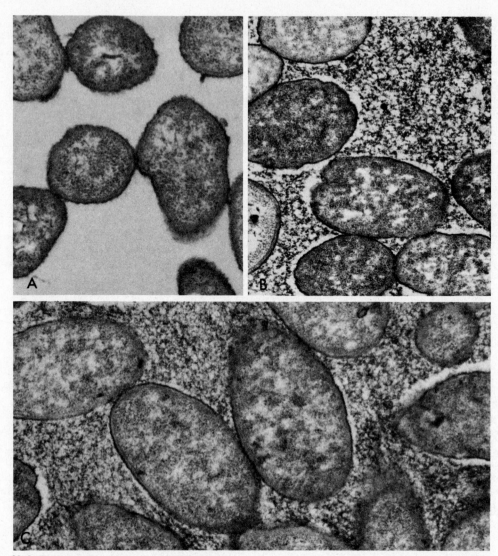

Figure 23–3. Electron micrograph of cells from colonies of *Yersinia pestis* grown on blood agar. *A*, 24 hours; *B*, 48 hours; *C*, 72 hours. The extracellular matrix is envelope Fraction 1; in this avirulent strain, the envelope antigen is not apparent after 24 hours of culture but is produced after 48 hours. Virulent strains produce extracellular Fraction 1, even in young cultures. (T. H. Chen, *et al.*, Infect. Immun. **11**:1382, 1975.)

plague bacillus is aerobic and facultatively anaerobic.

Sugar fermentations are variable, and a small amount of acid but no gas is produced. Three physiological varieties of the plague bacillus are distinguished, as shown in Table 23–2.

The primary foci of infection of variety *orientalis* are in India, Burma, and South China; this variety was the agent of oriental plague

Table 23–2. **Differentiation of *Yersinia pestis* Varieties**

	Variety		
Test	*orientalis*	*antigua*	*mediaevalis*
Acid from:			
Glycerol	−	+	+
Melibiose	−	−	+
Nitrate reduction	+	+	−

which caused the 1894 epidemic, and it is also responsible for sylvatic or wild rodent plague in the western United States. Variety *antigua,* probably the oldest, came from Transbaikalia, Mongolia, and Manchuria in Central Asia, moved west with the Aryan invasions, and followed the valley of the Nile into Central Africa, leaving foci that persist to the present time. It also moved back toward the Mediterranean in the sixth century and is believed to have been responsible for the Justinian plague that spread through the Roman Empire. It has since disappeared from Europe and has remained isolated in Africa. Variety *mediaevalis,* possibly arising by a slow transformation of variety *antigua,* spread from the Caspian Sea throughout the whole of Europe, causing the Black Death, and established endemic foci.

The plague bacillus does not exhibit any marked resistance to deleterious influences. Exposure to drying, particularly at higher summer temperatures, kills it within a short time. The bacillus is quite sensitive to the action of sunlight and chemical disinfectants. It is killed, for example, by 0.5 per cent phenol in 10 to 15 minutes and by heating to 55°C. in about the same time. Cultures kept in the refrigerator, however, remain viable over long periods. Although *Y. pestis* does not usually survive long outside the human body and disappears rapidly from water and buried cadavers, it may survive for some time in soils.

Toxins[35, 36]

At least two classes of toxins are produced by plague bacilli. The first of these is a lipopolysaccharide endotoxin, which is similar in pharmacological action to that produced by enteric bacilli. The endotoxin is antigenic, toxic for laboratory animals, evokes a pyrogenic response in rabbits, induces tolerance to *Salmonella* endotoxin, and produces both localized and generalized Shwartzman reaction in rabbits. In purified form, the endotoxin has an LD_{50} of 1 mg.; it has been calculated that sufficient amounts of the endotoxin can be produced *in vivo* to contribute to or account for death in infected experimental animals and for the toxicity observed in human disease.[53]

A second group of toxins is produced, and they appear to share some properties of both endotoxins and exotoxins. These are protein in nature but, unlike classical exotoxins, they do not appear to diffuse freely into the surrounding medium; they are released only after rupture or lysis of the bacterial cell and are a part of the cell membrane. These toxins, termed murine toxins, are active in rats and mice but are not toxic for guinea pigs, rabbits, or chimpanzees.

On local inoculation in mice, murine toxins produce edema, often followed by necrosis, and the general effects appear to be largely on the peripheral vascular system and liver to produce irreversible toxic effects when a lethal dose is given. The toxic action is antagonized by cAMP and by cholera toxin, which is known to elevate cAMP. It has been suggested that their action is similar to beta-adrenergic blocking agents, inhibiting the mobilization of free fatty acids.[5] The pathological condition induced in mice and rats is closely similar to that seen in infection, but this similarity is not observed in other animals.

The murine toxins have been prepared in highly purified form by ammonium sulfate fractionation and electrophoresis of extracts of acetone-dried bacilli. The toxicity is contained in two distinct protein components, designated toxins A and B, that may be separated by acrylamide gel electrophoresis. The two toxins have a mouse LD_{50} of 0.5 to 1.0 µg. Toxin A has a molecular weight of 240,000, while that of B is 120,000. Both toxins can be dissociated to low-molecular-weight subunits that retain the majority of the activity of the original preparation. The murine toxins are antigenic in rabbits, and high titers of specific antitoxins have been detected in the serum of plague patients. It is of interest to note that they are produced by avirulent, as well as virulent, *Y. pestis.* This is perhaps not surprising when it is recalled that virulence not only reflects the capacity to damage the host but also includes the ability to become established within that host.

The precise role of plague toxins in the pathogenesis of disease, particularly in humans, remains undefined, but it is possible that they contribute to the disease process.

Virulence[6, 48]

The question of virulence and its determinants in the plague bacillus remains an enduring one. Interest in matters such as variation, toxins, and antigenic structure has centered largely on the question of virulence. The usual S–R dissociation occurs, but the colonial morphology and associated properties are not related to virulence, since both S and R forms may be either virulent or avirulent. The plague bacillus is **antigenically homogeneous**; serotypes, in the conventional sense, do not occur. The antigenic structure is complex, however,

Table 23–3. **Virulence Determinants in *Yersinia pestis***

Fraction 1
VW antigens
Pesticin:coagulase:fibrinolysin
Hemin absorption
Purine synthesis

since more than 16 antigens are known to be present. Aside from the V and W antigens and the Fraction 1 envelope antigen discussed below, none of these antigenic components appears to be directly correlated with virulence. Virulence may be measured, in a practical sense, by the number of bacterial cells required to infect and kill experimental animals; thus, highly virulent strains of *Y. pestis* may have a mouse or guinea pig LD_{50} of fewer than 10 bacilli.

The factors associated with virulence have recently been clarified and are listed in Table 23–3. A polysaccharide-lipid component[19] contained in the envelope or capsule of the cell, designated **Fraction 1**, is associated with the resistance of the bacilli to phagocytosis. Although it is usually present in virulent and absent in avirulent bacilli, its role in virulence is questioned by the occurrence of mouse-virulent strains lacking or containing only small amounts of Fraction 1; such strains have been isolated in the laboratory as mutants and from some naturally occurring fatal infections of man. Further, bacilli may remain viable within neutrophils and macrophages after phagocytosis, raising some doubt regarding phagocytosis inhibition as an aggressive element.

Two antigens, designated **V** and **W**, appear to be invariably associated with virulence; they do not occur separately, but may vary in relative amounts. While the V and W antigens probably contribute to phagocytosis resistance, it is more likely that their virulence role is associated with the capacity for intracellular survival and multiplication following phagocytosis.

Virulent strains of plague bacilli produce a bacteriocin-like substance termed **pesticin**; such strains also show **coagulase** and **fibrinolytic** activity. These characters always occur together and are assumed to be genetically linked; coagulase and fibrinolytic action are believed to be related to lethality in the host, rather than to infectivity.

The **pigmentation** of virulent *Y. pestis* on hemin-containing mediums has been noted earlier; such strains also show pigmentation on ordinary mediums which contain the dye congo

red. Mutational loss of the ability to absorb hemin or dye results in loss of virulence, but such strains can be restored to full virulence in mice, provided ferrous iron is concomitantly inoculated.

Finally, plague bacilli which retain all of the above determinants of virulence but have mutationally lost the ability to **synthesize purines** have, thereby, lost their virulence. The effective block is the loss of guanosine monophosphate synthetase. When such purines are administered along with these nutritional mutants, virulence is restored.

PLAGUE[1, 25, 32, 41]

Plague in man appears most commonly in two forms, the **bubonic** or **glandular plague**, and **plague pneumonia**. In the bubonic type the symptom complex is characteristic, and diagnosis on clinical grounds is relatively simple. Following exposure, usually from the bite of an infected insect vector, the two- to five-day incubation period is succeeded by a sudden onset characterized by high fever and symptoms of generalized septicemic infection. Regional lymph nodes rapidly become painful, and the typical buboes appear. From the buboes bacilli pass over into the blood; in fatal cases the bacteria often multiply extensively in the blood. The case-fatality rate in bubonic plague is 60 to 90 per cent, and death generally occurs within 10 days of onset. During the plague epidemics in the Middle Ages subcutaneous hemorrhages seem to have been more prominent than at present, and the dark spots to which they give rise may have been the origin of the popular name "Black Death."

Plague pneumonia may occur secondarily to the glandular infection—21 per cent in one study.[30] Subsequent respiratory transmission from these infections gives rise to primary plague pneumonia in patient contacts. Pneumonic plague is almost always fatal in untreated cases. In this variety the sputum usually contains enormous numbers of plague bacilli, and the infection is spread from man to man by droplets. Because of this direct transmission, pneumonic plague is by far the more dangerous and rapidly spreading type. The extensive outbreak of pneumonic plague in Manchuria from 1910 to 1912 is said to have caused approximately 60,000 deaths, the case-fatality rate being practically 100 per cent. Although not so devastating, smaller plague outbreaks occur, as in Vietnam in the 1960s, when over 13,000 cases were reported in a five-year period. Both bubonic and pneumonic plague have been produced experimentally, giving diseases in monkeys which closely resemble the human infection.

Cases of mild plague, the so-called "pestis minor," are seen in some epidemics. Carriers in the classic sense probably do not exist; however, low numbers of asymptomatic contacts of plague cases have been found to carry the bacilli in their throats.

Epidemiology[2]

Plague is primarily a disease of **rodents** which is transmissible to man, giving rise to both sporadic cases and epidemics of disease. Susceptible rodents fall into two groups: domestic rodents, principally rats, and various wild rodents. Of the former, the black house and ship rat, *Rattus rattus,* and the less susceptible gray sewer rat, *R. norvegicus*, are most commonly involved. Natural infection also appears in a variety of other animals, including ground and tree squirrels, prairie dogs, and carnivores, such as cats, dogs, coyotes, and bobcats.

Although both the feces and urine of infected rats may contain plague bacilli, and animals may be infected by feeding upon others dead of the disease, the infection is most often transmitted by **fleas**. The Indian rat flea, *Xenopsylla cheopis,* is a common, and perhaps

the most effective, vector. Plague bacilli are present in the blood of infected rodents during the acute disease, as many as 100 million per ml., and fleas are infected by feeding on these animals.

When the plague bacilli are taken into the stomach of the flea, they multiply but do not spread to other parts of the body. On microscopic examination large masses of bacilli may be found in the infected flea, as seen in Figure 23–4. In some, the bacilli multiply so rapidly that the bacterial mass mechanically obstructs the proventriculus so that little or no food may pass. As the flea feeds, plague bacilli are mixed with the drawn blood of the host, and regurgitated into the bite. The bacilli are also discharged in the feces, and infection may occur by contamination of the bite wound with fecal pellets.

Sylvatic Plague[31]

As noted above, a wide variety of rodents are naturally infected with *Y. pestis*. This epizootic rodent disease, improperly but colorfully referred to as sylvatic plague, constitutes the natural reservoir of infection. In the United States wild rodent plague was first observed in California in 1908, and it has spread slowly eastward, reaching into Texas, Oklahoma, and Kansas. Indeed, most of the states west of the 100th meridian have reported the presence of

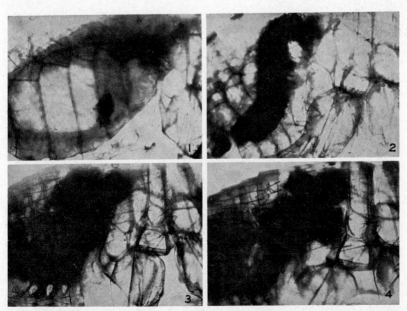

Figure 23–4. Plague bacilli in the infected flea; sections stained with methylene blue. The bacilli appear as dark stained masses. *1,* Flea on the ninth day after infection. *2,* Eighteenth day after infection; note the stomach and proventriculus packed with bacilli. *3,* Twenty-second day after infection; note the large mass of bacilli and the swollen proventriculus. *4,* Twenty-third day after infection; the proventriculus is further enlarged. (J. R. Douglas and C. M. Wheeler, J. Infect. Dis. **72**:18, 1943.)

sylvatic plague. It now constitutes one of the largest of the wild plague foci. Rodents such as prairie dogs, ground squirrels, wood rats, and mice are infected. There is evidence, too, that natural foci may be maintained in fleas, since infected fleas may live for one to four years in rodent burrows.

Although small pockets of sylvatic plague are present in many parts of the world, the major foci are now in Southeast Asia, North and South America, and Africa. In these areas, human cases of plague arise from human contact with the epizootic reservoir.

It is well known that wild plague exists in two kinds of endemic centers, temporary and permanent. The persistence of plague in these reservoirs depends upon the relative resistance of the rodent populations to the plague bacillus and the range of the individual animal species affected. Permanent reservoirs of infection are in relatively resistant wild rodents. If the rodent population is highly susceptible, the foci tend to be temporary and the disease dies out unless periodically reactivated by importation of the infection. Thus, the dynamics of the animal infection is determined by the balance between susceptible and resistant species, and

by their migratory habits. Infections in some foci tend also to be cyclical, with periodicities ranging from one or two years to a decade or more, possibly reflecting changes in the proportions of susceptible and resistant populations.

Transmission of plague among wild rodents is by ectoparasites, principally fleas. The infection may be passed by the infected vectors to domestic rodents or pets, such as dogs and cats.

Most cases of human plague are linked to the animal reservoirs, either by incursion of humans into the wild animal habitats or by entry of the reservoir hosts into human settlements. Infection is initially carried to man by ectoparasites of rodents, resulting in sporadic cases appearing in endemic areas. Although epidemic plague in man is now a rare occurrence, the bubonic type can be transmitted from person to person by human ectoparasites, notably the human flea, *Pulex irritans*. When human pneumonic plague develops, initial cases are usually secondary to the systemic disease, but subsequent transmission is by the aerosol route, resulting in explosive epidemics.

Although the number of human cases of

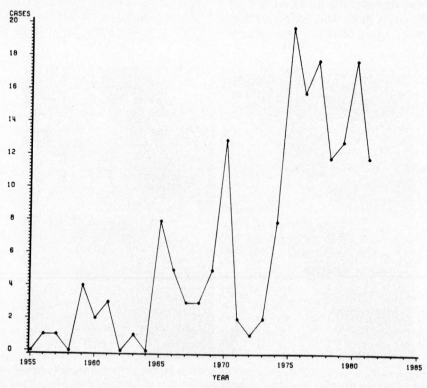

Figure 23–5. Reported cases of human plague in the United States, 1955–1981. Note the apparent 5-year periodicity. (Centers for Disease Control. Annual Summary 1981: reported morbidity and mortality in the United States. Morbidity and Mortality Weekly Report **30**, 1982.)

Table 23–4. **Human Plague Cases in the United States, 1960–1980***

Area	Number
Arizona	19
California	16
Colorado	10
Idaho	1
Nevada	3
New Mexico	90
Oregon	5
Texas	1
Utah	2
Wyoming	1
Total	148

*Centers for Disease Control, Annual Summary 1980: reported morbidity and mortality in the United States. Morbidity and Mortality Weekly Report **29**, 1981.

plague has remained low for many decades, the public health significance is unquestioned. Wild plague is extensive in many areas, and the general decline in incidence of human cases can be attributed to improved standards of living and to active epidemiological surveillance in the natural foci. On a worldwide basis, 505 cases of plague were reported in 1980, compared to more than 40,000 cases in 1950. In the United States, the number of cases has been small but has generally increased since 1965, as shown in Figure 23–5. Although the reasons for this increase are not clear, it may be due to greater activity of wild plague or to increased human incursion into the enzootic areas. Table 23–4 shows the distribution by states of human cases of plague in the United States from 1960 to 1980. New Mexico continues to report the greatest number of cases.

The prominent role of ectoparasites in transmission of plague, in both the wild and urban disease, points up the significance of control measures directed against these vectors. For example, human plague in India has disappeared, probably due to the extensive use of insecticides for malaria control. Control of domestic rats and wild rodents is more difficult but, ultimately, can prevent introduction of new infection and reduce probability of human infection.

Bacteriological Diagnosis[33, 49]

In man the bacilli are found in material aspirated from buboes; in cultures or smears of internal organs, especially the spleen; and in the sputum in pneumonic plague. The presence of gram-negative, bipolar-staining, ovoid bacilli is highly suggestive. Blood samples, taken late in the disease, should be cultured first in broth. Other material may be inoculated directly on blood agar and glycerol agar. Cultures are identified by cultural and biochemical characteristics and by agglutination in specific antiserum. The bacilli show some tendency to spontaneous agglutination, and the slide agglutination test is unsatisfactory. Isolated strains may be tested for the presence of virulence factors by recently developed and relatively simple methods. Because plague is characterized by rapid onset and short course, laboratory diagnosis is frequently retrospective. Postmortem diagnosis may be made by tapping the liver, lungs, and buboes with a syringe. The serous fluid is used for preparing smears; microscopic examination of these often gives almost unequivocal diagnosis, and fluorescent antibody staining may be useful when specimens are too grossly contaminated for culture. The hazards attendant to laboratory culture of *Y. pestis* should be clearly recognized.

Several serological tests for plague diagnosis have been developed, all using Fraction 1 antigen. A passive hemagglutination test has been the most extensively used, but an enzyme-linked immunosorbent assay (ELISA) and solid-phase radioimmunoassay (SPRIA) appear to be most sensitive.[24, 55] Serology has limited use as a diagnostic procedure, however, because titers reach useful levels only after one or two weeks following onset.[10]

Chemotherapy[9, 44]

Early treatment of plague is essential in view of the rapidity of the clinical course and should be instituted without waiting for laboratory confirmation of the diagnosis. Specific therapy in pneumonic plague, if begun within 15 hours, is usually successful. The drugs of choice are the tetracyclines, given in large doses. Streptomycin may be used in combination with other drugs, but in advanced cases should not be given in large doses because of the high risk of endotoxin shock. Penicillin is without effect on the plague bacillus. Individuals known to be exposed, as in laboratory accidents, should be given prophylactic antibiotics.

Immunity[12]

Recovery from plague confers a high degree of immunity to subsequent infection. Phagocytosis appears to be of primary importance in this immunity, functioning through opsonization to counteract the antiphagocytic properties of the envelope or capsule of the bacillus. It is probable that antibody to the envelope antigen, Fraction 1, plays a significant part in effective immunity, and that to the VW antigen complex may also be important. Antitoxic immunity does not contribute materially to effective immunity, and antitoxic serums are not protective.

Vaccines. A variety of vaccines have been utilized for protection of humans against plague. These have included killed cell suspensions, fractions of the bacilli, and attenuated live vaccines.

Vaccination of humans with either attenuated or killed vaccines has not always proved effective, although the killed vaccines used to immunize military forces in Vietnam apparently yielded solid immunity.[13] Vaccine use has reduced the mortality and incidence of bubonic but not pneumonic plague; the immunity appears to be short-lived.

The immunization of humans with Fraction 1 evokes a protective immune response, as measured by passive mouse protection tests, that appears to be of high order; unfortunately, delayed allergic reactions are also induced.

Inoculation with living attenuated bacilli produces immunity in experimental animals.[15] The use of such vaccines in man has been investigated in South Africa with encouraging results, and a similar vaccine used in Indonesia in more than 10 million inoculations was reported to be without untoward results.

YERSINIA PSEUDOTUBERCULOSIS

Yersinia pseudotuberculosis, like the plague bacillus, is a natural pathogen of rodents, especially guinea pigs; other natural reservoirs include domestic fowl. In guinea pigs it causes a fatal disease, with caseous swellings and nodules in various organs; these have been termed pseudotubercles and have given this bacterium its name.

The bacillus resembles the plague bacillus in many particulars, but may be differentiated from *Y. pestis* by its motility at 18° to 22°C., production of urease, and fermentation of rhamnose (Table 23–1). On deoxycholate-citrate agar it grows abundantly as large opaque colonies; *Y. pestis* grows only scantily as reddish pinpoint colonies on this medium. *Yersinia pseudotuberculosis* is less virulent for guinea pigs than the plague bacillus. A toxin is produced, but it differs antigenically from that produced by *Y. pestis* and has a wider host range, affecting rabbits and guinea pigs as well as rats and mice.

Yersinia pseudotuberculosis is separable into six serological groups, each with serotypes defined by somatic and flagellar antigens. Certain of the somatic antigens are shared with *Salmonella;* groups II and IV are agglutinated by the serum of persons infected by *Salmonella,* so that serodiagnostic reactions must be interpreted with caution. Many of the antigenic components are shared with *Y. pestis,* including the VW complex. As in the plague bacillus, VW antigens are associated with virulence.[3, 18]

Although human infections are rare, several have been reported in Europe and the United States. Most cases have been diarrheal in nature, often with mesenteric lymphadenitis that simulates appendicitis.[23, 39] Transmission appears to be peroral, resulting from close contact with infected animals; rabbits and guinea pigs have been the source of infection in several human cases.

YERSINIA ENTEROCOLITICA[6, 22, 50]

First described in 1933, *Yersinia enterocolitica* was not regarded as an important or widespread cause of human disease until a number of human cases were noted in the early 1960s in Europe. Within a decade thereafter, increasing numbers of human infection were recognized in the United States and Canada, and such infections are now considered to be worldwide in occurrence.

Yersinia enterocolitica resembles the other *Yersinia* in morphology and cultural characteristics. Like *Y. pseudotuberculosis,* it is motile, by peritrichous flagella, at 22°C. but not at 37°C. It may be distinguished from *Y. pseudotuberculosis* by the biochemical reactions listed in Table 23–1, by fermentation of sucrose, and by failure to ferment rhamnose. There is considerable biochemical variability among these bacilli, resulting in subdivision of the species into five biotypes based on biochemical reactions. *Yersinia enterocolitica* grows at 4°C., and its isolation from feces is facilitated by cold enrichment. Fecal specimens are suspended in buffered saline and incubated at 4°C. for several weeks before culture.

Antigenic Structure

The antigenic structure of *Y. enterocolitica* is complex, with O, H, and K antigens being present. At least 34 serotypes are designated, based on the possession of specific O antigens. Both serotype and biotype have epidemiological utility but, because of its complexity, serotyping is most reliably carried out in specialized reference laboratories. Surface VW antigens are produced, which are identical to those found in other *Yersinia*.[11]

Virulence

Spurred by the increasing medical significance of *Y. enterocolitica* and by the possible parallels with virulence of *Y. pestis,* investigators have energetically pursued studies on the determinants of virulence. In man, *Y. enterocolitica* infection is primarily intestinal, usually characterized by acute gastroenteritis. Observations on pathogenesis in animals reveal that virulent strains penetrate the epithelial lining of the intestine into the lamina propria and lymph follicles, with subsequent multiplication in mononuclear cells.[51]

In keeping with these observations, a number of virulence correlates have been proposed. Most virulent strains (1) adhere to epithelial cells and to cultured HeLa cells; (2) penetrate or invade HeLa cells and, perhaps, multiply intracellularly; (3) possess VW surface antigens; (4) resist the bactericidal action of normal serum;[40] and (5) produce a heat-stable enterotoxin.

It must be remembered that correlation with virulence does not establish a character as a virulence determinant, and even some of the correlates may be different expressions of the same character. Two of these properties seem to be established as virulence determinants— the production of VW antigens, which is plasmid-mediated, and the capacity to invade HeLa cells.[46]

Toxin

Clinical findings in *Y. enterocolitica* infections suggested that a toxin might be involved in pathogenesis. Enterotoxin production by many strains, particularly those associated with human infections, has been established, although its relationship to the human disease is still only suggestive.

The toxin, which is enterotoxigenic in the suckling mouse, is produced in cultures grown at 25°C. but not at 37°C. The enterotoxin is similar to the heat-stable enterotoxin (ST) of *Escherichia coli,* both in biological action and immunological properties. The toxin has a molecular weight of about 9700 daltons, is resistant to trypsin and protease, and is stable at 100°C. for 10 minutes. The minimum effective dose of purified toxin is approximately 25 ng. in suckling mice. The toxin is immuno-genic, evoking antitoxin that neutralizes both *Y. enterocolitica* toxin and *E. coli* ST.[37, 38] Its relationship to *E. coli* ST is further emphasized by similarity of action; both toxins, for example, stimulate guanyl cyclase, but not adenyl cyclase.[45]

Pathogenesis in Humans[4, 17, 28, 29]

In man, yersiniosis due to *Y. enterocolitica* is primarily an intestinal infection causing acute gastroenteritis with fever, abdominal pain, diarrhea, nausea, and headaches; stools occasionally contain blood. The disease occurs most often in children. Yersiniosis often mimics acute appendicitis and, in several instances, appendectomies have been performed. Although not common, septicemia has been reported, appearing most often in the young and in the elderly with underlying debilitating disease. In some instances, erythema nodosum and other skin manifestations, as well as arthritis, may follow the intestinal infection.

The bacilli are usually sensitive to sulfonamides, trimethoprim, tetracyclines, aminoglycosides, and co-trimoxazole, but not to ampicillin or other β-lactam antibiotics. Chemotherapy may be indicated in sepsis, but is not usually required for intestinal infections.

A number of animals are apparently infected with *Y. enterocolitica* and *Y. enterocolitica*-like bacteria. *Yersinia* have been found in aquatic ecosystems, *i.e.,* fish and fresh water, and in terrestrial animals, including domestic swine, cats, and dogs. A few human infections have been linked to household pets. It is likely that many sporadic cases in humans are associated with animal reservoirs. Epidemic outbreaks have been traced to food, including milk, and it is possible that contaminated water may be a transmission vehicle. Person-to-person spread is also a probable mode of transmission, exemplified by nosocomial outbreaks.[43]

Early in the disease, the microorganisms may be isolated from diarrheal stools, by cultivation on blood agar as well as on the usual mediums used for enteric bacteria. Later, serum agglutinins appear and these may aid in diagnosis; serological cross-reactions with *Brucella* and *Salmonella,* however, complicate the interpretation of these findings. The majority of isolates in the United States and western Canada are serotype O:8, while serotype O:3 predominates in eastern Canada, as it does in Europe and Japan.

Pasteurella[26]

The bacilli of the genus *Pasteurella* are gram-negative, asporogenous rods, usually exhibiting bipolar staining, that are, in many ways, similar to the plague and pseudotubercle bacilli (Fig. 23–6). The etiological agent of fowl cholera was among the first of them to be described and was the bacterium used by Pasteur—for whom the genus is named—in his early studies on immunity.

Pasteurella multocida
The group of animal diseases loosely designated as **hemorrhagic septicemias** and characterized by hemorrhagic lesions in the subcutaneous tissues, serous membranes, muscles, lymph glands, and internal organs are considered to be caused by a single species, *P. multocida*. Strains may differ widely in virulence and, seemingly, in host specificity.

These bacteria may be grown on conventional nutrient agar or in relatively simple synthetic mediums. Blood is not hemolyzed, although the colonies become darkened on blood mediums. They occur as distinct colonial types: smooth, mucoid, and rough.

The physiological and biochemical reactions that distinguish *P. multocida* from *Yersinia* and from other *Pasteurella* are shown in Table 23–1.

Most strains form polysaccharide capsules or envelopes and four serotypes, designated A, B, C, and D, are distinguished on the basis of these surface antigens. Serotyping may be accomplished by precipitin, capsular swelling, or passive hemagglutination reactions. Effective immunity is type-specific, and apparently is determined by opsonizing antibodies directed against the surface antigen.[56] A toxic lipopolysaccharide is immunogenic and induces partial protection in mice.[16] Type specificity is a property of the smooth colonial form; mucoid strains cannot be serotyped.

The pathogenicity of *P. multocida* is sometimes considered to be open to question because of the relatively common occurrence of

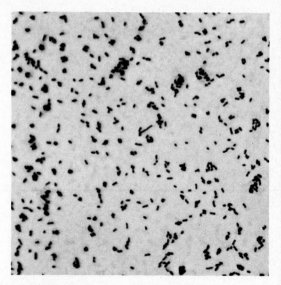

Figure 23–6. *Pasteurella multocida.* Smear from a pure culture. Fuchsin; × 1050.

the bacteria in normal animals. It appears, however, that randomly isolated strains vary widely in virulence, and those isolated from normal animals are usually of the avirulent, mucoid form. Virulence is associated only with the smooth form; host range and geographic distribution are, to a degree, related to the serotype. Type B, for example, is largely confined to Southeast Asia. The other types are associated with fowl cholera and bovine and swine pneumonias in the United States and Europe.

A number of human cases have been recorded. They commonly take the form of wound infections, frequently following dog and cat bites and scratches. Penicillin is the drug of choice in such cases, but even with intensive therapy, recovery is slow. The animal serotypes A and D tend to predominate in the human disease, reinforcing the suggestion that domestic animals constitute the sources of these infections.

Francisella tularensis

Tularemia is a disease particularly of rabbits and rodents that is transmitted to man either directly through the handling of the flesh of infected animals or indirectly through an insect vector. *Francisella tularensis* was discovered by McCoy and Chapin in 1912 in a plague-like disease of the California ground squirrel. Tularemia in man, however, is contracted largely from rabbits, either directly or indirectly by the bite of infected deer flies. Human cases

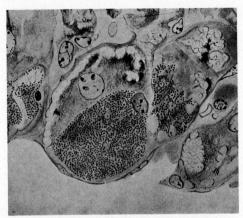

Figure 23–7. *Francisella tularensis* in hepatic cells of mouse. (Francis, Bull. Hygiene Lab. No. 130, 1922.)

have been observed throughout the continental United States and in many parts of Europe and Asia.

Morphology and Staining

In culture, *F. tularensis* is a minute, gram-negative pleomorphic rod 0.2 μm. in breadth and 0.3 to 0.7 μm. in length; the coccoid form predominates in young cultures and the bacillary form in older cultures. In smears from the spleens of infected mice or guinea pigs, the bacteria appear as coccoid forms in well-defined clusters (Fig. 23–7). Spores are not formed, and the microorganisms are nonmotile.

On solid mediums, *F. tularensis* forms minute, transparent, drop-like colonies that are mucoid in consistency and readily emulsifiable. Colonial variants, including those associated with virulence, are more sharply characterized when observed by oblique transmitted light.

This bacterium is somewhat difficult to stain; carbol-fuchsin, aniline gentian violet, or Giemsa may be used. Bipolar staining is often observed.

Physiology

Francisella tularensis differs sharply from *Pasteurella* and *Yersinia* in that it will not grow on ordinary mediums. It may be cultured on blood-glucose-cysteine agar or on chocolate-cystine agar. The microorganism is strictly aerobic and grows best at 37°C. A few carbohydrates are fermented with production of slight amounts of acid but no gas. Differential fermentations are of little value. The bacillus is killed by exposure to 56°C. for 10 minutes. It contains endotoxin and may possess a heat-labile toxin as well.

Two physiological varieties of *F. tularensis* are recognized. *Francisella tularensis* var. *tularensis* is distinguished by production of acid from glucose and possession of a citrulline ureidase system; it is the more virulent variety and is found in North America. *Francisella tularensis* var. *palaearctica* is less virulent and is not restricted in geographic range.

Pathogenicity

Two clinical types of tularemia are recognized: the **glandular** or **ulceroglandular** type, which is the more common, and the so-called **typhoidal** type. In the first instance the acute stage of the disease is characterized by headache, pains, and fever. A papule usually appears, frequently on a finger, where the bacilli presumably entered the body. This later breaks down and forms an ulcer. The axillary and epitrochlear glands become painful and swollen and may break down, discharging purulent material. In persons infected via the conjunctiva, ulcers form on the inner surfaces of the eyelids, and the cervical and preauricular glands may become tender and somewhat swollen. In the typhoidal type of the disease there are no local symptoms. A pleuropulmonary variety has been described which is easily confused with other types of pulmonary disease.[34]

During the first week of illness the bacilli may be present in the blood, but such cultures are only infrequently successful. It has been suggested that during the first week of the disease initial bacteremia occurs, which develops into septicemia in fulminating cases. Tularemia is characterized by **intracellular parasitism;** the bacilli have, in fact, been grown in tissue-cultured alveolar macrophages. Agglutinins are present in the blood in the second week of the disease and may persist in diminishing amounts for at least as long as 18 years after recovery. The average duration of the disease is two to four weeks. The case-fatality rate is low, about 5 per cent.

A variety of lower animals have been found to be naturally infected, including ground squirrels, rabbits, rodents, birds, and a number of carnivorous animals. In the western United States, a sheep infection, with mortality as high as 10 per cent, serves as a source of human infection.

Monkeys can be infected experimentally by inhalation of aerosols containing *F. tularensis.*[47] The LD_{50} in these animals ranges upward from 14 cells, depending upon aerosol particle size. The average incubation period is from

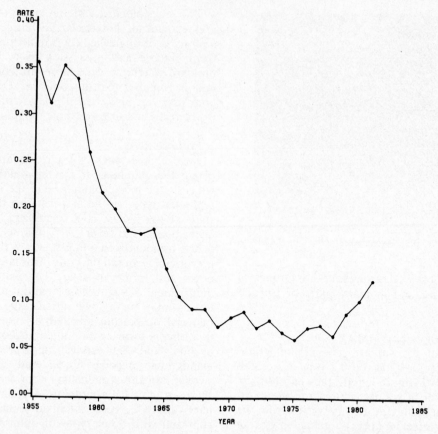

Figure 23-8. Reported cases of tularemia per 100,000 population in the United States since 1955. Increases since 1978 may reflect a long-term natural cycle in vectors and reservoirs. (Centers for Disease Control. Annual Summary 1981: reported morbidity and mortality in the United States. Morbidity and Mortality Weekly Report **30**, 1982.)

one to six days, followed by acute illness lasting up to 11 days; most animals survive and are bacteriologically negative within two months. Significant lesions are in the lower respiratory tract and include necrosis, pleural effusion, and adhesion; cervical and mandibular lymph nodes are often involved.

Epidemiology

As indicated above, tularemia is acquired by man from lower animals either directly or indirectly. Many infections are in hunters or others handling infected flesh; in these individuals the bacilli probably enter through minute abrasions of the skin. Eye infection also occurs, and was the first recognized type of human infection with this bacillus. These and other observations indicate that the infective dose for man is quite small.

Over 90 per cent of the human cases in this country are contracted from rabbits, and it is estimated that about 1 per cent of wild rabbits are infected. An outbreak in Vermont was, however, traced to infected muskrats. Asymptomatic infections doubtless occur, as shown by positive skin or serological tests of persons living in endemic areas and reporting no previous clinical infection.[21]

The infection is present in many wild animals; at least 48 kinds of naturally infected vertebrate animals are known. *Francisella tularensis* has also been found in streams and is perhaps associated with the epizootics occasionally observed in beavers. Waterborne epidemics have occurred in both Europe and Asia. In the United States infection of natural waters is relatively common in the northwestern states, and naturally occurring infections in beavers and muskrats are well known. In water and mud, the microorganisms may persist for many months, and evidence suggests that they may multiply there. The infection is also transmitted by the ingestion of infected tissue, and this may be a factor in the maintenance of the reservoir of infection in carnivorous animals.

The transmission of tularemia by an insect vector is common. In addition to the deer fly (*Chrysops discalis*), ticks of the genera *Dermacentor, Haemaphysalis,* and *Ixodes* may also carry it. In all probability wood ticks serve to disseminate the infection in the animal population. It is of particular interest that the tick infection is transmitted transovarially, *i.e.,* passed from the adult tick to the egg; both the larvae and the nymphs are infectious. Thus tularemia may be maintained in the insect population, and tickborne tularemia is an occupational hazard among farm workers in endemic locales.

Tularemia has been found in all parts of the United States, in Japan, and in Central Europe; extensive epidemics have also occurred in Russia. The strains of *F. tularensis* found in North America are generally more virulent than those found in Eurasia, and produce a more severe disease in humans. The incidence of tularemia in the United States since 1955 is shown in Figure 23–8.

Bacteriological Diagnosis[54]

When *F. tularensis* is present in sufficient numbers in exudates and tissues, it can be identified with facility by either direct or indirect fluorescent antibody staining.

Although not always successful, cultural isolation and identification is the best evidence of infection. A variety of clinical specimens are employed, including blood, exudate from the primary lesion, conjunctival scrapings, lymph node aspirates, and sputum. These should be inoculated onto blood-glucose-cysteine agar or enriched chocolate agar, such as Thayer-Martin medium. Characteristic minute, drop-like colonies may appear in one to five days, but a culture should not be recorded as negative in less than three weeks. In the event that cultures are negative, guinea pig inoculations can be performed, provided facilities are adequate for safety of personnel. Infected animals die in 5 to 10 days and exhibit characteristic pathology at autopsy.

Isolated cultures may be identified by serological means, either by agglutination in specific antiserum or by fluorescent antibody microscopy.

It should be noted that *F. tularensis* is a highly virulent microorganism with attendant hazards to laboratory personnel. A number of laboratory accidents have resulted in infections. The use of safety hoods and other precautions is essential.

Serological diagnosis of tularemia is usually reliable. All strains of *Francisella tularensis* are antigenically homogeneous; agglutinins normally appear late in the second week of the disease. Titers of 1:40 or greater in persons not previously infected are significant, but increasing antibody titers are more meaningful. *Francisella tularensis* shares somatic antigens with *Brucella,* so that agglutinin titers should be interpreted with caution.

Chemotherapy

The use of streptomycin, the most effective antibiotic for tularemia, has been credited with marked reduction of the mortality rate. Chemotherapy is complicated, however, by rapid acquisition of streptomycin resistance by *F. tularensis.* The tetracyclines are also effective, but chloramphenicol has only slight activity. Sulfonamides are completely ineffective.

Immunity

An attack of tularemia confers effective immunity, although occasional reinfections have been documented. The relationship of humoral antibodies to immunity is not certain, but evidence implies that they are not protective. A cell-mediated response is evident in man following immunization with attenuated vaccine, and it seems likely that effective immunity is of the cell-mediated type.[27] Humoral response does occur, however, and the presence of serum agglutinins is of importance in diagnosis and serological surveys, as mentioned earlier.

Prophylactic immunization with vaccines of killed organisms has been almost uniformly unsuccessful, presumably because little cell-mediated immunity is induced. A live attenuated vaccine has been used in laboratory personnel, which appears to offer protection against typhoidal tularemia and alters severity of the ulceroglandular type.[8]

Actinobacillus[26]

The microorganisms of the genus *Actinobacillus*, like *Pasteurella* and *Yersinia*, are small, ovoid, gram-negative, facultatively anaerobic bacilli. They are often found associated with actinomyces in certain actinomycotic infections

Actinobacillus lignieresii[54]

This nonmotile, nonbranching, nonacid-fast bacillus causes a disease of cattle resembling actinomycosis, with which it is frequently confused. Originally found in Argentina, *A. lignieresii* appears to be relatively common and has been recognized in Europe and the United States.

Granules, very similar to but smaller and more numerous than the "sulfur granules" of actinomycosis, are found in the thick pus from the lesions. These granules or colonies contain club-like forms radially arranged about a center composed of detritus and gram-negative bacilli. The microorganism is pleomorphic in cultures; coccoid and slender rods are found in smears from cultures in liquid mediums, while long curved forms are present in deep colonies in agar mediums. The bacilli are 0.4 μm. in diameter and 1 to 15 μm. in length.

Surface colonies on laboratory mediums are small, 0.5 to 1 mm. in diameter, smooth, glistening, convex, bluish-white, and delicate in appearance. In liquid mediums, such as serum-glucose broth, the growth consists of small grayish granules adhering to the sides of the tube and readily broken loose by shaking; the broth does not become turbid. The microorganism appears to be a strict parasite and grows very poorly or not at all except in mediums containing serum or whole blood. It is facultatively anaerobic and primary cultures are often more successful in fluid mediums or serum-glucose agar stab cultures, especially when incubated in an atmosphere containing 10 per cent carbon dioxide. Growth is apparent in 24 hours at 37°C., but is very slight at 20°C. Several carbohydrates are fermented with production of acid but no gas; hydrogen sulfide is formed, as is urease, but indol is not produced.

As indicated above, the disease in cattle closely resembles actinomycosis, differing in that the bones are seldom affected and the lesions are found in the soft tissues, the regional lymphatics commonly being involved; the subcutaneous tumors break down in time to form abscesses. The disease has been observed in both epizootic and sporadic form. A few cases of human infection have been reported; these apparently respond well to therapy with a combination of penicillin and streptomycin.

Actinobacillus equuli

This microorganism, very similar to *A. lignieresii*, causes suppurative diseases of horses and swine. It is differentiable from *A. lignieresii* by fermentation reactions and by its host range. The disease in man is indistinguishable from that due to *A. lignieresii*.

Actinobacillus actinomycetemcomitans

This bacillus has been observed and isolated from human cases of mixed infection with *Actinomyces*. It occurs as densely packed, gram-negative coccobacilli, contrasting with the gram-positive actinomycete mycelia in the interior of the sulfur granules. The significance of its presence in these human infections is open to question. In recent years, it has also been responsible for a number of other affections of man, primarily endocarditis, in which it is the sole etiological agent present.[7, 52]

REFERENCES

1. Almeida, C. R., *et al.* 1981. Plague in Brazil during two years of bacteriological and serological surveillance. Bull. Wld Hlth Org. **59**:591–597.
2. Akiev, A. K. 1982. Epidemiology and incidence of plague in the world, 1958–79. Bull. Wld Hlth Org. **60**:165–169.
3. Bölin, I., L. Norlander, and H. Wolf-Watz. 1982. Temperature-inducible outer membrane protein of *Yersinia pseudotuberculosis* and *Yersinia enterocolitica* is associated with the virulence plasmid. Infect. Immun. **37**:506–512.
4. Bouza, E., *et al.* 1980. *Yersinia enterocolitica* septicemia. Amer. J. Clin. Pathol. **74**:404–409.
5. Brown, S. D., and T. C. Montie. 1977. Beta-adrenergic blocking activity of *Yersinia pestis* murine toxin. Infect. Immun. **18**:85–93.
6. Brubaker, R. R. 1972. The genus Yersinia: biochemistry and genetics of virulence. Curr. Topics Microbiol. Immunol. **57**:111–158.
7. Burgher, L. W., G. W. Loomis, and F. Wave. 1973. Systemic infection due to *Actinobacillus actinomycetemcomitans*. Amer. J. Clin. Pathol. **60**:412–415.
8. Burke, D. S. 1977. Immunization against tularemia: analysis of the effectiveness of live *Francisella tularensis* vaccine in prevention of laboratory-acquired tularemia. J. Infect. Dis. **135**:55–60.
9. Butler, T. 1972. A clinical study of bubonic plague. Observations of the 1970 Vietnam epidemic with emphasis on coagulation studies, skin histology and electrocardiograms. Amer. J. Med. **53**:268–276.
10. Butler, T., and B. W. Hudson. 1977. The serological response to *Yersinia pestis* infection. Bull. Wld Hlth Org. **55**:39–42.

11. Carter, P. B., R. J. Zahorchak, and R. R. Brubaker. 1980. Plague virulence antigens from *Yersinia enterocolitica*. Infect. Immun. **28**:638–640.

12. Cavanaugh, D. C., and J. H. Steele (Eds.). 1974. Trends in research on plague immunization. J. Infect. Dis. (Suppl.) **129**:S1–S120.

13. Cavanaugh, D. C., *et al.* 1974. Plague immunization. V. Indirect evidence for the efficacy of plague vaccine. J. Infect Dis. (Suppl.) **129**:S37–S40.

14. Chen, T. H., and S. S. Elberg. 1977. Scanning electron microscope study of virulent *Yersinia pestis* and *Yersinia pseudotuberculosis* type 1. Infect. Immun. **15**:972–977.

15. Chen, T. H., S. S. Elberg, and D. M. Eisler. 1976. Immunity in plague: protection induced in *Cercopithecus aethiops* by oral administration of live, attenuated *Yersinia pestis*. J. Infect. Dis. **133**:302–309.

16. Ganfield, D. J., P. A. Rebers, and K. L. Heddleston. 1976. Immunogenic and toxic properties of a purified lipopolysaccharide-protein complex from *Pasteurella multocida*. Infect. Immun. **14**:990–999.

17. Gärtner, K. 1981. Yersinia-enterocolitica-Infektionen in Südwestdeutschland. Bericht über 580 bakteriologisch nachgewiesene Fälle. Münch. Med. Wochenschrift **123**:1498–1500.

18. Gemski, P., *et al.* 1980. Presence of a virulence-associated plasmid in *Yersinia pseudotuberculosis*. Infect. Immun. **28**:1044–1047.

19. Glosnicka, R., and E. Gruszkiewicz. 1980. Chemical composition and biological activity of the *Yersinia pestis* envelope substance. Infect. Immun. **30**:506–512.

20. Hall, P. J., *et al.* 1974. Effect of Ca^{2+} on morphology and division of *Yersinia pestis*. Infect. Immun. **9**:1105–1113.

21. Haug, R. H., and A. D. Pearson. 1972. Human infections with *Francisella tularensis* in Norway. Development of a serological screening test. Acta Pathol. Microbiol. Scand., Sect. B., **80**:273–280.

22. Highsmith, A. K., J. C. Feeley, and G. K. Morris. 1977. *Yersinia enterocolitica*: a review of the bacterium and recommended laboratory methodology. Hlth Lab. Sci. **14**:253–260.

23. Hubbert, W. T., *et al.* 1971. *Yersinia pseudotuberculosis* infection in the United States. Septicemia, appendicitis and mesenteric lymphadenitis. Amer. J. Trop. Med. Hygiene **20**:679–684.

24. Hudson, B. W., K. Wolff, and T. Butler. 1980. The use of solid-phase radioimmunoassay techniques for serodiagnosis of human plague infection. Bull. Pan Amer. Hlth Org. **14**:244–250.

25. Kaufmann, A. F., J. M. Boyce, and W. J. Martone. 1980. Trends in human plague in the United States. J. Infect. Dis. **141**:522–524.

26. Kilian, M., W. Frederiksen, and E. L. Biberstein. 1981. Haemophilus, Pasteurella, and Actinobacillus. Academic Press, London.

27. Koskela, P., and E. Herva. 1982. Cell-mediated and humoral immunity induced by a live *Francisella tularensis* vaccine. Infect. Immun. **36**:983–989.

28. Leino, R. 1981. Incidence of yersiniosis in Finland. Scand. J. Infect. Dis. **13**:309–310.

29. Mäki, M., *et al.* 1980. Yersiniosis in children. Arch. Dis. Childh. **55**:861–865.

30. Mann, J. M. 1979. Plague pneumonia. New Engl. J. Med. **300**:1276–1277.

31. Mann, J. M., *et al.* 1979. Endemic human plague in New Mexico: risk factors associated with infection. J. Infect. Dis. **140**:397–401.

32. Mann, J. M., *et al.* 1982. Peripatetic plague. J. Amer. Med. Assn **247**:47–48.

33. Martin, W. J., and J. A. Washington, II. 1980. *Enterobacteriaceae.* pp. 195–219. *In* E. H. Lennette, *et al.* (Eds.): Manual of Clinical Microbiology. 3rd ed. American Society for Microbiology, Washington, D.C.

34. Miller, R. P., and J. H. Bates. 1969. Pleuropulmonary tularemia. A review of 29 patients. Amer. Rev. Resp. Dis. **99**:31–41.

35. Montie, T. C., and S. J. Ajl. 1970. Nature and synthesis of murine toxins of *Pasteurella pestis*. pp. 1–37. *In* T. C. Montie, S. Kadis, and S. J. Ajl (Eds.): Microbial Toxins. Vol. III, Bacterial Protein Toxins. Academic Press, New York.

36. Montie, T. C., D. B. Montie, and D. Wennerstrom. 1975. Aspects of the structure and biological activity of plague murine toxin. pp. 278–282. *In* D. Schlessinger (Ed.): Microbiology—1975. American Society for Microbiology, Washington, D. C.

37. Okamoto, K., *et al.* 1981. Partial purification and characterization of heat-stable enterotoxin produced by *Yersinia enterocolitica*. Infect. Immun. **31**:554–559.

38. Okamoto, K., *et al.* 1982. Further purification and characterization of heat-stable enterotoxin produced by *Yersinia enterocolitica*. Infect. Immun. **35**:958–964.

39. Paff, J. R., D. A. Triplett, and T. N. Saari. 1976. Clinical and laboratory aspects of *Yersinia pseudotuberculosis* infections, with a report of two cases. Amer. J. Clin. Pathol. **66**:101–110.

40. Pai, C. H., and L. DeStephano. 1982. Serum resistance associated with virulence in *Yersinia enterocolitica*. Infect. Immun. **35**:605–611.

41. Pollitzer, R. 1954. Plague. Wld Hlth Org. Monogr. Ser., No. 22. Geneva.

42. Pollitzer, R. 1960. A review of recent literature on plague. Bull. Wld Hlth Org. **23**:313–400.

43. Ratnam, S., *et al.* 1982. A nosocomial outbreak of diarrheal disease due to *Yersinia enterocolitica* serotype O:5, biotype 1. J. Infect. Dis. **145**:242–247.

44. Report. 1970. WHO Expert Committee on Plague. Fourth report. Wld Hlth Org. Techn. Rep. Ser., No. 447. Geneva.

45. Robins-Brown, R. M., *et al.* 1979. Mechanism of action of *Yersinia enterocolitica* enterotoxin. Infect. Immun. **25**:680–684.

46. Schiemann, D. A., and J. A. Devenish. 1982. Relationship of HeLa cell infectivity to biochemical, serological, and virulence characteristics of *Yersinia enterocolitica*. Infect. Immun. **35**:497–506.

47. Schricker, R. L., *et al.* 1972. Pathogenesis of tularemia in monkeys aerogenically exposed to *Francisella tularensis* 425. Infect. Immun. **5**:734–744.

48. Straley, S. C., and R. R. Brubaker. 1982. Localization in *Yersinia pestis* of peptides associated with virulence. Infect. Immun. **36**:129–135.

49. Surgalla, M. J., E. D. Beesley, and J. M. Albizo. 1970. Practical application of new laboratory methods for plague investigations. Bull. Wld Hlth Org. **42**:993–997.

50. Swaminathan, B., M. C. Harmon, and I. J. Mehlman. 1982. A review. *Yersinia enterocolitica*. J. Appl. Bacteriol. **52**:151–183.

51. Une, T. 1977. Studies on the pathogenicity of *Yersinia enterocolitica*. I. Experimental infection in rabbits. II. Interaction with cultured cells *in vitro*. Microbiol. Immunol. **21**:349–363; 365–377.

52. Vandepitte, J., H. De Geest, and P. Jousten. 1977.

Subacute bacterial endocarditis due to *Actinobacillus actinomycetemcomitans*. Report of a case with a review of the literature. J. Clin. Pathol. **30**:842–846.

53. Walker, R. I. 1972. Detection of an endotoxin-like substance during human plague bacteremia. S. E. Asian J. Trop. Med. Publ. Hlth **3**:221–224.

54. Weaver, R. E., and D. G. Hollis. 1980. Gram-negative fermentative bacteria and *Francisella tularensis*. pp. 242–262. *In* E. H. Lennette, *et al.* (Eds.):

Manual of Clinical Microbiology. 3rd ed. American Society for Microbiology, Washington, D.C.

55. Williams, J. E., *et al.* 1982. Comparison of passive haemagglutination and enzyme-linked immunosorbent assay for serodiagnosis of plague. Bull. Wld Hlth Org. **60**:777–781.

56. Woolcock, J. B., and F. M. Collins. 1976. Immune mechanisms in *Pasteurella multocida*–infected mice. Infect. Immun. **13**:949–958.

Haemophilus and Bordetella

Haemophilus[1, 16, 34]

The genus *Haemophilus* is made up of a group of bacilli characterized by a nutritional affinity for constituents of fresh blood, including hemoglobin and related compounds, termed X factor; and heat-labile substances, probably NAD or NADP, called V factor. The requirement for one or both of these blood factors is a primary differential character for speciation of *Haemophilus*.

The hemophilic bacilli are facultatively anaerobic, small, gram-negative rods, usually coccoid in shape, but pleomorphism is common and is often manifest as filamentous and other aberrant shapes. Their taxonomic position is not yet certain; they are placed in the group of gram-negative, facultatively anaerobic bacilli along with the families Enterobacteriaceae and Vibrionaceae (Chapter 2). Seventeen species of *Haemophilus* are recognized; some are pathogenic for humans, others appear as part of the normal oral flora, while still others are found almost exclusively in animals. Table 24–1 lists those of medical importance along with their principal characteristics.

HAEMOPHILUS INFLUENZAE[15]

Haemophilus influenzae was isolated by Pfeiffer in 1892 and, until the early 1930s, was regarded by many as the etiological agent of epidemic influenza, since it was often found associated with that disease. Influenza is, however, caused by a virus, and *H. influenzae* is considered to be a secondary invader; the name influenzae has no etiological significance.

Morphology and Staining

The bacillus is one of the smaller pathogenic bacteria, rarely exceeding 1.5 μm. in length and 0.3 μm. in diameter. The ends of the cell are rounded; capsules, while not generally seen by microscopy, are present in smooth cultures. Pili are produced by most *H. influenzae;* these are responsible for hemagglutination of human type O erythrocytes and probably are responsible for oropharyngeal adherence and colonization.[13] Spores are not formed, and the bacilli are nonmotile. There is a marked tendency to produce filamentous and other anomalous cells

531

Table 24–1. **Principal Differential Characters of** *Haemophilus*

| Species | Growth Requirements | | | Catalase | Oxidase | Urease | Hemolysis |
	X Factor	V Factor	CO_2*				
H. influenzae	+	+	−	+	+	V†	−
H. haemolyticus	+	+	−	+	+	+	+
H. parainfluenzae	−	+	−	V	+	−	−
H. ducreyi	+	−	−	−	−	−	−
H. (Gardnerella) vaginalis	−	−	−	−	−	−	+
H. aphrophilus	+	−	+	−	−	−	−
H. aegyptius	+	+	−	−	+	+	−

*Increased (5 per cent) CO_2 required for growth.
†V = variable reaction.

in culture which is, to some degree, a characteristic of strains. Strains isolated from pathological processes are usually predominantly in the coccobacillary form, as shown in Figure 24–1; most workers regard these as "typical" and the longer, filamentous forms as "atypical."

On rabbit blood agar the colonies of *H. influenzae* are very small, rounded, discrete, and transparent, and may reach the size of a small pinhead. On Levinthal's medium, which contains blood extract, the colonies are somewhat larger, opaque, and flattened, and are iridescent when observed by oblique light. When blood agar is contaminated with other microorganisms, especially staphylococci, the colonies of *H. influenzae* in the vicinity of the contaminant may be considerably larger, more opaque, and of a grayish-white color, a phenomenon termed **"satellitism."**

These bacilli are somewhat more difficult to stain than are most bacteria; Loeffler's methylene blue for 5 minutes or dilute carbolfuchsin for 10 minutes is satisfactory. The bacilli are gram-negative.

Physiology

One of the more fastidious bacteria, *H. influenzae* requires, as noted above, the presence of blood in the culture medium. It has been found that two substances in blood are necessary to their growth: one, designated **X factor,** is heat-stable and associated with hemoglobin, and the second, **V factor,** is heat-labile and is found in yeast and various vegetable extracts as well as in whole blood. The satellite phenomenon noted above is due to the formation of this factor by other bacteria and its diffusion from the colony into the V factor–deficient medium.

The X factor of blood can be replaced by hemoglobin or heme. The iron protoporphyrins, or related compounds, are required for synthesis of enzymes involved in aerobic respiration; thus, some strains do not require X factor for anaerobic growth. It has been sug-

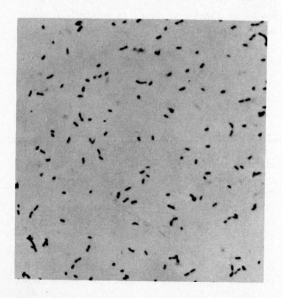

Figure 24–1. *Haemophilus influenzae,* pure culture. Note the variability from coccoid to bacillary form and the presence of longer filaments. Fuchsin; × 1050.

gested that heme is required for synthesis of catalase and can be replaced by cysteine, which would reduce peroxide and make catalase unnecessary.

The V factor may be replaced by NAD or NADP but not by nicotinic acid or its amide. Apparently the whole coenzyme molecule must be supplied, and it is assumed that this is the thermolabile substance represented by the V factor. Other growth requirements include pantothenic acid, thiamin, and uracil; some strains also require purine. Defined mediums will support the growth of some strains.

A number of mediums in addition to blood agar have been devised for the cultivation of these bacilli. Among the best of these for primary isolation is that of Levinthal. Levinthal's medium, as noted above, contains an extract of blood and supports good growth; it has the advantage of transparency. Blood agar, when prepared with rabbit blood, is satisfactory, but sheep and human blood are inhibitory for these bacilli and cannot be recommended. The bacillus grows luxuriantly on chocolate agar prepared by the addition of fresh blood to hot (90° C.) infusion agar, and yields heavy growth for agglutination and other purposes. Supplemented chocolate agar, with bacitracin to inhibit contaminants, is useful in primary isolation.

The optimum temperature for growth is 37° C. Growth is best under aerobic conditions, but the organism is facultatively anaerobic; some strains do not require X factor for anaerobic growth. Nitrate is reduced to nitrite. Some strains—about 50 per cent—form indole. Fermentation reactions are variable, some strains being inactive, while others ferment glucose and other carbohydrates. Biotypes are separated, based on the production of indole, urease, and ornithine decarboxylase.

The influenza bacillus shows little resistance to unfavorable environmental conditions. It is readily killed by drying and usually does not survive longer than 48 hours in dried sputum; it is destroyed by heating at 55° C. for one-half hour and by disinfectants. Even under favorable conditions, laboratory cultures soon die, but viability can be maintained by frequent subculture on chocolate agar. They may also be preserved by lyophilization or storage in the ultrafreezer.

Antigenic Structure

As tested by direct agglutination, *H. influenzae* is antigenically heterogeneous, and both rough and smooth forms occur; the smooth form is encapsulated and virulent. By means of the agglutination test, smooth encapsulated bacilli fall into six immunological types, designated a, b, c, d, e, and f; the surface antigens responsible are specific polysaccharides. One of these, the specific polysaccharide of type b, is a polyribose phosphate, containing ribose, ribitol, and phosphate as the principal constituents.[2] Diagnostically useful antiserums may be prepared for each of the *H. influenzae* types. Antigenic typing of these encapsulated strains may be accomplished by agglutination, by specific capsular swelling, by precipitin reaction using extracted polysaccharides, or by counterimmunoelectrophoresis.[23] Serotyping is of considerable practical importance, since almost all human infections are due to type b strains.

Many strains, even when freshly isolated, are in the rough, nonencapsulated state. By the agglutination test such strains are antigenically heterogeneous; the complete antigenic structure of *H. influenzae* has not yet been elucidated.

Influenza bacilli are immunologically related to several other microorganisms. Antiserum to type a, for example, reacts with the pneumococcal polysaccharide of type 6b; antiserum to type b also reacts with pneumococcus types 6 and 29 and with a variety of gram-positive bacteria that contain polyribitol-phosphate in their cell wall teichoic acids.[3]

Toxins

As in the case of many other bacteria, the cell substance of the influenza bacillus is toxic to experimental animals, mice in particular, upon parenteral inoculation. Toxic substances are produced in fluid cultures, are filterable, and may appear in appreciable quantities after six to eight hours' incubation. Similar culture filtrates, when used to treat tracheal organ cultures derived from rats, chick embryo, and human fetus, cause ciliostasis and epithelial cell damage.[6] It is possible that these toxic effects are due to endotoxin and that a true exotoxin is not formed.

MENINGITIS[5, 10, 19]

The pathogenicity of *H. influenzae* for man is well demonstrated by the occurrence of cases, most often in infants, of highly fatal meningitis. *Haemophilus influenzae* is apparently the sole invader and is found in pure culture in cerebrospinal fluid. Meningitis due to this microorganism is the most common form of septic meningitis, and almost all of these infections are due to type b. The disease occurs most often in children under two years of age. Prior to the 1960s, infections in infants under six months of age were not common, due to maternally transferred, bactericidal antibodies. Many mothers now lack such antibodies, with the result that their offspring are not protected at birth. It has been suggested that neonates are infected by the natural vaginal flora during birth.[24]

The long-term sequelae of *H. influenzae* meningitis are of serious concern. In survivors, perhaps as many as one-third exhibit **neurological** or **psychological sequelae,** including deafness, speech impairment, and behavioral anomalies, while a smaller proportion may be so seriously affected as to require custodial care.

Although *H. influenzae* was first isolated from cases of influenza and has been observed in a large proportion of cases, its relationship to this disease is that of a secondary invader. Indeed, in most respiratory infections, at least in adults, it seems probable that *H. influenzae* is rarely a primary agent of the disease. Moreover, experimental infections in animals indicate that viral respiratory infections can favor the development of *Haemophilus* meningitis.

While most infections are due to type b, other serotypes are sometimes involved and, on occasion, unencapsulated (untypable) strains may be responsible. Several of the *Haemophilus* species are found as normal oral flora in humans, and are rare causes of endocarditis. The normal inhabitants include both unencapsulated and encapsulated *H. influenzae* (other than type b), *H. haemolyticus*, *H. aphrophilus,* and *H. parainfluenzae.*

The exceptional virulence exhibited by type b strains as compared to other capsular serotypes is of interest, not only as it relates to pathogenesis but to humoral immunity as well. It appears that virulence of type b strains depends upon their resistance to the bactericidal effect of complement, so that they are not cleared from the tissues in unimmunized individuals.[31] Other serotypes, on the other hand, are sensitive to the action of complement, so that they are rapidly eliminated, even in the absence of specific antibody.[4]

Other Manifestations. While most infections with *H. influenzae* are manifest as meningitis, other clinical entities have been described that indicate the broad pathogenic potential of these bacilli. *Haemophilus influenzae* bacteremia has been observed in children, mostly occurring in those under 5 years, with epiglottitis as a common and serious clinical feature.[30] Occasional cases of pneumonia, cellulitis, septic arthritis, otitis media, and genitourinary and other localized infections may be caused by this bacterium.

Carriers

Individuals recovered from clinical infection with *H. influenzae* may remain nasopharyngeal carriers with a frequency of perhaps 2 to 5 per cent. As in meningococcal infections, the carrier rate is many times higher during localized epidemics. For example, in a closed population of children in a chronic disease ward, 24 per cent were found to carry *H. influenzae* type b, in spite of high levels of specific antibodies.[8] A high carrier rate in families also may presage the appearance of acute infection among its members.[33]

Immunity

Immunity to *H. influenzae* type b infections appears to be at least partially **type specific,** *i.e.,* associated with antibodies to the specific capsular polysaccharide. Antibody to the capsular polysaccharide of type b is responsible for complement activation and leads to bactericidal and opsonic activity. Thus, antibodies against the type b capsular substance could be expected to lead to immunity to most *H. influenzae* infections, since these are largely due to type b. Transient nasopharyngeal carriage or trivial respiratory infections with *H. influenzae* induces bactericidal antibody, and many adults possess such serum bactericidins.

As shown in field trials, immunization with type b polysaccharide vaccine induces a serum antibody response; the resulting immunity reduces the incidence of invasive disease. Unfortunately, the response does not regularly appear in children less than 18 months of age, so that a major high-risk group cannot be protected in this way.[26]

Recent investigations in animal models suggest that noncapsular antigens of the *H. influenzae* outer membrane can induce protective antibodies, thus offering some hope that vaccination is possible for human infants.[18]

Bacteriological Diagnosis[15]

Haemophilus influenzae in cerebrospinal fluid can often be detected and typed by direct microscopic examination. The spinal fluid should be centrifuged to concentrate the bacteria, which can then be gram-stained and typed with specific antiserum using the capsular swelling technique. Direct microscopic examination of other clinical specimens is not generally informative.

Blood, cerebrospinal fluid, or other clinical

specimens should be cultured directly on isolation mediums, since *H. influenzae* viability is rapidly lost upon drying or chilling. Both blood agar and supplemented chocolate agar should be inoculated. Sheep blood agar is inhibitory, but rabbit, guinea pig, or horse blood is satisfactory. Levinthal's medium is particularly recommended for culture of spinal fluid. The influenza bacillus grows as tiny dew-drop colonies with a bluish sheen; encapsulated strains show a characteristic iridescence on Levinthal's agar. Many laboratories employ the satellite phenomenon as a tentative identification scheme, by cross-inoculation with a streak of staphylococcus culture.

Isolates are identified by physiological characters such as those shown in Table 24–1. Serological typing is by agglutination or capsular swelling in the presence of type-specific antiserum.

Rapid diagnosis of *H. influenzae* infections is also possible by demonstrating the type-specific capsular polysaccharide in body fluids of infected individuals. Such tests are complex, however, and not usually available in clinical laboratories.

Chemotherapy

Chemotherapy has been of greatest interest in connection with meningitis, which in untreated cases is almost always fatal. Penicillin is not effective, but ampicillin, chloramphenicol, and tetracycline usually are. For several years ampicillin has been the drug of choice, but increased incidence of β-lactamase–producing, resistant strains prompts alternative use of chloramphenicol and tetracycline, antibiotics which appear to be of about equal efficacy.[7]

HAEMOPHILUS DUCREYI[14, 21]

Soft chancre or **chancroid** is a venereal disease transmitted by direct contact. The lesions, which are on the genitals or adjacent areas, are irregular ulcers which differ from the hard or Hunterian chancre—the primary lesion of syphilis—in that they are not indurated. Unlike syphilis, the infection remains localized, spreading no further than the neighboring lymphatics, which may become swollen to form secondary buboes in the groin.

The bacillus was found by Ducrey in 1890 in the purulent discharge from the lesion; he was able to transmit the disease by inoculating the skin of the forearm. The microorganism was obtained in pure culture by Besançon, Griffon, and le Sourd in the same year.

Ducrey's bacillus, *H. ducreyi,* is a short rod 1 to 1.5 μm. in length and 0.6 μm. in breadth. In smears from lesions it is generally ovoid, with a tendency to occur in parallel arrays; in broth culture longer chains may be observed. It is nonspore-forming and nonmotile. The bacillus frequently stains irregularly, and bipolar staining is often observed. It is stained by the usual aniline dyes and is gram-negative.

The bacillus is difficult to cultivate, growing only slowly on the most complex medium. For isolation from genital lesions or buboes, supplemented chocolate agar or rabbit blood agar, made selective with vancomycin, appears to support growth, but some strains may require incubation for up to 10 days; *H. ducreyi* requires X, but not V, factor. Cultures should be incubated under increased CO_2 tension; growth is improved by incubation at 33° C. Colonies are usually small, yellow-gray, and translucent. Identification is by physiological characters, as shown in Table 24–1.

There is little or no immunity in man. The chancroid is frequently multiple and is autoinoculable. Hypersensitivity, demonstrable as a reaction to the intradermal inoculation of killed bacilli, persists for many years. The disease may be successfully treated with the common drugs, with the exception of penicillin; chlortetracycline is regarded by many as the drug of choice, and streptomycin has given excellent results.

HAEMOPHILUS AEGYPTIUS

A small bacillus, first observed by Koch in Egypt in 1883, was successfully cultivated by Weeks in New York in 1887. Casually known as the Koch-Weeks bacillus, it is the etiological agent of a worldwide and highly contagious form of **conjunctivitis,** sometimes known as pinkeye. The disease occurs especially in tropical and subtropical climates and may assume epidemic form.

This bacillus is gram-negative, nonmotile, nonencapsulated, and sometimes shows bipolar staining. It is facultatively aerobic and requires both the X and V factors for growth. There is no hemolysis on blood agar, and the colonies are small and translucent, with a bluish tinge in transmitted light.

The Koch-Weeks bacillus is closely related to *H. influenzae* and has been regarded by some as a biotype of *H. influenzae,* since some

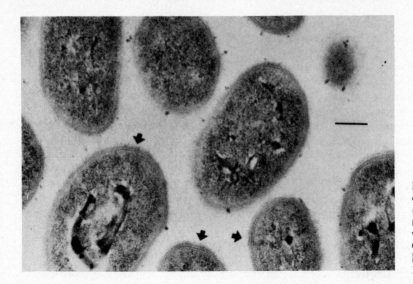

Figure 24–2. Electron micrograph of a thin section of *Haemophilus (Gardnerella) vaginalis*. Note the multilaminate nature of the cell wall (arrows). Bar = 50 nm. J. R. Greenwood, and M. J. Pickett, Internat. J. Syst. Bacteriol. **30:** 170, 1980.)

antigenic components are shared with this bacillus. These organisms, however, make up a closely related but heterogeneous serological group, distinct from nontypable *H. influenzae.* They are differentiated as *H. aegyptius.*

Haemophilus aegyptius produces conjunctivitis in man but not in laboratory animals. It has low virulence for mice and is highly virulent for 8-day, but not 12-day, chick embryos.

HAEMOPHILUS (GARDNERELLA) VAGINALIS[21, 27]

First described in 1953, the microorganism known for many years as *Haemophilus vaginalis* has been associated with **nonspecific human vaginitis.** The taxonomic position of *H. vaginalis* has been controversial for some time. Its classification as *Haemophilus* cannot be defended, nor can its classification as *Corynebacterium,* recommended by some, be accepted. A recent proposal[11] to transfer it to a new genus as *Gardnerella vaginalis* is gaining acceptance. It is placed here because many workers still use the *Haemophilus* classification.

The bacillus is small, nonencapsulated, nonmotile, and variable by Gram stain. Young cultures appear gram-positive, while older cultures are gram-negative; the cell wall shares many structural characteristics with gram-positive microorganisms, as shown in Figure 24–2.

It is somewhat more exacting in nutritive requirements than most other *Haemophilus* species, and grows best in the presence of blood. It does not, however, require either X or V factors. On primary isolation, it may be cultured on rich blood agar mediums incubated in an atmosphere of 5 per cent CO_2; colonies exhibit a diffuse β-hemolysis. *Haemophilus vaginalis* is biochemically inactive, exhibiting the physiological characters listed in Table 24–1.

The bacilli can be observed in stained smears of vaginal exudates, often attached to the surface of vaginal epithelial cells.

The bacilli are believed to stand in causal relationship to nonspecific vaginitis, either alone or in combination with vaginal anaerobes.

Bordetella

The *Bordetella* are a group of minute coccobacilli that superficially resemble *Haemophilus* and, at one time, were classified with them. They do not, however, require either X or V factors, although their growth is stimulated by blood because it reverses the toxicity of medium constituents. Unlike *Haemophilus,* *Bordetella* are strict aerobes. Three species of *Bordetella* are recognized; their salient characters are listed in Table 24–2. *Bordetella pertussis* is the predominant human pathogen, causing pertussis, or whooping cough; *B. par-*

Table 24–2. **Important Characters of Bordetella**

Species	Motility	Urease	Citrate Utilization	Nitrate Reduction	Growth On	
					Peptone Agar	Bordet-Gengou Agar
Bordetella pertussis	−	−	−	−	−	+*
Bordetella parapertussis	−	+	+	−	+†	+
Bordetella bronchiseptica	+	+	+	+	+	+

*Delayed, apparent only after 3 to 5 days.
†Medium becomes brown.

apertussis causes similar human infections. *Bordetella bronchiseptica* is found in animals, but only rarely causes human infections.

BORDETELLA PERTUSSIS

Bacilli resembling *H. influenzae* were reported by early observers as occurring in a large proportion of cases of whooping cough. A definitive description was provided in 1908 by Bordet and Gengou, who found in the bronchial exudate from whooping cough patients a characteristic short oval bacillus which grew feebly on a special medium they devised. The microorganism is known as *Bordetella pertussis* or, more casually, as the Bordet-Gengou bacillus.

Morphology and Staining

The Bordet-Gengou bacillus is a small ovoid rod from 0.5 to 1.0 μm. in length and 0.2 to 0.3 μm. in diameter. The majority of the bacteria occur singly, although they may occasionally be seen in pairs end to end; chains do not occur in smears of bronchial exudate, but short chains may be seen in liquid cultures. Their morphology is relatively constant, and there is not the tendency to the formation of thread-like and other aberrant forms exhibited by the influenza bacillus. *Bordetella pertussis* is nonmotile and nonspore-forming. The smooth form is encapsulated, but special stains are required for demonstration.

On the medium of Bordet and Gengou, the colonies are smooth, raised, and glistening, with a slightly metallic or pearl-like luster, and are larger and more opaque than are those of *H. influenzae;* incubation for 72 hours or more is required for their appearance and development. Upon further incubation they acquire a slight brownish color. A mucoid substance is abundantly produced by the culture, and growth is sticky and tenacious. On blood agar the colonies are surrounded by a narrow zone of hazy hemolysis.

While the bacilli are gram-negative, they usually stain poorly with the safranin counterstain. As in the case of *H. influenzae,* they may be stained with methylene blue or dilute carbol-fuchsin applied for 5 to 10 minutes. There is some tendency to bipolar staining.

Physiology

Bordetella pertussis is difficult to cultivate upon primary isolation. It can be grown on the Bordet-Gengou medium, which contains glycerol, potato extract, and up to 50 per cent defibrinated blood. The bacilli do not require the X and V factors that are essential to the development of *Haemophilus,* but blood serves to overcome the toxicity of fatty acids and other common medium constituents. The optimum temperature is 37° C., and the bacillus is strictly aerobic.

Bordetella pertussis is biochemically inactive. It does not form indol, does not reduce nitrates, and does not ferment any sugars. Its resistance is slight and of the same order as that of the influenza bacillus. It is, for example, killed by exposure to 55° C. for 30 minutes.

Bacilli somewhat different from *B. pertussis* have been isolated from a small proportion of whooping cough cases and are designated *B. parapertussis.* Unlike *B. pertussis* they grow readily on ordinary nutrient agar on primary isolation; other differences are listed in Table 24–2.

Toxins[28]

In the pathogenesis of whooping cough, the bacteria adhere to the ciliated epithelium and multiply at this location without invasion of tissues. Yet, profound biological changes in tissues accompany this colonization, many of which persist long after the responsible bacteria have been cleared. Observations of this kind suggested even to the earliest workers that microbial toxic products were involved in pathogenesis. In the intervening years at least three toxic products have been identified: (1) lipopolysaccharide, or endotoxin; (2) a heat-labile toxin described by Bordet and Gengou; and (3) pertussis toxin, exhibiting a variety of biological effects.

As in other gram-negative bacteria, **endotoxin** is present in the cell envelope. It is heat-stable and similar to classic endotoxins in pharmacological activity (Chapter 12). Antibodies to this lipopolysaccharide are specifically bactericidal to *B. pertussis* in the presence of complement, and these may behave as protective antibodies; the endotoxin probably does not play a role in pathogenesis of disease.

The **heat-labile toxin** is a protein, inactivated by heating at 56° C. It is found within the cell cytoplasm and is not spontaneously released from the cell. It apparently is present in the cell as a precursor and must be activated for toxicity to occur. Heat-labile toxin is convertible to toxoid, which is immunogenic and induces neutralizing antitoxin. Curiously, native toxin does not induce antitoxin. Heat-labile toxin, when released from lysed cells, is dermonecrotic and lethal. It has been implicated in the pathogenesis of whooping cough, but it apparently does not function as a protective antigen.

Most of the harmful effects in whooping cough appear to be attributable to a single protein exotoxin, termed **pertussis toxin** by Pittman. The biological manifestations of pertussis toxin include increased susceptibility to histamine, serotonin, and endotoxin (histamine-sensitizing factor, HSF); metabolic alterations (islet-activating toxin, IAP); and increased lymphocytic response (lymphocytosis-promoting factor, LPF). Although described independently, these activities reside in a single toxic entity. Pertussis toxin is (1) intermediate in heat stability, being inactivated at 80° C.; (2) convertible to toxoid by treatment with formaldehyde; and (3) neutralized by homologous antitoxin. Pertussis toxin is believed to be one of the major protective antigens in *B. pertussis*, and is responsible for the long-term immunity in whooping cough.

Variation and Antigenic Structure

Bordetella pertussis is generally in the smooth state when isolated from cases of whooping cough on optimal mediums. These freshly isolated, virulent strains are designated **phase I** and are presumed to be encapsulated. All *Bordetella* species share a common heat-stable O antigen (lipopolysaccharide), but the surface antigens responsible for agglutination reactions of smooth strains are thermolabile K antigens; these determine the serological reactivity of encapsulated phase I *Bordetella*. The

capsular antigen factors are designated by arabic numerals. Antigen factor 7 is common to all *Bordetella;* it is, therefore, a genus-specific antigen and is responsible for cross-reactions within the genus. The species specific antigen for *B. pertussis* is factor 1; serotypes are distinguished by two additional factors, 2 and 3. Recognized serotypes are 1,2,3; 1,2; and 1,3. The species specific antigen for *B. parapertussis* is factor 14, while that for *B. bronchiseptica* is factor 12.

Upon prolonged laboratory culture, even on blood agar, there appears to be a progressive loss of these surface K antigens; such strains have been designated **phases II, III,** and **IV.** These phases probably represent early stages in the S–R transformation. Although not obviously rough, phases III and IV strains have slightly altered colonial morphology and are less stable in saline suspension than phase I bacilli. These changes proceed to the obviously rough state with further alterations in colonial morphology, complete loss of capsular antigens, and loss of virulence.

Virulent strains of *B. pertussis* possess an additional surface antigen that agglutinates erythrocytes—termed **filamentous hemagglutinin**—and is likely an adhesin for attachment to ciliated host cells.

WHOOPING COUGH

Whooping cough is of worldwide occurrence, and it is estimated that a large proportion of the population suffer from it, in typical or atypical form, at one time or another. The typical disease is commonest in the lower age groups and is much more serious in children than in adults. Atypical and mild infections are more frequent than typical cases.

After an incubation period of about one week, the disease appears in three stages. The **catarrhal stage,** which lasts for about two weeks, begins with a mild cough and symptoms of an ordinary respiratory infection. It progresses in severity to a **paroxysmal stage** of 4 to 6 weeks' duration, characterized by rapid consecutive coughs and the deep inspiratory whoop. In the **convalescent stage** the number and frequency of paroxysms gradually decrease, and recovery is uneventful except that bronchial and lobar pneumonia and otitis media arise as complications, especially in children. Concurrent infections are frequent and in these patients the disease tends to be more severe. There is evidence, too, that adenovirus infections are reactivated by pertussis. The bacilli are present in large numbers in the respiratory tract in the catarrhal, and most contagious, stage and gradually disappear until they are rarely found after the fifth week.

Infection begins when *B. pertussis* attaches to the ciliated cells of the trachea (Figs. 24–3 and 24–4) and multiply in the ciliary spaces during the catarrhal stage. **Adherence** to the cilia and microvilli is by bacterial adhesins, possibly the hemagglutinins mentioned earlier. Pathological changes at the site of infection are minimal and temporary and do not result in invasion of tissues, although there may be mechanical interference with ciliary activity. It is likely that **systemic effects** in pertussis are mediated by toxic principles elaborated by the colonizing bacteria. The multiple biological activities ascribed to pertussis toxin make it the most likely candidate as the major toxin, accounting for many of the symptoms observed in whooping cough. Heat-labile toxin and endotoxic lipopolysaccharide may also contribute to the disease picture. The localization of the bacteria and especially the persistence of the paroxysmal cough after the bacteria are no longer detectable argue for the role of toxin in pathogenesis.

Many of these aspects of human disease are supported by observations in animal models, particularly organ cultures of chick and hamster tracheal rings. In this model, bacilli preferentially attach to the ciliated epithelial cells and induce cellular injury, as exemplified by ciliostasis with subsequent extrusion and loss of the ciliated cells from the epithelial layer. A bacterial product putatively responsible for these effects has recently been reported.[9] Nonciliated cells are not affected and there is no apparent injury to the epithelium. These effects are shown in Figure 24–5.

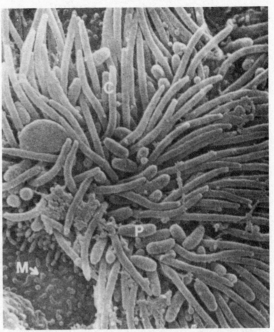

Figure 24–4. Scanning electron micrograph of *Bordetella pertussis (P)* infecting ciliated respiratory epithelial cells from a germ-free mouse 7 days after aerosol inhalation of a phase I strain. *C*, cilia; *M*, microvilli. (Y. Sato, *et al.,* Infect. Immun. **29**:261, 1980.)

Epidemiology

As a highly communicable upper respiratory infection, whooping cough is transmitted from infected cases by droplet infection, by fomites contaminated with nasal and oral secretions, and by direct contact. Control is complicated by the fact that communicability is greatest when the bacilli are present in greatest numbers in the passages of the upper respiratory tract, *i.e.*, during the catarrhal and early paroxysmal stages, when the disease is poorly recognized as such. Undiagnosed and atypical cases thus play an important role in the dissemination of the disease. The **age incidence** is marked, with almost all cases occurring in children. Sixty-two per cent of the cases in the United States in 1981 were in children less than one year of age. The incidence and mortality of whooping cough in this country between 1928 and 1981 are shown in Figure 24–6. Epidemiological studies on the prevalence of serotypes of *B. pertussis* have revealed a shift in recent years. The most prevalent type worldwide appears to be type 1,3, whereas in many areas prior to 1960, type 1,2 was most often encountered.[29]

Bacteriological Diagnosis[25]

Specimens for isolation and identification of *B. pertussis* are collected on nasopharyngeal

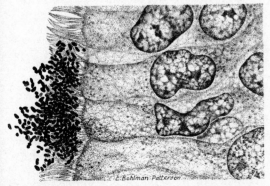

Figure 24–3. Whooping cough. Minute bacilli present in masses between cilia of two cells lining the trachea. About × 1500.

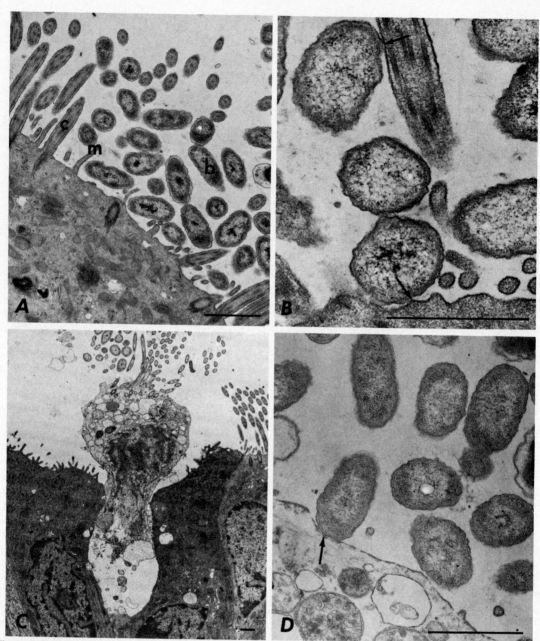

Figure 24–5. Electron micrographs of hamster trachea in organ culture infected with *Bordetella pertussis. A,* Luminal border of ciliated epithelial cell 24 hours postinfection. Bacteria *(b)* are located between cilia *(c)* and microvilli *(m). B,* Higher magnification showing close adherence of bacterial cells. *C,* Ciliated cells being extruded from epithelial layer 48 hours postinfection. Note normal ultrastructure of adjacent nonciliated cells. *D,* Higher magnification shows bacterial cells adherent to the degenerating ciliated cell. Bar = 1 μm. (A. M. Collier, L. F. Peterson, and J. B. Baseman, J. Infect. Dis. [Suppl.] **136:**S196, 1977.)

swabs; pernasal swabs give a higher proportion of positive cultures than postnasal. The swab, on thin flexible wire, is passed through the nostril into the nasopharynx and left there for two or three coughs before withdrawal. The specimen is inoculated onto Bordet-Gengou medium, both plain and containing antibiotics. Direct culture is recommended, but if trans-

port is required, casein hydrolysate medium may be employed. After inoculation of plates, swabs should be emulsified in casein hydrolysate medium and then examined for *B. pertussis* by direct immunofluorescent microscopy.

Colonies of *B. pertussis* on Bordet-Gengou medium appear after several days and are small, raised, glistening, and gray-white; they

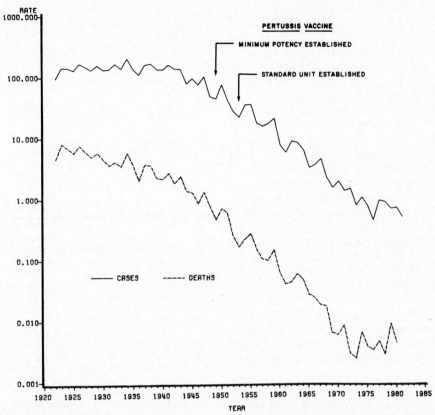

Figure 24–6. Incidence and mortality of whooping cough in the United States from 1922 to 1981. Rates shown are per 100,000 population. Most cases occur in children under one year of age. (Centers for Disease Control. Annual Summary 1981: reported morbidity and mortality in the United States. Morbidity and Mortality Weekly Report **30**, 1982.)

are often described as resembling a bisected pearl. They are larger and more opaque than those of *H. influenzae* and may be differentiated by hemolysis and growth in the absence of X and V factors. Suspicious colonies are picked for Gram stain and for serological identification by fluorescent-antibody staining. Physiological tests (Table 24–2) aid in the differentiation of *Bordetella* species.

Chemotherapy[32]

The chemotherapy of whooping cough is not so successful as that of many other infectious bacterial diseases, since the elimination of the pathogen does not always result in rapid clinical improvement. Nevertheless, antibiotic therapy reduces the severity and duration of the illness as well as eliminating secondary invaders in the respiratory tract. Antibiotics usually employed include chloramphenicol, ampicillin, erythromycin, and the tetracyclines.

Immunity[20, 22]

Recovery from whooping cough is accompanied by the development of immunity. Sec-

ond attacks occur only infrequently; they are very mild in children and more severe in adults. The immunological response includes the production of agglutinating, precipitating, bactericidal, and complement-fixing antibodies. Specific humoral antibodies do not appear until the third or fourth week of the disease and, consequently, are of limited diagnostic value.

Based upon admittedly incomplete knowledge of the pathogenesis of pertussis, the elements of effective immunity are beginning to emerge. Immune mechanisms would be expected to function in preventing attachment in the early stages of infection and later could act to neutralize the toxic bacterial metabolites that are responsible for systemic effects.

In the first instance, it has been proposed that IgA can act specifically to inhibit attachment and colonization. Vaccines prepared from hemagglutinating antigens afford significant protection against whooping cough, thus supporting this concept.

Prolonged immunity in pertussis is probably related to the production of antitoxin. Animal experiments reveal the presence of a protective antigen associated with *B. pertussis,* and this activity correlates well with the presence of pertussis toxin, leading to the presumption that antitoxin is responsible for the greater part of immunity. As noted earlier, protection is not associated with heat-labile toxin or with endotoxin. Protection by capsular antigens has not been directly established, but immunity in children usually correlates with levels of serum agglutinins.

Prophylactic Immunization. Whole cell, killed vaccines prepared from smooth phase I *B. pertussis* were introduced into general use in the 1940s. This was followed by a pronounced decline in both morbidity and mortality of pertussis (Fig. 24–6). Immunogenic potency of vaccines requires constant assay and control; in the United States, a standard test, using intracerebral challenge in the mouse, determines potency of the vaccine.

Pertussis vaccine is successfully combined with diphtheria and tetanus toxoids **(DPT vaccine)** to allow immunization against the three diseases simultaneously; the immune response is equal to that obtained with separate antigens.

There is little doubt that modern vaccines have been highly effective in controlling epidemic whooping cough. The present low incidence is, in large measure, due to their use. Such vaccines are not, however, without risk. In a small number of recipients, neurological complications have resulted from vaccine use. Nevertheless, analysis of the risk-benefit ratio supports the continuation of routine immunization programs to reduce the incidence and severity of pertussis.[12, 17] It is generally agreed, however, that the search must continue for a potent and less toxic vaccine.

REFERENCES

1. Albritton, W. L. 1982. Infections due to *Haemophilus* species other than *H. influenzae.* Ann. Rev. Microbiol. **36**:199–216.
2. Anderson, P., and D. H. Smith. 1977. Isolation of the capsular polysaccharide from culture supernatant of *Haemophilus influenzae* type b. Infect. Immun. **15**:472–477.
3. Argaman, M., T.-Y. Liu, and J. B. Robbins. 1974. Polyribitol-phosphate: an antigen of four gram-positive bacteria cross-reactive with the capsular polysaccharide of *Haemophilus influenzae* type b. J. Immunol. **112**:649–655.
4. Corrall, C. J., J. A. Winkelstein, and E. R. Moxon. 1982. Participation of complement in host defense against encapsulated *Haemophilus influenzae* types a, c, and d. Infect. Immun. **35**:759–763.
5. Dajani, A. S., B. I. Asmar, and M. C. Thirumoorthi.

1979. Systemic *Haemophilus influenzae* disease: an overview. J. Pediat. **94**:355–364.
6. Denny, F. W. 1974. Effect of a toxin produced by *Haemophilus influenzae* on ciliated respiratory epithelium. J. Infect. Dis. **129**:93–100.
7. Emerson, B. B., *et al.* 1975. *Hemophilus influenzae* type b susceptibility to 17 antibiotics. J. Pediat. **86**:617–620.
8. Glode, M. P., *et al.* 1976. An outbreak of *Hemophilus influenzae* type b meningitis in an enclosed hospital population. J. Pediat. **88**:36–40.
9. Goldman, W. E., D. G., Klapper, and J. B. Baseman. 1982. Detection, isolation and analysis of a released *Bordetella pertussis* product toxic to cultured tracheal cells. Infect. Immun. **36**:782–794.
10. Green, G. R. 1978. Meningitis due to *Haemophilus influenzae* other than type b: case report and review. Pediatrics **62**:1021–1025.
11. Greenwood, J. R., and M. J. Pickett. 1980. Transfer of *Haemophilus vaginalis* Gardner and Dukes to a new genus, *Gardnerella: G. vaginalis* (Gardner and Dukes) comb. nov. Internat. J. Syst. Bacteriol. **30**:170–178.
12. Grob, P. R., M. J. Crowder, and J. F. Robbins. 1981. Effect of vaccination on severity and dissemination of whooping cough. Brit. Med. J. **282**:1925–1928.
13. Guerina, N. G., *et al.* 1982. Adherence of piliated *Haemophilus influenzae* type b to human oropharyngeal cells. J. Infect. Dis. **146**:564.
14. Hammond, G. W., *et al.* 1980. Epidemiologic, clinical, laboratory, and therapeutic features of an urban outbreak of chancroid in North America. Rev. Infect. Dis. **2**:867–879.
15. Kilian, M. 1980. *Haemophilus.* pp. 330–336. *In* E. H. Lennette, *et al.* (Eds.): Manual of Clinical Microbiology. 3rd ed. American Society for Microbiology, Washington, D.C.
16. Kilian, M., W. Frederiksen, and E. L. Biberstein (Eds.). 1981. Haemophilus, Pasteurella and Actinobacillus. Academic Press, London.
17. Koplan, J. P., *et al.* 1979. Pertussis vaccine—an analysis of benefits, risk and costs. New Engl. J. Med. **301**:906–911.
18. Lam, J. S., *et al.* 1980. Immunogenicity of outer membrane derivatives of *Haemophilus influenzae* type b. Current Microbiol. **3**:359–364.
19. Levin, D. C., *et al.* 1979. Bacteremic Haemophilus influenzae pneumonia in adults. A report of 24 cases and a review of the literature. Amer. J. Med. **62**:219–224.
20. Manclark, C. R. 1981. Pertussis vaccine research. Bull. Wld Hlth Org. **59**:9–15.
21. Morse, S. A. 1980. Sexually transmitted diseases. pp. 344–349. *In* E. H. Lennette, *et al.* (Eds.): Manual of Clinical Microbiology. 3rd ed. American Society for Microbiology, Washington, D. C.
22. Mortimer, E. A., Jr., and P. K. Jones. 1979. An evaluation of pertussis vaccine. Rev. Infect. Dis. **1**:927–934.
23. Myhre, E. B. 1974. Typing of *Haemophilus influenzae* by counterimmunoelectrophoresis. Acta Pathol. Microbiol. Scand. Sect. B. **82**:164–166.
24. Nicholls, S., T. D. Yuille, and R. G. Mitchell. 1975. Perinatal infections caused by *Haemophilus influenzae.* Arch. Dis. Childh. **50**:739–741.
25. Parker, C. D., and C. C. Linnemann, Jr. 1980. *Bordetella.* pp. 337–343. *In* E. H. Lennette, *et al.* (Eds.): Manual of Clinical Microbiology. 3rd ed. American Society for Microbiology, Washington, D. C.

26. Peltola, H., *et al.* 1977. *Haemophilus influenzae* type b capsular polysaccharide vaccine in children: a double-blind field study of 100,000 vaccinees 3 months to 5 years of age in Finland. Pediatrics **60**:730–737.

27. Pheifer, T. A., *et al.* 1978. Nonspecific vaginitis. Role of *Haemophilus vaginalis* and treatment with metronidazole. New Engl. J. Med. **298**:1429–1434.

28. Pittman, M. 1979. Pertussis toxin: the cause of the harmful effects and prolonged immunity of whooping cough. A hypothesis. Rev. Infect. Dis. **1**:401–412.

29. Preston, N. W. 1976. Prevalent serotypes of *Bordetella pertussis* in non-vaccinated communities. J. Hygiene **77**:85–91.

30. Report. 1976. Haemophilus bacteraemia. Brit. Med. J. **2**:651.

31. Sutton, A., *et al.* 1982. Differential complement resistance mediates virulence of *Haemophilus influenzae* type b. Infect. Immun. **35**:95–104.

32. Trollfors, B., and E. Rabo. 1981. Whooping cough in adults. Brit. Med. J. **283**:696–697.

33. Turk, D. C. 1975. An investigation of the family background of acute haemophilus infections in children. J. Hygiene **75**:315–332.

34. Zinnemann, K. 1980. Newer knowledge in classification, taxonomy and pathogenicity of species in the genus Haemophilus. Zentbl. Bakt. I Abt. Orig. A **247**:248–258.

Pseudomonas and Legionella

Pseudomonas[8, 25]

The genus *Pseudomonas* is one of the larger groups of bacteria, comprising more than 80 recognized species; many more species have been proposed, but the taxonomic position of these is uncertain.

Casually known as pseudomonads, they are ubiquitous in distribution, being found in soil, water, and marine environments. Perhaps the most noteworthy property of this group is their **biochemical versatility.** They have been found to utilize a remarkable variety of organic substrates; some strains can use more than 100 organic compounds as the sole or principal source of carbon. Because of their biochemical diversity and habitat, they are significant agents in the mineralization of organic matter in natural environments. Microbial physiologists and geneticists have long found them to be an important tool in exploring the diverse pathways of biochemical degradation.

Many of the *Pseudomonas* species are pathogenic for plants, causing a variety of diseases and exhibiting host specificity in varying degrees. Others, perhaps because of their ubiquity, contaminate foodstuffs and are commonly associated with food spoilage.

Most pseudomonads are free-living, growing profusely and almost universally in soil or water. Fortunately, relatively few have pathogenic potential in man and animals, and even these must be considered to be opportunists with limited invasive potential. *Pseudomonas* are found with some regularity in the hospital environment, growing in a host of aqueous fluids, including ophthalmic solutions, dilute antiseptics, cleaning liquids, and water in flower vases, as well as on moist surfaces and in ventilation equipment. It is clear that this presents opportunities for nosocomial transmission of the opportunistic pathogens to hospitalized patients, who may be debilitated and susceptible.

One species, *P. aeruginosa*, is the predominant cause of pseudomonal infections in humans. It has limited invasive capacity, so that most infections occur in immunosuppressed or otherwise compromised hosts, but once established, *P. aeruginosa* causes serious and frequently life-threatening disease.

Two species, *P. pseudomallei* and *P. mallei*, are frankly pathogenic, particularly for animals, which serve as the reservoir for human infections caused by these species. Melioidosis, caused by *P. pseudomallei*, is rare in the United States but more common in the Pacific and Southeast Asia. It is typically a disease of

Table 25–1. **Representative Biochemical Reactions of the Medically Relevant** *Pseudomonas**

Test	P. aeruginosa	P. fluorescens	P. pseudomallei	P. mallei
Motility	+	+	+	–
No. of flagella	1	>1	>1	0
Acid from:				
Glucose	+	+	+	+
Lactose	–	–	+	+
Sucrose	–	V	+	–
Indophenol oxidase	+	+	+	V
Arginine dihydrolase	+	+	+	+
Pyoverdin	+	+	–	–
Growth at 42° C.	+	–	+	–

*Adapted from R. Hugh and G. L. Gilardi.[25]
Symbols: +, most strains positive; –, most strains negative; V, variable reactions.

animals, both domestic and wild, and human infections are more or less directly linked to these reservoirs. *Pseudomonas mallei* is the etiological agent of glanders, an equine disease that has been eliminated from North America but is still seen in other parts of the world.

Pseudomonas are strictly aerobic, gram-negative, usually straight bacilli. Most strains are motile either by a single polar flagellum or by a polar tuft of flagella; spores are not formed. Pseudomonads do not ferment carbohydrates, but may produce acids from some by oxidative metabolism. Many of the species produce pigments, some of which fluoresce when exposed to short-wavelength ultraviolet light. Nonfluorescent, water-soluble phenazine pigments are formed by some strains. One of these, pyocyanin, is produced by many strains of *P. aeruginosa* and has some differential significance. It is neither possible nor profitable to consider here the differentiation of species of *Pseudomonas*, since classification of this diverse group is based upon a multitude of phenotypic characters. Table 25–1 displays some of the characters that are employed to recognize the more relevant species. This listing is not exhaustive, and the appropriate identification of species requires a number of additional tests.

PSEUDOMONAS AERUGINOSA

Pseudomonas aeruginosa is the best known of the species of *Pseudomonas*. The blue or blue-green stains that sometimes appear on surgical dressings long ago attracted attention, and in 1860, even before the cause of the

phenomenon had been discovered, Fordos studied the pigment. In 1882, Gessard found that the pigment was a product of a specific microorganism, *P. aeruginosa,* which he isolated in pure culture.

Morphology and Staining
The cells of *P. aeruginosa* vary considerably in size but appear usually as small slender rods, 1.5 to 3 μm. long and 0.5 μm. in diameter. They are frequently united in pairs and short chains. There is a single polar flagellum by which the bacterium is actively motile. **Mucoid** strains contain a polysaccharide capsule or glycocalyx. The bacilli stain readily with aniline dyes and are gram-negative.

Colonies are large and spreading, with irregular edges and a butyrous consistency (Fig. 25–1). Pyocyanogenic strains (see below) produce a blue or blue-green pigment that diffuses into the medium. Mucoid strains exhibit characteristic colonial morphology (Fig. 25–2).

Physiology
Pseudomonas aeruginosa grows well on all of the common culture mediums and most rapidly at temperatures from 30° to 37°C. Aerobic conditions are required, although some anaerobic growth occurs in the presence of nitrate. In these circumstances, oxygen in nitrate serves as the electron acceptor. This bacterium is nonfermentative, although oxidation of glucose (and some other carbohydrates) leads to acid formation (see Table 25–1) in mediums high in carbohydrate and low in peptone. In common with other pseudomonads, a large number of organic substrates are utilized as carbon sources.

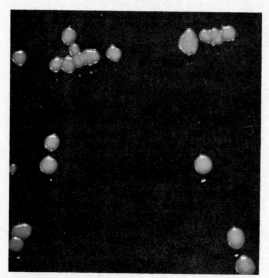

Figure 25–1. Colonies of *Pseudomonas fluorescens* on nutrient agar, 24-hour culture. ×3.

One of the most distinctive characters of *P. aeruginosa* is its production of one or more pigments, which do not color the colonies or other masses of growth but instead diffuse into the medium. Two separate kinds of pigment are formed. One, called **pyocyanin,** is a phenazine, deep blue in color, and not fluorescent; it can be extracted from aqueous solutions by chloroform. Fluorescent pigments are also produced: **pyoverdins** are yellow-green to yellow-brown, and **pyomelanin** is brown-black in color. The kinds of pigments produced, as well as their relative amounts, influence the coloration of the medium. Pyocyanin is unique to *P. aeruginosa*, but the fluorescent pigments are found in several other species as well.

Antigenic Structure

The antigenic makeup of *P. aeruginosa* was of questionable nature for many years. The species is antigenically diverse, possessing a variety of both H and O antigens. Antigenic analysis by a number of investigators has established several serotypes based on possession of different lipopolysaccharide O antigens, detected by agglutination reactions. There have been several antigenic schema proposed and used in many parts of the world,[22] but no one system has been universally adopted. It appears that about 17 serotypes can be differentiated in most of these typing systems. The O antigens found in *P. aeruginosa* seem to be specific for this species, *i.e.,* they do not occur in other *Pseudomonas* species; in addition, there is no cross-reactivity between serotypes of *P. aeruginosa*, indicating that each serotype possesses unique O antigens.

Although no O antigens are common to all or even most *P. aeruginosa* strains, there are several outer membrane antigens that seem to be closely related among serotype strains.[34] One **outer envelope protein** antigen, designated OEP, reportedly occurs in all strains of *P. aeruginosa* and thus constitutes a "common antigen" in this species.[21] Significantly, OEP appears to be a protective antigen, at least in animal infections.

Phage typing is also practiced by some and can be useful for epidemiological purposes. **Bacteriocin typing,** analogous to that used with

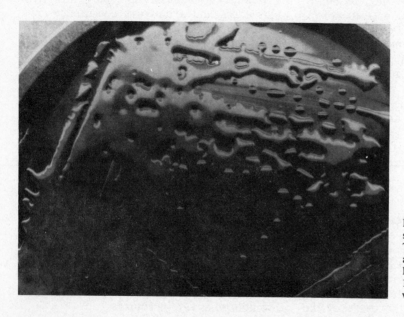

Figure 25–2. Colonies of mucoid strain of *Pseudomonas aeruginosa*. Twenty-four hour culture on blood agar. (R. S. Baltimore and M. Mitchell, J. Infect. Dis. **141**:238, 1980. Copyright 1980 by the University of Chicago.)

Shigella, also has wide currency. Bacteriocins, also called **pyocins** or **aeruginosins,** produced by strains of *P. aeruginosa,* are tested for their bactericidal activity against a series of sensitive indicator strains of *Pseudomonas.* Pyocin typing has been particularly valuable for tracing epidemic spread of nosocomial infections. A standard nomenclature simplifies the comparison of epidemiological patterns.[9]

Toxins[3]

Like other gram-negative microorganisms, *Pseudomonas* possess cell wall lipopolysaccharides with endotoxic and O antigen activity. The endotoxin is not so potent, however, as that produced by the enteric bacilli. Several minor toxins are also produced by *P. aeruginosa* with some strain variation. A leucocidin, which is active against polymorphonuclear leucocytes, is produced by a few strains. Slightly less than half of the clinical isolates produce hemolysis on blood agar plates, indicating synthesis of hemolysins. Heat-stable extracellular hemolysins are glycolipids,[26] while the heat-labile hemolysin is phospholipase C. Other minor cytotoxic proteins have also been described, but are not well characterized.[29, 35]

Exotoxin A.[43, 44] The *P. aeruginosa* toxin of greatest relevance to pathogenesis is exotoxin A. Like other microbial exotoxins, it is a protein of about 66,000 molecular weight and is convertible to toxoid by treatment with formalin or glutaraldehyde; its toxicity is specifically neutralized by antitoxin. Exotoxin A is a potent toxin, lethal in small amounts. For example, the LD_{50} of purified toxin in mice is about 60 to 80 ng. About 90 per cent of clinical isolates of *P. aeruginosa* are toxigenic, and toxin is produced *in vivo* in both clinical and experimental infections, suggesting a correlation with virulence and pathogenesis.

The injection of purified exotoxin A into animals results in liver lesions characterized by necrosis, cellular swelling, and fatty changes. These early events are succeeded by almost complete hepatocellular necrosis by 48 hours. Lesions in other organs include lung hemorrhages and kidney necrosis. These changes are associated with inhibition of protein synthesis in several organs, but especially in the liver. Most of these effects of toxin mimic those seen in animal infections by *P. aeruginosa.*

Exotoxin A has been found to act by **inhibiting protein synthesis** in a manner analogous to that of diphtheria toxin (Chapter 30). The toxin is thought to bind to specific receptors on target cell surfaces, with subsequent internalization by endocytosis; toxin internalization, but not binding, is calcium-dependent.[16]

In vitro studies indicate that the exotoxin A acts by catalyzing the adenosine diphosphate (ADP)-ribosylation of elongation factor 2 (EF2), using nicotinamide adenine dinucleotide (NAD) as the ADP-ribose donor. The reaction is summarized as follows:

$$NAD + EF2 \rightleftarrows ADP\text{-ribose-}EF2 + nicotinamide + H^+$$

The ribosomal protein, EF2, is inactivated in this reaction, and protein synthesis ceases. Thus, the enzymatically active portion of the toxin acts as an ADP-ribosyltransferase.

The intact, native toxin is a proenzyme with little activity in the *in vitro* reaction just described. It is converted to the active enzyme by reduction of two of its four disulfide bridges or by proteolytic cleavage to yield an active fragment of about 26,000 molecular weight.[28] The activated fragment does not exhibit toxicity for animals or tissue culture cells, presumably because it lacks the binding domain of the molecule. This leads to the further assumption that the intact toxin, after binding and internalization, is processed by cellular mechanisms to form the active enzyme.

The catalytic action of *Pseudomonas* toxin is strikingly similar to that of the diphtheria toxin, yet the two toxins are not alike in structure. They differ in immunological character, in target cell specificity, and in toxicity for animals. Although there may be homology in the active sites, it is clear that the peptides are otherwise quite different in structure.

Virulence[3, 21, 43, 44]

The metabolic versatility of *Pseudomonas* has been noted above. This versatility is also reflected in the number and kinds of microbial products that may serve as virulence determinants. Virulence determinants and their possible modes of action are listed in Table 25–2. It is apparent that many factors may come into play, and no single factor is responsible for virulence. Nevertheless, some have greater importance than others. Those of greatest relevance seem to be exotoxin A, proteolytic enzymes, and lipopolysaccharides. In the case of mucoid strains, which readily colonize the respiratory tract of cystic fibrosis patients, the capsular material may be of greater importance than in other infections. The production of hemolysins and leucocidins is probably not critical, and the presence of pili may be of greater significance for colonization of mucous

Table 25–2. **Possible Virulence Determinants in**
Pseudomonas aeruginosa

Product	Action
Exotoxin A	Prime virulence determinant; inhibits protein synthesis by ADP-ribosylation of elongation factor 2; produced by 90 per cent of strains.
Exoenzyme S	Action similar to that of exotoxin A; produced by only a few strains.
Proteolytic enzymes	Injections of purified enzymes cause hemorrhage and local lesions and destruction of elastin fibers of arteries; corneal damage and opacity when directly administered; complement destruction; act as aggressins to promote invasion; produced by most strains.
Lipopolysaccharides	Endotoxic; antiphagocytic.
Capsular material	Antiphagocytic; traps antibiotics by adsorption to polysaccharide; a glycolipoprotein fraction causes leucopenia; most prominent in mucoid strains.
Leucocidin	Destruction of leucocytes; produced by few strains.
Hemolysins	Glycolipids hemolyze erythrocytes by detergent-like action; phospholipase C induces hemorrhagic lesions.
Pili	Mediates adherence to host cells.
Flagella	Action not known; loss of flagella results in reduced virulence.
Pyochelin	Iron-binding siderophore; permits sequestration of iron; probably aids in regulation of exotoxin A synthesis; may be responsible for serum resistance.

membranes than for wound and burn infections.[42]

Most virulent strains produce exotoxin A, and, as noted above, the toxin is likely the prime factor in virulence. Animal studies with nontoxigenic strains suggest that the toxin is required for full virulence. Exotoxin A can be demonstrated in the tissues of infected animals; furthermore, administration of purified toxin reproduces many of the effects noted in *P. aeruginosa* infections. In infected humans, sufficient toxin is produced to induce a measureable antitoxin response, and the presence of antitoxin has been claimed to improve prognosis in the disease.

The proteolytic enzymes, particularly elastase and protease, also can mimic some of the effects seen in infection. These include hemorrhage in various tissues and corneal damage after instillation of the enzymes onto the incised cornea of rabbits. Infection studies indicate that strains lacking protease and elastase do not induce corneal damage in animals, and in animal burn models, toxigenic strains deficient in these enzymes were less virulent than the wild type. It is generally agreed that the proteolytic enzymes act as aggressins to enhance invasiveness.

Pathogenesis in Man[1, 10, 18]

For some time after its discovery, *P. aeruginosa* was generally regarded as a harmless saprophyte or, at most, as a microorganism of slight pathogenic power. In the past thirty years, however, it has become evident that the microorganism is causally associated with a great variety of infections. Such infections are usually nosocomial in nature, occurring in patients with compromised host defenses and related to changes in therapeutic modalities in modern hospitals.

In spite of its many virulence determinants, *P. aeruginosa* is regarded as an opportunistic pathogen, seldom capable of primary infection in normal, healthy individuals. In those with compromised defenses, however, the bacterium can gain a foothold in the host, leading to serious and life-threatening disease in these persons. As noted earlier, *P. aeruginosa* is a free-living microbial form capable of multiplying in environments not suitable for other microorganisms. In the hospital environment, in particular, it is encountered with some frequency in the absence of vigorous control measures. This microbial distribution, coupled with patient populations of low resistance, leads to the high incidence of nosocomial infections.

Patients at particular risk of *Pseudomonas* infection include those undergoing immunosuppressive therapy or invasive diagnostic and therapeutic procedures. Burn patients are frequently colonized, as are those with surgical or other wounds. In cystic fibrosis patients, pulmonary infection, usually with mucoid strains, occurs with regularity. Severe neutropenia predisposes to *Pseudomonas* infection; the reduced inflammatory response in these individuals may obscure the apparent seriousness of the infection.

Primary infections with *Pseudomonas* arise in the respiratory tract; urinary bladder; ears; and in burns, wounds, and surgical sites. *Pseudomonas* pneumonia, often bilateral, is a serious disease. Physical signs, such as cough and sputum, are usually modest, while fever is generally high. Mortality in pneumonia is often marked, approaching 80 per cent in most studies. The frequency of septicemia is high, except in cystic fibrosis patients. Septicemia is also the most serious sequel to other localized infections, with high mortality.

Since 1975, several outbreaks of *Pseudomonas* dermatitis have been recorded, usually associated with whirlpool baths contaminated with *P. aeruginosa*. The infection is characterized by a skin rash affecting the trunk and proximal extremities; normally, these infections are self-limiting.

Bacteriological Diagnosis[25]

Clinical specimens to be examined for *Pseudomonas* are usually cultured on blood agar (although blood is not required for growth) and on one of the less inhibitory selective mediums used for enteric bacilli, *e.g.*, MacConkey or eosin–methylene blue agar. Suspicious colonies are gram-stained and subcultured on Kligler iron agar or other mediums to establish the isolate as an aerobic, glucose nonfermenting, gram-negative bacillus. Pyocyanin production on noninhibitory mediums is presumptive evidence for *P. aeruginosa*. Nonpyocyanogenic isolates must be confirmed as *Pseudomonas* species by a battery of physiological and morphological tests.

Chemotherapy[4, 39]

Pseudomonas infections are difficult to treat; therapy, even with seemingly appropriate agents, is not uniformly successful. Antibiotic resistance by R-plasmid transfer from other *Pseudomonas* and enterobacteria is commonplace. Resistance to β-lactam antibiotics is effected by antibiotic exclusion, as in mucoid strains, or by formation of β-lactamases.

In spite of the appearance of resistance, β-lactam antibiotics of the penicillin and cephalosporin groups are widely employed in therapy, but are rarely effective when used alone. Combination therapy with a selected β-lactam antibiotic and one of the aminoglycosides is usually recommended.

Immunity

As noted in previous discussions, many of the cellular components and products of *Pseudomonas* induce immune protection in animals. For example, opsonic antibodies induced by capsular polysaccharides or by lipopolysaccharides offer some immunity against infection. Similarly, antibodies specific for the proteolytic enzymes and exotoxin A seem to protect animals against these products. Immunization with flagellar preparations is protective in the mouse burn model, presumably because the microorganisms are immobilized and fail to invade deeper tissues.[20]

Immunization with vaccines has not, however, been practiced in humans. Whole cell vaccines are toxic, and their usefulness is probably limited by the number of serotypes; component vaccines, using toxoids, capsular polysaccharides, or common protein antigens, might be expected to overcome this difficulty. It is evident, however, that the major groups at risk are those with impaired immune systems; whether immunization could be successful in these individuals is problematic.

PSEUDOMONAS MALLEI

Glanders is a disease seen, as a rule, only in the solipeds (the horse, mule, or ass) but is occasionally transmitted to other domestic animals, to wild animals, and to man. It has also been transmitted between humans in a few instances. The disease has been eradicated in the United States and Canada, although it still occurs occasionally in other parts of the world.

Morphology and Staining

The glanders bacillus, *P. mallei*, is a small rod, straight or slightly curved, usually with rounded ends and often of irregular contour, as shown in Figure 25–3. It is similar in morphology to other *Pseudomonas* species. In stains from pus, the bacilli are sometimes found within the leucocytes but more often are extracellular. There is no special arrangement in such smears, but in culture the bacilli may occur in pairs; in older cultures, filaments are produced with swollen ends in which true branching may be observed. The bacilli are nonmotile, nonencapsulated, and nonspore-forming.

Colonies on agar are small, round, convex, and amorphous in consistency. They are translucent and yellowish in color and, upon aging for 8 to 10 days, become opaque, sometimes developing a light brown center.

The glanders bacillus stains with ordinary aqueous aniline dyes, though not readily. Best results are obtained with Loeffler's alkaline methylene blue or Ziehl's carbol-fuchsin. The

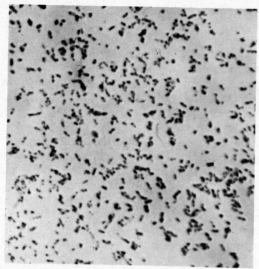

Figure 25–3. *Pseudomonas mallei* in pure culture. The generally poor staining is apparent, and bipolar staining may be observed in some of the cells. Methylene blue; ×1250.

bacilli are not acid-fast and are gram-negative. Cells from young cultures take the stain fairly uniformly, but those in older cultures stain irregularly, due to the accumulation of β-hydroxybutyrate granules. These lipid granules, which do not themselves stain with ordinary dyes, give the cells a beaded appearance after staining. The granules may be specifically stained with Sudan black B or iodine-fuchsin.

Physiology

Growth occurs on ordinary nutrient mediums but is poor and slow upon primary isolation. Forty-eight hours' incubation at the optimum temperature of 37°C. is generally necessary for the appearance on solid mediums of colonies 0.5 to 1 mm. in diameter. Representative physiological reactions of *P. mallei* are shown in Table 25–1.

The bacillus is but slightly resistant to adverse physical and chemical agents, being readily killed by heat (55°C. for 10 minutes) and disinfectants, such as hypochlorites, iodine, and mercuric chloride.

Pathogenicity for Lower Animals

Under natural conditions the horse is chiefly affected, but cases have been occasionally observed in the carnivora (cats, dogs, menagerie animals), goats, and sheep. Swine and pigeons are slightly susceptible, while cattle and goats are immune. In endemic areas, infected animals serve as the reservoir for human disease.

Pathogenicity for Man

In endemic areas, veterinarians and others having to do with the care of horses are the most liable to contract **glanders.** Freshly isolated cultures are highly virulent, and a number of fatal infections have occurred among laboratory workers. The acute form, with high fever and symptoms of a generalized infection, is the more common in man, most cases terminating fatally within two or three weeks, sometimes within a few days of their inception. Occasionally, the chronic form may appear and linger for months or even years, with spreading ulceration and other features closely resembling those observed in horses. Recovery from chronic glanders may take place, or the disease may pass into the acute stage.

In man the alimentary tract is not the ordinary channel of entrance; meat from glandered animals has been ingested without resulting infection. Infection probably occurs through the abraded skin. Unlike other *Pseudomonas,* it does not occur in soil or water and appears to be an adapted parasite of man and animals.

Bacteriological Diagnosis[25]

Cultural methods employed for the isolation and identification of *P. mallei* are similar to those used for other *Pseudomonas,* although it does not grow as readily on primary isolation as other species. *Pseudomonas mallei* is distinguished from other pathogenic pseudomonads by the properties listed in Table 25–1. Note that unlike most other species, *P. mallei* is not motile.

Chemotherapy

Glanders occurs so rarely in man that little is known concerning its chemotherapy. It has been reported that several chronic cases and laboratory infections were successfully treated with sulfadiazine.

Immunity

Permanent immunity to glanders can neither be conferred by an attack of the disease nor produced by artificial immunization. Chronic glanders can exist in the individual for years and is in no way a warranty against the sudden development of an acute attack.

PSEUDOMONAS PSEUDOMALLEI[24, 25, 36]

Melioidosis, caused by *P. pseudomallei,* is a disease similar to glanders in symptomatology.

The naturally occurring infection is primarily one of rodents. It appears to be endemic in the southwest Pacific area, *e.g.,* Burma, Thailand, Vietnam, Indonesia, and Australia, where it surfaces as a disease of domestic animals, including sheep, cattle, swine, and horses. It occurs in humans in these areas and, in rare instances, has been locally acquired in the Western Hemisphere.

Pseudomonas pseudomallei resembles other pseudomonads in morphology and staining. In contrast to *P. mallei,* it is motile, grows at 42°C., and liquifies gelatin; other physiological characters are shown in Table 25–1. Like the glanders bacillus, it may be difficult to isolate on primary culture, although growth is more vigorous. Colonies may be mucoid, smooth, or rough and wrinkled, with pigmentation that varies from a cream color to bright orange.

The bacillus is a free-living form and is found in moist soil and water in endemic areas. Human infection may be derived from animals or by soil contamination of wounds or abrasions.

Melioidosis in man[14, 37, 38] may assume many clinical forms. In otherwise debilitated persons, *e.g.,* diabetics, the initial manifestation is septicemia, with pulmonary symptoms and local abscesses. Such infections have high mortality rates. In chronic cases, the bacteria may be localized in any tissue. Serological evidence from studies in endemic areas indicates a substantial number of mild or latent infections.

The tetracyclines appear to be the most active of the chemotherapeutic agents when tested *in vitro*, and tetracycline alone or in combination with chloramphenicol has been used clinically with some success, provided treatment is prolonged—one to five months—to circumvent relapse.

Legionella[6, 30]

In the summer of 1976, an outbreak of severe respiratory illness occurred in a group of American Legion members attending a convention in Philadelphia. Promptly christened Legionnaires' disease in the press, it captured the attention of the public and became the subject of vigorous investigation by public health agencies. The epidemiological findings suggested a common source outbreak without person-to-person spread.

Intensive microbiological studies resulted in the isolation, by guinea pig inoculation, of a novel, gram-negative bacterium. These isolates were later cultivated in chick embryo yolk sac and in cell cultures. Ultimately, the bacteria were grown on complex bacteriological mediums. Retrospective studies, both bacteriological and serological, revealed that similar bacteria had been responsible for human infections at least as early as 1943. These bacteria are now classified in the genus *Legionella*, in the family Legionellaceae.

Classification and Taxonomy

Following the isolation of the Legionnaires' disease bacterium, the microorganism was intensively studied and compared to strains of early isolates of indeterminate taxonomy. It soon became obvious that similar, if not identical, bacilli had been responsible for earlier infections. Further, both sporadic cases and endemic outbreaks were soon ascribed to these bacilli. Bacteriological investigations demonstrated that these microorganisms, as judged by DNA homology, were unrelated to established bacterial genera. The name *Legionella pneumophila* was proposed, creating a new genus and family, Legionellaceae. Subsequently, additional species have been described. Each of these is genetically distinct, but the species show DNA relatedness. The presently recognized species are listed in Table 25–3, along with earlier synonymous designa-

Table 25–3. **The Species of *Legionella***

Species Name	Synonyms*
L. pneumophila	Legionnaires' disease bacterium (1976)
	OLDA (1947)
L. bozemanii	WIGA (1959)
L. micdadei	TATLOCK (1943)
	HEBA (1959)
	Pittsburgh pneumonia agent (1979)
	L. pittsburghensis
L. dumoffii	NY 23 (1979)
	TEX–KL (1979)
L. gormanii	LS–13 (1979)
L. longbeachae	*Legionella*-like organism (1981)

*Dates of original isolation are in parentheses.

Table 25–4. **Biochemical and Cultural Characters of *Legionella****

Test	L. pneum-ophila	L. boze-manii	L. micdadei	L. dumoffii	L. gormanii	L. long-beachae
Growth on:						
CYE agar†	+	+	+	+	+	+
F-G agar ‡	+	+	+	+	–	+
Blood agar	–	–	–	–	–	–
Fluorescence §	Y	BW	Y	BW	BW	Y
Browning ‖	+	+	–	+	+	+
Oxidase	+	–	+	–	–	W
Catalase	+	+	+	+	+	+
Hippurate hydrolysis	+	–	–	–	–	–
Gelatinase	+	+	+	+	+	+
β-Lactamase	+	+	–	+	+	V

*Adapted from R. M. McKinney, *et al.*[31] and G. K. Morris, *et al.*[32]
Symbols: Y, yellow; BW, blue-white; V, variable; W, weak.
†Charcoal yeast extract agar.
‡Feeley-Gorman agar.
§Fluorescence of colonies on solid medium examined by long wavelength (366 nm.) ultraviolet light.
‖Brown pigmentation in tyrosine-containing medium.

tions. Except for *L. gormanii*, all of the *Legionella* species have been directly associated with human infection. *Legionella gormanii* has been isolated from soil and has been linked serologically to human disease.[32] Immunological analysis has demonstrated six serogroups within *L. pneumophila* and two serogroups in *L. longbeachae*; only a single serogroup is recognized in each of the other species. The biochemical and cultural characteristics of *Legionella* species are listed in Table 25–4. Since *Legionella* are free-living soil and water forms, it can be expected that others will be described as more is learned of these fastidious, gram-negative bacilli.

Morphology and Staining
Legionella are small, aerobic, gram-negative rods, 0.5 to 0.7 μm. in diameter and generally about 2 μm. in length; they may be blunt or tapered in form. Longer filamentous bacilli are often present in cultures; usually these are less than 20 μm. in length, but are occasionally as long as 50 μm. The shorter forms are generally present in tissues (Fig. 25–4). The bacilli are motile (Fig. 25–5); most possess only a single polar flagellum, but subpolar and lateral flagella have been noted and flagella have been reported on bacilli observed in tissue sections. Pili or fimbriae are said to be present in some strains.

Although considered to be gram-negative, legionellae do not stain well by this stain. In tissue sections or smears they may be demonstrated by the Giménez rickettsial stain or by silver impregnation methods, such as the Dieterle stain. When stained by Sudan black B, fat vacuoles are noted; in transmission

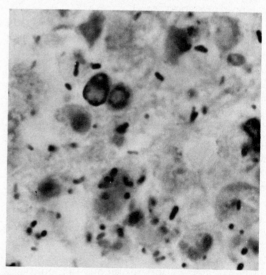

Figure 25–4. Lung section of patient from whom *Legionella* was isolated. Note the many small, blunt, pleomorphic intracellular and extracellular bacilli that stain with the modified Dieterle silver impregnation procedure. ×1500. (Courtesy of Dr. Francis W. Chandler.)

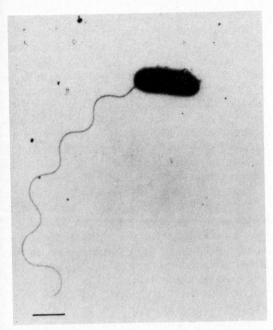

Figure 25–5. Electron photomicrograph of flagellated *Legionella pneumophila*, serogroup 1. Bar = 1 μm. (J. A. Elliott, and W. Johnson, Infect. Immun. **33**:602, 1981.)

electron microscopy of thin sections, the vacuoles are electron-lucent and resemble membrane-bound poly-β-hydroxybutyrate granules (Chapter 2).

Physiology[15]

Legionella are fastidious, aerobic bacilli, growing only on complex mediums; they do not grow on ordinary blood agar. The medium most often employed is a buffered charcoal yeast extract (BCYE) agar, which supports primary growth from clinical specimens. Tiny colonies, with a cut-glass appearance by oblique light microscopy, usually appear in 3 to 5 days. Chemically defined mediums have also been devised, containing amino acids and inorganic salts, but these are not suitable for primary isolation.

The biochemical and cultural reactions that characterize the several species of *Legionella* are shown in Table 25–4. Biochemically, these bacteria are relatively inactive except for the reactions shown. For example, urease is not formed, acid is not produced from carbohydrates, and neither lysine decarboxylase nor ornithine decarboxylase are present.

In contrast to most gram-negative bacteria, large amounts of branched chain fatty acids are present in cells, as demonstrated by gas-liquid chromatography. Based on the types and amounts of fatty acids present, three distinctive profiles are distinguished and are exemplified in *L. pneumophila, L. bozemanii,* and *L. micdadei.* The profiles of *L. gormanii* and *L. dumoffii* resemble *L. bozemanii,* while *L. longbeachae* resembles *L. pneumophila.*

Legionella are not resistant to the usual physical agents. They are rapidly killed at temperatures above 58°C.[33] and do not long survive in aerosols produced under conditions of low humidity.[2] Resistance to chemicals is variable; chlorine and other microbicides have been used to decontaminate air conditioning cooling towers.

Antigenic Structure[11]

Legionella cells contain two principal kinds of antigens. The flagellar antigens are not well characterized in most species. They are heat-labile proteins, and can be detected by slide agglutination of flagellated cells in specific antiserum. In *L. pneumophila,* the flagellar antigen is identical in all of the serogroups studied, viz., serogroups 1, 2, and 3. They have not proved suitable for identification or typing.

Located on the cell surface is a heat-labile, soluble antigen that has been employed for serological identification and grouping. The serospecific antigen is contained in a lipid-protein-carbohydrate complex on the cell surface and is detected by agglutination, coagglutination with staphylococcal protein A, and immunofluorescence microscopy.[40] The latter test is the most widely employed. Variations of this method are used to identify *Legionella* in tissue sections, exudates, or laboratory cultures; to detect specific antigen in clinical specimens; and to measure specific antibodies as an aid to serological diagnosis of legionellosis.

Within the species *L. pneumophila,* six serogroups are recognized, based on the presence of the group-specific, high-molecular-weight carbohydrate antigen, termed the F-1 antigen. In practice, *L. pneumophila* is identified using a polyvalent conjugated antiserum. Serogroup determination is by individual serogroup-specific antiserums. Similarly, two serogroups make up *L. longbeachae.*[5] Each of the other species is serologically homogeneous with respect to the cell surface antigen. It is of interest that immunization with the F-1 antigen from serogroup 1 *L. pneumophila* protects guinea pigs against serogroup 1 challenge, but not against serogroups 2, 3, or 4.[13] In addition to these serogroup antigens, a common antigen, possibly protein in nature, is found in all species.

Virulence

Considering their recent discovery, it is not surprising that virulence determinants in *Legionella* are not well delineated. It is evident that virulence is lost when strains are repeatedly subcultured on Mueller-Hinton medium, but not by culture on charcoal yeast extract agar. Virulence is restored, however, by chick embryo passage, by guinea pig passage, or by culture in human lung embryo fibroblast cells.[12, 41] Whether such observations reflect selection of virulent cells or enhancement of virulence is not known.

Legionella pneumophila is capable of intracellular parasitism, as indicated by its capacity to infect and multiply within fibroblasts, as noted above, and in macrophages and mononuclear cells.[23] It does not, however, multiply in polymorphonuclear leucocytes. The bacilli apparently do not activate the alternative complement pathway, and C3 is fixed only in the presence of specific antibody. Although opsonization by polymorphonuclear phagocytes is promoted by specific antibody and complement, ingested bacilli are not killed. The bacilli are, however, susceptible to the antimicrobial action of the myeloperoxidase-peroxide-halide system.[27] Virulence, then, may somehow be linked to the capacity for intracellular growth and failure to activate the alternative complement pathway.

Legionella contain an endotoxin with properties similar to that of other gram-negative bacteria, but which is not highly active biologically. In addition, the microorganism produces hemolysins, proteolytic enzymes, and a low-molecular-weight heat-stable **cytotoxin**. The latter may have some relevance to virulence. At concentrations not affecting viability of polymorphonuclear leucocytes, preincubation with the toxin impairs oxygen consumption and the oxygen-dependent sequelae of phagocytosis. These observations may explain the failure of leucocytes to destroy legionellae after phagocytosis.[17]

LEGIONELLOSIS[7]

Legionellosis in humans appears in two clinical forms. A pneumonic form, generally termed Legionnaires' disease, is a serious infection with significant mortality and relatively long incubation period. A nonpneumonic, febrile illness, called Pontiac fever, is self-limiting, nonfatal, and characterized by a short incubation period.

Legionnaires' Disease

The most serious and dramatic manifestation of *Legionella* infection is Legionnaires' disease, so called because it was the clinical entity manifest in the Philadelphia outbreak in 1976.

The chief clinical feature is a severe pneumonia with fever, malaise, chills, cough, dyspnea, myalgia, and headaches. The disease may occur as sporadic cases or in epidemic outbreaks, often under circumstances suggesting a common source of infection. The incubation period ranges between 2 and 10 days, with a median of 5 days.

Except for rare infections by other species, *L. pneumophila* is the etiological agent in most cases, and serogroup 1 outranks the other serogroups as the responsible agent. It has been estimated that serogroup 1 *L. pneumophila* causes about 1 per cent of the cases of pneumonia in the United States, or about 25,000 cases per year.

In epidemic outbreaks, the attack rate has been relatively low, 0.1 to 0.5 per cent, but the case-fatality ratios have been around 14 per cent; in sporadic cases, however, the case-fatality ratio has averaged about 19 per cent and, in 1980, was 25 per cent of reported cases in the United States. The groups at greatest risk are the elderly, particularly those above age 60; the immunosuppressed; and those with serious intercurrent disease. Males appear to be at risk; more than two-thirds of the cases in this country in 1981 were in males. As might be expected, a number of nosocomial infections have been recorded. Children are sometimes affected, but such infections seem to be uncommon.

As noted earlier, *Legionella* are found in soil and water, and most outbreaks appear to have been derived from these sources. The microorganisms have been isolated from the water of air conditioner cooling towers, and in several outbreaks these appear to have been the source of infection by **airborne transmission**. In other instances, outbreaks have occurred in the vicinity of recent soil excavations. There is no convincing evidence of person-to-person spread of the disease. The source of infection in sporadic cases is more difficult to document, but infections in hospitals have been traced to plumbing systems and to contaminated nebulizers. As shown in Figure 25–6, sporadic cases are seasonal, with greatest incidence in the period from July to September.

Although the greatest number of cases of legionellosis have been noted in the United

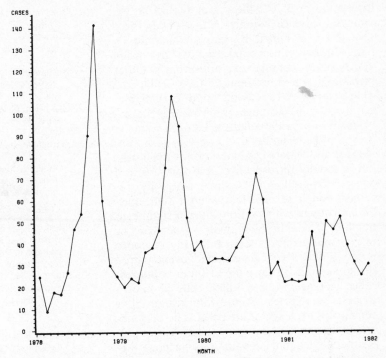

Figure 25–6. Reported cases of sporadic legionellosis in the United States, 1978–1981. Note the seasonality, with most cases having onset in the months from July to September. (Centers for Disease Control, Annual summary 1981: reported morbidity and mortality in the United States. Morbid. Mortal. Weekly Rep. **30** [54], 1982.)

States, infections have occurred in many other countries, suggesting worldwide distribution.

Pontiac Fever

Pontiac fever, in contrast to Legionnaires' disease, is a mild, self-limiting febrile illness without significant pulmonary involvement. After a short incubation period, generally about 36 hours, the disease is characterized by fever, malaise, chills, myalgia, and headache. The illness usually lasts from 2 to 5 days and recovery, although sometimes prolonged, is uneventful. As in Legionnaires' disease, *L. pneumophila* is the usual etiological agent.

Epidemics of Pontiac fever are uncommon; only two outbreaks have been recorded in the United States and most infections are seen as sporadic cases. The attack rate in epidemics is much higher than in the pneumonic form, averaging 95 to 100 per cent. The incidence of Pontiac fever is also much higher; it has been estimated, based on serological studies, that the incidence may be 100 times that of Legionnaires' disease.

The mode of transmission in epidemics is similar to that of Legionnaires' disease. It remains largely unknown in sporadic cases, but airborne transmission is assumed. For example, in one common source exposure of two individuals, one developed pneumonia, while the other developed the nonpneumonic form of disease. Both are infected with *L. pneumophila* serogroup 1.[19]

It is also important to note that many *Legionella* infections appear to be **asymptomatic**, as suggested by serological surveys. The incidence of such infection is only speculative, but antibody response is apparent in random populations, varying from 2 to 22 per cent.

Bacteriological and Serological Diagnosis[15]

Legionella are usually found in respiratory tissues and fluids. These include lung biopsies, pleural fluids, tracheal aspirates, and bronchial washings. Rarely, they may be recovered from blood.

Rapid diagnosis should be attempted by direct microscopy. Tissue smears or sections can be examined by appropriate staining, usually the Dieterle silver impregnation stain but the method is not specific; examination by Gram stain is not informative. Immunofluorescent staining using specific antibody conjugates is preferable and, if sufficient numbers of bacteria are present, can yield rapid and conclusive results.

Emulsified tissues or fluids may be cultured by plating to suitable mediums such as buffered charcoal yeast extract agar. Blood should be inoculated to diphasic bottles containing charcoal yeast extract medium. After 3 to 5 days incubation at 35°C., the plates should be examined for typical colonies. Smears from these should be examined by Gram stain and by direct immunofluorescent microscopy, using appropriate conjugated antiserum. Other physiological and biochemical tests (Table 25–4) are employed for identification. If available, both gas-liquid chromatography and DNA hybridization provide definitive identification.

Antibody response to *Legionella* is a convenient and widely used method for diagnosis, but is usually retrospective, due to the 3 to 4 weeks required for maximal antibody response. Single serum titers, even if high, must be interpreted with caution, since a significant number of healthy individuals—5 per cent or more—may exhibit titers. Antibody response is more definitively determined using paired serum samples in an indirect immunofluorescence test against heat-killed cells of known *Legionella* cultures. A fourfold rise in titer constitutes evidence of infection. The enzyme-linked immunosorbent assay (ELISA) test also has been recommended for this purpose; agglutination tests are less sensitive.

Chemotherapy

As noted earlier, most *Legionella* produce β-lactamase, so that cephalosporins and penicillin are not recommended as chemotherapeutic agents. The most effective antibiotics are the tetracyclines, erythromycin, and rifampin. Of these, erythromycin is the drug of choice and usually leads to rapid clinical improvement. To prevent relapses and reduce the period of convalescence, therapy with erythromycin should be continued for at least 3 weeks. Experience with tetracycline has not been uniformly successful. Although usually effective, there is potential for development of resistance to rifampin so that it is best used in combination therapy.

REFERENCES

1. Baltch, A. L., and P. E. Griffin. 1977. *Pseudomonas aeruginosa* bacteremia: a clinical study of 75 patients. Amer. J. Med. Sci. **274**:119–129.
2. Berendt, R. F. 1980. Survival of *Legionella pneumophila* in aerosols: effect of relative humidity. J. Infect. Dis. **141**:689.
3. Bergan, T. 1981. Pathogenetic factors of *Pseudomonas aeruginosa*. Scand. J. Infect. Dis. (Suppl.) **29**:7–12.
4. Bergan, T., A. Forsgren, and R. Norrby. 1981. Symposium on intensive therapy in Pseudomonas infections. Scand. J. Infect. Dis. (Suppl.) **29**:1–103.
5. Bibb, W. F., *et al.* 1981. Recognition of a second serogroup of *Legionella longbeachae*. J. Clin. Microbiol. **14**:674–677.

6. Blackmon, J. A., *et al.* 1981. Legionellosis. Amer. J. Pathol. **103**:427–465.
7. Broome, C. V., and D. W. Fraser. 1979. Epidemiologic aspects of legionellosis. Epidemiol. Rev. **1**:1–16.
8. Buchanan, R. E., and N. E. Gibbons (Eds.). 1974. Bergey's Manual of Determinative Bacteriology. 8th ed. The Williams & Wilkins Co., Baltimore.
9. Chadwick, P. 1976. A code of nomenclature for pyocin types of *Ps. aeruginosa*. Can. J. Publ. Hlth **67**:321–322.
10. Doroghazi, R. M., *et al.* 1981. Invasive external otitis. Report of 21 cases and a review of the literature. Amer. J. Med. **71**:603–614.
11. Elliott, J. A., and W. Johnson. 1981. Immunological and biochemical relationships among flagella isolated from *Legionella pneumophila* serogroups 1, 2, and 3. Infect. Immun. **33**:602–610.
12. Elliott, J. A., and W. Johnson. 1982. Virulence conversion of *Legionella pneumophila* serogroup 1 by passage in guinea pigs and embryonated eggs. Infect. Immun. **35**:943–946.
13. Elliott, J. A., W. Johnson, and C. M. Helms. 1981. Ultrastructural localization and protective activity of a high-molecular-weight antigen isolated from *Legionella pneumophila*. Infect. Immun. **31**:822–824.
14. Everett, E. D., and R. A. Nelson. 1975. Pulmonary melioidosis. Observations in thirty-nine cases. Amer. Rev. Resp. Dis. **112**:331–340.
15. Feeley, J. C., and G. W. Gorman. 1980. *Legionella*. pp. 318–324. *In* E. H. Lennette, *et al.* (Eds.): Manual of Clinical Microbiology. 3rd ed. American Society for Microbiology, Washington, D. C.
16. Fitzgerald, D., R. E. Morris, and C. E. Saelinger. 1982. Essential role of calcium in cellular internalization of *Pseudomonas* toxin. Infect. Immun. **35**:715–720.
17. Friedman, R. L., *et al.* 1982. The effects of *Legionella pneumophila* toxin on oxidative processes and bacterial killing of human polymorphonuclear leukocytes. J. Infect. Dis. **146**:328–333.
18. Frøland, S. S. 1981. Infections with *Pseudomonas aeruginosa* in the compromised host. Scand. J. Infect. Dis. (Suppl.) **29**:72–80.
19. Girod, J. C., *et al.* 1982. Pneumonic and nonpneumonic forms of legionellosis: the result of a common-source exposure to *Legionella pneumophila*. Arch. Intern. Med. **142**:545–547.
20. Holder, I. A., R. Wheeler, and T. C. Montie. 1982. Flagellar preparations from *Pseudomonas aeruginosa*: animal protection studies. Infect. Immun. **35**:276–280.
21. Homma, J. Y. 1980. Roles of exoenzymes and exotoxin in the pathogenicity of *Pseudomonas aeruginosa* and the development of a new vaccine. Japan. J. Exptl Med. **50**:149–165.
22. Homma, J. Y., *et al.* 1977. Serological typing of *Pseudomonas aeruginosa*—comparison of various antigenic schema. Japan. J. Exptl Med. **47**:195–201.
23. Horwitz, M. A., and S. C. Silverstein. 1981. Interaction of the Legionnaires' disease bacterium (*Legionella pneumophila*) with human phagocytes. I. *L. pneumophila* resists killing by polymorphonuclear leukocytes, antibody, and complement. II. Antibody promotes binding of *L. pneumophila* to monocytes but does not inhibit intracellular multiplication. J. Exptl Med. **153**:386–397; 398–406.
24. Howe, C., A. Sampath, and M. Spotnitz. 1971. The

Pseudomallei group: a review. J. Infect. Dis. **124**:598–606.

25. Hugh, R., and G. L. Gilardi. 1980. Pseudomonas. pp. 288–317. *In* E. H. Lennette, *et al.* (Eds.): Manual of Clinical Microbiology. 3rd ed. American Society for Microbiology, Washington, D. C.

26. Johnson, M. K., and D. Boese-Marrazzo. 1980. Production and properties of heat-stable extracellular hemolysin from *Pseudomonas aeruginosa*. Infect. Immun. **29**:1028–1033.

27. Lochner, J. E., *et al.* 1983. Effect of oxygen-dependent antimicrobial systems on *Legionella pneumophila*. Infect. Immun. **39**:487–489.

28. Lory, S., and R. J. Collier. 1980. Expression of enzymic activity by exotoxin A from *Pseudomonas aeruginosa*. Infect. Immun. **28**:494–501.

29. Lutz, F., S. Grieshaber, and I. Kaüfer. 1981. Cytotoxin from *Pseudomonas aeruginosa* in mice: distribution related to pathology. Toxicon **19**:763–771.

30. Meyer, R. D., and S. M. Finegold. 1980. Legionnaires' disease. Ann. Rev. Med. **31**:219–232.

31. McKinney, R. M., *et al.* 1981. *Legionella longbeachae* species nova, another etiologic agent of human pneumonia. Ann. Intern. Med. **94**:739–743.

32. Morris, G. K., *et al.* 1980. *Legionella gormanii* sp. nov. J. Clin. Microbiol. **12**:718–721.

33. Müller, H. E. 1981. Die Thermostabilität von *Legionella pneumophila*. Zentbl. Bakteriol. I **172B**:524–527.

34. Mutharia, L. M., *et al.* 1982. Outer membrane proteins of *Pseudomonas aeruginosa* serotype strains. J. Infect. Dis. **146**:770–779.

35. Nonoyama, S., *et al.* 1979. Inhibitory effect of *Pseudomonas aeruginosa* on the phagocytic and killing activities of rabbit polymorphonuclear leukocytes: purification and characterization of an inhibitor of polymorphonuclear leukocyte function. Infect. Immun. **24**:394–398.

36. Patamasucon, P., U. B. Schaad, and J. D. Nelson. 1982. Melioidosis. J. Pediat. **100**:175–182.

37. Rode, J. W., and D. D'A. Webling. 1981. Melioidosis in the Northern Territory of Australia. Med. J. Australia **1**:181–184.

38. Schlech, W. F., III, *et al.* 1981. Laboratory-acquired infection with *Pseudomonas pseudomallei* (melioidosis). New Engl. J. Med. **305**:1133–1135.

39. Slack, M. P. E. 1981. Antipseudomonal β-lactams. J. Antimicrob. Chemother. **8**:165–170.

40. Wilkinson, H. W., and B. J. Fikes. 1981. Detection of cell-associated or soluble antigens of *Legionella pneumophila* serogroups 1 to 6, *Legionella bozemanii*, *Legionella dumoffii*, *Legionella gormanii*, and *Legionella micdadei* by staphylococcal coagglutination tests. J. Clin. Microbiol. **14**:322–325.

41. Wong, M. C., *et al.* 1981. *Legionella pneumophila*: avirulent to virulent conversion through passage in cultured human embryonic lung fibroblasts. Current Microbiol. **5**:31–34.

42. Woods, D. E., *et al.* 1980. Role of pili in adherence of *Pseudomonas aeruginosa* to mammalian buccal epithelial cells. Infect. Immun. **29**:1146–1151.

43. Wretlind, B., and O. R. Pavlovskis. 1981. The role of proteases and exotoxin A in the pathogenicity of *Pseudomonas aeruginosa* infections. Scand. J. Infect. Dis. (Suppl.) **29**:13–19.

44. Young, L. S. 1980. The role of exotoxins in the pathogenesis of *Pseudomonas aeruginosa* infections. J. Infect. Dis. **142**:626–630.

CHAPTER 26

Bacteroides, Fusobacterium, Streptobacillus, and Calymmatobacterium

THE GRAM-NEGATIVE ANAEROBIC BACILLI	*Fusobacterium nucleatum* *Fusobacterium necrophorum*
BACTEROIDES	**STREPTOBACILLUS**
Bacteroides fragilis Group	*Morphology and Staining*
Bacteroides melaninogenicus-	*Culture*
asaccharolyticus Group	*Pathogenesis*
Other Bacteroides	**CALYMMATOBACTERIUM**
FUSOBACTERIUM	**(DONOVANIA)**

The Gram-Negative, Anaerobic Bacilli[3, 5]

A large group of nonspore-forming, gram-negative, anaerobic bacilli are normal inhabitants of the oropharynx, the urogenital tract, and the colon, where they may outnumber the aerobic flora. These microorganisms are opportunistic pathogens, sometimes associated with ulcerative processes of the mucous membranes, abscesses in tissues and organs, and septicemia. As obligate anaerobes they require special procedures for cultural isolation.

The taxonomic relationships of these bacteria have been somewhat controversial; the current Bergey classification places them in a single family, Bacteroidaceae, comprising three genera—*Bacteroides, Fusobacterium,* and *Leptotrichia* (Chapter 2). Those of greatest pathogenic potential are found in *Bacteroides* and *Fusobacterium; Leptotrichia* are rarely involved in human diseases. Table 26–1 lists the usual characters of *Bacteroides* and *Fusobacterium; Leptotrichia* will not be discussed here.

Morphologically, the Bacteroidaceae are heterogeneous, varying from slender rod forms, often tapered toward the ends (called fusiform bacilli), to filamentous and pleomorphic forms. These are illustrated in Figure 26–1.

The anaerobic bacilli that constitute the normal colonic flora will grow upon the usual laboratory mediums under appropriate anaerobic conditions. Others, associated with path-

ological processes in man, are generally more fastidious and require more complex mediums, usually enriched with blood. Some species will grow on defined mediums, usually requiring amino acids, glucose, vitamins, and other supplements.

The optimum pH is 6.3 to 7.0, and the optimum temperature for growth is 35° to 37° C. Completely anaerobic conditions are essential and growth is favored by the presence of carbon dioxide. The medium of choice for primary isolation is supplemented blood agar, often made selective by inclusion of vancomycin and kanamycin or gentamicin. The pigmentation of some *Bacteroides* is promoted by the use of laked blood in the medium. Relatively simple methods for the isolation and identification of the medically important members have been devised.[1, 3]

Table 26–1. **Usual Characters of *Bacteroides* and *Fusobacterium***

Bacteroides	*Fusobacterium*
Gram-negative	Gram-negative
Bacillus or coccobacillus	Bacillus
Obligate anerobe	Obligate anaerobe
Nonspore-forming	Nonspore-forming
Nonmotile	Nonmotile
Produce many fatty acids from peptones or carbohydrates	Produce butyric acid from peptones or carbohydrates

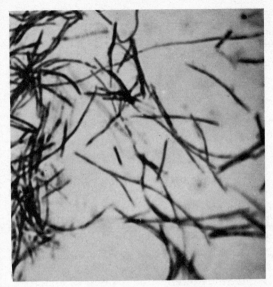

Figure 26–1. Fusiform bacilli in a stained smear from an anaerobic blood agar culture. × 1800. (Hemmens.)

At their usual site of colonization, the Bacteroidaceae rarely cause serious disease. It is only when they gain access to the tissues and organs that serious infection is initiated. Perhaps the most significant of these are intra-abdominal infections that arise from spillage of colonic contents into the tissues. Typically, these are mixed infections in which both aerobic and anaerobic microorganisms act synergistically to bring about suppurative disease. Bacteroidaceae are not all equally virulent and able to participate in infection. Indeed, of the several hundred anaerobic species that colonize the large bowel, only a few are associated with disease processes. Presumably, these possess virulence factors that are absent in the other varieties. *Bacteroides* of greatest clinical significance are found in the *B. fragilis* group, as discussed in the following section. It is evident that even in this group, virulence is limited, since the bacteria are seldom capable of initiating tissue infection except in the presence of other, usually aerobic, microorganisms.

BACTEROIDES[9, 11]

The anaerobic, gram-negative bacilli now known as *Bacteroides* were found by Veillon and Zuber in 22 cases of appendicitis in 1897. Subsequent studies have established their role in a variety of infections.

Bacteroides are separable into several large groups on the basis of cultural and morphological characteristics. The *B. fragilis* group contains several species that are bile-resistant, saccharolytic, and resistant to kanamycin and vancomycin; those of the *B. melaninogenicus-asaccharolyticus* group are bile-sensitive and pigmented; most other species are bile-sensitive and nonpigmented.

Bacteroides fragilis Group

Bacteroides of this group are the predominant flora of the intestinal tract. They are sometimes found in the genitourinary tract but seldom in the oropharynx. They are generally small, slender, nonmotile rods that stain poorly by the counterstain in the Gram stain. Capsules are formed, especially in virulent *B. fragilis* strains. Colonies are smooth, entire, and gray to white in color. The biochemical characters of the members of this group are shown in Table 26–2.

Bacteroides fragilis and, to a lesser extent, *B. thetaiotaomicron* are the most clinically relevant species and are particularly prominent in intra-abdominal sepsis. Considerable interest has developed, therefore, in the special properties that might explain the greater virulence of *B. fragilis*. Several factors appear to have significance in this regard. The **polysaccharide capsule** is undoubtedly involved in abscess formation, since the purified material

Table 26–2. Biochemical Characters of *Bacteroides fragilis* Group*

Species	Growth in 20% Bile	Esculin Hydrolysis	Catalase	Indole	Fermentation of		
					Glucose	Salicin	Trehalose
B. fragilis	+	+	+	−	+	−	−
B. diastonis	+	+	+	−	+	+	+
B. ovatus	+	+	−	+	+	+	+
B. thetaiotaomicron	+	+	+	+	+	−	+
B. uniformis	+	+	−	+	+	+	−
B. vulgatus	+	−	−	−	+	−	−

*Adapted from S. M. Finegold and D. M. Citron.[3]

Table 26–3. **Biochemical Characters of the *Bacteroides melaninogenicus-asaccharolyticus* Group***

Species	Growth in 20% Bile	Esculin Hydro-lysis	Pigment	Indole	Lipase	Glucose Fermen-tation
B. melaninogenicus						
subspecies *intermedius*	−	−	+	+	+	+
subspecies *melaninogenicus*	−	+	+	−	−	+
B. asaccharolyticus	−	−	+	+	−	−

*Adapted from S. M. Finegold and D. M. Citron.[3]

can induce abscesses in experimental animals; it may also promote adherence to tissue cells.[13] It is likely, too, that enzymes such as **proteases** and **lipases** also promote abscess formation. Another enzyme, **superoxide dismutase,** permits survival of *B. fragilis* in oxygenated tissues. *Bacteroides fragilis* isolated from clinical infections are significantly more sensitive to the bactericidal effects of serum than are fecal isolates or other *Bacteroides* species, suggesting that serum resistance is a virulence determinant.[2] It is of some interest that the surface lipopolysaccharide of *Bacteroides* is chemically incomplete as compared to that of enteric bacilli and does not possess the biological potency of endotoxins from these bacteria.

Bacteroides melaninogenicus-asaccharolyticus Group

The microorganisms of this group include two subspecies of *B. melaninogenicus—intermedius* and *melaninogenicus*—and *B. asaccharolyticus*. They are characterized by bile-sensitivity and the formation of a tan-to-black melanin pigment when they are grown on mediums that contain blood. In addition, their colonies exhibit deep red fluorescence when illuminated by ultraviolet light. The biochemical characteristics of this group of *Bacteroides* are shown in Table 26–3.

These microorganisms are a part of the normal microbial flora of the oropharynx, the urogenital tract, and the colon. Not surprisingly, they have been found in a number of opportunistic infections of the oral cavity, wounds, and the respiratory tract.

Other Bacteroides

The bile-sensitive, nonpigmented *Bacteroides,* as shown in Table 26–4, are more heterogeneous than the groups just discussed. They form a part of the normal microbial flora, with distribution similar to the *B. melaninogenicus-asaccharolyticus* group, but they are not as often encountered in human infections. In one study of infections caused by anaerobic bacteria, 22 per cent yielded one or more of these other *Bacteroides* species.[6] These included head and neck, pleuropulmonary, bacteremic, abdominal, urogenital, soft-tissue, and bone infections.

FUSOBACTERIUM[4, 8]

Although infections by many of the species of *Fusobacterium* have been recorded, most are due to one of two species—*F. nucleatum* or *F. necrophorum*. The ecological distribution of *F. necrophorum* is similar to that of the *Bacteroides,* and it causes similar types of infection. *Fusobacterium necrophorum* appears to be a more virulent microorganism and is capable of causing disseminated disease in humans.

Fusobacterium nucleatum

This fusiform bacillus is slender and tapered at each end, and exhibits little pleomorphism. The bacillus is gram-negative but tends to stain irregularly with aniline dyes. It is inhibited by the presence of bile in the medium, forms indole, and ferments fructose, but fails to

Table 26–4. **Biochemical Characters of the More Important Bile-Sensitive, Nonpigmented *Bacteroides***

Species	Growth in 20% Bile	Pigment	Esculin Hydrolysis	Indole	Urease	Fermentation of		
						Glucose	Lactose	Arabinose
B. ruminicola	−	−	+	−	−	+	+	+
B. ureolyticus	−	−	−	−	+	−	−	−
B. bivius	−	−	−	−	−	+	+	−
B. disiens	−	−	−	−	−	+	−	−
B. oralis	−	−	+	−	−	+	+	−

*Adapted from S. M. Finegold and D. M. Citron.[3]

ferment glucose or hydrolyze esculin. The bacterium is usually isolated on blood agar incubated anaerobically. Colonies on this medium are minute and often show hemolysis or green discoloration of the medium after exposure to air.

Fusobacterium necrophorum

This bacillus has been found in abscesses of the lung, liver, and other soft tissues, and in the blood stream. It is highly pleomorphic; slender bacilli may be found intermingled with filamentous and swollen forms, as shown in Figure 26–2. Although there is a marked tendency to irregular staining, the bacilli are gram-negative. Colonies growing on blood agar are often surrounded by a zone of green hemolysis that becomes apparent after the medium is exposed to oxygen. Its biochemical characters are similar to those of *F. nucleatum* except that fructose is not fermented and propionic acid is produced from lactic acid.

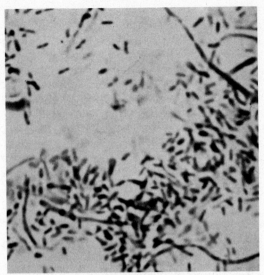

Figure 26–2. *Fusobacterium necrophorum.* The swollen and filamentous forms and poorly staining "ghost cells" are typical of the usual stained smear preparations. × 1000. (Dack.)

Streptobacillus[15]

A microorganism, known in the past by many names and now called *Streptobacillus moniliformis,* is the cause of an acute febrile illness sometimes given the descriptive name erythema multiforme. The disease in its usual form is acquired from an animal bite, usually by rats or mice, and the syndrome was first known as **rat-bite fever.** Transmission may also be effected by ingestion; an epidemic traced to consumption of contaminated milk was first noted in 1926 in Haverhill, Massachusetts, and this form of the disease came to be known as **Haverhill fever.** The name rat-bite fever is, however, more commonly used.

It should be noted that a clinically similar disease, known in Japan as sodoku, has also been called rat-bite fever, but it is caused by *Spirillum minor* (Chapter 32). There are, then, two types of rat-bite fever, with different etiological agents.

Morphology and Staining

Streptobacillus moniliformis is a gram-negative rod, usually about 1 μm. in breadth and 1 to 5 μm. in length, but often exhibiting considerable pleomorphism and irregular staining. A variety of morphological shapes are found in stained smears, including filamentous, bacillary, coccobacillary, swollen, and club-shaped cells. Filaments may exceed 100 μm. in length, and older cultures may fragment to yield coccobacillary cells.

Culture

Enriched mediums, containing blood, serum, or ascitic fluids, are required to support growth of the usually bacillary forms of *S. moniliformis.* Spontaneous L-phase variants have been found in some infections by this microorganism and require even more complex mediums for cultivation. Infusion mediums, supplemented with horse serum and yeast extract, permit growth of both bacillary and L-phase variants. Bacillary-phase colonies are entire, raised, and butyrous in consistency. L-phase colonies have the "fried-egg" appearance that is normally associated with *Mycoplasma* and other bacteria that lack cell walls (Chapter 35).

Pathogenesis

When the illness in man is contracted through a rat bite, the initial wound heals and is followed within 3 to 10 days by symptoms of toxemia. When the disease is acquired by ingestion, as in the milkborne epidemics, there is no initial lesion and the first evidence of infection is the toxic reaction—headaches, chills, vomiting, and general malaise. In either case, a cutaneous eruption appears, especially on the extremities, along with arthritis that is often severe in nature. The clinical resemblance to rat-bite fever of *Spirillum* etiology is quite close.

Streptobacillus moniliformis can be isolated by blood culture and has been found in the fluid of aspirated joints. The immune response to *S. moniliformis* infection takes the form of serum agglutinins, whose appearance has some diagnostic utility.

Streptobacillus moniliformis is a natural parasite of rats and mice, in which it colonizes the nasopharynx. Although usually of low viru-

lence for rats, it can assume pathogenicity for the rodent host, causing sporadic or epidemic disease. Man may acquire the infection by the bite of seemingly normal rats and probably almost all sporadic cases arise in this way. The distribution of the infection appears to be worldwide. In the United States, probably most instances of rat-bite fever are due to *Streptobacillus* rather than *Spirillum*. Several milkborne epidemics have been documented, likely arising from contamination of milk by rodents.

Calymmatobacterium (Donovania)[10, 12, 14]

Granuloma inguinale (granuloma venereum, Donovanosis) is an affliction characterized by a slowly progressive ulceration of the skin and mucous membranes of the genital region and rarely appears elsewhere. The initial lesion is a swelling, often in the groin, of a bubo, which later ruptures. Daughter lesions appear, discrete at first, but which subsequently spread and coalesce. The process may eventually involve the entire anogenital region, including the lower abdomen and buttocks, with development of a strong fetid odor. Little effective immunity appears to develop, at least not of sufficient magnitude to arrest the progress of the infection.

Bacillary bodies, stained by Wright's stain, were first observed by Donovan in 1905 in smears from lesions and in biopsy material (Fig. 26–3). The heavily encapsulated bacilli usually are found in the cytoplasm of phagocytes and present a characteristic appearance when stained by Wright's stain. The bacterial cells are blue or purple, usually with deeply staining polar granules, and are surrounded by a pink capsule. These have long been known as **Donovan bodies.**

The bacillus may be cultivated in the yolk sac of the developing chick embryo, but not on the chorioallantois. They may also be grown on enriched mediums, such as beef heart infusion, incubated at 37°C.

The microorganism, known for many years as *Donovania granulomatis,* has now been assigned to the genus *Calymmatobacterium,* as *C. granulomatis.* It is a short, plump, gram-negative bacillus, 1 to 2 μm. in length, often appearing in long filamentous chains; polar staining is a prominant character. Relatively heavy encapsulation is observed in prepara-

tions from lesions and is responsible for the mucoid character of yolk sac cultures and initial cultures on artificial mediums. Aside from its highly fastidious growth requirements, *C. granulomatis* closely resembles *Klebsiella* and, indeed, is related immunologically to these and other coliform bacilli.

Prior to isolation of *C. granulomatis* in pure culture, its causal relation to granuloma inguinale was only suggested by association. Immunological evidence supports an etiological role, however, since patients develop hypersensitivity to the specific cell substance and antibody is engendered to the capsular polysaccharide. The disease has also been reproduced by inoculation with lesion material and yolk sac cultures, but such attempts have not always been successful. Since it has not been possible to infect experimental animals other than the chick embryo, the etiological relation of *C. granulomatis* to granuloma inguinale cannot be regarded as completely established.

Donovanosis is generally regarded as a sexually transmitted disease, based in part upon the location of the lesions. For example, anogenital lesions are associated with rectal coitis, in both heterosexual and homosexual populations. It has been suggested that the organism is an inhabitant of the lower bowel and colonizes the genital region after contamination of abraded skin or membranes. It should be noted, however, that its occurrence in both sexual partners is uncommon.

Epidemiological evidence suggests that there is great individual variation in susceptibility and that natural resistance is of high order. This undoubtedly reflects the low invasiveness and virulence of *C. granulomatis.* Although widely distributed, the disease is uncommon

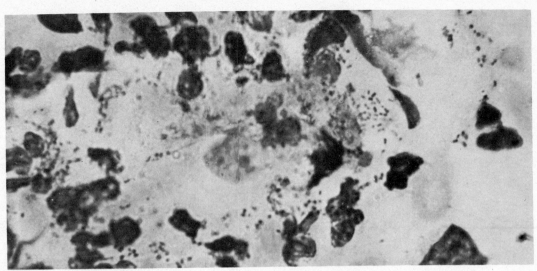

Figure 26–3. *Calymmatobacterium granulomatis* in a vaginal smear. The microorganisms are the small ovoid bodies both within polymorphonuclear leucocytes and lying free. Wright's stain; × 1200.

in temperate climates; endemic locations are primarily in hot and humid areas. In general, the epidemiology of granuloma inguinale is not well understood.

The disease may be successfully treated with several chemotherapeutic agents, including streptomycin and tetracyclines, although antibiotic resistance to the latter has been noted. Recently, co-trimoxazole has been reported to be particularly effective, with positive response in all patients treated.[7]

References

1. Allen, S. D., and J. A. Siders. 1980. Procedures for isolation and characterization of anaerobic bacteria. pp. 397–417. *In* E. H. Lennette, *et al.* (Eds.): Manual of Clinical Microbiology. 3rd ed. American Society for Microbiology, Washington, D.C.
2. Casciato, D. A., *et al.* 1979. Susceptibility of isolates of *Bacteroides* to the bactericidal activity of normal human serum. J. Infect. Dis. **140**:109–113.
3. Finegold, S. M., and D. M. Citron. 1980. Gram-negative, nonspore-forming anaerobic bacilli. pp. 431–439. *In* E. H. Lennette, *et al.* (Eds.): Manual of Clinical Microbiology. 3rd ed. American Society for Microbiology, Washington, D.C.
4. George, W. L., *et al.* 1981. Gram-negative anaerobic bacilli: their role in infection and patterns of susceptibility to antimicrobial agents. II. Little-known

Fusobacterium species and miscellaneous genera. Rev. Infect. Dis. **3**:599–626.
5. Hofstad, T. 1979. Serological responses to antigens of *Bacteroidaceae*. Microbiol. Rev. **43**:103–115.
6. Kirby, B. D., *et al.* 1980. Gram-negative anaerobic bacilli: their role in infection and patterns of susceptibility to antimicrobial agents. I. Little-known *Bacteroides* species. Rev. Infect. Dis. **2**:914–951.
7. Lal, S., and B. R. Garg. 1980. Further evidence of the efficacy of co-trimoxazole in granuloma venereum. Brit. J. Vener. Dis. **56**:412–413.
8. Langworth, B. F. 1977. *Fusobacterium necrophorum:* its characteristics and role as an animal pathogen. Bacteriol. Rev. **41**:373–390.
9. Macy, J. M., and I. Probst. 1979. The biology of gastrointestinal bacteroides. Ann. Rev. Microbiol. **33**:561–594.
10. Maddocks, I., E. M. Anders, and E. Dennis. 1976. Donovanosis in Papua New Guinea. Brit. J. Vener. Dis. **52**:190–196.
11. McGowan, K., and S. L. Gorbach. 1981. Anaerobes in mixed infections. J. Infect. Dis. **144**:181–186.
12. Morse, S. A. 1980. Sexually transmitted diseases. pp. 344–349. *In* E. H. Lennette, *et al.* (Eds.): Manual of Clinical Microbiology. 3rd ed. American Society for Microbiology, Washington, D.C.
13. Onderdonk, A. B., *et al.* 1978. Adherence of *Bacteroides fragilis* in vivo. Infect. Immun. **19**:1083–1087.
14. Rajam, R. V., and P. N. Rangiah. 1954. Donovanosis (granuloma inguinale, granuloma venereum). Wld Hlth Org. Monogr. Ser. No. 24, Geneva.
15. Rogosa, M. 1980. *Streptobacillus moniliformis* and *Spirillum minor.* pp. 350–356. *In* E. H. Lennette, *et al.* (Eds.): Manual of Clinical Microbiology. 3rd ed. American Society for Microbiology, Washington, D.C.

Bacillus—The Spore-Forming Aerobes

The spore-forming rod-shaped bacteria are divided into two groups on the basis of their relation to atmospheric oxygen. The genus *Bacillus* includes the aerobic forms; the anaerobic types are designated *Clostridium.* A very large number of species of *Bacillus* have been described, the majority of them from soil or dust. *Bacillus subtilis,* the type species, infects humans only rarely, while *Bacillus cereus* is a frequent cause of food poisoning (Chapter 36). With these two exceptions, *Bacillus anthracis,* the causative agent of anthrax, is the only member of this large group that is frankly pathogenic for man.

Bacillus anthracis

Primarily a disease of lower animals transmissible to man, anthrax is of particular historical interest, for it was in his study of this disease that Koch provided the first demonstration of the causal relation between a specific bacterium and an infectious disease. Although observed in animals dying of anthrax in 1850, the bacillus was first cultured by Koch in 1877; he also described its life history and reproduced the disease with a pure culture of the microorganism. The importance of this discovery in the development of bacteriology has been discussed elsewhere (Chapter 1).

Morphology and Staining

The anthrax bacillus is one of the largest of the pathogenic bacteria and ranges from 3 to 5 μm. in length and 1 to 1.25 μm. in breadth. The ends of the rod are often concave and somewhat swollen, so that the appearance of a chain of anthrax bacilli has been compared to a jointed bamboo pole. The cells occur singly and as end-to-end pairs or short chains in the body, but in culture long chains are formed (Fig. 27–1). Unlike most of the sporulating aerobic bacilli they are **nonmotile.**

Capsules may be found on the bacilli in smears from an infected animal but are not found in cultured cells except when grown on special mediums incubated under increased carbon dioxide tension. The capsular material is not polysaccharide as it is in many bacteria, but is a high-molecular-weight polypeptide composed exclusively of D-glutamic acid (the "unnatural" stereoisomer).

The anthrax bacillus also differs from other aerobic pathogenic bacteria in that it forms spores. Their diameter does not exceed that of the vegetative cell; hence, the spore-containing rod is not distorted. Spores are formed most abundantly at 32° to 35°C. and only under aerobic conditions, *i.e.,* not in the circulating blood of infected animals.

The bacilli are gram-positive; they stain readily, but often unevenly, with the usual aniline dyes. The granular material within the

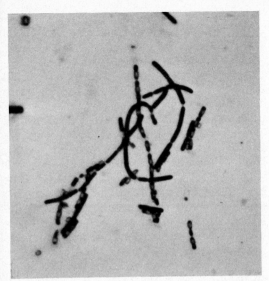

Figure 27–1. *Bacillus anthracis,* 48-hour culture on nutrient agar. The spores appear as unstained areas. Note the typical arrangement of the bacilli in coiled chains. Crystal violet stain; × 1200.

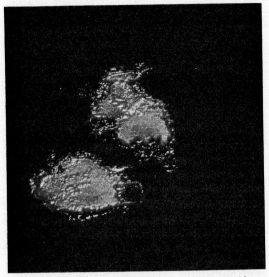

Figure 27–3. Colonies of *Bacillus cereus* var. *mycoides* on nutrient agar, 24-hour culture, × 3.

cell consists of fat, volutin, or glycogen. Spores are stained with difficulty but, after staining with hot carbol-fuchsin, are equally difficult to decolorize; hence, the vegetative cells may be decolorized and stained with a contrasting dye.

The colonies of the anthrax bacillus are irregular and have a curled or hair-like structure, giving what is sometimes called a "Medusa head" appearance (Fig. 27–2). On microscopic examination tangled coils of long chains of bacilli may be found. This colonial appearance is closely simulated by *B. cereus* and some other related saprophytic, aerobic, spore-forming bacilli (Figs. 27–3 and 27–4).

Physiology

The anthrax bacillus grows readily upon all the ordinary laboratory mediums, and growth is not improved by the addition of enriching substances; it can also be grown on simple synthetic mediums. The maximum growth temperature for most strains is 40°C., with an optimum at 37°C. The bacillus is aerobic and facultatively anaerobic.

The anthrax bacillus may be differentiated from other species of *Bacillus* without great

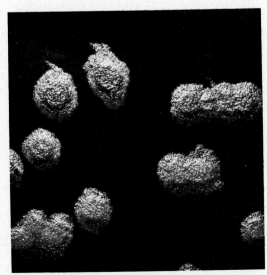

Figure 27–2. Colonies of *Bacillus anthracis* on nutrient agar, 24-hour culture. Note the large size and coarse texture suggestive of R variants. × 3.

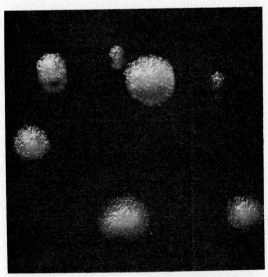

Figure 27–4. Colonies of *Bacillus subtilis* on nutrient agar, 24-hour culture. Note the resemblance to colonies of the anthrax bacillus. × 3.

difficulty and may be identified with a considerable degree of confidence by the aggregation of physiological and morphological characteristics; these are listed in Table 27–1.

Vegetative cells of the anthrax bacillus display no more than the usual resistance to deleterious influences, but the spores are relatively highly resistant, although not so resistant as the spores of *B. subtilis*. The bacilli have been isolated from naturally infected soil stored for as long as 60 years. Anthrax spores are usually destroyed by boiling for 10 minutes and by dry heat at 140°C. for three hours. Their resistance to disinfectants is variable, for 0.1 per cent mercuric chloride may fail to kill them in 70 hours, while oxidizing agents are much more effective; for example, 3 per cent hydrogen peroxide kills in one hour, and 4 per cent potassium permanganate in 15 minutes. In putrifying animal carcasses, vegetative cells are destroyed within a few days but spores are viable under such circumstances for many months. Thus, the eradication of anthrax cannot readily be accomplished by the elimination of animal reservoirs as in other animal diseases, such as brucellosis.

Toxins[9, 14]

Under ordinary conditions of culture the anthrax bacillus does not produce an exotoxin, nor is the cell substance of the microorganism toxic. Vaccines prepared with killed bacilli do not produce an effective immunity, and for many years the high virulence of the anthrax bacillus and the toxemia evident in infections were not understood. As pointed out elsewhere (Chapter 12), the discrepancy between the apparent atoxicity of a microorganism and the intoxication evident in the disease produced by it may be accounted for in two ways; *viz.*, toxicity may be produced by the microorganism only under the conditions of growth in the tissues of the infected animals, or the toxicity may be of host origin and produced by the infected tissues.

Table 27–1. **Characteristics that Differentiate Bacillus anthracis**[4]

Cellular and colonial morphology
Spores with diameter less than sporangium
Lack of motility
Capsule formation on bicarbonate agar
Failure to ferment xylose and arabinose
Growth under anaerobic conditions
Morphological changes induced by penicillin
Lysis by gamma phage
Immunofluorescence staining of both cell wall and capsule by *B. anthracis* conjugate

The former appeared to hold true in anthrax in that a toxic substance could be isolated from infected tissue. This was first shown in 1947, when a substance exhibiting inflammatory activity was isolated from tissues of infected animals. Subsequently, it has been shown that a toxin can be produced *in vitro* that is made up of several immunologically distinct protein components: an **edema factor (EF)**, a **protective antigen (PA)**, and a **lethal factor (LF)**. None of these is toxic when tested alone, but when the PA is combined with either EF or LF, the mixtures produce the edema (local) reaction or the lethal reaction, respectively. Recent evidence indicates that toxin production is mediated by a large, temperature-sensitive plasmid.[10]

It has recently been shown that EF is an **adenylate cyclase,** inactive as it occurs in *B. anthracis,* but activated when it enters susceptible eucaryotic cells.[8] A proposed model for the action of the anthrax toxin envisions PA as reacting with receptors on the host cell surface to produce changes that permit LF and EF to enter the cell. In the cytoplasm, EF is activated when it reacts with a heat-stable substance, probably calmodulin. Cyclic adenosine monophosphate (cAMP), formed by the enzyme (activated EF), leads to the edematous response. Thus, anthrax toxin is added to the growing number of bacterial products that elevate cAMP. Unlike cholera toxin and *Escherichia coli* enterotoxin, which activate host cell cyclase, EF is itself an adenylate cyclase.

Virulence

It was noted by Pasteur that prolonged cultivation of these bacilli at higher temperatures (42.5°C.) resulted in loss of virulence and the appearance of asporogenous variants. Virulence is not related, however, to the ability to form spores, for both asporogenous virulent strains and spore-forming avirulent strains may be produced. The loss of virulence is now explained by the finding, mentioned above, that toxin production is mediated by temperature-sensitive plasmids. Virulent strains may be cured of their plasmids by repeated culture at 42.5°C., and thus become nontoxigenic.[10] The production of toxin is, therefore, a prime virulence determinant.

Toxin production is necessary, but not sufficient, for virulence. Virulence is, in addition, partly dependent on the formation of the glutamyl polypeptide capsule. Virulent strains of *B. anthracis* produce the capsule *in vivo,* and also *in vitro* when grown under increased carbon dioxide tension on bicarbonate-containing mediums. Colonies grown in this way are mucoid in texture. These same strains appear rough, however, on ordinary mediums grown at atmospheric CO_2 concentrations, since capsular material is not produced. Occasionally, avirulent strains may be encapsulated, producing mucoid colonies in air culture, but these strains do not form toxins.

Pathogenicity for Lower Animals

In nature, anthrax is primarily a disease of cattle and sheep; horses and swine are susceptible but are less commonly affected. Wild deer and other gregarious herbivora are liable to occasional outbreaks. Although not a common disease in the United States, occasional outbreaks, usually derived from infected soil, occur in domestic animals. Human cases sometimes parallel these epidemics, generally appearing in individuals who work closely with infected animals. The incidence of animal (and human) disease is much greater in other parts of the world, particularly in countries with largely agricultural economies.

The smaller rodents are very sensitive to inoculation. Rabbits, guinea pigs, and white mice are susceptible in that order, and are fatally affected by the subcutaneous introduction of a very small number of virulent bacilli. Guinea pigs and mice are often used as experimental animals; white mice may succumb to inoculation with a single bacillus of a highly virulent strain. Carnivorous animals, though possessing greater resistance then the herbivora, are nevertheless susceptible, as several epidemics in zoological gardens have shown. Certain animals, *e.g.,* rats, possess a marked natural resistance to anthrax.

The route by which the bacilli enter the body exerts an important influence in both experimental and natural infections. Subcutaneous inoculation is the method most commonly practiced in experimental work and is almost uniformly fatal with the ordinary small laboratory animals. Feeding experiments show that administration of spore-free cultures even to highly susceptible animals is without result, owing to the destruction of the bacilli in the stomach. The feeding of spores, on the other hand, leads to infection of the more susceptible species, although not so certainly as in subcutaneous inoculation. Resistant species, such as swine, may be infected through the alimentary tract only with difficulty. Infection through the respiratory tract is possible in the experimental animal but is probably almost unknown in the lower animals under natural conditions.

In highly susceptible animals the disease is acute and runs a rapid course; the case fatality in cattle and sheep is about 80 per cent. It presents all the characteristics of typical septicemia, and local manifestations may be almost entirely absent. Enormous multiplication of the bacteria takes place in the blood and internal organs, and histological sections of the liver or spleen show the capillaries engorged with masses of bacteria. The spleen is a deep red color and greatly enlarged, hence the name splenic fever. The more resistant animal species do not develop this generalized infection, but the bacteria remain localized in an abscess or carbuncle and fail to spread through the body. Such natural resistance has been found, under experimental conditions, to be separable into two components: resistance to the establishment of an infection, *i.e.,* antibacterial resistance, and resistance to the toxin.

Under natural conditions cattle and sheep are infected through the alimentary tract by swallowing spores while grazing in infected pastures. As has been pointed out, spores are able to retain their vitality in soil for a long period, and pastures once infected may infect cattle after a lapse of as many as 30 years. In the United States contaminated feed, especially bone meal, has been responsible for the infection of livestock with anthrax. Hides imported from China and other countries where the disease prevails are not uncommonly contaminated with anthrax spores; in the United States several outbreaks of anthrax among cattle with some consequent cases of human infection have been traced to the overflowing of pasture land by streams receiving the drainage of tanneries.

HUMAN ANTHRAX[3]

Three routes of infection of human beings are known: (1) the skin, (2) the respiratory tract, and (3) the alimentary tract. The bacillus is almost always transmitted to man from lower animals, although human-to-human transmission may be possible.[6]

The persons most commonly affected are those having to do with cattle and their products, such as butchers, herdsmen, and handlers of hides, hair, and fleeces. Human anthrax is now an extremely rare occurrence in the United States. Only 17 cases were recorded between 1972 and 1981. This represents a significant reduction over the past 40 years, as shown in Figure 27–5. Although most cases of

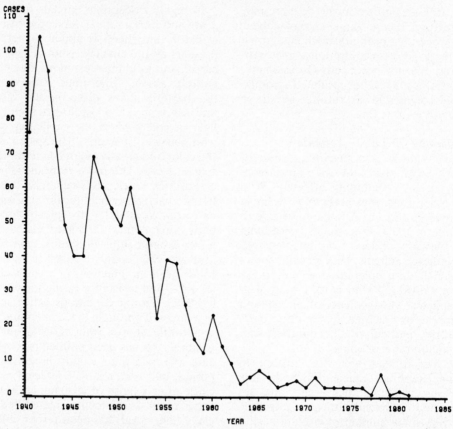

Figure 27–5. Reported cases of anthrax in the United States from 1940 to 1981. (Centers for Disease Control, Annual summary 1981: reported morbidity and mortality in the United States. Morbidity and Mortality Weekly Rep. **30**[54], 1982.)

anthrax are in those who work closely with animals, animal products have served to disseminate the microorganism. The incidence in those working with animal hides and bristles is significant, but consumers have also been infected from these products, due to the longevity of spores. Accordingly, international commerce involving these products is closely controlled, at least by developed nations.

Cutaneous Anthrax

The most common form of anthrax in the human subject is due to skin infection and usually takes the form of a localized boil or abscess, characteristically with a black eschar. The lesion often heals spontaneously but may progress to septicemia unless checked by incision or other surgical procedure, and may involve the central nervous system, causing meningitis. Owing to the relatively high resistance of man, septicemia does not often occur, especially if the carbuncle is incised and thoroughly drained. Lesions of all sizes may be produced, from a minute pustule to a large abscess.

Pulmonary Anthrax[2]

The pulmonary form of anthrax due to inhalation of the microorganisms is the most dangerous, although not the most common, variety of the disease in man. It was, at one time, an occupational disease among those handling and sorting wools and fleeces. The infection is contracted by inhalation of spores set floating in the air from the infected material; pulmonary anthrax is known in England as "woolsorters' disease."

Pulmonary anthrax is characterized by many of the symptoms of pneumonia and often passes into fatal septicemia or meningitis. In experimental airborne anthrax, a very few spores of virulent strains are infective. Inhaled spores are likely carried to the mediastinal lymph nodes, where they germinate to begin the infective process. From this focus, they enter the blood stream and are soon found in the spleen. It is thought that the bacilli, by virtue of their toxin, cause vascular injury with edema, hemorrhage, and thrombosis. It is of some interest that anthrax spores may occur in the nose and throat of healthy persons exposed to inhalation infection without subsequent development of the disease, and serological surveys have suggested the occurrence of subclinical infection.

Intestinal Anthrax

The alimentary tract, although the usual path of infection in domestic animals, is rarely so in man. In a few instances intestinal anthrax has been contracted through the medium of spore-infected food. Such cases occur among those who work with animal products and are probably due to handling food with uncleansed hands. Insufficiently cooked meat from anthrax-infected animals may also be a source of intestinal anthrax. The overall case fatality rate in untreated cases of anthrax of all types is probably around 20 per cent.

Bacteriological Diagnosis[4]

Anthrax bacilli are often presumptively identified by direct examination of material from the cutaneous lesion. The presence of typical gram-positive bacilli that exhibit immunofluorescent staining of both cell wall and capsule by *B. anthracis* conjugate is indicative of anthrax.

Isolation and identification of the microorganism from lesions, blood, or sputum provides definitive laboratory diagnosis. Blood culture is performed in the usual manner and subcultured to blood agar plates; other clinical specimens may be streaked directly. Typical colonies are selected for Gram stain and subjected to the identification procedures as outlined in Table 27–1.

Since there is no completely satisfactory selective medium for *B. anthracis,* heavily contaminated materials may be examined for these bacteria by animal inoculation, provided facilities are suitable and all materials can be autoclaved or decontaminated upon completion. Mice and guinea pigs die within 10 days after subcutaneous inoculation of anthrax bacilli; the enlarged and deep red spleen will contain enormous numbers of typical *B. anthracis.*

Chemotherapy

Prior to the development of the sulfonamides and antibiotics, anthrax was treated with only partial success by a combination of antiserum and arsenicals. While the number of treated cases is limited by the low incidence of the disease, sulfonamides appear to be effective chemotherapeutic agents, and penicillin remarkably so. In those instances in which the bacilli have been found to be penicillin-resist-

ant, the tetracyclines, streptomycin, and co-trimoxazole are satisfactory alternatives.

Immunity

Natural immunity, or resistance, of certain animal species is very high. This is a consequence, at least in part, of an anthracidal activity present in tissues and associated with a histone-like protein or polypeptide (Chapter 12).

Recovery from infection in the susceptible animal results in a solid immunity, and the serum contains protective antibody to high titer. Nevertheless, it has not been possible to produce any appreciable immunity to challenge inoculation by immunization with killed vaccines; effective immunity has resulted only from infection with attenuated strains or by inoculation with virulent, or partially virulent, strains in conjunction with protective antiserum. Both of these latter methods have been applied in animal immunization.

Following early examination of the immunological activity of *B. anthracis* products, a protective protein antigen was prepared and studied in some detail. This antigen is presumably the PA component of the holotoxin discussed earlier and is elaborated by the anthrax bacilli, or unencapsulated avirulent mutants, during growth. It is heat-labile and somewhat unstable, but can be preserved by lyophilization.

Effective immunity is produced by prophylactic inoculation with the protective antigen, in both man and animals, and is many times more effective in this regard than attenuated vaccines. A purified protein antigen of this nature is employed for immunization of high-risk occupational groups in the United States.

OTHER BACILLUS SPECIES

In the current Bergey classification, 22 species of *Bacillus* are accepted, with another 26 species of somewhat uncertain status.[1] Most *Bacillus* species are saprophytic soil forms and are of interest to the microbiologist in widely diverse ways. Morphogenesis and control of sporulation provides models for studies related to cell differentiation. Some, particularly *B. subtilis,* are important in the search for answers to questions in biochemical genetics. A significant number of *Bacillus* species produce antibiotic substances with importance in both medicine and biochemical research.[7] *Bacillus* species are frequently pathogenic for insects, and there is a burgeoning interest in the control

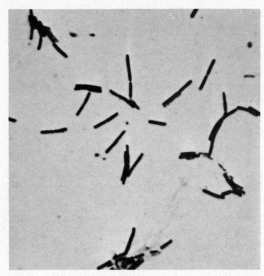

Figure 27–6. *Bacillus subtilis,* 24-hour culture on nutrient agar. No spores have formed as yet. Note the typical arrangement of the bacilli. Crystal violet stain; × 1200.

of insect pests, including insect vectors of disease, by infection with *B. thuringiensis* and *B. sphaericus.*[5, 11]

With the exception of *B. anthracis,* the pathogenic potential of these forms for man is slight at best. *Bacillus subtilis* is occasionally responsible for infection, particularly of the eye. *Bacillus* species have been reported as the etiological agent in a few cases of serious infections, including endocarditis, usually in drug addicts or in cancer patients.[13]

Bacillus cereus

This species has long interested medical microbiologists because it is quite similar to *B. anthracis* and, for many years, was difficult to differentiate from it. Although not pathogenic in the usual sense, *B. cereus* is a significant enterotoxin-producing agent responsible for a widespread food poisoning in humans; *B. cereus* food poisoning is discussed in Chapter 36.

It is also a rare opportunistic pathogen, causing meningitis, osteomyelitis, eye infections, and acute intestinal disease in drug abusers, neonates, and compromised patients.[12]

References

1. Buchanan, R. E., and N. E. Gibbons (Eds.). 1974. Bergey's Manual of Determinative Bacteriology. 8th ed. The Williams & Wilkins Co., Baltimore.
2. Dalldorf, F. G., A. F. Kaufmann, and P. S. Brachman. 1971. Woolsorters' disease. An experimental model. Arch. Pathol. **92**:418–426.
3. Dutz, W., and E. Kohout-Dutz. 1981. Anthrax. Internat. J. Dermatol. **20**:203–206.
4. Feeley, J. C., and C. M. Patton. 1980. *Bacillus.* pp. 145–149. *In* E. H. Lennette, *et al.* (Eds.): Manual of Clinical Microbiology. 3rd ed. American Society for Microbiology, Washington, D. C.
5. Hamon, J. (Reporter). 1981. Control of vectors by parasites and pathogens. Parasitology **82**(Pt. 4):117–129.
6. Heyworth, B., *et al.* 1975. Anthrax in the Gambia: a epidemiological study. Brit. Med. J. **4**:79–82.
7. Katz, E., and A. L. Demain. 1977. The peptide antibiotics of *Bacillus*: chemistry, biogenesis, and possible functions. Bacteriol. Rev. **41**:449–474.
8. Leppa, S. H. 1982. Anthrax toxin edema factor: a bacterial adenylate cyclase that increases cyclic AMP concentrations in eukaryotic cells. Proc. Natl Acad. Sci. USA **79**:3162–3166.
9. Lincoln, R. E., and D. C. Fish. 1970. Anthrax toxin. pp. 361–414. *In* T. C. Montie, S. Kadis, and S. J. Ajl (Eds.): Microbial Toxins. Vol. III, Bacterial Protein Toxins. Academic Press, New York.
10. Mikesell, P., *et al.* 1983. Evidence for plasmid-mediated toxin production in *Bacillus anthracis.* Infect. Immun. **39**:371–376.
11. Report. 1981. Mammalian safety of microbial agents for vector control: a WHO memorandum. Bull. Wld Hlth Org. **59**:857–863.
12. Shamsuddin, D., *et al.* 1982. *Bacillus cereus* panophthalmitis: source of the organism. Rev. Infect. Dis. **4**:97–103.
13. Tuazon, C. U., *et al.* 1979. Serious infections from *Bacillus* sp. J. Amer. Med. Assn **241**:1137–1140.
14. Wright, G. G. 1975. Anthrax toxin. pp. 292–295. *In* D. Schlessinger (Ed.): Microbiology—1975. American Society for Microbiology, Washington, D. C.

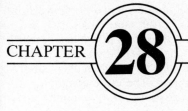
Clostridium—
The Spore-Forming Anaerobes

The group of anaerobic and microaerophilic sporulating bacilli includes a variety of forms. More than 300 species have been described, but only 61 of these are recognized as species of *Clostridium* in the most recent Bergey classification.[5] Some of these species are important in the production of organic solvents and other commercially useful metabolic products. A few, however, are pathogenic for man and lower animals, although their invasive capacity is generally quite limited. They are often found in the intestinal contents of man and animals as a part of the normal microbiota, but are widely distributed in soil and water. It is perhaps best to regard them as saprophytic soil microbes that may colonize the large bowel and, under some circumstances, act as opportunistic pathogens.

Because of their low invasiveness, these bacteria seldom cause disease in the absence of some precipitating factor or event. *Clostridium*

botulinum rarely causes infection of the tissues, while others, such as the tetanus bacillus, produce local infections when aided by traumatic injury to the tissues and, frequently, by the presence of other bacteria. Still others, exemplified by bacilli responsible for clostridial myonecrosis (gas gangrene), show pronounced invasive properties when once established, but the initial invasion is made possible by other factors, usually trauma and the presence of other bacteria.

The pathogenicity of the clostridia is, rather, attributable to their ability to form powerful exotoxins. In the case of botulism, the toxin is preformed outside the animal host and, since it is resistant to digestive enzymes, enters the body by absorption from the alimentary tract. In other cases, a focus of infection is established, and the toxin formed at that point may be disseminated. In some instances, such as gangrene, an extensive local destruction of tissue occurs, but in general, the diseases due to these bacilli are essentially toxemias.

The disease syndromes caused by clostridia are varied, depending on the species involved and the circumstances of infection or toxin ingestion. *Clostridium botulinum* is responsible for a serious and often fatal food poisoning, in which the preformed botulinum toxin is ingested in food. In infants, however, the toxin is formed during *C. botulinum* growth in the intestine to give rise to infant botulism after toxin absorption. Tetanus, or lockjaw, arises when *C. tetani* enters wounds and forms tetanus toxin, which is disseminated to target nerve tissue in the body. Clostridial myonecrosis, or gas gangrene, results from wound infections with one or more of a number of histotoxic clostridia. These form a variety of toxins that, in sum, result in the characteristic pathology; *C. perfringens* is the clostridial species most often encountered in gangrene. *Clostridium perfringens* appears to have varied potential, since it is also the cause of a common type of food poisoning (Chapter 36) as well as a rare, but more serious necrotizing infection of the small bowel. *Clostridium difficile* is the usual agent of pseudomembranous colitis, which ap-pears to be precipitated when other bowel flora are inhibited by certain antibiotics.

With the exception of *C. histolyticum*, which is microaerophilic, *Clostridium* are obligate anaerobes; they may be grown in deep cultures or in anaerobic jars. The more common pathogenic species are gram-positive, nonencapsulated bacilli, motile by peritrichous flagella; *C. perfringens*, however, is not flagellated and is therefore nonmotile. Spores are usually greater in diameter than the vegetative cell, and the spore-containing cells are spindle- or club-shaped. The spores of the tetanus bacillus are round and terminal; those of other clostridia are generally oval and subterminal. Two physiological types of clostridia are distinguished—one predominantly fermentative or saccharolytic and the other predominantly proteolytic; a number of volatile fatty acids are produced from carbohydrates or proteins. The useful characteristics of the more common pathogenic clostridia are shown in Table 28–1. Only the more important *Clostridium* species and their associated diseases will be discussed here; food poisoning syndromes due to *C. botulinum* and *C. perfringens* are treated in detail in Chapter 36.

Clostridium botulinum[29, 32]

Botulism was first observed in Germany in 1785. It was often associated with the consumption of sausages; hence the not altogether appropriate name botulism (Latin *botulus,* sausage). The causative bacterium, now called *Clostridium botulinum,* was isolated in 1896.

Morphology
Clostridium botulinum is a large, pleomorphic, gram-positive bacillus exhibiting wide variation in size, *viz.*, 0.3 to 1.3 μm. in breadth and 1.6 to 9.4 μm. in length (Fig. 28–1). It occurs singly, in pairs, and in chains. It is motile by four to eight peritrichous flagella. Spores are subterminal and oval; they distend the vegetative cell, often resulting in club-shaped cells.

Surface colonies on solid mediums incubated anaerobically are relatively large, 5 to 10 mm. in diameter; glistening; translucent at the edges

Table 28–1. **Morphological and Biochemical Characteristics of the More Important Pathogenic Clostridia**

Species	Spores	Capsule	Motility	Hydrolysis Gelatin	Hydrolysis Casein	Fermentation Glucose	Fermentation Lactose	Exotoxin
C. tetani	spherical, terminal	−	+	+	−	−	−	S
C. septicum		−	+	+	−	+	+	M
C. perfringens		+	−	+	−	+	+	M
C. novyi		−	+	+	−*	+	−	S
C. histolyticum	oval,	−	+	+	+	−	−	W
C. sporogenes	subterminal	−	+	+	+	+	−	−
C. difficile		−	+	+	−	+	−	M
C. botulinum		−	+	+	+*	+*	−	S
C. sordelli		−	+	+	+	+	−	M

*Most strains.
S = strong; M = moderate; W = weak.

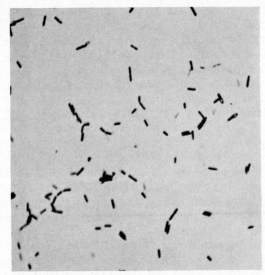

Figure 28–1. *Clostridium botulinum* type A from pure culture. Note the subterminal swollen spores and free unstained spores admixed with the vegetative cells. Fuchsin; × 1050.

with a thicker brownish center; filamentous; and hemolytic on blood agar.

Physiology

Clostridium botulinum grows on the usual laboratory mediums under strict anaerobic conditions. It may be grown also on synthetic mediums containing several amino acids. Mediums containing brain, meat, or coagulated proteins are blackened and digested; gelatin is liquified and milk is peptonized. Other differential reactions are listed in Table 28–1.

The spores of *C. botulinum* are highly resistant. They withstand 100°C. for up to 20 hours and autoclaving (121°C.) for as long as 20 minutes. The heat resistance of spores is of significance in the canning industry. Commercial processing of canned foods is designed to destroy the spores of these bacilli.

A potent exotoxin is formed that is unusually stable to heat, requiring 80°C. for 30 minutes or 100°C. for 10 minutes for destruction.

Types

Several types of *C. botulinum* are recognized based upon the different antigenic types of toxin produced, as shown in Table 28–2. Each of the toxins listed is immunologically distinct, except that there is some minor serological cross-reactivity between toxins E and F. Most human botulism is due to types A and B, with type E a distant third; a few cases have been ascribed to type G.[31]

Physiological and biochemical characteristics of *C. botulinum* strains do not always parallel the toxin-determined types, however. Type A strains, for example, are usually proteolytic, as are most type B strains found in the United States. European strains of type B, however, are usually nonproteolytic.

The distribution of *C. botulinum* is worldwide, and its principal habitat is soil. Both type A and proteolytic type B are found in soils in the United States. Type E appears principally in marine and fresh-water ecosystems and is the most prevalent type in Alaska. The predominant strain in Europe is nonproteolytic type B.

Toxins[27, 32]

Of the antigenically distinct types of toxin produced by *C. botulinum*, type A is the most potent, its toxicity exceeding that of all other known exotoxins. It has been estimated that a single LD_{50} dose for mice consists of slightly less than 5×10^6 toxin molecules and that ingestion of 7000 mouse LD_{50} units can induce botulism in humans.

In the natural state, botulinum toxins are high-molecular-weight complexes composed of a **neurotoxin** component combined with one or more nontoxic bacterial proteins. Type A

Table 28–2. **Types of *Clostridium botulinum***

C. botulinum Type	Antigenic Types of Toxin Produced	Disease
A	A	Botulism of man
B	B	Botulism of man
C_α	C_1 (predominant), C_2, D	Fowl botulism
C_β	C_2	Forage poisoning of cattle
D	D (predominant), C_1, C_2	Lamziekte of cattle
E	E	Botulism of man
F	F	Botulism of man
G	G	Botulism of man
Af	A (predominant), F	Unknown

toxin, for example, is a 900,000 dalton complex (also called **progenitor toxin**) made up of a nontoxic hemagglutinating protein of about 500,000 daltons and a neurotoxin of about 150,000 daltons. Other types of botulinum toxins are similar in makeup, but differ in the kinds of nontoxic proteins and the molecular weight of the complexes. The nontoxic portions of the complexes serve to protect the neurotoxin from the destructive effects of gastric proteinases and acid after oral administration.

The neurotoxin component can be separated from the progenitor complex in highly purified form; the separated neurotoxin is sometimes called **derivative toxin.** Neurotoxins from the several botulinum types have essentially the same pharmacological action and, although immunologically different, they are similar in structure. Neurotoxin is synthesized by *C. botulinum* as a single polypeptide chain, of about 150,000 daltons, with one or more intrachain disulfide linkages; this form of toxin has relatively low toxicity. The native neurotoxin is activated by trypsin, or by bacterial proteases having trypsin-like activity, to yield a molecule with enhanced toxic activity. In this reaction, the polypeptide chain is nicked to form two chains of unequal size—heavy (H) and light (L)—held together by interchain disulfide bonds.

Sugiyami has summarized these events and compared the activation process with that of the tetanus neurotoxin, as shown in Figure 28–2. Although the minimum molecular size required for toxicity is not yet established, there is some evidence that the H-chain is responsible for binding to target sites.

Both pure and crude botulinum toxin can be detoxified and converted to toxoid with formaldehyde. The formol toxin can be used for active immunization, as discussed later (see p. 576).

The botulinum neurotoxin causes **flaccid paralysis** of the muscles, acting on the peripheral nervous system, by blocking cholinergic transmission at the nerve-muscle junction. Paralysis develops in two steps. Toxin is first fixed to the surface of the nerve membrane, likely binding through the H-chain to specific receptors, possibly gangliosides. During this step the toxin is on the membrane surface and subject to neutralization by antitoxin. In the second step, which results in muscle paralysis, the toxin is translocated into or through the membrane to a site where it blocks the neurogenic **release of acetylcholine,** probably by impairing calcium-induced exocytosis. After translocation, toxin cannot be neutralized by antitoxin.

BOTULISM[11, 29]

In the generic sense, botulism is an intoxication. The botulinum toxins induce a flaccid

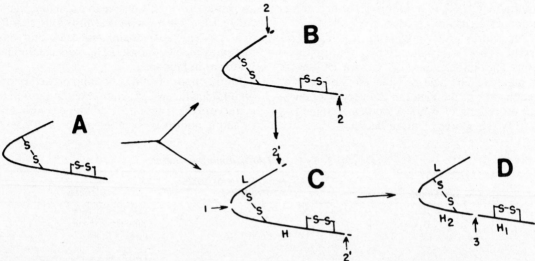

Figure 28–2. Molecular cleavages of botulinum and tetanus neurotoxins. Neurotoxin is synthesized intracellularly as a single peptide *(A).* Partial activation of the botulinum neurotoxin may result from action of SH-dependent protease at sites near to the end(s) of the chain *(B,* site 2). Nicking of the single chain by a nicking protease or trypsin at site 1 (C) forms a dichain molecule. The L-chain contains the original N-terminus of the molecule and is about one-third the molecular weight of the H-chain. It is not clear whether nicking alone results in activation of botulinal toxin. If not, activation probably results from enzymes acting at site 2′, just internal to site 2 *(A).* These alterations yield a maximally activated toxin. Further digestion *(D)* results in cleavage of the H-chain at site 3. (Sugiyama, H., Microbiol. Rev. **44:**419, 1980.)

paralysis of the muscles, resulting from blockage of transmitter release at nerve endings. The bilateral neuromuscular paralysis interferes with breathing and, ultimately, leads to death by **respiratory failure.** Observed symptoms include vomiting, constipation, ocular paresis, and pharyngeal paralysis. In fatal cases, death may occur within a day of the onset of symptoms or it may be delayed for as long as a week.

The manner in which the toxin is acquired determines the pathogenic form of botulism in humans: (1) botulinal food poisoning, (2) wound botulism, and (3) infant botulism. It is possible that infant botulism will prove to be the most common form of the disease.

Food Poisoning

The classical form of botulism is the food poisoning syndrome, in which the toxin is formed in food by growth of contaminating *C. botulinum*. Ingestion of the toxin gives rise to the disease. This syndrome is discussed in detail in Chapter 36.

In Europe, most cases have been due to the consumption of various kinds of preserved meats, such as sausages, ham, and potted goose or duck, while in the United States the incriminated foods for the most part have been home-processed foods, but with an increasing number traced to fish and fish products. There are surprisingly few cases in this country, in view of the wide distribution of *C. botulinum* in soils. In the United States, botulism is most commonly due to type A toxin. Rare cases of type E botulism have been associated with consumption of fish. Raw fish has been the vehicle in Japan, while smoked and canned fish have been incriminated in the United States.

Most cases of this form of botulism are due to consumption of toxin-containing food, and the epidemiology is typical of common-source outbreaks. The case-fatality rate is variable, probably depending largely on supportive therapy; in the period 1967 to 1975, it was 25 per cent, but had previously been as high as 60 to 70 per cent. Microbiologists have long been intrigued by the possibility that *C. botulinum* might colonize the intestine and produce toxin that could be absorbed, resulting in symptoms of botulism. If such cases occur in adults, they are rare, presumably because normal intestinal flora interfere with colonization and toxin production by *C. botulinum*. However, in a few cases of adult botulism, no food vehicle can be identified.

Wound Botulism

The invasive properties of *C. botulinum* are severely limited. Nevertheless, rare cases of botulism have been identified in which the microorganism has colonized wounds in mixed culture with other bacteria to produce toxin; absorption of the toxin is followed by neurological symptoms of botulism. Since the first report of wound botulism in 1943, 27 cases have been reported in the United States, most of these caused by type A.

Infant Botulism

Infant botulism was established as a disease entity in 1976 when *C. botulinum* organisms, toxin, or both were found in the stools of infants with neuromuscular weakness and constipation. Most recognized cases are characterized by weakness, hypotonia, hypoflexia, and cranial nerve dysfunction, usually preceded by constipation. Mild cases and inapparent infections are generally not recognized as botulism. The case-fatality rate is not particularly high, usually less than 4 per cent. A portion of cases of the sudden infant death syndrome are, however, judged to be infant botulism, based on the presence of *C. botulinum* in the bowel contents.

Children affected are almost always under six months of age, with a median age of 2.5 months. The physical diagnosis can be confirmed by demonstration of *C. botulinum* or toxin in the stools of the affected child.

Infant botulism is an **infective process** in which ingested spores of *C. botulinum* germinate and grow in the bowel. Toxin produced is then absorbed to give rise to the neurological symptoms. Large numbers of *C. botulinum* are sometimes found, ranging from 10^3 to 10^8 per gram of feces.[35] Type A infections are somewhat more frequent than type B; other types have not been reported.

As noted earlier, adults rarely, if ever, develop toxigenic intestinal infections with *C. botulinum*. Occurrence of such infections in infants is believed to be linked to the microbial ecology of the bowel. Adults are thought to possess intestinal microbial flora that interfere with colonization; interfering flora apparently are absent or in lower numbers in infants. This view is supported by animal studies showing that *C. botulinum* colonizes and produces toxin in the intestine of infant animals or germ-free adults, but that conventional adult animals are not colonized.

Infection sources for infants with botulism are largely unknown, although the consumption of honey, which is known to contain *C. botulinum* spores with some frequency, is associated with a portion of the cases studied. Potential sources also include dust and soil in the household or immediate vicinity.

Pathogenicity for Lower Animals

Many animals are subject to botulism under natural conditions. Types C and D appear to be associated exclusively with the disease in lower animals. Certain forms of forage poisoning in Australia, affecting horses and cattle, are botulism, as is the South African disease of cattle, lamziekte. Botulism of wild ducks and fowl, known as limberneck, is usually due to type C_α and has caused the deaths of thousands of waterfowl. In all of these animals, the toxin is ingested, arising from growth of the microorganism in forage materials. Experimental animals vary widely in susceptibility, but guinea pigs and mice are frequently used.

Immunity

Formol toxoid may be used as an immunizing antigen to produce an active immunity with circulating antitoxin present in the blood. Such immunizations are carried out in animals when economically feasible and advisable.

Humans may be immunized with fluid or alum-precipitated toxoid of type A or B, but naturally occurring botulism of man is so rare that active immunization is not feasible.

Antitoxin for prophylactic and therapeutic use in humans is produced by animal immunization with toxoid. These are usually trivalent, containing antitoxin against types A, B, and E, the types most prevalent in human disease. In botulinal food poisoning they have marked prophylactic value when administered before symptoms are evident, but their therapeutic efficacy has been slight. Antitoxic therapy is usually not indicated in infant botulism. As noted above, antitoxin is without effect after the toxin has been translocated into the neural cells, so that therapeutic failures may be attributable to the inevitable too-late administration.

Clostridium tetani

Tetanus is a disease of man and animals characterized by spasms of the voluntary muscles. The spasms are often most marked in the muscles of the jaw and neck, hence the name "lockjaw." The tetanus bacillus was first described in 1884 by Nicolaier; Kitasato isolated the microorganism in pure culture in 1889 and established its etiological relation to the disease. He also showed the inability of the tetanus bacillus to invade the blood stream and found the disease to be an intoxication. In 1890 von Behring and Kitasato laid the basis for antitoxic therapy when they discovered diphtheria and tetanus antitoxins.

Morphology

Individual tetanus bacilli are slender, gram-positive, sporulating rods with rounded ends; they are motile by many peritrichous flagella. Their common dimensions are 0.3 to 0.5 μm. in width and 2 to 5 μm. in length, but vegetative filaments of much greater length occur. Several of their morphological features are shown in Figure 28–3. The spore, which is without exosporium, is located subterminally, *i.e.*, near the end of the cell, and is larger in diameter than the sporangium, giving the cell a characteristic drumstick appearance. Surface colonies are flat, rhizoid, or even feathery, and frequently exceed 1 mm. in diameter. Later, the centers may become slightly raised. Colonies on blood agar show hemolysis.

Physiology

The tetanus bacillus grows well on ordinary mediums, provided low oxidation-reduction potential is maintained. The bacillus develops on infusion or peptone-containing mediums; broth mediums are frequently prepared by addition of chopped meat or brain tissue. To maintain anaerobic conditions, deep mediums are usually heated to expel dissolved oxygen and sealed by paraffin or petrolatum. If the depth is adequate, 7 to 12 cm., no special seal is required, especially for more viscous mediums. The temperature range for growth is between 14° and 43°C., with an optimum at 37°C.

The growth of *C. tetani* is influenced greatly by the presence of associated microorganisms. In sugar-free mediums it may be grown in mixed cultures upon the surface of culture mediums in contact with air, since the presence of aerobes may sufficiently lower the oxidation-reduction potential to permit growth. But in glucose broth the growth of the tetanus

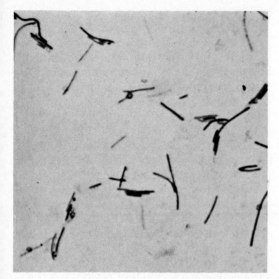

Figure 28–3. *Clostridium tetani* in pure culture. Young, actively growing culture showing beginning of spore formation. Note the refractile, unstained spores, the drumstick appearance when these are within the sporangium, and the tendency of the vegetative cells to remain attached end to end. Fuchsin; × 1150.

bacillus in mixed culture is likely to be inhibited by the acidic products of the associated bacteria.

In pure culture, glucose stimulates growth as in the case of other anaerobes, although glucose and other carbohydrates are not fermented by *C. tetani*. Sporulation is not inhibited by carbohydrates, as with the saccharolytic anaerobes; on the contrary, sporulation of the tetanus bacillus is accelerated in glucose broth. The tetanus bacillus is only weakly proteolytic; gelatin is slowly liquified, as are coagulated proteins, such as serum and egg white. Deep brain and meat mediums may be slightly softened, with some darkening. Biochemical reactions that permit differentiation from other clostridia are shown in Table 28–1.

The tetanus bacillus has been grown on synthetic mediums. Its growth requirements are relatively complex and include several amino acids, vitamins, purines, and oleic acid. Toxin production is best on complex mediums, usually containing both beef infusion and peptones.

Spores are readily formed in culture, usually in the late growth phases, beginning in about two days in cultures incubated at 37° C. The spores are highly resistant to physical and chemical agents. They remain viable for years when protected from light and excessive heat. Spores are destroyed by 5 per cent phenol only after 10 to 12 hours.

Antigenic Structure

The tetanus bacillus is antigenically heterogeneous, possessing a variety of cellular and flagellar antigens. A typing scheme has been described, but it has limited epidemiological value and is rarely practiced. Of the antigenic products of *C. tetani*, the neurotoxin—tetanospasmin—is of major importance. In contrast to *C. botulinum*, all toxigenic strains of *C. tetani* produce a **single immunogenic type** of the toxin.

Toxins[2, 19, 32]

The tetanus bacillus produces two toxins—**tetanospasmin** and **tetanolysin.** Tetanospasmin is the potent soluble toxin that affects the nervous system, while tetanolysin is a hemolysin. The former is by far the more important, but there is some evidence suggesting that tetanolysin may contribute to the pathogenesis of the disease. Although tetanospasmin is released from cells by autolysis and is found in the culture supernatant, it may also be extracted from the bacterial cells with molar sodium chloride.

Tetanospasmin has been extensively studied, both as to its chemical and physical nature and its action in the animal host. In aqueous solutions the toxin is unstable to both heat and light; it is, however, stable in the purified and dried form. Tetanospasmin occurs as a single antigenic type; it is an excellent antigen and gives rise to high-titer antiserum that neutralizes the biological activity of the toxin. The toxin is a protein and is destroyed by proteolytic enzymes; hence, it is inactive when given by mouth.

The tetanus neurotoxin is one of the most potent poisons known; its toxicity is of the same order of magnitude as those of *C. botulinum*. Tetanospasmin also resembles the botulinum neurotoxin in other ways (Fig. 28–2). It is synthesized as a single chain peptide of about 150,000 daltons with one intrachain disulfide linkage. Upon release from the cell by lysis, it is acted upon by bacterial enzymes to produce the nicked, dichain form held together by the disulfide bond. The H- and L-chains of tetanus toxin are similar in molecular weight to those of botulinal toxin; the H-chain of tetanus toxin is also believed to participate in toxin binding to target nerve cells. While the botulinal toxin in the single chain form is of low toxicity and requires activation to achieve maximum activity, tetanus toxin has the same toxicity in both the single chain and nicked dichain form.

There is still some uncertainty concerning the action of tetanospasmin. The toxin binds to the surface of neuronal cells, reacting with specific gangliosides through the H-chain portion of the molecule. Evidence strongly suggests that the receptor is structurally analogous to the receptor for thyrotropin on thyroid cell membranes. Since the action of tetanus toxin is on the spinal cord, it must be transported from the adsorption site on the nerve endings. The toxin moves centripetally from the peripheral nerve endings to the central nervous system by retrograde, intra-axonal transport. The details of toxin action are the subject of many investigations, but it appears that convulsant action on the central nervous system arises from presynaptic action that interferes with the release of inhibitory neurotransmitters, *viz.*, glycine and gamma-aminobutyric acid. There is evidence, too, that the toxin can induce flaccid paralysis by action similar to that of botulinal toxin.

TETANUS

Tetanus is essentially an intoxication. The bacilli set up a localized infection, and the toxin formed there is disseminated through the body and gives rise to the symptom complex characteristic of the disease. Bacillemia may occur very rarely, but has been produced experimentally. The bacilli generally gain entrance to the tissues by means of a deep dirty wound which may be relatively small, so small sometimes as to escape serious attention. The widespread occurrence of the tetanus bacillus would seem inconsistent with the relative infrequence of tetanus infection, but mere introduction of the bacillus into the body is not sufficient to produce the disease; the microorganisms must find favorable conditions for proliferation at the site of penetration. Experimentally, pure cultures of vegetative cells or spores that have been freed from toxin cannot proliferate in uninjured tissues, but simultaneous inoculation with common saprophytes or with irritant chemicals, such as calcium salts or lactic acid, enables the bacilli to grow and form toxin. A sufficiently low oxidation-reduction potential is necessary for the growth of the bacilli and it is likely that the potential of normal tissues is too high to allow multiplication, but is reduced by injury.

The **tonic spasms** characteristic of tetanus usually begin at the site of infection, and the initial symptoms may include headache and stiffness of the neck. The spasms may remain localized in mild infections, but usually they are general and involve the whole somatic muscular system; death is usually by respiratory failure. Postmortem findings are insignificant; other than a moderate congestion, the organs show no pathological changes and the initial lesion may, of course, be inapparent or small.

The incubation period of tetanus is variable and may range from 2 to 50 days. The case-fatality rate is inversely related to the incubation time; it may be as high as 70 to 80 per cent or as low as 15 to 20 per cent. Death, if it occurs, follows relatively soon after the appearance of symptoms; the dictum of Hippocrates, "Such persons as are seized with tetanus die within four days, or if they pass these they recover," still stands. When the disease has a prolonged incubation period, a less sudden development of symptoms, and consequently a more favorable prognosis, it is sometimes termed "chronic."

Tetanus continues to be a highly fatal disease. The case-fatality rate in the United States in 1978 was 37 per cent, a figure much lower than in many developing countries. The rate has diminished over time, and can undoubtedly be reduced still further by adoption of modern supportive and therapeutic measures, such as paralysis induction and artificial ventilation.[7]

The number of cases of tetanus in the United States steadily declined before 1976, but has remained relatively stable since then (Fig. 28–4). The reduction was due primarily to immunization programs, and the residual cases are likely in those not reached by immunization programs. This view is supported by the observation that most cases appear in individuals over 50 years of age (Fig. 28–5).

As late as 1925, postoperative or surgical tetanus accounted for as much as 10 per cent of the cases, but this has become relatively rare. The disease may also be associated with uncommon circumstances; for example, tetanus among drug addicts, due to the use of contaminated drugs or unsterilized needles or syringes, has been observed in large cities in the United States.

By far the most common kind of tetanus in the developed countries is that following injury, even apparently minor or trivial injury, which facilitates the growth of the anaerobic bacilli. This kind of tetanus tends to occur in rural males, especially children.

Neonatal tetanus, or tetanus of the newborn, is most often a consequence of infection of the umbilicus through septic midwifery. The disease is, therefore, especially common in under-

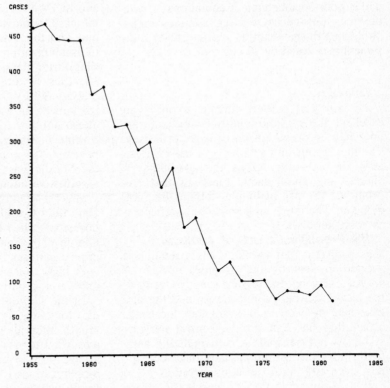

Figure 28–4. Reported cases of tetanus in the United States, 1955–1981. After a steady decline from 1955 to 1976, the number of cases has been stable, probably reflecting inadequate vaccination coverage in higher age groups (Fig. 28–5). (Centers for Disease Control, Annual summary 1981: reported morbidity and mortality in the United States. Morbidity Mortality Weekly Rep. **30**[54], 1982.)

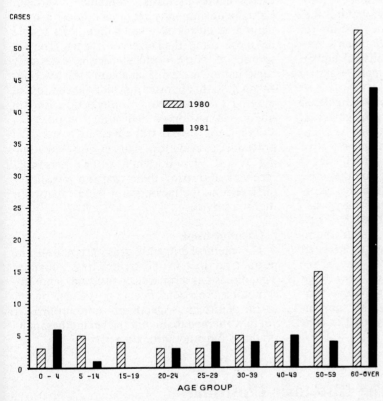

Figure 28–5. Reported cases of tetanus, by age group, in the United States, 1980 and 1981. (Centers for Disease Control, Annual summary 1981: reported morbidity and mortality in the United States. Morbidity Mortality Weekly Rep. **30**[54], 1982.)

*EXCLUDES UNKNOWN AGES.

developed countries and among those living under poor socioeconomic conditions. Under these circumstances it often assumes major public health significance, with mortality rates sometimes exceeding 80 per cent.

Immunity

As indicated earlier, tetanus toxin is an excellent antigen, and high-titer antitoxic serums may be prepared, particularly in horses. The therapeutic and prophylactic use of horse antitoxin, however, raises the possibility of allergic and anaphylactic reactions that has promoted the use of human tetanus immune globulin. The latter appears to be as effective as horse antitoxin.[3, 28]

The Prophylactic Use of Antitoxin.[16, 20, 28] It is probable that in many cases tetanus is averted in man by the prophylactic use of antitoxin. Even if the disease is not prevented, the incubation period is delayed, and the disease may be very mild or remain localized. Toxin that has entered the central nervous system is not neutralized by circulating antitoxin, however; symptoms may therefore appear even after antitoxin administration.

Passive immunization is necessarily transient, since the foreign immunoglobulin is metabolized by the recipient. The half-life of horse serum globulin in man has been calculated to be 7 to 14 days, while that of human globulin, as in antitoxin of human origin, is about four weeks.

From time to time attempts are made to passively immunize the newborn by maternal immunization during pregnancy, via transplacental antibody.[24] This can be a highly effective procedure, and it has been suggested that if all females aged 10 years were given one dose of toxoid at that time and every five years thereafter, neonatal tetanus would disappear.

The Therapeutic Use of Antitoxin.[25, 36] Tetanus antitoxin appears to have limited therapeutic value under most conditions. It has been reported, however, that mortality may be reduced somewhat by the use of very large amounts of antitoxin. Intrathecal administration has been successfully used, with substantial decrease in mortality as compared to conventional administration.

Active Immunization.[4, 8] Beginning in World War II, active immunization was adopted by the armed services of France, Britain, and the United States. The effectiveness of immunization is substantiated by the fact that during the period from 1942 to 1945, only 16 cases of tetanus occurred in the United States military forces; 9 of these were in unimmunized individuals. In contrast, in the Japanese military forces, which did not practice routine immunization, the rate was about 10 per 100,000 wounded. British experience in the Middle East war zone similarly indicated an effective immune response.

Several types of immunizing toxoid are available; **fluid toxoid,** requiring three immunizing doses; **adsorbed toxoid,** precipitated with aluminum phosphate and requiring only two immunizing doses; and an **adsorbed** preparation with **high concentration of toxoid.** The latter may require only a single dose.

In the United States, guidelines for immunization suggest three inoculations at two-month intervals in early infancy, followed by a fourth after 1½ years, and a final inoculation at age 4 to 6 years. The vaccine for these immunizations is normally an **adsorbed diphtheria-tetanus-pertussis** combined vaccine. Permanent immunity requires a booster inoculation of adsorbed tetanus-diphtheria toxoid no more often than every 10 years. The response to booster inoculation is extremely rapid in persons giving an anamnestic reaction, so much so that booster inoculation with toxoid may be substituted for prophylactic antitoxin under circumstances indicating prophylaxis. Prophylactic toxoid was given as a standard procedure to American military personnel during World War II, while British personnel received antitoxin; there was no significant difference in the incidence of tetanus between the two services.

Chemotherapy

The chemotherapeutic drugs are not an important adjunct in the treatment of tetanus. The disease is primarily a toxemia, and the symptoms are a consequence of damage by the toxin. Antitoxin is mandatory to neutralize as yet uncombined toxin, but the chemotherapeutic drugs have no antitoxin activity.

The Histotoxic Clostridia

Most species of *Clostridium* are considered to be saprophytic, free-living bacteria found in soil and water. Some of these are also found in the intestine of man and animals as commensals, and their numbers in soil are increased by contamination with fecal matter.

Although these normally saprophytic microorganisms have limited invasive capacity, many are capable of colonizing injured tissues when they are introduced into open wounds. Under these circumstances, their capacity to form a variety of exotoxins leads to further invasion of tissues and can result in the syndrome of **gas gangrene** or **clostridial myonecrosis.**

Many clostridial species can participate in this infection, but the most commonly found are *C. perfringens, C. novyi,* and *C. septicum.*

CLOSTRIDIUM PERFRINGENS

Since its original isolation by Achalme in 1891, this bacillus has been known by several names; there is still some variation in terminology. It is designated *Clostridium welchii* in England and *C. perfringens* by American workers.

Morphology

Clostridium perfringens is a plump, nonmotile, gram-positive rod of variable length, occurring singly and in chains (Fig. 28–6). Polysaccharide capsules are usually present in preparations made from the organs or body fluids. Spores are formed sparingly and only in the absence of fermentable carbohydrates; they are subterminal and do not swell the vegetative cell in which they are formed.

Physiology

Clostridium perfringens is a strict anaerobe and grows readily in deep brain and meat infusion mediums. Growth in sugar-free mediums is restricted. Optimum conditions are provided by mediums containing fermentable carbohydrates, but such cultures are often short-lived because of the reduced spore formation and the destructive action of the formed acids on the vegetative cells. Brain and meat mediums are not blackened normally, but the presence of metallic iron produces a distinct discoloration. Gelatin is liquefied, but coagulated serum or egg is not digested. Other characteristics are listed in Table 28–1.

Nutritive requirements are complex, although it may be grown on synthetic mediums if supplied with most of the amino acids and B vitamins, purines, pyrimidines, glucose, and salts.

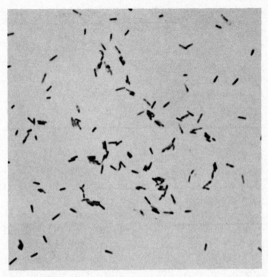

Figure 28–6. *Clostridium perfringens* from pure culture. Note the relatively smaller size of these bacteria and the subterminal spores. Fuchsin; × 1050.

Types

Serological identification of *C. perfringens* based on cellular antigens is not practical because of the number of cross-reacting antigens. However, *C. perfringens* types are distinguished on the basis of elaborated filtrate antigens, *i.e.*, substances released by the cell, many of which are toxic; each of these is antigenically distinct. The prinicipal toxins produced by the types of *C. perfringens* are listed in Table 28–3.

The vast majority of human disease caused by *C. perfringens* is due to type A, but animal infections with this type are rare. Type C is primarily an animal pathogen, but some strains of type C cause a necrotizing enterocolitis in man, which is now largely confined to New Guinea. The remainder of *C. perfringens* types are animal pathogens, rarely encountered in human infections. Unless otherwise specified, *C. perfringens* is taken here to mean type A.

Toxins[6, 30]

The α-toxin has been of greatest interest, since it is most closely associated with the virulence of *C. perfringens* type A in wound infections and is the chief lethal toxin of these strains. The α-toxin is a calcium-dependent phospholipase C, with lethal and hemolytic properties. It is a zinc metalloenzyme of 35,000 daltons, which hydrolyzes membrane-associated lecithin sphingomyelins. Because of its calcium-dependency, it is inhibited by phosphate. The *in vivo* effect of the α-toxin is the

Table 28–3. **Principal Toxins Produced by** *Clostridium perfringens* **Types**

Activity of Toxin	Designation	Produced by Type				
		A	B	C	D	E
Hemolytic, lethal necrotizing	α	+	+	+	+	+
Lethal, necrotizing	β	–	+	+	–	–
Lethal, necrotizing	ε	–	+	–	+	–
Lethal, activated by protease	ι	–	–	–	–	+
Enterotoxin	—	+	V*	V	–	–

*V = variable with strain.

destruction of erythrocytes, platelets, and leucocytes and weakening of muscle cell plasma membranes.

Clostridium perfringens type A also produces an 80,000 dalton collagenase, designated κ-toxin, that acts as a virulence factor. It attacks collagen in the connective tissues that support muscle fibers, resulting in muscle destruction. It does not appear to be as important as α-toxin, for while antiserum to the latter alone is protective, that to κ-toxin is not. In addition to these major toxins, many strains also produce hyaluronidase (μ-toxin), deoxyribonuclease (ν-toxin), and an oxygen-labile hemolysin (θ-toxin).

In general, the toxins formed by *C. perfringens* type A appear to account in large measure for the observed histopathology of wound infection. Comparison of the histopathology of naturally occurring infection in man, in experimentally infected animals, and in normal human muscle exposed to culture filtrates *in vitro* has shown that the changes are substantially the same in all three.

Type C strains of *C. perfringens* produce a lethal and necrotic toxin designated β-toxin. The β-toxin is considered to be central to the pathogenesis of necrotizing enterocolitis in that it damages intestinal villi, permitting attachment of *C. perfringens,* and brings about necrosis of the gut wall.

Enterotoxin. The association of *C. perfringens* with a type of food poisoning prompted a search for a filterable enterotoxin produced by this bacterium. Food-poisoning strains do, in fact, produce a heat-labile exotoxin, active in cell-free form in the rabbit ileal loop model, which causes diarrhea in monkeys and humans after oral administration. The enterotoxin, which is formed during sporulation by many, but not all, type A strains as well as some type C and D strains, is a protein of about 34,000 daltons; it has been purified by a variety of procedures. The enterotoxin is not immunologically related to the other toxins of *C. perfringens* discussed above. Type A strains producing the toxin are also capable of pro-

ducing gangrene under experimental conditions; enterotoxin, however, probably does not play a role in pathogenesis of gaseous gangrene. *Clostridium perfringens* food poisoning is fully discussed in Chapter 36.

Pathogenicity for Man

In addition to their role in *C. perfringens* food poisoning and gangrene, the bacilli are sometimes observed in closed abscesses; in uterine infections; in affections of the gastrointestinal, genitourinary, and biliary tracts; and in rare septicemic conditions. *Clostridium perfringens* is a normal inhabitant of the human intestine and is constantly present in low numbers.

As noted earlier, a necrotizing jejunitis, **enteritis necroticans** or pig-bel, is associated with pig-feasting in the highland regions of New Guinea. Pig-bel is caused by β-toxin producing strains of *C. perfringens* type C. This geographical restriction is associated with the dietary habits of the natives. The microorganisms, consumed in inadequately cooked pork, grow and produce toxin in the intestine. The β-toxin responsible for the pathogenesis is sensitive to tryptic digestion, but sweet potato, usually consumed with the pork, contains a trypsin-inhibitor so that the β-toxin is not inactivated as it is in other populations.

CLOSTRIDIUM NOVYI

The anaerobe now known as *C. novyi* was first described by Novy in 1894 as a cause of animal infection. *Clostridium novyi* is noteworthy because it is perhaps the second most important cause of clostridial myonecrosis. The Bergey designation of *C. novyi* is synonymous with *C. oedematiens* used by European workers.

Morphology

Clostridium novyi is a large, relatively thick gram-positive rod, 2.5 to 10 μm. in length and 0.8 to 1 μm. in breadth, and occurs singly and

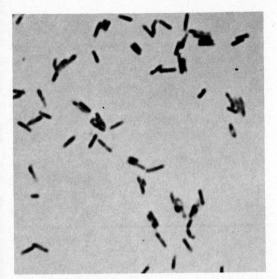

Figure 28–7. *Clostridium novyi* from pure culture. The slight tendency to curvature is apparent in some of the vegetative cells. Note the subterminal spores and the absence of large numbers of free spores. Fuchsin; × 1200.

in chains (Fig. 28–7). Its numerous spiral flagella, which often become entangled in "bouquets," have been emphasized in nearly all of the published descriptions. The rod is nonmotile under ordinary conditions of examination, for movement is markedly inhibited in the presence of air. Subterminal spores are produced but sparsely as a rule and best in nonfermentable mediums.

Surface colonies are extremely delicate; they are flat, transparent, and bluish gray, with irregular contours, and exhibit slight hemolysis on blood agar.

Physiology
Clostridium novyi is a strict anaerobe and grows well at 37°C. in ordinary mediums and especially abundantly in the presence of a fermentable sugar. Meat and brain are not darkened; indeed, the former may be turned slightly pink or bleached. Gelatin is liquefied, but coagulated serum and egg are not digested. Differential properties are found in Table 28–1.

Toxins
Three types of *C. novyi*—A, B, and C—are distinguished, based primarily on toxins and other biologically active antigens released into the culture medium. Altogether, eight of these antigenic components or toxins have been described and their distribution distinguishes the antigenic types. The principal toxins and their distribution are listed in Table 28–4. European workers include a fourth type, D, but in the Bergey classification this type is separated as *C. histolyticum* (Table 28–4; Fig. 28–8). *Clostridium novyi* strains found in human disease, *i.e.*, gas gangrene, are usually of types A and B; these are also the types that produce the lethal α-toxin. Among the toxins produced by the histotoxic clostridia, *i.e.*, those responsible for gas gangrene, α-toxin of *C. novyi* is the most powerful and is the principal virulence factor in this species.

Pathogenicity for Man
Clostridium novyi is a relatively frequent participant in the gas gangrene syndrome. The disease is characteristically a toxemia, although septicemia is not rare. In pure infections there is less tissue destruction than with *C. perfringens* or *C. septicum;* postmortem findings include massive localized edema, with neither the extensive gas production of the former nor the sanguineous necrosis of the latter.

Antitoxin, produced by immunization of animals, has prophylactic and, to some extent, therapeutic value, and is now represented in several polyvalent antiserums for anaerobic infections.

CLOSTRIDIUM SEPTICUM

Clostridium septicum was isolated in 1877 by Pasteur, who called it "vibrion septique." A similar organism was isolated by Koch in 1881, but it is not known if they are identical. This microorganism is a prominent member of the histotoxic clostridia causing gas gangrene.

Table 28–4. **Principal Toxins of *Clostridium novyi* and *Clostridium histolyticum***

Action of Toxin	Designation	C. novyi Type			C. histolyticum
		A	B	C	
Lethal, necrotizing	α	+	+	−	−
Hemolytic, necrotizing, lecithinase	β	−	+	−	+
Hemolytic, lecithinase	γ	+	−	+	−

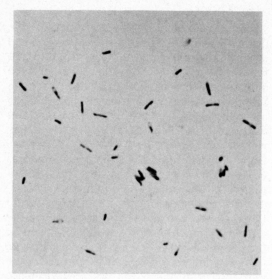

Figure 28–8. *Clostridium histolyticum* from pure culture. Note the characteristic short rods with rounded ends and the clostridial subterminal spores. Fuchsin; × 1050.

Morphology

Clostridium septicum (Fig. 28–9) is a grampositive, sporulating, spindle-shaped rod or filament, and in young cultures it is motile, with many peritrichous flagella. The ends are slightly rounded and the spores, which are oval, are usually subterminal and swell the vegetative cell prior to their release. Spores are formed only in mediums not containing fermentable carbohydrate in excess. Surface colonies are irregular, large, raised, translucent, and gray.

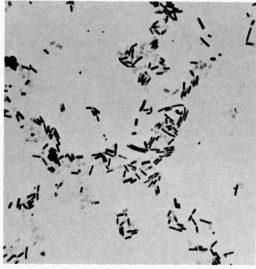

Figure 28–9. *Clostridium septicum* from pure culture. The tendency to form elongated vegetative cells is apparent. Fuchsin; × 1050.

Physiology

This microorganism is a strict anaerobe and develops readily in deep brain or tissue mediums, producing gas rather abundantly. These mediums are not discolored even in the presence of metallic iron. Gelatin is liquefied, but coagulated serum and other proteins are not digested or blackened. Table 28–1 lists the properties of differential value.

Antigenic Structure and Toxin

Strains of *C. septicum* are immunologically related but distinct. Six groups can be distinguished on the basis of somatic and flagellar antigens. The principal toxin found is immunologically distinct but is a relatively weak lethal agent. When injected into animals it produces a gelatinous edema and some local necrosis of the tissues. The toxin has a specific cardiac action in the cat and rabbit, producing a fall in systemic and a rise in venous blood pressure, and in the cat a specific constriction of the pulmonary and coronary circulations, with edema of the lungs and loss of fluid from the circulation. This lethal necrotic toxin, or *C. septicum* α-toxin, is an oxygen-labile hemolysin. A deoxyribonuclease (β-toxin) attacks the nuclei of rabbit leucocytes. Hyaluronidase is formed also and is sometimes referred to as the γ-toxin.

Pathogenicity

Clostridium septicum does not occur in gaseous gangrene of man as frequently as some of the other anaerobic bacilli, but it has been found both alone and in mixed cultures. *Clostridium septicum* is strikingly pathogenic for many laboratory animals, in which the bacteria develop rapidly, producing gas and a reddish, serous edema. They invade the adjacent tissues and the circulation, producing septicemia, which is usually fatal within 24 to 48 hours; sublethal doses do not produce observable reaction.

Antitoxin serums that are prophylactic and, to some degree, curative may be prepared by immunizaiton of animals with *C. septicum* toxin. The antiserums do not have the high antitoxin content that is found in antitetanic serums. Polyvalent commercial serums for prophylactic and therapeutic use in wound infections often contain *C. septicum* antitoxin.

CLOSTRIDIAL MYONECROSIS[18]

Clostridial myonecrosis, often called **gas gangrene,** is a syndrome that includes rapid necrosis of muscle tissue with little inflammation and with production of gas in the tissues. It often follows dirty lacerated wounds, especially those involving fractures. It is a characteristic complication of war wounds; knowledge of this affliction was largely developed during World War I. But the disease is by no means rare in civilian life; injuries in automobile accidents are responsible for many cases of gangrene. Certain forms of peritonitis, appendicitis, intestinal obstruction, puerperal sepsis, and postoperative infections (particularly after laparotomy) are etiologically closely related to it.

The trauma usually, and probably necessarily, preceding the development of gangrene results in a local area of tissue anoxia, anaerobic oxidation of carbohydrate continues, and the local reducing potential drops to levels permitting growth of the obligate anaerobes. Under the conditions of increasing acidity, the catheptic enzymes of the muscle tissue are activated, and free amino acids accumulate as a consequence of the proteolysis to provide an adequate nutrient medium for the invading microorganisms.

Gangrene is usually a **mixed infection,** and both aerobic and anaerobic bacteria may be isolated from a single gangrenous lesion. The aerobic and facultatively anaerobic forms, such as streptococci and coliform bacilli, are not primarily concerned in the development of the pathological process but may contribute indirectly to it by lowering the oxidation-reduction potential. The gangrenous process is, rather, a consequence of the activity of the sporulating obligate anaerobes and the exotoxins produced by them. In the fulminating form of gaseous gangrene the muscle tissue becomes filled with gas and with a serosanguineous exudate, the character of which depends upon the properties of the associated microorganisms.

Clostridum perfringens is the most important

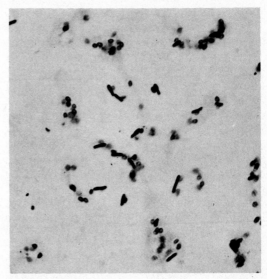

Figure 28–10. *Clostridium sporogenes* from pure culture. Note the close morphological resemblance of this species to the pathogenic forms. Fuchsin; × 1050.

cause of gas gangrene and is found either alone or mixed with other anaerobes in the majority of cases. Tissue injury is probably essential for the initiation of infection, but once the bacilli are established they rapidly invade the surrounding tissues.

Other clostridia found with some frequency in myonecrosis are *C. novyi* and *C. septicum;* occasionally other clostridia are isolated, including the nonpathogenic *C. sporogenes* (Fig. 28–10).

It is evident that the bacteriology of gas gangrene is complicated, and while there is in effect a typical form of the disease, it is not always produced by the same organism; it is frequently due to several associated agents, and it often is the complex result of the combined action of anaerobic bacilli with various other bacteria that play an indeterminant accessory role.

Clostridium difficile[13, 26, 34]

First described in 1935 as a normal inhabitant of the intestinal tract of infants, *Clostridium difficile* was not recognized as a significant pathogenic *Clostridium* until 1977. It has subsequently been established as the predominant, perhaps the sole, etiological agent of a form of pseudomembranous colitis associated with the use of antibiotics.

Morphology[5]
Clostridium difficile is a large gram-positive bacillus, forming oval subterminal spores—later becoming terminal—of lesser diameter than the parent sporangium. The bacilli are motile by peritrichous flagella. Colonies on solid mediums are large, circular, convex, translucent, and white with a matte surface.

Physiology

This microorganism grows moderately in ordinary mediums, with or without carbohydrates, under strict anaerobic conditions. It hydrolyzes gelatin but casein is not digested. Growth occurs over the temperature range of 25° to 45°C., with an optimum of 30° to 37° C. Other differential reactions are listed in Table 28–1.

Clostridium difficile can be isolated with facility on mediums containing cycloserine and cefoxitin as selective agents. Freshly isolated strains exhibit fluorescence when illuminated with ultraviolet light. Antigenic toxins are formed that are causally linked to the colitis and are neutralized by their antitoxins.

Toxins[14, 17, 33]

Culture filtrates of *C. difficile* are toxic when injected into experimental animals and will also produce cecitis when introduced intracecally into guinea pigs. The latter mimics penicillin-induced cecitis in guinea pigs caused by *C. difficile*. Recently, it has been found that these effects are due to two immunologically distinct toxins, designated A and B. Their properties, as currently known, are summarized in Table 28–5. Although the details of toxin activity are largely derived from studies in animal models, available data strongly suggest that these toxins, acting in concert, are responsible for the symptoms observed in human cases of antibiotic-associated pseudomembranous colitis. Toxins are produced by most, if not all, strains of *C. difficile*.

Animal Models[1, 9, 10]

As early as 1943, it was noted that the administration of antibiotics to guinea pigs and other laboratory animals often resulted in a fatal enterocolitis. For many years, deaths were ascribed to overgrowth of intestinal gram-negative bacteria leading to bacteremia. In 1977, studies on clindamycin-induced colitis in

Table 28–5. **Properties of the Toxins of Clostridium difficile**

Property	Toxin A	Toxin B
Cytotoxicity in tissue culture	±	+
Lethality for mice	+	+
Acid-labile	+	+
Heat-labile	+	+
Trypsin-sensitive	+	+
Fluid response in ileal loop	+	−
Mouse protection by antiserum to:		
A + B	+	+
A	+	−
B	−	+
Molecular weight ($\times 10^5$ daltons)	4.5 to 5.0	3.6 to 4.7

Data from several authors.[14, 17, 33]

hamsters led to the conclusion that the disease is caused by toxin-producing strains of *C. difficile*. It is now established that the condition can be induced by a variety of antimicrobial agents, including ampicillin, cephalosporins, erythromycin, gentamicin, and vancomycin.

Following antibiotic administration, hamsters develop enterocolitis with hemorrhagic cecitis as the principal lesion. Concomitantly, there is alteration of the intestinal flora, generally with reduction of gram-positive bacteria and an increase in several clostridia, including *C. difficile*. Examination of the cecal contents reveals significant amounts of a cytopathic toxin produced by *C. difficile*. The disease can be reproduced in normal animals, *i.e.*, those untreated with antibiotics, by injection of cell-free supernatants of *C. difficile* cultures.

The relevance of *C. difficile* toxins is exemplified by immunization with toxoids prepared from toxins A and B. Immunization with a mixture of toxoids A and B protects hamsters against clindamycin-induced colitis. Immunization with either toxoid A or toxoid B does not fully protect such animals.[15] It appears, therefore, that both toxins participate in pathogenesis.

It is now accepted that the enterocolitis of laboratory animals induced by antibiotics is attributable to toxins produced by *C. difficile* colonizing the cecum. Induction by antibiotics is generally believed attributable to changes in the normal flora. In untreated animals, the normal flora are thought to inhibit colonization by *C. difficile*. This view is supported by the rarity of *C. difficile* isolations from untreated animals. Alternatively, the normal flora may inhibit toxin synthesis by *C. difficile* or may interfere with toxin action. For example, the supernatant from lactobacillus cultures will inactivate *C. difficile* toxins *in vitro*, possibly by action of acidic metabolic products that inactivate the toxin.

These animal models have been pivotal in elucidation of the elements of a similar affliction of humans. Nevertheless, many questions remain unanswered. For example, clindamycin-induced cecitis in hamsters can be delayed or aborted by administration of vancomycin. Thus, the disease can be both induced and prevented by antibiotics to which *C. difficile* is sensitive.

PSEUDOMEMBRANOUS COLITIS[13, 26]

Pseudomembranous colitis in humans was first described in 1893, in a patient following surgery. It was little more than a medical curiosity until the advent of the antibiotic era in the early 1940s. In the ensuing years, the disease was noted following therapeutic use of antibiotics and was ascribed to overgrowth of intestinal bacteria, *e.g.,* gram-negative bacilli or staphylococci. It was not until 1977, following renewed interest in the animal infections just cited, that *C. difficile* was incriminated as the predominant etiological agent.

Although the affliction has been precipitated by surgery and other gastrointestinal procedures, *e.g.,* multiple enemas or nasogastric intubation,[23] the antecedent event is almost always the administration of **antimicrobial drugs.** This led to the designation of the disease as antibiotic-associated pseudomembranous colitis. During the 1970s, the colitis was most often linked to the use of clindamycin, lincomycin, or ampicillin, but it is now clear that a number of antibiotics can induce the disease, irrespective of their action against *C. difficile* as judged by *in vitro* testing.

Although the incidence varies widely, antibiotic treatment initiated for other infections can induce the disease syndrome. Onset may follow soon after beginning antibiotic administration or it may be delayed. Symptoms range from a mild diarrhea to the typical pseudomembranous colitis, with watery and often bloody diarrhea, abdominal pain, and fever. Histological examination reveals inflammation of the colonic mucosa, with ulceration and formation of a pseudomembrane composed of fibrinogen, mucosal cell debris, and leucocytes. These symptoms may continue for several weeks in untreated cases. Proctoscopic examination detects multiple raised plaques, 2 to 5 cm. in diameter, adherent to the edematous, friable colonic mucosa.

Pathogenesis of the disease is believed to be quite similar to that of the animal infection. There is disturbance of the normal microbial flora of the large bowel, permitting colonization and overgrowth of *C. difficile;* in severe cases the number of *C. difficile* may reach 10^9 per gram of feces. Toxin production by these bacteria and its absorption then leads to the histological changes and the observed symptomatology. Both *C. difficile* and toxin can usually be detected in the fecal contents. It is assumed that both toxins A and B are involved in pathogenesis, based on their action in animal infections; toxin B, but not toxin A, has been found in intestinal contents from human cases. The failure to detect toxin A may only reflect technical difficulties, however.

Epidemiology

The incidence of pseudomembranous colitis varies greatly, being dependent on both geographical location and the patient population studied. Reported incidence has ranged from one or two cases per 10,000 treated patients to as high as 10 to 20 per cent. This is perhaps not surprising in view of the natural history of the disease, wherein two independent variables must be simultaneously matched, *i.e.,* antibiotic administration must coincide with the presence of *C. difficile* in the host, before disease can evolve.

It appears that *C. difficile* does not easily colonize the intestinal tract of adults. Limited studies on adult populations in the United States suggest a low colonization rate, about 3 per cent, whereas in Japan, isolation rates exceeding 10 per cent have been reported.[21] Hospital populations, particularly in hospitals where cases of colitis have occurred, may exhibit greater carriage rates than the general population. Failure to isolate *C. difficile* in normal individuals may not preclude existing colonization, since isolation methods do not detect fewer than about 100 *C. difficile* per gram of feces.

Colonization rates in healthy infants appear to be much higher than in adults. Although colonization of infants is often sporadic, rates as high as 64 per cent have been reported.[12] The rate of carriage is generally highest in those 1 to 8 months of age. Whether the lower carriage rates in adults reflects developing immunity or a maturing normal bowel flora that inhibits colonization with the microorganism has not been established.

A major unanswered question in the epidemiology of pseudomembranous colitis is the source of infecting *C. difficile.* The low incidence in some populations suggests that they are endogenous in origin, *i.e.,* antibiotic therapy permits intestinal overgrowth of resident clostridia. On the other hand, clustering of cases seen in some hospital populations may be due to acquisition of the microorganisms from the environment at about the time of antibiotic administration.

Chemotherapy

Treatment of pseudomembranous colitis may be either nonspecific or specific. Certainly, the appearance of colitis should be a signal to discontinue the inducing drug. If diarrhea is severe, therapeutic replacement of fluid and electrolytes may be warranted. Specific therapy is directed toward the eradication of *C. difficile*. Orally administered vancomycin has been successful in most instances, giving prompt clinical improvement. The microorganisms are generally sensitive to the drug; since the drug is poorly absorbed by this route and is well tolerated, high fecal concentrations can be achieved. Occasional relapses do occur, however, after vancomycin treatment. It is thought that the drug is inactive against the clostridial spore, so that they may germinate after therapy is discontinued and recolonize the bowel before its normal flora is completely reestablished.[22]

Immunity

The toxins of *C. difficile* are immunologically distinct and induce protective antitoxin when toxoids are used to immunize animals. Antitoxin, when premixed with toxin, neutralizes toxicity for animals. Toxin is rapidly bound to target cells in tissue cultures, and within a few minutes becomes insusceptible to the neutralizing effects of antitoxin. Thus, it appears unlikely that passive administration of antitoxin would have therapeutic effect in humans. The status of active immune mechanisms in humans has not been assessed, but antitoxin has been detected in the serum of young adults who are colonized with *C. difficile*.[21]

Presumably, active immunization of humans with toxoids is a possibility, but definition of the at-risk population would be difficult and immunization is probably not feasible.

It is some practical interest that similar toxins are produced by *C. sordelli*, one of the clostridia sometimes found in gas gangrene. Indeed, early studies in the pathogenesis of the disease were greatly aided by the observation that the cytopathic toxin in pseudomembranous colitis was neutralized by polyvalent gas gangrene antitoxin; the specific fraction was subsequently determined to be the *C. sordelli* antitoxin. Although the toxins from *C. sordelli* and *C. difficile* may not be identical, their immunological relationships are very close.

Bacteriological Diagnosis

The diagnosis of pseudomembranous colitis is facilitated by the isolation of *C. difficile* and the detection of toxin in the fecal contents.

Several selective mediums have been devised for isolation of *C. difficile*. These are generally complex mediums, such as blood agar, containing cycloserine and cefoxitin as selective agents. Primary colonies of *C. difficile* grown on these mediums exhibit fluorescence when exposed to ultraviolet light. Isolation plates are incubated under strict anaerobic conditions.

The presence of toxin in stool can be detected by tissue culture assays. Stool specimens are centrifuged, filtered to remove bacteria, and added to tissue cultured cells; almost all cell lines have proved to be susceptible to the toxin. Within a few hours the cultured cells begin to exhibit cytopathic changes. The specificity of the toxin is established by the absence of cytopathogenic changes in control cultures containing *C. sordelli* antitoxin. This antitoxin is more readily available than *C. difficile* antitoxin and has essentially the same immunological specificity, as noted above.

REFERENCES

1. Bartlett, J. G., *et al.* 1979. Colitis induced by *Clostridium difficile*. Rev. Infect. Dis. **1**:370–378.
2. Bizzini, B. 1979. Tetanus toxin. Microbiol. Rev. **43**:224–240.
3. Blake, P. A., *et al.* 1976. Serologic therapy of tetanus in the United States, 1965–1971. J. Amer. Med. Assn **235**:42–44.
4. Breman, J. G., *et al.* 1981. The primary serological response to a single dose of adsorbed tetanus toxoid, high concentration type. Bull. Wld Hlth Org. **59**:745–752.
5. Buchanan, R. E., and N. E. Gibbons (Eds.). 1974. Bergey's Manual of Determinative Bacteriology. 8th ed. The Williams & Wilkins Co., Baltimore.
6. Duncan, C. L. 1975. Role of clostridial toxins in pathogenesis. pp. 283–291. *In* D. Schlessinger (Ed.): Microbiology—1975. American Society for Microbiology, Washington, D.C.
7. Edmondson, R. S., and M. W. Flowers. 1979. Intensive care in tetanus: management, complications, and mortality in 100 cases. Brit. Med. J. **1**:1401–1404.
8. Edsall, G. 1976. Problems in the immunology and control of tetanus. Med. J. Australia **2**:216–220.
9. Fekety, R., *et al.* 1979. Antibiotic-associated colitis: effects of antibiotics on *Clostridium difficile* and the disease in hamsters. Rev. Infect. Dis. **1**:386–396.
10. Fekety, R., *et al.* 1980. Studies on the epidemiology of antibiotic-associated *Clostridium difficile* colitis. Amer. J. Clin. Nutrition **33**:2527–2532.
11. Feldman, R. A. (Ed.). 1979. A seminar on infant botulism. Rev. Infect. Dis. **1**:607–700.
12. Holst, E., I. Helin, and P.-A. Mårdh. 1981. Recovery of *Clostridium difficile* from children. Scand. J. Infect. Dis. **13**:41–45.
13. Kallings, L. O., R. Möllby, and C. E. Nord (Eds.). 1980. Antibiotic associated colitis and *Clostridium difficile*. Scand. J. Infect. Dis. (Suppl. 22), 52 pp.
14. Libby, J. M., and T. D. Wilkins. 1982. Production of antitoxins to two toxins of *Clostridium difficile* and immunological comparison of the toxins by cross-neutralization studies. Infect. Immun. **35**:374–376.
15. Libby, J. M., B. S. Jortner, and T. D. Wilkins. 1982. Effects of the two toxins of *Clostridium difficile* in antibiotic-associated cecitis in hamsters. Infect. Immun. **36**:822–829.

16. Lowbury, E. J. L., *et al.* 1978. Prophylaxis against tetanus in non-immune patients with wounds: the role of antibiotics and of human antitetanus globulin. J. Hygiene **80**:267–274.

17. Lyerly, D. M., *et al.* 1982. Biological activities of toxins A and B of *Clostridium difficile*. Infect. Immun. **35**:1147–1150.

18. MacLennan, J. D. 1962. The histotoxic clostridial infections of man. Bacteriol. Rev. **26**:177–274.

19. Mellanby, J., and J. Green. 1981. How does tetanus toxin act? Neuroscience **6**:281–300.

20. Morgan, W. J., *et al.* 1981. Tetanus prophylaxis and accidental wounds. Scottish Med. J. **26**:24–26.

21. Nakamura, S., *et al.* 1981. Isolation of *Clostridium difficile* from the feces and the antibody in sera of young and elderly adults. Microbiol. Immunol. **25**:345–351.

22. Onderdonk, A. B., R. L. Cisneros, and J. G. Bartlett. 1980. *Clostridium difficile* in gnotobiotic mice. Infect. Immun. **28**:277–282.

23. Pierce, P. F., *et al.* 1982. Antibiotic-associated pseudomembranous colitis: an epidemiologic investigation of a cluster of cases. J. Infect. Dis. **145**:269–274.

24. Rahman, M., *et al.* 1982. Use of tetanus toxoid for the prevention of neonatal tetanus. 1. Reduction of neonatal mortality by immunization of non-pregnant and pregnant women in rural Bangladesh. Bull. Wld Hlth Org. **60**:261–267.

25. Sanders, R. K. M., *et al.* 1977. Intrathecal antitetanus serum (horse) in the treatment of tetanus. Lancet **1**:974–977.

26. Silva, J., Jr., and R. Fekety. 1981. Clostridia and antimicrobial enterocolitis. Ann. Rev. Med. **32**:327–333.

27. Simpson, L. L. 1979. The action of botulinal toxin. Rev. Infect. Dis. **1**:656–659.

28. Smith, J. W. G., D. R. Laurence, and D. G. Evans. 1975. Prevention of tetanus in the wounded. Brit. Med. J. **3**:453–455.

29. Smith, L. DS. 1977. Botulism. The Organism, Its Toxins, The Disease. Charles C Thomas, Springfield, Ill.

30. Smith, L. DS. 1979. Virulence factors of *Clostridium perfringens*. Rev. Infect. Dis. **1**:254–260.

31. Sonnabend, O., *et al.* 1981. Isolation of *Clostridium botulinum* type G and identification of type G botulinal toxin in humans: report of five sudden unexpected deaths. J. Infect. Dis. **143**:22–27.

32. Sugiyama, H. 1980. *Clostridium botulinum* neurotoxin. Microbiol. Rev. **44**:419–448.

33. Sullivan, N. M., S. Pellett, and T. D. Wilkins. 1982. Purification and characterization of toxins A and B of *Clostridium difficile*. Infect. Immun. **35**:1032–1040.

34. Symposium. 1979. Antibiotic-associated colitis. pp. 255–279. *In* D. Schlessinger (Ed.): Microbiology—1979. American Society for Microbiology, Washington, D.C.

35. Wilcke, B. W., Jr., T. F. Midura, and S. S. Arnon. 1980. Quantitative evidence of intestinal colonization by *Clostridium botulinum* in four cases of infant botulism. J. Infect. Dis. **141**:419–423.

36. Young, L. S., F. M. LaForce, and J. V. Bennett. 1969. An evaluation of serologic and antimicrobial therapy in the treatment of tetanus in the United States. J. Infect. Dis. **120**:153–159.

CHAPTER 29

Listeria and Erysipelothrix

LISTERIA MONOCYTOGENES	**ERYSIPELOTHRIX**
Morphology and Staining	**RHUSIOPATHIAE**
Physiology	*Morphology and Staining*
Antigenic Structure	*Pathogenicity for Lower Animals*
Toxins	*Pathogenicity for Man*
Pathogenicity	
Listeriosis in Man	

Listeria monocytogenes[1, 3, 5]

The microorganism now known as *Listeria monocytogenes* had undoubtedly been isolated from diseased lower animals and man prior to 1926, but without sufficiently precise characterization to allow its identification. In that year it was described as the etiological agent of an epizootic among laboratory rabbits and guinea pigs, which was characterized in part by a monocytosis. What proved to be the same microorganism was isolated the following year from gerbils in South Africa. These isolates were later recognized as the same species, which, after a varied taxonomic history, was ultimately given the name *Listeria monocytogenes*, by which it continues to be known. Although several species of *Listeria* are listed in Bergey,[4] the status of most is uncertain, and only *L. monocytogenes* is of medical significance.

Morphology and Staining[4]

Listeria monocytogenes is a nonsporulating, nonencapsulated rod. In very young cultures it is found in bacillary form, 0.5 μm. by 1 to 2 μm. (Fig. 29–1), later becoming predominantly coccoid, the form in which it is usually observed. In old cultures or cultures of the rough form, filaments 6 to 20 μm. in length occur. The arrangement of the cells is not characteristic; they may be found singly, in pairs sometimes at acute angle to one another, and in short chains.

In young cultures the bacilli are invariably gram-positive, but as the culture ages the Gram reaction becomes irregular. Some of the conventional simple stains, *e.g.*, methylene blue, are not satisfactory, and the Gram stain or Giemsa stain should be used, especially for tissue sections.

These bacteria are motile, a characteristic which, among others, distinguishes them from *Erysipelothrix;* motility is demonstrable by swarming on soft agar culture at 20°C. as well as by direct observation. When grown at room temperature they are peritrichously flagellated, but when cultured at 37°C. usually only a single polar flagellum is demonstrable.

On solid mediums, *e.g.*, tryptose, blood, or

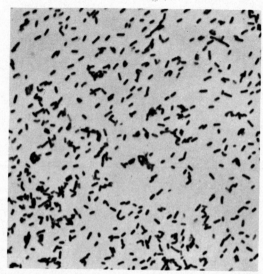

Figure 29–1. *Listeria monocytogenes.* Smear from a pure culture. Fuchsin; × 1050.

serum agar, minute opaque colonies appear in 24 to 48 hours, becoming larger with raised edges on continued incubation. There is a very small zone of β-hemolysis; occasional strains show much greater hemolytic activity on sheep blood agar that is correlated with lecithinase activity of the strain. Two main types of variants are found, one more translucent and less hemolytic, which is agglutinable in saline but retains antigenicity; the other is typically rough.

Physiology

These bacteria are best grown, especially on primary isolation, on relatively rich mediums and under reduced oxygen and increased CO_2 tension. Growth occurs at neutral or slightly alkaline reactions, and these bacteria are unusual in their ability to grow well at high pH, up to 9.6, and in the presence of 10 per cent sodium chloride. Growth is relatively slow in liquid mediums in the absence of fermentable carbohydrate, and may be delayed for one to two weeks or may not occur at all when the inoculum is small; this probably accounts for some failures to isolate *Listeria* from pathological material. When fermentable carbohydrate, *e.g.*, glucose, is included in the medium, growth is much more rapid, but as the pH falls to 5.6 or less, the bacteria die out in two to three days. Enrichment occurs when the specimen is allowed to stand for several weeks or months in the refrigerator, owing presumably to the ability of these bacteria to grow slowly at such low temperatures; therefore, subsequent subculture may be successful when immediate culture was not. *Listeria* are similar in some respects to *Erysipelothrix;* the cultural and morphological characteristics that serve to separate them are shown in Table 29–1.

Table 29–1. **Cultural and Morphological Characters of *Listeria* and *Erysipelothrix***

Test	*Listeria monocytogenes*	*Erysipelothrix rhusiopathiae*
Acid from:		
Glucose	+	+
Fructose	+	+
Mannitol	+	−
H_2S production*	−	+
Nitrate reduction	−	−
Esculin hydrolysis	+	−
Catalase	+	−
Hemolysis	β	α
Motility	+	−

*In triple-sugar-iron agar.

Table 29–2. **Antigenic Structure of *Listeria monocytogenes****

Serotype	Antigens	
	Somatic (Heat-Stable)	Flagellar (Heat-Labile)
1a	I, II, (III)	A, B
1b	I, II, (III)	A, B, C
2	I, II, (III)	B, D
3a	II, (III), IV	A, B
3b	II, (III), IV	A, B, C
4a	(III), (V), VII, IX	A, B, C
4b	(III), V, VI	A, B, C
4ab	(III), V, VI, VII, IX	A, B, C
4c	(III), V, VII	A, B, C
4d	(III), VI, VIII	A, B, C
4e	(III), V, VI, VIII, IX	A, B, C

*Modified from M. L. Gray and A. H. Killinger, Bacteriol. Rev. **30**:309, 1966.

Antigenic Structure

Detailed antigenic analysis of *L. monocytogenes* reveals both heat-labile flagellar antigens and heat-stable carbohydrate-containing somatic antigens. These allow differentiation of four main serotypes, designated 1, 2, 3, and 4, and the subdivision into subtypes. The antigenic structure of these serotypes is shown in Table 29–2. Most clinical isolates are of serotypes 1a, 1b, and 4b. Immunological cross-reactions occur with a number of other bacteria, including strains of *Streptococcus faecalis, Staphylococcus aureus, Escherichia coli,* and various *Corynebacterium* species. The serodiagnosis of *Listeria* infection using paired serums from patients is, then, not reliable, for rise in titer to *Listeria* antigen may occur in infections with other microorganisms.

Toxins

Infection of animals with *L. monocytogenes* is characterized by monocytosis; these cells may constitute up to 30 per cent of the total white cell count by the fourth day of experimental infections in rabbits. This response is due, in large part, to the presence of a **monocytosis-producing agent** in the microorganism.[6] It is a lipid, liberated by mechanical disruption of the cells, and is extracted by certain organic solvents. The activity is correlated with virulence, for it is present in large amount in freshly isolated virulent strains, decreases rapidly coincident with decline in virulence on serial culture on laboratory mediums, and may be restored by animal passage. The partially purified material produces an effect on the hematopoietic system substantially identical with that which occurs in experimental infection, but it does not appear to be otherwise toxic. An **oxygen-labile hemolysin** is produced that has pronounced cardiotoxic activity and may play a prominent role in the observed intoxication of listeriosis.[10]

Pathogenicity

Naturally occurring listeriosis of lower animals and man is apparently worldwide in distribution, though most of the reported cases have been in the United States and Western Europe. Infections in lower animals, particularly domestic animals, are common, and many hundreds of human cases have been recorded as well. It is probable that others are missed because the disease cannot be diagnosed with certainty on clinical grounds alone and because of failure to isolate the microorganism.

Of the common experimental animals, the mouse and rabbit appear to be among the most susceptible, and fatal infection is readily produced by intravenous or intraperitoneal inoculation. Freshly isolated smooth strains of *L. monocytogenes* appear to be almost invariably virulent; virulence is, however, readily lost by culture on laboratory mediums.

Listeriosis in Man[2, 7–9]

Human listeriosis was first described in 1926. At that time, recognized cases resembled infectious mononucleosis. This form of the disease is now rare, as are the cutaneous and oculoglandular syndromes. Listeriosis is now most often seen as central nervous system infection, as bacteremia, and, rarely, as endocarditis. Most cases appear either in neonates or in the elderly, and tend to be opportunistic in nature.

Infections in neonates are the most common, appearing in two clinical syndromes. **Early-onset listeriosis** in infants is generally septicemic, while the **late-onset form** is usually meningitic, with greatest incidence in infants less than one month of age. Listerial meningitis in infants is a serious infection with case-fatality ratios approaching 30 per cent. The septicemic infections may be considered opportunistic and are often associated with obstetrical complications or colonization of the genital tract of the mother.

Most listerial infections of adults occur in the elderly, usually those over 60 years of age. In this group, meningitis is the usual clinical form. In middle-aged adults, listerial meningitis is sometimes found in cancer patients, but is otherwise rare in this group. Mortality rates of the meningitic form are about 30 per cent, but may be twice as high in cancer patients.

Bacteremia does not seem to be as clearly age-related as meningitis, nor is its fatality rate as high. Sepsis occurs primarily in cancer patients, in the immunosuppressed, and in alcoholics. A significant association with pregnancy has also been noted. Endocarditis due to *Listeria* is occasionally seen, usually in patients with preexisting cardiac lesions. It does not differ clinically from endocarditis due to other bacteria.

Of particular interest is the greater incidence of listeriosis in renal transplant recipients. This group is at risk from all forms of listeriosis, but meningitis is the most common. Susceptibility in these patients appears to be linked to the use of corticosteroids that depress the cell-mediated immune response.

Listeriosis in humans has no distinctive clinical manifestations that permit diagnosis on clinical grounds, so that isolation and identification of *Listeria* is an important aid to diagnosis. Asymptomatic carriage of *L. monocytogenes* has been frequently noted, especially in the intestine and genital tract. Clinical specimens, such as blood, cerebrospinal fluid, and genital tract secretions may be cultured on conventional mediums, and isolates identified by the characteristics listed in Table 29–1.

Several antibiotics have been recommended for treatment of listeriosis, including penicillin, ampicillin, tetracyclines, and erythromycin. High doses of penicillin or ampicillin have often been successful in the meningitic form. Bacteremia is more benign and reportedly resolves without antimicrobial therapy.

Erysipelothrix rhusiopathiae[13]

Microorganisms similar to the actinomycetes have been found to be the causative agents of swine erysipelas; they also infect man, and the disease produced is termed **erysipeloid** to distinguish it from erysipelas of streptococcal etiology. It is generally agreed that the etiological agents of these infections, although given a variety of names in the past, are either identical or closely related varieties of the same species; they are now given the name *Erysipelothrix rhusiopathiae* and are considered to be related to *Listeria monocytogenes*.

Morphology and Physiology

Erysipelothrix rhusiopathiae occurs in two rather well-defined morphological types usually designated smooth and rough. The smooth type appears as a small, slender, sometimes slightly curved, nonmotile, nonsporulating, gram-positive rod. Long chains of bacilli and filaments, sometimes beaded and showing swollen areas, are present in smears of the rough form. Both stain readily and sometimes irregularly with deeply staining granules (Fig. 29–2). Colonies of the smooth form on solid mediums are round, convex, amorphous, water-clear, and small, perhaps 0.1 mm. in diameter, and broth cultures are uniformly turbid. The rough form produces larger colonies with a granular, curled appearance like that of very small colonies of anthrax bacilli, while growth in liquid mediums is in the form of flocculent, hair-like masses with little or no turbidity. The most characteristic growth is in gelatin stab cultures; bead-like colonies appear along the line of inoculation from which lateral filamentous growth occurs, resembling a test-tube brush.

The organism is microaerophilic but will grow under aerobic or anaerobic conditions; growth appears on the usual infusion mediums with 24 hours' incubation at the optimum temperature of 30°C. Green discoloration, or α-hemolysis, is seen on blood agar. Other cultural and morphological characteristics are listed in Table 29–1.

Erysipelothrix rhusiopathiae is somewhat more than ordinarily resistant to chemical and physical agents. The organism is known to survive for long periods in soil and probably is not destroyed by methods used in meat preservation, such as smoking, salting, and pickling. It is probably because of this survival of the organisms that endemic areas experience recurrences of the disease year after year.

Pathogenicity for Lower Animals

The principal animal reservoir of *E. rhusiopathiae* is domestic swine. In addition to the cutaneous form of swine erysipelas, animals may also exhibit septicemia, endocarditis, and arthritis. The microorganisms are excreted in great numbers in the feces, and the disease is spread by healthy carriers as well as diseased animals. Swine erysipelas has been of very great economic importance in Europe and is also found in the United States. The organism is pathogenic, too, for a variety of birds, and in the United States turkeys are most often seriously affected; cyanosis is a prominent feature and is evident in the "blue comb." It has also been found in wild rats, which should perhaps be considered as a reservoir of infection and possibly a source of the human disease.

Pathogenicity for Man

Human infection with *E. rhusiopathiae* is well known. A septicemic type with diffuse erythema is rare in man,[11] and only a very few instances have been reported. A chronic form with endocarditis and polyarthritis is also very rare.[12] **Erysipeloid,** the usual type of infection, is an erythematous-edematous lesion, with local lesions commonly developing on the fingers or hand from an abrasion where the microorganism enters. The lesion, although spreading, almost never extends beyond the wrist. There is some swelling and a marked erythema of the lesion and sometimes local arthritis and regional adenitis. The disease is usually self-limiting and terminates within a month. The organism may be cultivated from biopsy specimens taken from the advancing edge of the lesion.

Human infection can almost invariably be traced to contact with animals and animal products, such as meat, hides, bones, and manure, or to fish and shellfish. The disease is, therefore, associated with certain occupations, occurring in persons working in kitchens with raw meat and fish. In the United States, contact with live fish and crustacea appears to be a major source of infection.

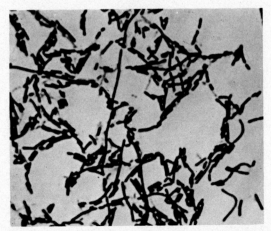

Figure 29–2. *Erysipelothrix rhusiopathiae,* pure culture. Note the similarity of this microorganism to the actinomycetes. × 1000. (Kral.)

REFERENCES

1. Albritton, W. L., *et al.* 1980. *Listeria monocytogenes.* pp. 139–142. *In* E. H. Lennette, *et al.* (Eds.): Manual of Clinical Microbiology. 3rd ed. American Society for Microbiology, Washington, D. C.

2. Albritton, W. L., G. L. Wiggins, and J. C. Feeley. 1976. Neonatal listeriosis: distribution of serotypes in relation to age at onset of disease. J. Pediat. **88**:481–483.
3. Bojsen-Møller, J. 1972. Human listeriosis. Diagnostic, epidemiological and clinical studies. Acta Pathol. Microbiol. Scand., Sect. B., Suppl. No. 229. 157 pp.
4. Buchanan, R. E., and N. E. Gibbons (Eds.). 1974. Bergey's Manual of Determinative Bacteriology. 8th ed. The Williams & Wilkins Co., Baltimore.
5. Gray, M. L., and A. H. Killinger. 1966. *Listeria monocytogenes* and listeric infections. Bacteriol. Rev. **30**:309–382.
6. Holder, I. A., and C. P. Sword. 1969. Characterization and biological activity of the monocytosis-producing agent of *Listeria monocytogenes*. J. Bacteriol. **97**:603–611.
7. Larsson, S. 1979. Epidemiology of listeriosis in Sweden 1958–1974. Scand. J. Infect. Dis. **11**:47–54.
8. Nieman, R. E., and B. Lorber. 1980. Listeriosis in adults: a changing pattern. Report of eight cases and review of the literature, 1968–1978. Rev. Infect. Dis. **2**:207–227.
9. Skidmore, A. G. 1981. Listeriosis at Vancouver General Hospital, 1965–79. Can. Med. Assn. J. **125**:1217–1221.
10. Sword, C. P., and G. C. Kingdon. 1971. *Listeria monocytogenes* toxin. pp. 357–377. *In* S. Kadis, T. C. Montie, and S. J. Ajl (Eds.): Microbial Toxins. Vol. IIA, Bacterial Protein Toxins. Academic Press, New York.
11. Townshend, R. H., A. E. Jephcott, and M. H. Yekta. 1973. Erysipelothrix septicaemia without endocarditis. Brit. Med. J. **1**:464.
12. Volmer, J., and G. Hasler. 1976. Erysipelothrix-Endokarditis. Deut. Med. Wschr. **101**:1672–1675.
13. Weaver, R. E. 1980. *Erysipelothrix*. pp. 143–144. *In* E. H. Lennette, *et al.* (Eds.): Manual of Clinical Microbiology. 3rd ed. American Society for Microbiology, Washington, D. C.

Corynebacterium

Corynebacterium diphtheriae[2]

As a clinical entity diphtheria dates from the observations of Bretonneau in 1826. The diphtheria bacillus was observed and described by Klebs in 1883, and was isolated by Löffler in the following year. Löffler expressly disclaimed the assumption that his bacillus was the causal agent of diphtheria, in part because he found it in the throat of a healthy child, and in part because he did not find it in all cases of what were apparently clinical diphtheria. The significance of his findings is now clear, however, for it is known that other bacteria, such as streptococci, can produce a condition in the throat closely resembling diphtheria and that the diphtheria bacillus may be present in the nasopharynx of carriers. Further investigations by other workers indicated that the bacillus was always present in the typical false membrane of diphtheria. In 1888 Roux and Yersin showed that this bacillus formed a soluble toxin that reproduced the characteristic symptoms of diphtheria and thus demonstrated its etiological relation to the disease. The diphtheria bacillus is the most important member of the genus *Corynebacterium*, which includes very many species—saprophytic forms as well as those producing disease in animals and plants.[2, 5]

Morphology and Staining[5]
The diphtheria bacillus is a slender rod ranging from 1 to 6 μm. in length and 0.3 to 0.8 μm. in breadth. The bacilli are highly pleomorphic; in addition to the straight or slightly curved rods, club-shaped and long filamentous forms are often observed. Near the completion of cell division, a movement designated as snapping occurs, and the bacilli may remain attached at sharp angles to one another in a palisade or picket-fence arrangement; groups of these cells are said to resemble Chinese letters.

The diphtheria bacillus tends to stain irregularly. Some cells stain solidly, others take the stain more deeply in transverse bands to give a barred appearance, and in still others deeply staining metachromatic or Babès-Ernst granules are found. This irregular staining is apparent with Löffler's alkaline methylene blue or with toluidine blue. The bacillus is not encapsulated and is nonmotile.

In stained smears the appearance of diphtheria bacilli is highly characteristic. They may not be identified on morphological grounds alone, for many of the pseudodiphtheria bacilli, or diphtheroids, also stain irregularly and are similarly pleomorphic. The diphtheria bacillus is gram-positive but decolorizes more readily than most of the gram-positive bacteria.

Surface colonies on blood agar are small, raised, translucent, and gray (Fig. 30–1). On differential mediums containing potassium tellurite, colonies of the diphtheria bacillus are

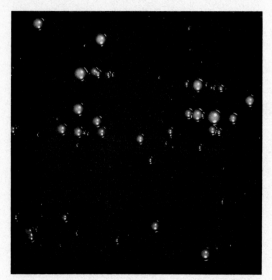

Figure 30–1. Colonies of *Corynebacterium diphtheriae* on blood agar. Note the smooth, raised, translucent appearance and relatively small size. × 2.

dark gray or black because of the reduction of tellurite and are readily differentiated from those of contaminating bacteria. Tellurite reduction apparently occurs within the bacterial cell. It should be noted that microscopic morphology may not be characteristic in smears made from tellurite medium cultures.

Physiology[9]

The optimum growth temperature for the diphtheria bacillus is 34° to 36°C., and it grows well at 37°C.; growth will take place over the range from 15° to 40°C. An alkaline reaction, in the pH range of 7.8 to 8.0, is required and free access to air is essential, for growth under anaerobic conditions is sparse.

In primary isolation the diphtheria bacillus is best cultivated on enriched mediums. Growth is rapid on Löffler's serum medium, an infusion medium containing glucose and coagulated serum. Minute but visible colonies appear after 12 to 24 hours' incubation. A variety of differential and selective mediums have been used extensively, all of which contain potassium tellurite and, usually, cystine. As indicated above, the characteristic morphology of the diphtheria bacillus is not always seen in smears from colonies on tellurite mediums; therefore, in some laboratories both Löffler's medium and a differential tellurite medium are inoculated. The former is used for microscopic examination if typical colonies appear on the differential medium.

The diphtheria bacillus can be cultivated on ordinary nutrient and infusion mediums.

Growth is somewhat scanty on the former but good on fresh meat infusions and on heated blood, or chocolate, agar. The biochemical reactions that aid in differentiation from other *Corynebacterium* are listed in Table 30–1.

In ordinary culture mediums the diphtheria bacillus may remain viable for relatively long periods. In diphtheritic membrane, it may survive for several months. Although virulence is ordinarily reduced by continued culture on laboratory mediums, some strains remain fully virulent, *i.e.,* toxigenic, on prolonged cultivation. The bacilli are unusually susceptible to heat; a suspension or broth culture is killed by holding at 58°C. for 10 minutes. In diphtheritic membrane they are considerably more resistant.

Antigenic Structure

Although the diphtheria toxin is apparently immunologically identical in all strains, the diphtheria bacilli are heterogeneous with respect to cell antigens. They contain heat-stable somatic antigens, which appear to be polysaccharide in nature, and heat-labile surface protein antigens.[17] The former have little differential value, and the agglutinative types that have been described depend upon the protein antigens. There is some correlation between agglutinative types and the **mitis-intermedius-gravis** colonial types, but such agglutinative types have little significance to the disease, although antibacterial immunity is considered by some to be a possible element in effective immunity (see below).

Toxins[2, 4, 22]

The diphtheria bacillus elaborates a potent exotoxin that, in cell-free form, reproduces the toxic manifestations of diphtheria. Although there is some evidence that invasiveness of the diphtheria bacillus may be separated from toxigenicity, virulence is essentially synonymous with toxigenicity, and the measure of virulence is a test for the formation of toxin.

The production of toxin is markedly influenced by environmental and nutritive conditions. A slightly alkaline reaction, pH 7.8 to 8.0, is essential, since acid pH inhibits toxin formation; aerobic conditions are also necessary. Maximum amounts of toxin are found after 7 to 10 days' incubation at 36°C. to 37°C. The protein toxin is unstable at pH 6.0 or less, and is heat-labile.

The critical factor for toxin formation is not the quality of the usual nutrients, but is rather the concentration of iron in the medium; the optimum iron concentration is 0.14 μg. per

Table 30–1. Biochemical Reactions of Selected *Corynebacterium* Species*

Species	Catalase	Nitrate Reduction	Urease	Gelatinase	Acid from: Glucose	Maltose	Trehalose
C. diphtheriae	+	+	–	–	+	+	–
C. ulcerans	+	–	+	+	+	+	L
C. hofmannii	+	+	+	–	–	–	–
C. xerosis	+	+	V	V	+	+	–
C. pseudotuberculosis	+	V	V	V	+	+	–
C. equi	+	+	–	–	–	+	–
C. haemolyticum	–	–	–	–	+	+	V
JK bacteria	+	–	–	–	L	L	L

*Adapted from several authors.[5,9]
Symbols: V, variable; L, late fermentation.

ml.; 5.0 μg. per ml. almost completely inhibits its formation. Iron concentrations optimal for growth exceed the optimum for toxin production. Toxin release lags behind growth and begins rapid accumulation in the medium when the bacterial population has reached near-maximal levels.

Toxin Production and β-Phage. In 1951 the remarkable observation was made that toxin production in virulent *C. diphtheriae* is dependent upon the presence of a lysogenic bacteriophage in the bacterium. Only those strains lysogenic for β-phage were capable of toxin production, and nontoxigenic strains could be converted to toxigenicity by lysogenization. The phage gene, **tox⁺**, codes for the production of the protein toxin; so far as is known, the gene serves no essential viral function. In the lysogenic state, the integrated prophage is quite stable and is retained without significant loss, *viz.,* the PW 8 strain, after many years in culture, is still highly toxigenic.

It is of interest that some 60 years after the etiology of diphtheria had apparently been fully established, it became evident that more than one microorganism is involved and the disease can be considered to be of dual etiology.

Nature and Action of the Toxin.[14] The diphtheria toxin is a potent poison, though not as potent as the botulinum toxin. It has been highly purified and is a single polypeptide chain of 62,000 daltons. The lethal dose of purified toxin for man and animals is of the order of 130 ng./kg. of body weight. The dose-response curve in the guinea pig is very steep, so much so that the MLD assay for potency, adopted many years ago and persisting to the present, is practical.

The pharmacological activity of the toxin is quite characteristic, and the essential features of diphtheria are experimentally reproduced with the toxin alone. Degenerative changes are produced in the heart muscle, kidneys, liver, and peripheral nerves. The pathological condition in the adrenals of the guinea pig is accentuated and characteristic. The immediate cause of death in the acute disease is heart failure; damage to peripheral nerves accounts for the post-diphtheritic paralysis observed in man and in guinea pigs receiving near-fatal doses of toxin.

At the cellular level, diphtheria toxin is cytotoxic for certain cells in tissue culture. The initial effect in these cells is an enzymatic **inhibition of protein synthesis.** This enzymatic activity resides in only a portion of the diphtheria toxin molecule, designated **fragment A.**

When the intact toxin is treated with trypsin, it is cleaved or "nicked" at only one point in the chain, so that two polypeptide chains result; these chains are held together by an interchain disulfide linkage. If "nicked" toxin is then reduced, the two peptide fragments, A and B, are disjoined. Fragment A is the amino-terminal fragment and is the smaller, with molecular weight of about 22,000 daltons. Neither fragment alone is toxic for intact cells, but reduced fragment A exhibits enzymatic activity in broken cell preparations.

It is now clear that the **fragment B** portion of the toxin functions only in a binding capacity in that it possesses recognition sites for glycolipid receptors on the plasma membrane of toxin-sensitive cells. Cells from animals that are insensitive to diphtheria toxin, such as those of rats and mice, apparently lack the toxin-binding sites on their cell membranes. After the toxin is bound to the cell surface, the A fragment must enter the cell. The precise mechanism for this is not completely understood. It could traverse the plasma membrane directly, or it could enter the cell by endocytosis, being taken into intracellular vesicles, which then fuse with lysosomes. The latter mechanism appears to be the most likely. By either route, diphtheria toxin is believed to form transmembrane channels through which fragment A enters the cell cytosol.

In the cytoplasm, **fragment A** assumes an active configuration and catalyzes the transfer of adenosine diphosphoribose (ADP-ribose) from nicotinamide adenosine dinucleotide (NAD) to elongation factor 2 (EF-2). Elongation factor 2, a protein found in all eucaryotic cells, functions in protein synthesis by catalyzing the translocation of the growing peptide chain on the ribosome. When EF-2 is ADP-ribosylated, however, it is inactive in this regard, and protein synthesis is inhibited. The substrate for fragment A activity is a histidine derivative, named **diphthamide,** contained in EF-2.

The mechanism of diphtheria toxin action is strikingly similar to that of toxin A of *Pseudomonas aeruginosa* (Chapter 25) and has parallels with the action of cholera toxin (Chapter 21) and the enterotoxin of *Escherichia coli* (Chapter 18).

Cord Factor. In addition to the classic diphtheria toxin just described, *C. diphtheriae* produces a toxic glycolipid which is lethal for mice and which disrupts mouse mitochondria. This substance, trehalose-6,6'-dicorynemycolate, is similar to the mycobacterial cord factor (Chapter 31), both in general structure and pharmacological activity, and reinforces the presumed close relationship between coryne-bacteria and mycobacteria.

Biotypes

Morphological types of the diphtheria bacillus were first described in 1931. These were of very considerable interest when first observed, for there appeared to be an association, especially in England, between the type and the degree of severity in the clinical manifestations of the disease. Those designated as the *gravis* and *intermedius* types were found in severe cases of diphtheria, and the *mitis* type in the milder cases. The association was less clear on the Continent, and there appeared to be little or no correlation in the United States, where the *mitis* type occurs much more frequently and perhaps only 1 per cent of the strains are of the *gravis* type. The toxins produced by the three types are immunologically identical. The three types also appear to be equally virulent for the guinea pig. It is more or less generally agreed that the differentiation of these types is not significantly related to clinical severity but has been useful from an epidemiological point of view. Bacteriophage types generally correlate with these biotypes; phage typing may yield some additional fine distinctions of value in defined epidemics.[26]

These types may be differentiated by their colonial form on tellurite mediums (Table 30–2, Fig. 30–2). Colonial differences are also apparent on certain other mediums. On fresh blood agar the *mitis* type is usually hemolytic, although a filterable hemolysin is not produced; the *intermedius* type is nonhemolytic, and the *gravis* type usually so.

There is some association between colonial type and the morphology of the bacillary forms (Figs. 30–3 and 30–4). Those of the *gravis* type show one or two deeply staining areas, the remainder of the cell staining very lightly; metachromatic granules are seldom observed. Bacilli of the *mitis* variety stain irregularly and contain very many well-developed metachromatic granules. The *intermedius* forms have the familiar barred appearance.

Not all strains showing the morphological and biochemical characteristics of these types are virulent, *i.e.*, toxigenic, diphtheria bacilli. Since virulent diphtheria bacillus is differentiated on the basis of the formation of immunologically specific toxin, it is apparent that *mitis, gravis,* and *intermedius* types of nontoxigenic bacilli occur and are avirulent. Both toxigenic and nontoxigenic variants may be present in a single infection.[6]

DIPHTHERIA

Historically, diphtheria has been a disease primarily of children. As the prevalence of the disease has decreased in recent years (Fig. 30–5), there has been an increased number of cases in the older age groups, particularly in those over 30 years of age (Fig. 30–6). This

Table 30–2. **Characteristics of the Diphtheria Bacillus Types**

Type			mitis	intermedius	gravis
Morphology	Microscopic		Usually long, with many metachromatic granules—80 per cent typical	Usually barred, club forms common—80 per cent typical	Short, evenly staining—50–60 per cent typical
	Colonial	Tellurite	Small, round, smooth, convex, black with grayish periphery	Small, flat, dull, gray, raised center	Large, irregular, dull, gray, raised center, radial striations
		Chocolate	Smooth, semiopaque, glistening	Flat, dry, opaque, slight greenish zone	Flat, dry, matte, opaque
		Broth	Uniform turbidity, sometimes slightly granular, soft pellicle	Finely granular turbidity	Granular, flakes, pellicle—variable
Physiology	Fermentation of	Glycogen	−	−	+
		Starch	−	−	+
	Hemolysis		+	−	±

A   B   C

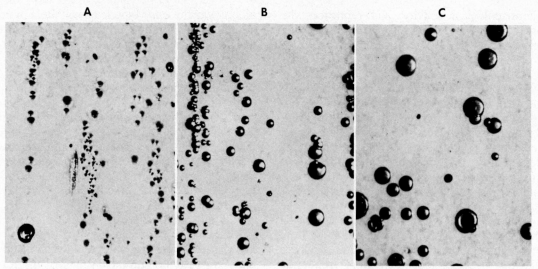

Figure 30–2. The types of the diphtheria bacillus on chocolate tellurite agar. *A, mitis* type; note the characteristic raised, small black colony. *B, intermedius* type; the lighter color, beginning radial striation, and small size are apparent. *C, gravis* type; the gray color, larger size, raised center, and radial striation are evident.

age distribution is associated with the rise and fall of immunity. Infants are usually protected by passive immunity of maternal origin.[20] As this immunity wanes with age, the child becomes more susceptible in the absence of artificial immunization or immunizing subclinical infections. In the United States and other countries where artificial immunization of preschool children is widely practiced, the lower incidence of the disease in children and young adults is probably due to this measure rather than to inapparent, immunizing infections. Since the disease has become relatively uncommon in this country, reinforcement of childhood immunity by subclinical infection is reduced, so that by early adulthood, immunity again wanes; the disease has, therefore, become more common in the older age groups. In other geographical areas where artificial immunization is not so widely applied, and where the prevalence remains high, naturally acquired immunity by infection, both overt and covert, is probably more important in protection of the older population and greater incidence is noted in children and young adults.

Diphtheria in humans is typically a local

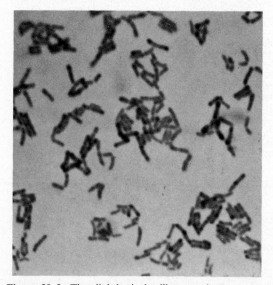

Figure 30–3. The diphtheria bacillus, *gravis* type, pure culture on blood agar. Note the bipolar staining and the club-shaped forms. The lightly stained cells with deeply stained areas are characteristic of *gravis* morphology. Methylene blue stain; × 1200.

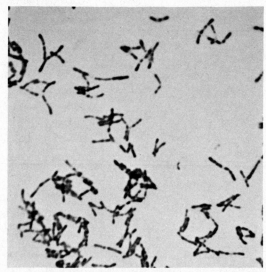

Figure 30–4. The diphtheria bacillus, *intermedius* type, pure culture on blood agar. Note the irregular staining and barred appearance characteristic of this variety. Methylene blue stain; × 1200.

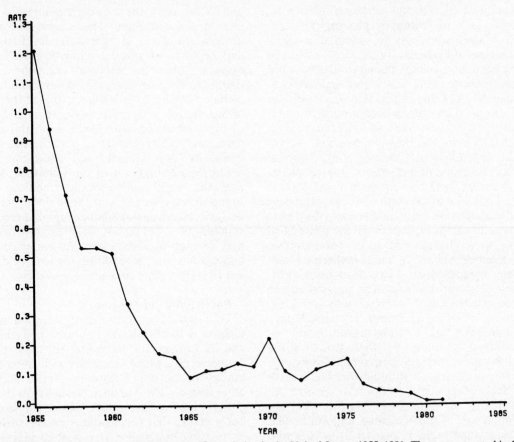

Figure 30–5. Reported cases of diphtheria per 10^5 population in the United States, 1955–1981. The cases reported include both cutaneous and noncutaneous diphtheria; the increase in rate beginning in 1973 and reaching a peak in 1975 is composed entirely of cutaneous cases. The number of such cutaneous cases has decreased rapidly since 1975. (Centers for Disease Control, Annual summary 1981: reported morbidity and mortality in the United States. Morbid. Mortal. Weekly Rep. **30**[54], 1982.)

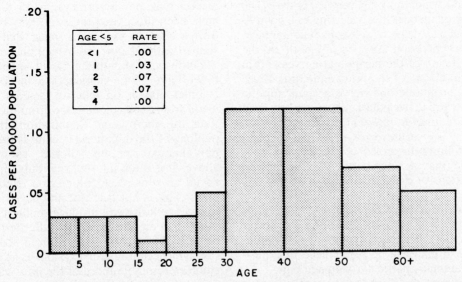

Figure 30–6. Age incidence of diphtheria in the United States, 1976. Note the increase beginning after about age 20 and the relatively high rates in the older population. (Centers for Disease Control, Annual supplement. Morbid. Mortal. Weekly Rep. **25**, 1976.)

infection of the mucous surfaces, usually occurring as a **membranous pharyngitis;** occasionally the lesions may be laryngeal or nasal. **Cutaneous diphtheria,** once rare, has been increasing, particularly among children in rural areas or those living under poor sanitary conditions.[3, 7] Although such skin infections do not often exhibit generalized diphtheritic toxemia, they do constitute a source of respiratory tract infection. Ulcerative skin lesions, sometimes appearing in epidemic form in tropical areas, are called **desert sore** or **tropical ulcer.**

The chief local consequence of infection is a degeneration of the epithelial cells, extending to the underlying tissue and accompanied by a profuse fibrinous exudation. In the pharyngeal form, these changes lead to the formation on the mucosal surface of the **diphtheritic membrane,** composed of fibrin, dead tissue cells, leucocytes, and bacteria. The membrane can be so extensive as to interfere with breathing, even necessitating intubation or tracheotomy.

Diphtheria bacilli rarely invade tissues beyond the local lesion, but their growth in the diphtheritic membrane is accompanied by production of the toxin. Although diphtheria toxin probably plays a part in the formation of the membrane, its systemic effects following absorption are by far the most important; like tetanus, diphtheria is essentially a toxemia. The organs most severely affected are the kidneys, heart, and nerves.

A variety of lesions may be found in the kidneys, acute interstitial nephritis being the most common. The lesions in the heart consist commonly of a fatty degeneration in the muscle fibers, which may be very extensive. The diphtheritic myocarditis occurring as a complication usually leaves no permanent damage. Fatty degeneration also occurs both in the myelin sheath of the peripheral nerves and in the white matter of the brain and cord. These changes in muscle and nerve account for the serious cardiac weakness often observed in diphtheria and the frequent occurrence of the more or less extensive paralysis that so commonly follows an attack of the disease. It is probable that a small amount of toxin can cause extensive damage in these tissues.

Animal Models of Diphtheria

Diphtheria is not a natural disease of lower animals, but the general symptoms of diphtheria seen in man can be reproduced in experimental animals, particularly guinea pigs.

The subcutaneous inoculation of a guinea pig with a sufficient amount of a young broth culture or toxic filtrate will produce death in one to four days, the time depending upon the size of the inoculum. The animal becomes obviously ill 12 to 18 hours after inoculation, and nephritic symptoms, paralytic manifestations, and other characteristics of human diphtheria are often observed. Postmortem findings include edema and possibly necrosis at the site of inoculation, congestion of the regional lymphatics and abdominal viscera, a pleural exudate, and, characteristic of diphtheritic toxemia in this animal, an enlarged and hemorrhagic condition of the adrenals. As a rule, the bacilli remain localized and are not found in large numbers in the internal organs of the infected animal. Guinea pigs that receive smaller doses and do not die by the fourth day may develop paralytic symptoms and cachexia and die later on, a condition obviously different from the acute toxemia.

Bacteriological Diagnosis[9]

To establish a diagnosis of infection with diphtheria bacilli, the bacillus must be isolated and its toxigenicity demonstrated, since nontoxigenic *C. diphtheriae* occurs with some frequency in the upper respiratory tract and in other lesions. The specimen is taken on a swab, either plain or previously dipped in sterile horse serum that is coagulated on the surface by twirling in a flame. It is best to inoculate two mediums, Löffler's serum agar and cystine-tellurite agar; if only a single medium can be used, tellurite is preferable. A blood agar plate should be inoculated as well, both for the isolation of diphtheria-like colonies and to provide for the cultivation of hemolytic streptococci that may be present. After the plates have been inoculated the swab may be rolled over a slide to prepare a smear that is then stained with alkaline methylene blue.

Colonies of diphtheria bacilli appear in 18 to 24 hours. If the characteristic black or gray colonies appear on tellurite, smears may be made from such colonies and from the Löffler slant for microscopic examination; the morphology of the diphtheria bacillus is frequently not characteristic on tellurite, as indicated above. It is often inferred that only diphtheria bacilli grow as black colonies on tellurite medium. This is not true, for any bacterium that reduces tellurite will produce similar colonies; other than diphtheria bacilli, tellurite-reducing bacteria from the nose and throat are usually staphylococci or micrococci, and as a rule their colonies resemble those of the *mitis* variety of diphtheria bacillus but are blacker.

The Virulence Test. If morphologically typical bacilli are found, toxigenicity must be tested by animal inoculation or by *in vitro* toxigenicity tests. The growth from a Löffler slant is suspended in neutral broth and injected subcutaneously into each of two guinea pigs, one of which receives 1000 units of diphtheria antitoxin. The diphtheria bacillus will kill the unprotected pig in three to five days, and autopsy will show local edema and the characteristic hemorrhagic enlarged adrenals, while the protected animal will survive.

An *in vitro* virulence test based on the gel-diffusion technique has been widely applied. It consists essentially of growth of the bacterial strain under consideration on an agar plate in which antitoxin has been placed in a well or trench in the agar medium, or a strip of filter paper soaked in antitoxin is laid on the agar surface. The toxin diffusing from the growth forms a line of specific precipitate with the antitoxin diffusing from the reservoir or paper strips.[10] The use of tissue cultures has been proposed, in which HeLa cell monolayers are overlaid with agar and then inoculated with the suspect culture;[16] toxin production is indicated by death of the sensitive eucaryotic cells.

Immunity

Immunity to diphtheria resulting from a frank attack of the disease, a subclinical infection, or prophylactic inoculation is essentially an antitoxic immunity, *i.e.,* immunity to the disease rather than to the infection *per se.* Although the diphtheria toxin is of overriding importance, there is evidence that other toxic substances formed by diphtheria bacilli may contribute to the pathogenesis of the disease, and the question of the significance of an antibacterial immunity is one of perennial interest. The latter is complicated by the serological heterogeneity of the diphtheria bacilli noted above. Effective immunity is, however, generally considered to be primarily antitoxic in nature.

The Schick Test. Immunity to diphtheria may be measured by the amount of circulating antitoxin present in a given individual. The Schick skin test was devised for this purpose; in practice, a standard amount of diphtheria toxin[1] is injected intradermally. In nonimmune individuals the toxin gives rise to local erythema followed by necrosis and desquamation, and the reaction is said to be positive. If the person is immune, however, the toxin is neutralized by the antitoxin present in the recipient. The characteristic skin reaction does not then develop, and the Schick test is negative.

The question of whether the Schick test indicates a degree of immunity such that subsequent infection is highly improbable is one that cannot be answered *a priori*. Experience has shown, however, that it is pragmatically sound to assume that a Schick-negative person is, for all practical purposes, immune. It should be pointed out, however, that antitoxic immunity bears no relation to the carrier state; pharyngeal carriage of virulent *C. diphtheriae* is unaffected by antitoxin level or Schick reaction.

Prophylactic Immunization[19, 21, 24]

It was early observed that experimental animals can be immunized to diphtheria by the injection of living cultures of the bacilli after a protective dose of antitoxic serum, by the inoculation of toxin neutralized with antitoxin, or, more practically, by the administration of toxoid.

Toxoid. The use of formol toxoid as an immunizing agent was introduced by Ramon in 1923 and has been widely adopted. Potent toxin, when treated with small amounts of formalin at 37°C. for one month, loses its toxicity but retains antigenicity and is a highly efficient immunizing agent. The administration of this material in three doses renders 95 per cent of recipients Schick-negative.

Alum-Precipitated Toxoid. Toxoid precipitated with small amounts of potassium alum is superior to ordinary formol toxoid (fluid toxoid) as an immunizing agent. Toxoid is adsorbed to the insoluble precipitate (it may be redissolved in sodium citrate or sodium tartrate) and remains in the subcutaneous tissue for a considerable time, to provide a prolonged antigenic stimulus. In spite of this, a single inoculation is not sufficient—as little as 11 per cent Schick conversion has been observed, together with a tendency to reversion—but two inoculations are as effective as three of fluid toxoid.

The immunizing agent in current use is combined with tetanus toxoid and *Bordetella pertussis*—the diphtheria-tetanus-pertussis vaccine (DPT)—and is administered early in life.[15] It is currently recommended that three doses of DPT be administered during the first few months of life, an additional dose at one year, and a final dose at about age six years. Alum toxoid, like fluid toxoid, rarely induces untoward reactions, and these usually resolve without permanent sequelae.[8]

Passive Immunity

Susceptible, *i.e.,* Schick-positive, individuals may be passively immunized to diphtheria by the injection of antitoxic horse serum or purified preparations of antitoxin. Such immunity is of relatively short duration and is not effective for longer than two or three weeks at the most.

The Therapeutic Use of Antitoxin. Serum therapy is more successful in diphtheria than in any other disease, and there is no question of its efficacy in reducing case-fatality rates. As in the case of tetanus and botulism, the therapeutic administration of antitoxin cannot bring about repair of tissues already damaged by toxin. Early administration is therefore essential, and there is progressive increase in the case-fatality rate with each day's delay. There is no limit, beyond the volume, to the number of units that may be safely injected. Antitoxin is generally administered intramuscularly but in severe cases may be given intravenously. It is without effect when given by mouth.

Epidemiology

The epidemiology of diphtheria is considerably better understood than that of any other disease, in part because the causative agent can be isolated with relative facility from infected individuals, and in part because the Schick test allows the differentiation of immunes and nonimmunes. As in the case of other respiratory diseases, infectious material leaves the body in the secretions of the nose and throat, is transmitted from man to man by contact or infective droplets, and enters the body via the mouth and nose. Furthermore, the diphtheria bacillus is disseminated not only by persons with the disease but also through the agency of healthy carriers in whom there is no clinical evidence of infection. Unlike many of the diseases of the respiratory tract, diphtheria is an immunizing disease and prolonged or repeated contact with the bacillus results in the development of a solid immunity to clinical manifestations of diphtheria.

Immunity and Susceptibility. Schick testing indicates that while susceptibility is generally low in the first six months of life, owing to passive immunization with maternal antibody, the proportion of Schick-positives increases rapidly and is at a maximum in children under four or five years of age, then gradually declines in an unimmunized population in areas where the disease is prevalent. When immunization of children is widely practiced, the effective levels of antitoxin in the population decline at about age 15 in some groups, but not in others, presumably as a consequence of a greater carrier rate in the latter.

Carriers. As indicated above, healthy individuals may harbor both virulent and nontoxigenic diphtheria bacilli in their throats. These carriers need not be either immune or convalescent and are, for the most part, casual or temporary carriers.

The prevalence of diphtheria carriers is not known with certainty. It probably varies with season, and is higher when cutaneous lesions are present in the population. Since both toxigenic and nontoxigenic C. diphtheriae are found in carriers, there is the possibility of phage conversion of nontoxigenic strains. Further, since antitoxic immunity has no antibacterial effect, carriage of C. diphtheriae can occur in Schick-negative individuals. The carrier state may be eliminated, however, by treatment with antimicrobials, such as erythromycin or penicillin. Erythromycin resistance of C. diphtheriae has been noted, however, and is associated with the presence of a large plasmid.[25]

The Control of Diphtheria

It will be obvious from these considerations that diphtheria is widely disseminated in the human population and cannot be controlled by the isolation of carriers or, except in a strictly limited sense, by quarantine of cases. The diphtheria bacillus is especially sensitive to erythromycin, but antibacterial therapy cannot replace immunotherapy in diphtheria.

The control of diphtheria is a matter of immunization, and if a sufficiently large proportion of the susceptible population is rendered immune, the prevalence of clinical diphtheria should decrease. In early studies, it was found that the immunization of 50 per cent or more of the children of school age, 5 to 14 years, did not produce a drop in the incidence of diphtheria in a number of large American cities, but when 30 per cent or more of the preschool children were immunized there was a definite reduction in the incidence of diphtheria, not only among these children but in the community as a whole. It is commonly assumed that immunization of 70 per cent of children suffices to control epidemic diphtheria. Other as yet unknown factors are involved also, for the disease persists in relatively high incidence in some well-immunized communities or groups.

To what extent prophylactic inoculation and the therapeutic use of antitoxin have influenced the decline in diphtheria is problematical. It is believed by some that the present decline is in part a continuation of a periodic trend that has accelerated in the past several decades.

Other Corynebacteria

Microorganisms morphologically closely similar to and frequently indistinguishable from the diphtheria bacillus are found in man and lower animals; many *Corynebacteria* are plant pathogens and others are free-living saprophytes. Of the 30 recognized species, only a few are known to infect humans. Except for *C. diphtheriae,* those that occur in man are casually known as diphtheroids; they often are a part of the normal flora and, on occasion, are responsible for infections and disease. The more important of these are listed in Table 30–1, along with properties that serve to separate them from the diphtheria bacillus.

Corynebacterium ulcerans[18]

This is the only *Corynebacterium* other than *C. diphtheriae* that is known to produce diphtheria toxin; presumably, toxigenic strains are lysogenized with β-phage. *Corynebacterium ulcerans* is a pleomorphic form, usually coccoid, that produces few metachromatic granules; colonies on cystine-tellurite medium may resemble *C. diphtheriae.* It is often found as a part of the normal pharyngeal flora, and toxigenic strains have been the cause of a diphtheria-like disease in humans, but it is generally mild. The infection reportedly has been associated with consumption of cows' milk.

Corynebacterium haemolyticum[11]

The taxonomic position of this species is uncertain; possibly it is related to streptococci. Microscopically, it resembles *C. diphtheriae* but hemolysis is usually seen on blood agar and growth is poor on tellurite medium. *Corynebacterium haemolyticum* is occasionally found as the causative agent in pharyngeal infections, often accompanied by maculopapular rash.

Corynebacterium xerosis[23]

This microorganism resembles the diphtheria bacillus and is a part of the normal flora of the pharynx and skin. It has been isolated from a form of conjunctivitis known as xerosis, but its presence is probably that of a contaminant. It has been found in a few cases of invasive infection as an opportunistic pathogen.

Corynebacterium hofmannii

Also known as *C. pseudodiphtheriticum,* this bacillus is closely similar to the diphtheria bacillus in cellular and colonial morphology (Fig. 30–7). It is a common inhabitant of the nasopharynx and, aside from rare cases of endocarditis, it is essentially nonpathogenic. It does not form toxins and can be distinguished from *C. diphtheriae* by toxigenic tests as well as by physiological properties.

JK Group[12, 27]

Diphtheroid strains, known as group JK bacteria, commonly colonized the skin and rectum of hospitalized patients, particularly following antibiotic therapy. Most patients have serious underlying diseases, so that infections with the JK bacteria often are of a serious nature with high fatality rates. Nosocomial infections have included bacteremia, meningitis, pyelonephritis, peritonitis, wound infection, and abscesses. Most strains are sensitive to vancomycin and it is said to be the drug of choice.

Animal Pathogens

A number of species of corynebacteria are pathogenic for lower animals; some of these infect humans on rare occasion. *Corynebacterium bovis* has been found in endocarditis, otitis media, and skin infections; *C. equi* has been isolated from human pulmonary and bacteremic infections in compromised hosts.

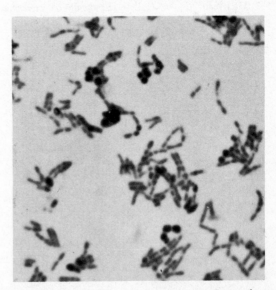

Figure 30–7. *Corynebacterium hofmannii.* Smear from pure culture stained with alkaline methylene blue. Note the irregular staining, club-shaped forms, and general close resemblance to *C. diphtheriae.* × 2000.

REFERENCES

1. Barile, M. F., R. W. Kolb, and M. Pittman. 1971. United States standard diphtheria toxin for the Schick test and the erythema potency assay for the Schick test dose. Infect. Immun. **4**:295–306.
2. Barksdale, L. 1970. *Corynebacterium diphtheriae* and its relatives. Bacteriol. Rev. **34**:378–422.
3. Belsey, M. A., and D. R. LeBlanc. 1975. Skin infections and the epidemiology of diphtheria: acquisition and persistence of *C. diphtheriae* infections. Amer. J. Epidemiol. **102**:179–184.
4. Bonventre, P. F. 1975. Diphtheria. pp. 272–277. *In* D. Schlessinger (Ed.): Microbiology—1975. American Society for Microbiology, Washington, D.C.
5. Buchanan, R. E., and N. E. Gibbons (Eds.). 1974. Bergey's Manual of Determinative Bacteriology. 8th ed. The Williams & Wilkins Co., Baltimore.
6. Chang, D. N., G. S. Laughren, and N. E. Chalvardjian. 1978. Three variants of *Corynebacterium diphtheriae* subsp. *mitis* (Belfanti) isolated from a throat specimen. J. Clin. Microbiol. **8**:767–768.
7. Cockcroft, W. H., W. J. Boyko, and D. E. Allen. 1973. Cutaneous infections due to Corynebacterium diphtheriae. Can. Med. Assn J. **108**:329–331.
8. Cody, C. L., *et al.* 1981. Nature and rates of adverse reactions associated with DPT and DT immunizations in infants and children. Pediatrics **68**:650–660.
9. Coyle, M. B., and L. S. Tompkins. 1980. Corynebacteria. pp. 131–138. *In* E. H. Lennette, *et al.* (Eds.): Manual of Clinical Microbiology. 3rd ed. American Society for Microbiology, Washington, D.C.
10. Davies, J. R. 1974. Elek's test for toxigenicity of corynebacteria. pp. 1–7. Publ. Hlth Lab. Serv. Monogr. Ser. No. 5.
11. Fell, H. W. K., *et al.* 1977. *Corynebacterium haemolyticum* infections in Cambridgeshire. J. Hygiene **79**:269–274.
12. Fraser, D. W. 1981. Bacteria newly recognized as nosocomial pathogens. Amer. J. Med. **70**:432–438.
13. Gauvreau, L., *et al.* 1977. Épidémie de diphtérie survenue sur la côte Nord du St-Laurent à l'automne de 1974. Can. Med. Assn J. **116**:1279–1283.
14. van Heyningen, S. 1981. Diphtheria toxin: which route into the cell? Nature **292**:293–294.
15. Immunization Practices Advisory Committee, Centers for Disease Control. 1981. Diphtheria, tetanus, and pertussis. Guidelines for vaccine prophylaxis and other preventive measures. Ann. Intern. Med. **95**:723–728.
16. Laird, W., and N. Groman. 1973. Rapid, direct tissue culture test for toxigenicity of *Corynebacterium diphtheriae*. Appl. Microbiol. **25**:709–712.
17. Lazar, I. 1968. Serological relationships of corynebacteria. J. Gen. Microbiol. **52**:77–88.
18. Meers, P. D. 1979. A case of classical diphtheria, and other infections due to *Corynebacterium ulcerans*. J. Infection **1**:139–142.
19. Miller, L. W., *et al.* 1972. Diphtheria immunization. Effect upon carriers and the control of outbreaks. Amer. J. Dis. Child. **123**:197–199.
20. Nathenson, G., and B. Zakzewski. 1976. Current status of passive immunity to diphtheria and tetanus in the newborn. J. Infect. Dis. **133**:199–201.
21. Nelson, L. A., *et al.* 1978. Immunity to diphtheria in an urban population. Pediatrics **61**:703–710.
22. Pappenheimer, A. M., Jr. and D. M. Gill. 1973. Diphtheria. Science **182**:353–358.
23. Porschen, R. K., Z. Goodman, and B. Rafai. 1977. Isolation of *Corynebacterium xerosis* from clinical specimens. Infection and colonization. Amer. J. Clin. Pathol. **68**:290–293.
24. van Ramshorst, J. D., T. K. Sundaresan, and A. S. Outschoorn. 1972. International collaborative studies on potency assays of diphtheria and tetanus toxoids. Bull. Wld Hlth Org. **46**:263–276.
25. Schiller, J., N. Groman, and M. Coyle. 1980. Plasmids in *Corynebacterium diphtheriae* and diphtheroids mediating erythromycin resistance. Antimicrob. Agents Chemother. **18**:814–821.
26. Toshach, S., A. Valentine, and S. Sigurdson. 1977. Bacteriophage typing of *Corynebacterium diphtheriae*. J. Infect. Dis. **136**:655–660.
27. Young, V. M., *et al.* 1981. The emergence of coryneform bacteria as a cause of nosocomial infections in compromised hosts. Amer. J. Med. **70**:646–650.

31

Mycobacterium

The genus *Mycobacterium* includes a number of species, some pathogenic for man or animals, some opportunistically pathogenic, and others essentially saprophytic. Mycobacteria are characterized by (1) large amounts of lipid in the cell soma, thus exhibiting acid-fast staining (Chapter 2); (2) relatively slow, or very slow, growth rates; and (3) cellular morphology that sometimes includes branching and production of long filamentous forms. The occurrence of filaments and true branching indicate the relationship of mycobacteria to the higher fungi. While mycobacteria are not usually stained by Gram's method, the morphological fine structure of the cell wall is commensurate with that of gram-positive bacteria.

Among the pathogenic mycobacteria, those that cause tuberculosis in man are best known.

Two quite similar species are responsible for the disease—*Mycobacterium tuberculosis* (the human tubercle bacillus) and *Mycobacterium bovis* (the bovine tubercle bacillus). Other species of mycobacteria engender a tuberculosis-like disease of man, but because they differ from the classical tubercle bacilli, they are referred to as "atypical" or "anonymous" mycobacteria. While this terminology is unfortunate from the taxonomic viewpoint, it is generally accepted. The human leprosy bacillus, *Mycobacterium leprae,* and the rat leprosy bacillus, *Mycobacterium lepraemurium,* make up the third pathogenic group. *Mycobacterium leprae* differs from other members of this genus in that it is noncultivable, *i.e.,* it does not grow on laboratory mediums, because of special, and presently unknown, growth requirements.

The Tubercle Bacilli[1, 34]

Tuberculosis is an ancient disease of man and is still one of the most widespread. Its infectious nature was suspected by Fracastorius in the early part of the sixteenth century, and

in 1865 Villemin showed that the disease could be transmitted by the inoculation of tuberculous material. It was in 1882 that Koch demonstrated the tubercle bacillus by special staining methods, isolated and grew it in pure culture, and reproduced the disease by inoculation with the bacilli.

Morphology and Staining

The tubercle bacilli are slender, sometimes slightly curved, rods 0.2 to 0.6 μm. in diameter and 1 to 4 μm. in length. They occur singly but are often found in small groups, sometimes in compact masses in which the individual bacilli cannot be distinguished. The bacilli of the human variety tend to be somewhat longer and more slender than those of the bovine type, but the morphology of both is variable, and no distinction can be made on this basis. Branched forms are rarely seen in mammalian varieties. The bacillary form is generally retained in the tissues; in culture longer filamentous forms are sometimes seen together with swollen or club-shaped cells resembling the diphtheria bacillus. The tubercle bacillus is nonmotile and nonspore-forming.

The granular structure of individual cells is marked. Cytoplasmic granules often occur in abundance and may even give the stained cell the appearance of a chain of cocci. These include metachromatic granules, composed of polyphosphate, and lipid granules that stain with lipophilic dyes.

The tubercle bacilli are not stained by those methods that are effective with other bacteria, for there is marked resistance to the penetration of dyes into the cell because of the presence of relatively large amounts of cellular lipids.

The cells may be stained in two or three minutes by steaming carbol-fuchsin or by 18 hours' exposure to the dye at room temperature. Once stained, the bacilli are difficult to decolorize and resist the action of alcohol and dilute solutions of mineral acids and for that reason are termed "**acid-fast**." Retention of the fuchsin is considered to be, in part, a matter of permeability (Chapter 2). The bacilli may be demonstrated by Ziehl-Neelsen staining, in which the smear is stained with hot carbol-fuchsin, decolorized with acid alcohol, and counterstained with a dye of contrasting color, such as methylene blue (Figs. 31–1 and 31–2). The bacilli may also be stained with carbol-auramine, a dye that fluoresces a brilliant yellow in weak ultraviolet light. Non-acid-fast bacilli are sometimes seen in young cultures.

In broth cultures without wetting agents there is a thick, wrinkled skin of surface growth, tending to spread up the sides of the flask; masses of bacilli may become detached

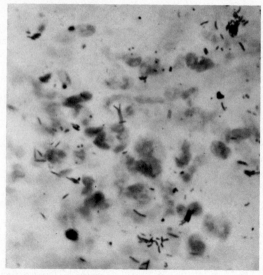

Figure 31–1. *Mycobacterium tuberculosis.* Acid-fast stained smear of tuberculous sputum. × 1050.

and sink to the bottom as a lumpy sediment. Growth on the surface of solid mediums is generally dry and granular, with nodular, heaped-up areas, as shown in Figure 31–3. On the usual mediums, *M. tuberculosis* usually produces a buff- or cream-colored growth, but *M. bovis* is not pigmented.

Physiology[32, 42]

The tubercle bacilli are obligately aerobic, although *M. bovis* may be microaerophilic on primary isolation. Tubercle bacilli grow best at 37°C. and not at all below 30°C. or above 42°C. Growth is relatively slow, and four to

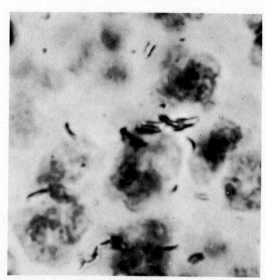

Figure 31–2. Tubercle bacillus. Acid-fast stained smear of pus from a liver abscess in a rhesus monkey. × 2600.

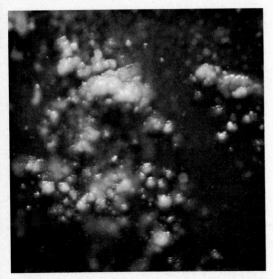

Figure 31–3. Colonies of the human variety of the tubercle bacillus. H-37 strain, on Löwenstein's medium, at five weeks' incubation, × 5.

six weeks are generally required for abundant growth, although minute colonies may appear in eight to 10 days.

Enriched mediums are required for primary isolation. The more complex mediums usually contain eggs, potato flour, and glycerol; malachite green is added to inhibit the growth of contaminants. Perhaps the best known and most widely used are the Löwenstein-Jensen and Petragnani mediums. Many workers prefer some variant of the Middlebrook medium; these usually contain salts, vitamins, cofactors, oleic acid, catalase, albumin, glycerol, and sometimes glucose and casein hydrolysate.

The human variety of the tubercle bacillus grows more abundantly than the bovine variety on these mediums, and for that reason it is termed "**eugonic**" and the bovine type "**dysgonic**." These two varieties also differ in that glycerol markedly favors the growth of *M. tuberculosis* but does not so affect *M. bovis*. Egg yolk reportedly contains a lipid growth factor, but it appears to stimulate rather than be essential to growth.

Following primary isolation, mycobacteria are less fastidious in subculture and grow much more readily and upon simpler mediums. The human tubercle bacillus grows well on ordinary nutrient agar or broth containing glycerol (2 to 5 per cent) and has been cultivated in a variety of synthetic solutions. Growth is facilitated and occurs diffusely throughout liquid mediums in the presence of certain water-soluble lipids, such as Tween 80 (a polyoxyethylene derivative of sorbitan monooleate),

which act as dispersing agents. Dispersal and rapid growth may also be attained by vigorous shaking during incubation. The bovine type grows poorly on Tween-containing mediums and is benefited only slightly by the presence of glycerol.

Table 31–1 lists the properties of *M. tuberculosis* and *M. bovis* that serve to differentiate them from one another and from other medically important mycobacteria. There may be some strain variation in these properties, however. For instance, strains of *M. tuberculosis* that are isoniazid resistant may be catalase-negative and avirulent for guinea pigs.

Mycobactin.[26] Iron is an essential trace element for the growth of mycobacteria, as it is for many bacteria. The mycobacterial mechanism for iron transport, however, appears to be unique. These microorganisms produce a lipid-soluble iron chelator, mycobactin, that is present in the cell envelope and has high affinity for iron; it serves as a mediator of iron transport and internalization. Mycobactin has been suggested as a virulence determinant, in that it permits mycobacteria to compete more effectively for available iron in host tissues (Chapter 12).

Growth in Cell Culture.[9, 22] The growth of tubercle bacilli in cultures of animal cells has been of interest since the early studies of Maximov on the pathogenesis of such infections. Established cell lines, macrophages, and human tissue explants, such as spleen and liver, have been employed. In many instances, *in vitro* infection models have been used for differentiation of strains with respect to virulence. When mycobacteria are inoculated into tissue cultures, they are internalized and lie in cytoplasmic vacuoles within the host cells. It has been consistently observed that within

Table 31–1. **Properties of Tubercle Bacilli**

Mycobacterium tuberculosis	Mycobacterium bovis
Acid-fast bacilli	Acid-fast bacilli
Slow growth rate	Slow growth rate
Rough colonial form	Thin, rough colonial form
Buff or cream pigmentation	Not pigmented
Eugonic	Dysgonic
Stimulated by glycerol	Not stimulated by glycerol
Catalase weakly positive (heat-sensitive)	Catalase weakly positive (heat-sensitive)
No growth at 24° or 45° C.	No growth at 24° or 45° C.
Niacin produced	Niacin not produced
Nitrate reduced	Nitrate not reduced
Urease produced	Urease produced
Virulent for guinea pigs	Virulent for guinea pigs

these vacuoles virulent strains grow more rapidly than avirulent; appreciable growth obtains in three to five days with concurrent destruction of the host cells. In infected macrophages, it has been reported that living, virulent *M. tuberculosis* inhibits the fusion of lysosomes with the bacillus-containing phagosomes, whereas inhibition of fusion by attenuated strains is not so pronounced.[23] Thus, the virulent strain would be expected to show greater viability and intracellular growth, since exposure to the bactericidal lysosomal enzymes is reduced. The factor responsible for fusion inhibition may be cyclic AMP produced by the phagocytized bacteria.

Chemical Composition[21]

The chemical composition of mycobacteria has been more intensively investigated than most bacteria. Mycobacteria are of particular interest because of their **high lipid content**— up to 40 per cent of the dry weight of the cell—and the unique nature of the lipid components. Cellular proteins, which include tuberculins, constitute another major class of mycobacterial components; polysaccharides, aside from those in the glycolipids, are found in relatively small amounts.

Because of their relationship to cellular physiology and virulence, the lipids of mycobacteria are of particular interest. Many of the lipids are associated with the cell wall structure and are responsible, in part, for such mycobacterial characteristics as acid-fast staining, hydrophobicity, and slow growth rates. Only a few of the more important mycobacterial lipid classes will be mentioned here:

1. The phospholipids of mycobacteria include cardiolipin, phosphatidylethanolamine, phosphatidylinositol, and mannophosphatidyl inosides. The fatty acid substituents of these phospholipids are varied; among those found are the well-known palmitic, linoleic, and linolenic acids. Also found are phthioic and tuberculostearic acids, fatty acids that are unique to mycobacteria.

2. The mycolic acids, a family of α-alkyl, β-hydroxyl fatty acids are found as constituents in a number of other lipids and as a part of the mycobacterial cell wall, often esterified with arabinose. Mycolic acids constitute a major part of the cell wall lipids. Their nature and location account for the acid-fast staining reactions of mycobacteria.

3. The glycolipids are varied in nature, and include the mycolic acid-containing cord factor (6,6' dimycoloyl-α-D-trehalose) and related sulfolipids, acylglucoses, and several mycosides of complex structure. One of the latter, mycoside C, is reported to act as a receptor for specific mycobacteriophages. Other glycolipids found in mycobacteria are toxic

for experimental animals and induce granuloma formation.[36]

4. The complex peptidoglycolipid, wax D, contains arabinose, galactose, glucosamine, muramic acid, mycolic acid, and amino acids; it may be extracted from mycobacterial cells with chloroform. Wax D exhibits a variety of biological activities, the best known being its behavior as an adjuvant in the immune response, and induction of interferon.

Lipid-containing extracts of mycobacteria appear to be physiologically active. Unsaponifiable wax fractions apparently stimulate multiplication of undifferentiated connective tissue cells; phthioic acid induces a proliferation of epithelioid cells.

Polysaccharide mixtures, containing immunologically active and inactive substances, have been isolated from mammalian tubercle bacilli, but their significance is not as yet understood. The protein constituents of the cell appear to be the most important immunologically and have been studied in connection with the preparation and activity of the various tuberculins.

Cord Factor. The tendency of tubercle bacilli to grow in filaments, or cords, in liquid culture has been thought to be associated with the virulence of human and bovine varieties of the microorganism. On treatment with petroleum ether, the filaments break up, and a lipid substance is extracted which is acid-fast and toxic to leucocytes and to mice. The chemical nature of this substance, termed cord factor, has been established, as noted above. While its association with virulence is not altogether clear, since it is also found in saprophytic mycobacteria and in attenuated strains, it does exhibit a variety of interesting biological activities that may be relevent to pathogenesis and immunity. These include: (1) stimulation of macrophages to increased phagocytosis and lysosomal enzyme activity;[51] (2) lethal toxicity for mice, associated with the destruction of mitochondrial membranes; (3) adjuvancy;[43] (4) activation of the alternative complement pathway;[33] and (5) induction of granuloma formation.

Resistance

Although having much the same degree of resistance to heat as the vegetative cells of other bacteria, the tubercle bacilli are relatively highly resistant to drying, chemical disinfectants, and other environmental factors, very likely as a consequence of their lipid content. The bacilli may remain viable in sputum for weeks or months; if it is completely dried so that particles are capable of floating as dust in the air, bacilli may be infective for 8 to 10 days. Under these conditions they may survive 100°C. for an hour but are killed in the usual way by moist heat. Phenol penetrates the bacilli only slowly, and a 5 per cent solution requires 24 hours to kill the bacilli in sputum. The action of other disinfectants is similarly retarded, and hypochlorites and certain synthetic detergents have almost no effect on these bacteria.

A number of different kinds of substances are active against the tubercle bacilli, including streptomycin, p-aminosalicylic acid (PAS), sulfones, thiosemicarbazones, and certain pyrimidine derivatives such as isoniazid. These substances are extremely useful for chemotherapeutic purposes.

Antigenic Structure[6]

With the increasing prominence of the atypical mycobacteria as causative agents of human disease, immunological differentiation of the tubercle bacilli has assumed greater significance. Unfortunately, the methods used for serological differentiation of other bacteria, e.g., agglutination, have not been successful with the tubercle bacilli.

The sharing of antigenic components, not only among the mycobacteria, but with corynebacteria and nocardia as well, is evident from immunochemical studies on culture filtrates and extracts of mycobacterial cells. It is well known, for example, that immunological cross-reactions, demonstrable as tuberculin hypersensitivity, are common among mycobacteria. Immunoelectrophoretic analyses of cell fractions reveal that mycobacteria contain multiple antigens whose characterization is complicated by the physical and chemical methods used for fractionation. The cell wall of mycobacteria contains antigenic proteins, peptides, and polysaccharides. The polysaccharides include arabinolactan and arabinomannan; the latter appears to be a surface antigen that promises to be useful in the serological differentiation of species. Unfortunately none of the available immunochemical methods are yet suitable for routine use, but these studies are expected to provide a detailed antigenic mosaic of the pathogenic mycobacteria that will clarify the taxonomic position of the individual species.

Variation

The tubercle bacilli exhibit considerable variation, some resulting from environmental and cultural conditions, while others represent more permanent changes. The latter include mutations that result in loss of virulence or resistance to drugs.

Colonial variation is usually associated with environmental changes, since prompt alteration of colonial appearance results on transfer to a new medium. For example, colonies growing in the presence of ether extract of egg yolk are smooth and markedly different from the usual colonial type, but the effect is only temporary.

Variation of the L type also occurs, and L forms have been noted in infected individuals. These usually assume the bacillary form on conventional culture mediums. L forms are probably not infective, per se, but become so after reversion in vivo.[35]

Attenuation of Virulence. A strain of M. bovis was attenuated in virulence by Calmette, who subcultured it repeatedly over a period of 13 years. This strain is designated as **BCG (bacille Calmette-Guérin)** and has been of particular interest in connection with active immunization against tuberculosis, since it establishes infection in the human or animal host, but does not give rise to clinically apparent disease. The attenuation of virulence appears to be a permanent change, but the nature of the change is completely unknown. There are undoubtedly multiple changes in the microorganism, since marked differences are apparent in the infectivity of BCG cultures carried in different laboratories. Although BCG fails to induce disease in normal hosts, it can do so in those that are immunodeficient.

Drug Resistance.[28] Like other bacteria, the tubercle bacilli may become resistant to some chemotherapeutic drugs in vitro and in vivo. The latter is more common with these bacteria than with others, because of the nature of the disease and the prolonged treatment required. Furthermore, resistance to certain of the effective drugs, streptomycin and isoniazid in particular, is especially prone to occur. Isoniazid resistance in pathogenic mycobacteria is accompanied by a loss of catalase activity, while some catalase activity persists in resistant saprophytic mycobacteria. There is evidence that the latter contain two catalase systems, one of which is not isoniazid sensitive.

The practical importance of drug resistance depends upon the drug and its toxicity. For example, a blood level of 10 to 15 μg. per ml. of streptomycin may be attained, and sensitive strains are inhibited in vitro by 0.5 μg. per ml.; slightly resistant strains by 2 to 4 μg. per ml.; moderately resistant strains by 200 to 400 μg. per ml.; and more than 50,000 μg. per ml. is required to inhibit the growth of highly resistant strains. Blood levels of isoniazid of 3 μg. per ml. may be attained, and sensitive strains are inhibited by 0.025 μg. per ml. in vitro. Thus, a proportionately higher resistance must occur in the case of isoniazid than of streptomycin to allow growth in achievable therapeutic concentrations. The assay of drug sensitivity is complicated by the slow growth of the bacilli, and more rapid methods have been devised that are based on the use of suspensions of bacilli and indicators of oxidative metabolism, such as reazurin or tetrazolium.

The facility with which resistance to a single chemotherapeutic agent develops is such that for practical purposes it is necessary to reduce the development of drug resistance by the use of combinations of drugs. If a resistant strain arises as a consequence of the selection of a chance mutant by the drug-containing environment, and if resistance to one drug is independent of that to another, the probability of occurrence of a double mutant is the product of the two mutation rates and becomes extremely small. The development of drug resistance *in vivo* is in fact markedly inhibited by the use of two drugs in combination. Resistant strains do not exhibit other significant differences from the sensitive parent strain except in the case of those resistant to isoniazid, which are appreciably less virulent though still capable of producing fatal disease in man.

TUBERCULOSIS[16, 19, 31, 40]

One hundred years after Robert Koch's discovery of the tubercle bacillus, tuberculosis is still the most important specific communicable disease in the world. It is estimated that 10 million new cases of tuberculosis appear each year in the developing countries and at least 3 million persons die of the disease. In the technically advanced countries the incidence is much less than this. In the United States, more than 53,000 cases and over 11,000 deaths were reported in 1961; these figures had been reduced to 27,000 and 1,770 in 1980. Even so, it remains as the leading cause of death among the specific communicable diseases.

Both *M. tuberculosis* and *M. bovis* cause tuberculosis in humans. The human variety is practically always responsible for pulmonary tuberculosis in adults and is usually found in children also. The bovine variety may occur occasionally in the pulmonary form in children but is more often found in infections of other tissues. Mixed infections are rare. In the United States, most cases of tuberculosis are due to *M. tuberculosis*; infections due to *M. bovis* have largely disappeared with the institution of control measures directed against infections in cattle.

Routes of Infection

The tubercle bacillus may enter the body by way of the respiratory tract, the alimentary tract, the genitourinary tract, the conjunctiva, or the skin.

The respiratory tract is the most frequent and most important route of infection, and the facility with which this occurs is demonstrable under both controlled and natural conditions. The coarser infectious particles in inspired air are filtered and deposited on the nasal, buccal, and pharyngeal mucosal surfaces. In most instances, however, infectious particles in aerosols and dust are sufficiently small that they enter the alveoli and adhere to these mucous surfaces. Following deposition, tissues are penetrated to establish a primary focus of infection. From this primary focus, the bacilli may be disseminated, first to regional lymph nodes and later to other tissues. These events are diagrammatically represented in Figure 31–4.

Primary infection by the alimentary tract is a consequence of the ingestion of the bacilli in infected food, most commonly milk. This type of transmission is rare in technologically advanced countries, but still occurs in some developing countries where *M. bovis* infection of cattle is endemic. Secondary infection of this type is sometimes seen, particularly in children, by swallowing tuberculous material of respiratory origin. Following penetration of the mucous membranes of the alimentary tract, the bacilli are found in the regional lymph nodes.

Primary infection of the genitourinary tract is possible, but under natural conditions rarely occurs. Infection through the conjunctiva takes place readily under experimental conditions; its frequency under natural conditions is not known, for the cervical lymph nodes, where the infection would first appear, are readily infected by other channels. Infection through the skin is through abrasions or other traumatic injury and is rare, but has resulted in verruca tuberculosa (pathologist's wart) or lupus vulgaris.

Dissemination of Infection[12, 14]

Tubercle bacilli are disseminated through the body from primary or secondary foci by way of the lymphatics or blood stream. The blood stream may also be invaded directly through erosion of a vessel wall by a focus of infection. The bacilli are transported throughout the body by the blood and give rise to **acute miliary tuberculosis** or other extrapulmonary manifestations. Practically every organ

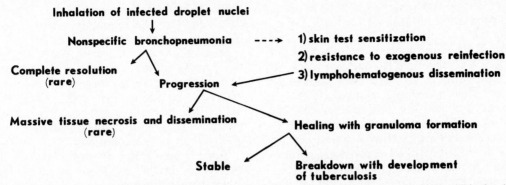

Figure 31–4. Events in aerosol infection with tubercle bacilli. Infection begins with the deposition of bacilli in the alveolus and development of an asymptomatic area of bronchopneumonia. From this primary focus, bacilli reach the regional lymph nodes. Subsequent lymphatic drainage delivers bacilli to the circulation and other organs. Progression of the pulmonary infection can result in clinically apparent infection. In most instances, healing occurs, with granuloma formation. If the granuloma later breaks down, the bacilli multiply and clinical tuberculosis results. (A. G. Robbins, and D. E. Snider, Jr., New Engl. J. Med. **302**:1441, 1980.) (Reprinted by permission of the New England Journal of Medicine.)

and tissue of the body may be invaded by tubercle bacilli.

Tuberculosis in humans is most commonly the pulmonary form—more than 85 per cent of the cases in the United States are of this type—but there is considerable variation by age, sex, race, and geographical location. In developed countries, there has been a general decline in the incidence of pulmonary tuberculosis, but extrapulmonary disease has not followed this pattern. Extrapulmonary disease is manifest as tuberculosis of the abdomen, bones and joints, genitourinary system, meninges and central nervous system, lymphadenitis, and other disseminated infection. Most cases of tuberculosis occur in adults, and in recent years it has become a disease of the elderly. Almost one-third of the cases, both pulmonary and extrapulmonary, occur in those over 65 years of age. Some types of extrapulmonary disease occur with high frequency in the young, however. In one study, over one-fourth of meningeal and central nervous system tuberculosis occurred in children under 5 years of age.

The Tubercle

Following the initial "seeding" of the tubercle bacilli, there follows a cellular immune response to the microorganism, as discussed in a later section (Immunity). One of the consequences of this response is the formation of granulomas, called tubercles, that serve to contain the proliferating microorganisms. Small tubercles, plainly visible to the naked eye, are so uniformly observed in advanced infections that their presence has given the name to the disease.

The young tubercle probably originates from fixed cells surrounding the invading bacilli. Elongated epithelioid cells develop in concentric layers and come to form the substance of the tubercle. Giant cells with multiple nuclei soon appear in the developing tubercle. During this process, polymorphonuclear leucocytes and later lymphocytes, cluster around the periphery of the tubercle. Degeneration of the tubercle eventually sets in and the central portion becomes necrotic; this is followed by caseation and then softening of the caseous mass.

In some cases calcium is deposited in the tubercle, converting it to a hard, dry, friable body that may become encapsulated and completely walled off from surrounding tissues. In other instances, however, this healing process is not complete, and there is instead an extension with coalescence and the formation of large confluent masses. If erosion of a blood vessel occurs, large numbers of bacilli can be discharged into the blood. Multiple secondary foci can result, with formation of small tubercles of the size of millet seeds, giving rise to acute miliary tuberculosis.

Predisposing Factors

Infection with tubercle bacillus is exceedingly common in endemic areas. At one time, there were few adults, particularly those living in cities, who escaped infection. Tuberculosis is a disease associated with confinement and crowding, situations in which opportunities for transmission are much greater. Apparently the human host has little resistance to infection, yet the developing immune response is remarkably effective in containing the infection, so that clinical tuberculosis develops in only a small proportion of those infected (Fig. 31–4).

The tendency to develop clinically apparent disease is therefore associated with factors that interfere with the effective immune response. These predisposing factors include such things as nutritional inadequacy, particularly protein deficiency; intercurrent infections; climate and exposure; alcoholism; and chronic fatigue.

In individuals exposed to dust and particulates, there is a marked occupational predisposition to the pulmonary disease. The constant inhalation of almost any kind of dust results in increased incidence; silica dusts appear almost specifically to predispose to tuberculosis.

It has long been suspected that there are familial or hereditary tendencies to tuberculosis in man. Resistance to infection in experimental animals is to some degree genetically determined, but the conclusive demonstration of a similar phenomenon in man is difficult owing to both a long generation time and the inability to carry out appropriate genetic experiments. The incidence of new infection in tuberculous families is considerably greater than in the general population, but whether this is a consequence of increased risk alone or, in part, of genetically determined factors is not clear. There is some indication that increased susceptibility and severity of tuberculosis of blacks is associated with certain HLA phenotypes. In any case the disease itself is not inherited, and congenital tuberculosis occurs only rarely.

The relation of earlier infection to clinical tuberculosis in the adult has been a matter of considerable interest, and it has been suggested that pulmonary tuberculosis of the young adult may, in many instances, be a consequence of the reactivation of an earlier, quiescent infection. Tuberculosis in the adult may also be a consequence of reinfection rather than of a flaring up of the healed or partially healed lesions from earlier infection. A considerable period, possibly years in some instances, may elapse between reinfection and the appearance of tuberculosis in clinical form.

Epidemiology

In humans, tuberculosis is largely an **airborne infection** and its transmission is facilitated by close contact. Infection is not synonymous with disease, however; in most instances clinical tuberculosis does not occur—the primary lesion heals and the infection is not transmitted. The evidence of infection in these individuals is provided by a positive tuberculin test (see Immunity, page 616) in an otherwise well individual.

In a 1972 study, 21.5 per cent of adults 25 to 74 years of age were tuberculin-positive.[13] The prevalence of positive reactions by age and sex are shown in Figure 31–5. These figures may be approximately compared to the reported cases of tuberculosis in all age groups of 15.79 per 10^5 population in 1972.

In the United States, there are marked racial differences in the incidence of tuberculosis. Cases in nonwhite males are remarkably higher than all other groups, particularly after early adulthood (see Fig. 12–3, page 337). Nonwhite death rates have also been higher than in the white population. Whether higher death and case rates are attributable to environmental conditions or to racial differences in susceptibility has not been determined.

Tuberculosis has been decreasing at a steady and relatively rapid rate since 1850 or thereabouts, as indicated by the decline in the death rate from this disease. As in the case of some other diseases, the decline set in before the discovery of the bacterial etiology of infectious disease and hence is not entirely attributable to the practice of preventive measures. Nevertheless, decline in death rates during the past several decades has been greatest in the Western countries.

There is no simple explanation for this observed decline in both morbidity and mortality.

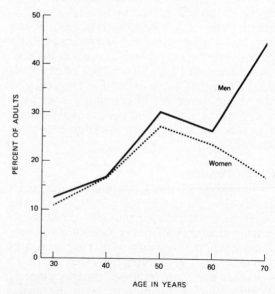

Figure 31–5. Prevalence of tuberculin-positive skin tests among adults, by age and sex: United States, 1971–72. (A. Engel, and J. Roberts, Vital Health Statistics, Series 11, No. 204, 1977.)

Among the factors of undoubted importance are (1) the identification and chemotherapy of active cases to reduce the source of infection; (2) improvement of living conditions, both environmental and nutritional; and (3) immunization of the population. Such a decline is usually taken as a manifestation of the inability of a disease to maintain itself and leads to predictions of its eventual disappearance. Indeed, in relatively closed populations, where appropriate control measures are initiated, both morbidity and mortality can be markedly reduced. Nevertheless, eradication is an elusive goal, at least partly because of the great number of inactive and unrecognized infections that may persist for a lifetime. Although the risk of reactivation diminishes with time, the possibility for development of active tuberculosis continues.

Bacteriological Diagnosis[42]

Tubercle bacilli are usually discharged from the infected individual in sputum and urine and may be demonstrated in these materials as well as in gastric washings, spinal fluid, or infected tissues, depending on the location of the infection. Of specimens from these sources, those obtained by gastric lavage are of particular value in respiratory tuberculosis in children, who tend to swallow sputum. Results must be interpreted with caution because of the presence of saprophytic acid-fast bacilli in the gastrointestinal tract derived from the ingestion of foods, especially fruit, on which these forms occur. The presence of the bacilli may be shown, either directly or after concentration, by examination of stained smears, culture, and guinea pig inoculation.

As a rule, some method of concentration is desirable, for not less than 100,000 bacilli per ml. must be present before there is a reasonable chance of finding them by microscopic examination. The relatively greater resistance of the tubercle bacillus allows treatment of the specimen with a variety of digestive agents, e.g., acetyl–cysteine–alkali, sodium hydroxide, or benzalkonium chloride–trisodium phosphate, to destroy contaminants and digest the viscous sputum to facilitate concentration by centrifugation. The sediment is used to prepare smears for direct examination and to inoculate culture mediums and guinea pigs.

Smears are usually stained by the Ziehl-Neelsen method or by analogous fluorochrome staining. The demonstration of acid-fast bacilli allows a provisional diagnosis but does not indicate whether they are virulent tubercle bacilli. Their presence in urine specimens in particular must be interpreted with caution because of the frequent occurrence of the smegma bacillus, Mycobacterium smegmatis, which is also acid-fast.

A variety of mediums, generally containing glycerol and egg, may be used for culture, the particular medium varying from one laboratory to another. Characteristic colonies of tubercle bacilli appear after about three weeks' incubation. Extended incubation, to as long as five months, may give a few additional positive cultures. Culture is not identification, of course, and acid-fast bacilli that grow like the tubercle bacilli are occasionally found in nontuberculous lesions. Identification is by the properties listed in Table 31–1.

Guinea pigs are inoculated in the groin or in the muscle of the thigh. If a reasonable number of tubercle bacilli have been inoculated, enlargement of the regional lymphatics may be noted in two or three weeks, the pig becomes emaciated by four to six weeks and usually dies not long after that. With very small numbers of bacilli, evidence of the infection may be delayed two or three weeks longer. At autopsy the regional lymph nodes will be found to be enlarged and filled with caseous material. Necrotic areas in the spleen and liver are characteristic of the gross pathology in this animal; tubercles are seldom seen, and the lungs are only slightly affected and the kidneys almost never. Tubercle bacilli may be cultured from the lesions and found in acid-fast-stained smears. Some workers tuberculin-test the animals before inoculation and again three to four weeks afterward, the development of hypersensitivity indicating infection.

With respect to culture and animal inoculation with M. tuberculosis and M. bovis, a precautionary note is in order. Laboratory manipulation of cultures and experimental infections of small animals represent serious infection hazards and should be undertaken only if adequate safety can be assured and only by trained personnel.

Chemotherapy

Effective chemotherapy of tuberculosis requires that the chemotherapeutic agent be diffusible into the tuberculous process and have specific antibacterial activity. In addition, the necessity for administration over relatively long periods accentuates the problems of toxicity and the development of drug resistance by the microorganism. While the ideal chemotherapeutic agent for this disease has not been found, a number of drugs of reasonable efficacy are now available. These fall into two groups, *viz.*, the synthetic compounds and the antibiotics.

The Synthetic Antitubercular Drugs. There are several groups of these agents; those best known are the sulfones, the aminohydroxybenzoic acids, and the pyrimidine carboxylic acid derivatives. The observation that sulfanilamide affects the progress of experimental tuberculosis led to the preparation and trial of related compounds. Of these, the sulfones, 4,4'-diaminodiphenyl sulfone and its derivatives, were found to be partially effective chemotherapeutic agents. All are toxic, the most common effect being on the erythrocytes. These drugs are now rarely used.

The observation that benzoates and salicylates stimulate the respiration of the tubercle bacillus *in vitro* provided the basis for the discovery of the chemotherapeutic activity of *p*-aminosalicylic acid. This substance is of low toxicity and is readily absorbed from the gastrointestinal tract. It has appreciable chemotherapeutic activity when given alone, but its greatest utility is in combination with other drugs.

A number of pyrimidine derivatives, isonicotinic acid hydrazide (isoniazid) and related compounds such as the isopropyl derivatives, are available under a number of proprietary names; they are widely used and are effective chemotherapeutic agents, although isoniazid has some hepatotoxicity.

More recently introduced is ethambutol, a butanol derivative of minimal toxicity, which has been found effective, particularly in combination with other drugs.

Antibiotics. Streptomycin was the first of the antibiotics to be used for the therapy of tuberculosis; along with rifampin it continues to be widely employed. Most other antibiotics that are effective in the treatment of acute infectious diseases are not entirely satisfactory, although kanamycin or cycloserine are occasionally used.

To minimize the occurrence of drug-resistant variants, chemotherapeutic agents for treatment of tuberculosis are commonly used in combination. Moreover, if resistant varieties arise during therapy, or if retreatment is required, an entirely new set of agents is recommended. Of the drugs available for treatment in the United States, the primary drugs, isoniazid and rifampin, are effective and of low toxicity. Secondary drugs usually less effective and of greater toxicity include ethambutol, *p*-aminosalicylic acid, pyrazina-

mide, and streptomycin. Recommended and widely used combinations are isoniazid–rifampin, isoniazid–streptomycin, and isoniazid–ethambutol.

These and other combinations are highly effective and, in most instances, can be self-administered. Effectively treated patients are said not to represent a significant risk to contacts, so that hospitalization is not usually required and patients are often treated on an outpatient basis.

Antibacterial Activity in Vivo. The chemotherapeutic efficacy of antitubercular drugs is dependent upon the nature and stage of the infection. For example, in early infection, growth of the bacilli is largely intracellular and the bacilli are little affected by streptomycin and PAS, which do not readily penetrate macrophages. Isoniazid, pyrazinamide, and rifampin can enter macrophages to affect the phagocytized bacilli. In tuberculous lesions the bacilli grow most densely at the periphery of the caseous zone, and as the lesion expands they are engulfed in caseous material and lie dormant. Such dormant bacilli are not appreciably affected by some of the drugs, and the concentration of drug is lower in such lesions than in the blood. Thus, a focus of infection may persist in the individual undergoing chemotherapy and result in relapse, and possibly infection with drug-resistant bacilli, when therapy is discontinued.

Immunity[2, 34, 48]

The immune response to the presence of tubercle bacilli is indicated by the appearance of agglutinins, precipitins, opsonins, and complement-fixing antibodies in the serum. This response is not marked, however, for these antibodies are present only in low titers.

This humoral immune response is of little more than passing interest, since protection against infection is almost entirely due to cell-mediated immunity. The most readily observable consequence of the cell-mediated immune response is the development of a **delayed-type hypersensitivity** to certain components of the bacterial cell. This hypersensitivity is associated with protection against infection, as shown by Koch's early experiments. Koch demonstrated that subcutaneous inoculation of normal guinea pigs with tubercle bacilli does not elicit an immediately observable effect, but in 10 to 14 days a nodule develops at the inoculation site, which breaks down to a persistent tuberculous ulcer; the regional lymph nodes then become swollen and caseous. In animals previously infected with tubercle bacilli, however, inoculation in this manner is characterized by an indurated area developing within a day or two, followed by slight necrosis and formation of a rapidly healing shallow ulcer. This superinfection does not result in tubercle formation or invasion of the regional lymphatics, and the animal is therefore resistant to the second infecting dose of the tubercle bacilli. This has come to be known as the **Koch phenomenon.**

It is now accepted that the protective response, and the accompanying hypersensitivity, is of the cell-mediated type; neither protection nor hypersensitivity may be passively transferred by antibody, but normal animals may be rendered immune to infection and hypersensitive to cell components (tuberculin) by transfer of lymphoid elements from immune animals.

The cellular immunity acquired by infection or active immunization generally is not as complete as that observed in diseases in which protection is associated with a humoral response. Immunity to tuberculous infection develops relatively slowly and is not apparent until the primary infection is of some weeks' standing or unless very large numbers of bacilli are administered. Experimental studies in guinea pigs have shown that the infective dose for immunized animals is about 1000-fold greater than that for normal animals. Hypersensitivity develops in animals after infection with virulent or attenuated bacilli, or after inoculation with large numbers of killed bacilli; but sensitization with bacillary components is difficult. For example, when given alone neither tuberculin nor wax D can induce hypersensitivity but when they are administered together they will do so; wax D presumably acts as an adjuvant. It is of some theoretical interest that hypersensitivity induced in this way is not accompanied by protection against infection.

Tuberculin. The sensitive animal will react, in skin tests, to injection of the soluble cell substance of the tubercle bacillus, preparations of which are called tuberculin. Tuberculin is usually prepared from the human variety, though that of the bovine variety is practically as active in infections caused by *M. tuberculosis.* A number of tuberculins have been prepared, but most are variations of the original preparation by Koch.

The first of these, usually designated old tuberculin (OT), consisted of a filtrate of a glycerol broth culture concentrated by evaporation on a water bath (the activity is heatstable). Although used for many years as a reagent for hypersensitivity testing, OT has

disadvantages of instability and variability. Modern tuberculin preparations are usually prepared from culture filtrates of bacilli grown in synthetic medium and purified by precipitation with trichloroacetic acid; these are designated **PPD (purified protein derivative)** or PPD–S to indicate the standard *M. tuberculosis* tuberculin.

At best, tuberculin is a heterogeneous mixture of proteins of low to moderate molecular weight. Analysis of tuberculin preparations by electrophoresis has revealed a great number of protein bands, some of which elicit skin reactions.[29] Tuberculins are active, not only in skin reactions, but also in the correlated *in vitro* reactions of cell-mediated immunity, including stimulation of lymphocyte mitogenesis.[5]

The Tuberculin Reaction. Three types of reaction may be elicited in the sensitized, *i.e.,* infected, animal by the injection of tuberculin. In addition to a local inflammatory reaction at the site of inoculation, there is a focal reaction manifest as an acute congestion around tuberculous foci that, if marked, may aggravate the pathological process, and a constitutional reaction in which the temperature rises to a peak of 102° to 104°F. and subsides in 12 to 18 hours. In man the constitutional reaction also includes malaise, pain in the limbs, and perhaps vomiting, dyspnea, and other symptoms. These reactions do not appear in normal animals. The primary utility of tuberculin is to detect delayed hypersensitivity to the tubercle bacillus, which is, in turn, an indicator of infection. Such reactions must be interpreted with caution, since infection with other mycobacteria may yield a positive tuberculin reaction (see below, Atypical Mycobacteria).

The diagnostic tuberculin test in man is generally a skin test. In the Mantoux test, the most commonly used, graded doses of tuberculin are injected intradermally, usually beginning with 5 tuberculin units (TU) and ranging upward to 100 TU or more. Tuberculin is biologically standardized in infected guinea pigs, and the 5 TU dose is equivalent to 0.1 μg. of the international standard for mammalian-type PPD (PPD–S). A patch test has been introduced by Volmer; small squares of filter paper are impregnated with tuberculin of increased strength, dried and taped to the cleansed skin of the sternum or upper margin of the trapezius. The patch test appears to be somewhat less sensitive than the intradermal test.

A **positive test** is indicated by an induration of 10 mm. or more following administration of 5 TU intradermally. Reactions of 5 to 9 mm.

are considered **doubtful**, while those less than 5 mm. are **negative.** Reactivity may be temporarily depressed under some conditions, especially in the incubation and early stages of measles, presumably due to suppression of the immune response. It was formerly believed that once established, hypersensitivity persisted essentially throughout life, and that the tuberculin reaction was of limited value in the adult. It is now apparent, however, that reversion to a negative reaction usually follows elimination of the infection, as by chemotherapy. Reversion is now more commonly seen, reflecting a reduction in prevalence of the disease and, therefore, in the risk of reinfection.

The Mechanism of Immunity.[4] The protective immune reaction in tuberculosis, as well as several other chronic diseases marked by intracellular infection, is quite different from that observed in acute infectious diseases. In the latter, protection is associated with the presence of humoral antibodies that act to neutralize toxins, to promote phagocytosis, or, with the aid of the complement system, to kill the invading microorganism. Although antibodies may be formed in tuberculosis, they are not protective. Rather, protection of the host is associated with a cellular response. Infection with these microorganisms confers a definite protection against superimposed tubercular infection; while the host is not capable of entirely eliminating the original infection, the effects of pathogenesis may be minimized. Two theories have been advanced to explain the mechanism of effective immunity in tuberculosis. These differ in the relative importance assigned to the specificity of effective immunity and in the role played by delayed hypersensitivity.

Immunity in tuberculosis is immunologically acquired, *i.e.,* the cell-mediated immune compartment is stimulated, with lymphocyte proliferation and the consequent activation of macrophages. **Activated macrophages** are characterized by their increased lysosomal enzyme content and perhaps other microbicidal properties that are believed to permit them to dispose of the intracellular tubercle bacilli in a more effective way. It is clear that lymphocyte stimulation is a specific immunological event, since it is rapidly and specifically recalled upon subsequent exposure to the homologous antigen, in this case the tubercle bacillus. Activated macrophages are, however, active in a nonspecific way, since they are more microbicidal, not only toward tubercle bacilli, but also toward a variety of other microorganisms.

Thus, resistance is specifically engendered, but is, to a degree, nonspecific in action. In the naturally infected host, resistance to reinfection develops simultaneously with delayed hypersensitivity to tuberculoproteins; this hypersensitivity is the most obvious response to infection. In the view of many investigators, the development of hypersensitivity is indicative of effective immunity. It is commonly observed, for example, that in those individuals giving a positive tuberculin reaction, living cells are usually free of tubercle bacilli and the bacteria are present in necrotic areas separated by an avascular barrier, while in infected individuals that show a negative reaction, tubercle bacilli are found in great numbers in living tissue.

Others take a somewhat different view of the immunology of tuberculosis, based on findings that resistance and delayed hypersensitivity are dissociable phenomena. Youmans[52] and his colleagues have shown that immunization with ribosomal fractions of mycobacterial cells induces a protective response, but without inducing tuberculin hypersensitivity. It has been reported that host protection is associated with the production, by specifically stimulated lymphocytes, of a lymphokine, termed mycobacterial growth inhibitory factor (MycoIF), which acts on macrophages to bring about specific inhibition of intracellular multiplication of tubercle bacilli. This lymphokine is different from the macrophage inhibition factor (MIF), a lymphokine that mediates tuberculin hypersensitivity. It would therefore appear that immunity following natural infection with tubercle bacilli may involve both specifically and nonspecifically stimulated macrophages, and that the former are possibly more effective in resistance.

Active Immunization.[10, 38, 39] The possibility of active immunization against tuberculosis has been of great interest since the discovery of the microorganism. In human immunization, the vaccines most widely used have been suspensions of either living attenuated tubercle bacilli or killed bacilli. The newer ribosomal vaccines are of great theoretical interest, but have not yet been tested in man.

The attenuated bovine strain of Calmette, BCG, has been regarded as the most promising immunizing agent and has been extensively studied. It was originally given as an oral vaccine in France in the early 1920s. However, the combination of inadequate statistical data and an incident in Germany (in which a virulent strain was inadvertently substituted for the vaccine strain, resulting in tuberculosis in inoculated persons) put it into disrepute. Nevertheless, immunization with BCG was further studied in the Scandinavian countries, beginning in 1925 in Sweden and in 1927 in Norway and Denmark.

There is a large body of evidence supporting the conclusion that such immunization gives an appreciable degree of protection against childhood tuberculosis, but whether it protects against infection later in life is not so clear. There is great likelihood, however, that even if infection with virulent tubercle bacilli is not prevented, immunization with BCG does inhibit the generalized spread of the infection. Although the early history of BCG vaccination was somewhat tarnished, the safety of BCG vaccination is essentially unquestioned. There is no evidence of reversion to virulence, and while progressive disease in immunocompromised recipients is possible and has been occasionally reported, the overall safety record has been exceptional.

Immunization has been very generally applied in Scandinavian countries (where its effect on the decline in tuberculosis is probably overestimated), less so in Europe, and in only a restricted way in the United States. While a general program of immunization may serve as a control measure in areas in which the disease is widespread and where the general application of chemotherapy and isolation is not practical, it appears to have only limited utility in this country, as in groups exposed to unusual risk of infection.

Useful and effective BCG vaccines must be prepared from strains of greatest protective potency and preserved so as to maintain highest viability. Freeze-dried vaccines, which maintain viability for long periods without refrigeration, have been developed. The vaccine is usually administered intracutaneously, and a positive tuberculin reaction appears in 6 to 10 weeks in over 90 per cent of those inoculated. The hypersensitivity lasts about four years, though in some persons there is reversion in as little as one year. On the assumption that a positive tuberculin reaction is indicative of immunity, reversion is taken to mean that reinoculation is required.

Pathogenicity for Lower Animals

Tuberculosis of lower animals living under natural conditions is probably very rare. Animals in captivity, however, may contract the infection with some facility; tuberculosis is found in animals kept in zoos and in monkeys kept in the laboratory for experimental purposes. Domestic animals may be similarly affected. Many different animals may be infected experimentally with one or another of the types of tubercle bacilli.

Domestic Animals. The most commonly infected domestic animals are cattle, pigs, and chickens. The disease in cattle has the greatest relevance to human tuberculosis, since cattle have served as reservoirs for *M. bovis* infections. Cattle are infected with the bovine type of tubercle bacillus almost exclusively; they are not completely resistant to the human type, as Koch originally thought, but infection is accomplished with some difficulty. The proportion of cattle infected increases with advancing age and, in the absence of control measures, may reach 70 to 90 and possibly 100 per cent in animals kept in stalls. The natural infection is generally of a chronic, slowly progressive nature. The lymphatics are most frequently involved and may be the only tissues to show lesions; the lungs are also commonly affected. Lesions on the pleura have a peculiar characteristic appearance, the so-called perlsucht disease. The liver, spleen, and kidneys are less frequently involved, infection of the mammary glands is not uncommon, and tubercle bacilli may be excreted in the milk in the absence of detectable lesions of the mammae. In the United States tuberculous infection in cattle is rigorously controlled, with extensive annual tuberculin testing.

Experimental Animals. Experimental animals vary in their susceptibility to the varieties of the tubercle bacillus and in the type of infection produced. The guinea pig is highly susceptible to both bovine and human bacilli, and death follows the subcutaneous injection of even small doses in 6 to 15 weeks. The lymphatic glands, spleen, and liver are most affected, the lungs only slightly, and the kidneys never. The necrotic areas in the spleen and liver are the most striking feature of the gross pathology and are peculiar to the guinea pig. True tubercles are seldom seen except in the very early stages of the disease.

Rabbits are highly susceptible to infection with the bovine bacillus, but quite resistant to the human variety. This difference has been used as a means of distinguishing *M. tuberculosis* from *M. bovis* but is now supplanted by cultural methods. Injection of bovine bacilli produces a generalized infection that terminates fatally in two to three months. On autopsy, tubercles may be found in the spleen and liver, but the lesions are most marked in the lungs and kidneys and may even be confined to them.

The Atypical Mycobacteria[3, 8, 42, 50]

Acid-fast bacilli other than the tubercle bacilli have been found in association with human disease from time to time, but have been isolated with greater frequency in recent years as more intensive bacteriological isolation procedures have been practiced. In the past, when such "nontubercle bacilli" were isolated from pulmonary disease they were usually disregarded, since they were thought to be "contaminating saprophytes." As their relationship to disease became increasingly recognized, there was a tendency to refer to them as atypical (with reference to the "typical" tubercle bacilli), "anonymous," or "unclassified" mycobacteria. While none of these is ideal from the purely taxonomic view, the term atypical mycobacteria has gained such wide currency that it will be used here.

The atypical mycobacteria are found in man in the absence of disease, admixed with tubercle bacilli in tuberculosis infections, and as the causative agent in several types of infection, including a tuberculosis-like pulmonary disease. The pulmonary illness closely simulates tuberculosis, but endobronchitis seems to be more common and there is somewhat more nonspecific inflammation and fibrosis. Similarly, the pathology of lymphatic infections resembles that of tuberculosis infection, including calcification in later stages, but the infected nodes tend more often to be necrotic and suppurative in character. Most studies have indicated that pulmonary and disseminated infections with the atypical mycobacteria tend to follow injury to the tissues, as in the case of miners and others in dusty occupations, or after the use of cortisone and immunosuppressive agents; these observations strongly suggest that impairment of defense mechanisms is antecedent to invasion.

A granulomatous type of cutaneous disease, called **swimming pool granuloma,** is well recognized and is usually attributable to *Mycobacterium marinum,* a free-living marine organism; the disease, often preceded by injury,[15] is acquired by exposure to salt or brackish waters, and occasionally from aquariums containing the microorganism. Rarely, other mycobacteria, such as *Mycobacterium scrofulaceum,* are responsible agents. Other skin infections, in the form of a necrotizing ulcer known as **Buruli ulcer,** are common in Africa and are usually caused by *Mycobacterium ulcerans.* Wound infections have also reportedly been caused by *Mycobacterium fortuitum* and *Mycobacterium chelonei,* although these species are more often found in pulmonary disease.

The atypical mycobacteria differ from tubercle bacilli in that they are not pathogenic for the guinea pig, are generally resistant to the usual antituberculosis chemotherapeutic agents, grow more rapidly, and are often pigmented. Runyon has divided the atypical mycobacteria into four groups, based largely on pigment production and growth rate. Their classification and disease potential are shown in Table 31–2. They are immunologically related to the tubercle bacilli and infections are accompanied by delayed hypersensitivity to tuberculin. Many attempts have been made to distinguish such infections from tuberculosis by skin testing. A number of individuals infected with atypical mycobacteria give small reactions to standard tuberculin, and a larger number react to second-strength PPD–S. In efforts to improve specificity, sensitins have been prepared from many strains of the Runyon groups—PPD–B from a strain of *M. intracellulare* (Battey bacillus), PPD–Y from a strain of *M. kansasii,* PPD–A from *M. avium,* PPD–G from the Gause strain of Runyon Group II, and a variety of other strains. Such studies have not been as informative as anticipated, although they may have some application in childhood infections.

In contrast to the tubercle bacilli, many of the atypical mycobacteria can be serotyped by the agglutination reaction. The greatest number of serological varieties are distinguished in

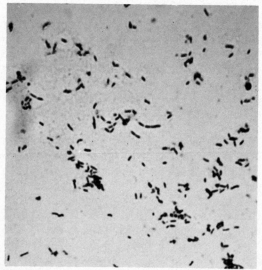

Figure 31–6. Atypical mycobacterium, *Mycobacterium avium.* Acid-fast stain of a smear from a pure culture. × 1050.

Table 31–2. **The Atypical Mycobacteria**

Runyon Classification		Mycobacterium Species	Predominant Disease in Man
Group	*Description*		
I	Photochromogens. Produce bright yellow pigment in presence of light. Rough colonies produced after 14 to 21 days.	M. kansasii	Pulmonary disease resembling tuberculosis, but usually milder.
		M. marinum (balnei)	Swimming pool granuloma; lesions usually on skin of extremities.
		M. simiae	Pulmonary disease, very rare in man.
II	Scotochromogens. Produce reddish-orange pigment, independent of light. Smooth colonies produced after 10 to 14 days.	M. scrofulaceum	Lymphadenitis in children.
		M. szulgai	Pulmonary disease.
III	Nonphotochromogens. Usually non-pigmented; if produced, pigment is weak and light-independent. Require 14 to 21 days for growth.	M. avium M. intracellulare }	Chronic pulmonary disease.
		M. xenopi	Pulmonary disease.
IV	Rapidly growing. Some pigmented. Colonies produced in 5 to 7 days.	M. fortuitum M. chelonei }	Skin abscesses; pulmonary disease.
		M. ulcerans	Buruli ulcer of skin.

M. intracellulare (25 serovars), while 3 serovars of *M. avium* and 3 of *M. scrofulaceum* are recognized. In many cases serology does not parallel cultural properties, so that some strains, morphologically and biochemically identifiable as *M. avium* or *M. intracellulare,* are serotyped as *M. scrofulaceum* and *vice versa.* Thus, it is a popular convention to designate complexes, *e.g.,* the *M. avium–M. intracellulare–M. scrofulaceum* (MAIS) complex. Serological typing is ·not necessary for management of disease, but has found utility in epidemiology of disease caused by atypical mycobacteria.

There is considerable variation in the geographical distribution of these bacilli. In the United States, atypical mycobacteria represent about one-third of the isolates from human infections with mycobacteria. The MAIS complex is most often isolated, representing just over 20 per cent of total isolates.[20]

The prevalence of atypical mycobacterial infections is not known with certainty. The available evidence from skin sensitivity testing indicates that the infection rate is considerably higher than that of tuberculosis,[49] but the clinical disease is much rarer, perhaps 1 to 5 per cent of the number of tuberculosis cases.

Mycobacterium leprae[37, 47]

Like tuberculosis, leprosy is an ancient disease of man. The first accurate description of the disease in India was in the Sushruta Samhita about 600 B.C.; it was known in Egypt in the time of the Pharaohs, and in China in the fifth century B.C. Perhaps more prevalent in antiquity, it is now most common in Central Africa, India, Japan and other Asiatic countries, and the South Pacific. The disease is prevalent in South America, with endemic centers in Brazil, Colombia, and Argentina. In the world there are more than 3.5 million registered patients, and probably more than 12 million total cases.

Leprosy has been introduced into the United States with varying consequences. In Hawaii, Louisiana, Florida, and Texas the imported cases have established foci in which the disease has a tendency to perpetuate itself, while in California and the central northwestern states it tends to die out. Elsewhere in the United States transmission is so rare as to be negligible. Many of the cases in this country are segregated in the United States Public Health Service Hospital in Carville, Louisiana, while others live, for the most part, in Hawaii, Texas, California, and New York. Although relatively rare in the United States, there has been a marked increase in the number of reported cases of leprosy since 1957 (Fig. 31–7).

Leprosy bacilli were first found by Hansen

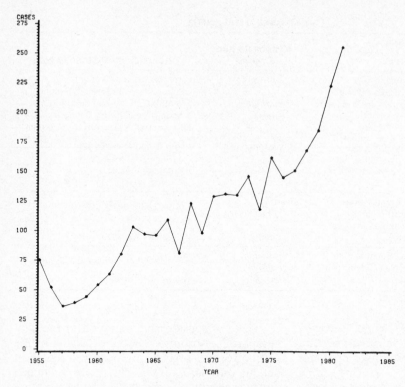

Figure 31–7. Reported cases of leprosy in the United States, 1955–181. (Centers for Disease Control, Annual summary 1981: reported morbidity and mortality in the United States. Morbidity and Mortality Weekly Rep. **30**, 1982.)

in 1872 in the round epithelioid cells generally known as lepra cells; his observation was one of the first of pathogenic bacteria.

Morphology and Staining

Morphologically, the leprosy bacilli closely resemble the tubercle bacilli. They are long (up to 8 μm.), slender rods, usually straight, but sometimes slightly curved; club-shaped forms are found occasionally. They are non-motile and do not produce spores. They generally occur within the cells but are sometimes found free in the lymph spaces. Their arrangement within the cells is characteristic, several bacilli usually being grouped together in bundles like packets of cigars (Fig. 31–8). Capsules are present on cells that are presumed to be viable, but are destroyed by hot carbol-fuchsin generally used for staining.

The staining reaction of these microorganisms is similar to that of the tubercle bacilli. They stain somewhat more readily than the latter, and also decolorize more quickly with acids, but the difference is not great enough for differentiation. Both evenly and unevenly staining cells are found in diagnostic smears, and only the former are considered to be viable on the basis of the mouse footpad infection. The presence of large numbers of bacilli within the cells, together with the clinical features of the disease, makes it possible to distinguish

leprosy bacilli from tubercle bacilli without difficulty. Because of their acid-fast staining characteristic and their morphological resemblance to the tubercle bacilli and similar bacteria, these bacilli are included with the mycobacteria and designated *Mycobacterium leprae*. Deoxyribonucleic acid homology, how-

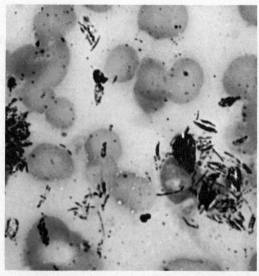

Figure 31–8. The leprosy bacillus. Acid-fast stained smear from a skin lesion. Note the characteristic tendency to parallel arrangement of the bacilli in packets. × 1800.

ever, indicates a close genetic relationship to *Corynebacterium*.[24]

Cultivation

Unsuccessful attempts to cultivate Hansen's bacillus on artificial mediums were made for years by bacteriologists all over the world, with a few reporting positive results. In most instances acid-fast bacilli have been cultivated, and there are at present a number of cultures in various laboratories labeled *M. leprae*. It seems highly improbable that these cultures truly represent leprosy bacilli; it is more likely that they are nonpathogenic mycobacteria and are best grouped with the saprophytic acid-fast forms such as the smegma and timothy bacilli. There have been, however, a number of reports of persistence, possibly with a few cell divisions, in tissue culture.

LEPROSY

Leprosy is a chronic inflammatory disease of man that may be manifest in two distinct types of disease—**tuberculoid** and **lepromatous**—but intermediate types are also recognized. The type of disease is to a large degree determined by effectiveness of the cell-mediated immune response. In tuberculoid leprosy, the more benign form of the disease, the cellular immunity is minimally effective and the disease is localized, affecting primarily the skin and nerves; it progresses more slowly than the lepromatous type, with an average case duration of about 18 years. In lepromatous leprosy little or no immunity develops and the disease is more generalized, with greater numbers of skin lesions and with less neural damage, at least in the early stages. Lepromatous leprosy is, then, more acute in nature and is characterized by the development of masses of granulation tissue. The typical lesion of leprosy, the so-called **leproma,** appears in different parts of the body and, by growth and coalescence, produces the distortion and mutilation that has marked the leper as a pariah in many societies.

The microorganisms are found in the lesions of both forms of leprosy; they occur in enormous numbers in the lepromatous type, and less abundantly in tuberculoid leprosy. Very few bacilli are observed outside body cells; within cells they are located in the cytoplasm but do not invade the nucleus. While the skin and peripheral nerves are the site of localization and growth in tuberculoid leprosy, almost any site may be invaded in the lepromatous variety; the more common sites, in addition to skin and nerves, are the upper respiratory tract, kidneys, eyes, liver, spleen, and blood stream.

Experimental Infections[45, 46]

Until the early 1960s, it had not been possible to produce lesions, with multiplication of leprosy bacilli, in experimental animals, so that studies on the host-parasite relationships lagged behind that of other diseases. Shepard, in 1961, found that leprosy bacilli grew *in vivo* when injected into the footpads of mice. This was later followed by the production of lepromatous leprosy in mice and rats immunosuppressed by thymectomy and irradiation. This animal model has permitted studies on growth rates of *M. leprae,* measurement of virulence, drug prophylaxis and therapy, and immunity induced by BCG immunization. The success of the mouse footpad model, as well as similar infections produced in ears and footpads of hamsters, apparently stems from the fact that optimum growth temperature for leprosy bacilli is lower than normal body temperature.

These remained the only animal models available until the observation, in the early 1970s, that the armadillo develops nodular lesions in which the bacilli grow to tremendous numbers.[25] This animal is a suitable host because of its low body temperature and, presumably, weak cellular immunity. Subsequently, an alternative model became available when nude mice were shown to develop "lepromatous" leprosy when inoculated with *M. leprae* from leprosy patients.[27] The large numbers of bacilli recoverable from infected animals has provided impetus for physiological and antigenic studies of the bacillus. It is of some interest that the armadillo appears to be naturally infected with *M. leprae,* or an indistinguishably similar mycobacterium.

Transmission

Until the development of the footpad infection in mice to fulfill Koch's postulates, the etiology of leprosy remained clouded. The indirect supporting evidence of the contagiousness of the infection tended not to be convincing, owing in part to the prolonged incubation period of the disease and in part to the practical difficulties in carrying out controlled studies in areas where the morbidity rate is sufficiently high. Field studies in Madras have given evidence of the man-to-man transmission of the disease and of the greater infectivity of the lepromatous type. In studies in the United States, where the disease is sufficiently rare as not to cast doubt on the origin of the infection, there is indication of much greater risk in family contacts.

The contagious nature of the disease is supported by several lines of evidence. First, considerable success has attended the isolation and segregation of the leprous patient. A Norwegian experience showed that a careful, but not unduly rigorous, system of separation was accompanied by a significant diminution in the number of cases. Second, children living in close association with leprous parents, particularly those with lepromatous leprosy, tend to show much higher prevalence of the disease. There is rapidly accumulating evidence, too, that leprosy is, like tuberculosis, a disease with a high degree of transmission, but a relatively low attack rate in endemic areas.

Immunological studies in endemic areas indicate that those living in such areas for a year or more develop a specific immunological response, but without overt clinical illness; 50 per cent of those with occupational or case contacts respond similarly.[18] These subclinical infections are considerably more common in endemic areas than are frank clinical cases.[17] Whether such covert infections represent an infection source is not yet known.

The manner of transmission of leprosy is uncertain. The bacilli may be found in nasal secretions—in tremendous numbers in cases of lepromatous leprosy, but in lesser numbers in borderline or indeterminant leprosy. The number excreted per day approximates that in tuberculosis and may exceed 10^8 bacilli.[7] The excreted bacilli survive drying and exposure, and remain viable for 1 to 2 days. While the opportunity for air- or insectborne dissemination obtains, it is not established that the respiratory tract is the portal of entry for leprosy bacilli.

For diagnostic purposes, microscopy is most useful. Acid-fast staining or immunofluorescence methods may be applied to nasal smears or to scrapings from skin lesions. Diagnosis of subclinical infections may be accomplished by lymphocyte-transformation or by leucocyte migration inhibition test.[17]

Chemotherapy[11, 41]

The similarities between the acid-fast bacilli observed in leprosy and tubercle bacilli inevitably suggested the use of the drugs effective in tuberculosis in the chemotherapy of leprosy. Of these the sulfones have been the most satisfactory, usually providing relatively rapid clinical improvement and slower bacteriologi-

cal improvement. There is some tendency to relapse following cessation of chemotherapy and inadequate or intermittent therapy has resulted in the appearance of bacterial drug resistance. Diaminodiphenyl sulfone (DDS) or diacetyldiaminodiphenyl sulfone (DADDS) are considered to be the chemotherapeutic agents of choice. The sulfones are also important in the epidemiology of leprosy, since treatment reduces the likelihood of person-to-person spread of the disease. Clofazimine appears to be as effective as the sulfones with the advantage that drug resistance has not been encountered. Rifampin is the most rapidly acting of the antileprosy drugs, but does not completely rid the body of all bacilli; resistance has been noted on occasion. As in tuberculosis, the use of drug combinations is recommended to minimize appearance of drug resistance.

Immunity[44]

In perhaps no other disease are the subtleties of the immune response so clearly tied to immunity and to the clinical spectrum of disease. While there is an antibody response in leprosy, it is apparently not effective in rendering the host immune to the disease; the effective immune response is associated with cell-mediated immunity.

Man appears to be highly resistant to disease caused by *M. leprae*. Although subclinical infections occur with some frequency in endemic areas, as noted above, rarely do these develop into clinical disease. It is generally believed that subclinical infections are contained by an effective cell-mediated immune response. In those persons who develop clinical disease, the relative effectiveness of cellular immunity determines the type of leprosy that ensues. If the individual exhibits a partially effective immunity, the disease assumes the tuberculoid form, with relatively few lesions and accordingly low numbers of bacilli in the tissues; few microorganisms are shed in the nasal secretions and this form of the disease is relatively noncontagious. At the other extreme is the lepromatous form of the disease, in which there is defective cellular immunity; no protection is apparent and the microorganisms are widely disseminated in many organs; the number of lesions is also much greater than in tuberculoid leprosy. The bacilli reach tremendous numbers in the tissues and are shed in nasal secretions in quantities that constitute an infection hazard to contacts of such cases. It is remarkable that the bacillary load in lepromatous leprosy shows so little toxicity to the host; leprosy, even in the lepromatous form, is a relatively benign process that may take years to terminate fatally. Intermediate gradations of these two extremes occur—the variations of borderline leprosy.

Figure 31–9 presents a diagrammatic representation of the specific immune responses to an intracellular parasite such as *M. leprae.* These same responses are present in infections by the tubercle bacilli and the atypical mycobacteria causing disseminated disease.

The immune defect in lepromatous leprosy appears to be located in the T-cell function. It is specifically related to *M. leprae,* since there is diminished capacity to develop hypersensitivity to many antigens, but this defect is more pronounced with antigens of *M. leprae.* The B-cell function is unimpaired, however, as antibody response to a variety of antigens appears to be unaffected in leprous individuals. Indeed, antibodies produced against *M. leprae* antigens are thought to lead to an antibody-mediated reaction found in some cases of leprosy with high concentrations of bacilli in the tissues—*erythema nodosum leprosum.* This reaction, thought to be an immune complex syndrome, is characterized by painful erythem-atous subcutaneous nodules. Borderline patients may exhibit another type of tissue damage that is a cell-mediated hypersensitivity—the **lepra reaction.**

Specific immunoprophylaxis, which requires sufficient numbers of bacilli for vaccine production, has not been possible in leprosy because of the inability to cultivate the organism on artificial mediums. There is, however, evidence of an immunological relationship to other mycobacteria, and there appears to be a mutual exclusion between leprosy and tuberculosis infections. With the successful application of BCG vaccination against tuberculosis as well as the common sensitivity of tuberculous and leprous persons to tuberculin, the question immediately arose as to the possibility of protection against leprosy by BCG vaccine. That this might hold true was indicated by the protection afforded by BCG vaccine against the mouse footpad infection and by scattered data on family contacts. A long-term study of childhood vaccination carried out in Burma by the World Health Organization failed, however, to show protection—an example of the failure of results obtained by animal experimentation to apply to human disease.

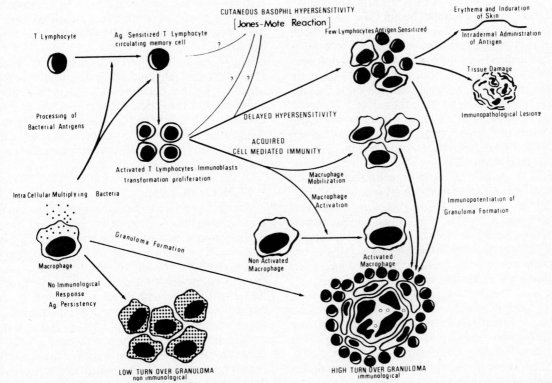

Figure 31–9. Diagrammatic representation of the specific immune responses to infection by obligate intracellular bacteria and the development of acquired cellular resistance, delayed hypersensitivity and granuloma formation. (P. Sansonetti, and P. H. Lagrange, Rev. Infect. Dis. **3**:422, 1981.) (Published by the University of Chicago Press. © 1981, The University of Chicago.)

The search for a successful vaccine must, therefore, center on the use of cultivable mycobacteria with close antigenic relationship to *M. leprae,* or on *M. leprae* derived from infected armadillos, to furnish sufficient antigenic material for vaccine preparation.

Lepromin. The hypersensitivity developed by leprous persons may be demonstrated by the intradermal inoculation of material prepared from leprous nodules or animal-derived *M. leprae.* Two reactions are observed, one early and occurring after three or four days, and one later, appearing three to four weeks after inoculation. The first is the **Fernandez reaction** and the second the **Mitsuda reaction.** The Mitsuda reaction is regarded by some workers as an expression of immunity, but it is nonspecific in that it also occurs in tuberculosis and is induced by immunization with BCG.

Other Mycobacteria

Mycobacterium lepraemurium

A native disease of wild rats, commonly known as rat leprosy and characterized by enormous numbers of acid-fast bacilli present in the lesions, was described by Stefansky in 1903 as occurring in wild rats in Odessa. The disease was observed in the same year by Dean, who later showed it to be transmissible. It has since been observed in wild rats all over the world.

The acid-fast bacilli closely resemble the leprosy bacillus in size and shape and are found intracellularly but not as often in the packet arrangement of parallel bacilli. *Mycobacterium lepraemurium* had not, until recently, been cultivated on artificial mediums. Nakamura and colleagues, however, have reported successful cultivation.[30] Growth also occurs in tissue-cultured cells and in cell-impermeable diffusion chambers maintained in the mouse or on monolayer petri dish cultures of mouse peritoneal macrophages, suggesting that an intracellular environment may not be essential for *in vivo* growth.

The disease may be transmitted to white rats, mice, and guinea pigs by inoculation with pieces of infected tissue. Wild mice are relatively insusceptible, and subcutaneous inoculation results in only a transient granuloma. The experimental infection is a relatively benign process. A local, circumscribed lesion develops following subcutaneous inoculation which becomes palpable in four to five weeks and eventually develops to a large tumorous mass ulcerating on the surface and persisting throughout the life of the rat. The earliest lesions in the other organs do not appear before four to six months, and the animal dies only after a year or more.

Murine leprosy caused by *M. lepraemurium* has many parallels to human leprosy due to *M. leprae,* particularly in the elements of the immune response. Murine leprosy has, therefore, served as a useful model for this kind of disease.

Mycobacterium paratuberculosis

A chronic enteritis of cattle usually terminating fatally is caused by an acid-fast bacillus closely resembling *Mycobacterium avium.* The disease is sometimes called Johne's disease and the organism Johne's bacillus after its discoverer. The disease only remotely resembles tuberculous infection. The lesions in the intestinal wall are proliferative, and the granulomatous tissue may contain epithelioid cells and occasionally giant cells, but there is no caseation.

The disease appears to be widespread in the United States. Infected cattle become hypersensitive to the bacillary substance, and filtrates of cultures produce a skin reaction analogous to the tuberculin reaction which is designated the "johnin reaction." No case of human infection with *M. paratuberculosis* has been recorded.

The Vole Bacillus

An acid-fast bacillus responsible for an epizootic, chronic infection of the field vole, *Microtus agrestis,* that resembles tuberculosis was discovered by Wells in 1937. Named *Mycobacterium microti,* it closely resembles the tubercle bacillus culturally, though it forms no pigment and growth is not enhanced by glycerol. It is pathogenic for both guinea pigs and rabbits, considerably more so for the latter, but is not pathogenic for fowls. The microorganism has been of particular interest because tuberculin sensitivity is induced, though it produces only a localized and retrogressive infection when inoculated in small doses in guinea pigs and calves; preliminary experiments on its use in prophylaxis have given suggestive results.

Saprophytic Acid-Fast Bacilli

Included in this category are the well-known timothy bacillus, *Mycobacterium phlei,* found in soil, on grasses, and elsewhere in nature; the "butter bacillus," *Mycobacterium butyricum;* and *Mycobacterium smegmatis,* which is, however, a parasite found in both male and female smegma. The smegma bacillus is often difficult to distinguish from the tubercule bacillus on morphological grounds, and confusion of the two may have considerable practical importance in the diagnosis of suspected cases of tuberculous infection of the urinary tract. It is, it may be noted, also found in the urine and may contaminate fecal specimens. The saprophytic bacilli all grow much more rapidly than the tubercle bacilli, and neither they nor the acid-fast bacilli isolated from cold-blooded animals are pathogenic for guinea pigs and rabbits, or at best only feebly so.

REFERENCES

1. Barksdale, L., and K.-S. Kim. 1977. *Mycobacterium.* Bacteriol. Rev. **41:**217–372.
2. Chaparas, S. D. 1982. Immunity in tuberculosis. Bull. Wld. Hlth. Org. **60:**447–462.
3. Chapman, J. S. 1977. The Atypical Mycobacteria and Human Mycobacteriosis. Plenum Medical Book Co., New York.
4. Crowle, A. J., and M. May. 1981. Preliminary demonstration of human tuberculoimmunity in vitro. Infect. Immun. **31:**453–464.
5. Daniel, T. M., and C. F. Hinz, Jr. 1974. Reactivity of purified proteins and polysaccharides from *Mycobacterium tuberculosis* in delayed skin test and cultured lymphocyte mitogenesis assays. Infect. Immun. **9:**44–47.
6. Daniel, T. M., and B. W. Janicki. 1978. Mycobacterial antigens: a review of their isolation, chemistry, and immunological properties. Microbiol. Rev. **42:**84–113.
7. Davey, T. F., and R. J. W. Rees. 1974. The nasal discharge in leprosy: clinical and bacteriological aspects. Lepr. Rev. **45:**121–134.
8. Davidson, P. T. (Ed.). 1981. International conference on atypical mycobacteria. Rev. Infect. Dis. **3:**813–1097.
9. Edelson, P. J. 1982. Intracellular parasites and phagocytic cells: cell biology and pathophysiology. Rev. Infect. Dis. **4:**124–135.
10. Eickhoff, T. C. 1977. The current status of BCG immunization against tuberculosis. Ann. Rev. Med. **28:**411–423.
11. Ellard, G. A. 1974. Growing points in leprosy research. 4. Recent advances in the chemotherapy of leprosy. Lepr. Rev. **45:**31–40.
12. Enarson, D. A., *et al.* 1980. Non-respiratory tuberculosis in Canada: epidemiologic and bacteriologic features. Amer. J. Epidemiol. **112:**341–351.
13. Engel, A., and J. Roberts. 1977. Tuberculin skin test reaction among adults 25–74 years, United States, 1971–1972. Vital Hlth Statistics, Series 11, No. 204. DHEW Publication No. (HRA)77-1649.
14. Farer, L. S., A. M. Lowell, and M. P. Meador. 1979. Extrapulmonary tuberculosis in the United States. Amer. J. Epidemiol. **109:**205–217.
15. Feldman, R. A., M. W. Long, and H. L. David. 1974. *Mycobacterium marinum*: a leisure-time pathogen. J. Infect. Dis. **129:**618–621.
16. Glassroth, J., A. G. Robbins, and D. E. Snider, Jr. 1980. Tuberculosis in the 1980s. New Engl. J. Med. **302:**1441–1450.
17. Godal, T. 1974. Growing points in leprosy research. 3. Immunological detection of sub-clinical infection in leprosy. Lepr. Rev. **45:**22–30.
18. Godal, T., and K. Negassi. 1973. Subclinical infection in leprosy. Brit. Med. J. **3:**557–559.
19. Goldstein, R. S., *et al.* 1982. Tuberculosis—a review of 498 recent admissions to hospital. Can. Med. Assn. J. **126:**490–492.
20. Good, R. C. 1980. Isolation of nontuberculous mycobacteria in the United States, 1979. J. Infect. Dis. **142:**779–783.
21. Goren, M. B. 1972. Mycobacterial lipids: selected topics. Bacteriol. Rev. **36:**33–64.
22. Goren, M. B. 1977. Phagocyte lysosomes: interactions with infectious agents, phagosomes, and experimental perturbations in function. Ann. Rev. Microbiol. **31:**507–533.
23. Hart, P. D'A., and J. A. Armstrong. 1974. Strain virulence and the lysosomal response in macrophages infected with *Mycobacterium tuberculosis.* Infect. Immun. **10:**742–746.
24. Imaeda, T., W. F. Kirchheimer, and L. Barksdale. 1982. DNA isolated from *Mycobacterium leprae*: genome size, base ratio, and homology with other related bacteria as determined by optical DNA-DNA reassociation. J. Bacteriol. **150:**414–417.
25. Kirchheimer, W. F., and E. E. Storrs. 1971. Attempts to establish the armadillo (*Dasypus novemcinctus* Linn.) as a model for the study of leprosy. I. Report of lepromatoid leprosy in an experimentally infected armadillo. Internat. J. Lepr. **39:**693–702.
26. Kochan, I. 1973. The role of iron in bacterial infections, with special consideration of host-tubercle bacillus interaction. Curr. Topics Microbiol. Immunol. **60:**1–30.
27. Kohsaka, K., *et al.* 1979. Experimental leprosy with nude mice. Japan. J. Lepr. **48:**37–41.
28. Kopanoff, D. E., *et al.* 1978. A continuing survey of tuberculosis primary drug resistance in the United States: March 1975 to November 1977. A United States Public Health Service cooperative study. Amer. Rev. Resp. Dis. **118:**835–842.
29. Laguerre, M., and R. Turcotte. 1975. Purification and characterization of tuberculin-active components from BCG. Can. J. Microbiol. **21:**2019–2027.
30. Nakamura, M. 1975. Improvement to the NC-5 medium for culturing *Mycobacterium lepraemurium* (ND-5 medium). Kurume Med. J. **22:**67–70.
31. Powell, K. E., and L. S. Farer. 1980. The rising age of the tuberculosis patient: a sign of success and failure. J. Infect. Dis. **142:**946–948.
32. Ramakrishnan, T., P. S. Murthy, and K. P. Gopinathan. 1972. Intermediary metabolism of mycobacteria. Bacteriol. Rev. **36:**65–108.
33. Ramanathan, V. D., J. Curtis, and J. L. Turk. 1980. Activation of the alternative pathway of complement by mycobacteria and cord factor. Infect. Immun. **29:**30–35.
34. Ratledge, C. 1976. The physiology of mycobacteria. Adv. Microbial Physiol. **13:**115–244.
35. Ratnam, S., and S. Chandrasekhar. 1976. The pathogenicity of spheroplasts of *Mycobacterium tuberculosis.* Amer. Rev. Resp. Dis. **114:**549–554.

36. Reggiardo, Z., and A. K. M. Shamsuddin. 1976. Granulomagenic activity of serologically active glycolipids from *Mycobacterium bovis* BCG. Infect. Immun. **14**:1369–1374.
37. Report. 1977. WHO Expert Committee on Leprosy. Wld Hlth Org. Tech. Rep. Ser., No. 607, Geneva.
38. Report. 1980. Vaccination against tuberculosis. Wld Hlth Org. Tech. Rep. Ser., No. 651, Geneva.
39. Report. 1980. BCG vaccination policies. Wld Hlth Org. Tech. Rep. Ser., No. 652, Geneva.
40. Report. 1982. Tuberculosis control. Wld Hlth Org. Tech. Rep. Ser., No. 671, Geneva.
41. Report. 1982. Chemotherapy of leprosy for control programmes. Wld Hlth Org. Tech. Rep. Ser., No. 675, Geneva.
42. Runyon, E. H., *et al.* 1980. *Mycobacterium.* pp. 150–179. *In* E. H. Lennette, *et al.* (Eds.): Manual of Clinical Microbiology. 3rd ed. American Society for Microbiology, Washington, D.C.
43. Saito, R., *et al.* 1977. Adjuvancy (immunity-inducing property) of cord factor in mice and rats. Infect. Immun. **16**:725–729.
44. Sansonetti, P., and D. H. Lagrange. 1981. The immunology of leprosy: speculations on the leprosy spectrum. Rev. Infect. Dis. **3**:422–469.
45. Shepard, C. C. 1971. The first decade in experimental leprosy. Bull. Wld Hlth Org. **44**:821–827.
46. Storrs, E. E. 1974. Growing points in leprosy research. 1. The armadillo as an experimental model for the study of human leprosy. Lepr. Rev. **45**:8–14.
47. Symposium. 1976. Symposium on leprosy. Southern Med. J. **69**:969–996.
48. TenDam, H. G., *et al.* 1976. Present knowledge of immunization against tuberculosis. Bull. Wld Hlth Org. **54**:255–269.
49. Wijsmuller, G., and P. Erickson. 1974. The reaction to PPD–Battey. A new look. Amer. Rev. Resp. Dis. **109**:29–40.
50. Wolinsky, E. 1979. Nontuberculous mycobacteria and associated diseases. Amer. Rev. Resp. Dis. **119**:107–159.
51. Yarkoni, E., L. Wang, and A. Bekierkunst. 1977. Stimulation of macrophages by cord factor and by heat-killed and living BCG. Infect. Immun. **16**:1–8.
52. Youmans, G. P. 1975. Relation between delayed hypersensitivity and immunity in tuberculosis. Amer. Rev. Resp. Dis. **111**:109–118.

CHAPTER 32

The Spirochetes

In the early history of microbiology, spiral and curved microorganisms were grouped together under various names such as *Spirochete, Spirillum,* and *Vibrio.* With the advent of modern observational methods, *e.g.,* electron microscopy, it became evident that the flexuous spirochetes possess a fundamentally different morphology and fine structure from the rigid spiral and curved bacteria. Accordingly, they are placed in the family Spirochetaceae (Chapter 2).

For a period of time, the spirochetes were considered to be intermediate between the true bacteria and protozoa. Their procaryotic nature is now accepted, however, and they are known to differ from the protozoa in the lack of anterior-posterior polarity, absence of a nuclear membrane, presence of muramic acid as a cell wall constituent, and sensitivity to antibacterial antibiotics and lysozyme. Unlike most other bacteria, their cell wall is not ordinarily rigid and their motility is a function of cell structures other than typical external flagella.

While some spirochetes may be grown on artificial mediums, many are cultivable only with difficulty or not at all; thus, the biochemical and cultural reactions used for the differentiation of other bacteria are not applicable. Their characterization rests almost entirely on morphology and has been greatly facilitated by electron microscopy; in the parasitic varieties, host and vector specificity also have differential value.

Structure of Spirochetes[9, 19, 23]

The basic spirochetal structure is the helically shaped **protoplasmic cylinder,** composed of the cytoplasm enclosed in a cytoplasmic membrane, surrounded by a thin peptidoglycan layer. The morphological distinction between the cytoplasmic membrane and the glycan layer is not obvious, and the combined structure is often referred to as the peptidoglycan-membrane complex. Aside from its spiral shape, the cell wall of the protoplasmic cylinder is similar to that of gram-negative cells and its structure correlates with the observed gram-

629

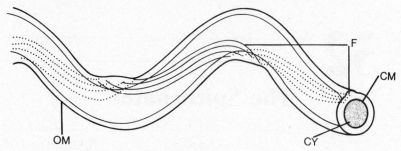

Figure 32–1. Diagrammatic representation of a generalized basic structure of spirochetes. *OM,* outer membrane; *CM,* cytoplasmic membrane-peptidoglycan complex; *CY,* cytoplasm; *F,* axial fibrils.

negative staining character of spirochetes. Loosely or tightly apposed over the protoplasmic cylinder is an **outer membrane** or **envelope** that is elastic and fragile; it is apparently essential to the integrity of the cell, since reaction of specific antibodies with outer envelope antigens, in the presence of complement, is bactericidal. Lying between the outer envelope and the peptidoglycan-cytoplasmic membrane complex are one or more **axial fibrils,** structures which resemble the external flagella of other bacteria and are believed to be associated with motility. Individual fibrils, like flagella, are made up of a filament (usually sheathed), hook, and basal body (Chapter 2). The fibrils are inserted into the cytoplasmic membrane near the ends of the cell and extend along the protoplasmic cylinder, beneath the outer envelope. Those originating from opposite ends of the cell may overlap near the central region. The basic structure of spirochetes is shown diagrammatically in Figure 32–1.

Spirochetes vary greatly in length, from a minimum of 2 μm. to a maximum of about 500 μm. but the pathogenic spirochetes rarely exceed 25 μm. Some of the slender spirochetes have been considered to be filterable because they pass through bacteriological filters, probably by an active boring motion through the channels and pores. As a group the spirochetes are unusually sensitive to drying, and are killed by most disinfectants. They do not form spores and are killed by heating at 60° C. for 30 minutes.

The family Spirochetaceae is divided into five genera whose principal features are outlined in Table 32–1. The spirochetes pathogenic for humans are in the genera *Treponema, Borrelia,* and *Leptospira.*

Borrelia: The Relapsing Fever Spirochetes[7, 9, 10, 22]

The relapsing fevers are a group of closely related infections characterized clinically by an initial pyrexia of three to four days' duration, followed by successive relapses at intervals of a few days. Relapsing fevers are widely distributed and occur in practically every country of the world. The microorganisms responsible for these diseases are spiral forms that were first observed by Obermeier in 1873 in the blood of patients with European relapsing fever.

Morphology
The basic structure of *Borrelia* is that described earlier, with 15 to 20 axial fibrils wound around the protoplasmic cylinder. These fibrils are believed to be responsible for locomotion, possibly by inducing a kind of rotatory motion. The cells are helical in shape, with 3 to 10 somewhat coarse and uneven coils. All are 0.2 to 0.5 μm. in diameter by 3 to 20 μm. in

length and the various species cannot be distinguished from one another by their morphology. They are best stained by the Romanowsky method or some modification, such as Giemsa; in contrast to other spirochetes, however, they are stained by aniline dyes. Figures 32–2 and 32–3 illustrate the staining and morphology of several relapsing fever spirochetes.

Cultivation
The spirochetes of relapsing fever had not been grown in pure culture until 1971, when *B. hermsii* was successfully cultured under microaerophilic conditions in a complex medium.[24] Subsequently, other *Borrelia* have been cultivated, including *B. recurrentis, B. parkeri, B. turicatae,* and *B. hispanica.*

Limited physiological studies indicate that some *(B. duttonii)* derive energy from homolactic fermentation of glucose, forming lactate

Table 32–1. **The Genera of Spirochetaceae and Their Principal Features**

Genus	Features
Spirochaeta	Characteristically large (up to 500 μm. in length) spirals with two axial fibrils. They are free-living, usually found in H₂S-containing mud, polluted water, and sewage; they are anaerobic or facultatively anaerobic. The type species is *Spirochaeta plicatilis.*
Cristispira	Cells are not as long as *Spirochaeta* (up to 150 μm.); they possess more than 100 axial fibrils, which, if detached from the protoplasmic cylinder, give rise to the crista, a membranous appendage wound around the cylinder. They have not yet been grown in pure culture. *Cristispira* are commensals, frequently found in mollusks. The type species is *Cristispira pectinis.*
Treponema	Slender, flexuous spirals (0.09 to 0.5 μm. by 5 to 20 μm.), with one or more axial fibrils. Most are closely adapted parasites of man and animals. The genus includes the etiological agents of syphilis *(T. pallidum)*, yaws *(T. pertenue)*, and pinta *(T. carateum)*, together with parasitic forms of limited or no pathogenicity, often occurring as a part of the normal flora of the mouth, intestine, or urogenital tract. Cultivable species are obligately anaerobic. The type species is *Treponema pallidum.*
Borrelia	Spirals similar in size to *Treponema*, with 15 to 20 axial fibrils. Includes the agents causing relapsing fevers of man and spirochetoses of cattle and fowl. *Borrelia* also are found in insect vectors, usually ticks and lice. They are anaerobic or microaerophilic. The type species is *Borrelia anserina.*
Leptospira	Spiral forms similar in size to *Treponema*, with two axial fibrils; the cells frequently exhibit hooked ends. *Leptospira* cause infectious jaundice and various febrile conditions of man and animals. The human disease is commonly derived from infected animal reservoirs. Some are free-living in aquatic environments. The type species is *Leptospira interrogans.*

via the Embden-Myerhof pathway. Cultivable borreliae require lipids for growth, metabolizing lysolecithin to fatty acids, choline, inorganic phosphate, and glycerol.

Classification

The relapsing fever spirochetes are assigned to the genus *Borrelia*. It is not clear to what extent the relapsing fever spirochetes can be divided into species; in many cases, it is probable that those given species rank are, in fact, only strains or varieties. The recognized species are immunologically heterogeneous and unstable in that they are modified in antigenic character by residence in different vectors or mammalian hosts. Cross protection tests, therefore, are not useful. The Bergey classification is based upon the natural animal reservoir hosts and the vectors responsible for transmission. Nineteen species are delineated, most of which are pathogenic for man and are transmitted by ticks of the genus *Ornithodoros* or by the human body louse. Borreliae responsible for diseases in birds, cattle, and horses are transmitted by other vectors.

RELAPSING FEVER

Relapsing fever is an ancient disease; one of the first epidemics, described by Hippocrates, occurred 2000 years ago on the island of Thasos, but was not mentioned again for many centuries. Historically, there was a tendency to confuse relapsing fever with louseborne typhus fever, which had similar geographical distribution. The Yellow Plague that followed the pandemic of bubonic plague in the time of Justinian was probably relapsing fever, as was an epidemic in Ireland in 664. Presently, relapsing fever occurs sporadically in various parts of the world.

The relapsing fevers constitute a group of closely related diseases. The spirochete observed by Obermeier was that of **European** or **epidemic relapsing fever,** a disease recognized

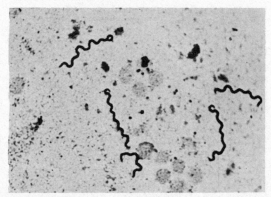

Figure 32–2. *Borrelia recurrentis* in a blood smear from an infected rat. Fontana stain; × 1160.

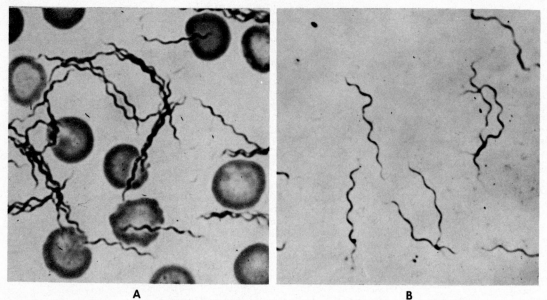

A   **B**

Figure 32–3. Relapsing fever spirochetes. *A, Borrelia duttonii* of Central African relapsing fever. *B, Borrelia duttonii* of East African relapsing fever. × 2000. (Kral.)

in the early part of the eighteenth century that has at times prevailed extensively in parts of Europe.

The causal microorganism of the epidemic disease is designated *B. recurrentis* and is transmitted by the louse *Pediculus humanus* subspecies *humanus*. A second type, **endemic relapsing fever,** is transmitted by *Ornithodoros* ticks. One of many *Borrelia* species may be responsible, and each is carried by its specific tick vector. Thus, the geographical distribution of the disease and its specific borrelial agent is determined by the vector distribution; the vectors and geographical distribution of the relapsing fever borreliae are detailed in Table 32–2.

All forms of relapsing fever are clinically identical. The onset is sudden, with chills, fever, and severe headache; muscular and joint pains are frequently observed, and there is a moderate enlargement of the spleen and liver; jaundice is commonly seen. The fever ends suddenly by crisis in three or four days. Successive relapses occur at intervals of 2 to 14 days, and the period of relapse varies from a few hours to longer than the primary fever; the number of relapses varies. Spirochetes may be found in the blood during the paroxysms. The case fatality in European relapsing fever is not high, perhaps 4 to 5 per cent; there are no characteristic findings at autopsy.

The relapsing fevers are effectively treated with a variety of antibiotics, including penicillin, erythromycin, and the tetracyclines. Treat-

ment with many of the antibiotics is, however, frequently followed by symptoms of endotoxin shock—the **Jarisch-Herxheimer reaction.** Presumably, the rapid destruction of spirochetes engendered by vigorous antibiotic treatment releases endotoxin, sometimes resulting in death of the patient.

Rats and mice may be experimentally infected; ordinarily these infections are inapparent in that there are no observable symptoms, but successive relapses, or "attacks," are evidenced by the appearance of the spirochetes in the blood, beginning two to four days after inoculation. They are present for two to three days, disappear, and reappear three or four days later in a second attack. Usually only two or three such relapses occur, the spirochetes becoming fewer and persisting for shorter times in the successive relapses. Experimental disease may also be produced in monkeys, and its course is very similar to that in man.

Natural infection of lower animals occurs with some frequency in endemic areas, and there is much evidence to support the hypothesis that small mammals, especially rodents, constitute a natural reservoir of the tickborne infection. A wide variety of wild animals may be infected, although susceptibility varies considerably among animal species; there is also variation in the virulence of spirochetal strains.

It is of considerable epidemiological importance that a reservoir of infection is maintained in tick vectors by **transovarial** transmission from one generation to the next. Transovarial

Table 32–2. **Pathogenic Borreliae, Their Vectors and Geographical Distribution**

Borrelia	Vector	Geographical Distribution	Human Disease
B. recurrentis	*Pediculus humanus*	Ethiopia, Sudan, South America; may become cosmopolitan	Epidemic relapsing fever
B. duttonii	*Ornithodoros moubata*	East and South Africa	Often severe endemic relapsing fever
B. hispanica	*O. erraticus erraticus*	Mediterranean, Middle East, Northern part of Africa	Endemic relapsing fever
B. persica	*O. tholozani (papillipes)*	Middle East, Central Asia	Endemic relapsing fever
B. latyschewii	*O. tartakovskyi*	Central Asia ⎱	Usually mild endemic relapsing
B. caucasica	*O. verrucosus*	Caucasian area ⎰	fever
B. venezuelensis	*O. rudis (venezuelensis)*	South America	Endemic relapsing fever
B. dugesii	*O. dugesi*	Western part of the Americas	Endemic relapsing fever in Central and South America
B. turicatae	*O. turicata*	Western U.S., part of Midwest U.S., Central and South America	Usually mild endemic relapsing fever
B. parkeri	*O. parkeri*	Canada, Western U.S.	Endemic relapsing fever
B. hermsii	*O. hermsi*	Western U.S.	Often severe endemic relapsing fever
B. crocidurae	*O. erraticus sonrai*	Middle East, Africa	In rodents; seldom, mild human disease
B. theileri	{ *Rhipicephalus evertsi* *Boophilus microplus*	Africa ⎱ Australia ⎰	Cattle and horse spirochetoses
B. anserina	*Argas persicus* and others	Cosmopolitan; at present not in the U.S.	Fowl spirochetosis

infection of the louse has not been observed, however.

Immunity

Following infection, agglutinins as well as lytic and spirocheticidal antibodies may be found in the serum. Usually the immunity following recovery from an attack of relapsing fever is of short duration, but occasionally a more solid immunity may develop. The latter is often attributed to a persistence of the infection, *i.e.,* an immunity to superinfection, possibly due to cellular immunity.

Relapse appears to be basically an immunological phenomenon and is related to the **antigenic instability** of the spirochetes. Following initial infection with *Borrelia*, the host responds with the production of spirocheticidal antibodies against the infecting strain. Most of the spirochetes are then killed, but some are resistant, presumably because they express different antigens on the cell surface. This new serological variety then multiplies and a relapse occurs. Subsequent relapses occur as new serological varieties appear in sequence and are eliminated. As expected, spirochetes isolated from successive relapses differ serologically from the spirochetes of earlier attacks. In *Borrelia carteri* infections, for example, as many as nine different serotypes have been distinguished. After any particular type appeared in an animal it never reappeared in the

further course of the disease in the same animal. Two North American varieties, *B. turicatae* and *B. parkeri,* have been shown to contain three antigenic components, A, B, and C, of which B is shared and invariant, while A and C are both strain- and relapse-specific. *Borrelia hermsii* occurs as four major serotypes, designated O, A, B, and C, which appear in that sequence in rats infected with the O serotype, but infection with a relapse serotype tends to revert to the O serotype. Relapse serums are protective against both initial attack and relapse, whereas attack serum protects against attack but not relapse strains.

Laboratory Diagnosis[7]

The spirochetes of relapsing fever can usually be demonstrated in patients' blood during the onset of a relapse by direct microscopic examination or by animal inoculation. Either the usual blood smear or a thick film similar to that used for the detection of malarial parasites may be used. The films are air-dried and stained with Giemsa; Wright's stain is satisfactory for thin films. Spirochetes may also be found in fresh wet preparations by darkfield examination. Alternatively, Kelly's medium may be inoculated with fresh blood and observed at intervals for the presence of spirochetes by darkfield microscopy. Mice or rats may be infected by intraperitoneal inoculation of patients' blood; these infections in animals are followed by darkfield examination of blood samples. Immunological methods of diagnosis are not adaptable to routine use and are not widely applied.

Epidemiology

The relapsing fever spirochetes are blood rather than tissue parasites, and the infection is transmitted by blood-sucking insects. Two epidemiological types of the disease are distinguished, one **tickborne** and usually representing transmission to man from an animal reservoir of infection, and the other **louseborne** and spread from man to man. The geographical distribution of the two epidemiological types is illustrated in Figure 32–4.

Tickborne relapsing fever is the only type that occurs in the United States; endemic foci are in Arizona, California, Colorado, Idaho, Oregon, Texas, and possibly in Montana, Utah, and Washington. As a rule, only sporadic cases are seen. On occasion, however, multiple cases appear, as among 27 employees and 35 tourists at the North Rim of the Grand Canyon in 1973.[6] In this outbreak infection appeared to be linked to ticks and rodents present in rustic cabins used for overnight lodging in the park.

Vectors for transmission in the United States are *Ornithodoros turicata, O. parkeri,* and *O. hermsi; O. dugesi* transmits the infection in tropical America but apparently not in the United States; *O. rudis* is regarded as the most

important vector in the tropics in this hemisphere. The traditional vector, and the most common in West Africa, is *O. moubata.*

Infection in the tick may persist for long periods; survival in starved ticks for as long five years, and in refed ticks for six and one-half years has been reported. In addition, the infection can persist in the insect vector for at least five generations by ovarial transmission.

The spirochetes are present in the coxal fluid, saliva, and feces of infected ticks. Of these, the first two appear to be the more important in transmission of the infection to man. For example, *O. moubata,* an excellent vector, secretes coxal fluid copiously while feeding, thus making possible infection of the bite, while *O. hermsi* does not pass coxal fluid while feeding and is a less effective vector. The relative importance of direct introduction of the spirochete into the bite by infected saliva is not altogether clear. It is probable that infection of the bite by contaminated feces occurs occasionally.

European relapsing fever is transmitted from man to man by the human body louse, *Pediculus humanus,* and has the epidemiological characteristics of louseborne disease. In contrast to the tickborne infection, the bite is not infected by the secretions of the louse; rather, the infected louse must be crushed on the skin and the spirochetes present in the body fluids contaminate the bite. The fingers may become contaminated by crushing infected lice and transmit the infection by scratching.

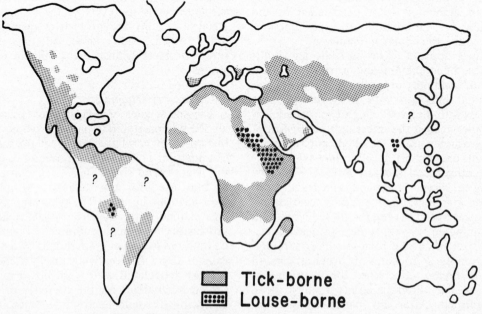

☐ **Tick-borne**
▦ **Louse-borne**

Figure 32–4. The global distribution of relapsing fever.

Treponema and the Treponematoses[9, 19, 22, 23]

Spirochetes of the genus *Treponema* are indistinguishable from *Borrelia* by the usual microscopic morphology (Fig. 32–5), but the pathogenic forms are set apart from the relapsing fever spirochetes by the kinds of diseases they cause. The human pathogenic forms are *Treponema pallidum,* the causative agent of syphilis; *Treponema pertenue,* the causative agent of yaws; and *Treponema carateum,* the causative agent of pinta. Nonpathogenic *Treponema* are a part of the normal flora. In spite of perennial reports to the contrary, it is not likely that the pathogenic *Treponema* have been grown in artificial mediums.

The pathogenic species of *Treponema* make up a group of interrelated microorganisms, separable only by differences in the kinds of diseases they produce. Conversely, the infections with these microorganisms, known collectively as the treponematoses, are at the same time both similar, as with respect to the immune response, and differentiable by the character of the clinical disease. The treponematoses fall into four groups; *viz.,* syphilis, which is divided into the venereal and nonvenereal forms; yaws, or tropical syphilis; and pinta, or pintid yaws.

A disease similar to syphilis was present on the China coast in ancient times; the Biblical plague of Moab is thought to have been syphilis; and syphilitic infection apparently occurred in Eastern Europe prior to the fifteenth century. Venereal syphilis, or "morbus gallicus," occurred in epidemic form in Europe after the return of Columbus from the Americas, and some believe that this form of treponematosis was introduced from the Western Hemisphere. There is evidence, however, that syphilis had already invaded Europe from the East before Columbus. Syphilitic infection also seems to persist in nonvenereal form following epidemics of venereal syphilis. With improving economic and sociological conditions, the disease tends to die out, but nonvenereal syphilis persists at the present time in the Near East, in Africa, and in Central Europe, and occurred in epidemic form in Chicago as late as 1949.

The earliest description of a yaws-like disease appeared in 1558 in Brazil; the disease as known today was identified in the seventeenth century in the West Indies and in Brazil in the eighteenth century; it is now known to be ubiquitous in tropical regions. Pinta is more recently identified as a treponematosis occurring in Mexico, Cuba, and adjacent areas; the spirochetal etiology was established in 1938.

While the differences among these diseases are thought to require consideration of them as separate entities, the differences are not much greater than those between venereal syphilis in the Middle Ages and present-day venereal syphilis. The similarities are more striking than the differences, leading to a "unitarian" view of the treponemal infections in which the several clinical manifestations are considered to be variations on a central theme.

Cultivation[13, 35]

The *in vitro* cultivation of *T. pallidum* was first reported in 1909 and has been followed by many similar reports since that time. Nevertheless, these cultivated strains appear not to have been virulent *T. pallidum* and are usually referred to as host-associated *Treponema.* It is generally accepted that *T. pallidum* has not yet been cultivated in pure culture in artificial mediums.

The cultivable strains of *Treponema* share antigenic components with *T. pallidum* and have been useful in physiological and serological studies. These cultivable strains are considered to be biotypes of either *T. phagedenis* or *T. refringens.* The best known are the Reiter and Kazan biotypes of *T. phagedenis.* Genetic studies, based on DNA sequence homology, confirm the existence of three genetically distinct groups: (1) the noncultivable pathogenic treponemes, including *T. pallidum* and *T. pertenue;* (2) *T. phagedenis;* and (3) *T. refringens.*[27, 28]

Although it cannot be cultivated, *T. pallidum* is capable of infecting experimental ani-

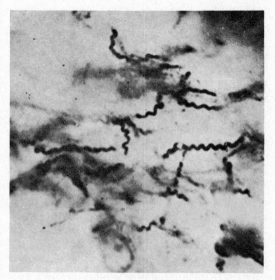

Figure 32–5. *Treponema pallidum* in stained (silver impregnation) smear. × 3000. (Kral.)

mals, especially rabbits. Testicular infections of these animals can yield considerable numbers of viable spirochetes for physiological and metabolic studies. In suitable mediums, rabbit-derived *T. pallidum* will survive for extended periods, but is not actually cultivated. The strain most often used in physiological experiments is the virulent Nichols strain of *T. pallidum*. It retains virulence for rabbits and also for man, *viz.*, inoculation of 57 Nichols strain spirochetes infected 4 of 8 nonsyphilitic human volunteers, while the ID_{50} for rabbits was 23 spirochetes.

The past decade has seen renewed interest in the physiology and metabolism of *T. pallidum* that has been spurred by techniques permitting *in vitro* survival of the spirochete. For example, such studies have demonstrated that *T. pallidum,* unlike the cultivable treponemes, is microaerophilic and possesses a functional electron transport system. Physiological and metabolic studies have yielded information that can be expected to lead to eventual cultivation of *T. pallidum*.

For several years, investigators have attempted to cultivate *T. pallidum* in tissue cultures of animal cells. These efforts were not successful until 1981, when virulent *T. pallidum* (Nichols strain) was first found to replicate in rabbit epithelial cell cultures;[11, 12] these findings have been independently confirmed.[30]

Tissue culture infections have yielded information on virulence and attachment. Virulent *T. pallidum,* but not avirulent treponemes, adhere to mammalian cells in culture and rapidly attain intracellularity.[14] Adherence to mammalian cells is through a terminal end structure of the spirochete which appears to anchor the spirochete to a cell membrane receptor site (Fig. 32–6); the spirochetes retain motility after attachment, with observable waving and flexing.[18]

The treponemas are extremely fragile microorganisms and die out quickly outside the body. They are destroyed by soap and water or by drying, and are unusually susceptible to heat; suspensions of infected rabbit testicle are sterilized at 41.5° C. in one hour and in two hours at 41° C., but the cultivable strains may remain viable in culture mediums kept at 37° C. for as long as a year. The viability of *T. pallidum* is of interest in connection with the possibility of transmission of syphilis by infected blood; although occasional transmission has occurred in this way, the risk is not great with blood from blood banks, for the spirochete dies out in three or four days at refrigerator temperature and quite rapidly in lyophilized plasma.

Pathogenicity for Animals

Syphilis may be transmitted to anthropoid apes, such as the chimpanzee and gibbon, and, with less certainty, to monkeys. Inoculation by scarification of the genitals or eyebrows results in development of a primary chancre followed in a few weeks by the appearance of lesions of secondary syphilis.

Rabbits may be infected by inoculation of the anterior chamber of the eye, and intratesticular inoculation or implantation produces orchitis. Intrascrotal inoculation produces a primary chancre, followed by generalized lesions characteristic of secondary syphilis. A generalized infection may be produced by intravenous inoculation of very young rabbits. The spirochetes remain alive indefinitely in the lymphatics and may be obtained by excision of a popliteal gland.

The rabbit has been the experimental animal of choice, and the reaction to intradermal inoculation has allowed the differentiation of strains of *Treponema* with respect to pathogenicity. A small inoculum suffices to infect, and multiplication occurs exponentially after 24 to 48 hours, with the production of a mass of microorganisms and a visible lesion. The generation time is estimated to be about 30 hours.

Immunity

The humoral immune response in treponematosis is twofold. The antibody-like activity, designated **reagin,** has wide diagnostic utility. It characteristically reacts in complement fixation and flocculation tests with nonspecific cardiolipin prepared from normal tissues, and its titer is correlated with the status of the clinical disease, disappearing when cure by chemotherapy is effected. The other is a **specific antibody** response to antigens present in the infecting spirochetes, demonstrable as spirochetal immobilization and other phenomena. A cellular immune response also develops and, in the rabbit, is apparently the protective response; available information in human infections indicates that the cellular immune response may be depressed as a consequence of treponemal infection. There appears to be no immunological difference between the spirochetes of venereal syphilis, nonvenereal syphilis, yaws, and pinta, and all of these diseases give positive reactions to the same diagnostic tests. *Treponema pallidum* shares common antigens with the Reiter biotype of *T. phage-*

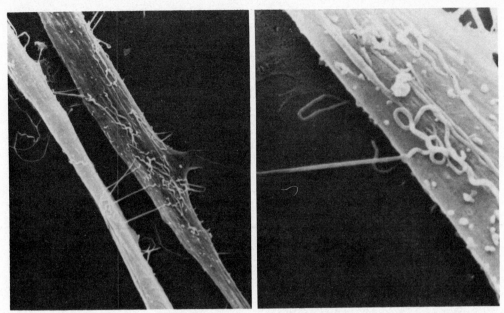

Figure 32–6. Scanning electron micrographs showing adherence of *Treponema pallidum* to rabbit testicular cells in tissue culture. *Left,* Single treponemes are shown attached by their terminal ends to host cell surfaces and bridging the gap between two testicular cells (× 3500). *Right,* Similar association of host and treponeme (× 11,200). (N. S. Hayes, *et al.,* Infect. Immun. **17**:174, 1977.)

denis, with *T. denticola,* and with *T. zuelzerae,* but they may be differentiated from one another by the use of absorption or blocking procedures, and by application of fluorescent antibody methods.

TREPONEMA PALLIDUM[15, 22, 23]

Syphilis[33]

Syphilis, by far the most intensively studied of the treponematoses, occurs in two forms— **venereal syphilis,** the best known, and **nonvenereal,** or **endemic, syphilis.** The two are epidemiologically distinct in that transmission is almost always sexual in the first instance, but in the second the infection is transmitted both by direct nonsexual contact and indirectly by the common use of eating and drinking utensils among children and adolescents. Consistent with this, the primary lesion is usually on the genitalia in venereal syphilis, but the first lesion in the childhood disease is on the oral mucous membranes.

The prevalence of syphilis is not known with certainty. The number of cases reported annually in the United States has shown wide fluctuation. It was highest in the early 1940s, but showed a steady decline until 1955, coincident with the application of penicillin therapy. The case rate increased again until it reached a more or less steady state in the early 1960s. Beginning in 1977, there has again been an increase in the case rate each year (Fig. 32–7). Congenital syphilis has declined markedly since 1950, and reached an all-time low in 1978. The trend in congenital syphilis expectedly follows the trend of primary and secondary syphilis in women (Fig. 32–7).

Two aspects of syphilis epidemiology are noteworthy. The first is the disproportionately high number of cases in homosexual and bisexual males. In the early 1970s, a study in England, Scotland, and Wales revealed that 42 per cent of males reported with primary and secondary syphilis were homosexual. A similar study in the United States in 1974 indicated that 34 per cent of males reported with syphilis were either homosexual or bisexual; in 1980 this figure had grown to 47 per cent.[32] The second feature of importance, and possibly related to the first, is the predominance of syphilis in urban areas. In 1981, large cities constituting 26 per cent of the population accounted for more than 61 per cent of the reported cases of syphilis.

The Disease in Man
Syphilis is a disease of protean manifestation, but it assumes relatively well-defined clinical stages. Congenital syphilis is best regarded separately.

Primary Stage. Following the penetration

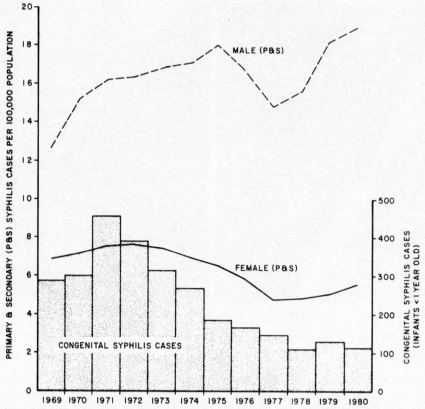

Figure 32–7. Primary and secondary syphilis case rates by sex and number of cases of congenital syphilis in the United States, 1969–1980. (Morbidity and Mortality Weekly Rep. **30**:441, 1981.)

of the skin or mucous membranes, *T. pallidum* rapidly invades tissues. The initial or primary lesion, which is clinically an ulcer, appears 10 to 30 days following infection. Often called the **Hunterian chancre,** after the author who first described it accurately, it is also called hard chancre or sore. It is indolent, has a hard floor, and is solitary if concurrent invasion by treponemas has not occurred in another locus. Treponemas may be demonstrated in the "serum" expressed from the chancre.

Although the primary stage may appear to be a localized infection, evidence from both rabbit and human infections indicate that dissemination of the treponemes begins almost immediately after entry; they appear in the draining lymph nodes in a very short time and are spread to other tissues within hours.

At the same time, the treponemes multiply at the point of entry, forming the characteristic chancre. Although early multiplication is without tissue damage, hemorrhage, vascular damage, and necrosis results within a few days, with accumulation of mucoid material in the chancre. This material is thought to be hyaluronic acid and chondroitin sulfate, and contributes to the morphology of the lesion. The chancre heals within a few weeks, but the disseminated infection continues.

Secondary Stage. The generalized nature of the syphilitic infection becomes apparent during this phase, which develops four to eight weeks after the appearance of the primary lesion but which may be delayed for a year or more, particularly in insufficiently treated patients. Cutaneous lesions of varied appearance and duration; bone, joint, and eye lesions; enlargement of the lymph nodes; and other phenomena occur. Treponemas are present in large numbers, not only in the lesions and mucous membranes but also in the blood, although they are difficult to demonstrate.

As in the primary stage, an effective immune response leads to healing of the lesions, but the spirochetes are not necessarily eliminated. The effectiveness of the immune response is indicated by the observation that only about one-fourth of patients develop secondary syphilis, and of these only about one-half progress to the tertiary stage.

Tertiary Stage. This stage may last for many years. Cutaneous ulcerations and gummatous lesions of the viscera develop. Their localization and extent determine the clinical symptomology, which may be quite unclear. Treponemas are present in tertiary lesions, but only in small numbers best demonstrated by silver impregnation methods.

Neurosyphilis.[20] This may develop during the third, or even second, stage. In most instances, however, neurosyphilis is a manifestation of late tertiary syphilis and was formerly termed quaternary or parasyphilitic disease. Tabes dorsalis and general paresis are the most frequent clinical forms. Treponemas may be found in the central nervous system.

Latent Syphilis. In some instances, the primary lesion is not noticed or is misdiagnosed, and, in addition, both primary and secondary stages may be overlooked. In other instances, latency develops after unusually severe primary and secondary symptoms, with a manifest state developing at a later time. Latency may, perhaps, be regarded as the result of a sustained or temporary biological balance between host and parasite.

Congenital Syphilis. Treponema may readily infect the fetus *in utero;* during the fifth month of pregnancy the placenta reaches a developmental stage that permits transmission of the spirochetes to the fetus. Syphilis may result in a cessation of the development of the fetus, premature birth of a dead fetus may take place, or the pregnancy may continue to term. Perinatal death due to syphilis is not a rare event. If the infant survives, it may or may not have manifest syphilis. Late congenital syphilis with clinical symptoms appearing as late as 10 to 20 years of age has been described. In many instances, however, the child is born with generalized syphilis and with lesions characteristic of the secondary state—treponemas are numerous in the affected organs in such instances. Third-generation congenital syphilis has been reported but is very rare.

Virulence

The virulence factors of *T. pallidum* are incompletely understood, and will probably remain so until the treponemes have been cultivated and can be studied without the interfering presence of host components.

Two virulence factors have been proposed. The first is a mucopolysaccharide surface component, or capsule, of *T. pallidum* that is believed to protect the cell from oxygen toxicity and from the deleterious effects of antibody against outer membrane components. The second is a mucopolysaccharidase that is said to be the bacterial receptor mediating adherence to host cells by interacting with hyaluronic acid on the host cell membrane. By virtue of its enzymatic activity, it also provides the treponeme with N-acetyl-D-glucosamine, which is utilized in synthesis of the capsular substance. The specificity of the adherence ligand is believed to account for the tissue and organ specificity observed in treponemal infection; its enzymatic activity would lead to degradation of the hyaluronic acid ground substance providing structural support for blood vessels, and result in the pathology of the syphilitic lesion.

Immunity[15, 29, 31]

At the present time syphilis is not so severe a disease in man as it was in the early sixteenth century. Whether this is an expression of an adaptive response on the part of man with the development of a low degree of natural immunity or a decrease in virulence of the spirochete, is not known; possibly both may have occurred.

In the immune response to syphilitic infection there is a marked apparent insusceptibility to reinfection; this is illustrated by the fact that a second chancre may be produced by reinfection prior to the appearance of the first chancre, but after the first chancre has appeared further reinfection does not produce another initial lesion. It is commonly stated that man, once infected, is refractory to reinfection and that reinfection occurs only very rarely. Immunity, therefore, superficially resembles that in tuberculosis and is similarly a manifestation of cell-mediated immunity. It is apparent, however, that the developed immunity is not completely protective in that elimination of the original infecting spirochetes does not always ensue. This may be due to suppression of cell-mediated immunity that is expressed in early stages of *T. pallidum* infection. Thus, delayed hypersensitivity manifest as a delayed-type skin reaction appears only in the later stages of disease.

Infection with *T. pallidum* also induces a humoral response, with the appearance in the serum of antilipoidal reagins as well as antibodies against specific *T. pallidum* antigens. The protective role of these antibodies is uncertain. Spirochetes are immobilized and killed by specific antibodies in the presence of complement, but passive immunization of rabbits with immune serum does not confer immunity to challenge, although the development of lesions is suppressed or delayed. It has been suggested that the mucopolysaccharide capsule, which is well developed *in vivo,* interferes with the action of bactericidal antibodies.

Serodiagnosis[2, 25]

Primary syphilis is generally diagnosed on a clinical basis, aided by the demonstration of spirochetes in chancre fluid by darkfield microscopy. However, the early primary lesion is usually painless, and if it occurs at sites other than the external genitalia, it may be overlooked. Furthermore, the chancre usually heals within a few weeks, even in untreated cases, and the individual may not seek medical aid. Nevertheless, the generalized spread of spirochetes is inexorable, even from the earliest stages of infection, and many untreated infections progress to later stages. Accurate diagnosis in these latter stages usually requires demonstration of the humoral immune response to the spirochetal infection—the serodiagnostic tests.

The humoral response is of two kinds, *vis.,* the appearance of reagins (not to be confused with the reagins of immediate hypersensitivity), and antibodies engendered against the specific antigenic substances present in the spirochete. The reaginic antibodies have been widely used for diagnostic purposes, employing the so-called nontreponemal serological tests. The specific, or treponemal, tests are now usually employed as confirmatory diagnostic aids to overcome the difficulties of nonspecificity associated with nontreponemal serology; they are not substitutes for these simpler procedures, however.

A complement-fixation test was proposed by Wassermann and his co-workers in 1906 as an immunologically specific reaction, using an aqueous extract of syphilitic fetus, containing large numbers of spirochetes, as the antigen. It was soon found, however, that the antigen in these extracts was not derived from the spirochetes, since extracts of normal tissue were equally reactive with syphilitic serums. Not long after the development of the Wassermann complement-fixation test, it was observed that syphilitic serums also produce a flocculation when mixed with Wassermann-type antigen.

The reactive substance present in tissue extracts has subsequently been found in a great variety of normal tissues and other biological materials. It has been identified as a phospholipid and given the name **cardiolipin,** since it is consistently present in beef heart muscle.

Reaginic antibodies are immunoglobulins that typically appear as a consequence of syphilitic infections (as well as other conditions) and react with cardiolipin in serological tests. Since they are not directed specifically against the spirochetes, their appearance was enigmatic until recently. It is now apparent that they are autoantibodies, engendered by infection but formed against components in mitochondrial membranes, probably cardiolipin. Diagnostic tests that utilize the cardiolipin antigen have long been known as reagin tests, but their designation as lipoidal antigen tests is gaining currency.

Types of Reagin Tests. Probably no serological reactions have been studied as intensively as the complement-fixation and precipitation tests for syphilis. The techniques have been modified and refined by many workers to increase sensitivity and specificity. Reaginic antibodies are not specific for syphilis, since they appear also in a number of other diseases, such as leprosy, malaria, and lupus erythematosus.

At the present time, the complement-fixation tests are rarely used in the United States because of their complexity and difficulties in standardization and control. Although many precipitation tests have been devised and used over the years, only a few are in common use today. Among these are the Venereal Disease Research Laboratory (VDRL) slide tests, the Rapid Plasma Reagin (RPR) card test, and the Automated Reagin Test (ART). The ART is most useful for screening large numbers of serums, but all are more or less equivalent in sensitivity.

Specific Treponemal Tests. Any serological test making use of spirochetal antigen, and thus having immunological specificity in the conventional sense, should be much more precise than lipoidal antigen tests. Antigen for specific treponemal tests is generally a suspension of the Nichols strain of *T. pallidum* prepared by extraction of infected rabbit testicular tissue. In the *T. pallidum* immobilization tests (TPI), living, motile spirochetes are specifically immobilized in the presence of antibody and complement under anaerobic conditions. The TPI test has been extensively applied and critically tested, and found to be highly specific. It is, however, technically complex and expensive; for these reasons, it has been largely supplanted by other specific treponemal tests.

Fluorescent treponemal antibody tests are now more generally used, particularly when combined with an absorption procedure to remove antibodies not specific to *T. pallidum*—the fluorescent treponemal antibody absorption (FTA–ABS) test. In this procedure, the patient's serum is absorbed with the cultivable Reiter strain of *T. phagedenis* to remove antibodies to shared and, therefore, nonspecific antigens. The absorbed serum is reacted with nonviable, Nichols strain *T. pallidum;* if the serum contains specific antibody, it reacts with antigens on the spirochetal surface and may be detected by the indirect fluorescent antibody technique, using labeled antihuman globulin. Although more complex than the reagin tests, the FTA–ABS test is highly satisfactory when carefully standardized and controlled.

More recently, a simple and inexpensive treponemal test has been devised—the treponemal hemagglutination (TPHA) test. In this procedure, tanned erythrocytes are sensitized with treponemal antigens derived from the Nichols strain. When these react with specific antibody to the spirochete antigens, the erythrocytes are agglutinated. The specificity may be improved by preliminary serum absorption with Reiter treponemes; for simplicity, the test has been adapted for microtitration. TPHA is as specific and sensitive as other specific antibody tests and may prove superior to cardiolipin tests for screening purposes.

The wide variety of serodiagnostic tests is an expression of the continuing search for a completely reliable test, but it is probable that no single test will suffice in the face of complications of therapy, biological false positive and negative reactions, and the like. The usual practice has been to employ the VDRL or TPHA test for screening purposes and to test reactive serums by FTA–ABS.

The Effect of Therapy. The specific treponemal tests often remain positive long after apparently effective chemotherapy. On the other hand, the majority of individuals undergoing therapy in time become serologically negative to the cardiolipin type of test, and this response is usually taken as an indication of the efficacy of treatment. The time required to attain negativity is variable and depends upon the individual; the stage of the disease; the course of therapy, especially if continuous or intermittent; and the sensitivity of the serological test used. No general statement of any precision is possible, therefore, but it is usually said that the majority of persons with primary or early secondary syphilis become negative within a few months after the usual therapeutic regimen. Others may remain positive for many months and a certain small proportion remain positive indefinitely. The last is spoken of as Wassermann-fast, reagin-fast, or seroresistant syphilis. Seroresistance is generally believed to indicate a failure to completely eradicate the spirochetes in persistent foci of infection.

Specificity and False Reactions. The presence of insufficient antibody accounts for many false-negative reactions and occurs in several stages of the disease, especially in early primary syphilis (a positive reaction usually does not develop until two to three weeks after infection) and late syphilis which is latent or localized. Particular problems are posed by neurosyphilis and ocular syphilis, in which negative serological tests are frequent despite the presence of treponemas in the infected organs.

False-positive reactions may be a result of technical error or may be biological in nature. When reaginic serodiagnostic tests are employed, a certain proportion of individuals that are nonsyphilitic, but suffering from other infections, give positive tests. For example, it is reported that 4 to 10 per cent of cases of malaria are positive. *Brucella* infection and other febrile diseases occasionally produce isolated or repeated positive reactions, as do the collagen diseases.

False reactions occur less commonly with the specific tests using treponema or treponemal antigen. The specific treponemal tests, as well as those employing cardiolipin, are, however, almost always positive in other treponematoses. Because of their specificity, the treponemal tests have their greatest utility when the technically simpler cardiolipin reactions give equivocal results.

Chemotherapy[42]

The chemotherapy of syphilis, like that of tuberculosis, has been of great interest for many years. The use of arsenicals in syphilis was one of the earliest examples of infectious disease chemotherapy. Penicillin, to which the spirochetes are exquisitely sensitive, was first used in human infections in 1943 and remains today as the treatment of choice. The efficacy of penicillin therapy is, however, dependent upon the stage and nature of the disease and the dose/time relationship. Primary syphilis, in which relatively few treponemes are present, is most amenable to therapy. In later stages, the disease is more refractory and dose/time relationships are increasingly important. As related in Chapter 5, penicillin acts upon growing bacterial cells by interference with the synthesis of peptidoglycans in the cell wall. Thus, penicillin therapy in syphilis requires adequate serum levels of penicillin for prolonged periods because of the long generation time (30 to 33 hours) of the spirochetes. These levels are most easily attained by the use of repository or long-acting penicillin, such as procaine penicillin G in aqueous or oil suspension. In both primary and secondary syphilis, penicillin treatment is almost always successful; in late syphilis, the success rate is somewhat diminished and requires increased doses of antibiotic. So far as can be established, however, *T. pallidum* has not developed resistance to penicillin during several decades of therapeutic use.

One of the consequences of chemotherapy in syphilis is the occurrence of the **Jarisch-Herxheimer reaction.** Although not usually serious, symptoms of toxicity are observed in 50 to 80 per cent of the cases of primary syphilis treated with antibiotics or arsenicals. The reaction is very rarely encountered, however, during treatment of late syphilis. Toxicity is believed due to the drug-induced lysis of large numbers of spirochetes, with release of toxic substances, possibly lipopolysaccharides of the outer sheath.

Penicillin therapy is sometimes contraindicated because of individual hypersensitivity to the drug. In such cases, the alternative drugs include the broad-spectrum antibiotics, such as the tetracyclines and erythromycin. These have been used with generally satisfactory results, and their efficacy is close to that of penicillin.

NONVENEREAL SYPHILIS[33]

Nonvenereal or endemic syphilis (also known as bejel) occurs in foci in many parts of the world under various local names. It occurs in Southeast Asia, in Africa, and with some frequency in eastern Europe (Fig. 32–8). In the last area, prior to mass treatment under WHO auspices, patients with the disease made up as much as 5 per cent of the population, but recent surveys indicate that active infections have been almost eradicated.[17]

The disease is an epidemiological rather than clinical entity, occurring, as indicated earlier, largely in children and within families. There appears to be little or no basis for separating the diseases occurring in widely separated foci from one another or from venereal syphilis.

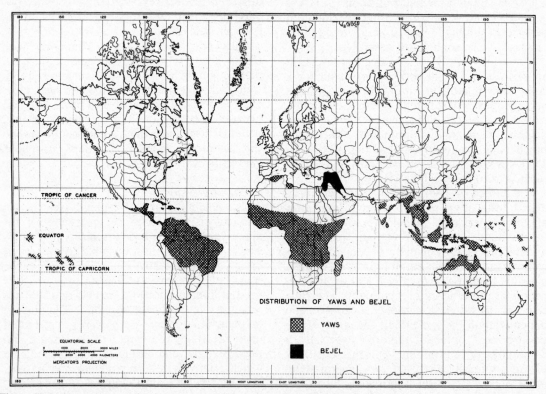

Figure 32–8. The world-wide distribution of yaws and nonvenereal syphilis (bejel). (Redrawn from map prepared by Army Medical Intelligence. Based on Goode *Base Map* No. 201M. By permission of the University of Chicago Press.)

Clinical differences between venereal and non-venereal syphilis, *viz.*, the relative rarity of primary lesions and congenital manifestations in the latter, seem to be a consequence of the mode of transmission and age distribution of the disease rather than of differences in the pathogenicity of the causative microorganism.

The first manifestations of the infection are most commonly mucous patches in the mouth; skin lesions also occur and include anogenital condylomata. The oral and skin lesions show the presence of spirochetes upon darkfield examination, as do the lesions found on the nipples of mothers infected by their children. In most individuals latency occurs after the early stages, with subsequent development of tegumentary lesions, including gummatous destruction of the skeleton, which are indistinguishable from those of venereal syphilis. The causative microorganism is *T. pallidum*, and the disease is effectively treated with repository penicillin.

TREPONEMA PERTENUE

YAWS[21, 33]

Yaws, or frambesia tropica, is a tropical disease found in the West Indies, tropical Americas, equatorial Africa, the Pacific Islands, and some tropical regions of the Far East (Fig. 32–8). The incidence may be as high as 5 to 20 per cent. It is prevalent in rural rather than urban areas and associated with low economic status. Primary infection is more common in children than in adults. The causative agent is *T. pertenue* (Fig. 32–9), which was described by Castellani in 1905.

The spirochete is found in the serous exudate of the cutaneous lesions and in the lymphatics. It may be demonstrated in Giemsa-stained smears or by darkfield examination of fresh preparations and is morphologically indistinguishable from *T. pallidum*.

The disease in man is characterized by a papular eruption. The prevailing site of infection is the lower leg and foot. A general malaise precedes the appearance of the initial lesion, which is practically always extragenital and takes the form of a single papule or a small group of them. The papule enlarges to a diameter of 3 to 4 mm., the thickened epidermis cracks, and the fungoid mass beneath exudes a seropurulent fluid. The mass enlarges to 3 to 5 cm. in diameter and the lesion is termed a yaw. When the infection occurs on the sole of the foot, it is known as crab yaws or wet crab yaws. It eventually dries, leaving only a scar. Six weeks to three months after the primary lesion appears, a secondary eruption occurs which is similarly preceded by a general malaise. The lesions are of the same general character as the primary lesion, appearing on the extremities and neck, and at the juncture of the skin and mucous membrane about the nose, mouth, and anus. Tertiary lesions similar to those of syphilis are said to be rare. The serological tests for syphilis are positive, and in some endemic areas, such as New Guinea, where the incidence is particularly high, up to 75 per cent of the population show positive TPI tests.[16] In certain stages, as in late secondary eruption, differential diagnosis may be very difficult.

Yaws has been produced by inoculation of monkeys and rabbits. The infection in rabbits with *T. pertenue* is similar to that with *T. pallidum,* but relatively few spirochetes are found in the lesions, multiplication is arrested early, and the inflammatory reaction is slight.

The human disease is seldom venereal, and the most common mode of transmission is contact between individuals. Trauma of the skin usually precedes infection, and the ability of the spirochete to penetrate the intact skin is questionable; biting flies may also transmit the disease.

Yaws is successfully treated with penicillin, and the tetracyclines may also be effective. The change to seronegativity is usually not as rapid as in effectively treated syphilis, possibly because the disease is usually of longer standing.

The eradication of yaws is an achievable public health goal. Mass treatment campaigns in the Western Hemisphere have effectively reduced the number of cases so that yaws is a public health problem only in a few areas; similar findings obtain in other endemic areas, but the disease has shown recrudescence when public health surveillance has been relaxed.

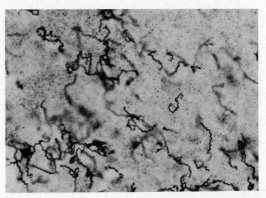

Figure 32–9. *Treponema pertenue* in biopsy specimen. Krajian-Erskine silver impregnation stain.

The relationship of yaws to syphilis is very close, the points of difference being the non-venereal transmission of yaws, the differences between the yaw and the indurated Hunterian chancre, and the relative infrequency of visceral and tertiary lesions. Yaws is regarded by many as a tropical type of syphilis, differing from endemic syphilis as a result of environmental factors. There is evidence of cross-immunity between syphilis and yaws in that the two diseases tend to be mutually exclusive.

TREPONEMA CARATEUM

Pinta

Pinta, known in Mexico as "mal de pinto" and in Colombia as "carate," is clinically a skin disease in which dyschromic changes occur in patches, which may be discrete and small or large and confluent. In color they are gray, bluish gray, or pinkish; eventually they become white. The disease has long been confined to the Western Hemisphere, but due to mass treatment campaigns in the endemic areas, it is now found only in a few areas in Mexico, Central America, and Colombia.

Etiology

For many years this disease was of uncertain etiology. Herrejon suggested in 1927 that the disease was caused by a spirochete, but it was not until 1938 that spirochetes were first demonstrated. The spirochete is widely, but not universally, known as *Treponema carateum*.

The spirochetes are found in material taken from early cutaneous lesions and in that aspirated from lymph nodes. *Treponema carateum* stains with Giemsa and by the usual silver impregnation methods used for *T. pallidum* (Fig. 32–10) and may be found by darkfield examination of fresh material. Morphologically it is indistinguishable from the spirochete of syphilis, and the serological tests of syphilis, both lipoidal and treponemal, are generally positive in pinta. Attempts to cultivate *T. carateum* have failed, but chimpanzees have been successfully infected; the histopathology of the lesions is remarkably similar to that of the human disease. The experimental disease in human volunteers also has been studied in considerable detail.

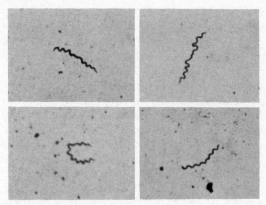

Figure 32–10. Various forms of *Treponema carateum*. Krajian-Erskine silver impregnation stain.

The Disease in Man

In the experimental infection the incubation period is from 7 to 20 days, with the initial lesion being a papule which appears at the site of inoculation. During the primary stage of the disease, the papule spreads peripherally to form a squamous, erythematous patch reaching a diameter of 1 cm. in four or five weeks. It continues to spread, varying considerably in appearance, and may be lichenoid or psoriasiform. There is less inflammatory reaction than in either syphilis or yaws. In about five months the secondary stage begins with the appearance of secondary lesions, occurring about the initial papules and elsewhere on the body. Progressive hyperpigmentation occurs, and depigmentation, resulting in varied hues, follows in the third stage; keratosis and superifical atrophoderma become apparent. The lipoidal antigen tests are almost always negative in the primary stage, positive in something over half the cases in the secondary stage, and practically always positive in the tertiary stage. Correspondingly, superinfection is readily produced in the first stage but not in the third stage; syphilitic individuals may be infected without difficulty. Pinta may be successfully treated with penicillin.

Transmission

Experimental human infections have shown that serous fluid from the early lesion is highly infectious when placed on abraded skin. Contact infection appears to be a likely mode of spread, but flies have been suspected of transmitting the disease.

Leptospira and Leptospirosis[9, 19, 22, 23, 41]

Leptospirosis is the name applied to infections caused by the immunologically heterogeneous spirochetes of the genus *Leptospira*. Although the leptospiroses have been assigned a variety of names related to geographical distribution and differ somewhat in their clinical manfestations, they are probably best considered as a single clinical disease. The pathogenic leptospira are contained in the genus *Leptospira interrogans,* along with saprophytic varieties. The latter are usually referred to as *Leptospira biflexa,* although the Bergey classification recognizes only the single species. The parasitic *L. interrogans, i.e.,* those responsible for leptospirosis, are divided into several serological groups and these are, in turn, separated into serotypes.

Morphology

Leptospira differ from *Treponema* and *Borrelia* species in that their spirals are very fine and close, one or both ends of the cell may be hooked, and the individual cells are smaller. They are usually less than 0.3 μm. in breadth and 6 to 10 μm. in length, although exceptional forms as long as 25 to 30 μm. may be observed. The axial filament is applied along one side of the tightly coiled protoplasmic cylinder and enclosed by the outer membrane. A slime layer is often adherent to the external surface of the outer membrane. The axial filament is composed of two axial fibrils, each attached subterminally at opposite ends of the cylinder. The outer membrane is thick and almost transparent and appears in the darkfield as a narrow clear zone or halo and, in certain stained preparations, as a grayish or unstained halo. Representative morphology of leptospira is illustrated in Figure 32–11. The mechanism of locomotion is more complex than in the treponemas; the hooked ends of the cell are probably involved and they appear to rotate while the body of the cell remains stationary. The small diameter and active motility of *Leptospira* allow penetration of bacteriological filters; thus, contaminated materials are often filtered before primary isolation to separate the leptospires from other bacteria.

Cultivation

The *Leptospira* are the most **readily cultivable** of the spirochetes; most may be grown in mediums containing peptone and beef extract, supplemented with 10 per cent sterile rabbit serum, or serum albumin and fatty acids. For blood culture, one or two drops of blood are

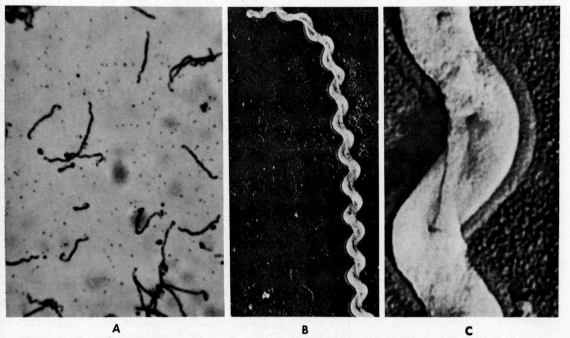

A **B** **C**

Figure 32–11. Leptospira morphology. *A,* Conventional stained smear of Leptospira, serogroup Pomona. *B, C,* Electron micrographs of chromium-shadowed spray preparations of Leptospira, serogroup Icterohaemorrhagiae. *B,* × 12,500; *C,* × 125,000. (C. F. Simpson and F. H. White, Electron microscope studies and staining reactions of leptospires. J. Infect. Dis. **109**:243, 1961.)

generally added to 5 ml. of medium and incubated for as long as 28 days; larger amounts of blood may be inhibitory. *Leptospira* are obligately aerobic, with an optimum growth temperature of 30° C. Many of the parasitic strains have been cultivated on chemically defined mediums. *Leptospira* require long-chain fatty acids, which provide both energy and carbon sources for growth; thiamin and vitamin B_{12} are also required. Those tested do not ferment sugars and are indifferent to the presence of carbohydrates in the medium. A number of cultural properties allow the differentiation of most pathogenic and nonpathogenic strains. The former are frequently hemolytic, oxidase-positive, and are not inhibited by 5-fluorouracil or 8-azaguanine. The two groups also differ in nutritive requirements, susceptibility to copper sulfate, and ability to grow in CO_2-free air and in the presence of aniline dyes.

When leptospira are grown on the surface of appropriate solid mediums, two different colony types are apparent. One type produces a small, relatively opaque colony, while the other forms a larger translucent colony ranging from 1 to 4 mm. in diameter.

Cultures are maintained in liquid or soft agar mediums, usually covered with a thin layer of paraffin oil to retard evaporation. The cultures are incubated at 28° to 30° C. for one to two weeks, during which time leptospiral growth appears as a band of turbidity a few millimeters below the surface. They may be preserved by ultrafreezing, but not by storage at −20° C. or by lyophilization.

Antigenic Structure

The leptospira are excellent antigens; agglutinating, lytic, and complement-fixing antibody is produced to high titer and persists in recovered individuals, thus allowing diagnosis of past infection. The serogroups of pathogenic *L. interrogans* are differentiable and are characterized on an immunological basis by agglutination reactions and the serotypes by cross-agglutinin absorption.

Both serogroups and serotypes have been given place or descriptive names, implying species rank, but no formal classification within this group is firmly established. Eighteen serogroups have been proposed, with more than 180 serotypes. For example, serogroup Icterohaemorrhagiae includes 18 serotypes, serogroup Canicola has 10 serotypes, and so on; new types are constantly reported and added to the list. Serotypes responsible for human infection in the United States include *copenhagen, canicola, pomona, autumnalis, grippotyphosa, wolffi, djatzi,* and *patoc.*[1]

These immunological forms appear to be quite stable, although antigenic changes can be produced by cultivation in antiserum. There are minor cross-reactions with some other microorganisms, notably *Shigella.* Immunity to experimental infection is largely group-specific, with only occasional cross-protection between groups.

Pathogenicity

The pathogenic leptospirae are parasites of lower animals, including wild rodents and a variety of domestic animals. Of the latter, pigs, dogs, and, in some areas, cattle, are probably the most important quantitatively. Unlike *Borrelia,* they are not primarily blood parasites, although they may be found in the blood as early as the first day and perhaps as late as the fourteenth day of the disease. Characteristically, the leptospira localize in the kidneys and are excreted in the urine.

Human infection is acquired from lower animals by contact with infectious urine or water contaminated with infected urine, or by direct contact with infected tissue. In the first instance, the source of infection is most often rodents, dogs, swine, or cattle; outbreaks often have a common source, such as contaminated water, and the microorganisms usually enter the host through abraded skin. In the second, domestic animals, especially swine and cattle, serve as a source of infection for slaughterhouse workers, veterinarians, herdsmen, and the like.

Leptospiral infections in man are all closely similar and are characterized by a febrile reaction; anemia; jaundice, which may be generalized or confined to the sclera; hemorrhage; and infection of the kidneys, causing acute nephritis and, later, chronic lesions. **Weil's disease** or **infectious jaundice,** is the classic example of leptospirosis and has been known for many years.

Infections with leptospira are much more common than has been generally realized. In many instances these are acquired through contact with mice and other infected rodents, and, since the infection often occurs in connection with work in cultivated fields and similar rural areas, the disease is variously known as swamp fever, field fever, harvest fever, and the like. Leptospirosis is given place names also, such as Mossman fever and Pomona fever, but infection is much more widespread than this would suggest.

Recovery from the disease is accompanied

by the appearance of specific antibody and the development of effective immunity. Prophylactic inoculation with leptospiral vaccines has been applied for many years in both man and animals. Two or more serogroup strains are generally included and protection is elicited against the disease entity, but not against infection *per se*. Whether or not this protection is associated with agglutinating antibodies is not clear.

Laboratory Diagnosis[1]

The laboratory diagnosis of leptospirosis is based upon detection and isolation of the infecting microorganisms and upon the immune response to the infection. In man the bacteria may be isolated from the blood early in the disease by culture or by inoculation of young guinea pigs or weanling hamsters. The experimental animal infection may be substantiated by demonstration of the leptospira in the tissues, especially in the kidney, but, in general, animal inoculation gives a smaller proportion of positive results than does culture.

The immune response is assayed as leptospiral agglutination (observed with the dark-field microscope), as lysis in the presence of complement, or by complement-fixation tests. The agglutination-lysis titers range from 1:400 to 1:100,000, and the complement-fixation titers from 1:32 to 1:256. A fourfold or greater rise in antibody titer in paired serums is regarded as diagnostic, but in some portion of cases, demonstrable antibody is not present. The immune response in infection is ordinarily of sufficiently broad specificity that the serological identity of the infecting microorganism is not deducible from it, and for precise identification the leptospira must be cultured and typed serologically.

Chemotherapy

Penicillin, the tetracyclines, and erythromycin are somewhat effective in the early stages of experimental infections, and the last two, as well as streptomycin, may have some effect on the kidney infection. In general, chemotherapy of human leptospiral infections has been disappointing.

HUMAN LEPTOSPIROSIS[26]

The causative agent of infectious jaundice in man was first isolated in Japan in 1914 and in Germany in the following year. In the ensuing years, *Leptospira* have been found in all parts of the world as the causative agent of febrile illnesses, some of which are characterized by jaundice. The etiological agents of these diseases are considered to be serologically distinct groups of *L. interrogans*. Table 32–3 lists these leptospiral diseases, their distribution, and their reservoir hosts. The more severe infections, in which jaundice is usually seen, are most often caused by members of serotype *icterohaemorrhagiae*, and are of worldwide distribution.

Geographical separation of the leptospiroses is obviously not sound, for some serogroups are encountered in widely separated regions and diseases given different names are caused by *Leptospira* of the same immunological group.

In the United States, the disease is relatively rare. There have been fewer than 100 cases per year reported since 1967, but it is probably underdiagnosed. The microorganisms most often found have been those of serogroups Icterohaemorrhagiae, Canicola, and Autumnalis.

The Disease in Man

The incubation period is 6 to 12 days, and the high initial fever is followed by nausea, vomiting, epistaxis, headache, and muscular pains, and there may be moderately severe bronchitis. Jaundice, or Weil's syndrome, characterizes the more severe infections, particularly with serotype *icterohaemorrhagiae*, but is seen in less than half of the cases. Convalescence is slow, and weakness may persist for months.

The leptospira are distributed throughout the body in the first week of illness and may be demonstrated by inoculating guinea pigs with blood, but are rarely seen by microscopy. After the first week they are present in the urine and may continue to be excreted for four to five weeks. There is some evidence that the case fatality is reduced by treatment with antiserum. In fatal cases death usually occurs during the second or third week, but occasionally as early as the end of the first week. The case-fatality rate is variable; it has varied from 4.6 to 32 per cent in Japan and has been about 10 per cent in the Netherlands and as high as 25 per cent in Scotland. At autopsy the leptospira are found in almost all the organs and tissues in those dying during the initial febrile stage; if death occurs in the second week or later, they are rarely found elsewhere than in the kidneys. Acute renal failure is the most common immediate cause of death.

Immunity

Recovery from the disease is accompanied by the development of a solid immunity, and a specific lysin is present in the blood which persists in detectable amounts for several

Table 32–3. **The More Important Leptospiroses***

Serogroup	Disease in Man	Important Animal Reservoirs	Infections in Other Animals	Geographical Distribution
Icterohaemorrhagiae	Weil's disease	*Rattus norvegicus*, other rodent species	Dog, pig, cattle, horse	Worldwide
Canicola	Canicola fever	Dog	Pig, cattle	Worldwide
Pomona	Pomona fever, swineherd's disease	Pig, cattle, *Mus musculus, Apodemus agrarius*	Dog, horse, opossum, raccoon, skunk, wildcat	Worldwide
Grippotyphosa	Mud fever, Schlammfieber, field fever	*Microtus arvalis, Evotomys glareolus, Cricetus* spp., *Apodemus sylvaticus*	Cattle, horse, dog, raccoon, goat	Worldwide
Autumnalis (Akiyami A)	Hasami fever, Fort Bragg fever	*Microtus montebelli, Apodemus speciosus, Bandicoota* spp.	Dog, opossum, raccoon, cattle	S.E. Asia, Japan, U.S.
Bataviae	Indonesian Weil's disease, rice-field fever	*Rattus norvegicus, Micromys minutus, Rattus rattus*	Dog, cat	S.E. Asia, Europe, Africa, Japan
Australis A (Ballico)	Cane-field fever	*Rattus conatus, Apodemus flavicollis, Rattus rattus culmorum*	Dog, cattle, raccoon, opossum, hedgehog	Australia, U.S., Europe, S.E. Asia, Japan
Australis B	Cane-field fever	*Rattus rattus, Isoodon* spp.	–	Australia, S.E. Asia, Europe
Sejroe	Feldfieber B	*Mus musculus, Apodemus sylvaticus, Apodemus agrarius, Microtus* spp.	Cattle (?), dog, pig	Europe, U.S. (?)
Hebdomadis	Nanukayami Akiyami B, seven-day fever	*Microtus montebelli*	Dog, cattle	Japan
Pyrogenes	Leptospirosis febrilis	*Rattus rattus, Rattus brevicaudatus*	–	S.E. Asia, Japan
Ballum	–	*Mus musculus*, opossum	*Rattus norvegicus*, skunk, raccoon, wildcat, pig	U.S., Europe, Israel
Hyos (Mitis)	Swineherd's disease	Pig	Cattle	U.S., Europe, Australia, South America, New Zealand

*Compiled by Colonel M. B. Starnes, Walter Reed Army Medical Center.

years. Agglutinins appear in the convalescent stage, sometimes to very high titer, but the relation of demonstrable antibody and effective immunity is far from clear. Prophylactic inoculation has given encouraging results.

Transmission

The animal reservoir of infection is related to geographical distribution of the disease and the serogroup involved. Rodents are important reservoirs in most parts of the world, but are not the primary reservoir in the United States, being replaced by dogs and domestic animals, such as swine and cattle. Reservoirs of infection also occur in wild animals such as skunks, raccoons, mongooses, muskrats, opossums, and nutrias, as shown by both serological evidence and the isolation and identification of leptospira. The animal infections may be detected by darkfield examination of urine and kidney emulsion, by culture, or by animal inoculation.

The leptospira are discharged in the urine of infected animals and are transmitted to man via stagnant water contaminated with urine. The disease is to some extent occupationally related, occurring in field and farm workers, coal miners, sewer workers, and others in contact with contaminated water. There is evidence, however, that occupational relationships, at least in the United States, are waning; a significant proportion of the cases occur in children, students, and housewives and are often avocationally related, as among swimmers. The manner in which the spirochetes enter the body is not known, but very possibly it is through minute cuts and abrasions in the skin or via the alimentary tract after ingestion.

Lyme Disease[37, 39]

A skin disorder termed **erythema chronicum migrans,** characterized by a small annular papule expanding centrifugally to exhibit a wide border with central clearing, was first observed in Europe in 1908. It was subsequently reported throughout Europe and in the United States in 1970. During this time the etiology of the disease was not known, although evidence suggested an infectious agent transmitted by certain ticks.

In 1975, a cluster of cases appeared in southeastern Connecticut, centering in the community of Lyme, Connecticut. Intensive investigation of this outbreak led to the recognition of Lyme disease, or Lyme arthritis, a multisystem disorder that usually begins with the unique skin lesions of erythema chronicum migrans and is later followed by joint, neurological, and cardiac manifestations. The disease is linked to the bite of **ixodid ticks** and has been observed in Europe, the United States, and Australia.

Etiological Agent[3, 4, 8, 40]

Both the skin lesions of erythema chronicum migrans and the later manifestations of Lyme disease appear to be due to a **cultivable spirochete,** transmitted by *Ixodes* ticks and possibly by mosquitos in some localities.

Spirochetes have been isolated from human cases of disease and from *Ixodes* ticks, mice, raccoons, and deer. The isolates are all closely similar in cultural requirements, morphology, and antigenic makeup. The spirochetes are morphologically similar to *Treponema.* Cells are irregularly coiled with tapered ends and possess 6 to 8 axial fibrils located beneath the outer membrane; the cell diameter is about 0.2 μm. and ranges from 4 to 30 μm. in length. Cellular morphology of spirochetes isolated from *Ixodes* ticks is shown in Figure 32–12.

Growth of the spirochete is accomplished on cell-free, complex mediums, such as modified Kelly's medium containing peptones, gelatin, bovine serum, rabbit serum, and other supplements. The spirochete has been successfully cultivated from blood and skin lesions of patients with Lyme disease, although recovery sometimes has required one or more blind passages in the medium. Growth is demonstrated by darkfield microscopy of the culture fluid; the generation time of the spirochete is about 12 hours. Immunological studies have demonstrated that the spirochetes isolated from infected individuals, ticks, and small mammals are antigenically similar, but are not immunologically related to other well-known pathogenic spirochetes of the genera *Borrelia, Treponema,* or *Leptospira.* A classification for these new microorganisms has not yet been established.

The Disease in Man

It has been noted that the skin disease erythema chronicum migrans, or ECM, was first observed in Europe and has been reported from Scandinavia, Russia, and the United States. The lesion usually appears weeks or months following the bite of ticks, beginning as a papule that expands to form a red ring up to 30 cm. in diameter; the central portion often clears, but concentric rings may also form within the original ring. Multiple lesions sometimes occur and are thought to be attributable to multiple tick bites. The skin lesions may be accompanied by fever, headache, fatigue, and regional adenopathy. Some patients subsequently exhibit meningitis and peripheral neuropathy.

Prior to 1975, there were no reports that ECM was followed by arthritis and cardiac abnormalities. The outbreak that occurred in Lyme and nearby communities was characterized by brief but recurring episodes of asymmetric oligoarticular swelling and pain in the large joints, particularly the knee; about 25 per cent of the patients reported antecedant ECM. A few patients also develop cardiac

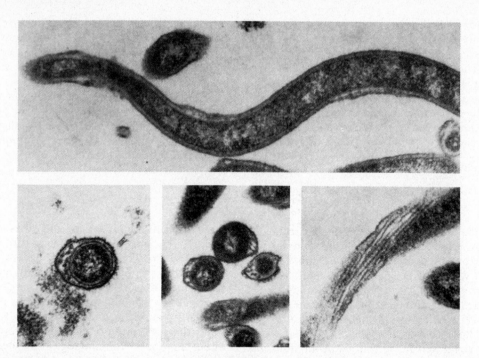

Figure 32–12. The morphology of the *Ixodes* spirochete. Note the several axial fibrils located between the cell wall and outer membrane. (A. C. Steere, *et al.,* New Engl. J. Med. **308**:733, 1983.) (Reprinted by permission of the New England Journal of Medicine.)

abnormalities, commonly atrioventricular block. Thus, Lyme disease typically begins with ECM and is followed by arthritis and, sometimes, carditis. Some of these manifestations are thought to be due to immune-complex injury. Most cases of Lyme disease have been reported in the United States, but a few cases have been recorded in Europe and Australia.

The putative etiological agent of both ECM and Lyme arthritis is the spirochete described above. The spirochete has been observed in some, but not all, patients; it has been cultivated in the laboratory; and an experimental disease resembling ECM has been produced by inoculation of rabbits. Further, antibodies are produced in patients with Lyme disease that react specifically with the cultured spirochetes. Thus most of the requirements of Koch's postulates have been satisfied.

Epidemiology[5, 36]

The distribution of ECM and Lyme disease is apparently determined by the occurrence of infected arthropod vectors.

The European vector appears to be ticks of the *Ixodes ricinus* complex. These ticks inhabit most areas where ECM is endemic, and studies in one area of Switzerland have shown that as many as 36 per cent of collected ticks harbor

the spirochete. Further, there is evidence for transovarial infection of tick progeny. Experimental studies have also shown that infected *I. ricinus* can transmit the infection to rabbits. Since ECM has been reported from areas of Scandinavia that do not have ticks, it is likely that other vectors can also transmit the disease; mosquitos are likely candidates.

In the United States, the responsible vectors for the spirochete appear to be *Ixodes dammini* and *I. pacificus*. Three distinct foci of the disease are noted in this country: along the northeastern coast from Massachusetts to Maryland, in Wisconsin, and in California and Oregon. The distribution of Lyme disease in the northeast and central regions correlates with that of the tick *I. dammini,* while disease in the western region correlates with the ranges of *I. pacificus*. Both of these tick species are members of the *Ixodes ricinus* complex. As in the case of the European vector, the spirochete may be transovarially passed to the offspring.

Ixodes dammini is naturally infected with the spirochetal agent of Lyme disease. In several surveys of tick populations in the northeastern United States, the proportion of infected ticks has ranged from 19 to 61 per cent. It has also been proposed that small mammals may serve as reservoir hosts for the spirochete. Both white-footed mice and white-tailed deer are known to be naturally infected with the spirochete, and *I. dammini* can become infected by feeding on these animals.

Chemotherapy[38]

Although the number of cases treated has not been large, several antibiotics appear to be effective in treatment of erythema chronicum migrans. The skin lesion usually resolves within 3 to 10 days after initiation of penicillin therapy. Tetracyclines appear to have similar efficacy, and erythromycin somewhat less.

The efficacy of antibiotic therapy for subsequent disease states—carditis, neuropathy, and arthritis—is somewhat less clear. In some cases, oral penicillin G appears to prevent or attenuate the arthritis; in the other disease states, response to antibiotic therapy has been disappointing. These results are perhaps to be expected if the late manifestations are due to immune complex formation.

Spirillum minor and Rat-Bite Fever[34]

There are two distinct kinds of disease which may follow the bite of rats; both are designated rat-bite fever. One, *Streptobacillus moniliformis* infection, is discussed elsewhere (Chapter 26). The other, known in Japan as "sodoku," is caused by a spiral microorganism, first discovered in 1916.

The spiral microorganism of rat-bite fever (Fig. 32–13) was originally assigned to the *Spirochaeta*, but it is currently known as *Spirillum minor*. It is not cultivable in artificial mediums and is shorter than the recognized spirochetes (0.2 to 0.5 μm. by 2 to 5 μm.); is relatively rigid; and possesses polar tufts of external flagella that give it a rapid darting motion, unlike the flexible undulating movements of spirochetes.

Following the bite of an infected rat, the original wound heals, but after an incubation period of 10 to 22 days, the area becomes inflamed and painful. Fever, swelling of the lymph glands, skin eruptions, and other symptoms occur. The fever is of the relapsing type, with paroxysms at fairly regular intervals, usually about once a week, which continue to recur for one to three months or longer. The case-fatality rate varies from 2 to 10 per cent.

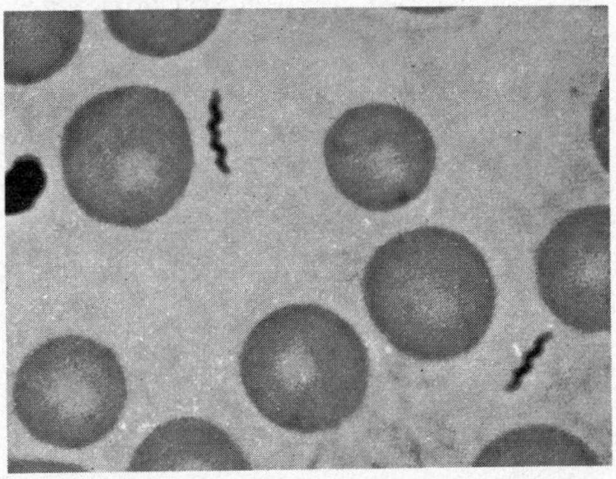

Spirillum minor has been found in the swollen local lesions of the skin and the enlarged lymph glands and, rarely, in the circulating blood. Guinea pigs and mice may be infected by the inoculation of blood or fluid expressed from the local lesions. Rats are not the only vector of the infection, for cases of what is apparently the same disease have been traced to bites of other wild rodents, cats, dogs, and pigs.

The disease has long been known in Japan and has been reported from many localities all over the world, with a few cases observed in the United States. What proportion of the earlier reported cases were *Streptobacillus* infections is, of course, unknown. Of 40 cases reported from 1931 to 1940, the spirillum was demonstrated by animal inoculation in 17; of these, 11 resulted from rat bite and the remainder had a history of mouse bite, cat bite or scratch, contact with dogs, or trauma without known animal contact. There is little doubt that the affection is more common than appears from the records, for cases occur sporadically and their true nature has probably gone unrecognized.

Not a great deal is known of the immune response to infection other than that a spirillicidal antibody is produced that is also responsible for immobilization of the spirilla in immune serum. A positive Weil-Felix reaction of the OX–K type (Chapter 33) is produced in experimental animals, but the antigen shared with these strains of *Proteus* is distinct from that responsible for the spirillicidal antibody.

Arsenicals have been used chemotherapeutically in the past, and the bacteria are sensitive to penicillin and the broad-spectrum antibiotics; penicillin-tetracycline therapy was found to be highly effective in one instance.

Figure 32–13. *Spirillum minor* in blood of an inoculated mouse. (Van Sandt.)

References

1. Alexander, A. D. 1980. *Leptospira.* pp. 376–382. *In* E. H. Lennette, *et al.* (Eds.): Manual of Clinical Microbiology. 3rd ed. American Society for Microbiology, Washington, D.C.

2. Balows, A., J. C. Feeley, and H. W. Jaffe. 1976. Laboratory diagnosis of treponematoses (with emphasis on syphilis). pp. 201–208. *In* R. C. Johnson (Ed.): The Biology of Parasitic Spirochetes. Academic Press, New York.

3. Barbour, A. G., S. L. Tessier, and W. J. Todd. 1983. Lyme disease spirochetes and ixodid tick spirochetes share a common antigenic determinant defined by a monoclonal antibody. Infect. Immun. **41**:795–804.

4. Benach, J. L., *et al.* 1983. Spirochetes isolated from the blood of two patients with Lyme disease. New Engl. J. Med. **308**:740–742.

5. Bosler, E. M., *et al.* 1983. Natural distribution of the *Ixodes dammini* spirochete. Science **220**:321–322.

6. Boyer, K. M., *et al.* 1977. Tick-borne relapsing fever: an interstate outbreak originating at Grand Canyon National Park. Amer. J. Epidemiol. **105**:469–479.

7. Burgdorfer, W. 1980. *Borrelia.* pp. 383–388. *In* E. H. Lennette, *et al.* (Eds.): Manual of Clinical Microbiology. 3rd ed. American Society for Microbiology, Washington, D.C.

8. Burgdorfer, W., *et al.* 1983. Erythema chronicum migrans—a tickborne spirochetosis. Acta Tropica **40**:79–83.

9. Canale-Parola, E. 1977. Physiology and evolution of spirochetes. Bacteriol. Rev. **41**:181–204.

10. Felsenfeld, O. 1971. Borrelia. Strains, Vectors, Human and Animal Borreliosis. Warren H. Green, Inc., St. Louis.

11. Fieldsteel, A. H., D. L. Cox, and R. A. Moeckli. 1981. Cultivation of virulent *Treponema pallidum* in tissue culture. Infect. Immun. **32**:908–915.

12. Fieldsteel, A. H., D. L. Cox, and R. A. Moeckli. 1982. Further studies on replication of virulent *Treponema pallidum* in tissue cultures of SflEp cells. Infect. Immun. **35**:449–455.

13. Fitzgerald, T. 1981. *In vitro* cultivation of *Treponema pallidum:* a review. Bull. Wld Hlth Org. **59**:787–812.

14. Fitzgerald, T. J. 1977. Interaction of *Treponema pallidum* (Nichols strain) with cultured mammalian cells: effects of oxygen, reducing agents, serum supplements, and different cell types. Infect. Immun. **15**:444–452.

15. Fitzgerald, T. J. 1981. Pathogenesis and immunology of *Treponema pallidum.* Ann. Rev. Microbiol. **35**:29–54.

16. Garner, M. F., R. W. Hornabrook, and J. L. Backhouse. 1972. Prevalence of yaws on Kar Kar Island, New Guinea. Brit. J. Vener. Dis. **48**:350–355.

17. Grin, E. I., and T. Guthe. 1973. Evaluation of a previous mass campaign against endemic syphilis in Bosnia and Herzegovina. Brit. J. Vener. Dis. **49**:1–19.

18. Hayes, N. S., *et al.* 1977. Parasitism by virulent *Treponema pallidum* of host cell surfaces. Infect. Immun. **17**:174–186.

19. Holt, S. C. 1978. Anatomy and chemistry of spirochetes. Microbiol. Rev. **42**:114–160.

20. Hooshmand, H., M. R. Escobar, and S. W. Kopf. 1972. Neurosyphilis. A study of 241 patients. J. Amer. Med. Assn **219**:726–729.

21. Hopkins, D. R. 1977. Yaws in the Americas, 1950–1975. J. Infect. Dis. **136**:548–554.

22. Johnson, R. C. (Ed.). 1976. The Biology of Parasitic Spirochetes. Academic Press, New York.

23. Johnson, R. C. 1977. The spirochetes. Ann. Rev. Microbiol. **31**:89–106.

24. Kelly, R. 1971. Cultivation of *Borrelia hermsii.* Science **173**:443–444.

25. Luger, A. 1981. Diagnosis of syphilis. Bull. Wld Hlth Org. **59**:647–654.

26. Martone, W. J., and A. F. Kaufmann. 1979. Leptospirosis in the United States, 1974–1978. J. Infect. Dis. **140**:1020–1022.

27. Miao, R., and A. H. Fieldsteel. 1978. Genetics of *Treponema:* relationship between *Treponema pallidum* and five cultivable treponemes. J. Bacteriol. **133**:101–107.

28. Miao, R. M., and A. H. Fieldsteel. 1980. Genetic relationship between *Treponema pallidum* and *Treponema pertenue,* two noncultivable human pathogens. J. Bacteriol. **141**:427–429.

29. Miller, J. N. 1976. Potential for vaccine for venereal diseases. Bull. N.Y. Acad. Med. **52**:986–1003.

30. Norris, S. J. 1982. In vitro cultivation of *Treponema pallidum:* independent confirmation. Infect. Immun. **36**:437–439.

31. Pavia, C. S., J. D. Folds, and J. B. Baseman. 1978. Cell-mediated immunity during syphilis. Brit. J. Vener. Dis. **54**:144–150.

32. Report. 1981. Syphilis trends in the United States. Morbid. Mortal. Wkly. Rep. **30**:441–444, 449.

33. Report. 1982. Treponemal infections. Wld Hlth Org. Tech. Rep. Ser., No. 674, Geneva.

34. Rogosa, M. 1980. *Streptobacillus moniliformis* and *Spirillum minor.* pp. 350–356. *In* E. H. Lennette, *et al.* (Eds.): Manual of Clinical Microbiology. 3rd ed. American Society for Microbiology, Washington, D.C.

35. Smibert, R. M. 1976. Cultivation, composition and physiology of avirulent treponemes. pp. 49–56. *In* R. C. Johnson (Ed.): The Biology of Parasitic Spirochetes. Academic Press, New York.

36. Steere, A. C., and S. E. Malawista. 1979. Cases of Lyme disease in the United States: locations correlated with distribution of *Ixodes dammini.* Ann. Intern. Med. **91**:730–733.

37. Steere, A. C., *et al.* 1977. Erythema chronicum migrans and Lyme arthritis. Ann. Intern. Med. **86**:685–698.

38. Steere, A. C., *et al.* 1980. Antibiotic therapy in Lyme disease. Ann. Intern. Med. **93**:1–8.

39. Steere, A. C., *et al.* 1980. Lyme carditis: cardiac abnormalities of Lyme disease. Ann. Intern. Med. **93**:8–16.

40. Steere, A. C., *et al.* 1983. The spirochetal etiology of Lyme disease. New Engl. J. Med. **308**:733–740.

41. Sullivan, N. D. 1974. Leptospirosis in animals and man. Australian Vet. J. **50**:216–223.

42. Willcox, R. R. 1981. Treatment of syphilis. Bull. Wld Hlth Org. **59**:655–663.

The Rickettsias

The casual name rickettsia is generally applied to a group of very small, gram-negative coccobacilli of the genera *Rickettsia* and *Coxiella* that are the etiological agents of several human infections. These include typhus fevers; spotted fevers and related diseases; tsutsugamushi disease of the Far East; and Q fever, first found in Australia and now known to occur throughout the world. *Rochalimaea* are also commonly included with the rickettsiae on epidemiological grounds, although they differ from *Rickettsia* and *Coxiella* in that they are cultivable on artificial mediums. Clearly similar microorganisms are the causal agents of animal diseases; *Ehrlichia* is typically a canine pathogen and *Cowdria* is the etiological agent of heartwater disease in cattle. Neither of the latter two is pathogenic for man.

Related to the rickettsiae are the *Bartonella*, which cause a human disease known as Oroya fever or verruga peruana, depending upon its clinical form, occurring in South and Central America. Similar microorganisms are found in both vertebrates and invertebrates, either as causative agents of animal diseases or as nonpathogenic, sometimes mutualistic, parasites of insects. More distantly related are the *Chlamydia,* which are considered in the following chapter (Chapter 34). The classification of the rickettsias is outlined in Chapter 2.

Rickettsias of human infection were first observed by Ricketts in 1909; the microorganism he found in association with Rocky Mountain spotted fever is now designated *Rickettsia rickettsii.* The typhus rickettsia was found by da Rocha Lima in 1916 in the bodies of lice taken from typhus fever patients. He named the agent *Rickettsia prowazekii,* in honor of Ricketts, who had died in 1910 of typhus fever during an investigation of that disease, and von Prowazek, another early worker who had died of typhus.

Rickettsia, Rochalimaea, and Coxiella[4, 15, 16, 23, 24]

The rickettsiae are of special interest, not only as the causative agents of human disease, but also because they are perhaps among the simplest of bacterial forms, and were once considered transitional between bacteria and viruses. They are, however, procaryotes with the morphological and structural details characteristic of gram-negative bacilli and are thus

Table 33–1. **Rickettsiae Pathogenic for Humans**

	Species	Mole % G + C*	Intracellular Location	Antigenic Structure	Usual Vector
Typhus group	Rickettsia prowazekii Rickettsia typhus (mooseri) Rickettsia canada (?)	29 29 29	Cytoplasm; found free and within phago-lysosomes	Group- and species-specific antigens	Lice, fleas
Spotted fever group	Rickettsia rickettsii Rickettsia sibirica Rickettsia conorii Rickettsia australis Rickettsia akari	33	Cytoplasm and nucleus; found free and within phagolysosomes	Group- and species-specific antigens	Ticks, mites
Scrub typhus group	Rickettsia tsutsugamushi	—	Cytoplasm, found free and within phago-lysosomes	Species-specific antigens; strains heterogeneous	Mites
	Coxiella burnetii	43–45	Cytoplasm; found in phagolysosomes	Two antigenic phases (I, II)	Ticks
	Rochalimaea quintana	39	Not intracellular	Homogeneous	Lice

*Guanine plus cytosine content of DNA.

quite different from the viruses. As described elsewhere (Chapter 12), bacteria may be arranged in a series, from the purely saprophytic nonpathogenic forms through those which are saprophytic but pathogenic because they form potent toxins, to the closely adapted parasites which make up the majority of the disease-producing bacteria. Many of the latter have fastidious nutritive requirements, reflecting limitations in synthetic abilities. Certain forms, especially *Francisella tularensis,* grow within the host cells but are cultivable on artificial mediums. Others, such as the leprosy bacillus and the spirochetes of syphilis, have not been grown on lifeless mediums.

The rickettsiae are set apart from other bacteria by their inability to grow, with rare exceptions, in the absence of the living host cell, necessitating culture in the embryonated egg or in some form of tissue culture. While it is a reasonable inference that they are dependent upon the host cell for essential metabolic reactions rather than essential metabolites, the rickettsiae do show limited metabolic activity and resemble other bacteria in having a similar cell structure and multiplying by transverse binary fission. It is relevant that infections with rickettsiae and the related *Chlamydia* are susceptible to treatment with antimicrobial chemotherapeutic drugs, while the diseases of viral etiology are not.

Classification

In general, the rickettsiae pathogenic for man fall into four broad groups. Three of these are well defined with respect to immunological character and pathogenicity: the rickettsiae

responsible for the typhus fevers, those of the spotted fever group, and the agent of scrub typhus. Some confusion arises in the spotted fever group of diseases because of the use of names such as "tick typhus." Rickettsiae causing Q fever *(Coxiella)* and trench fever *(Rochalimaea)* are set apart from the other rickettsiae, and make up a miscellaneous group. These relationships are summarized in Table 33–1.

The rickettsiae of these groups are classified in the family Rickettsiaceae and are contained in the genera *Rickettsia, Rochalimaea,* and

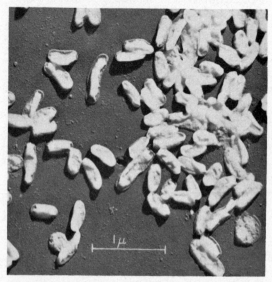

Figure 33–1. Transmission electron micrograph of Q fever rickettsiae purified by elution from a cellulose anion exchanger. The method of preparation has partially collapsed the individual cells, but their bacillary morphology is evident. (B. H. Hoyer et al., Science **127**:859, 1958.)

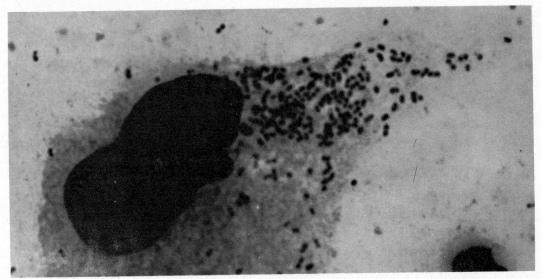

Figure 33–2. The rickettsiae of tsutsugamushi in scrapings from a mesothelial surface of an infected guinea pig. Note the coccobacillary forms, often paired, and their intracellular location. × 2000.

Coxiella. All are transmitted by blood-sucking insects—lice, ticks, fleas, and mites. Humans are incidental hosts for these rickettsiae, except for those causing louseborne typhus fever and, possibly, trench fever. With the exception of *Rochalimaea,* they are obligate intracellular parasites; only *Rochalimaea* has been cultivated in artificial mediums in pure culture. The degree of relatedness among the rickettsiae is inferred by the guanine plus cytosine content of their DNA; data for several species are shown in Table 33–1 and suggest that typhus fever and spotted fever groups are closely related, while *Coxiella* and *Rochalimaea* are more distantly related to *Rickettsia.*

Morphology and Staining[3, 14]

These microorganisms may appear as either coccobacillary or bacillary forms. The smallest are *Coxiella,* with average dimensions of 0.25 × 1 μm.; intermediate in size are *Rickettsia* of the typhus group (0.3 × 1.2 μm.); and the largest are those of the spotted fever group (0.6 × 1.2 μm.). Figure 33–1 shows the typical bacillary shape. Within infected host cells, rickettsiae occur singly, in pairs, and often in dense masses (Fig. 33–2); some species are found only in the cytoplasm (Fig. 33–3), while others replicate in the nucleus as well.

The rickettsiae are gram-negative bacteria, but stain poorly or not at all by this method. They stain readily, however, with Giemsa, Macchiavello, or Giménez stains; the latter is considered the most suitable. *Rickettsia tsutsugamushi* appears reddish black when stained by the Giménez stain; all other rickettsiae are brilliant red.

Fine Structure. Rickettsiae possess a well-defined cell wall, with fine structure commensurate with that of **gram-negative bacteria.** Comparative electron microscopy of the *Rickettsia* has revealed some variation in cell wall fine structure, as shown diagrammatically in Figure 33–4.

It has long been suspected that rickettsiae possess a **slime layer,** based on the loss of soluble antigens from the cells during purification. The presence of a slime layer, or cap-

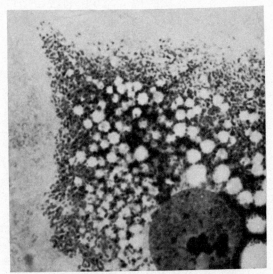

Figure 33–3. *Rickettsia prowazekii* in an infected cell from chick endoderm cultured *in vitro.* Most of the cytoplasm of the cell is occupied by rickettsiae. × 1500. (Weiss.)

Typhus and Spotted Fever Groups

Scrub Typhus Group

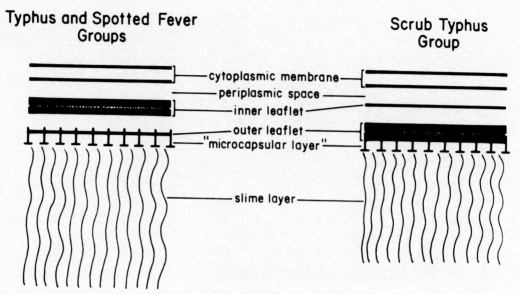

cytoplasmic membrane
periplasmic space
inner leaflet
outer leaflet
"microcapsular layer"
slime layer

Figure 33–4. Diagrammatic representation of the cell membrane, cell wall, and external layers of the rickettsiae. (D. J. Silverman and C. L. Wisseman, Jr., Infect. Immun. **21**:1020, 1978.)

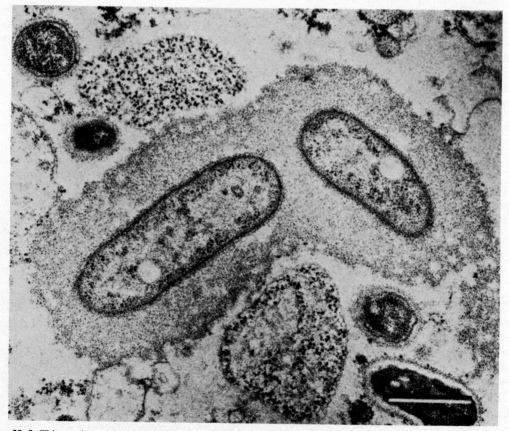

Figure 33–5. Thin section of *Rickettsia prowazekii* showing cells surrounded by a large slime layer. The preparation was stabilized by antityphus serum. Bar=0.5 μm. (D. J. Silverman et al., Infect. Immun. **22**:233, 1978.)

sule, has now been established by ruthenium red staining and by antibody stabilization prior to electron microscopy (Fig. 33–5). This slime layer is probably polysaccharide in nature.

Although most rickettsiae show no more than the usual variation in cell size, *Coxiella* have recently been shown to undergo a developmental cycle that involves the production of two principal cell types—designated **large** and **small cell variants.**[11] The small cell variant has a more dense cytoplasm and narrower periplasmic space than the large cell variety. Both variants are capable of division and are infectious for host cells. In the developmental cycle, tiny multilayered dense bodies form in the large cell variety, are released by lysis, and then reorganize into the small cell variety, which then either divides or enlarges into the large cell type (Fig. 33–6). The small dense bodies have been likened to spores of other bacteria in that they are more resistant than the parent cell, but their designation as "spores" may not yet be warranted.

Physiology

With the exception of *Rochalimaea*, rickettsiae grow only within living eucaryotic cells. It is logical to assume that they are dependent on the host cell for required substrates or synthetic machinery. Yet studies on rickettsiae separated from host cells indicate that they possess some metabolic capability. They are not energy parasites, being capable of generating ATP by metabolism of substrates such as glutamate, but they can also transport and capture exogenous ATP. Glutamate and, in some cases, succinate are oxidized via the Krebs cycle, with production of ATP. A variety of other enzymatic activities have been identified, including glutamate-oxaloacetate transaminase and a flavin-iron-cytochrome system. They are also capable of synthesizing both proteins and lipids in small amounts.

Rickettsiae are easily inactivated when stored in the absence of a metabolizable substrate. This inactivation is reflected in loss of physiological activity, infectivity, toxicity, and hemolytic capacity. These losses appear to result from temporary physiological changes; reactivation takes place when the microorganisms are further incubated with NAD, coenzyme A, or ATP, restoring infectivity and physiological, toxic, and hemolytic activities. It has also been shown that rickettsiae in starved ticks are avirulent, but virulence is regained when the ticks are fed a blood meal.

Growth of Rickettsiae

The trench fever rickettsia, *Rochalimaea quintana*, is unique in that it may be cultivated on artificial mediums containing blood, since heme is a required substrate. It also differs from other members in that it occurs extracellularly in its host vector and probably also in man.

The other rickettsiae, *Rickettsia* and *Coxiella*, grow only within eucaryotic host cells. In embryonated hen's eggs they grow readily and profusely in the yolk sac, and this method of cultivation is the most widely used. Growth obtains also on the chorioallantoic membrane, but the numbers produced are small.

Rickettsiae may be grown in various kinds of tissue culture as well. The mode of **penetration** into host cells is of considerable theoretical interest as a part of the mechanism of pathogenesis; only viable rickettsiae are able to penetrate and they must be capable of energy-yielding metabolism. Penetration of the host cell differs, therefore, from the somewhat passive phagocytosis observed with other bacteria; it is termed **induced phagocytosis,** since rickettsiae induce and have an active role in the process.

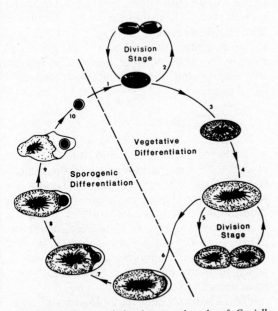

Figure 33–6. Proposed developmental cycle of *Coxiella burnetii* within phagolysosomes. After phagocytosis, small dense bodies or small cell variants are present in phagolysosomes *(1)*. Activation by acid pH initiates multiplication *(2)*. Alternatively, the small cell variant differentiates into the large cell variant *(3 and 4)*, which then multiplies *(5)* or begins differentiation, resulting in unequal cell division *(6)*. Successive stages *(7 to 9)* lead to the production of the small dense body (or "spores"), which are released by cell lysis *(10)*. (T. F. McCaul and J. C. Williams, J. Bacteriol., **147**:1063, 1981.)

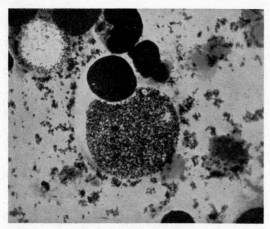

Figure 33–7. Rickettsiae of Q fever in a smear of skin exudate. Note the macrophage packed with enormous numbers of the rickettsiae. × 1125.

Soon after entry into the host cell, the rickettsiae lie within phagolysosomes in the cytoplasm. *Coxiella* are able to multiply profusely in these vacuoles (Fig. 33–7), exhibiting some resistance to the lysosomal hydrolases and being stimulated by the low pH of this environment. *Rickettsia,* on the other hand, are not able to withstand the rigors of the phagolysosomal environment, and must escape into the cytoplasm if they are to survive. The ability to escape from the vacuole is apparently associated with a phospholipase and is directly related to virulence; avirulent strains are unable to leave the phagolysosome and are destroyed.

Subsequent events in intracellular growth vary with *Rickettsia* groups and species. The typhus fever rickettsiae multiply only in the cytoplasm and do not invade the nucleus. *Rickettsia prowazekii* multiplies rapidly, becoming very numerous in the cytoplasm; lysis of the host cell eventually occurs and the rickettsiae are released (Fig. 33–8). On the other hand, spotted fever rickettsiae not only multiply in the cytoplasm of infected cells, but also invade and multiply in the nucleus. Early in the infection process, *R. rickettsii* escapes from the host cell through the plasma membrane, so that relatively few accumulate in the cytoplasm. During the later stages of intracellular growth, however, *R. rickettsii* may cause extensive cytopathology, including host cell lysis.[20]

Like typhus fever rickettsiae, *R. tsutsugamushi* rapidly escapes from the phagolysosome and replicates in the cytoplasm. It then moves to the cell surface and is extruded through the host cell membrane by a budding process. In doing so, it is enveloped by host plasma membrane. When these enveloped forms infect a new host cell by phagocytosis, the coat is shed as they escape from the vacuole (Fig. 33–9).

The intracellular multiplication of rickettsiae requires metabolizing, but not necessarily growing, host cells. Irradiated cells, for example, are fully capable of supporting intracellular growth of these microorganisms, as are enucleated cells.[21] In egg embryo yolk sac, *Coxiella* continue to grow for up to two days after death of the embryo, but typhus and spotted fever rickettsiae do not, and their numbers decline after death of the embryo.

Resistance

The resistance of the rickettsiae to deleterious influences is generally of the same order as that of the more delicate bacterial vegetative cells. They are killed by the usual disinfectants and by heating at 55 to 60° C. for 30 to 60 minutes. The Q fever rickettsiae are sturdier than the other members and viability is retained for some months at room temperatures; they are the most resistant to heat, and may survive 63° C. for 40 minutes. This relative resistance may be associated with the presence of the small dense bodies produced during the growth cycle. These and the typhus rickettsiae are relatively resistant to drying. *Coxiella* persist for considerable periods in viable infectious form in the airborne state, and typhus rickettsiae survive and remain infectious in infected louse feces.

Pathogenicity

The rickettsiae appear to be well-established parasites of arthropods, and there is good evidence for the acarinid origin of the rickettsial diseases. Except for lice, they are not pathogenic for the insect vectors that transmit them, and, in fact, the infection is congenital in insects undergoing an incomplete metamorphosis, *e.g.,* ticks. They also appear to be well adapted to certain animals, especially rodents, which in many instances constitute a natural reservoir of infection.

The characteristic pathological changes found in rickettsial disease result from host cell penetration and subsequent multiplication of the microorganisms within the endothelial cells of the small blood vessels throughout the body. In the case of typhus fever, these pathological changes are especially prominent in the skin and brain. As the number of affected cells expands, thrombosis follows injury to the lining of small vessels. Inflammatory cells ac-

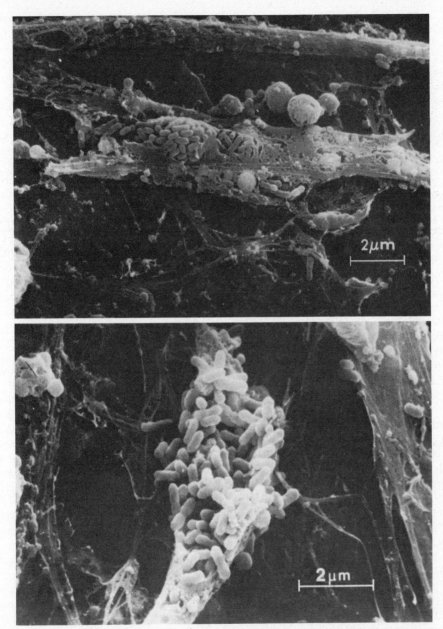

Figure 33–8. Scanning electron micrograph of chicken fibroblast cells infected with *Rickettsia prowazekii. Top,* generalized breakdown of the cells of the monolayer. *Bottom,* release of rickettsia from a disintegrating host cell. (D. J. Silverman, C. L. Wisseman, Jr., and A. Waddell. Infect. Immun. **29**:778, 1980.)

cumulate around areas of affected vessels and, in severe infections, *e.g.,* those of spotted fever, the smooth muscle cells of the vessel may be involved; the resulting extensive thrombosis can lead to necrosis.

Toxicity. Two kinds of rickettsial toxicity are demonstrable. One is associated with the presence of **endotoxin,** while the other is seen as **cytotoxicity** for several kinds of animal cells.

In common with endotoxin from other gram-negative bacteria, that of rickettsiae is lipopo-lysaccharide in composition and possesses many of the biological activities that characterize endotoxins of the Enterobacteriaceae.[19] In *Coxiella* the lipopolysaccharide of the virulent phase I cells is complete, while that found in the less virulent phase II organisms is incomplete and is probably analogous to the core lipopolysaccharide of rough enteric bacilli.[18]

Rickettsiae are cytotoxic for a variety of cell types. The cytotoxic effects are not attributable to a soluble toxin, but appear to result from

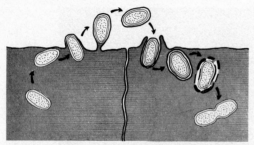

Figure 33–9. Hypothetical scheme for infection of *Rickettsia tsutsugamushi* in mouse mesothelial cells. Rickettsiae multiplying in the cytoplasm move to the cell surface, acquire a host-membrane coat, and bud from the surface. After phagocytosis by new cells, they escape from the phagosome as the vacuole membrane and host membrane coat disintegrate. Cytoplasmic multiplication completes the cycle. (E. P. Ewing, Jr., *et al., Infect. Immun.* **19**:1068, 1978.)

events associated with rickettsial contact, adherence, and penetration into susceptible host cells. Cytotoxicity is directly proportional to the number of rickettsiae present and is correlated with their viability. Most agents that destroy infectivity also reduce toxicity; ultraviolet irradiation is an exception, selectively reducing infectivity without affecting cytotoxicity.

Cytotoxicity is exemplified by the hemolysis of human, sheep, and rabbit red blood cells, but not those of a number of other species. Hemolysis requires viable rickettsial cells with intact energy-generating systems. Rickettsiae adsorb to the erythrocyte surface at receptor sites containing glycerophospholipids; red blood cell lysis then results from phospholipase A activity, but the origin of the enzyme is not clear. It may be a rickettsial enzyme, or the rickettsiae may activate a latent erythrocyte enzyme.[26]

Cytotoxic effects are also manifest in tissue cultures and in intact animals. Cellular injury results from massive infection by rickettsiae that damages the integrity of the plasma membrane. In tissue cultures, plaques are formed on monolayer cultures of L cells, and injury to these cells involves phospholipase activity, as in hemolysis. The injection of large numbers of rickettsiae into mice leads to acute toxicity and death, arising from similar membrane alterations in the endothelial cells of the small blood vessels.

It now seems reasonably well established that pathogenesis of rickettsial infections is associated with the penetration of host cells, and subsequent intracellular growth, by large numbers of rickettsiae. Many of the features

of rickettsial infection are also consistent with endotoxic activity of lipopolysaccharide.

Experimental Infections. Although more resistant to rickettsial infection than humans, guinea pigs may be infected by intraperitoneal inoculation. Most animals exhibit a febrile attack in 7 to 12 days, but the disease is often not fatal. With several varieties of rickettsia, a characteristic **orchitis** or **scrotal reaction** is produced, in which a fibrinous exudate is formed in the scrotal sac and many cells packed with rickettsiae may be found. This reaction has differential value for some of the rickettsiae.

Model experimental infections have been established in the silvered leaf-monkey *(Presbytis cristatus)* with *R. tsutsugamushi* that are sometimes fatal. Other laboratory animals (rats, mice, rabbits, dogs, and cats) are more resistant and may show no outward manifestations of disease, though infection is established.

Chemotherapy[16]

Several chemotherapeutic agents have proved effective in this group of diseases, including chloramphenicol and the tetracyclines. The most widely used today is doxycycline, a derivative of tetracycline. It has been reported that a single dose of doxycycline is effective in most cases of louseborne typhus or scrub typhus; the other rickettsioses require several daily doses of the antibiotic. Q fever does not respond as rapidly as other rickettsial infections, and endocarditis and chronic *Coxiella* infections may demand prolonged therapy, possibly several months. These drugs are rickettsiostatic, so that relapses sometimes occur with chloramphenicol but uncommonly with tetracyclines. Rickettsiae are not susceptible to penicillin, although this agent has been used to control secondary bacterial infections.

Drug-resistant strains of rickettsiae have not been encountered in nature, but resistant strains have been developed in the laboratory.

Antigenic Structure

Although the immunochemistry of rickettsiae is only now becoming clear, immunological differences have provided one of the major means for their separation. Historically, two principal kinds of antigens have been studied. One of these, soluble and probably associated with the slime layer, is usually responsible for group-specific reactions. The second kind, revealed after extensive washing or purification of the cells, is likely a part of the outer membrane and generally carries species specificity; many of the antigens of this series are probably proteins.

In the typhus group, the group antigen is a soluble antigen, and there is cross-reactivity between the three species constituting this group—*R. prowazekii, R. typhi,* and *R. canada*—but little or no cross-reactivity with other *Rickettsia*. Each species, on the other hand, possesses species-specific protein antigens demonstrable with washed cells.

A similar antigenic structure is noted in the spotted fever group. All members possess a unique group-reactive soluble antigen. Each species is defined by species-specific antigens, although there may be some interspecies cross-reactions, even when washed cells are used as antigen.

In *R. tsutsugamushi,* a species-specific soluble antigen is analogous to the group-specific antigens of the typhus and spotted fever groups. There is, however, immunological heterogeneity in this species when washed cells are employed as the test antigen.

Coxiella are quite different from the *Rickettsia* in antigenic structure. The principal antigen is a lipopolysaccharide, and *Coxiella* of phase I, analogous to the S form of other gram-negative bacteria, are antigenically homogeneous. There is no immunological cross-reaction with other rickettsiae. Similarly, *Rochalimaea quintana* appears to be immunologically homogeneous and does not share antigenic components with other rickettsiae.

Immunity

Recovery from an attack of rickettsial disease usually confers a solid immunity. In at least some instances, this is associated with the prolonged survival of the microorganisms in the body, as indicated by the occurrence of Brill-Zinsser disease and the demonstration of tsutsugamushi rickettsiae in clinically recovered individuals.

The development of artificial immunization procedures will be considered later, but it may be noted here that the immune response is manifest by the appearance of antibodies against both somatic and capsular antigens of rickettsiae, as well as antibody neutralizing the toxicity of rickettsiae.

The antibody response in rickettsial infection is only partially protective against subsequent challenge. Antibody is not rickettsiacidal, but does promote phagocytosis, and this leads to significant, but not complete, intracellular destruction of the microorganism. Effective immunity is more closely linked to the cell-mediated immune compartment. A cellular immune response is exemplified by the activation of macrophages that are enhanced in their capacity to destroy the invading microorganism; effective immunity in animals can, therefore, be adoptively transferred by lymphoid elements. Thus, it appears that both humoral and cellular immune responses are operative in protection, but that complete immunity is dependent upon the latter.

In certain of the rickettsioses, antibodies are produced that agglutinate some strains of *Proteus*. This apparently anomalous response, observed by Weil and Felix in 1915, has had considerable diagnostic utility. They found that a strain of *Proteus vulgaris,* which they designated X-2, was agglutinated by serum of typhus patients, and another strain, designated X-19, was similarly agglutinated but to much higher titer. The reactive *Proteus* antigen is a part of the somatic O antigen complex and these strains of *Proteus* are commonly termed OX strains. This agglutination test, the **Weil-Felix reaction,** is specific for the typhus group of fevers, serums from other rickettsial diseases agglutinating to low titer or not at all. The agglutination of *Proteus* is due to shared polysaccharide sequences in the lipopolysaccharide O antigen of the typhus rickettsiae and the X strains of *Proteus*.

Another immunological variety of *Proteus,* the OX-K strains, was found to be agglutinated by serums from infections with *R. tsutsugamushi,* but not by typhus serums. This, coupled with the OX-19 type, makes possible the division of rickettsial diseases into three groups: the typhus group, in which OX-19 is agglutinated; the tsutsugamushi group, in which OX-K is agglutinated; and the spotted fever group, which is indeterminate in that neither type of *Proteus* is agglutinated to high titer. A classification of the rickettsial diseases on this basis is given in Table 33–2.

The *Proteus* agglutinin is only a part of the rickettsial antibody response. It is not identical to the specific rickettsial agglutinin, for the latter appears earlier, persists longer, and has some protective capacity. Furthermore, the specific opsonin remains in typhus serums after adsorption with *Proteus* cells.

Specific Serological Reactions. Although it has been extremely useful, the Weil-Felix reaction is not a specific reaction and is not completely reliable. An accurate method of serological diagnosis and identification should be based on true immunological specificity

Table 33–2. **Immunological (Weil-Felix) Grouping of Rickettsial Diseases**

Immunological Group		
OX-19	*OX-K*	*Indeterminate*
OX-19 + + + + OX-2 + OX-K –	OX-19 – OX-2 – OX-K + + + +	OX-19 + OX-2 + OX-K +
Classic, European typhus Brill-Zinsser disease Endemic murine typhus	Tsutsugamushi disease Scrub or rural typhus Sumatran mite fever	Spotted fever São Paulo typhus Fièvre boutonneuse South African tick fever Kenya typhus Indian tick typhus North Asian tick typhus

through the use of rickettsial antigens. Specific *in vitro* serological reactions became practical only after rickettsiae were cultivated in the yolk sac of chicken embryos and, later, in tissue cultures. Using these rickettsial antigens, serological tests have been developed that permit better serodiagnostic tests for rickettsial diseases as well as improved immunological differentiation of rickettsiae.

The commonly used serological tests include direct agglutination of rickettsiae in suspension, complement fixation, indirect hemagglutination, latex agglutination, and indirect immunofluorescence. Of these, the last is the most satisfactory but is not universally available.

Laboratory Diagnosis[14]

Laboratory diagnosis is an indispensable adjunct to the identification of diseases of rickettsial etiology and involves two general kinds of procedures: (1) identification of the causative agent by morphological and immunological means, and (2) serological detection of serum antibody. The latter also allows retrospective diagnosis and estimation of the prevalence of infection by serological surveys.

Rickettsiae can be isolated from blood and tissues by inoculating guinea pigs or mice. Rickettsiae in these experimental infections can be identified by their morphological characters and by immunofluorescence microscopy, as described below. However, such isolation procedures are of limited diagnostic utility because of technical complications and inherent dangers to personnel; isolation should only be attempted in reference laboratories using appropriately collected and transported specimens. Unlike other rickettsiae, *Rochalimaea quintana* can be cultivated in artificial mediums containing blood.

The microorganisms can often be demonstrated in stained infected tissues or cells ob-

served microscopically; suitable stains include Giménez, Macchiavello, and Giemsa. The typical morphology of the principal groups has been described earlier (p. 655). Unfortunately, these stains do not offer reliable differentiation from other bacteria of similar size and shape.

Of greater value for detection and identification of rickettsiae in tissues is direct immunofluorescent microscopy. Group-specific antiserum, labeled with fluorescent dye, is reacted with smears of infected tissues and observed by fluorescence microscopy. This technique has proved successful in identification of rickettsiae in skin biopsies from spotted fever patients.

By far the most commonly used diagnostic tests are the serological procedures that detect patients' antibody response to rickettsial infection. The assays employed include the Weil-Felix reaction as well as the serological tests that employ specific rickettsial antigens. These serological tests must, however, be interpreted with some caution. In certain endemic areas, members of the population may possess serum antibodies against *R. rickettsii, R. typhi,* and *C. burnetii,* arising from previous subclinical or mild infections. Furthermore, some groups have received immunizations with typhus or Rocky Mountain spotted fever vaccines and may exhibit serum antibodies. It is obvious that a single titration for antibodies in such individuals can be misleading. This is overcome by antibody titration of paired serums—one acute and the other convalescent—to demonstrate a rise in antibody titer.

The Weil-Felix Reaction. For a number of years the Weil-Felix reaction has been widely used in diagnosis because it is readily performed in any clinical laboratory. False reactions arise, however, due to the nonspecificity of the reaction, and the test requires rigid controls for reproducibility.

The Weil-Felix test offers presumptive evidence for the typhus fever group of infections when both *Proteus* OX-2 and OX-19, but not OX-K, are agglutinated. Presumption of scrub typhus is indicated by agglutination of *Proteus* OX-K, but not the other strains. Because normal serums sometimes show low agglutinin titers, a minimum titer of 1:160 in initial serums, with fourfold rise in titer in subsequent serum samples, may be significant. Agglutinins usually appear as early as five to seven days and generally reach peak titer by the end of the second or third week.

Some rickettsial infections fail to yield positive Weil-Felix reactions, including Q fever, rickettsialpox, and, often, Brill-Zinsser disease. Some scrub typhus patients also fail to develop agglutinins to *Proteus* OX-K. While the spotted fevers are indeterminate in reaction, on occasion they exhibit significant titers. False-positive reactions sometimes arise in other febrile conditions, including infections with *Proteus, Pseudomonas, Borrelia,* and *Salmonella typhi.*

Specific Serological Reactions. It is apparent that serological tests employing rickettsial antigens are more specific than *Proteus* agglutination, and their use has expanded with the availability of suitable rickettsial antigens. Two types of tests are now widely used: complement fixation and rickettsial agglutination.

Complement fixation is the most useful specific serological test and is applicable to all rickettsioses except scrub typhus, in which the multiplicity of types limits the application of the test. Complement-fixing antigens are available for phase II of *C. burnetii* and for the typhus and spotted fever groups; in the latter groups, the test cannot differentiate disease caused by the individual species. Complement-fixing antibodies usually become apparent, with titers of about 1:8, during the second week after onset of disease and increase markedly during convalescence. In Q fever, complement-fixing antibodies against phase II antigens arise early and reach high titers, while antibodies to phase I antigens appear much later and the titer is usually low. Subacute endocarditis due to *Coxiella* is, however, an important exception; complement-fixing antibodies to phase I antigen occur in high titer.

Rickettsial agglutination, using purified antigen and usually modified as a microagglutination test, is at least comparable in sensitivity and specificity to complement fixation. It has the advantage of simplicity and ease of performance, but the required antigens are not routinely available at present. This test has greatest utility in *Coxiella* infections; in contrast to complement fixation, agglutinins to both phase I and phase II antigens appear early in the disease.

Other serological tests have been devised, including indirect immunofluorescence microscopy, indirect hemagglutination, and latex agglutination, but these are not usually available in clinical laboratories.

THE TYPHUS FEVERS[2, 16, 24, 25]

The typhus fevers constitute a group of closely related infections that occur in various parts of the world. The incubation period is 5 to 18 days, and the clinical picture is essentially the same in all the typhus fevers, though the severity of the disease varies widely. In typical cases there is an initial violent headache which persists with the onset of chills and higher fever. A macular eruption appears soon after the fourth day, which remains until defervescence. Crisis occurs at about the twelfth day, and recovery may be more or less complete at the end of another two weeks, though the cough which develops may persist, and mental vigor may remain impaired for some time. Complications include typhus gangrene, which is probably associated with the circulatory disturbances arising during the disease; a highly fatal bronchopneumonia; otitis media; and typhus encephalitis. Death rarely occurs before the end of the first week. The case fatality is highly variable; it has been as great as 70 per cent in some epidemics, and 20 to 30 per cent is not uncommon; it is much lower, perhaps 5 per cent, in sporadic cases. Typhus is almost always a considerably milder disease in children than in adults.

Two species of *Rickettsia* are responsible for these diseases, and are characteristically found in the cytoplasm but not in the nucleus of invaded cells. They are associated with two epidemiologically different types of typhus fever. One is the classic European or epidemic typhus in which the etiological agent is *R. prowazekii*. The other is murine typhus, sometimes called endemic typhus, and the causative rickettsia is *R. typhi (R. mooseri)*. As indicated earlier, each is immunologically homogeneous, and strains from all parts of the world appear to be substantially identical. These rickettsiae may be distinguished from one another by complement fixation and contain both common and individual antigens.

Rickettsia canada is considered to be a member of the typhus group, although its intranuclear growth and occurrence in ticks are char-

Table 33–3. **Rickettsial Diseases of Man**

	Name of Rickettsia	Disease	Geographical Distribution
Typhus group	*Rickettsia prowazekii*	Epidemic typhus (classic, European, louseborne typhus)	Africa, Asia, C. and S. America
		Brill-Zinsser disease	N. America, Europe
		Sylvatic typhus	N. America
	Rickettsia typhi	Murine typhus (endemic typhus, fleaborne typhus)	Worldwide
Spotted fever group	*Rickettsia rickettsii*	Spotted fever (Rocky Mt. spotted fever)	North America
		São Paulo typhus	Brazil
		Tobia fever	Colombia
	Rickettsia sibirica	North Asian tick typhus	Northern Asia
	Rickettsia conorii	Boutonneuse fever (Marseilles or Mediterranean fever)	Mediterranean littoral
		Indian tick typhus	India
		Kenya typhus	East Africa
		South African tick-bite fever	South Africa
		Siberian tick typhus	Central Asia
	Rickettsia australis	North Queensland tick typhus	Australia
	Rickettsia akari	Rickettsialpox	Urban localities in N.E. United States and in USSR
Scrub typhus group	*Rickettsia tsutsugamushi*	Tsutsugamushi disease	Japan, Korea, China, USSR,
		Japanese river fever	Philippines, S.E. Asia,
		Kedani fever	India, Indonesia,
		Scrub typhus	N. Australia
		Rural typhus	
	Coxiella burnetii	Q fever	Worldwide
	Rochalimaea quintana	Trench fever (Wolhynian fever; five-day fever)	Europe, Africa, N. America

acteristics usually associated with the spotted fever rickettsiae. There is serological evidence of human infection with *R. canada* that clinically resembles spotted fever. The occurrence of *R. canada* in ticks is significant in that it suggests a tick reservoir of infection and may account for positive reactions of serums with group antigen in the absence of typhus.

EPIDEMIC LOUSEBORNE TYPHUS FEVER

The classic form of typhus fever is the louseborne typhus of Central Europe, which persists in endemic foci in Asia, Africa, and Central and South America; it has occasionally broken out in major epidemic form from time to time during periods of stress. The disease is associated with overcrowding and has been termed "camp fever" and "jail fever." Epidemics have occurred in both civil and military populations during time of war and may become very extensive; for example, it is estimated that 315,000 persons died of typhus in Serbia in 1915 and that 25 million cases occurred in Russia from 1917 to 1921. Fortunately, louseborne typhus is relatively rare today, and only a few thousand cases are reported annually. More than 95 per cent of these are found in North Africa and only a few hundred cases are noted each year in South America.

Although *R. prowazekii* has been found in a few domestic and wild animals, it is essentially a **human infection**; in most instances the animal reservoirs are only temporary and probably do not play a role in the epidemiology of the disease. An exception may exist, however, in the newly described sylvatic typhus discussed below.

The disease is transmitted by the **human body louse**, *Pediculus humanus*. The head louse may also transmit the infection, but its importance in the spread of the disease is not established. During the febrile stage of the

Table 33–3. **Rickettsial Diseases of Man** (*Continued*)

Vectors	Vertebrate Reservoir	Experimental Infections and Observations	Weil-Felix Group
Human body louse	Man	Guinea pig (fever only)	OX-19
Fleas Rat louse	Wild rats Field mice	Guinea pig (fever and scrotal swelling)	OX-19
Ixodid ticks	Incomplete evidence indicates: foxes, small rodents, dog, opossum (S. America)	Guinea pig (fever and severe scrotal reaction with necrosis)	Indeterminate
Ixodid ticks	Domestic animals and rodents	Guinea pig (fever and scrotal swelling)	Indeterminate
Ixodid ticks	Dog Rodents	Guinea pig (fever and scrotal swelling)	Indeterminate
Ixodid ticks	Rat? Marsupials?	Guinea pig (fever and scrotal swelling)	Indeterminate
Mouse mite	House mice	Mouse (ascites, splenomegaly, death)	Indeterminate
Trombiculid mites	Wild rodents	Mouse (ascites, splenomegaly, death)	OX-K
Ixodid ticks	Bandicoot (Australia) Human infections occur from direct or indirect contact with infected sheep, cattle, goats	Guinea pig (fever only)	None
Human body louse	Man	None	None

disease, rickettsiae are present in the blood, and the louse is infected when it feeds. In the louse the rickettsiae infect the cells lining the gut, multiply, and are discharged in the feces after rupture of the infected cells; lice become infective in six to eight days at 32° C. The salivary glands are not infected, congenital transmission of the infection does not occur, and the louse is eventually killed by the infection.

Most human infections are probably acquired by contamination of the louse bite with infected feces, but infection via the mucous membranes is possible. The rickettsiae persist in viable form in dried material such as louse feces, and accidental laboratory infections have occurred following inhalation of infectious materials.

Although bedbugs and ticks have been experimentally infected, it is probable that the louse is the sole vector of the disease under natural conditions.

Brill-Zinsser Disease

Following an initial attack of epidemic typhus, a few individuals may continue to harbor *R. prowazekii* as a **latent infection.** Relapses sometimes occur in these infections, to give rise to a mild type of typhus, known as recrudescent typhus or Brill-Zinsser disease. The second attack may appear within a few years after the initial infection, but may be delayed for several decades. The disease was at one time present in cities along the Atlantic coast of the United States, but has largely disappeared; presumably the disease was imported from Europe. It has also been found in Australia among immigrants from Central Europe. Brill-Zinsser disease is now the only form of *R. prowazekii* infection that appears in Europe.

It has been proposed that the latent form of the disease can serve as an interepidemic reservoir for louseborne epidemic typhus, since lice become infected by feeding upon such individuals. Thus, in lice-infested populations, latent infections could provide the starting point of epidemics.

Sylvatic Typhus[8, 12, 17]

In the 1970s, a sylvatic form of *R. prowazekii* infection was described among flying squirrels *(Glaucomys volans)* in the eastern United States. *Rickettsia prowazekii* from this widespread natural infection are indistinguishable from human strains of the microorganism. The sylvatic infection appears to be transmitted among the squirrel population by the flying squirrel louse.

Following this discovery, a few cases of human *R. prowazekii* infection began to appear in the eastern United States, with distribution consistent with the range of the flying squirrel. These were the first indigenous cases of this type of typhus in the United States in over 50 years. At least a few of the human cases appear to be directly linked to squirrels. The seasonal incidence of the disease, with greatest frequency in the winter months, is coincident with the tendency of squirrels to seek warmth in the attics of dwellings. It is now considered likely that sylvatic typhus is a new epidemiological type of classic typhus, transmitted to humans from an infected animal reservoir.

Immunization

The low incidence of epidemic louseborne typhus in the United States and the efficacy of chemotherapy do not argue for immunization programs, and vaccination is not currently practiced. Vaccines are used, however, in areas where the disease is prevalent. These vaccines are prepared from either inactivated or attenuated *R. prowazekii*.

Inactivated vaccines are composed of *R. prowazekii* grown in the yolk sac of chicken embryos and inactivated with formalin. This was the vaccine used by the United States Army during World War II, and is credited with modifying the course of the disease and reducing mortality.

An attenuated vaccine can be produced from the Madrid E strain of *R. prowazekii*, which is avirulent for guinea pigs and other laboratory animals. This vaccine, used in human volunteers in endemic areas, induces signifi-

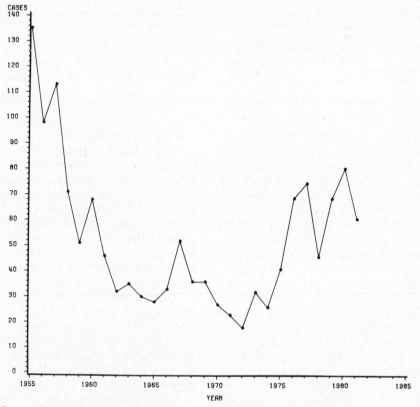

Figure 33–10. Reported cases of murine typhus in the United States, 1955–1981. (Centers for Disease Control, Annual summary 1981: reported morbidity and mortality in the United States. Morbidity and Mortality Weekly Report **30,** 1982.)

cant humoral antibody response and an effective immunity that persists for six years or more.

Murine Typhus

Murine typhus is a type of typhus fever that is closely related to classic typhus. The disease, caused by *Rickettsia typhi,* is more widely distributed than louseborne typhus and occurs throughout the world. It is typically a disease of rodents, principally rats, and is transmitted in the reservoir host population, and to man, by fleas and lice; it is frequently known as fleaborne or endemic typhus.

Murine typhus prevails in the southern United States and in Mexico, where it is known as tabardillo. In these localities it is found in rats and transmitted by the rat flea, *Xenopsylla cheopis,* and the rat louse, *Polyplax spinulosus.* Unlike classic louseborne typhus, which has tended to occur in explosive epidemics, murine typhus appears in small outbreaks and sporadic cases. This disease may, at times, be transmitted by the human louse and, when a case occurs by transmission from rats in a community where lice are found in abundance, it has been suggested that murine typhus may become an epidemic louseborne infection. Such infections occur from time to time in Mexico. Some degree of control of the disease is possible by reduction of rat and rat flea populations.

In the United States prior to 1946, murine typhus occurred with considerable frequency. In 1945, for example, more than 5000 cases and 214 deaths were recorded in 44 states. The number of cases has since declined, as detailed in Figure 33–10.

Clinically, murine typhus does not differ appreciably from the classic European type. It is sometimes said that the European disease is likely to be more often fatal, but this does not appear to be true; both forms are equally fatal in epidemic form and relatively mild in endemic form.

Differences between *R. prowazekii* and *R. typhi* are demonstrable but not great. The murine rickettsiae produce a necrotic scrotal reaction in guinea pigs, while the European variety does not; the murine variety may be carried indefinitely in mice without alteration, but the European variety tends to degenerate; the rickettsial pneumonia and intraperitoneal multiplication in rats with the production of enormous numbers of rickettsiae may be produced by the murine variety but not by the European type alone. Immunological differences between the two are slight, but they may be differentiated by the complement fixation test. Recovery from either infection results in a solid and lasting immunity to both, but the attenuated *R. prowazekii* strain E vaccine yields only partial and unpredictable protection against murine typhus. There is no vaccine currently available for murine typhus.

THE SPOTTED FEVERS

The rickettsiae of the spotted fever group are considerably more heterogeneous than those of the typhus fever group. They are immunologically related, but may be differentiated by appropriate serological procedures. In contrast to the typhus fever group, these rickettsiae are found within the nucleus as well as in the cytoplasm of invaded cells.

With the exception of *Rickettsia akari,* which causes the miteborne rickettsialpox, all are transmitted by **ixodid ticks**; these spotted fevers are often termed tick fevers or tickborne typhus fevers. The New World, or American, spotted fevers are due to infection with *R. rickettsii;* in the United States the disease is known as Rocky Mountain spotted fever and, clinically, is the most severe of the rickettsioses. The tickborne typhus fevers of the Old World are generally milder infections and are caused, in different localities, by *R. siberica,* *R. conorii,* or *R. australis.* These species are similar to *R. rickettsii,* but are immunologically differentiable.

Rocky Mountain Spotted Fever[5]

Rocky Mountain spotted fever is almost always initiated by the bite of an infected tick. Following an incubation period of 2 to 14 days, onset is sudden, with severe headache, chills, fever, aching, and nausea. After 2 to 6 days of fever, a macular rash generally is seen, first on the extremities, particularly the palms and soles, and later extending to other parts of the body and becoming maculopapular. Neurological symptoms are common during fever. Death, if it occurs, is usually near the end of the second week and is due to toxemia, vasomotor weakness, shock, or renal failure.

Rocky Mountain spotted fever apparently first occurred in the United States about 1873 on the west side of the Bitterroot Valley of Montana. It was essentially limited to the Rocky Mountain regions until about 1930, when an increasing number of cases were recognized in the South Atlantic states. Since that time, the incidence in the West has markedly declined, while it has increased in the South Central and South Atlantic states, particularly in the Piedmont area of the Carolinas and Virginia. In 1981, an all-time high of almost 1200 cases were reported in the United States. Figure 33–11 shows the increase in case rates that have occurred in this country since the late 1960s.

In the western regions, the reservoir hosts for *R. rickettsii* are rodents and small mammals, including voles, mice, chipmunks, ground squirrels, and rabbits. The predominant vector is the **wood tick**, *Dermacentor andersoni.* A number of other ixodid ticks may maintain the infection in animals, but they seldom feed on humans.

In the eastern United States, the animal reservoirs include voles and mice, and the vector is the **American dog tick,** *Dermacentor variabilis.* It is possible that the lone star tick, *Amblyomma americanum,* is also a vector in the southern areas.

The infection in ticks is congenital, *i.e.,* ovarially transmitted from one generation to the next, and serves to maintain the rickettsiae outside of the animal hosts, at least for several generations. It should be noted that in starving ticks the rickettsiae appear to be avirulent, *i.e.,* they are not capable of infecting an animal host. As the tick ingests a blood meal, the rickettsiae are reactivated and become virulent. This is believed to explain the finding that the bite of a tick does not result in infection unless the tick has attached and fed for several hours.

The case-fatality rate of spotted fever has been highly variable and, in past years, has ranged up to 90 per cent in some areas, such as the Bitterroot Valley. In the period from 1975 to 1977, the overall death rate from Rocky Mountain spotted fever was 5.2 per cent, but in those over 40 years of age it reached 11 per cent.[7] By 1981 the overall mortality rate had dropped to 3.4 per cent. The fall in case-fatality rates is undoubtedly due to the effectiveness of broad-spectrum antibiotic therapy as well as increased clinical awareness and improved diagnostic aids.

Spotted fever was transmitted to guinea pigs and monkeys by Ricketts in 1907. Guinea pigs show a febrile reaction, the spleen is enlarged, and the necrotic scrotal reaction occurs. *Rickettsia rickettsii* is immunologically related to the typhus rickettsiae, but the titer of cross-reaction in the complement fixation test is not high enough to cause confusion; there is also a small degree of cross-protection between the two.

Other Spotted Fevers

Closely similar tickborne diseases have been observed in Central and South America; in Central America and Brazil it is known as São Paulo typhus and in Colombia as Tobia fever. The causative rickettsiae are very closely re-

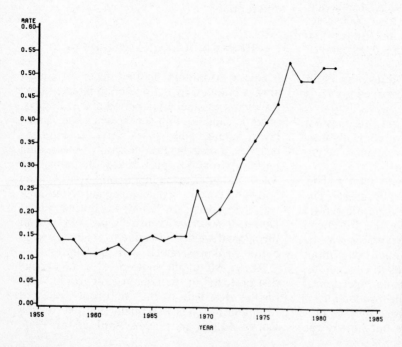

Figure 33–11. Incidence of Rocky Mountain spotted fever in the United States from 1955 to 1981—reported cases per 100,000 population. (Centers for Disease Control, Annual summary 1981: reported morbidity and mortality in the United States. Morbidity and Mortality Weekly Report **30**, 1982.)

lated to, if not identical with, *R. rickettsii*. There seems to be no doubt that these diseases are spotted fever, and they are often collectively referred to as American spotted fever.

Immunization

A solid immunity is associated with recovery from spotted fever, and some prophylactic immunity may be produced by inoculation with vaccine. The current vaccine, a killed suspension of rickettsiae grown in yolk sac culture, produces an effective immunity in experimental animals such as guinea pigs; it is only partially protective in humans, however, modifying the course of disease but failing to protect completely in a large proportion of individuals.

OTHER TICKBORNE TYPHUS FEVERS

There are a number of diseases of rickettsial etiology that are closely related to the American spotted fevers. These are generally known as tick typhus or tick fever and identified by the locality in which they are observed. The causative rickettsiae have been shown in some cases to be closely related to, but apparently not identical with, *R. rickettsii*, while others that are not this well known show clinical and epidemiological features which suggest a closely similar etiology.

Boutonneuse Fever

This disease, also known as fièvre boutonneuse and Marseilles fever, is prevalent in the Mediterranean area and is caused by *R. conorii*. This rickettsia is immunologically similar to, but separable from, *R. rickettsii* by serological methods. Cross-protection is practically complete in convalescent guinea pigs, but immunization with *R. conorii* vaccine will not protect against *R. rickettsii* infection, and immunological differences are also demonstrable by the complement fixation test.

The animal reservoir of infection is the dog, and the disease is transmitted by the tick, *Rhipicephalus sanguineus*, in which the infection is congenital. The disease is milder than American spotted fever, with a case-fatality rate of 1 to 2 per cent. It is distinguished clinically by regional adenopathy and by the small, local, indurated lesion with a necrotic center which develops at the site of the tick bite and is known as the eschar or tâche noire.

The tick-bite fevers of Africa, including Kenya fever or Kenya typhus and South African tick fever, together with Indian tick typhus, appear to be the same disease as boutonneuse fever, although there is no eschar in Kenya fever. In Africa the infection is found in a number of ixodid ticks of the genera *Haemaphysalis, Amblyomma,* and *Rhipicephalus*. While these vectors constitute a reservoir of infection, there is also evidence that a reservoir may be present in wild rodents.

North Queensland Tick Typhus

This disease, occurring in Australia, was first described in 1946. The causative rickettsia is immunologically related to the spotted fever group but is sufficiently distinct that it has been designated *R. australis*. The evidence for tick transmission suggests that *Ixodes holocyclus* is a vector of the disease.

Siberian Tick Typhus

This is a relatively mild rickettsial disease, occurring in Central Asia and extending to the eastern coast of Siberia. The causative rickettsia is closely related to, but differentiable from, *R. conorii* and has been called *R. sibirica*. The disease is believed to be transmitted by several ticks, including *Haemaphysalis* and *Dermacentor*.

RICKETTSIALPOX[1]

Rickettsialpox was first observed in New York City in 1946, when 124 cases were reported, and subsequently has been found in urban areas on the eastern seaboard of this country. It has also been reported to occur in urban areas in Russia, and the organism has been isolated from wild rodents in Korea. The disease is a mild febrile illness, characterized by an eschar at the site of infection, and a varicelliform rash. It is rarely if ever fatal.

The causative agent is *R. akari*, a member of the spotted fever group immunologically related to, but distinguishable from, *R. rickettsii*. The animal reservoir of infection is the wild house mouse, *Mus musculus,* and the disease is transmitted by the mite *Allodermanyssus sanguineus*. The causative agent has been isolated from mice and mites as well as from patients' blood, and the human infection is apparently acquired from the bite of infected mites. *Rickettsia akari* is pathogenic for both wild and laboratory mice, and for the guinea pig, in which a febrile disease and scrotal reaction are produced.

Rickettsia akari is readily cultivable in the embryonated hen's egg, in the amnionic cavity or the yolk sac. Yolk sac antigen fixes complement in the presence of patient's serum, but also cross-reacts with spotted fever antibody.

SCRUB TYPHUS[22]

A disease of rickettsial etiology prevalent in the Far East is known in Japan as tsutsugamushi disease (dangerous bug disease), Japanese flood fever, or Kedani fever; in Sumatra as mite typhus; and in Malaya as rural or scrub typhus. The disease is very similar to spotted fever in its distribution and clinical picture but differs in the latter respect in that there is a primary sore and adenitis as in fièvre boutonneuse; symptoms include headache, orbital pain, maculopapular rash, and fever. As in spotted fever, the case-fatality rate varies widely, from 0.5 per cent to perhaps as high as 60 per cent in some areas such as Korea.

The causative microorganism is *Rickettsia tsutsugamushi.* Strains are closely related immunologically but are readily differentiated by complement fixation. There seems, however, to be no clear serological differentiation into types, and the strains also differ in virulence and in degree of adaptation to egg culture. Those commonly used as antigens are the Gilliam, Kato, and Karp strains. Serums from some cases react predominantly with one type or another, while others exhibit about the same titer with all three. *Rickettsia tsutsugamushi* may be grown in the yolk sac or chorioallantois of the chick embryo, in tissue culture, and in the lungs of rats.

Experimental animals recovered from nonfatal infection show practically complete cross-immunity among strains of *R. tsutsugamushi.* Immunization with vaccine is a difficult matter, however, for apparently subcutaneous inoculation does not protect, but intraperitoneal vaccine protects against intraperitoneal challenge. Formalinized tissue culture vaccine or rat lung vaccine has been used for successful immunization of experimental animals. Vaccines of killed organisms are ineffective in man, but an effective immunity has been produced with vaccine of living rickettsiae given together with chloramphenicol to provide protection against illness. At present, however, active prophylactic immunization of man is not practical because of lack of cross-protection between the various strains of *R. tsutsugamushi.*

Scrub typhus occurs over a wide area in the Asiatic Pacific region. It appears to persist as an infection of rodents and of trombiculid mites (chiggers) and is transmitted to man by mites, in which the microorganism is ovarially transmitted. The vertebrate host and insect host and vector differ somewhat from place to place. Rodent hosts include rats, mice, and shrews; vectors are usually species of *Leptotrombidium.* The mites occur in low, damp areas of grass, underbrush, and scrub, and along the uncultivated banks of rivers; the infection is thus restricted to certain localities. In the temperate climate of Japan the disease has a seasonal incidence, but in tropical regions there is no strict seasonal distribution of the human disease.

Q FEVER[9, 13]

Q fever was described in Australia in 1937 as occurring in slaughterhouse workers, and the causative agent was shown to be a rickettsia. What proved to be a closely similar, if not identical, microorganism was isolated in the United States from ticks, and the disease it produced in guinea pigs was called Nine-Mile fever. When the Australian and American strains proved to be substantially identical, the disease was called American Q fever in this country, but since the microorganism has been found to be of worldwide occurrence, the geographical designations have been dropped.

The causative microorganism, *Coxiella burnetii,* is set apart from the other rickettsiae in a number of its characteristics. It is not toxic, is more resistant to heat and drying than the other rickettsiae, and is unique within the group in that arthropod transmission is not an essential link in its dissemination. It is immunologically distinct from the other rickettsiae. In general, it appears to be sufficiently different from the other rickettsiae causing human disease to justify giving it independent generic status.

Like most other rickettsiae, it grows profusely in the yolk sac of the embryonated egg and may be cultivated in various kinds of tissue cultures. Guinea pigs may be infected, and the infection is either symptomless or accompanied only by a febrile reaction, but there is a specific immunological response. *Coxiella burnetii* occurs in **two antigenic phases.** The naturally occurring, virulent phase I contains the full antigenic complement of the somatic O antigen, whereas phase II, which arises under conditions of laboratory cultivation, lacks the specific polysaccharide sequences that characterize the complete LPS. Phase II may revert to phase I after animal passage. The variation from phase I to phase II is accompanied by reduction in virulence and increased susceptibility to phagocytosis and is analogous to S–R variation in other bacteria. All phase I *Coxiella burnetii* appear to be antigenically homogeneous; phase I antigen has higher protective potency as vaccine.

The Disease in Man

The disease in man is a febrile respiratory illness, with an incubation period of 14 to 26 days. The infection is usually acquired by **inhalation of infectious material**, although transmission by blood transfusion has been reported. It characteristically takes the form of atypical pneumonia and is responsible for an appreciable portion of illness diagnosed clinically as primary atypical pneumonia; pneumonic involvement is demonstrable by x-ray examination in even mild cases. Convalescence is apt to be protracted. There is often evidence of liver involvement, headache is a prominent symptom, and there is no rash. *Coxiella burnetii* has recently been shown to cause subacute endocarditis; as noted earlier, endocarditis requires more vigorous antibiotic therapy than the respiratory infection. Complement-fixing antibody is present in convalescent serums, and delayed hypersensitivity may develop.

The human disease is widespread, occurring in all major geographical areas, as shown both by diagnosed illness and by the prevalence of serum antibody found in surveys. The largest number of cases has been reported from North America and various parts of Europe, especially from Germany and the Mediterranean area. The number of cases reported in this country probably does not reflect the true incidence, since the disease is not nationally notifiable. Since 1948, an average of 39 cases per year has been reported to the Centers for Disease Control.[6] A number of these infections have been laboratory-associated.

Infection in Lower Animals

The Australian studies showed the existence of a relatively intricate host-parasite relationship. In Australia, *C. burnetii* is maintained in wild animals, especially bandicoots, and is transmitted by *Haemaphysalis* and *Ixodes* ticks. Cattle may be infected by these ticks and, in turn, cattle ticks become infected. The rickettsiae occur in large numbers in the feces of infected ticks and survive for long periods in the dry state. The contamination of cattle hides with such infected feces, and the inhalation of this dust, is regarded as the probable mechanism of infection of slaughterhouse workers in Australia. The disease also occurs among slaughterhouse workers in the United States.

Infection in dairy cattle is very widespread over the United States, with herd infection rates ranging from 1 to 65 per cent. *Coxiella burnetii* is constantly present in the milk from such herds, and is shed into the environment in infected placentas at parturition. Inapparent infection in dairy workers, as reflected serologically, is substantial and parallels the incidence of infection in cattle. Pasteurization of milk suffices to destroy the *Coxiella*, but the margin of safety is very narrow, and the microorganism is occasionally found in pasteurized milk.

The infection is maintained in sheep herds by contamination of the environment by milk and infected placentas taken at lambing time; the latter is reflected in the seasonal increase of human disease. It is probable that infection occurs by inhalation of contaminated dust. There is also serological evidence for the occurrence of reservoirs of infection in domestic fowl and wild birds, and their ectoparasites.

TRENCH FEVER

In the course of World War I a specific infection became known by the name of trench fever or Wolhynian fever. It is said to have caused almost one-third of all the illness in some of the armies in northern France. It appeared again in World War II in the German army in Russia. It has a long incubation period (6 to 22 days); the most constant symptom is pain in the legs; the fever is often high and of the relapsing type. Recovery is the rule. Experimentally, the disease can be transmitted to healthy individuals by the intravenous injection of whole blood taken from patients.

Natural transmission is chiefly, if not solely, through the **body louse.** The bites of infective lice appear to be the most important element in producing trench fever, but the infectious agent is also present in the excreta and may enter through abrasions in the skin caused by scratching. The infectious agent is present in the urine of patients and is said to remain active for a long period in dry louse feces and dried urine.

The association of rickettsiae with the disease was established in 1919; the causative agent, known as *Rochalimaea quintana*, has been cultured on blood agar, with both erythrocytes and serum contributing essential nutrients. The disease has been reproduced in human volunteers and monkeys with such cultures but not as yet in other experimental animals. Patients' serums agglutinate rickettsiae and diagnosis is based on the louse-feeding test, or xenodiagnosis.

In the original studies it was found that the blood remains infectious for lice, and the lice for human volunteers, for some months after disappearance of symptoms. Subsequently it has been found that the infection may persist for years, with relapse as long as 19 years after the initial illness.

Bartonella[10]

Included in the order Rickettsiales are several hemotropic bacteria that grow in blood and appear to have an affinity for erythrocytes during infection; most of these are animal pathogens, but at least one, *Bartonella bacilliformis,* causes disease in humans. Two genera, *Bartonella* and *Grahamella,* make up the family Bartonellaceae. These bacteria are coccobacillary in shape and are transmitted by infected arthropod vectors; unlike most of the rickettsiae, however, they are cultivable on artificial mediums. *Grahamella* are natural parasites of small mammals, while *Bartonella* affect only humans.

A number of other related organisms are classified in several genera of the family Anaplasmataceae, including *Anaplasma, Hemobartonella,* and *Eperythrozoon* as the principal animal pathogens. These microorganisms are transmitted by arthropod vectors and have not been grown on artificial mediums. A variety of domestic and wild animals are naturally infected.

BARTONELLA BACILLIFORMIS

Oroya fever, an infectious anemia, and **verruga peruana**, a disease characterized by miliary or nodular skin eruptions, have existed for centuries in certain districts in Peru and have recently been found in Colombia and Ecuador. It was shown by Carrión, through fatal self-inoculation, that the two are stages or manifestations of a single disease which is now commonly known as Carrión's disease. The etiological agent is a small pleomorphic bacillus that was first observed by Barton in 1905 and was later named *Bartonella bacilliformis.*

Morphology and Staining
Bartonella bacilliformis is a small, motile, aerobic, gram-negative bacillus 0.2 to 0.5 μm. in diameter and 1 to 2 μm. in length. It is slightly curved and occurs singly, end-to-end in pairs, and in short chains. A rounded ovoid form, 0.3 to 1.0 μm. in diameter, also is seen in pairs and in groups. The bacillus stains reddish-violet with Giemsa, sometimes showing a reddish-purple granule at one end of a bluish rod. In culture, a unipolar tuft of flagella may be formed.

Physiology
This microorganism was first cultivated in semisolid leptospira medium and later in tissue culture and in the developing chick embryo, though it could not be carried in serial transfer in the latter. Sparse growth occurs on cystine-glucose-blood agar, and apparently heme is required while NAD is not. Relatively little is known of its physiology; it is not biochemically active and grows at 28° to 37° C.

Pathogenicity for Man
As indicated above, the disease is seen in two forms: the systemic form, in which the red cells are infected, and the histoid cutaneous form. The two may exist independently, coexist, or appear sequentially. The usual course is the appearance of the systemic form followed by the cutaneous form if the former is not fatal. The first is a severe, often fatal, febrile anemia, with an incubation period of about three weeks. The anemia is thought to be due to the direct action of the microorganisms on the erythrocytes, including hemolysis, and to tissue hemorrhage. The fever is of an irregular remittent type, and pain in the bones, joints, and head is common. The case-fatality rate is 20 to 40 per cent, death occurring two to three weeks after onset. With recovery, the eruptive stage of the disease may appear and persist for two to three months. Whether it follows the systemic form or is the primary clinical manifestation of infection, this stage is characterized by a miliary or nodular eruption; the former is by far the more common. The miliary eruption usually appears on the face and extremities, in the form of a macule that becomes nodular and eventually disappears, leaving no scar. The nodular type of eruption

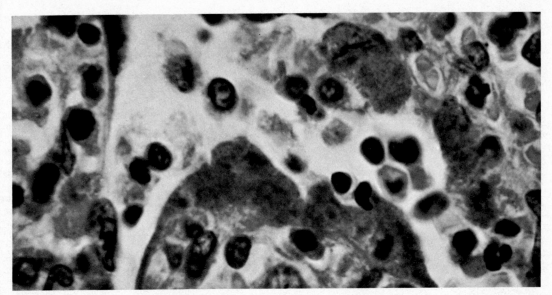

Figure 33–12. *Bartonella bacilliformis* in human spleen. Note the huge numbers of the microorganisms packed into the lining cells. Giemsa; × 1450. (Humphreys.)

develops more slowly; the nodules may become 2 to 3 cm. in diameter and have a tendency to become strangulated. They are formed by the proliferation of endothelial cells and fibroblasts, and show a marked tendency to hemorrhage.

Bartonella cells are found in large numbers within erythrocytes in Oroya fever and may be demonstrated in Giemsa-stained blood smears. In both forms of the disease they are found in the tissue macrophages, especially the vascular endothelial cells of the lymphatics, spleen, and liver, often in large clusters within individual cells (Fig. 33–12). The infection is frequently complicated by *Salmonella* infection to give a high mortality. It is reported that blood cultures are frequently positive in the systemic infection, but it is not clear whether this is a reliable method of diagnosis. The disease has been treated successfully with chloramphenicol and tetracycline.

Epidemiology

Bartonellosis is strictly limited geographically, being, so far as is known, exclusively American and tropical, occurring in the Andes mountains at elevations between 500 and 3000 m. It appears that man is the only naturally infected vertebrate host; the reservoir of infection is thought to be asymptomatic individuals who carry the microorganisms in their blood, and carrier rates of 5 to 10 per cent have been reported in endemic areas. It is transmitted by *Phlebotomus* in Peru, but whether other arthropods, such as *Dermacentor,* are natural vectors is not known.

Immunity

It is generally said that recovery from an attack of either form of the disease confers a solid immunity to both. With the cultivation of *B. bacilliformis,* it has been possible to study the occurrence of circulating antibody and to investigate the possibilities of prophylactic immunization. Agglutinins may be demonstrated during the early stages of the disease but, in spite of the lasting immunity, almost always disappear with the subsidence of clinical symptoms. Their diagnostic significance is not as yet known.

Pathogenicity for Animals

In general, experimental animals appear to be highly resistant to infection with *B. bacilliformis.* Both the eruptive and systemic forms of the disease have been produced in rhesus monkeys, the latter form in splenectomized animals.

REFERENCES

1. Brettman, L. R., *et al.* 1981. Rickettsialpox: report of an outbreak and a contemporary review. Medicine **60**:363–372.
2. Brezina, R., *et al.* 1973. Rickettsiae and rickettsial diseases. Bull. Wld Hlth Org. **49**:433–442.

3. Buchanan, R. E., and N. E. Gibbons (Eds.). 1974. Bergey's Manual of Determinative Bacteriology. 8th ed. The Williams & Wilkins Co., Baltimore.

4. Burgdorfer, W., and R. L. Anacker. 1981. Rickettsiae and Rickettsial Diseases. Academic Press, New York.

5. Burgdorfer, W. 1977. Tick-borne diseases in the United States: Rocky Mountain spotted fever and Colorado tick fever. A review. Acta Tropica **34**:103–126.

6. D'Angelo, L. J., E. F. Baker, and W. Schlosser. 1979. Q fever in the United States, 1948–1977. J. Infect. Dis. **139**:613–615.

7. D'Angelo, L. J., W. G. Winkler, and D. J. Bregman. 1978. Rocky Mountain spotted fever in the United States, 1975–1977. J. Infect. Dis. **138**:273–276.

8. Duma, R. J., et al. 1981. Epidemic typhus in the United States associated with flying squirrels. J. Amer. Med. Assn **245**:2318–2323.

9. Hall, C. J., et al. 1982. Laboratory outbreak of Q fever acquired from sheep. Lancet **1**:1004–1006.

10. Kreier, J. P., and M. Ristic. 1981. The biology of hemotropic bacteria. Ann. Rev. Microbiol. **35**:325–338.

11. McCaul, T. F., and J. C. Williams. 1981. Developmental cycle of Coxiella burnetii: structure and morphogenesis of vegetative and sporogenic differentiations. J. Bacteriol. **147**:1063–1076.

12. McDade, J. E., et al. 1980. Evidence of Rickettsia prowazekii infections in the United States. Amer. J. Trop. Med. Hygiene **29**:277–284.

13. Meiklejohn, G., et al. 1981. Cryptic epidemic of Q fever in a medical school. J. Infect. Dis. **144**:107–113.

14. Ormsbee, R. A. 1980. Rickettsiae. pp. 922–933. In E. H. Lennette, et al. (Eds.): Manual of Clinical Microbiology. 3rd ed. American Society for Microbiology, Washington, D.C.

15. Philip, R. N., et al. 1980. Rickettsiology conference. J. Infect. Dis. **141**:112–118.

16. Report. 1982. Rickettsioses: a continuing disease problem. Bull. Wld Hlth Org. **60**:157–164.

17. Russo, P. K., et al. 1981. Epidemic typhus (Rickettsia prowazekii) in Massachusetts: evidence of infection. New Engl. J. Med. **304**:1166–1168.

18. Schramek, S., and H. Mayer. 1982. Different sugar compositions of lipopolysaccharides isolated from phase I and pure phase II cells of Coxiella burnetii. Infect. Immun. **38**:53–57.

19. Schramek, Š., R. Brezina, and J. Kazár. 1977. Some biological properties of an endotoxic lipopolysaccharide from the typhus group rickettsiae. Acta Virol. **21**:439–441.

20. Silverman, D. J., and C. L. Wisseman, Jr. 1979. In vitro studies of rickettsia-host cell interactions: ultrastructural changes induced by Rickettsia rickettsii infection in chicken embryo fibroblasts. Infect. Immun. **26**:714–727.

21. Stork, E., and C. L. Wisseman, Jr. 1976. Growth of Rickettsia prowazeki in enucleated cells. Infect. Immun. **13**:1743–1748.

22. Traub, R., and C. L. Wisseman, Jr. 1974. The ecology of chigger-borne rickettsiosis (scrub typhus). J. Med. Entomol. **11**:237–303.

23. Weiss, E. 1973. Growth and physiology of rickettsiae. Bacteriol. Rev. **37**:259–283.

24. Weiss, E. 1982. The biology of rickettsiae. Ann. Rev. Microbiol. **36**:345–370.

25. Weyer, F. 1978. Progress in ecology and epidemiology of rickettsioses. Acta Tropica **35**:5–21.

26. Winkler, H. H., and E. T. Miller. 1980. Phospholipase A activity in the hemolysis of sheep and human erythrocytes by Rickettsia prowazeki. Infect. Immun. **29**:316–321.

34

Chlamydia

The microorganisms now known as *Chlamydia* were first described in 1907, in association with trachoma, a human eye infection. The trachoma agent was long considered to be protozoan, but in the 1920s, when a similar microorganism was found to cause psittacosis, it was concluded that these were large viruses. Definitive studies in the 1960s led to the now-accepted view that they are procaryotic in nature and, like rickettsiae, are gram-negative, obligately intracellular bacteria.

Chlamydiae resemble rickettsiae in a number of respects. They stain in a similar fashion, but chlamydiae are slightly smaller, falling just within the limits of optical resolution; they are obligate intracellular parasites; multiplication is by binary fission; the cell wall is like that of gram-negative bacteria; and they are sensitive to antibiotics effective against other bacteria. On the other hand, they differ from rickettsiae and other bacteria by a relatively complex growth cycle. Their resemblance to rickettsiae has led to classification with these microorganisms (Chapter 2). They are formally classified within the family Chlamydiaceae in the genus *Chlamydia*. Two species, *Chlamydia trachomatis* and *Chlamydia psittaci,* compose the genus. These resemble one another closely, and it is believed that they may have emanated from a common ancestral form by association with different host species. There is, however, only slight DNA homology between the two species.

Chlamydiae are ubiquitous parasites in a variety of vertebrate hosts. *Chlamydia psittaci* is primarily an animal pathogen, affecting both domestic and wild mammals as well as a great number of birds and fowl. Man is only incidentally infected by this species; most human infections are due to the avian strains of *C. psittaci*, particularly those from psittacine birds and domestic fowl. Mammalian strains apparently have only low virulence for humans, since human infections due to these strains are relatively rare despite undoubtedly frequent exposure.

In contrast, *Chlamydia trachomatis* appears to be confined to the human host, in which it produces several kinds of illness that includes trachoma and other ocular infections, lymphogranuloma venereum, arthritis, genital infections, and neonatal pneumonia.

675

The Biology of Chlamydiae[1, 5, 11, 12]

Chlamydiae are **obligately intracellular bacteria,** *i.e.,* they grow only within eucaryotic host cells. They are set apart from similar bacteria by an intricate developmental cycle that characterizes their growth in parasitized cells. Within infected cells, the microorganisms occur in intracytoplasmic inclusion bodies or vesicles. During morphological development of chlamydiae in these vesicles, two types of particles are observed: a small, dense particle—the elementary body—and a larger, less dense form—the reticulate body. The comparative fine structure of these two forms is shown in Figure 34–1.

Developmental Cycle and Morphology

The mature, infectious, stable form of chlamydiae is the **elementary body** (Fig. 34–2). It is spherical in shape and ranges from 200 to 400 nm. in diameter. The elementary body consists of a central nucleoid, compact and electron-dense, enclosed within a cell wall that is similar in construction to that of other gram-negative bacteria; the peptidoglycan of the cell wall does not, however, contain muramic acid as in other gram-negative bacteria. Both elementary and reticulate bodies possess regular arrays of surface projections (Fig. 34–3). Although their function is not known, they apparently do not mediate adherence to host cells.[8]

The genome of the elementary body is smaller than that of most other bacteria. The molecular weight of the genomic DNA is about 6.6 to 9.5 × 10[8] daltons with 6 to 8 × 10[5] base pairs, which is roughly equivalent to that of

rickettsiae, and less than one-fourth the size of *Escherichia coli* DNA.

The developmental cycle of chlamydiae begins when the infectious elementary body contacts specific receptors on the surface of susceptible host cells. The bacterial ligand is a heat-labile surface component of the elementary body, while the host cell receptor is a trypsin-sensitive site on the cytoplasmic membrane. After attachment, the elementary body is internalized by a process akin to phagocytosis. Chlamydiae play an active role in this internalization process, since they induce phagocytosis even in nonprofessional cells that do not normally engulf particles. Upon entry, the elementary bodies are enveloped within phagosomes, but these do not fuse with lysosomes at this stage; lysosomal fusion is inhibited by the viable chlamydiae and is directed by the chlamydial surface antigens.

During the next 6 to 8 hours, the elementary bodies undergo a type of reorganization that is discernible by the formation of a new morphological form, called **reticulate,** or **initial,** bodies. Reticulate bodies are larger, 0.8 to 1.0 μm. in diameter, are less electron-dense, and are rich in RNA. This form is metabolically active, synthesizing proteins and other macromolecules and multiplies by binary fission, forming microcolonies within vesicles that are called **inclusion bodies** (Figs. 34–4 and 34–5). Reticulate bodies are less stable than elementary bodies and are not infectious for other host cells. About 20 hours into the cycle, some of the reticulate bodies condense and mature, forming new elementary bodies. The host cell is apparently not damaged until late in the

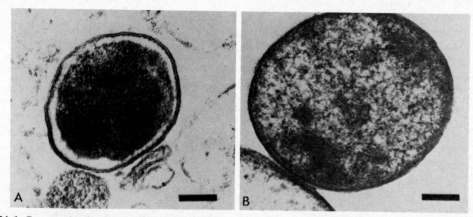

Figure 34–1. Comparative fine structure of the elementary body *(A)* and the reticulate body *(B)* of *Chlamydia trachomatis.* Bars = 0.1 μm. (R. B. Clark *et al.,* Infect. Immun. **38**:1273, 1982.)

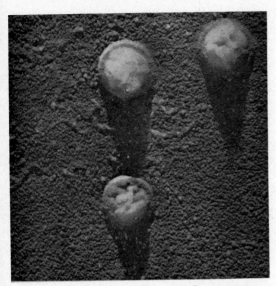

Figure 34–2. Shadow-cast electron micrograph of *C. psittaci* (feline pneumonitis agent). Note the collapse of the spherical particle in the dried preparation, showing the dense central mass and the outer limiting membrane. × 30,000. (Moulder and Weiss.)

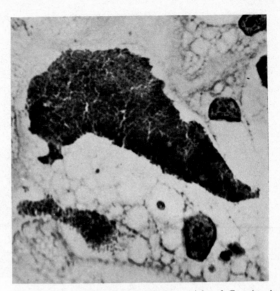

Figure 34–4. A mature intracellular vesicle of *C. psittaci* in chick endodermal cell culture. May-Gruenwald-Giemsa stain; × 432. (Weiss.)

cycle, when lysosomal fusion begins to occur. The vesicle then disintegrates, liberating new elementary bodies to begin the cycle once more. The properties of both elementary and reticulate bodies are listed in Table 34–1.

Chlamydial elementary bodies stain readily with aniline dyes. With Macchiavello stain they appear red, while the immature reticulate bod-

ies and surrounding dense ground substance, are stained blue. Later in the growth cycle, the matrix becomes less dense, so that blue reticulate bodies and red elementary bodies are seen against the pale blue background of the matrix. When stained with Lugol's iodine, the inclusion bodies of the two species are differentially stained. Those of *C. trachomatis* are usually brown in color, due to the presence in the matrix of a carbohydrate, probably glycogen; *C. psittaci* inclusion bodies do not stain with iodine.

Physiology and Cultivation

Chlamydiae are considered to be **energy parasites** in that they utilize ATP produced by the host cell. In addition, host cells contribute essential precursors for chlamydial synthetic reactions, and some host synthetic machinery

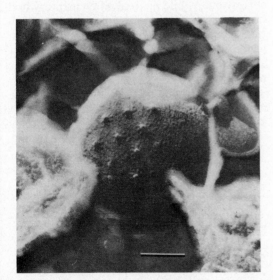

Figure 34–3. Electron photomicrograph of a frozen and deep-etched preparation of elementary body of *Chlamydia psittaci*. Note the surface projections arising from the center of a "flower structure" composed of a radial arrangement of several leaves. Bar = 100 nm. (A. Matsumoto, J. Bacteriol. **151**:1040, 1982.)

Table 34–1. **Properties of Elementary and Reticulate Bodies of *Chlamydia****

Property	Elementary Body	Reticulate Body
Size	0.2 to 0.4 μm.	0.6 to 1.0 μm.
Rigid cell wall	+	−
Extracellular stability	+	−
Metabolic activity	−	+
Infectivity	+	−
Replication	−	+
RNA:DNA ratio	< 1	3–4
Toxicity	+	−

*Adapted from J. Schachter and H. D. Caldwell, Ann. Rev. Microbiol. **34**:285, 1980.

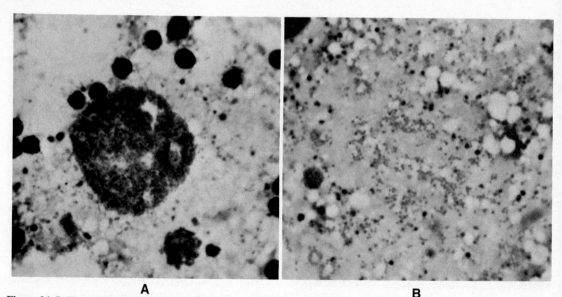

A   **B**

Figure 34–5. The elementary bodies of *Chlamydia trachomatis* in egg culture. *A,* An intracellular aggregate representing a "colony" of the microorganism; *B,* extracellular particles. Macchiavello stain; × 1330. (M. L. Tarizzo and B. Nabli, Bull Wld Hlth Org., **27**:741, 1962.)

may be utilized as well. Chlamydiae do, however, exhibit a limited number of independent metabolic activities.

Like rickettsiae, chlamydiae can be cultivated in the chicken embryo yolk sac. Such methods are difficult and cumbersome, however, and the study of these microorganisms was greatly advanced when it was established that they can be grown in a variety of cells in tissue culture. Cell cultures that have proved satisfactory include McCoy cells, a mouse fibroblast cell line; HeLa cells, from human cervical cancer; and BHK-21, a baby hamster kidney cell line.

Intracellular chlamydial growth is not dependent upon replication of the host cells. Indeed, the growth of *C. trachomatis* is enhanced if the host cell population is rendered metabolically inactive by ultraviolet irradiation or by chemical treatment with cytostatic agents, such as iododeoxyuridine or cyclohexamide, before infection.

Classification

Two species are recognized in the genus *Chlamydia* and are differentiated on the basis of sulfonamide resistance, staining of intracellular inclusions by iodine, guanosine plus cytosine content of their DNA, and, to some extent, host range, as shown in Table 34–2. Although *C. trachomatis* primarily affects humans, strains that cause rodent pneumonitis have been noted. Within each species, subspecies are differentiated on the basis of their antigenic structure, as discussed below.

Toxicity

The toxicity of chlamydia can be demonstrated either by injection of large numbers of elementary bodies into experimental animals or by exposure of animal cells in culture to chlamydiae. Toxicity is not due to released toxins, but is associated with cellular events related to attachment and induced phagocytosis of the elementary bodies. In experimental animals, death follows the inoculation of large numbers of active (or ultraviolet irradiated) chlamydiae, while heat-killed elementary bodies have no effect. Animal toxicity is neutralized by specific antiserum, presumably by interfering with attachment. Chemotherapeutic agents, on the other hand, are without effect on toxicity.

Exposure of animal cells in culture to chlamydiae at high multiplicities—more than 1000 infective particles per host cell—results in cytotoxicity, and such cell cultures are usually

Table 34–2. **Differential Characters of the Chlamydia**

Character	C. trachomatis	C. psittaci
Sensitivity to sulfonamides	+	−
Inclusion staining by iodine	+	−
Mole % G + C*	44–45	41
Usual host range	Humans	Mammals, birds

*Guanine plus cytosine content of DNA.

destroyed within 20 hours. Use of lower infective doses extends the time required for death of the cell culture. In some circumstances, occasional cells may survive the infection and become persistently infected with a cryptic form of chlamydiae; such cells are not subject to superinfection with exogenous chlamydiae.[6, 7]

Cellular death, whether in intact animals or in tissue cultures, does not require multiplication of the infective agent, but is related to phagocytic events and is likely due to multiple lesions produced in the plasma membrane during phagocytosis.

In the later stages, chlamydial development within eucaryotic cells is accompanied by release of lysosomal enzymes into the host cell cytoplasm, which also leads to cytopathogenic effects.[13]

There is reason to believe that chlamydial toxicity may contribute significantly to the pathogenesis of disease, as in the induction of hemorrhage and edema in the lungs.

Antigenicity

All chlamydiae share antigens specific to the genus. The dominant group-specific antigen of this kind is a heat-stable, acidic lipopolysaccharide that resembles *Salmonella* lipopolysaccharide. The antigen reacts in the **complement fixation reaction**, and this has been the serological test most often employed for serodiagnosis. Complement-fixing antibodies against the group-specific antigens are induced in systemic infections, except in infants, but do not reach diagnostically useful levels in trachoma, inclusion conjunctivitis, or urethritis. Furthermore, large segments of the general population exhibit low complement fixation titers against the antigen.

Both *C. trachomatis* and *C. psittaci* possess antigen complexes that seem to be species-specific. These are, for the most part, proteins and are heat-labile. Those of *C. psittaci* are not well known, but in *C. trachomatis*, the predominant species antigen, apparently shared by all strains except the mouse pneumonitis agent, is a heat-labile, membrane-associated protein. The species-specific antigens can be detected by fluorescent antibody methods, by immunodiffusion, or by indirect hemagglutination.

The relevance of species-specific antigens to protection is suggested by the fact that antibody to these antigens protects animals against chlamydial toxicity. Incubation of elementary bodies with homologous strain antibody prior to inoculation into mice neutralizes their toxicity. Only small amounts of protective and neutralizing antibody are found in convalescent serums, so that such tests have no diagnostic value.

It is apparent that all chlamydiae are antigenically complex, and a number of serotypically specific antigens have also been noted; unfortunately, information on these antigens is somewhat sketchy and conflicting. *Chlamydia psittaci* is composed of many different serological varieties, but these are not well known and differentiation has not proved useful. Fifteen serotypes of *C. trachomatis* are recognized. The antigens responsible for serotype specificity are varied in nature; many appear to be proteins, but some may be lipoidal haptens. Antibodies to these serotype antigens are produced in most infections and can be titrated by microimmunofluorescence. Such determinations are valuable in seroepidemiology, but have little utility in diagnosis.

Laboratory Diagnosis[10]

In spite of the clinical importance of chlamydial infections, the more sophisticated laboratory procedures to aid in diagnosis are not routinely available.

With a few exceptions, to be discussed later in connection with specific infections, serological tests to detect antibody response to infection have not been particularly informative. Complement fixation may be useful in some systemic infections, such as lymphogranuloma and psittacosis, but not, as noted earlier, in other chlamydial infections.

Direct cytological methods, as by Giemsa stains of conjunctival scrapings, are most useful in inclusion conjunctivitis of neonates, but less sensitive for other infections. Direct cytological methods are improved by use of fluorescent antibody staining.

The most satisfactory and sensitive aid to diagnosis is the **direct isolation** and cultivation of the causative agent. Although cultivation in chicken embryo yolk sac has been used, it is slow, cumbersome, and of relatively low sensitivity. The method of choice is by cultivation in tissue culture systems, usually nonreplicating McCoy cells, *e.g.,* those treated with iododeoxyuridine or cyclohexamide. Infection of these cells with chlamydiae requires intimate contact with the host cell, so that the inoculum must be centrifuged onto cell monolayers to promote contact and infection. After 48 to 72 hours' incubation, the monolayer cells are examined for chlamydial inclusions by Giemsa, iodine, or fluorescent antibody staining. Antibiotics, such as streptomycin, are used to inhibit contaminants. *Chlamydia psittaci* and the lymphogranuloma venereum strains of *C. trachomatis* are able to infect adjacent cells during growth, so that plaques or other evidence of cytopathogenesis can be observed after incubation for 5 to 10 days.

Unfortunately, the isolation methods just described can be carried out only in laboratories with tissue culture capabilities; thus, isolation in this way is not routinely available in clinical laboratories. In any case, manipulations of *C. psittaci* are exceedingly hazardous and require appropriate isolation facilities to minimize infection hazards for laboratory personnel.

Chemotherapy

Chlamydiae are effectively suppressed in culture by rifampin, tetracyclines, and erythromycin. Penicillin has an appreciable but lesser effect, while aminocyclitols are not effective. These drugs are primarily growth inhibitory, and drugs effective *in vitro* may not be clinically useful.

All chlamydial infections respond to tetracycline, and resistance has not been reported. Erythromycin has also been successfully used, as has sulfisoxazole for *C. trachomatis* infections. It should be recognized that chlamydial infections are **intracellular**, with a tendency to become **latent** or **persistent**; short-term therapy is, therefore, not recommended. Tetracyclines, administered in 1-gram doses for 14 to 21 days is usually recommended, but sometimes must be repeated. Therapy for shorter periods may result in temporary clinical improvement followed by relapse. In the case of trachoma, intermittent local application of antibiotic ointments may be indicated, and should be carried out for at least six months.

Chlamydia trachomatis Infections[5, 9, 11, 12]

With the exception of a few strains causing rodent pneumonitis, *Chlamydia trachomatis* is typically a human pathogen with man as the sole natural host. Although *C. trachomatis* strains are immunologically related to one another, a number of serotypes can be differentiated, and there is some correlation of serotype with the different disease entities. On the basis of biological behavior and serology, two distinct groups of *C. trachomatis* can be recognized.

The group usually responsible for the sexually transmitted disease lymphogranuloma venereum is casually known as the LGV group. These are considered to be somewhat more invasive than the other members, perhaps related to their greater avidity for host cell receptors; they fall into three serotypes—L_1, L_2, and L_3.

The second group is associated with a variety of ocular and genital tract infections and comprises 12 serotypes, the trachoma–inclusion conjunctivitis (TRIC) agents. Those causing hyperendemic trachoma—TRIC serotypes A, B, Ba, and C—are transmitted by direct, usually nonsexual, contact. The remaining TRIC serotypes—D, E, F, G, H, I, J, and K—are responsible for a variety of disease conditions. Many of these are sexually transmitted, including genital tract infections in both sexes and inclusion conjunctivitis in adults. In neonates, infection is usually acquired at birth from infected mothers and may occur as inclusion conjunctivitis or neonatal pneumonia. These relationships are summarized in Table 34–3.

Table 34–3. **Human Diseases Caused by**
Chlamydia trachomatis

Group	Predominant Serotypes	Disease
LGV	L_1, L_2, L_3	Lymphogranuloma venereum
TRIC	A, B, Ba, C	Trachoma
TRIC	D through K	Inclusion conjunctivitis (adult and neonatal) Genital tract infections (nongonococcal urethritis, epididymitis, cervicitis, salpingitis) Neonatal pneumonia

LYMPHOGRANULOMA VENEREUM

Lymphogranuloma venereum (LGV) is a venereal disease caused by microorganisms of the *C. trachomatis* complex. The disease is also known as climatic bubo, tropical bubo, lymphopathia venereum, and lymphogranuloma inguinale. Although described as a clinical entity in 1913, it was not until the 1930s that its microbial etiology was recognized. During this period the application of immunological methods allowed the grouping of various genital diseases, such as elephantiasis of the female pudenda and inflammatory rectal strictures, into a disease of common etiology.

The affection tends to occur in tropical regions, because of socioeconomic rather than climatic conditions, but its true incidence is not known with any certainty because it is usually not reportable. It is known to be prevalent in South America, the West Indies, Africa, and Southeast Asia. In developed countries it appears in homosexual men and in travelers returning from endemic areas.

The microorganism is morphologically indistinguishable from other *C. trachomatis* and undergoes the developmental cycle in host cells previously described. The chlamydial agents of LGV share the group antigen of other chlamydia, but are unique in immunotype; three are recognized by microimmunofluorescence, designated L_1, L_2, and L_3, and are thereby differentiated from other *C. trachomatis* strains. Rarely, strains of *C. psittaci* are found as etiological agents of this clinical entity. Lymphogranuloma venereum is clinically distinct, and apparently occurs only in man, the sole natural host. While mice, monkeys, and embryonated eggs may be infected experimentally, the microorganism does not infect birds.

Pathogenicity for Man[3]
Following the initial wide dissemination of the microorganism in the blood, spinal fluid, and other tissues, the primary lesion appears within a few days. It takes the form of a vesicular or herpetiform lesion usually occurring on the coronal sulcus of the penis in males or on the posterior portions of the labia, vaginal wall, or cervix in women, and may also be found within the urethra and in the anal region. The vesicle breaks down to leave a shallow ulcer that is not indurated and heals without scarring; the lesion is painless and is frequently overlooked.

The second stage of the disease is an invasion of the lymphatics. The regional nodes, commonly inguinal and also pelvic in the female, become enlarged and painful to form the bubo. In half or more of cases these suppurate and may continue to drain for a long time. In this stage general as well as local symptoms occur, including fever and general aches; in some cases arthritic and conjunctival symptoms and signs of involvement of the central nervous system may occur.

The third stage is a urethrogenitoperineal syndrome. The structural changes include nondestructive elephantiasis of the labia and clitoris in the female (esthiomene) and of the penis and scrotum in the male; the rectum and anus may become involved with the development of rectal stenosis and stricture. The disease can be successfully treated with sulfonamides or the tetracyclines; resistance to sulfonamides, but not to tetracyclines, has been described.

Model Infections
The human disease is reasonably well reproduced in the monkey when the microorganism is inoculated into the prepuce, lymph nodes, or rectal tissue, with development of typical inflammatory reactions. Monkeys may also be infected by the intraperitoneal, intraocular, or intranasal routes, but not by intravenous or intracerebral inoculation. Unlike other *C. trachomatis* strains, the LGV agents are lethal for mice when injected intracerebrally and are capable of cell-to-cell transmission in tissue cultures to form plaques. LGV agents may be differentiated from other strains by these characters, as well as by immunofluorescence.

Immunity
Effective immunity to this disease appears to be an infection immunity associated with continued presence of the infectious agent. Experimental inoculation of an infected individual gives a hypersensitivity reaction similar to the Frei test (see below) but does not lead to the appearance of the initial vesicular lesion or an inflammatory response in the regional lymphatics.

An immune response is evident by the appearance of complement-fixing antibody after two to four weeks and the development of a hypersensitivity to the microbial substance. The complement fixation reaction is positive with serums from individuals infected with other chlamydia, but may be made more specific by preliminary adsorption of the serum with heterologous antigen; syphilitic serums may be nonspecifically positive. It is often not possible to obtain serum early in the disease, but a titer of 1:32 in conjunction with typical clinical findings is regarded as diagnostic, and an increasing titer has greater value. Specific antibody response can be detected by the microimmunofluorescence test.

Hypersensitivity was observed by Frei in 1925, occurring as a typical delayed reaction following intradermal inoculation of the microorganism. It was, in fact, the application of this reaction, the **Frei test**, that led to the identification of apparently diverse genital diseases, which had been known for many years, as manifestations of infection with this microorganism. Hypersensitivity develops one to six weeks after infection and probably remains positive for the life of the individual. The Frei test is relatively insensitive, however, and is no longer regarded as useful in diagnosis.

Epidemiology

The disease occurs in many tropical regions and is found largely in persons of low socioeconomic status. Indigenous infections in the United States are often in homosexual males.[2] Lymphogranuloma is usually, though not necessarily, transmitted by sexual intercourse. Infection of the eye with an oculoglandular syndrome is known, and primary infection may occur in the mouth with painless vesicular lesions and swelling of the tongue, followed by infection of the glands of the neck. Occasional accidental infections occur, as in hospital orderlies infected while cleaning patients and in surgeons infected during removal of infected lymph glands. Control of the disease is difficult because it is not ordinarily reportable.

TRACHOMA

Trachoma and inclusion conjunctivitis are similar diseases of the external eye which are caused by microorganisms of the *Chlamydia trachomatis* complex. This subgroup is sometimes referred to as the TRIC (*t*rachoma-*i*nclusion *c*onjunctivitis) group of agents. Naturally occurring infections are found only in man, and the host-specificity is sharp in experimental infections, which are similar to but generally milder than those in man and can be produced only in certain primates. Although trachoma is a specific infection with *C. trachomatis*, a major part of pathogenesis is due to superimposed bacterial infection.

Trachoma is an ancient disease and is referred to in some of the earliest known writings. It occurs in the Mediterranean area, especially in North Africa and the Middle East, and in Southeast Asia. In the United States it is principally found in a mild form among American Indians. Incidence is greatest, up to 90 per cent, in Egypt and in the Middle East, and 4 to 5 per cent of the residents of many areas are blind as a result of trachoma.[4] It is the leading cause of preventable blindness in the world.

There has been evidence of the microbial etiology of trachoma and inclusion blennorrhea, since the work of the Trachoma Commission in the early 1930s. The agent can be isolated and grown in yolk sac of embryonated eggs (Fig. 34–4) and in various types of tissue culture. In morphology and other growth characteristics it resembles closely the other microorganisms of this group. The agent of trachoma is a part of the TRIC complex of *C. trachomatis* and thus is related antigenically, through the group antigen, to other chlamydia. The TRIC agents are, however, separable into immunotypes by microimmunofluorescence. Immunotypes A, B, Ba, and C are those most often found in the hyperendemic trachoma of Africa and Asia characterized by eye-to-eye transmission. Other immunotypes in the TRIC complex are generally found in inclusion conjunctivitis and genital infections in Europe and the Americas (see below). The disease is approximately reproduced in various primates by infection with the trachoma agent; strain differences in virulence are sometimes observed.

Pathogenicity for Man

When the disease develops slowly, the first sign of infection is a slight ptosis of the lids, and there is follicular hypertrophy of the upper tarsal conjunctiva. When the disease develops rapidly in a fulminating form, there is an inflammatory reaction characterized by a papillary or follicular hypertrophy of the conjunctiva and a mucopurulent exudate; secondary bacterial infection is common, occurring in 50 per cent or more of cases. Intracytoplasmic inclusion bodies are found in the conjunctival and corneal epithelial cells in expressed follicular material. They are most numerous in the cells of the superficial layers of epithelium from the upper tarsal and upper limbus areas.

The disease progresses with vascularization of the cornea and pannus formation and secondary cicatrization of the cornea; partial or total blindness may result.

The disease is treated by systemic administration of tetracyclines, erythromycin, rifampicin, or sulfonamides. Tetracycline is the drug of choice in most instances but, as noted earlier, requires long-term therapy to achieve consistent cure. Mass treatment campaigns in endemic areas rely heavily on topical therapy, usually employing erythromycin ointment. As with systemic drugs, therapy must be persistent.

There appears to be little or no effective immunity, since reinfection or relapse is not uncommon. While vaccines have offered some short-lived protection, hypersensitivity may develop and lead to more severe disease; no practically useful vaccine is available. The complement fixation test is not sufficiently sensitive or specific for diagnostic purposes, but microimmunofluorescence permits detection of type-specific antibody response.

INCLUSION CONJUNCTIVITIS

Inclusion conjunctivitis is a benign conjunctivitis found in newborns and in adults. It differs clinically from trachoma in that pannus and scarring of the cornea are not observed; the disease is self-limiting and persistent chronic infections are rare, but infections lasting for some months or even as long as a year have been seen in adults.

The microorganism was isolated initially in the yolk sac of embryonated eggs by blind passage, with eventual adaptation to the egg. The organism may be grown in cell culture and appears to be closely related in all respects to the trachoma agent. The immunotypes most often involved are not those seen in trachoma, but are usually of types D through K.

Although overtly a disease of the eye, the infection is, in fact, derived from the genitourinary tract. Infants acquire the disease at birth from a genitourinary tract infection of the mother. In adults, the disease is most often acquired from infected genital tract secretions, and thus is considered to be sexually transmitted. Genitourinary tract infections may be asymptomatic in women, but often produce urethritis in men.

Neonatal Infections
Inclusion conjunctivitis of the newborn, or inclusion blenorrhea, usually appears after an incubation period of 5 to 14 days. The onset of the disease is sudden and characterized by an acute infiltration of the conjunctiva of the lower lid and a purulent exudate. The conjunctival epithelium is infiltrated with polymorphonuclear cells and contains basophilic intracytoplasmic inclusion bodies indistinguishable from those of trachoma. The demonstration of these bodies in epithelial scrapings has diagnostic significance. Occasionally the disease is severe, with the formation of transient pseudomembranes. The acute stage persists for perhaps two weeks and then gradually subsides, but the cornea does not return to normal for some months and may show evidence of infiltration for as long as a year.

Chlamydial inclusion conjunctivitis is the most common form of neonatal infectious conjunctivitis, with a high rate of attack in infants born of infected mothers. It has been estimated that 40 to 50 per cent of infants who are exposed develop this form of the disease.

Pneumonia. Infants with inclusion conjunctivitis often harbor chlamydiae in the nasopharynx and upper respiratory tract, as shown by cultural studies. The risk of chlamydial pneumonia in such infants is significant; a high proportion of cases of neonatal pneumonia, perhaps 30 to 50 per cent of those developing in the first six months of life, is due to *C. trachomatis*.

The pneumonia syndrome is characterized by an afebrile course, with a slowly developing distinct cough resembling pertussis, but without the inspiratory whoop; other than occasional vomiting and cyanosis, clinical findings are sparse. Antecedent conjunctivitis is present in only about 50 per cent of the pneumonia cases. Unlike conjunctivitis, high titers of serum antibodies to *C. trachomatis* are demonstrable by immunofluorescence in the pneumonic infection; serum IgM concentrations are virtually always elevated.

The pneumonia syndrome responds to erythromycin therapy, but relapses sometimes occur after therapy is discontinued.

Adult Conjunctivitis
The disease in adults differs in that it is an acute follicular conjunctivitis with little discharge and a mild periauricular adenopathy. The follicles have the same appearance as those found in trachoma, but the hypertrophy is more marked in the lower lid, there is an absence of corneal change, and, on microscopic examination, the follicular material does not show necrotic changes. It may, however, be difficult to differentiate from other forms of acute follicular conjunctivitis, and clinical diagnosis must be confirmed by the presence of inclusion bodies. The adult disease is also self-limited, resolving spontaneously without residual corneal or conjunctival changes; the disease in adults tends to persist longer than in the infant.

The adult disease is of greatest prevalence in sexually active young adults. In most cases it is an **autoinfection**, transferred to the eye by infected genital tract discharges. Some cases are contracted by swimming in pools that are inadequately chlorinated, and the disease has been called swimming pool conjunctivitis; it has also been reported in occupationally exposed medical personnel. Treatment is by oral tetracycline or erythromycin.

GENITAL TRACT INFECTIONS

The association of inclusion conjunctivitis with genital infections, as discussed in the foregoing section, is now well authenticated and it is clear that the ocular disease is transmitted by genital contact. These observations have stimulated interest among clinicians and epidemiologists concerning the possible role of chlamydial agents in urethritis in the absence of eye disease.

Nongonococcal urethritis (NGU), often termed nonspecific urethritis (NSU), is a common illness in Britain and the United States, probably exceeding gonorrhea in prevalence. A large number of these NGU cases cannot be accounted for by the usual causes. Although mycoplasmas (Chapter 35) are often found in association with this type of urethritis, evidence for their etiological role is not completely convincing. There is, however, evidence that a significant portion of NGU infections are due to chlamydial strains of the TRIC complex and that these infections are sexually transmitted. Chlamydial isolations and serological studies indicate that 40 per cent or more of primary nongonococcal urethritis in men is due to chlamydiae; in a significantly high number of cases, their female sexual partners also harbor the microorganism in the cervix. Infected women probably carry the microorganism for long periods, although genitourinary signs of disease are usually minimal or absent.

In a number of instances, **postgonococcal urethritis** follows penicillin therapy that elimi-nates the gonococcal infection. Like nonspecific urethritis, postgonococcal urethritis does not respond to penicillin, but is effectively treated with tetracyclines, thus suggesting specific microbial etiology. *Chlamydia* have been isolated from a significant number of these cases and it is usually assumed that the two infections are acquired at the same sexual exposure.

Chlamydial genital tract infection in males is ordinarily manifest as urethritis, sometimes complicated by epididymitis. The possibility of latent or inapparent infections cannot, however, be dismissed.

In women, chlamydia are frequently recovered from the cervix, particularly in those attending clinics for sexually transmitted diseases. It is clear that chlamydiae are associated with mucopurulent cervical inflammation, but cervical infections are often not clinically apparent. Chlamydiae are also a likely cause of nongonococcal pelvic inflammatory disease and, possibly, perihepatitis. Chlamydial infections in women are not as evident as those in males, so that infected women may serve as a partially hidden reservoir of the sexually transmitted disease.

Chemotherapy

Treatment of chlamydial genital tract infections can be highly successful. Tetracycline, sulfisoxazole, and erythromycin are effective, provided treatment extends over 14 to 21 days. In many cases, both sexual partners are infected, and concomitant treatment of the consort is recommended to prevent reinfection.

Chlamydia psittaci Infections[8, 11]

Psittacosis, or parrot fever, was first observed in Switzerland in 1880. For many years it was regarded as an unimportant disease of possible *Salmonella* etiology. In 1929 and 1930 it appeared in many parts of the world as a disease acquired for the most part from South American parrots. The elementary bodies were described in 1930; their nature and etiological relation to the disease were established in the early 1930s, largely through the work of Bedson and his colleagues.

During that decade it also became apparent that exotic imported psittacine birds are not the only source of infection and, in fact, that a domestic reservoir of infection occurs in many avian species, including gulls and other sea birds, pigeons, ducks, turkeys, and chick-ens. The 1938 epidemic of pneumonitis in the Faroe Islands, for example, was associated with widespread infection in fulmar petrels. Although often traced to psittacine birds, human disease in the United States and Europe is usually found in those occupationally exposed to domestic fowl, especially turkeys and ducks.

A variety of similar microorganisms have been isolated from lower animals and from human cases of pneumonitis. These are now considered to be strains of a single species, *Chlamydia psittaci.*

The pneumonitis in man was originally called psittacosis because it appeared to be acquired largely from psittacine birds; the term ornithosis was introduced when the broader base of the infection reservoir became apparent. Ornithosis, while not yet universally used, has gained increasing acceptance as a more inclusive term especially for disease in, and acquired from, other than psittacine birds.

Pathogenicity for Man

Pneumonitis produced in man by these avian chlamydiae is essentially the same regardless of the source of infection. The incubation period is one to two weeks, and the onset may be sudden or insidious. The symptoms include chills and fever, photophobia, headache, anorexia, sore throat, nausea, and vomiting. A dry cough develops which persists and may become more severe; cyanosis and low blood pressure are frequent; and disorientation, apathy, insomnia, and occasional delirium indicate involvement of the central nervous system. The extent of the lung involvement is usually not apparent except by x-ray examination, which shows patchy areas of consolidation in one or both lungs. The organism may be found in the blood during the first week of the disease and in the scanty sputum after the lungs are involved. Autopsy findings are clearly indicative of the generalized nature of the infection. The case-fatality rate was about 20 per cent in 1929 and 1930, dropped to about 10 per cent with the recognition of mild cases by serodiagnostic methods, and has been further reduced by therapy with tetracyclines.

Pathogenicity for Lower Animals

Naturally acquired infection is not uncommon among certain lower animals and, as a latent infection, occurs with even greater frequency.

Birds. The natural hosts of these microorganisms among the birds include parrots, parakeets, and budgereegahs; infections appear in no fewer than 31 species of the parrot family. Other birds such as canaries, finches, and sparrows contract the disease when exposed to infected psittacine birds; naturally occurring latent infection among pigeons appears to be relatively common, and microorganisms of the same group are found in doves, petrels, gulls, and egrets. The domestic chicken is naturally infected, though not commonly, and spontaneous infection, possibly derived from wild birds such as gulls and at times assuming epidemic form, occurs in turkeys and ducks.

Natural infections in birds are frequently nonfatal, and there is reason to suspect a reservoir of latent infection of considerable proportions. Infected birds excrete the infectious agent in the droppings, and dried fecal material is an important source of airborne infection.

Mammals. A number of mammals are infected with closely similar microorganisms in a latent form, and such infections may be activated to give a clinically apparent, and possibly fatal, disease. The mammalian strains of *C. psittaci,* although widespread infective agents in animals, apparently have little pathogenic potential in humans. Only rare instances of human infection with these strains have been reported, including ocular, respiratory, and urogenital infections;[14] such infections are more reminiscent of those caused by *C. trachomatis.*

Other mammals develop clinically apparent infections with microorganisms of this group, producing pneumonia of swine, meningopneumonitis of opossums, bovine encephalitis, ewe abortion, and cat distemper. The last, feline pneumonitis, has been widely used for experimental studies.

Immunity

As indicated above, the immune response results in the appearance of complement-fixing, protective, and antitoxic antibodies, varying with the host species. Complement-fixing antibody appears in 10 days to 2 weeks and hypersensitivity a week or two later. Effective immunity appears to be a part of infection immunity and dependent upon the continued presence of the infectious agent. Some attempts have been made to produce a prophylactic immunity in man by the use of vaccines, but with disappointing results.

Laboratory Diagnosis[10]

Infection with these microorganisms may be established by isolation of the infectious agent from blood, sputum, or lung tissue taken at autopsy. The organism is best grown in treated McCoy cell cultures (p. 679), in which inclusions can be identified by Giemsa stain or by immunofluorescent staining. *Chylamdia psittaci* is differentiated by the properties listed in Table 34–2. *Chlamydia psittaci* of avian origin will also grow well in the brain of mice after intracerebral inoculation or in liver and spleen following intraperitoneal challenge.

Serodiagnosis. The serological procedure used for diagnosis of *C. psittaci* infections is most commonly the complement fixation test. A rise in titer usually occurs within 10 days to 2 weeks, but may be delayed by chemotherapy. A fourfold rise in complement fixation titer to the group antigen is diagnostically significant.

Microimmunofluorescence titration, if available, is more sensitive than complement fixation.

Epidemiology

In the human disease the infectious agent usually enters the body via the respiratory tract. As indicated earlier, it is most often acquired from an avian reservoir of infection, usually indirectly by inhalation of dried infectious material such as feces, and less commonly by direct contact with infected birds. Psittacine birds are the best known of these reservoirs, and infection appears to be common among wild parrots and parakeets. It may assume clinical form in caged birds and is generally endemic in aviaries and in breeding colonies of pigeons and ducks. Under some circumstances the infection may be transmitted directly from man to man, as shown by a number of well-documented infections in hospital or nursing personnel; these are derived from infected patients. The highly virulent nature of the microorganism is evident from the number of laboratory infections that have occurred.

The incidence of the disease is largely an expression of risk. This factor accounts for its predominance in owners of pet birds and bird fanciers, and its tendency to occur as an occupational disease among professional handlers and breeders of birds. Control of the reservoir of infection in psittacine birds by quarantine has had some small success, but control generally depends upon avoiding sufficiently intimate contact with the animal reservoirs of endemic infection.

The disease is relatively rare in the United States. About 120 to 140 cases per year have been reported since 1978, representing about a twofold increase over the average during the period from 1960 to 1969. This increase is principally due to outbreaks among workers in turkey-processing plants.

REFERENCES

1. Becker, Y. 1978. The Chlamydia: molecular biology of procaryotic obligate parasites of eucaryotes. Microbiol. Rev. **42**:274–306.
2. Bolan, R. K., *et al.* 1982. Lymphogranuloma venereum and acute ulcerative proctitis. Amer. J. Med. **72**:703–706.
3. Hopsu-Havu, V. K., and C. E. Sonck. 1973. Infiltrative, ulcerative, and fistular lesions of the penis due to lymphogranuloma venereum. Brit. J. Vener. Dis. **49**:193–202.
4. Majčuk, J. 1976. Trachoma control in the Eastern Mediterranean region. Wld Hlth Org. Chron. **30**:97–100.
5. Mårdh, P.-A., B. R. Møeller, and J. Paavoneno (Eds.). 1982. *Chlamydia trachomatis* in genital and related infections. Scand. J. Infect. Dis. Suppl. 32, pp. 1–199.
6. Moulder, J. W., N. J. Levy, and L. P. Schulman. 1980. Persistent infection of mouse fibroblasts (L cells) with *Chlamydia psittaci:* evidence for a cryptic chlamydial form. Infect. Immun. **30**:874–883.
7. Moulder, J. W., S. L. Zeichner, and N. J. Levy. 1982. Association between resistance to superinfection and patterns of surface protein labeling in mouse fibroblasts (L cells) persistently infected with *Chlamydia psittaci.* Infect. Immun. **35**:834–839.
8. Potter, M. E., A. K. Kaufmann, and B. D. Plikaytis. 1983. Psittacosis in the United States, 1979. Morbid. Mortal. Wkly Rep. (Surveillance Summaries) **32** (Suppl. 1):27SS–31SS.
9. Report. 1981. Nongonococcal urethritis and other sexually transmitted diseases of public health importance. Wld Hlth Org. Tech. Rep. Ser., No. 660, Geneva.
10. Schachter, J. 1980. Chlamydiae (psittacosis-lymphogranuloma venereum-trachoma group). pp. 357–364. *In* E. H. Lennette, *et al.* (Eds.): Manual of Clinical Microbiology. 3rd ed. American Society for Microbiology, Washington, D.C.
11. Schachter, J. 1978. Chlamydial infections. (in three parts.) New Engl. J. Med. **298**:428–435; 490–495; 540–549.
12. Schachter, J., and H. D. Caldwell. 1980. Chlamydiae. Ann. Rev. Microbiol. **34**:285–309.
13. Todd, W. J., and J. Storz. 1975. Ultrastructural cytochemical evidence for activation of lysosomes in the cytocidal effect of *Chlamydia psittaci.* Infect. Immun. **12**:638–646.
14. Wachendörfer, G., and W. Lohrbach. 1982. Säugetier Chlamydien: neuere Erkenntnisse zur Humanpathogenität. Münch. Med. Wschr. **124**:127–130.

CHAPTER

The Mycoplasmas

At the turn of the century, Nocard and his colleagues isolated a unique microorganism from cattle suffering from a contagious form of pleuropneumonia. The causative microorganism was exacting in its growth requirements and could be cultivated only on mediums supplemented with bovine or rabbit serum. Subsequently, a number of similar forms, both parasitic and saprophytic, have been found. Because of their obvious relationship to the bovine pleuropneumonia organism, they were known for many years as pleuropneumonia-like organisms, or more simply as PPLO. Such trivial names are now less commonly used with the advent of a more formal classification,[4] in which they are separated from the true bacteria and placed in a new class, Mollicutes, with several families and genera. These are known informally and collectively as mycoplasmas.

The mycoplasmas are unique in that they **do not possess the distinctive cell wall** of true bacteria. The cytoplasm is surrounded by a plasma membrane, the outermost structure of the cell. They are the **smallest** of the cellular microorganisms, generally measuring 0.2 to 0.3 μm. in diameter and rarely exceeding 1.0 μm. The cell size approaches the minimum for a free-living cell, being barely adequate to contain the genome and synthetic machinery necessary to carry out the metabolic and synthetic functions required of a minimal reproductive unit.

Mycoplasmas are said to be **highly pleomorphic.** A great variety of morphological types have been described, including long filaments, sometimes branched and starlike; small coccoid or teardrop forms; ringlike structures; and large, sometimes vacuolated, round bodies. The multiplicity of shapes is due, in part, to cellular plasticity resulting from the absence of a rigid cell wall. This deficiency also leads to increased fragility of the cells, so that some of the configurations that have been observed are probably artifacts arising from cultural, preparative, and staining conditions.

The Biology of Mycoplasmas[1, 2, 11, 13, 16, 20]

Because of their unusual physical structure, the mycoplasmas are considered to be different from bacteria and are thus placed in a separate class—the Mollicutes. Within the class, two families are recognized: the Mycoplasmataceae, which are characterized by a requirement for cholesterol or other sterols, and the Acholeplasmataceae, which do not require sterols. Mycoplasmataceae comprises two genera, *Mycoplasma* and *Ureaplasma,* while *Acholeplasma* is the only genus in the Acholeplasmataceae. More than 50 species of *Mycoplasma,* one of *Ureaplasma,* and about 7 of *Acholeplasma* are recognized. The taxon-

Table 35–1. **Taxonomy and Properties of the Principal Mycoplasmas***

Classification	Genome Size (Mdaltons)	G + C† %	Cholesterol Requirement	Urea Hydrolysis
Mycoplasmataceae				
Mycoplasma	400–500	23–41	+	–
Ureaplasma	410–480	27–30	+	+
Acholeplasmataceae				
Acholeplasma	950–1110	31–34	–	–

*Adapted from S. Razin, Microbiol. Rev. **42**:414, 1978, and J. Maniloff, Ann. Rev. Microbiol. **37**:477, 1982.
†Guanine plus cytosine content of DNA.

omy and properties of these microorganisms are summarized in Table 35–1. The mycoplasmas are a diverse and heterogeneous group of microorganisms in their physiology and antigenic makeup, as well as in their pathogenic potential. Although some are free-living saprophytes, most are closely adapted parasites, occurring not only as commensals or pathogenic agents in vertebrates but also as agents of disease in insects and plants. The animal parasites are, for the most part, classified as *Mycoplasma* and *Ureaplasma; Acholeplasma* are of minor importance in this regard and will not be discussed in detail.

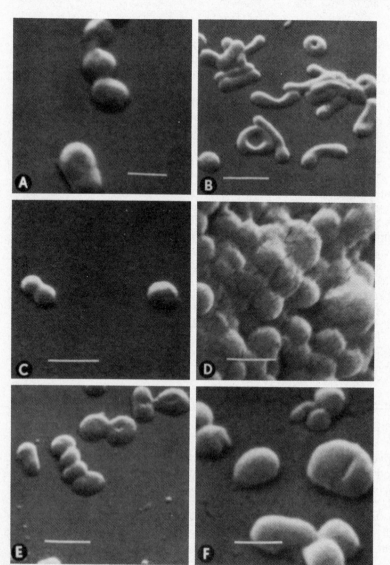

Figure 35–1. Scanning electron photomicrographs of mycoplasma. *A, Mycoplasma gallinarum*, showing spherical and rod-shaped cells. Bar = 0.5 μm. *B, M. meleagridis*, with circular, spherical, and rod-shaped cells. Bar = 1 μm. *C. Acholeplasma laidlawii* of coccoid morphology. Bar = 1 μm. *D, M. bovirhinis*, showing spherical cells in cluster. Bar = 1 μm. *E, M. bovis*, showing spherical, coccobacillary, and rod-shaped morphology. Bar = 1 μm. *F, M. bovigenitalium*, with spherical, coccobacillary, and rod-shaped cells. Bar = 0.5 μm. (J. E. Gallagher and K. R. Rhoades, J. Bacteriol. **137**:972, 1979.)

Morphology and Staining

The development of newer cytological techniques with improved culture and fixation methods permits more accurate delineation of morphology. There now appears to be a certain constancy of morphology in individual species. The morphological groups include coccoid cells; filamentous cells, occasionally branched; and either filamentous or teardropshaped cells with terminal structures. Some of these morphological forms are displayed in Figure 35–1; comparative sizes are shown in Figure 35–2. **Terminal structures,** seen primarily in *Mycoplasma pneumoniae* and *Mycoplasma gallisepticum,* are of special interest. In the human pneumonia organism, the terminal structure appears to be an organelle for specific attachment to host epithelial cells (Figs. 35–3 and 35–4) and is also thought to be responsible for the peculiar motility of these microorganisms (see below).

The mode of reproduction of mycoplasmas has been controversial, at least partly because of the inadequacy of early preparative and observational methods, and partly because of the inevitable confusion arising from their plasticity. There is now widespread agreement that the basic mode of reproduction is similar to that in bacteria and other procaryotes, *i.e.,* binary fission. Although budding is frequently seen, it is considered to be analogous to binary fission, but with unequal distribution of the cytoplasmic contents to the two daughter cells. In the filamentous forms, cell division is not fully synchronized with nuclear division. Nuclear division leads to the formation of long filaments that are eventually multinucleate and without transverse septae; as cell division is initiated, the filaments fragment, producing a series of coccoid elements.

One of the unusual qualities of these microorganisms is their ability to pass through filters that retain bacteria. They are described as filterable, a property they share with viruses. Many mycoplasmas will pass through membrane filters with an average pore diameter (APD) of 0.22 μm., provided that high filtration pressure is applied; under less stringent pressures, however, they are retained by membrane filters with APD of 0.45 μm. These filtration characteristics are thought to be associated with the plastic nature of the cell, *i.e.,* they are "squeezed" through the very small pores by high pressure. The normal cell size, however, is larger than these filtration data would imply, being of the order of 125 to 300 nm. or more in the coccoid forms, while filamentous cells range from 1 or 2 μm. to as much as 150 μm. in length.

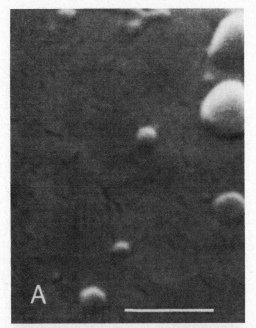
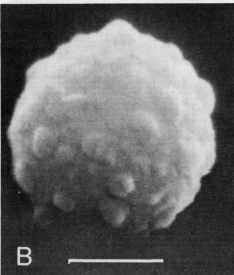

Figure 35–2. Scanning electron photomicrograph showing relative sizes of two mycoplasmas. *A*, Spherical particles of *Mycoplasma bovigenitalium*, 0.125 μm. in diameter. *B*, Large spherical particle of *M. bovirhinis*, 2.25 μm. in diameter. Bars = 1.0 μm. (J. E. Gallagher and K. R. Rhoades, J. Bacteriol. **137**:972, 1979.)

The animal mycoplasmas do not possess flagella, but motility has been noted in a few species. The mechanics of motility are not certain, but adherence to surfaces such as glass is required for its demonstration, and it has been suggested that alternate release and attachment of the cell to a surface, possibly by the terminal structure noted above, may be the underlying mechanism.

As the smallest cellular life form, the ultrastructure of mycoplasma is not complex, at

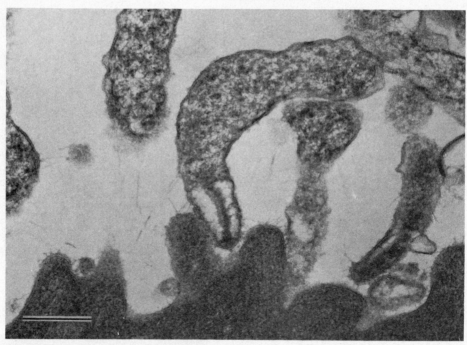

Figure 35–3. *Mycoplasma pneumoniae* in hamster tracheal ring organ culture (72 hr.), showing the filamentous morphology of the microorganisms. Note that the specialized terminal structure touches a nonciliated cell. Bar = 0.2 μm. (M. H. Wilson and A. M. Collier. J. Bacteriol, **125**:332, 1976.)

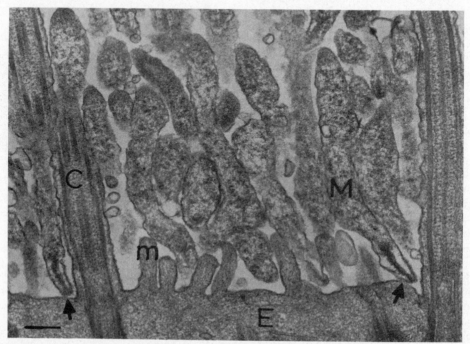

Figure 35–4. *Mycoplasma pneumoniae* in hamster tracheal ring organ culture after 72 hr. Note that the terminal structure (arrows) of the *Mycoplasma* (*M*) lies in close apposition to the bases of the cilia *(C)* and microvilli *(m)* of the epithelial layer *(E)*. Bar = 0.2 μm. (M. H. Wilson and A. M. Collier, J. Bacteriol. **125**:332, 1976.)

least in comparison to bacterial cells. Mycoplasmas are procaryotic with a circular chromosome of double-stranded DNA; the genome size is said to be about one-fifth that of *Escherichia coli,* thus limiting their capacity for metabolic and synthetic processes. The cytoplasm apparently contains no membranous organelles, although ribosomes are present as cytoplasmic granules; mRNA and tRNA are also present. The outermost membrane is a trilaminar cytoplasmic membrane, built of protein and lipid. Many of the mycoplasmas possess a polymeric capsule, demonstrable by ruthenium red staining. The chemical structure of the capsule is variable among species, but is probably carbohydrate in most instances. Thus, they resemble bacteria except for their smaller size, relative simplicity of structure, and absence of cell wall.

Mycoplasmas are considered to be gram-negative, but they stain poorly or not at all by ordinary staining procedures. In tissues, they may be stained, albeit poorly, with Giemsa stain.

On primary isolation, or upon attempted culture in a slightly different medium, broth cultures sometimes show no detectable evidence of growth and may be carried along by "blind passage" for several transfers before obvious growth is seen. Some strains show a uniform opalescence, while others exhibit a granular type of growth. The property of some strains to grow as small colonies, appearing as flakes attached to the side of the tube, is of some differential value. In any case, visible growth is very slight, and almost all workers with these organisms have found it necessary to carry along an uninoculated tube of medium for comparison.

The colonies upon agar surfaces are usually not detectable before two or three days' incubation. The typical mycoplasma colony is small, 10 to 600 μm. in diameter, and generally has a characteristic morphology—the so-called "fried egg" colony that exhibits a dense center with a thin, translucent periphery, as shown in Figure 35–5. The cells in the center of the colony are drawn into the agar matrix and grow downward into the medium. The peripheral zone is not always evident; some species exhibit no peripheral zone, while its presence in others is dependent upon cultural conditions. As an example, crowded colonies on plate cultures often show no translucent zones. Extremely small colonies, from about 10 to 25 μm. in diameter, are characteristic of some mycoplasmas (Fig. 35–6); strains displaying

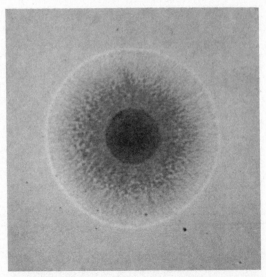

Figure 35–5. Colony of *Mycoplasma salivarium* showing "fried egg" appearance with dense center and translucent periphery. × 500. (Courtesy of Dr. John Griffin.)

such tiny colonies have, therefore, been called T-mycoplasmas. Oily droplets are often observed in mycoplasma colonies; these have been found, in some cases at least, to be cholesterol already present in the medium. Pseudocolonies, once thought to be mycoplasma colonies, are composed of insoluble soaps arising from mechanical disturbance of the medium surface; it is said that these are readily differentiated from true mycoplasmal colonies by experienced observers.

Physiology

Growth of these microorganisms requires infusion or digest mediums enriched by the addition of serum in relatively large amounts. The animal and human mycoplasmas are regularly cultivable on beef heart infusion mediums containing peptone and enriched with heat-stable factors present in serum. **Cholesterol** is required by *Mycoplasma* and *Ureaplasma* species, but not by *Acholeplasma,* and the serum supplement provides the necessary cholesterol and other required lipids. This requirement for cholesterol is unique among bacteria and is related to the peculiar function of the plasma membrane in these wall-less forms. Cholesterol is thought to aid in regulating fluidity of the membrane. Some mycoplasmas tolerate a relatively wide pH range, but others die out at pH 7.0 and below and require a pH of 7.8 to 8.0 for growth. The saprophytic varieties will grow at 22°C., with an optimum at 30°C., but the parasitic ones require 37°C.

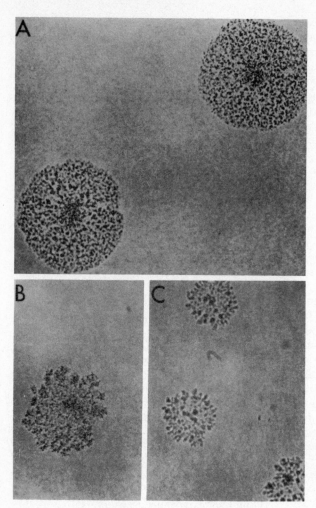

Figure 35–6. Colonies of *Ureaplasma urealyticum. A*, Colonies after five days' growth in 100 per cent CO_2. Central and peripheral zones are evident. × 240. *B* and *C*, Colonies showing convoluted borders and dark granules that appear after medium becomes alkaline upon exposure to air. *B*, × 240; *C*, × 100. (S. Razin *et al.*, J. Bacteriol. **130**:464, 1977.)

Growth occurs both aerobically and anaerobically but is less abundant in most strains under anaerobic conditions.

Fairly heavy inoculums are necessary, whether for primary isolation or for subculture. In transferring agar cultures, a small section of the medium is cut out and dropped into liquid mediums or rubbed onto another plate. Curiously, their primary isolation is, as a rule, accomplished more readily than their maintenance. These microorganisms may also be grown on the chorioallantoic membrane of the egg embryo. They can be cultivated in tissue cultures, but do not usually produce cytopathic effects. Their presence in tissue cultures, though grossly inapparent, may complicate the use of such substrates for the growth of animal viruses.

Glucose is usually fermented, but the pH seldom drops below 7.0 owing to death of the organisms at this point; the addition of other sugars may inhibit growth. In general, fermentations and other biochemical characteristics have minimal differential value.

The heat resistance of some strains is of the same order as that of most bacteria, while others appear to be more frail and are killed by exposure to 45°C. for 15 minutes. Although not as sensitive as bacterial protoplasts, they are disrupted by extreme changes in the osmotic environment; it is thought that the presence of lipids in the cytoplasmic membrane furnishes some osmotic stability. Cultures remain viable for a month or more, even at 37°C., in mediums without added carbohydrate and sealed with petrolatum. They may also be preserved by lyophilization or by storage at −70°C. or below.

Antigens

The mycoplasmas are not as antigenically complex as the bacteria that contain cell walls and associated antigens. For the most part, the different named species are antigenically distinct, although minor cross-reactions sometimes occur, depending in part on the particular serological test employed. Complement fixation is widely applied and is generally useful in distinguishing the several *Mycoplasma* species. Somewhat more specific and sensitive is a test for growth inhibition by specific antiserum. Filter paper discs impregnated with specific antiserum are placed on the surface of plates previously inoculated with mycoplasma culture; growth inhibition by antiserum occurs in a manner analogous to the disc antibiotic assay. The antigenic structure of these microorganisms may also be adduced from the pattern of solubilized antigens separated by gel electrophoresis, a method not widely employed with bacteria because of their antigenic complexity.

By use of the more sensitive and specific techniques, several of the mycoplasma species have been shown to be divisible into serotypes. For instance, at least two serotypes of the bovine pleuropneumonia organism, *Mycoplasma mycoides,* may be distinguished, while *Ureaplasma urealyticum* is quite heterogeneous with a number of serotypes.[17]

In addition to the cellular antigens, at least one species, *Mycoplasma neurolyticum,* produces a neurotoxin. The toxin is a protein with apparent molecular weight in excess of 200,000 daltons; it is immunogenic and induces neutralizing antitoxin.

Adherence and Pathogenesis[6]

Mycoplasmas, unlike most other pathogenic bacteria, do not invade the tissues or bloodstream. Rather, they colonize the cell surfaces of the respiratory and genitourinary tracts, rarely penetrating the cells of the epithelial lining. Essential to their parasitism is the capacity to adhere closely to eucaryotic cells through specific binding sites on the bacterial surface. The mycoplasmas adhere to a wide variety of cell types, including erythrocytes, epithelial cells, macrophages, and spermatozoa.

The resulting close association between the mycoplasma and host cells is thought to be relevant to other events in pathogenesis. The mycoplasma gain a nutritional advantage from metabolites that are concentrated at the host cell surface; they probably can also utilize lipids and cholesterol contained in host cell membranes. Their colonization and multiplication may thus be enhanced by the availability of nutrients and essential metabolites.

With the exception of the neurotoxin produced by *M. neurolyticum,* mycoplasma are not known to produce powerful exotoxins.

Cellular and organ damage induced by these microorganisms must, therefore, have a different basis. Several possible modes of pathogenesis have been proposed, many predicated upon the intimate cellular association following adherence. Possibly the most important of these pathogenic mechanisms is the elaboration by the mycoplasma of toxic metabolic products.

Several species of *Mycoplasma* produce hydrogen peroxide as a metabolic product. Normally, tissue catalases would be expected to destroy this product, but the close adherence of mycoplasma at the cell membrane surface is thought to lead to locally high concentrations of hydrogen peroxide that damage the host cell membrane. Ammonia, produced by *Ureaplasma* during hydrolysis of urea, has been identified as a cytopathogenic factor for bovine oviduct organ explants. In addition to these toxic metabolic products, certain soluble bacterial antigens are believed to have toxic properties. These include the capsular galactan of *M. mycoides,* causing hemorrhage and blood pressure changes, and a mycoplasmal lipoglycan that reportedly has some toxic properties resembling those of endotoxins.

Attachment may be important, too, in other aspects of infection and pathogenesis. The attachment of genital mycoplasmas to spermatozoa is thought to facilitate the transport and dissemination of these microorganisms in the female genital tract. The infection of spermatozoa may also affect fertility by reducing sperm motility, but this issue is not resolved.

The attachment of mycoplasma to host cells is specific, and is related to host cell receptors and complementary binding sites on the bacterial surface. Some mycoplasmas, such as *M. pneumoniae,* possess a specialized polar structure[14, 22] that appears to be important in adherence (Figs. 35–3 and 35–4). The bacterial ligand mediating adherence is a protein, occurring in high concentration in the terminal organelle.[3] The principal receptor site on host cell membranes most likely contains sialyl residues, since it is sensitive to the action of neuraminidase. Since neuraminidase treatment of host cells does not completely abrogate adherence, other receptors, as yet unidentified, are also postulated.

Chemotherapy[9, 19]

Because the mycoplasmas have no cell wall, antibiotics affecting cell wall synthesis, such as penicillin, are without effect. Although increased drug resistance has been noted, chemotherapy with tetracycline is usually effective, as is erythromycin.

Mycoplasmal Infections[5, 8, 18, 21]

The mycoplasmas are only weakly pathogenic for man and animals. Many are common inhabitants of the mucous membranes of the upper respiratory or genitourinary tracts, usually as commensals, but capable of disease initiation under conditions of host stress or intercurrent disease. Several are, however, frankly pathogenic for animals, and are usually responsible for respiratory infections. Only three species have been incriminated in human mycoplasmoses, although several others are found as commensals. Table 35–2 lists the species of *Mycoplasma* and *Ureaplasma* that are etiological agents of human and animal disease.

RESPIRATORY DISEASE

Interest in *Mycoplasma* was greatly stimulated by the demonstration of the etiological relation of one of these agents to human pneumonia. The human disease, primary atypical pneumonia, was characterized as a clinical entity in the 1940s. Although a number of microbial agents can be responsible for the syndrome, a significant portion are due to *Mycoplasma pneumoniae*.

Primary Atypical Pneumonia
Mycoplasmal infection of the respiratory tract is generally a benign disease, with upper respiratory tract symptoms, tracheitis, and bronchitis. Many infections are subclinical in nature and most probably go unrecognized. After an incubation period of two to three weeks, early symptoms of headache, fever, chills, and malaise are followed by sore throat and a dry, unproductive cough; after about a week, mucoid sputum is produced.

Only about 3 to 10 per cent of infected persons develop clinically apparent pneumonia. Nevertheless, these account for up to 20 per cent of pneumonia cases in the general population, indicating the widespread distribution of the infection. The young are most often affected, incidence being greatest in those 5 to 19 years of age; younger children seldom develop severe disease. Although cases of primary atypical pneumonia may occur throughout the year, peak incidence is during the fall and winter. Respiratory transmission is the rule, the microorganism being disseminated by coughing during the acute stages of the disease. Transmission is facilitated by close contact and is greatest in families, schoolchildren, military personnel, and other groups subject to crowded conditions.

Although respiratory illness caused by *M. pneumoniae* is generally mild, a few fatal cases have been noted. Moreover, extrapulmonary complications are sometimes evident. The latter are manifest as cardiovascular disturbances, neurologic syndromes, arthritis, and a multi-

Table 35–2. **The Pathogenic Mycoplasmas**

Species	Cholesterol Required	Acid from Glucose	Hydrolysis of		Pathogenicity
			Urea	Arginine	
Mycoplasma pneumoniae	+	+	–	–	Primary atypical pneumonia of humans
Mycoplasma hominis	+	–	–	+	Possible pathogen in urogenital tract of humans
Ureaplasma urealyticum	+	–	+	–	Possible pathogen in urogenital tract of humans
Mycoplasma mycoides	+	+	–	–	Pleuropneumonia of cattle and goats
Mycoplasma gallisepticum	+	+	–	–	Respiratory disease of fowls
Mycoplasma neurolyticum	+	+	–	–	Neurological (rolling) disease of mice
Mycoplasma pulmonis	+	+	–	–	Infectious catarrh of rodents
Mycoplasma hyopneumoniae	+	+	–	–	Enzootic pneumonia of swine
Mycoplasma agalactiae	+	–	–	–	Contagious agalactia of sheep, goats, and cattle
Mycoplasma arthritidis	+	–	–	+	Purulent arthritis of rats

plicity of rashes. Many of these complications are thought to be related to immunologic disturbances, including immune complex formation and production of autoantibodies.

Respiratory infections by *M. pneumoniae* respond somewhat slowly to treatment with erythromycin or tetracycline. These antibiotics relieve most symptoms within three to four days, but the microorganisms are not completely eliminated from the tissues, and lung lesions are slow to resolve.

Immunity

Infection with *M. pneumoniae* induces a formation of complement-fixing, growth-inhibiting, and precipitating antibodies. Whether these antibodies are associated with protection against subsequent infection is uncertain, but much of the available evidence indicates that they are not, although such antibodies do promote phagocytosis.[15] While the significance of serum antibodies is in doubt, there is some interest in the protective effect of IgA antibodies in respiratory secretions. Challenge experiments in human volunteers suggest that secretory antibody is related to resistance to *M. pneumoniae* infections; a similar suggestion arises from animal experiments. Although not extensively studied, a cell-mediated immune response may also be tied to effective immunity. In populations of children, antigen-reactive lymphocytes become increasingly detectable as resistance to *M. pneumoniae* infection develops.[10] It has also been observed that mice with defective cell-mediated immune response are more susceptible to infection and disseminated disease than normal animals.

Laboratory Diagnosis[12]

The diagnosis of mycoplasmal pneumonia is materially aided by the isolation of *M. pneumoniae* in culture or by significant rises in specific antibody titer. Isolation procedures are, however, slow and are generally more useful for epidemiological studies than for diagnosis of individual cases.

Material from the respiratory tract, preferably sputum or throat washings, is inoculated onto a complex medium containing peptone, yeast dialysate, serum, and, usually, penicillin and thallium acetate to control bacterial contaminants. Cultures should be incubated aerobically and observed microscopically for typical mycoplasma colonies for at least one month before discarding as negative. Isolates may be tentatively identified by colonial appearance, hemolysis, and biochemical reactions (Table 35–2). Confirmation is achieved by demonstration of growth inhibition of isolates by specific antiserum.

Mycoplasma pneumoniae tends to be set apart from the other *Mycoplasma* species in that it grows relatively slowly, forming granular colonies with translucent peripheral zones, and produces hemolysis of red blood cells; unlike the bacterial protein hemolysins, however, the hemolytic principle of *M. pneumoniae* is hydrogen peroxide. *Mycoplasma pneumoniae* must be differentiated from *M. salivarium* and *M. orale,* commensal species commonly found in the respiratory tract. The latter two species, in contrast to *M. pneumoniae,* hydrolyze arginine and grow reasonably well under microaerophilic or anaerobic conditions.

Serological testing of patients' serum for *M. pneumoniae* antibodies is usually by complement fixation, using lipid antigen extracted from *M. pneumoniae* cells. A fourfold or greater rise in titer between acute and convalescent phase serums is of diagnostic significance.

In many cases of mycoplasmal pneumonia—33 to 75 per cent—serum antibodies are engendered that agglutinate type O human erythrocytes at 4°C., but not at 37°C. These **cold hemagglutinins** appear after about seven days and reach peak titer in about one month. Although they are nonspecific, cold agglutinins have found some diagnostic utility because the test is rapid and simple to perform.

GENITAL INFECTIONS

Mycoplasmas are common inhabitants of the genital tract, most occurring as commensals without disease association. Two species, *Mycoplasma hominis* and *Ureaplasma urealyticum* (T-mycoplasmas), are frequently isolated, however, and there is some evidence that these genital mycoplasmas have pathogenic potential in humans.

Two patterns of genital colonization with mycoplasmas are evident. About one-third of infants are colonized at birth with *U. urealyticum,* and a lesser number with *M. hominis,* presumably occurring during passage through the birth canal. This colonization does not persist, and most are free of genital mycoplasmas by the beginning of puberty. Recolonization, resulting from sexual contacts, occurs after puberty, so that young adults are significantly colonized. Colonization rates as high as 75 per cent have been reported in women having several sexual partners; somewhat lower rates are found in sexually active males. The high frequency of colonization in normal adults has complicated efforts to establish the role of these mycoplasmas in genital tract infections.

Nongonococcal Urethritis

The role of *U. urealyticum* and *M. hominis* in nongonococcal urethritis of males is still controversial. As noted earlier (Chapter 34), *Chlamydia trachomatis* is responsible for less than 50 per cent of such infections, leaving more than 50 per cent of unknown etiology. Like *Chlamydia,* the mycoplasmas are sensitive to tetracycline, and this antibiotic is usually effective in treatment of nongonococcal urethritis. Nevertheless, controlled studies suggest that *U. urealyticum* is etiologically associated with some cases of urethritis and can cause this illness in human volunteers.

Infection in Women

The evidence for an etiological role for mycoplasmas in infections of the female genital tract is somewhat tenuous. Although *M. hominis* is often found in association with cervicitis or vaginitis, its importance in these affections is not yet established; *Ureaplasma* does not seem to be involved. Some cases of nongonococcal pelvic inflammatory disease may be due to the genital mycoplasmas, and *M. hominis* may be the cause of postpartum fever and fever after abortion. Delineation of the role of mycoplasmas in genital tract infections of females must await definitive and controlled studies.

Other Infections

It has been suggested that mycoplasmas may be responsible for a variety of other disorders. *Mycoplasma hominis,* but not *U. urealyticum,* seems to be responsible for some cases of pyelonephritis, while *Ureaplasma* may be linked to chorioamnionitis and low birth weight of infants.

RELATION TO BACTERIAL L FORMS[7, 20]

In the early 1930s, Klieneberger-Nobel, at the Lister Institute, isolated a microorganism from rats that was first thought to be a mycoplasma but was later shown to be a spontaneously arising, cell wall–free variant of *Streptococcus moniliformis*. It is presently known that such spontaneous variants, now called L

forms, occur in several bacterial species and may be induced in others by substances that inhibit or interfere with cell wall synthesis. The induced forms usually are osmotically sensitive and, in such cases, must be maintained in mediums containing serum and with increased concentrations of salts or sugars for osmotic protection. These induced L forms will often revert to the bacterial phase when the inducing agent is removed; occasionally, however, they remain in the L phase and are then termed **stable L forms.**

When the L form does not demonstrate extreme osmotic fragility, as in the case of the original isolate, it is maintained on the same type of mediums supporting growth of mycoplasmas, and, in fact, such forms are similar to mycoplasmas in colonial morphology, filterability, and insensitivity to antibiotics affecting cell wall synthesis. It was perhaps inevitable that the discovery of L forms would lead to the proposal that mycoplasmas arise from a bacterial parent by loss of the ability to synthesize cell wall constituents. The discovery that *M. pneumoniae* infection induces antibody that agglutinates certain streptococci lent further credence to this view. The controversy continued over almost three decades and was only resolved by application of DNA hybridization. In each case where there was a suspected relationship between a mycoplasma and a putative parent bacterial phase, significant DNA homology could not be demonstrated. While such negative findings cannot be regarded as predictive that no such relationships will be found, the likelihood seems to grow smaller and smaller.

In any case, the significance of L phase bacteria must be judged not on their relationship to mycoplasmas but, in the present context at least, as bacterial forms that may play pathogenic roles.

L forms are known to be present in certain infections, particularly those of the urinary tract. This is not surprising, since the hypertonicity of this environment might protect osmotically fragile cells. Such L forms may arise spontaneously or as a result of penicillin therapy, and they may persist at this location. There is also some indication that L forms may be present in the blood in *Salmonella* infections and in brucellosis; in both of these cases they may arise as a consequence of antibody-complement action on the cell wall. Although these observations are interesting and suggestive, the pathogenicity of cell wall–deficient bacteria is not yet established, and clearly needs further study.

REFERENCES

1. Archer, D. B. 1981. The structure and functions of the mycoplasma membrane. Internat. Rev. Cytol. **69**:1–44.
2. Barile, M. F., et al. (Eds.). 1982. Current topics in mycoplasmology. Rev. Infect. Dis. **4** (May/June Suppl.):S1–S228.
3. Baseman, J. B., et al. 1982. Molecular basis for cytadsorption of Mycoplasma pneumoniae. J. Bacteriol. **151**:1514–1522.
4. Buchanan, R. E., and N. E. Gibbons (Eds.). 1974. Bergey's Manual of Determinative Bacteriology. 8th ed. The Williams & Wilkins Co., Baltimore.
5. Cassell, G. H., and B. C. Cole. 1981. Mycoplasmas as agents of human disease. New Engl. J. Med. **304**:80–89.
6. Cassell, G. H., et al. 1978. Pathobiology of mycoplasmas. pp. 399–403. In D. Schlessinger (Ed.): Microbiology—1978. American Society for Microbiology, Washington, D.C.
7. Clasener, H. 1972. Pathogenicity of the L-phase of bacteria. Ann. Rev. Microbiol. **26**:55–84.
8. Embree, J. E., and J. A. Embil. 1980. Mycoplasmas in diseases of humans. Can. Med. Assn J. **123**:105–111.
9. Evans, R. T., and D. Taylor-Robinson. 1978. The incidence of tetracycline-resistant strains of Ureaplasma urealyticum. J. Antimicrob. Chemother. **4**:57–63.
10. Fernald, G. W., A. M. Collier, and W. A. Clyde, Jr. 1975. Respiratory infections due to Mycoplasma pneumoniae in infants and children. Pediatrics **55**:327–335.
11. Furness, G., et al. 1976. Morphology, ultrastructure, and mode of division of Mycoplasma fermentans, Mycoplasma hominis, Mycoplasma orale, and Mycoplasma salivarium. J. Infect. Dis. **134**:224–229.
12. Kenny, G. E. 1980. Mycoplasmata. pp. 365–370. In E. H. Lennette, et al. (Eds.): Manual of Clinical Microbiology. 3rd ed. American Society for Microbiology, Washington, D.C.
13. Maniloff, J. 1983. Evolution of wall-less prokaryotes. Ann. Rev. Microbiol. **37**:477–499.
14. Muse, K. E., D. A. Powell, and A. M. Collier. 1976. Mycoplasma pneumoniae in hamster tracheal organ culture studied by scanning electron microscopy. Infect. Immun. **13**:229–237.
15. Powell, D. A., and W. A. Clyde, Jr. 1975. Opsonin-reversible resistance of Mycoplasma pneumoniae to in vitro phagocytosis by alveolar macrophages. Infect. Immun. **11**:540–550.
16. Razin, S. 1978. The mycoplasmas. Microbiol. Rev. **42**:414–470.
17. Robertson, J. A., and G. W. Stemke. 1982. Expanded serotyping scheme for Ureaplasma urealyticum strains isolated from humans. J. Clin. Microbiol. **15**:873–878.
18. Stanbridge, E. J. 1976. A reevaluation of the role of mycoplasmas in human disease. Ann. Rev. Microbiol. **30**:169–187.
19. Stopler, T., C. B. Gerichter, and D. Branski. 1980. Antibiotic-resistant mutants of Mycoplasma pneumoniae. Israel J. Med. Sci. **16**:169–173.
20. Symposium. 1978. Cellular and molecular biology of mycoplasma and bacterial L-forms. pp. 387–415. In D. Schlessinger (Ed.): Microbiology—1978. American Society for Microbiology, Washington, D.C.
21. Taylor-Robinson, D., and W. M. McCormack. 1980. The genital mycoplasmas. (In two parts.) New Engl. J. Med. **302**:1003–1010; 1063–1067.
22. Wilson, M. H., and A. M. Collier. 1976. Ultrastructural study of Mycoplasma pneumoniae in organ culture. J. Bacteriol. **125**:332–339.

CHAPTER 36

Bacterial Food Poisoning

INTOXICATION FOOD POISONING	INFECTION FOOD POISONING
BOTULISM	SALMONELLA FOOD POISONING
STAPHYLOCOCCAL FOOD POISONING	VIBRIO HAEMOLYTICUS FOOD POISONING
CLOSTRIDIUM PERFRINGENS FOOD POISONING	*Shellfish and Disease*
BACILLUS CEREUS FOOD POISONING	

In preceding chapters, frequent references have been made to the importance of food and water in the transmission of infectious agents. In many instances, food serves simply as a vehicle for the transmission of disease, as in the case of parasitic, viral, and bacterial enteric infections. In addition to these, however, other types of illness may result from the ingestion of food, including that group of affections designated as food poisoning. The types of illnesses that are associated with ingestion of foods are summarized in Table 36–1.

Although the distinction between foodborne diseases and bacterial food poisoning is not always clear-cut, the clinical manifestations associated with bacterial food poisoning proper almost always include vomiting, diarrhea, enteritis, and a greater or lesser degree of prostration. In addition, cases of food poisoning often occur in clusters and are traceable to the common consumption of a specific foodstuff. Certain diseases, such as cholera and bacillary dysentery, sometimes exhibit these clinical and epidemiological characteristics, but are not generally considered to be food poisoning in the accepted sense. The categories of bacterial food poisoning listed in Table 36–1 are those that are generally recognized.

Although a number of the food-associated illnesses listed in Table 36–1 are not bacterial in origin, their clinical character may simulate bacterial food poisoning, and this possibility must be considered in any attempt to ascertain the etiology of a given outbreak. Hypersensitivity to a given food substance, for example, is frequently manifest as vomiting, and an outbreak confined to a family may be the result of a familial tendency; similarly, the gastrointestinal disturbances following the ingestion of naturally poisonous foods such as toadstools or foods contaminated with poisons such as arsenic or cyanide are often indistinguishable from those induced by some bacterial toxins.

Table 36–2 outlines the salient features of the recognized bacterial food poisoning illnesses. The comparative reported incidence of these illnesses in the United States from 1972 to 1978 is summarized in Table 36–3.

Intoxication Food Poisoning[3, 6, 17]

Poisoning by food containing toxic substances of bacterial origin is very common. The term "ptomaine poisoning," often still used by laymen in the United States, is a misnomer that is both misleading and inaccurate. The organic bases such as putrescine, cadaverine, methylamine, and the like, called ptomaines, will result from the bacterial decomposition of protein, but are not toxic when given by mouth. Neither are the other decomposition products toxic *per os*. While a partially decomposed food may be esthetically unattractive, the innocuous nature of the products of decomposition is obvious when one considers the advanced state of decomposition reached by some cheeses. On the contrary, toxicity is attributable to the presence of substances synthesized by bacteria whose presence may or may not be associated with obvious evidence of decomposition of the food substance.

BOTULISM[8, 11]

Botulism is a highly fatal form of food poisoning resulting from the ingestion of food containing protein toxins produced by *Clostridium botulinum*, an anaerobic, spore-forming bacillus. *Clostridium botulinum* strains are separated into types, designated by capital letters, on the basis of the immunological specificity of their toxins; individual strains produce only a single antigenic type of toxin (see Chapter 28). The toxins produced are neurotoxins and are among the most potent poisons known.

Clostridium botulinum is commonly found in soil and marine sediments as well as in the feces of both warm- and cold-blooded animals. Except in rare cases of wound botulism, the microorganism rarely, if ever, directly infects adults. In infants, however, colonization of the intestine is believed to result in synthesis of toxin to give rise to infant botulism (Chapter 28). In adults, food poisoning is the principal illness produced by this species.

Clostridia from soil represent the major source of contamination of food, especially in the case of *C. botulinum* types A and B. Type E botulism, on the other hand, is often associated with the consumption of fish and fish products, and the bacilli have been isolated from fish in many areas of the continental United States and Alaska. A rare sixth type, type F, has been isolated from salmon from the Columbia River, from crabs in Virginia, and from venison.

Although many foods may be contaminated with *C. botulinum*, a series of circumscribed events must occur before food poisoning results. First, there must be an opportunity for the microorganisms to grow and, since they are obligate anaerobes, anaerobic conditions must prevail. These opportunities are most often provided in preserved foods prepared so that the heat-resistant spores are not destroyed, and which are sealed to exclude free

Table 36–2. Bacterial Food Poisoning

Agent	Type	Common Vehicles	Usual Incubation Period	Prominent Features
Clostridium botulinum	Intoxication	Home canned foods; some commercial foods, including fish, meats, and soup	12–36 hr.	Nausea, emesis, abdominal pain, weakness, dysphagia, dysarthria, blurred vision
Staphylococcus aureus	Intoxication	Pastries, custards, salads, meats, dairy products	1–6 hr.	Nausea, emesis, abdominal pain, diarrhea
Clostridium perfringens	Intoxication	Inadequately cooked meats and poultry, gravies; foods often reheated	8–12 hr.	Abdominal pain, diarrhea, sometimes nausea
Bacillus cereus	Intoxication	Cereal and cereal products, potatoes	1–6 hr.*	Abdominal pain, diarrhea, emesis
Salmonella	Infection	Shellfish, meats, dairy products, eggs	12–24 hr.	Diarrhea, fever, some emesis and nausea
Vibrio parahaemolyticus	Infection	Shellfish	12–24 hr.	Abdominal pain, nausea, emesis, diarrhea, often chills and fever

*In some outbreaks, the incubation period and symptoms resemble *C. perfringens* food poisoning.

Table 36–3. **Outbreaks and Cases of Bacterial Food Poisoning in the United States, 1972 to 1978***

Agent	No. of Outbreaks	No. of Cases
Clostridium botulinum	104	279
Staphylococcus aureus	281	10,388
Clostridium perfringens	70	4573
Bacillus cereus	13	369
Salmonella	261	16,172
Vibrio parahaemolyticus	12	1125

*Data from H. E. Sours and D. G. Smith, J. Infect. Dis. **142**:122, 1980.

oxygen. Appropriate conditions frequently obtain in cold-packed, home-canned foods; some inadequately processed commercially canned foods; sausages in casings; or smoked fish sealed in plastic wraps. Second, a period of incubation is required to permit growth and toxin elaboration. This offers little difficulty, for such processed foods are thought to be preserved and are stored, often for considerable periods of time, without refrigeration. Under these circumstances, growth and toxin formation occur with perhaps only slight, if any, overt evidence of spoilage. Although the botulinum toxins are heat-labile and are destroyed by boiling for about 10 minutes, many of the foods are consumed without terminal cooking. Botulinum toxins are not destroyed by the action of proteolytic enzymes of the digestive tract and, in fact, the native protein toxin is activated by trypsin.

Botulism outbreaks occur in groups of small numbers of cases—the individuals who consume the toxin-containing foods. Botulism of types A and B in the United States most often involves home-canned foods, particularly neutral foods such as green beans, which are difficult to sterilize and may have been preserved by the cold-pack method. Such outbreaks tend to occur in rural areas. Outbreaks of type E botulism are usually associated with fish and fish products. In Canada and Alaska, the foods often incriminated are whale meat, fish, crabs, and shrimp, often consumed raw, as well as fermented salmon eggs.[4] A raw fish preparation, izushi, has been the most common vehicle in Japan. Uncooked fish has also been involved in outbreaks in the United States; in one instance, botulism resulted from consumption of smoked whitefish from the Great Lakes which had been packed in plastic bags and distributed through a supermarket chain. Over the past several decades, commercially canned foods have been occasionally incriminated in botulism outbreaks, sometimes traced to canned fish.

A typical history of a botulism outbreak usually includes the serving of the food at fault, some agreement that it tasted a bit peculiar, with the remainder being discarded. Symptoms of toxemia usually begin within 12 to 36 hours, depending upon the amount of toxin ingested. Among the symptoms commonly observed are gastroenteritis with nausea and vomiting, abdominal pain, muscle weakness, and some difficulty in swallowing and focusing the eyes. The fatality rate is quite high, and death is usually due to respiratory failure. Antitoxin is effective but only prophylactically, since symptoms are the result of neurological damage which antitoxin cannot repair. In nonfatal cases, recovery is slow and prolonged.[13] There is no immunological cross-reactivity among the several toxin types, except for subtypes of type C. Successful use of antitoxin depends upon identification of the toxin type and administration of appropriate specific antiserum or, more commonly, administration of trivalent antitoxin against the prevalent A, B, and E types. For confirmation of botulism outbreaks, the food, if available, is injected into experimental animals, some of which are passively protected by antitoxin, and the animals observed for typical symptoms; the microorganism may also be isolated and identified on the basis of its toxigenicity. Figure 36–1 shows the reported cases and deaths in the United States for the period 1960 to 1980.

Botulism in the United States is usually due to type A, or B, with an increasing number of outbreaks due to type E. Type E predominates in Canada, Alaska, Japan, and Scandinavia. In Europe, most cases are of type B origin, while type A predominates in the continental United States. The geographical distribution in the United States is striking: almost all type A outbreaks occur west of the Mississippi River, while type B outbreaks are usually east of the Mississippi River.

STAPHYLOCOCCAL FOOD POISONING[8]

Like botulism, staphylococcal food poisoning is a consequence of the ingestion of foods containing preformed toxins, in this case the enterotoxins produced by strains of *Staphylococcus aureus* (Chapter 14). Not all strains of

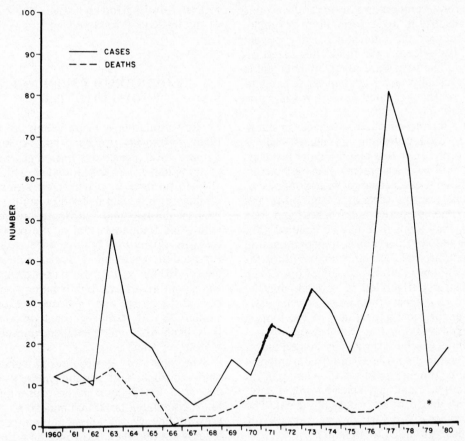

Figure 36–1. Reported cases and deaths due to foodborne botulism in the United States, 1960 to 1980. (Centers for Disease Control, Annual summary 1980: reported morbidity and mortality in the United States. Morbidity and Mortality Weekly Report, Vol. 29, 1981.)

S. aureus, however, produce enterotoxin. Most enterotoxigenic strains are lysed by group III phages, but there are no other distinguishing morphological or physiological characteristics associated with enterotoxin production.

The staphylococcal enterotoxins have been prepared in highly purified form, and are found to be single-chain polypeptides with molecular weights between 28,000 and 35,000 daltons. Five well-characterized immunological types of enterotoxin are now recognized, designated by capital letters. The types may be differentiated by gel diffusion tests and other serological assays, but they do not appear to differ from one another in toxicity. The toxins are highly active; the effective dose of purified material for man is of the order of 1 to 4 μg. Monkeys are also susceptible to toxin administered by the oral route, but the effective dose is perhaps tenfold that required to elicit a response in man. A gastroenteritis is produced, and the outward symptoms are similar to but less marked than those in man.

Enterotoxigenic strains of staphylococci may elaborate one or two types of toxin. In the United States, Canada, and the United Kingdom, present evidence indicates that most food poisoning strains produce either type A or both types A and D.

Staphylococci are widely distributed in nature. Strains involved in food poisoning usually originate from the normal bacterial flora of the anterior nares and skin or from skin lesions of food handlers. It is estimated that 15 to 20 per cent of the population are carriers of enterotoxigenic staphylococci, but this estimate may be low.

Staphylococci are introduced into foods and, if circumstances permit, the microorganisms multiply and produce toxins. Contamination of the food frequently occurs after cooking. Such foods are then held at temperatures which permit staphylococcal growth. Proper refrigeration, *i.e.,* at temperatures below 45° F., will prevent growth and toxigenesis, while prolonged incubation of contaminated food at room temperature or on food warming tables results in toxin formation. Staphylococci, but not the enterotoxin, may be destroyed by reheating the food after initial incubation. The toxins are relatively heat-stable and not usually inactivated in these circumstances, so that reheated foods can still cause food poisoning.

Most often incriminated as vehicles in staphylococcal food poisoning are meats such as hams, corned beef, and poultry; dairy products such as milk and ice cream; prepared salads, particularly those prepared with potatoes or macaroni; pastries such as cream puffs and eclairs; and prepared sandwiches and box lunches. Any foods that may be handled after cooking and are thus subject to contamination and which are held at warm temperatures for several hours before consumption, even though later refrigerated or cooked, may be regarded as suspect. In most cases, the taste, odor, and physical appearance of the food is not altered by staphylococcal growth.

The illness is characterized by sudden onset, usually within 2 to 6 hours after consumption of toxin-containing foods, and symptoms include nausea, vomiting, and abdominal pain, often with diarrhea; fever does not occur. The mortality rate is very low, and recovery usually is complete within 24 to 48 hours.

The identification of an outbreak of food poisoning as staphylococcal in etiology has largely been inferential, i.e., the vehicle is defined on epidemiological grounds and is found on culture to contain enormous numbers of staphylococci, sometimes exceeding 10^9 microorganisms per gram. Ordinarily, human volunteers or monkeys are not available to test either the toxicity of the food or the toxigenicity of the isolated staphylococci. However, by use of gel diffusion, reverse passive hemagglutination, or other serological tests, toxin production by isolated staphylococci can be detected. Toxins in food may be assayed by enzyme-linked immunosorbent assay (ELISA),[20] by serological testing of toxins recovered from food by solvent extraction,[16] or by affinity chromatography.[7]

Staphylococcal food poisoning is common in the United States; from 1972 through 1978, 281 outbreaks with more than 10,000 cases were reported, representing almost 40 per cent of the outbreaks of bacterial foodborne disease of known etiology and 28 per cent of the cases.[18] A large number of small outbreaks occur, especially in family groups, and are not reported. In England and Wales, the incidence of staphylococcal food poisoning is very much less.

CLOSTRIDIUM PERFRINGENS FOOD POISONING[9, 10]

The sporulating obligate anaerobe, *Clostridium perfringens (welchii)* type A, long recognized as a causative agent of gaseous gangrene (Chapter 28), was found by McClung in 1945 to produce food poisoning in man. The etiology of this kind of food poisoning is now well established and outbreaks are reported with some frequency. During the period 1972 to 1978, 70 outbreaks with 4573 cases were reported in the United States, representing almost 10 per cent of the bacterial food poisoning outbreaks and slightly more than 12 per cent of the cases;[18] the incidence in England is similar. As with staphylococcal food poisoning, it is likely that mild, smaller outbreaks are seldom reported.

Symptoms of gastroenteritis—abdominal pain, diarrhea, and possibly nausea—usually appear 8 to 12 hours after consumption of foods containing large numbers of *C. perfringens,* of the order of several millions per gram; fever is not observed and vomiting is rare. The foods most often involved include meats, poultry, and gravies. A typical outbreak begins with the preparation of bulky foods such as turkeys or large roasts which are cooled slowly after cooking and held at ambient temperatures for a period of time; in many cases, the food is reheated before serving. *Clostridium perfringens* spores, present as contaminants in the original food, are not destroyed by cooking and may even be activated by cooking or reheating. Heating also drives off the dissolved oxygen, creating anaerobic conditions that promote the vegetative growth of the bacilli during the extended cooling period.

The essential element in *C. perfringens* food poisoning is the production of a heat-labile, protein enterotoxin by the microorganism. The toxin resembles the cholera enterotoxin in that it mediates the movement of water and ions from the tissues into the lumen of the bowel to produce diarrhea. Toxin is formed during sporulation of the bacilli and is released from the sporangium at lysis, along with the mature spore.[5] Available evidence indicates that sporulation and, therefore, toxin production does not take place in the food but occurs primarily in the large intestine after ingestion of the large numbers of vegetative cells contained in the food. It is unlikely that foods support sporulation and toxin production, but instead offer excellent opportunities for vegetative growth. In this respect, then, *C. perfringens* food poisoning differs from that caused by *C. botulinum* and staphylococci, in which the toxins are preformed in the food before consumption.

Enterotoxin may be detected by biological assay or serological methods. Biological assays for toxin include the ligated ileal loop response and the skin vascular permeability test in rabbits. These techniques may be applied to establish the presence of the toxin in stools or the toxigenic potential of isolated strains. Such tests are not, however, performed routinely in epidemiological studies; to establish the etiology of an outbreak, it is only necessary to show the presence of large numbers of *C. perfringens* in the suspected food and in the stools of patients.

Only *C. perfringens* types A and C are known to produce enterotoxins, and only type A is of major public health importance in food poisoning incidents. Even within these types, not all strains are toxigenic and there seem to be no differential characteristics of food poisoning strains. Food poisoning strains also may produce gas gangrene under experimental conditions, and there appears to be no basis for separating *C. perfringens* strains into the food poisoning and the gas gangrene, or classic, strains.

BACILLUS CEREUS FOOD POISONING[10]

Although food poisoning caused by *B. cereus* is not of great public health importance in the United States, it occurs with somewhat greater frequency in Canada, England, and other parts of Europe. In the years 1972 to 1978, only 13 outbreaks involving 369 cases were reported in the United States.[18] Food poisoning due to *B. cereus* was first described in Europe in the early 1950s; in these early reports, the outbreaks resembled those caused by *C. perfringens*—viz., an incubation time of about 12 hours and symptoms of abdominal pain and diarrhea. A variety of foods were incriminated, including cereals and cereal products, potatoes, rice, vegetables, and meats. Since about 1971, however, most incidents have followed a somewhat different pattern. In these later outbreaks, the incubation period has been shorter (1 to 6 hours); the foods involved have been predominantly cereals, usually rice; and the symptoms have included emesis, or vomiting.

Bacillus cereus food poisoning has some similarity to that caused by staphylococci in that one or more enterotoxins are produced by the bacilli growing in the foodstuffs. Man suffers the disease after consumption of food containing preformed toxin. The aerobic spore-forming bacilli survive the usual cooking temperatures; when the cooked foods are then held at room temperature, the microorganisms multiply and elaborate enterotoxin. The fact that cereals are often naturally contaminated with *B. cereus* spores accounts for the frequent incrimination of these foods in outbreaks. Cereals also provide the nutritive requirements for the bacilli, which may reach levels of several millions per gram of food.[15, 22]

The *B. cereus* enterotoxin, produced during logarithmic growth of the microorganisms, is apparently protein in nature, since it is destroyed by pronase and trypsin; it is also inactivated by heating at 56°C. for 5 minutes. The toxin acts to induce fluid accumulation in ligated rabbit ileal segments and alters skin vascular permeability.[19] Recent reports indicate that several toxins may be formed, one or two being responsible for diarrhea, one for mucosal damage, and one for emesis.[14, 23]

This type of food poisoning may be most effectively controlled by the simple practice of refrigerating foods after initial cooking. The toxin, if present, and the vegetative bacterial cells are also destroyed by adequately heating the foods before consumption.

The observation that two forms of foodborne illness may be caused by *B. cereus* has not yet been satisfactorily explained. Recent studies, however, indicate that certain flagellar serotypes of *B. cereus* (types 1, 3, and 5) were associated with outbreaks characterized by a shorter incubation period and vomiting, and involving rice as a vehicle, whereas other serotypes (2, 6, 8, 9, and 10) were found in incidents in which the longer incubation period and diarrhea were prominent features. The possibility that multiple toxins are involved gains credence from the report that *B. cereus* cultures grown on rice but not on other mediums induce vomiting when given to monkeys.[14]

Infection Food Poisoning

It is questionable whether enterotoxins are produced by other kinds of bacteria that are associated with food poisoning syndromes characterized by the presence of large numbers of microorganisms in foods incriminated on epidemiological grounds. For the present, the association of these microorganisms with food-borne illnesses may be considered to be food-borne infections, as opposed to the foodborne intoxications discussed above.

Infection food poisoning is characterized by sudden onset, vomiting, diarrhea, and, usually, fever. The symptoms are of limited duration and usually subside in two to three days. This kind of disease resembles intoxication food poisoning, except that the incubation period is longer (12 to 24 hours rather than 1 to 6 hours) and fever is frequently a symptom. The great majority of outbreaks of this kind represent infections with species of *Salmonella* other than the typhoid bacillus and, although they are commonly known as *Salmonella* food poisoning, are in fact infections of the gastrointestinal tract. In recent years, still another foodborne infection of this nature, that produced by *Vibrio parahaemolyticus,* has been increasing in public health importance. Other bacteria, including streptococci, coliforms, and other gram-negative bacilli, have occasionally been implicated as etiological agents of similar kinds of food poisoning, but more by circumstantial than by definitive evidence.[21]

SALMONELLA FOOD POISONING

With the exception of *Salmonella typhi,* any of the *Salmonella* are potentially capable of causing *Salmonella* food poisoning (Chapter 19). Epidemiological studies, however, indicate that relatively few serotypes are usually encountered, and these vary somewhat in geographical distribution. In the United States, the serotypes most frequently isolated have included *typhimurium, enteritidis, newport,* and *heidelberg,* with *typhimurium* by far the most prevalent single serotype (see Table 19–5, p. 469).

As noted above, the ingestion of food containing large numbers of these organisms frequently results in diarrhea, fever, nausea, and emesis. It has not been firmly established that enterotoxins are responsible for the disease symptoms, although the synthesis of vascular permeability factors and enterotoxin have been reported. It is probable that actual infection of the gastrointestinal tract takes place, as indicated by the somewhat longer incubation period, the typical febrile response, and the shedding of bacteria in the feces. The case-fatality rate is quite low, and severe illness generally occurs only in those with intercurrent disease or in the elderly or very young.

Almost any kind of food may serve as a vehicle, probably because of the widespread occurrence of *Salmonella*. In general, the vehicles are tissues from infected animals or foods subject to contamination by animal or human fecal wastes. In almost all instances, the consumed food is raw or inadequately cooked. The classical sources of infection include fish, shellfish, meats, unpasteurized milk, and eggs. Both *typhimurium* and *enteritidis* serotypes are commonly carried by rats and mice, and it is probable that in many cases these rodents are responsible for the contamination of food. In others, the source of infection may be a human carrier and in many cases of meat poisoning it has been found that the meat was from a diseased animal.

As in the case of staphylococcal and other food poisoning, there is usually a history which includes a possible, or probable, source of contamination and storage of the contaminated foods under conditions permitting bacterial growth. The identification of the microbial agent found in the food is a routine laboratory procedure, involving isolation and identification by conventional cultural and serological methods (Chapter 17). As would be expected from the mode of transmission, *Salmonella* gastroenteritis exhibits sharp seasonal incidence in the United States with the greatest numbers of cases occurring in the warmer months.

VIBRIO PARAHAEMOLYTICUS FOOD POISONING[1, 2]

Food poisoning caused by this organism was first recognized in Japan in 1951, where it was associated with the consumption of raw seafoods. The etiological agent is a halophilic marine vibrio and was the first marine microorganism incriminated as a human pathogen. The ubiquity of this vibrio in warm coastal waters is now recognized, and since the early

1970s, it has been increasingly found as a food poisoning agent throughout the world; outbreaks almost invariably involve seafood as the vehicle of infection.

Consumption of raw or partially cooked seafood contaminated with the vibrios may result in acute gastroenteritis of sudden onset, with abdominal pain, nausea, vomiting, diarrhea, and often chills and fever. The median incubation period ranges from about 13 to 23 hours. The disease tends to show seasonal variation, with greatest incidence during the warmer months, at the time when vibrio colonization of marine forms is most pronounced.

While there are conflicting reports concerning the production of enterotoxins by *V. parahaemolyticus,* there is yet no certain evidence that such toxins are produced, although a possible analogy with toxins of the cholera vibrio is obvious.

As in *Salmonella* food poisoning, it is likely that the vibrios initiate gastrointestinal infection, as indicated by the incubation period and the occurrence of vibrios in diarrheal stools. The infective dose for man is probably fairly large, but the vibrios grow rapidly at moderate temperatures in contaminated seafood and easily reach infective numbers in a relatively short time.

Shellfish and Disease

Shellfish, including oysters, clams, and mussels, have been responsible for transmission of a number of enteric diseases, including infectious hepatitis, enteric fevers, and various kinds of infection food poisoning. Shellfish become contaminated from pollutants in the water in which they are grown or stored. They are commonly eaten in an uncooked or partially cooked condition, which facilitates transmission of disease. Although the pathogenic microorganisms are destroyed by adequate cooking, in many instances the accepted methods for preparation of seafoods are insufficient for this purpose. In the course of breathing and feeding, shellfish filter large quantities of water and readily take up bacteria from their environment, in effect, concentrating any pathogens present. They are similarly contaminated with viruses, as indicated epidemiologically by the occurrence of foodborne epidemics of infectious hepatitis. Various enteroviruses, including ECHO and Coxsackie viruses, have been isolated from oysters taken from contaminated waters. Under experimental conditions, oysters take up poliovirus and Coxsackie virus,

and these have been found to persist for as long as 28 days.

Most imbibed bacteria, however, appear to pass through the gastrointestinal tract and are discharged in about 5 hours. The rapidity with which many bacteria are passed through shellfish suggests the possibility that these marine animals may be cleansed of infection by storage in clean or even chlorinated water. The possibility is not only feasible but has been practiced in some instances. Under these conditions, there is evidence that coliforms are essentially eliminated in 4 days. However, these practices may need to be re-evaluated in light of findings that oysters experimentally infected with *S. enteritidis* serotype *typhimurium* continued to excrete this organism for periods up to 14 days.[12]

REFERENCES

1. Barker, W. H., Jr., and E. J. Gangarosa. 1974. Food poisoning due to *Vibrio parahaemolyticus.* Ann. Rev. Med. **25**:75–81.
2. Barrow, G. I. 1974. Microbiological and other hazards from seafoods with special reference to *Vibrio parahaemolyticus.* Postgrad. Med. J. **50**:612–619.
3. Collee, J. G. 1974. Bacterial challenges in food. Postgrad. Med. J. **50**:636–643.
4. Dolman, C. E. 1974. Human botulism in Canada (1919–1973). Can. Med. Assn J. **110**:191–200.
5. Duncan, C. L. 1973. Time of enterotoxin formation and release during sporulation of *Clostridium perfringens* type A. J. Bacteriol. **113**:392–396.
6. Foster, E. M. 1978. Foodborne hazards of microbial origin. Fed. Proc. **37**:2577–2581.
7. Genigeorgis, C., and J. K. Kuo. 1976. Recovery of staphylococcal enterotoxin from foods by affinity chromatography. Appl. Environ. Microbiol. **31**:274–279.
8. Gilbert, R. J. 1974. Staphylococcal food poisoning and botulism. Postgrad. Med. J. **50**:603–611.
9. Hauschild, A. H. W. 1975. Criteria and procedures for implicating Clostridium perfringens in foodborne outbreaks. Can. J. Publ. Hlth **66**:388–392.
10. Hobbs, B. C. 1974. *Clostridium welchii* and *Bacillus cereus* infection and intoxication. Postgrad. Med. J. **50**:597–602.
11. Hughes, J. M., *et al.* 1981. Clinical features of types A and B food-borne botulism. Ann. Intern. Med. **95**:442–445.
12. Janssen, W. A. 1974. Oysters: retention and excretion of three types of human waterborne disease bacteria. Hlth Lab. Sci. **11**:20–24.
13. Mann, J. M., *et al.* 1981. Patient recovery from type A botulism: morbidity assessment following a large outbreak. Amer. J. Publ. Hlth **71**:266–269.
14. Melling, J., *et al.* 1976. Identification of a novel enterotoxigenic activity associated with *Bacillus cereus.* J. Clin. Pathol. **29**:938–940.
15. Mortimer, P. R., and G. McCann. 1974. Food-poi-

soning episodes associated with *Bacillus cereus* in fried rice. Lancet **1**:1043–1045.

16. Reiser, R., D. Conaway, and M. S. Bergdoll. 1974. Detection of staphylococcal enterotoxin in foods. Appl. Microbiol. **27**:83–85.

17. Riemann, H., U. C. Davis, and F. Bryan. 1979. Foodborne Infections and Intoxications. 2nd ed. Academic Press, New York.

18. Sours, H. E., and D. G. Smith. 1980. Outbreaks of foodborne disease in the United States, 1972–1978. J. Infect. Dis. **142**:122–125.

19. Spira, W. M., and J. M. Goepfert. 1975. Biological characteristics of an enterotoxin produced by *Bacillus cereus*. Can. J. Microbiol. **21**:1236–1246.

20. Stiffler-Rosenberg, G., and H. Fey. 1978. Simple assay for staphylococcal enterotoxins A, B, and C: modification of enzyme-linked immunosorbent assay. J. Clin. Microbiol. **8**:473–479.

21. Taylor, W. R., *et al.* 1982. A foodborne outbreak of enterotoxigenic *Escherichia coli* diarrhea. New Engl. J. Med. **306**:1093–1095.

22. Todd, E., *et al.* 1974. Two outbreaks of *Bacillus cereus* food poisoning in Canada. Can. J. Publ. Hlth **65**:109–113.

23. Turnbull, P. C. B. 1976. Studies on the production of enterotoxins by *Bacillus cereus*. J. Clin. Pathol. **29**:941–948.

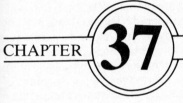

CHAPTER 37

Normal Flora and Oral Microbiology

Indigenous Microflora of Humans[1, 3, 12, 22, 23, 27]

Throughout the history of medical microbiology, attention has largely focused on the frankly pathogenic bacteria—those whose presence in the host almost invariably signals disease. The microbiologist has been primarily concerned with the isolation and identification of the pathogenic microorganisms, including their differentiation from the nonpathogenic bacteria that are found in the human host. Knowledge of the nonpathogenic microorganisms was then ancillary to that of the disease-producing forms; rarely were studies directed specifically toward the normal microflora of the human host. The understanding of infectious diseases that has evolved over the past several decades now emphasizes the importance of those microorganisms that normally colonize the human host without disease production. Many of those once considered to be innocuous members of the normal flora are now known to be potentially pathogenic under certain circumstances, leading to renewed interest in the indigenous microflora and their possible role in both health and disease.

The healthy fetus *in utero* is essentially free of microorganisms. The infant is exposed to the microflora of the vagina during birth and to the microorganisms present in the environment almost immediately thereafter. Within a few hours the oral and nasopharyngeal flora of the neonate are established, and within a day or so the resident microflora of the lower intestinal tract appear. These are not entirely random events, for colonization follows more or less predictable and characteristic patterns. In the neonate, for example, bifidobacteria and lactobacilli appear in the lower intestinal tract within the first day and are followed by colonization with anaerobic cocci within a week, irrespective of environmental factors. Nevertheless, development of indigenous flora is to a degree affected by external influences. Breastfed infants develop a colon microflora containing large numbers of bifidobacteria, but fewer clostridia, enterobacteria, and enterococci than are found in infants who are given formulas based on cow's milk. The indigenous microflora show some fluctuation during life, influenced by anatomic and physiologic maturation. In the oral cavity, for instance, gram-negative anaerobic bacteria and *Streptococcus sanguis* are rare before the teeth have erupted, but appear in high frequency afterwards.

It is apparent that microorganisms in great variety abound in the environment and that the human host is exposed to these from the moment of birth. Relatively few of these bacteria, however, are capable of colonizing on the skin and mucous membranes. Some may be regarded as **transients,** present on the body as contaminants but soon eliminated by mechanical means. Others are able to establish and multiply on the exposed body surfaces to become the **indigenous,** or **normal, microflora.** They probably possess adhesins that permit adherence to cells and other body surfaces of the host through receptor-ligand interactions, as described in Chapter 12.

The indigenous microflora rarely possess the virulence factors that permit invasion of host tissues. Colonization by these microorganisms is therefore limited to certain body sites—skin and adjacent mucous membrane surfaces. Resident microflora are found in the mouth, tonsils, nasal passages, and oropharynx, but not in the esophagus, stomach, and upper parts of the small intestine. A large and varied bacterial population is established in the large intestine and, in smaller numbers, in the distal ileum. A few bacteria are sometimes observed in the respiratory tract, but are regarded as transients; the lower respiratory tract is not colonized in healthy individuals. The external genitalia, the anterior urethra, and vagina possess a normal resident bacterial population, but the posterior urethra and other parts of the genitourinary tract are generally sterile.

Activities of the Normal Microflora

Studies on gnotobiotic animals reveal that while the normal flora are not essential to the well-being of the host, several beneficial effects of indigenous bacteria are noteworthy. It is likely, for instance, that some of the colon microflora synthesize vitamins K or B *in situ;* these bacterial products are then absorbed to provide some of these essential nutrients to the host.

Because of the complex ecological associations at sites of colonization, opportunities arise for a number of competitive events among the constituent flora. For example, metabolic products of some may be antagonistic to others in the population. Ammonia production leads to local increases in pH that are inimical to the growth of some species. In other instances, population dynamics of the resident flora are regulated by microbial products with antibiotic action or bacteriocins produced by gram-negative bacteria. Microbial competition for attachment sites on the mucous membranes also serves to prevent or inhibit colonization by pathogenic forms.

Antibodies are often produced by the host in response to the antigens of the normal flora. When these are cross-reactive against antigens of the pathogenic bacteria, as they frequently are, immune protection against the pathogenic bacteria is engendered. This is thought to be the origin of many of the "natural" antibodies active against disease-causing bacteria.

The normal microbiota are not always beneficial to the host, however. Some members of the resident flora can give rise to disease when the natural defenses are compromised, as by immunosuppressive drugs or intercurrent disease. In other instances, activities of the normal flora are obvious, but not of a serious nature, as when microbial skin residents give rise to rancid body odors by lipolytic action on constituents of apocrine sweat.

Knowledge of the composition and activities of the indigenous microflora is admittedly fragmentary, owing to the complexities of interaction among the members and the tremendous variations in numbers and kinds of microorganisms. It has been estimated that more than 300 bacterial species are harbored in the oral cavity, and about 500 species are found in the large intestine. These estimates may be low, for many of the morphological types seen by microscopy cannot be cultivated. Moreover, the composition changes with climate, personal hygiene, diet, and environmental variations.

SKIN[10, 20, 21]

In contrast to other body sites, the microflora of the skin is restricted to a relatively few kinds of microorganisms. The predominant bacteria include the diphtheroids, *e.g.,* *Corynebacterium* and *Propionibacterium,* and the staphylococci. Less numerous are the nonhemolytic and α-hemolytic streptococci, *Micrococcus,* and *Clostridium;* gram-negative bacilli are rare. The principal yeasts are *Pityrosporum,* while *Candida* and *Torulopsis* appear in fewer numbers.

There is considerable variation in the total numbers of bacteria resident on the skin, ranging from about 10^1 to 10^6 per sq. cm., with greatest numbers generally appearing at skin sites that are typically moist; anaerobes usually outnumber the aerobic forms.

Acne

The role of normal skin microflora in the etiology of acne is controversial, but much circumstantial evidence relates some of these microorganisms, particularly *Propionibacterium acnes* to this affliction. Acne usually develops at puberty, probably arising from noninflamed whiteheads and progressing to inflamed pustules, papules, and nodules. Certainly many factors are involved in the genesis of the lesions, but many believe that *Propionibacterium acnes* may contribute to the inflammatory response by formation of biologically active substances.

UPPER RESPIRATORY TRACT

The indigenous microflora of the upper respiratory tract are largely confined to the mouth, throat, and nasal passages. Other anatomic areas, such as the nasal sinuses, larynx, and the respiratory tree are generally without resident flora and are normally sterile except for occasional transient microorganisms.

Mouth [2, 3, 8, 24]

The oral cavity offers a beneficial environment for the continuous growth of microorganisms. The saliva is particularly important in this respect, carrying nutrients to the microorganisms growing on the epithelial and tooth surfaces and in the gingival crevice; saliva also serves to flush away microbial cells and products, which are then swallowed. Because of salivary flow, microorganisms in the oral cavity must adhere tightly to the surfaces, or find sanctuary in the gingival crevice, to avoid being washed away.

Several hundred bacterial species have been found as components of the oral flora; many of these are capable of anaerobic growth. Indeed, the anaerobic bacteria generally outnumber the aerobes by a ratio of 10:1 or more. Bacterial concentrations in saliva may reach 10^8 to 10^9 colony forming units per ml., while concentrations as high as 10^{10} per ml. are found in gingival scrapings. Table 37–1 lists some of the bacteria commonly observed in the mouth. Many of these exhibit site preferences, to be discussed more fully in the following section on oral microbiology.

Pharynx

The normal flora of the pharynx is not as varied as that found in the mouth, and numbers are not as great. Nevertheless, a great many bacteria have been found at this site, as shown in Table 37–2. It is also noteworthy that several frankly pathogenic forms are sometimes isolated from healthy individuals, *viz.*, *Neisseria meningitidis*, *Streptococcus pyogenes*, and *Streptococcus pneumoniae*. In some cases these may represent temporary or convalescent carriers.

Table 37–1. **Bacteria Found in the Oral Cavity.***

Actinomyces	Leptotrichia
Arachnia	Micrococcus
Bacillus	Mycoplasma
Bacterionema	Neisseria†
Bacteroides	Pasteurella
Bifidobacterium	Peptococcus
Borrelia	Peptostreptococcus
Campylobacter	Propionibacterium
Clostridium	Proteus
Corynebacterium	Pseudomonas
Enterobacter	Rothia
Escherichia	Selenomonas
Eubacterium	Spirillum
Fusobacterium	Staphylococcus
Haemophilus†	Streptococcus†
Klebsiella	Treponema
Lactobacillus	Veillonella†

*In addition, *Candida*, *Entamoeba*, and *Trichomonas* are found.
†Predominant bacteria.

Nose

Only a relatively few bacteria regularly colonize the nasal passages. Staphylococci, including *S. aureus*, are found with some regularity. Corynebacteria are sometimes found, as are neisseriae and streptococci.

ALIMENTARY TRACT [6, 11, 25, 26]

The normal flora of the gastrointestinal tract are established within a few days after birth and are thought to be derived principally from the vaginal and gastrointestinal flora of the mother. Throughout life, additional microorganisms are introduced from a variety of environmental sources. Whether introduced microorganisms establish as a part of the normal flora is dependent upon a number of factors, many of which are incompletely understood. The predominant flora of the gastrointestinal tract are shown in Table 37–3.

Few, if any, bacteria colonize the stomach, duodenum, jejunum, and proximal ileum. Bacteria in foods and saliva are introduced into

Table 37–2. **Microorganisms Commonly Isolated from the Pharynx**

Actinomyces	Klebsiella
Bacteroides	Mycoplasma
Branhamella	Neisseria
Campylobacter	Peptococcus
Candida	Peptostreptococcus
Corynebacterium	Proteus
Enterobacter	Selenomonas
Fusobacterium	Staphylococcus
Haemophilus	Streptococcus
	Veillonella

Table 37–3. **Predominant Bacteria of the Gastrointestinal Tract**

		Location		
Microorganism	Stomach	Duodenum and Jejunum	Ileum	Colon
Bacteroides			+	+
Bifidobacterium			+	+
Clostridium			+	+
Eubacterium				+
Fusobacterium			+	+
Lactobacillus	+	+		
Streptococcus	+	+		
Coliforms			+	+

the stomach, but most are rapidly destroyed by gastric acids, so that luminal contents in the stomach and upper small intestine rarely contain more than 10^4 bacteria per ml.; most of these are aciduric, facultatively anaerobic, gram-positive bacteria of the genera *Streptococcus* and *Lactobacillus*.

Marked changes in the intestinal microflora begin in the lower portion of the ileum. The numbers of gram-negative bacteria increase and soon outnumber the gram-positive forms. Coliforms appear with regularity, along with increasing numbers of obligately anaerobic bacteria—*Bacteroides, Bifidobacterium, Fusobacterium,* and *Clostridium*. The composition of the normal flora is qualitatively similar to that of the luxuriant flora of the colon, but the numbers are generally fewer, usually less than 10^9 per ml.

The bacterial content of the colon is essentially that of the feces. Most of the intestinal bacteria are present in the colon, with numbers sometimes reaching 10^{13} per gram, although 10^{10} to 10^{12} per gram is usually quoted; they constitute about one-third of the fecal mass. The anaerobic bacteria of the colon usually outnumber the facultative forms by a factor of 10^2 to 10^4.

Control Mechanisms

It has been noted that the colonization and growth of bacteria in the upper small intestine is negligible, being held in check by a variety of factors, some of host origin and others associated with microbial interactions.

The host factors of major importance in limiting bacterial overgrowth are gastric acid and peristalsis. Not only does gastric acid destroy most bacteria entering the stomach, but the lower pH serves to inhibit the growth of all but a few of the survivors. Thus, achlorhydric individuals usually have greater numbers of bacteria in the upper small intestine. Similarly, individuals with decreased or ineffective peristalsis do not rapidly clear bacteria from the intestine, resulting in greater bacterial content.

Several bacterial activities probably aid in regulating microbial populations. The facultative forms, by utilizing available oxygen, create an environment suitable for growth of obligate anaerobes and promote their colonization. In other instances, some strains are killed or inhibited by bacteriocins or antibiotic substances produced by others in the ecosystem. Metabolic products, such as the short-chain fatty acids formed by anaerobes, also suppress bacterial growth, thus limiting microbial populations.

Perturbations in the microbial population, particularly overgrowth in the small bowel, may have clinically apparent consequences. The appearance of an abnormal bacterial population, especially an increase in anaerobes in the small bowel, results from achlorhydria, stasis of luminal content, and malnutrition. The abnormal flora often are associated with chronic malabsorption of fats, carbohydrates, or vitamin B_{12}—a condition known as **blind loop syndrome,** or more descriptively as **contaminated small bowel syndrome.** Fat malabsorption is believed to be associated with deconjugation of bile salts by anaerobic bacteria, thus interfering with their fat-solubilizing properties and resulting in steatorrhea. The presence of large numbers of intestinal bacteria may also interfere with absorption of vitamin B_{12}, since this vitamin is bound to the bacteria and becomes unavailable to the host. Carbohydrate malabsorption is possibly related to the metabolic breakdown of carbohydrates by intestinal bacteria. An etiological role for the abnormal bacterial flora in this syndrome is supported by the observation that the symptoms are ameliorated when the microbial flora are reduced by antibiotic therapy. It has also been suggested that tropical sprue, a similar malabsorption syndrome, is due to bacterial overgrowth; it, too, responds to antimicrobial therapy.

GENITOURINARY TRACT

The inhabited areas of the genitourinary tract include the external genitalia, the anterior urethra, and the vagina. Most other areas do not usually have an indigenous microflora and are generally sterile. Many different bacteria have been isolated from the genitourinary tract, but because of frequent contamination, particularly by fecal flora, many of these are probably transients.

The external genitalia are often inhabited by streptococci, staphylococci, mycobacteria, enteric bacilli, corynebacteria, mycoplasmas, anaerobic gram-negative bacilli, and yeasts. The anterior urethra, in both sexes, is colonized by similar flora. The numbers of microorganisms are not as great as in some other sites, *e.g.,* the mouth and colon.

Vagina[9, 13, 14]

The vagina represents a unique ecosystem of the human body, subject to hormonal influences and the events of menstruation, pregnancy, and parturition. The normal cervical-vaginal microflora assume great importance, owing to infections by many of these microorganisms that follow trauma, *e.g.,* parturition, surgery, and malignancy.

The most prevalent of the normal microflora are the lactobacilli and diphtheroids. Also found with some frequency are the aerobic and anaerobic cocci, *e.g.,* staphylococci and groups B and D streptococci; *Gardnerella; Bacteroides,* especially *B. disiens* and *B. bivus;* and *Escherichia.* Those occasionally present include other enteric bacilli, *Fusobacterium, Bifidobacterium, Eubacterium, Veillonella, Clostridium,* and *Candida.* Total microbial counts average about 10^9 per ml. of vaginal fluid, with anaerobes usually outnumbering aerobes.

Although the vaginal microflora are relatively constant, composition may be influenced by hormonal changes, pregnancy, parturition, menstruation, and surgery. Lactobacilli are most prevalent after puberty and before menopause, and increase temporarily during pregnancy. The anaerobic bacteria decrease during pregnancy and following estrogen administration in postmenopausal women. Trauma to the genital tract may lead to microfloral changes, including proliferation of anaerobes and enteric bacilli.

Oral Microbiology[4, 7, 8, 17, 24]

The oral cavity represents a complex microbial ecosystem subject to many variations that affect the makeup and succession of the oral microbiota.

During the life of the host, the occurrence of several major anatomic changes alter the habitat, effecting changes in the microbial communities of the oral cavity. In the predentulous infant, only soft tissue surfaces are present, and the resident bacteria are largely those that can adhere to and colonize epithelial cells. Later, with eruption of the teeth, hard surfaces appear with crevices, fissures, and other cryptic recesses that offer different types of habitat. Throughout life, oral architecture is subject to additional alterations such as changes in the arrangement of the teeth, the introduction of artificial materials, the development of carious lesions, and the loss of dentition.

More rapid, and less predictable, alterations result from environmental factors, including diet, salivary composition and flow rate, hormonal influences, quality of dental hygiene, and use of antimicrobial agents.

The number and kinds of bacteria in the oral environment are profoundly affected by this multiplicity of habitats. Initial colonization is dependent upon the ability of the bacteria to adhere to surfaces in the oral cavity and resist dispersion by salivary flow and mastication. Adhesion, as noted in Chapter 12, is determined by bacterial adhesins interacting with specific receptor sites on epithelial or enamel surfaces. Adherence of bacteria to epithelial surfaces is usually direct, *i.e.,* the bacterial ligand combines with a host cell surface component. Additional factors come into play when bacteria adhere to the enamel and dentinal surfaces of the teeth. Of paramount importance in this regard are the salivary glycoproteins, which rapidly and strongly bind to enamel surfaces of the teeth. These glycoproteins also interact with many bacteria, so that bacterial adherence to tooth surfaces is often through their affinity for this intermediate substance. Salivary glycoproteins, binding to bacterial surfaces, also provide a mechanism for coaggregation of different bacteria in the oral cavity, resulting in communal associations between a variety of bacteria on tooth surfaces.

Bacterial colonization of enamel surfaces of the teeth is not subject to the same forces that control mucosal epithelial cell colonization. Bacteria adherent to mucosal cells in the oral cavity are continuously lost by the normal desquamation of surface cell layers, whereas bacteria colonizing the hard surfaces are not removed and reach enormous numbers. Moreover, the affinity of bacteria for the enamel surfaces is exceedingly strong in comparison to their affinity for epithelial cell surfaces; if teeth are immersed in saliva for one minute, bacteria adhere so strongly that they are removed only by such measures as ultrasonic treatment. At certain of the oral colonization sites, the bacteria are effectively protected from mechanical removal. In the fissures of the occlusal surface of the teeth and in the gingival sulcus, *i.e.,* the crevice between the tooth and gums, bacteria are not easily removed by mechanical forces; those colonizing such protected sites do not therefore require the same strong adherence factors as bacteria that colonize the exposed smooth tooth surfaces. The diversity of bacterial cell types observed in colonization sites on the teeth is, to a great extent, due to cell-to-cell binding, mediated either by salivary glycoproteins or by bacterial products such as extracellular polysaccharides.

It is not likely that significant bacterial growth occurs in the salivary fluids. Rather, the salivary microflora represent transients that are shed into the saliva from colonization sites in the oral cavity, such as the tongue and tooth surfaces.

It should be apparent that initial colonization and the development of microbial communities in the many sites of oral colonization are dependent on bacterial, host, and environmental factors. The composition of microbial communities also varies with their location. Microorganisms initially colonizing a particular site must possess adhesins that can bind to receptors at that location. After initial flora are established, microbial interactions become increasingly important in development of microbial communities, facilitating or inhibiting the attachment and growth of other microorganisms. Metabolic products of one microbial type may provide nutrients for others, alterations in pH may favor some and inhibit others, while the growth of aerobic forms can lower the oxidation-reduction potential to levels suitable for anaerobic bacteria. Thus, the oral cavity comprises a variety of smaller ecosystems, each with a more or less distinctive flora that, within limits, changes with time and environmental conditions.

DENTAL PLAQUE AND ORAL DISEASES

The masses of bacteria that accumulate on teeth are termed dental plaque (Fig. 37–1). This consists of enormous numbers of bacteria embedded in a plaque matrix composed of extracellular bacterial polysaccharides and

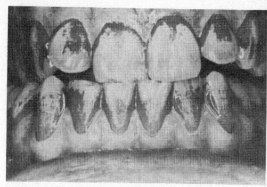

Figure 37–1. Dental plaque on the teeth of an individual who had not brushed for 72 hours. Plaque has been stained with erythrocin. (R. J. Gibbons and J. van Houte, Bacterial adherence and the formation of dental plaques. *In* E. H. Beachey (Ed.), Bacterial Adherence. Chapman and Hall, London, 1980.)

macromolecules of host origin. Plaque formation is an important antecedent event in the etiology of the two major oral diseases—dental caries and periodontal disease.

Formation of Plaque

Newly cleaned teeth are rapidly covered by a strongly adherent thin film of acidic glycoproteins, termed the **acquired pellicle.** These glycoproteins, present in saliva, are specifically adsorbed to hydroxyapatite, a crystalline salt of calcium phosphate that is the major constituent of tooth enamel. The presence of the pellicle promotes subsequent adherence of many bacteria to the tooth surface.

Plaque formation begins with the selective adherence of certain bacteria to the tooth surface. As these bacteria multiply, a plaque matrix is formed, followed by incorporation and growth of a variety of other bacterial species. The microbial constitution of dental plaque is markedly influenced by the site of colonization. **Supragingival plaque,** occurring in occlusal fissures, on buccal and lingual smooth enamel surfaces, and between the teeth, possesses a different microbial makeup from the **subgingival plaque** that occurs in the gingival sulcus. Thus, many bacteria are capable of colonizing tooth surfaces, but to different degrees, and are variously affected by a number of environmental and host variables.

Only relatively few of the bacteria that can colonize the dental surfaces are capable of initiating or contributing to oral disease. Streptococci and certain of the gram-positive filamentous bacteria, such as *Actinomyces,* are the predominant members of the plaque flora associated with caries and periodontal disease.

Of central importance in the initial colonization of the coronal surfaces are the oral streptococci, principally *Streptococcus mutans.* Bacteria can associate with the tooth surface by electrostatic forces, but available evidence indicates a more specific process, probably through bacterial ligand-receptor interactions. Initial adherence of oral streptococci and other bacteria to the pellicle-coated hydroxyapatite is a relatively weak association, and is reversible.

This weak association must be augmented by additional adhesive interactions if plaque formation is to proceed. Because *S. mutans* is believed to be the principal bacterial species initiating caries formation, factors that promote its accumulation on teeth have received greatest attention. Experimental studies in animals first indicated that *S. mutans* would form extensive plaque accumulations when the diet contained large amounts of sucrose. Under these circumstances the microorganisms synthesized large amounts of extracellular polysaccharides, including glucans and fructans. One of the glucans, characterized by predominantly α-1,3 linkages and relative insolubility in aqueous mediums, is considered to be the major determinant in adherence and colonization. The glucan is formed by action of an *S. mutans* enzyme, **glucosyl transferase,** which catalyzes the formation of the polymer from glucose moieties of sucrose. Both the insoluble glucan (termed mutan) and glucosyl transferase (GTF) participate in the sucrose-dependent adhesive interactions of *S. mutans* at the tooth surface.

Mutan, synthesized by *S. mutans* GTF, is first bound to protein receptors on the bacterial surface. Aggregation of bacterial cells then takes place when GTF molecules interact with the cell-bound glucans on adjacent cells, forming GTF-glucan complexes and permitting cross-linking within the matrix. Although some other bacteria, including oral streptococci, can produce extracellular polysaccharides, they do not readily form plaque, presumably because they lack the ability to bind glucans to the cell surface.

These adherence mechanisms are sufficient to initiate plaque formation by *S. mutans,* but as plaque matures, other bacterial species are incorporated, resulting in a heterogeneous mixture of bacterial types. Presumably these arise from complex interrelations in which there is cell-to-cell adherence between species. This **coaggregation** is often highly specific and likely is due to receptor interactions of diverse nature. These are frequently striking, as in the case of "corncob" formations resulting from coaggregation of oral streptococci with filamentous bacteria, such as *Actinomyces, Fusobacterium,* and *Bacterionema* (Figs. 37–2 and 37–3). In many instances, however, other bacteria interact with or become entrapped in the glucan matrix.

The formation of subgingival plaque probably does not require the strong adherence characterizing coronal plaque formation. Presumably weaker adherence factors, such as fimbriae, may be sufficient to promote colonization in these protected sites.

DENTAL CARIES[5]

The production of dental caries is indisputably due to the action of oral microorganisms.

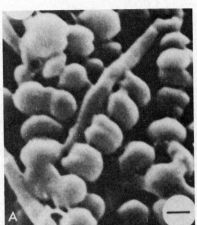
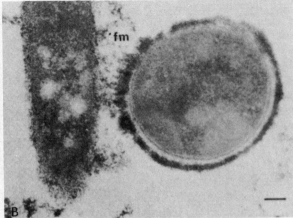

Figure 37–2. Electron photomicrograph of "corncobs" formed *in vitro* by coaggregation of *Fusobacterium nucleatum* and *Streptococcus sanguis. A,* Scanning electron photomicrograph; *B,* transmission electron photomicrograph showing fimbriae *(fm).* (P. Lancy, Jr., *et al.,* Infect. Immun. **40**:303, 1983.)

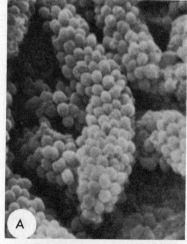

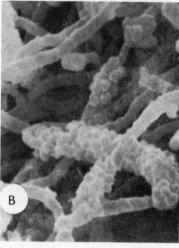

Figure 37–3. Scanning electron photomicrograph showing formation of "corncob" structures by adherence of cocci to filamentous bacteria. (R. J. Gibbons and J. van Houte, Bacterial adherence and the formation of dental plaques. *In* E. H. Beachey (Ed.), Bacterial Adherence. Chapman and Hall, London, 1980.)

Although its infectious nature is not always appreciated, it ranks as one of the most prevalent infectious diseases. While it is not life-threatening, the disease has important social and economic consequences.

Dental caries arises when bacterial products create localized lesions on the tooth surfaces. The deposition of the masses of bacteria in dental plaque begins the process of tooth decay. The microorganisms ferment carbohydrates of the diet, principally sucrose, forming lactic and other organic acids. The physical nature of plaque inhibits diffusion, resulting in localized high concentrations of acidic products at the enamel or dentin surface. The hydroxyapatite crystals are solubilized and the carious lesion is formed, with subsequent loss of the organic matrices of enamel and dentin.

Although carious lesions may occur on the smooth enamel surfaces, more often they are seen in fissures and pits of the occlusal surfaces and in sheltered areas between the teeth and in the gingival crevices. At these sites, adherent microorganisms of plaque are best protected from mechanical removal.

The complexity of the oral microflora has complicated studies to determine the specific bacteria that are responsible for dental caries; certainly no one microoganism can be said to cause the disease. Nevertheless, most evidence indicates that in caries of the enamel surfaces, the microorganism usually initiating the condition is *Streptococcus mutans*. In the presence of sucrose, the most cariogenic dietary factor, *S. mutans* colonization is promoted by the production of mutan and GTF. Furthermore, *S. mutans* produces copious amounts of lactic acid from sucrose and certain other carbohydrates, and is the most aciduric of the oral streptococci. This is not to say that other plaque bacteria do not contribute to the process. Lactobacilli are probably secondary invaders in carious lesions, producing additional lactic acid by their metabolism; possibly other oral streptococci, such as *S. sanguis,* are similarly involved.

As noted earlier, plaque that forms in the gingival sulcus is different in makeup. Filamentous bacteria, including *Actinomyces,* are more often observed, with increased numbers of anaerobic bacteria, such as fusobacteria. Although *S. mutans* can initiate root surface caries, other bacteria appear to be of greater importance in inducing lesions of the cemental surface and in periodontal disease.

Control of Caries[15, 18]

Recognition of the etiology of dental caries permits a rational approach to prevention and control. Many of the proposed control measures are intended to inhibit or reduce colonization by bacteria, especially *S. mutans*.

Caries activity can be markedly reduced by the simple expedient of restricting dietary sucrose or altering the manner of its consumption; caries is promoted, for example, by frequent ingestion of sucrose. Substitution of noncariogenic sweeteners, such as sorbitol or other sugar substitutes, is known to restrict plaque formation.

Adherence of *S. mutans* can also be inhibited by use of enzymes that degrade the glucan of the plaque matrix. Dextranases (α-1,6 glucanases) are reportedly effective in animals, but results in humans have been equivocal. On the other hand, limited trials with α-1,3 glucanases are more encouraging.

It has been suggested that cariogenic bacteria could be eliminated by use of antibiotics. Although these have been successfully employed to reduce or eliminate oral plaque organisms, their use on a long-term basis is both unwise and impractical.

One of the more effective methods of caries control is by ingestion of fluoridated water or fluoride dietary supplements. Fluoride levels of 1 part per million in drinking water have been shown to effect a 50 per cent reduction of the caries rate in permanent teeth. Topical application of fluoride is less effective, and fluoride-containing toothpastes have little beneficial effect in this regard.

The possibility that immunization with cariogenic bacteria, *e.g., S. mutans,* could protect against caries has long been an attractive hypothesis. Indeed, protection against caries by antibody has been established in a variety of animal systems. Systemic immunization with *S. mutans* lowers the caries rate in rodents, inducing both serum IgG and salivary IgA responses. Similarly, oral immunization, inducing only salivary IgA, results in caries protection. The significance of antibodies in immunity is also exemplified by the protection engendered against caries in rats that are fed colostrum or milk from immunized dams. Presumably, effective immunity rendered by antibodies to *S. mutans* can result from inhibition of GTF activity or by reaction with surface antigens mediating adherence.

The possibility that serum antibodies to *S. mutans* may cross-react with heart muscle antigens has inhibited attempts to immunize with conventional systemic vaccines, but the potential for oral immunization, stimulating only secretory IgA antibodies, remains as a possible alternative. Furthermore, purified virulence antigens, such as GTF or cell surface antigens, may offer other avenues for vaccine development.

PERIODONTAL DISEASE[3, 16, 19, 24, 28]

Suspension of all oral hygiene measures for a period of several weeks results in a massive accumulation of supragingival plaque that progresses to the margin of the gingiva and culminates in the formation of subgingival plaque. The presence of bacteria in the gingival sulcus engenders an inflammatory response in the underlying connective tissue that characterizes gingivitis.

Gingivitis

This condition arises as a consequence of the alterations in the composition of the accumulating plaque. As plaque begins to form, the primary bacterial colonizers are the gram-positive cocci and rods. After a few days, fusobacteria and actinomycetes appear in greater number, followed by motile bacteria, including vibrios and spirochetes. Thus, within a week or 10 days, the plaque flora progress from a relatively simple composition to one that is exceedingly complex, with a significant population of gram-negative and anaerobic bacteria. These bacteria generally occur in zones within the plaque; the gram-positive cocci adhere to the tooth surface and are overlaid with a zone of adherent gram-negative and motile bacteria. Bacterial enzymes and metabolic products are responsible for the inflammatory host response.

Although gingivitis does not always progress to destructive lesions of the periodontium, the loss of soft and hard tissue that characterizes periodontitis is almost always preceded by gingivitis. Periodontal disease is generally taken to include both gingivitis and periodontitis.

Periodontitis

The extension of supragingival plaque into the gingival crevice to form subgingival plaque is accompanied by further alterations in bacterial composition. In the relatively stagnant environment of the gingival sulcus, gram-negative anaerobes are predominant, including *Bacteroides, Fusobacterium,* and *Capnocytophaga.* As the bacteria of subgingival plaque proliferate, the depth of the sulcus increases, with destruction of gingival tissue, periodontal fibers, and alveolar bone, giving rise to periodontitis.

Bacteria in the periodontal lesion, or periodontal pocket, do not invade the adjacent tissues. Rather, bacterial products accumulate and diffuse into surrounding tissues, inducing the severe inflammation. Among the bacterial products associated with pathogenesis are enzymes (collagenase, hyaluronidase, deoxyribonuclease, and proteinases), endotoxin, and metabolic products (*e.g.,* organic acids, ammonia, and hydrogen sulfide). In addition to the direct action of these substances, bacterial products may indirectly stimulate destructive host responses, such as release of endogenous enzymes from lysosomes and stimulation of immunopathological mechanisms.

Although the bacteria responsible for periodontal disease do not generally invade the tissues, one condition, known as **acute necro-**

tizing ulcerative gingivitis (ANUG), represents a destructive invasion of soft tissues by plaque microorganisms. This disease appears to be associated with the presence of large numbers of fusobacteria and spirochetes in the subgingival plaque.

Control of Periodontal Disease

Since periodontal disease does not occur in the absence of plaque, control of the disease is possible by reduction of plaque. This can be accomplished by vigorous and effective oral hygiene procedures, such as those employed for control of dental caries, including brushing and the use of toothpicks, dental floss, water irrigation devices, and, possibly, antimicrobial mouth rinses.

REFERENCES

1. Burman, L. G. 1980. Influence of antimicrobial agents on host-parasite interactions. Scand. J. Infect. Dis., Suppl. 24, pp. 179–187.
2. Carlsson, J. 1980. Symbiosis between host and microorganisms in the oral cavity. Scand. J. Infect. Dis., Suppl. 24, pp. 74–78.
3. Evaldson, G., et al. 1982. The normal human anaerobic microflora. Scand. J. Infect. Dis., Suppl. 35, pp. 9–15.
4. Gibbons, R. J., and J. van Houte. 1980. Bacterial adherence and the formation of dental plaques. pp. 61–104. In E. H. Beachey (Ed.): Bacterial Adherence. Chapman and Hall, London.
5. Gibbons, R. J., and J. van Houte. 1975. Dental caries. Ann. Intern. Med. 26:121–136.
6. Gracey, M. S. 1981. Nutrition, bacteria and the gut. Brit. Med. Bull. 37:71–75.
7. Hamada, S., and H. D. Slade. 1980. Mechanisms of adherence of Streptococcus mutans to smooth surfaces in vitro. pp. 105–135. In E. H. Beachey (Ed.): Bacterial Adherence. Chapman and Hall, London.
8. Hamada, S., and H. D. Slade. 1980. Biology, immunology, and cariogenicity of Streptococcus mutans. Microbiol. Rev. 44:331–384.
9. Hammann, R. 1982. A reassessment of the microbial flora of the female genital tract, with special reference to the occurrence of Bacteroides species. J. Med. Microbiol. 15:293–302.
10. Holland, K. T., E. Ingham, and W. J. Cunliffe. 1981. A review: the microbiology of acne. J. Appl. Microbiol. 51:195–215.
11. Isaacs, P. E. T., and Y. S. Kim. 1979. The contaminated small bowel syndrome. Amer. J. Med. 67:1049–1057.
12. Isenberg, H. D., and B. G. Painter. 1980. Indigenous and pathogenic microorganisms of humans, pp. 25–39. In E. H. Lennette, et al. (Eds.): Manual of Clinical Microbiology. 3rd ed. American Society for Microbiology, Washington, D.C.
13. Larsen, B., and R. P. Galask. 1980. Vaginal microbial flora: practical and theoretical relevance. Obstet. Gynecol. (Suppl. 5) 55:100S–113S.
14. Larsen, B., and R. P. Galask. 1982. Vaginal microbial flora: composition and influences of host physiology. Ann. Intern. Med. 96:926–930.
15. Leverett, D. H. 1982. Fluorides and the changing prevalence of dental caries. Science 217:26–30.
16. Löe, H. 1981. The role of bacteria in periodontal diseases. Bull. Wld Hlth Org. 59:821–825.
17. McGhee, J. R., and S. M. Michalek. 1981. Immunobiology of dental caries: microbial aspects and local immunity. Ann. Rev. Microbiol. 35:595–638.
18. Newbrun, E. 1982. Sugar and dental caries: a review of human studies. Science 217:418–423.
19. Newman, M. G. 1979. The role of Bacteroides melaninogenicus and other anaerobes in periodontal infections. Rev. Infect. Dis. 1:313–323.
20. Noble, W. C., and D. A. Somerville. 1974. Microbiology of Human Skin. W. B. Saunders Co., Ltd, London.
21. Pitcher, D. G. 1978. Aerobic cutaneous coryneforms: recent taxonomic findings. Brit. J. Dermatol. 98:363–370.
22. Rosebury, T. 1962. Microorganisms Indigenous to Man. McGraw-Hill, New York.
23. Rotimi, V. O., and B. I. Duerden. 1981. The development of the bacterial flora in normal neonates. J. Med. Microbiol. 14:51–62.
24. Russell, C., and T. H. Melville. 1978. A review: bacteria in the human mouth. J. Appl. Bacteriol. 44:163–181.
25. Savage, D. C. 1977. Microbial ecology of the gastrointestinal tract. Ann. Rev. Microbiol. 31:107–133.
26. Simon, G. L., and S. L. Gorbach. 1982. Intestinal microflora. Med. Clinics North Amer. 66:557–574.
27. Skinner, F. A., and J. G. Carr (Eds.). 1974. The Normal Microbial Flora of Man. Academic Press, London.
28. Socransky, S. S. 1977. Microbiology of periodontal disease—present status and future considerations. J. Periodontol. 48:497–504.

Virology

CHAPTER 38

Fundamentals of Animal Virology

Preston H. Dorsett, Ph.D.

The viruses constitute a unique group of infectious agents that are distinguished from other microorganisms by certain inherent characteristics. Initially viruses were set apart in that they would pass through bacteriological filters; hence the term "filterable virus." Although most viruses are smaller than other microorganisms, small size is only one such feature. The viruses are **obligate intracellular parasites** consisting of a single type of nucleic acid, either DNA or RNA, surrounded by a **capsid** or shell composed of proteins. They may have an **envelope** composed of a lipid-containing unit membrane and glycoproteins **(spike proteins).** The viruses do not reproduce by binary fission. Since they themselves do not contain the components essential for production of macromolecules, viral component parts are synthesized via the macromolecular-synthesizing machinery of the host cells. The virus particle then is assembled by a process of **self-assembly** in which the component parts aggregate into the proper configuration. The complete particle is termed the **virion.**

Virion Morphology[15]

Compared to most microorganisms, the virus particle is small. Viruses range in size from about 20 to 25 nm. for the parvoviruses and picornaviruses, respectively, to 200 to 300 nm. for the poxviruses, which are resolvable by light microscopy.

Early electron micrographs showed that virus particles occurred in various shapes. The poxviruses were seen as brick-shaped, most of the plant viruses were rod-shaped, the bacterial viruses showed a more elaborate, tailed structure, and most animal viruses were approximate spheres. However, improved fixation and staining methods and the advent of negative staining techniques have allowed the visualization of the physical structure of most of the viruses. It became apparent that the viral nucleic acid surrounded by its protein coat or capsid took the form of either a **helix** or an **icosahedron.** This complex was termed a **nucleocapsid.** The capsid was found to be composed of subunits or **capsomers.** Later, by chemical techniques, the capsomers were shown to be composed of multiple polypeptide chains that had aggregated to form the morphological units. The subunits formed from a single polypeptide chain were termed **structural units,** and capsomers are therefore polymers of structural units. Structural units are used to construct the helical capsids, whereas capsomers are used to build the more complex icosahedral capsids. The virion may be made up of the nucleocapsid alone, or the nucleocapsid may be surrounded by an envelope that contains spike-like glycoproteins. The envelope is acquired by **budding** through a cellular membrane. The nomenclature of virus morphology is given in Table 38–1. The viruses can be grouped into five categories based on their morphology and nucleocapsid symmetry. These groups are shown schematically in Figure 38–1, and electron micrographs of the various morphologies are shown in Figures 38–2, 38–3, and 38–4.

Naked Icosahedral Viruses

These viruses consist of an icosahedral nucleocapsid, and initially were thought to be spherical. High-resolution electron microscopy has delineated the icosahedral symmetry. Examples are the papovaviruses, picornaviruses, and adenoviruses.

Enveloped Icosahedral Viruses

The virion of this group consists of an icosahedral nucleocapsid surrounded by an envelope. Examples of the enveloped icosahedral viruses are the herpesviruses and togaviruses.

Naked Helical Viruses

These viruses appear to be long rods; however, they consist of an RNA genome inter-

Table 38–1. **Nomenclature of Viral Morphology**

Virion	The mature infectious virus particle.
Capsid	The protein shell that encloses and protects the viral nucleic acid.
Structural units	A morphological unit of the capsid that is composed of a single polypeptide chain. The structural units for the helical capsids.
Capsomer	The morphological unit of the icosahedral capsid, which consists of aggregated structural units.
Core	The internal part of the virus particle which consists of the nucleic acid and closely associated proteins.
Nucleocapsid	The structure composed of the capsid containing the nucleic acid or core.
Spike proteins	Viral glycoproteins that project from the envelope.
Envelope	The viral membrane, consisting of a lipid bilayer containing spike proteins.

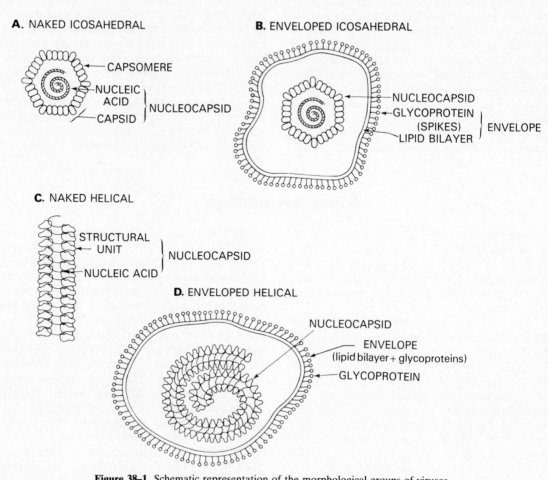

A. NAKED ICOSAHEDRAL

CAPSOMERE
NUCLEIC ACID
CAPSID
} NUCLEOCAPSID

B. ENVELOPED ICOSAHEDRAL

NUCLEOCAPSID
GLYCOPROTEIN (SPIKES)
LIPID BILAYER
} ENVELOPE

C. NAKED HELICAL

STRUCTURAL UNIT
NUCLEIC ACID
} NUCLEOCAPSID

D. ENVELOPED HELICAL

NUCLEOCAPSID
ENVELOPE (lipid bilayer + glycoproteins)
GLYCOPROTEIN

Figure 38–1. Schematic representation of the morphological groups of viruses.

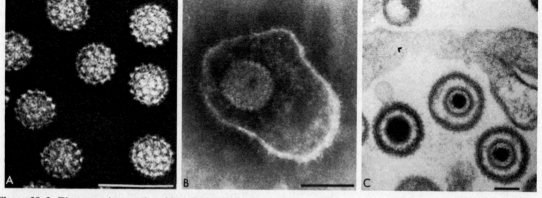

Figure 38–2. Electron micrographs of icosahedral viruses. *A*, Negative stain of human papilloma virus. (Courtesy of A. Howatson.) *B*, Negative stain of a herpes simplex virus. (Courtesy of R. W. Darlington.) *C*, Thin section of herpes simplex showing the core, capsid, and envelope. (Courtesy of M. Rodriguez.) The bars represent 100 nm.

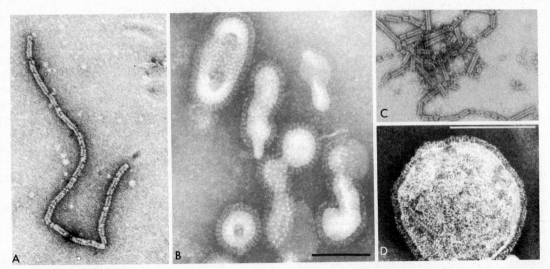

Figure 38–3. Electron micrographs of helical viruses. *A*, Negative stain of the Newcastle disease virus nucleocapsid showing the helical symmetry. *B*, Negative stain of influenza A virus. *C*, Negative stain of Sendai nucleocapsid. *D*, Negative stain of measles virus. The bars represent 100 nm. (*A, B*, and *C*, Courtesy of R. W. Darlington; *D*, courtesy of M. Dubois-Dalcq.)

twined within protein structural units to form a helix. The naked helical viruses are composed of a rigid helical nucleocapsid. Although none of the animal viruses are in this group, many plant viruses are. Examples are bacteriophage M13 and tobacco mosaic virus.

Enveloped Helical Viruses

Viruses in this group consist of a flexible helical nucleocapsid surrounded by an envelope. The nucleocapsid may be coiled into a pleomorphic ball within the envelope, but the helical symmetry can be demonstrated after

disruption of the virion envelope to release the nucleocapsid. Morphologically, the virions may appear as rods or spheres; hence, they are pleomorphic. Examples are the orthomyxoviruses and the paramyxoviruses.

Complex Viruses

Some viruses do not fit into any of the above categories due to the complexity of the virion. Examples are the poxviruses and some of the bacteriophages. The poxviruses, the most complex of the animal viruses, do not have a discernible nucleocapsid structure.

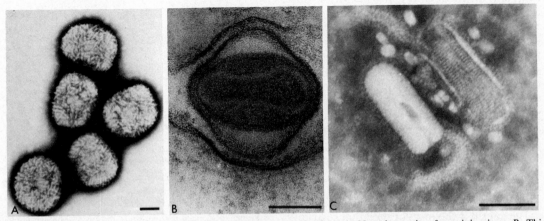

Figure 38–4. Electron micrographs of viruses with complex morphology. *A*, Negative stain of vaccinia virus. *B*, Thin section of vaccinia virus. *C*, Negative stain of vesicular stomatitis virus. The bars represent 100 nm. (*A* and *B*, Courtesy of S. Dales; *C*, courtesy of R. W. Darlington.)

Composition and Structure of Virus Particles

The virion contains a core composed of the nucleic acid and associated proteins (core proteins). The core is sheathed in a capsid, which may or may not be enveloped.

NUCLEIC ACID

A virus contains either RNA or DNA, never both. The nucleic acid present may be **single-** or **double-stranded,** and many possible types have been demonstrated, including linear and covalently closed circular DNA and segmented RNA. For example, the reoviruses contain segmented double-stranded RNA, and the influenza virus genome is segmented single-stranded RNA. Segmented DNA genomes have not yet been demonstrated. Viruses containing single-stranded RNA may be classified according to whether the RNA is of the same polarity as messenger RNA, *i.e.,* (+)RNA, or whether the RNA is of opposite polarity to mRNA, or (−)RNA. This is characteristic of the particular virus. In contrast, the single-stranded DNA viruses that infect vertebrates, the parvoviruses, may contain the two complementary strands of DNA in separate virions, both of which appear to be infectious. The single-stranded DNA phages contain DNA of the same polarity. Some of the linear DNA's can form closed circles by annealing cohesive ends or by association of identical terminal ends. These circular DNA forms may be of special advantage in replication.

The amount of nucleic acid per virion ranges from 1 or 2 per cent to about 35 to 45 per cent, and the number of genes per virion varies from four to eight for the smaller viruses to more than 200 for the poxviruses. It is apparent that most viruses enter the host cell with a limited amount of nucleic acid with which to specify all of the necessary functions. Thus, it is imperative that viruses utilize their genetic material efficiently. This is accomplished by using host cell machinery when possible and by using multiple identical protein subunits to form the capsid.

CAPSID

The capsid is the protein shell that surrounds the genome and protects it from the environment. In the nonenveloped viruses, the capsid contains the attachment proteins that interact with receptors on the host cell during viral attachment. Whether the capsid symmetry is helical or icosahedral, the capsid is formed by the association of many subunits. As already mentioned, the subunits for the helical viruses usually consist of a single polypeptide chain and are termed **structural units.** The subunits of the icosahedral viruses usually consist of more than one polypeptide chain and are termed **capsomers.** The use of identical subunits to form the capsid conserves the viral genetic material, since the same gene can be transcribed and translated to yield multiple capsid polypeptides.

Helical Capsids

The helical capsid resembles a cylinder with the RNA wound in a helix and encased by the structural units of the capsid (Fig. 38–5). The diameter of these capsids is determined by the structural units, and the length is governed by the length of the genome. The helical capsid has a single rotational axis of symmetry which passes through the center of the cylinder. Helical capsid formation initiates with the structural units aggregating to form a flat, nonhelical disc containing two rings of structural units. This disc then becomes associated with the

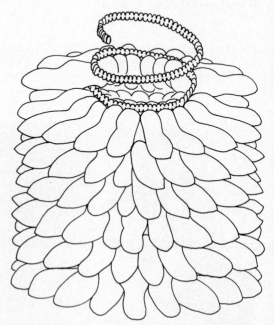

Figure 38–5. Schematic representation of a helical nucleocapsid. The RNA lies in a groove formed by the association of the structural units where it is protected from the environment. (Redrawn from Klug, A., and Caspar, D. L., Adv. Virus Res. **7:**274, 1960, with permission of the authors and publisher.)

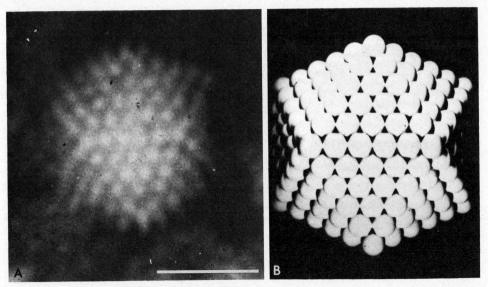

Figure 38–6. *A*, Negative stain of adenovirus showing the capsomer arrangement of two triangular faces. *B*, A model of an adenovirus capsid demonstrating the arrangement of the capsomers to form the faces and vertices of the capsid. Two triangular faces and two vertices are clearly evident. The bar represents 50 nm. (From Horne, R. W., *et al.*, J. Molec. Biol., **1**:85, 1959, with permission of the authors and publisher.)

viral RNA after which the disc shifts to produce a helix and the capsid is completed by the association of capsomers along the RNA.

Icosahedral Capsids

The icosahedron is geometrically more complex than the cylinder, and it is not easy to envision why this shape is favored and how the capsomers associate to form the icosahedral capsid. The icosahedron has 20 triangular faces, 12 vertices, and 30 edges (Fig. 38–6). Each icosahedron has a fivefold rotational axis of symmetry that passes through each vertex, a threefold rotational axis that passes through the center of each triangular face, and a twofold rotational axis that passes through the middle of each edge formed by the triangular faces. Thus, the icosahedron is characterized as having 5:3:2 rotational symmetry. An octahedron and a tetrahedron have 4:3:2 and 3:3:2 rotational symmetry, respectively. The icosahedral shell is the most efficient and stable geometric form that can be constructed from identical basic units. As demonstrated by the geodesic domes of Buckminster Fuller, the icosahedron can be constructed from two units, hexagons and pentagons. The hexagons form the flat triangular faces and the pentagons form the vertices of the icosahedron. Both have the same edge length and can be built from the same basic subunits. The icosahedral capsids are constructed similarly with capsomers which consist of associated structural units. The icosahedron has structural advantages not possessed by the other two regular polyhedra, the tetrahedron and the octahedron. The vertices of the octahedron are squares and those of the tetrahedron are triangles. The angles of the square and the triangle are much sharper than those of the pentagon and therefore cause more strain on the fit of the subunits when the capsomers are composed of identical structural units. The advantage of a vertex capsomer composed of a pentamer rather than a trimer or tetramer is maximized. Also, the bonds that exist between the capsomers on the edges of the icosahedron presumably are the same as those between the identical capsomers on the faces. These bonds must flex somewhat to allow the angle of the edge. The edge angle of the icosahedron is less than that of the octahedron or tetrahedron and therefore places less strain on these flexible bonds. Electron micrographs show that the capsomers located on the faces of the icosahedron are surrounded by and interact with six capsomers, whereas those on the vertices have five neighboring capsomers (Fig. 38–6). The face capsomers have been termed **hexons** and the vertex capsomers **pentons**. Figure 38–6 shows an electron micrograph and a model of an adenovirus. The capsomers are visible, showing the hexons and pentons.

Each polypeptide chain of the capsid, helical or icosahedral, is coded by the viral genome. The size and morphology of the capsid depend on the primary amino acid sequence of these polypeptide chains which constitute the cap-

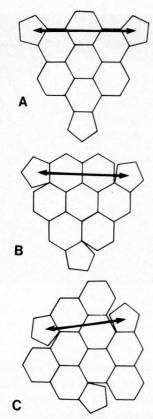

Figure 38–7. Examples of the arrangement of capsomeres to form the triangular faces of an icosahedron. *A*, Capsomeres arranged so that X = 3 and N = 3. *B*, Capsomeres arranged so that X = 1 and N = 4. *C*, Capsomeres arranged in a "skew" so that X = 7 and N = 1.

somers or structural units, and are characteristic for each virus. The number of capsomers that constitute the icosahedron can be varied, but must be 12, 32, 42, 92, 162, 252, and so

forth. Again, this is characteristic for each virus. The formula of Horne and Wildy[16] states that the number of capsomers is $10x (n - 1)^2 + 2$, where x is a constant and n is the number of capsomers whose centers lie on a straight line between two fivefold symmetry axes (vertices). This is diagrammed in Figure 38–7, and includes both vertex capsomers. The constant x is derived from geometric laws and is referred to as the **packing order.** For animal viruses, x may be 1, 3, or 7. Figure 38–7 shows how the capsomers may be arranged to form triangular faces. The dashed lines show the number of capsomers through which the line between the pentons located on the vertices will pass. The adenovirus illustrated in Figure 37–6 has 252 capsomers ($x = 1$, $n = 6$), of which 12 are pentons that constitute the vertices and 240 are hexons that form the triangular faces. The icosahedron formed when $x = 7$ is a unique type in which the triangular faces are "skewed." Such "skewed" icosahedrons are found infrequently in the viruses.

ENVELOPE

The viral envelope, acquired by budding through a cellular membrane, consists of a lipid bilayer membrane containing viral glycoproteins. The glycoproteins are coded by the virus, whereas the lipid is of cellular origin. Cellular glycoproteins are virtually excluded from the viral envelope. Budding may occur at any of the cell membranes and is characteristic of the virus. For example, the herpesviruses bud through the nuclear membrane and the rhabdoviruses bud through the cell membrane.

Classification of Animal Viruses

Viral classification has presented some unique problems to the taxonomist, since it has been difficult to establish evolutionary and phylogenetic relationships among viruses. Initially, viruses were classified and named on the basis of host specificity, and were separated into subgroups according to the type of disease produced. The names frequently were derived from the disease produced, from the tissue of isolation, from the mode of transmission, or from the geographic site of isolation. Hence, there are polioviruses, which cause poliomyelitis; adenoviruses, which were isolated from adenoid tissue; arboviruses, which require an arthropod vector; and Coxsackie viruses, which were isolated in Coxsackie, New York.

It is clear that the code of bacterial nomenclature is not strictly applicable to viral nomenclature. Similarly, the viruses cannot be classified on the basis of the nature of the disease or of the organ most frequently involved. The problem of classification has been referred to the Internal Committee on Taxonomy of Viruses of the International Association of Microbiological Societies. This committee has recommended family and genera names for most of the virus groups. A classification has been proposed and accepted that incorporates these recommendations[29] and is summarized in Tables 38–2, 38–3, and 38–4. The viruses have been subdivided into families and genera based on the following criteria: (1)

Table 38–2. **Classification of Viruses with a DNA Genome***

Capsid symmetry	Icosahedral	Icosahedral	Icosahedral	Icosahedral	Icosahedral	Complex
Presence or absence of envelope	Naked	Naked	Naked	Enveloped	Enveloped	Complex Envelope
Site of envelopment				Cytoplasm	Nucleus	Cytoplasm
Reaction to ether	Resistant	Resistant	Resistant	Sensitive	Sensitive	Resistant
Number of capsomers	32	72	252	1500	162	
Diameter of viron (nm.)	18–26	45–55	70–90	130	100–200	250–300
Genus names	Parvovirus; Adeno-associated virus group	Papillomavirus; Miopapovavirus	Mastadenovirus; Aviadenovirus	Iridovirus	Varicellavirus; Simplexvirus; Cytomegalovirus; Lymphocryptovirus	Orthopoxvirus; Leporipoxvirus; Parapoxvirus
Typical members	Kilham rat virus; Adeno-associated virus, type 1	Human wart virus; Simian virus 40, JC virus	Human adenovirus type 1; CELO virus	African swine fever virus	Varicella zoster virus; Herpes simplex virus; Cytomegalovirus; Epstein-Barr virus	Vaccinia virus; Myxoma virus; ORF virus
Family names	Parvoviridae	Papovaviridae	Adenoviridae	Iridoviridae	Herpesviridae	Poxviridae

*Adapted from Melnick, J. L., Prog. Med. Virol. **28**:208, 1982.

Table 38–3. **Classification of Viruses with an RNA Genome***

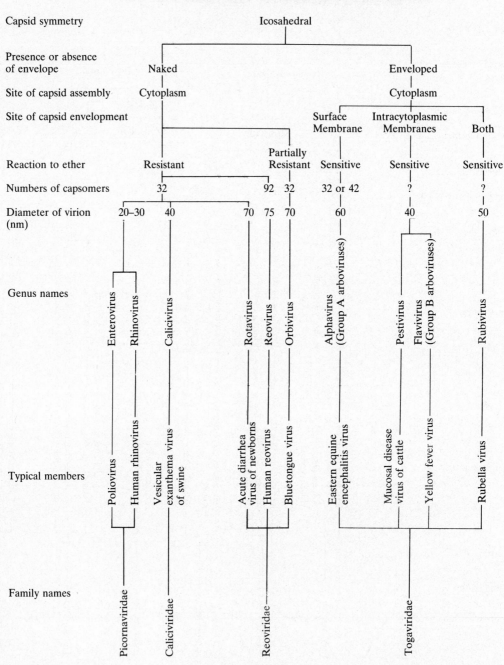

Capsid symmetry	Icosahedral							
Presence or absence of envelope	Naked			Enveloped				
Site of capsid assembly	Cytoplasm			Cytoplasm				
Site of capsid envelopment				Surface Membrane	Intracytoplasmic Membranes	Both		
Reaction to ether	Resistant		Partially Resistant	Sensitive	Sensitive	Sensitive		
Numbers of capsomers	32		92 32	32 or 42	?	?		
Diameter of virion (nm)	20–30 40	70	75 70	60	40	50		
Genus names	Enterovirus Rhinovirus	Calicivirus	Rotavirus Reovirus Orbivirus	Alphavirus (Group A arboviruses)	Pestivirus Flavivirus (Group B arboviruses)	Rubivirus		
Typical members	Poliovirus Human rhinovirus	Vesicular exanthema virus of swine	Acute diarrhea virus of newborns Human reovirus Bluetongue virus	Eastern equine encephalitis virus	Mucosal disease virus of cattle Yellow fever virus	Rubella virus		
Family names	Picornaviridae	Caliciviridae	Reoviridae		Togaviridae			

*Adapted from Melnick, J. L., Prog. Med. Virol. **28**:208, 1982.

Table 38–4. **Classification of Viruses with an RNA Genome***

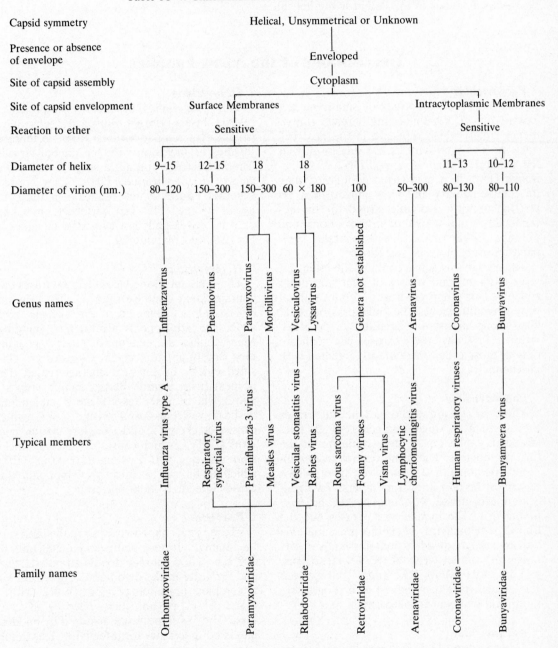

*Adapted from Melnick, J. L., Prog. Med. Virol. **28**:208, 1982.

type of nucleic acid in the virion, (2) capsid symmetry, (3) presence or absence of an envelope, (4) sites of capsid assembly and envelopment, (5) size and shape of the virion, and (6) number of capsomers for the icosahedral viruses or diameter of the helix for the helical viruses. These physical characteristics allow the viruses to be subdivided into 17 families. Viruses whose genome and symmetry have yet to be determined should likewise fit into this scheme.

Descriptions of the Virus Families

Parvoviridae

This family is composed of small, naked, icosahedral, DNA-containing viruses (*parvo* means small) which replicate in the host cell nucleus. The parvoviruses are unique in that the genome is single-stranded DNA. The genomic DNA in a parvovirus population may be complementary and may anneal after extraction to form a double strand, or the genomic DNA may consist of strands of only one polarity. Either of the strands contains sufficient information to be infectious.

The *Parvovirus* genus contains the latent rat virus (Kilham) and viruses of mice and other rodents. This group of viruses initiates normal productive infections. The "adeno-associated" virus group consists of "satellite" or defective viruses. Typically, these viruses can replicate only in those cells concomitantly infected with an adenovirus.

Papovaviridae

These viruses are naked icosahedral viruses that contain a single molecule of double-stranded, cyclic DNA; they replicate in the host cell nucleus. The name derives from *pap*-illoma, *po*lyoma, and *va*cuolating agent, which describes the best known members. Two genera are recognized, *Miopapovavirus* and *Papillomavirus*. The human wart viruses and the Shope papillomavirus of rabbits are papilloma viruses. *Miopapovavirus* contains mouse polyomavirus, simian virus 40 (SV40), BK virus, and JC virus. SV40, BK, and JC viruses are related and have been linked with progressive multifocal leukoencephalopathy in man.

Adenoviridae

These viruses are naked icosahedral viruses that contain linear double-stranded DNA. They replicate in the host cell nucleus. Two genera are recognized, *Aviadenovirus* (avian) and *Mastadenovirus* (human). Thirty-three serotypes of human adenoviruses have been isolated, all of which share a common antigen. The adenoviruses are associated with respiratory tract and eye infections.

Iridoviridae

This virus family has been exemplified by several insect viruses; however, subsequent isolation of similar viruses from vertebrates justifies its inclusion with the animal viruses. The iridoviruses contain a single linear molecule of double-stranded DNA. They are icosahedral viruses which replicate in the cytoplasm of the cell. The vertebrate members may be enveloped; however, the envelope is not acquired by budding.

Herpesviridae

These are enveloped icosahedral viruses that contain linear double-stranded DNA. The nucleocapsid is assembled in the nucleus, after which the envelope is acquired by budding. Many genera are recognized. There is no common family antigen, and the viruses are classified chiefly by physical characteristics. The herpesviruses include herpes simplex types 1 and 2, which cause "fever blisters" and genital herpes; varicella-zoster virus (VZ), which causes chickenpox and shingles; cytomegalovirus (CMV), which causes cytomegalic inclusion disease; and Epstein-Barr virus (EB), which is linked to Burkitt's lymphoma and causes infectious mononucleosis.

Poxviridae

These brick-shaped viruses are the largest of the animal viruses, being about 200 nm. by 300 nm. They contain double-stranded DNA and replicate in the cytoplasm. The virion has a complex morphology (Fig. 38–4), with a dense central portion surrounded by an envelope. The envelope is not acquired by budding and is not necessary for infectivity. This family contains the causative agents for smallpox, vaccinia, and molluscum contagiosum, and for many animal diseases, including myxoma and fibroma of rabbits. Some insect viruses are morphologically similar to the poxviruses.

Picornaviridae

These are naked icosahedral viruses that contain linear single-stranded RNA and replicate in the cytoplasm. The name is derived from *pico,* which means small, and RNA. The genome is (+)RNA. The *Enterovirus* genus contains the polioviruses, which cause poliomyelitis; the Coxsackie viruses, which cause many illnesses, including pericarditis and myocarditis; and the echoviruses, which cause febrile illness and the common cold. The *Rhinovirus* genus contains the rhinoviruses that are etiological agents for many common colds.

Reoviridae
These viruses have a double icosahedral capsid and a genome of 10 segments of double-stranded RNA (dsRNA). The reoviruses replicate in the cytoplasm. Three genera are recognized: *Reovirus* contains viruses that cause minor febrile illness, *Rotavirus* contains agents that cause gastroenteritis, and *Orbivirus* contains the viruses that cause such diseases as bluetongue and Colorado tick fever.

Togaviridae
The togaviruses contain linear single-stranded (+)RNA and replicate in the cytoplasm. The icosahedral nucleocapsid is assembled in the cytoplasm, after which an envelope is acquired by budding through the cell membrane. The viruses formerly classified as arboviruses (*arthropod bor*ne) are in this family. Four genera are recognized: *Alphavirus* contains Western, Eastern, and equine encephalitis viruses, Simliki Forest virus, Sindbis virus, and others; *Flavivirus* contains St. Louis and Japanese encephalitis viruses, yellow fever virus, and others; *Rubivirus* contains rubella virus; and *Pestivirus* contains hog cholera virus.

Orthomyxoviridae
The orthomyxoviruses (*myxo* means mucus) consist of a single genus, *Influenzavirus.* The genome is linear single-stranded (−)RNA that exists as eight segments, and the virion contains an RNA transcriptase which catalyzes synthesis of RNA from an RNA template. The helical nucleocapsid is assembled in the cytoplasm and the envelope is acquired by budding through the cell membrane. The replicative cycle involves both the nucleus and the cytoplasm. The influenza viruses are pleomorphic and as such are difficult to size. Types A, B, and C have been separated on the basis of immunological reactivity.

Paramyxoviridae
The virion is an enveloped helical nucleocapsid and the genome is linear single-stranded (−)RNA. The host cell cytoplasm and nucleus may be involved in replication and nucleocapsid assembly, and the envelope is acquired by budding through the cell membrane. An RNA transcriptase is associated with the virion. The *Pneumovirus* genus contains respiratory syncytial virus; the *Paramyxovirus* genus contains Newcastle disease, mumps, and parainfluenza viruses; and the *Morbillivirus* genus contains measles virus.

Rhabdoviridae
These "bullet-shaped" viruses contain linear single-stranded (−)RNA, and the virion contains an RNA transcriptase. The nucleocapsid matures in the cytoplasm and buds through the cell membrane. Two genera are recognized. The *Vesiculovirus* genus contains vesicular stomatitis virus, and the *Lyssavirus* genus contains rabies virus.

Retroviridae
This family contains the RNA tumor viruses (former genus *Leukovirus*). The virion contains linear single-stranded (+)RNA. The genome is enclosed in a helical nucleocapsid, which in turn is enclosed in an icosahedral capsid. This structure is then enveloped by budding through the cell membrane. The virion contains an RNA-dependent DNA polymerase (reverse transcriptase). There are three subfamilies: the *Oncovirinae* contains the RNA tumor virus group, the *Spumavirinae* contains the foamy agents, and the *Lentivirinae* contains visna viruses and other related viruses.

Arenaviridae
These are pleomorphic enveloped viruses containing a (−)RNA genome. The symmetry of the nucleocapsid is unknown. The nucleocapsid is assembled in the cytoplasm, and the envelope is acquired by budding through the cell membrane. In thin sections, characteristic electron-dense granules are apparent in the nucleocapsid, hence the name (*arena* means sand). The envelope contains closely spaced spike proteins. Members of the arenaviruses are lymphocytic choriomeningitis virus (LCM), Lassa fever virus, and the "Tacaribe" complex. These viruses cause chronic infections in rodents; however, Lassa fever virus also causes a severe disease in man.

Coronaviridae
These viruses contain single-stranded (+)RNA. The helical nucleocapsid is assembled in the cytoplasm and acquires an envelope

by budding into cytoplasmic vacuoles. The envelope spike proteins have a characteristic, club-shaped morphology. This family contains a single genus, *Coronavirus*, which contains human respiratory coronaviruses, mouse hepatitis virus, avian infectious bronchitis virus, and others. There are 21 serotypes of human coronaviruses which are the etiological agent for some common colds.

Bunyaviridae

These viruses contain segmented single-stranded (−)RNA genomes. The genome exists in three segments. The helical nucleocapsid is coiled and is assembled in the cytoplasm, after which the virion matures by budding from the Golgi and the endoplasmic reticulum membranes. The bunyaviruses include over 90 serological types. Members of this group are LaCrosse virus, unileukemia virus, California encephalitis virus, Lumbo virus, and many others.

Unclassified Viruses

Hepatitis Viruses. Experiments involving human volunteers established that serum hepatitis and infectious hepatitis were of viral etiology. Only recently have the agents been described. Type A, or infectious hepatitis, is caused by a small, nonenveloped virus that contains an RNA genome. The virus particle is 27 nm. in diameter and appears to be icosahedral. This virus most likely will be classified as a picornavirus, since it closely resembles the enteroviruses. It probably will be classified as enterovirus 72. Type B, or serum hepatitis, is also caused by a virus. The agent in question, termed the **Dane particle,** is 42 nm. and con-

tains an electron-dense core of 27 nm., surrounded by a surface coat (not an envelope) that is 7 nm. thick. The characteristic **"Australia antigen,"** or hepatitis B surface antigen (HBsAg), is associated with the coat. The core contains circular double-stranded DNA. The hepatitis B virus and related animal viruses apparently represent a distinct virus family.

Subacute Spongiform Virus Encephalopathies. Kuru and Creutzfeldt-Jakob disease in man is caused by a virus that is similar to the etiological agents of scrapie and transmissible encephalopathy of mink. These diseases have been classified in a group of virus-induced slow infections called subacute spongiform virus encephalopathies. This has led to the recognition of a new group of viruses which possess unconventional physical and chemical properties and biological behavior.[13] These agents are not recognizable as viruses by electron microscopy. They appear as vesicular membranes without a core or capsid. In fact, they have been postulated to be self-replicating membrane fragments. They are sensitive to most membrane disrupting agents, but are resistant to formaldehyde, β-propiolactone, nucleases, heat, and ultraviolet radiation. Nonhost proteins have not been demonstrated in partially purified preparations. As such, they do not fit into any family of viruses and may represent a new class of microorganisms.

The Marburg Agent. This virus was isolated from an outbreak among laboratory personnel who had handled imported monkeys. The virion contains RNA and morphologically resembles the rhabdoviruses in that one end is rounded. However, the virus is highly pleomorphic, with long cylindrical forms predominant.

Propagation of Viruses

Viruses are obligate intracellular parasites. Therefore, any substrate used for virus propagation must consist of living cells. The commonly used systems are (1) cell cultures, (2) embryonated eggs, and (3) laboratory animals.

Cell Culture

The demonstration that cells could be grown or maintained *in vitro* opened the door to modern virology. As soon as cell cultures were established, virologists had reasonably homogenous host cell systems in which to propagate viruses. Such cultures were not susceptible to the host factors of stress, hormone activities,

and natural defense mechanisms. The cell culture technology also provides systems for the quantitative analysis of viruses, similar to those used with the bacteriophages.

Primary cell cultures are obtained directly from tissues. A tissue fragment is dispersed into constituent cells with proteolytic enzymes, such as trypsin and collagenase, after which the cells are suspended in an isosmotic medium containing amino acids, vitamins, and serum. The cell suspension is placed in a container, such as a bottle, Petri plate, or tube, and the cells are allowed to settle and attach to the container surface. Once attached, the cells undergo mitosis until a confluent monolayer of cells covers the vessel surface. At this time, cell division ceases due to contact inhibition, and the monolayer can be maintained for relatively long periods (30 to 60 days).

Cells grown *in vitro* usually exhibit **epithelioid** or **fibroblastic morphology.** The epithelioid cells are flat and stellate, whereas the fibroblastic cells are long and narrow, with tapering ends (Fig. 38–8). The fibroblastic cells tend to be aligned in parallel arrays in the cell monolayer.

Primary cultures can be subcultured a limited number of times to produce secondary cultures. This is accomplished by removing the cells from the vessel surface with trypsin or a chelating agent, after which the cell suspension is dispensed into new containers. Primary and secondary cultures contain the same number of chromosomes as the parent cells and are termed diploid. These cultures have a finite lifetime and usually cease growth after two or three serial subcultures. Some secondary cultures, however, retain the ability to undergo division over many serial subcultures. These cultures have then produced a **cell strain,** which retains the growth characteristics and morphology of the secondary culture. These cells also are diploid. Although cell strains can be subcultured many more times than the secondary cultures, they also have a limited *in vitro* growth capability. After characteristic numbers of serial subcultures, the cells undergo senescence and the cell strain is lost. Cell strains of human origin usually undergo about 50 subcultures, after which the cells die.

In some instances, continued subculture of a cell strain may be selective for an altered cell that is capable of infinite growth *in vitro*. These cells grow faster than the cell strains, show deviation from the diploid number of chromosomes, and are termed **cell lines.** Such cell lines are aneuploid and usually contain chromosomal abnormalities. After continued subculture, the cell lines assume the characteristics of transformed cells. These cell lines usually then are neoplastic; they have lost the property of contact inhibition and tend to orient in a random pattern in culture.

Primary and secondary cells must be subcultured at high cell densities in order to initiate a new culture. Similarly, cell strains also must

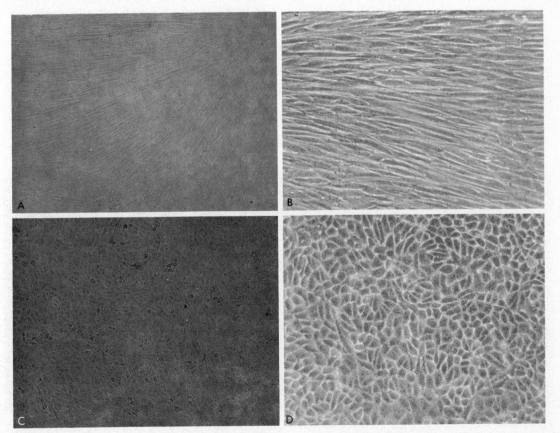

Figure 38–8. Monolayers of fibroblastic and epithelioid cells. *A*, Unstained fibroblastic cells. *B*, Phase microscopy of unstained fibroblastic cells. *C*, Unstained epithelioid cells. *D*, Phase microscopy of unstained epithelioid cells.

be subcultured at relatively high cell densities. However, cell lines can be transferred at low cell density, so a **clone** of cells can be obtained that originated from a single cell in the cell line. Cells from cell strains also can be cloned; however, the percentage of cells that yield clones is very low. In established cell lines, the cloning percentage may approach 100 per cent. Such cloning techniques are useful for isolating genetically pure cell cultures.

Cultured cells can be stored for many years frozen in liquid nitrogen ($-196°C$). Dimethylsulfoxide or glycerol may be added to prevent damage to the cell membrane. Since cells undergo mutation and selection while in culture, freezing provides a method of preserving a particular cell type or strain.

Embryonated Eggs

Embryonated eggs provided a suitable cell system for virus propagation before the advent of cell culture techniques. Viruses can be propagated in the amnionic, allantoic, chorionic, or yolk sac membranes. Usually embryos of 5 to 14 days are used, since the embryo of this age is easily visible but has not developed adult characteristics. The use of embryonated eggs has largely been discarded in favor of cell culture except for some viruses, such as the influenzaviruses, which grow best in the embryonated egg.

Laboratory Animals

Since cell cultures are easier to handle and provide a more controlled substrate, the use of laboratory animals has almost ceased. However, some studies require intact animals. For example, some Coxsackie viruses and togaviruses require animal inoculation for isolation, and most of the "slow" viruses can be studied only in a suitable animal model.

Visualization of Viral Replication in Cell Cultures

The visual effect of virus growth in a cell culture ranges from no detectable change to complete destruction of the cells. The cellular pathology caused by virus replication is termed **cytopathic effect (CPE).** The CPE is characteristic for a particular virus–host cell system, and often is an important diagnostic aid. Virus-induced CPE can be grouped into the following categories: (1) Syncytia formation (Fig. 38–9B)—a **syncytium** consists of a giant multinucleated cell that is a result of fusion of contiguous cells in the monolayer. This type of CPE is characteristic of the paramyxoviruses. (2) Cell necrosis and lysis (Fig. 38–9C)—the infected cells become pyknotic and granular. They lose their flat, stellate shape, become rounded, detach from the vessel surface, and float free in the medium. This type of CPE is characteristic of the enteroviruses. (3) Cellular clumping (Fig. 38–10)—the cells do not fuse, but remain clumped together in clusters. (4) Cellular inclusion body forma-

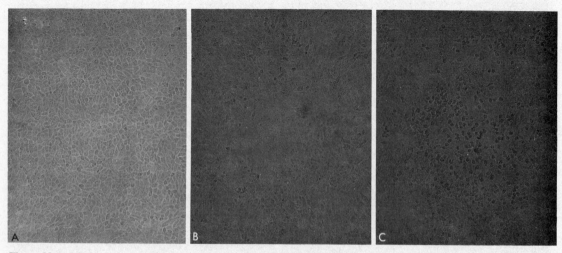

Figure 38–9. Viral cytopathic effect in epithelioid cell cultures. A, Uninfected Vero cell cultures. B, Vero cell culture infected with measles virus showing a syncytium. C, Vero cell culture infected with poliovirus type 3, showing typical enterovirus cytopathic effect. (Unstained preparations.)

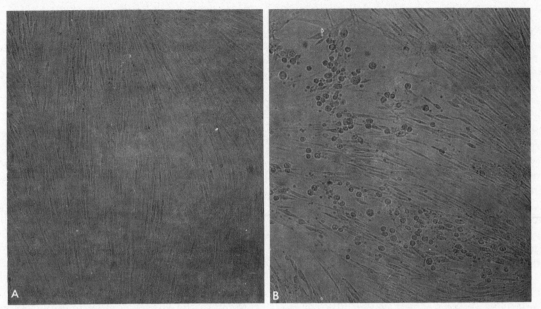

Figure 38–10. Viral cytopathic effect in fibroblastic cells. *A*, Uninfected Flow-7000 cell culture. *B*, Flow-7000 cell culture infected with herpes simplex type 2. (Unstained preparations.)

tion—in some virus–host cell systems, the viral replication becomes compartmentalized. These compartments show specific staining characteristics and are termed **inclusion bodies.** They may be the site of viral replication, or they may represent aggregates of viral particles or subparticles. Frequently, they are of diagnostic importance. For example, if cell scrapings taken from a skin pustule resembling those of chickenpox or smallpox show intranuclear inclusion bodies, the diagnosis of chickenpox can be made. Smallpox also exhibits characteristic inclusion bodies, but they are intracytoplasmic rather than intranuclear.

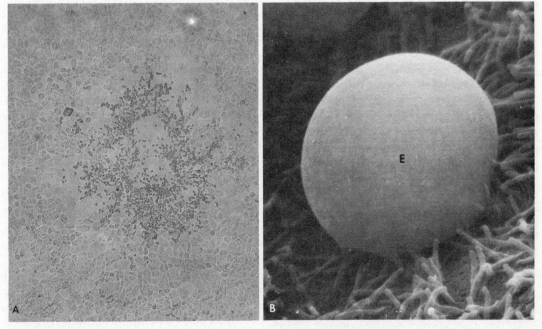

Figure 38–11. Hemadsorption of erythrocytes to Vero cells infected with measles virus. *A*, Unstained preparation showing adsorption of the erythrocytes to the cells around the periphery of the syncytium. *B*, Scanning electron micrograph showing an erythrocyte *(E)* adsorbed to the villi projecting from the infected cell. *(B*, courtesy of B. Rentier.)

In some virus–host cell systems, the virus replication causes new antigens to be expressed on the cell surface. This is typical of the enveloped viruses. Some of these antigens have an affinity for receptors on erythrocytes and the infected cells then acquire the ability to adsorb erythrocytes onto their cell membranes. This is termed **hemadsorption** (Fig. 38–11) and is characteristic of cells infected with orthomyxoviruses, paramyxoviruses, and togaviruses. Specific antiserum against the virus can be used to block the hemadsorption and thus identify the virus.

Visualization of viral antigens also can be accomplished with immunofluorescent staining techniques, in which specific antiviral antibody coupled with a fluorescent dye is used to locate the antigens (Fig. 38–12).

The replication of one virus in a cell may inhibit the replication of a second virus in that same cell. A virus which causes little or no CPE may be detected by interference with a second virus which produces a characteristic CPE in that cell. For example, African green monkey kidney cells infected with rubella virus do not exhibit CPE or hemadsorption; however, they are resistant to infection with echovirus, which normally produces characteristic enterovirus CPE. The rubella virus–infected cells can be identified by their failure to propagate echovirus.

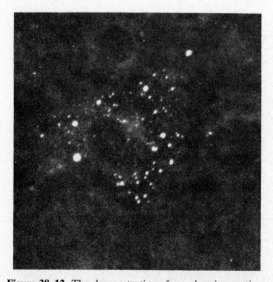

Figure 38–12. The demonstration of measles virus antigen in a Vero cell culture by fluorescent antibody staining. The fluorescein-labeled antibody has reacted with the viral antigen and will fluoresce yellow green. The fluorescence is shown here as white. Discrete areas of antigen localization are evident. (Courtesy of M. Ferguson.)

ASSAY OF VIRUSES

Virus particles in a suspension can be quantitated by chemical and physical means, but virions must be quantitated by infectivity assay.

Particle Counts

The number of virus particles of a characteristic morphology can be enumerated by use of the electron microscope. The most common method is to mix the virus suspension with a known number of latex spheres. The two types of particles then can be counted and the number of virus particles in the suspension can be calculated from the ratio of latex spheres to virus particles. This technique enumerates both infectious and noninfectious particles.

Hemagglutination

Many of the viruses contain multiple copies of viral proteins in the capsid or envelope that can bind to receptors on erythrocytes from specific species, *i.e.,* hemagglutinins. Such viruses can be quantitated by the agglutination of these erythrocytes. Typically, the erythrocytes are added to serial dilutions of a virus suspension, after which the erythrocyte-virus complex is allowed to form and settle. The complex will settle, forming a diffuse, salmon-colored pattern in the bottom of a tube or well, whereas free erythrocytes settle to form a dark compact button. The erythrocyte species that can be agglutinated vary with the virus and the conditions used; however, the mechanism is the same. The virus particle is multivalent and it attaches to two erythrocytes by the binding of the viral hemagglutinin molecules to membrane receptors. If enough virus is present, the erythrocytes are bound into lattice-like aggregates. These aggregates then settle to the bottom of the tube, where they remain in a complex. Nonaggregated erythrocytes also settle to the bottom; however, they slide to the center of the tube bottom to form a pellet. The **hemagglutinating titer (HA)** is the reciprocal of the last dilution showing complete hemagglutination. The HA test also can be used to identify a particular virus. After the HA has been quantitated, the virus in question is allowed to react with a monospecific antiserum. If the antiserum reacts with the virus, subsequent HA activity will be inhibited. This is termed the **hemagglutination-inhibition test (HI),** and it is routinely used in research and diagnostic laboratories.

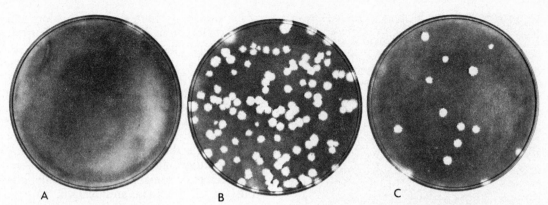

Figure 38–13. Plaque assay of simian hemorrhagic fever virus, a togavirus. *A*, Uninoculated. *B*, Inoculated with a 10^{-4} dilution of virus. *C*, Inoculated with a 10^{-5} dilution of virus. The plaques are the clear areas in the cell monolayer where the cells have been destroyed.

Some viruses, particularly the myxoviruses and paramyxoviruses, contain a neuraminidase as a structural protein. Since the cell membrane receptors typically are mucoproteins with *N*-acetylneuraminic acid (NANA) residues, this enzyme can hydrolyze a NANA residue from the receptor and thus free the virus from the erythrocyte. This enzymatic activity can be minimized by conducting the HA assay at 0° to 4°C.

Plaque Assays

This technique makes the effect of replication of a single virus particle visible, and it yields precise quantitation of viral infectivity. In this method, serial dilutions of a virus suspension are inoculated onto confluent monolayers of susceptible cells. After adsorption of the virus the monolayer is covered with medium containing a gelling agent such as agar or methylcellulose. The gelled medium restricts the spread of released progeny particles such that only neighboring cells are infected and each infectious particle produces a focus of infection called a **plaque**. Visualization of the plaque caused by cytocidal viruses can be accomplished by staining the noninfected cells so that the plaques appear as clear areas against a dark background. To obtain the titer, the plaques on the assay plates are counted and the number is adjusted by the dilution factor. The resultant virus titer usually is expressed as **plaque-forming units (PFU)** per volume. Since each plaque is initiated by one infectious particle, the plaque titer is the infectivity titer. A typical plaque assay is shown in Figure 38–13. Many viruses do not produce a cytocidal effect in cell cultures. Noncytocidal virus plaques may be visualized by employing

techniques such as hemadsorption, immunofluorescence, or interference. Some viruses, such as the poxviruses, can be plaque-assayed in the absence of a gelled medium. These viruses spread from cell to cell and release only small amounts of progeny virus into the medium.

Oncogenic viruses can be assayed by measurement of their ability to cause cell transformation. Normal cells possess the property of contact inhibition such that the cells grow as a monolayer. Cells transformed by the oncogenic viruses are not contact-inhibited and grow as multilayered masses (Fig. 38–14). Thus, the transforming activity of these viruses can be assayed by measuring the number of foci of transformed cells. This is expressed as **focus-forming units (FFU)** per unit volume.

Pock Assays

Poxviruses can be assayed by inoculation of the virus onto the chorioallantoic membrane of a 10 to 12 day chick embryo. The replication of the virus produces characteristic localized lesions **(pocks)**, which are gray-white against the transparent chorioallantoic membrane. Each pock arises from infection by a single infectious particle, and is analogous to a plaque. This method has largely been replaced by the plaque assay.

Quantal (Endpoint) Assays

The infectivity of some viruses cannot be measured by the plaque assay, and a quantal assay system must be used. Since quantal assays do not enumerate the infectious particles but only measure the presence of infectivity, this assay is not as precise as the plaque assay. In this method, serial dilutions of the virus

Figure 38–14. Normal rat kidney cell monolayer infected with Rous sarcoma virus. The transformed cells are growing in a multilayered focus or colony.

suspension are inoculated into susceptible test systems. The test system may be cell cultures, embryonated eggs, or animals. After a suitable incubation period, the test systems are observed for evidence of viral infection. The highest dilution that causes an effect must contain at least one infectious unit. The virus titer usually is expressed as the 50 per cent infectious dose (ID_{50}) and is the reciprocal of the dilution necessary to infect 50 per cent of the test systems. The accuracy of this method depends on the total number of test systems inoculated with each dilution. Since it may not be appropriate to use large numbers of test systems (such as animals), a method was devised by Reed and Meunch[33] for estimating 50 per cent endpoints with relatively few test units. This method uses all of the units employed in the titration and thereby increases the validity of the calculated endpoint.

COMPARISON OF THE DIFFERENT ASSAY METHODS

When a virus suspension is assayed by different methods, the titer will vary acording to the method. Each assay measures a specific property, hence, the sensitivity may vary greatly. The assays of infectivity are the most sensitive, and generally these assays yield approximately the same result. However, the statistical precision depends on the number of test units employed. For example, if the PFU titer is calculated by counting 50 plaques at a given dilution, the quantal assay must employ 50 test units per dilution to achieve equal precision.

The infectivity titer very rarely approaches the particle count. For example, a virus suspension may have a particle count of 10^{10} particles/ml., and have an infectivity titer of 10^8 PFU/ml. The ratio of the infectivity titer to the total number of virus particles is the efficiency of infection for that virus. This varies widely depending on the virus and the host system. In most cases, it is far less than one, which means that most of the viral particles do not initiate infection. These particles may be defective or some may be potentially infectious yet fail to initiate an infection.

QUANTITATIVE ASPECTS OF INFECTION

When a virus suspension is added to a cell culture, the random attachment of the virions to the cells will result in individual cells being infected with different numbers of virions. The percentage of the cells which receive 1, 2, and so forth virions can be determined and is a function of the multiplicity of infection (m), which is the input average number of virions per cell. The proportion (%) of cells infected by k virions is defined by the Poisson distribution:

$$P(K) = \frac{e^{-m}m^k}{k!} \tag{1}$$

To calculate the percentage of cells receiving *0* particles ($k = 0$), this equation becomes:

$$P(0) = e^{-m} \tag{2}$$

The m required to infect a given proportion of the cells also can be calculated. For example, calculate the m required to infect 95 per cent of the cells in a culture. This would result in 5 per cent of the cells being uninfected.

$$
\begin{aligned}
P(0) &= 5\% = 0.05 \\
\text{From equation (2):} \quad m &= ln\ P(0) \\
m &= ln\ (0.5) = 3
\end{aligned}
$$

These equations assume that all cells in a population are equivalent and can be infected with the same efficiency. Although the cells in any population do differ, the predicted values are usually close to the observed values. In some cases, a variable may significantly affect the efficiency of infection, and the predicted values then would be grossly inaccurate. For instance, cell age or cell cycle phase may alter the ability of the cell to adsorb virus.

If the plaque assay for infectivity is to be accurate, each plaque must originate from a cell infected with one virion. From the Poisson distribution, it is evident that when m is very small, the percentage of cells receiving multiple virions is negligible. In the plaque assay, m is on the order of 10^{-4} to 10^{-6}; thus, the number of plaques equals the number of infectious particles.

Biochemistry of Virus Replication

REPLICATIVE CYCLE

When an infectious virus particle encounters a susceptible cell, a series of molecular events is initiated which culminates in the release of progeny virus. The molecular biology of the viral replicative cycle has been investigated by biochemical techniques using **one-step** (single-cycle) growth conditions. In such experiments, the inoculum virus is added to susceptible cells and allowed to adsorb, after which unadsorbed virus is removed or neutralized with specific antiserum. Thus, the replicative events occur simultaneously in the majority of the cell population and can be detected more easily.

Since a virus is a piece of genetic material surrounded by a protective coat, propagation depends on entry into a susceptible cell, uncoating of the nucleic acid, and expression of the genetic information. The nucleic acid must be replicated and must direct synthesis of viral proteins, after which the virus can be assembled and ultimately released from the cell. The replicative cycle can be divided into four merging steps: (1) adsorption, (2) penetration and uncoating, (3) eclipse (biosynthesis), and (4) maturation and release. The specific biochem-ical processes that occur in each phase depend on the characteristics of the virus and the host cell. A schematic representation of viral growth curves is shown in Figure 38–15, and the steps during replication are indicated. Although the curves differ in shape for viruses that are released by cell lysis and for those that are extruded from the cell, the relative sequence of events is the same. This figure also demonstrates the necessity of using one-step experimental conditions in order to delineate the steps of the replicative cycle.

ADSORPTION (ATTACHMENT)

Adsorption of a virus to a cell depends on interactions between attachment proteins on the virus and receptor sites on the cell. Attachment involves electrostatic bonds between the viral proteins and the receptors, and it is temperature-independent. The adsorbed virus often can be recovered in infectious form by interfering with the virus-receptor complex. For example, poliovirus can be eluted from the cells by treatment with high salt or low pH, whereas influenza viruses, which attach to

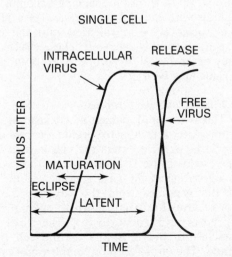

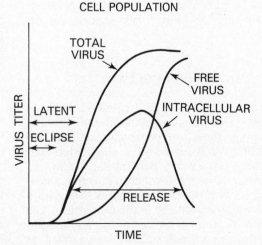

Figure 38–15. Schematic representation of virus replication in a single cell and in a cell population. Infection was initiated at zero time, and the viral infectivity was monitored at intervals and expressed as the virus titer.

a mucoprotein receptor in the cell membrane, can be recovered by treatment with neuraminidase. After neuraminidase treatment, the cells undergo a transient period when they are no longer able to adsorb influenza virus.

Attachment to a cell receptor appears to be required for infection for all viruses except poxviruses, which attach to a variety of cells and to any appropriately charged surface. Indeed, there may not be a cellular receptor for this virus. In contrast, poliovirus receptors have been isolated from susceptible cells and are glycoprotein complexes. These receptors were not found on cells which were not susceptible to poliovirus infection. Additional evidence supporting the necessity of virus-receptor interaction comes from studies with infectious nucleic acids. All primate cells contain receptors for poliovirus, whereas nonprimate cells do not contain these receptors and do not propagate poliovirus. However, if the poliovirus capsid is disrupted and the genomic RNA is isolated, the RNA can enter primate and nonprimate cells. Such RNA is capable of bypassing the need for receptors and infecting nonprimate cells, which then produce infectious poliovirus. This demonstrates that the capacity to adsorb virus governs the susceptibility of most cells to a given virus.

The presence or absence of virus receptors on a given cell type depends on the species, the tissue of origin, and the physiological state of the cells. For example, primary cells from human brain, spinal cord, and intestine adsorb poliovirus but primary cells from kidney, lung, and muscle do not. However, the vaccine strains of poliovirus are prepared in human kidney cells. Apparently, this receptor is not expressed in the kidney tissue in the host, but culture *in vitro* changes the normal organismal controls and the kidney cells express this receptor.

PENETRATION AND UNCOATING

These steps are often treated as separate entities. However, penetration may initiate uncoating. Therefore, penetration and uncoating will be considered as a single step that embraces two events. Penetration of the animal viruses does not involve an injection mechanism as with the bacteriophages. The virion or the nucleocapsid enters the cell, after which the capsid proteins are removed. The mechanisms of penetration can be summarized as follows:

Direct Passage

Nonenveloped viruses may penetrate the cell by direct passage through the cell membrane. After attachment to the cell membrane via the receptors, the virus passes directly through the membrane without forming a phagocytic vacuole. Once in the cytoplasm, the capsid is removed by cellular proteolytic enzymes and the genome is liberated. Electron micrographs have documented direct penetration of the cell membrane by adenoviruses and picornaviruses.

Penetration and uncoating may begin at the point of attachment to the cell receptors. After attachment, the virus may undergo a conformational change that is the initiation of uncoating. This has been demonstrated with the picornaviruses. After adsorption, the genome of the externally situated virions becomes sensitive to RNase, which indicates that the capsid has lost its structural integrity. Such virus also exhibits a change in antigenicity. The interaction between the virus and the receptor apparently induces a rearrangement of the viral capsomers. The virus then enters the cell by phagocytosis or by passing directly through the cell membrane, after which the genome is liberated into the cell cytoplasm.

Fusion

Some enveloped viruses enter the cell by fusion of the viral envelope with the cell membrane. Such membrane fusion is pH-dependent and occurs optimally when the environmental pH is less than 6. This has been demonstrated with paramyxoviruses and herpesviruses. Electron microscopy of these viruses has shown that the viral envelope and the cell membrane fuse so that the virion envelope becomes contiguous with the cell membrane. As a result, the nucleocapsid is released into the cytoplasm, where it is uncoated. These viruses also may enter the cell by viropexis, so both mechanisms may be used.

Endocytosis or Viropexis

This is the predominant mechanism of virus entry. After attaching to specific receptor sites, the virus particle enters the cell in a vacuole or vesicle. Little is known about the process of uncoating of the viral genomes or the exit of the genomes from the vesicles. Semliki Forest virus has been shown to enter the cell by adsorptive endocytosis.[14] The virus first attaches to the receptors on the cell membrane. The virus-receptor complex moves into a "coated pit" which pinches off to form a coated vesicle. The coated vesicles then lose their clathrin coat and fuse with endosomes and lysosomes. After fusion with the lysosomes, the pH of the vesicle becomes acid which triggers the fusion of the viral envelope with the vesicle membrane, thereby releasing the nucleocapsid into the cytoplasm. The genome then is released from the capsid proteins by host cell proteolytic enzymes. It is not certain whether other viruses utilize similar mechanisms for release from the phagocytic vesicle into the cytoplasm.

The uncoating of the poxviruses involves a different and unique mechanism. The poxviruses enter the cell by viropexis and the outer membrane is subsequently removed from the particle. The virus cores then are released from the phagocytic vesicle into the cell cytoplasm. Virus-specific messenger RNA is transcribed from the viral DNA by a virion RNA polymerase. This messenger RNA is translated to produce the enzyme(s) that are necessary to liberate the viral DNA from the core.

ECLIPSE (BIOSYNTHESIS)

Once the process of uncoating has begun, the infectious virus cannot be recovered from the infected cell. It is said to be in eclipse. Later, after progeny has been assembled, infectivity can be recovered. Thus, the time from the initial loss of infectivity until the appearance of progeny is the **eclipse phase** (see Fig. 38–15). It is now known that biosynthesis of the viral components occurs during the eclipse phase. Once the components have assembled to produce mature virions, viral infectivity can be detected and the eclipse phase is over. The **latent phase** is the time span after the initial loss of infectivity until progeny can be recovered in a cell-free form. The latent phase contains the eclipse phase plus the time required for the release of the virus particles from the cell (Fig. 38–15). For a virion to replicate, the genome must be reproduced in multiple copies, specific enzymes must be synthesized, and quantities of the capsid proteins must be synthesized. The most important biosynthetic events are genome replication, messenger RNA (mRNA) transcription, and translation and maturation of viral proteins. The mechanisms involved in these processes may be the same as those of the eukaryotic host cells. Some viruses, however, employ molecular mechanisms that apparently are unique. It is important to understand the molecular

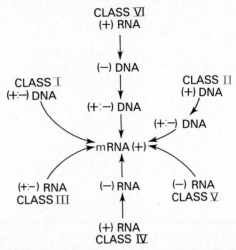

Figure 38–16. Classification of viruses on the basis of the method of the genome replication and messenger RNA transcription. $(+:-)$ RNA or $(+:-)$ DNA refers to double-stranded RNA or DNA. (From Baltimore, D., Bacteriol. Rev., **35**:236, 1971. Redrawn with permission from the author and publisher.)

biology of viral replication so that these unique events can be identified, since it is here that the action of chemotherapeutic agents must be focused, in order to attack selectively the viral mechanisms. The viruses can be divided into six general classes based on the nucleic acid type and the method of mRNA synthesis.[2] Messenger RNA is defined as the RNA that binds to ribosomes and codes for protein synthesis. This mRNA is termed positive RNA, $(+)$RNA. Negative strand RNA, $(-)$RNA, is anti-message in polarity and does not code for protein synthesis. The distinctive biochemical features of gene transcription and gene product synthesis and maturation will be discussed for each group. Figure 38–16 shows the routes of synthesis of mRNA for each virus class.

Class I
These viruses contain double-stranded DNA (dsDNA), either linear or circular, as the genome. The papovaviruses contain nonpermuted covalently closed circular dsDNA and the adenoviruses, herpesviruses, and poxviruses contain nonpermuted linear dsDNA. Representative examples of replication for each group will be discussed. A diagram of Class I virus replication is shown in Figure 38–17.

The genomes of many of the smaller DNA viruses and some RNA viruses have been completely sequenced. This was made possible by the discovery and description of action of **restriction endonucleases,** enzymes which

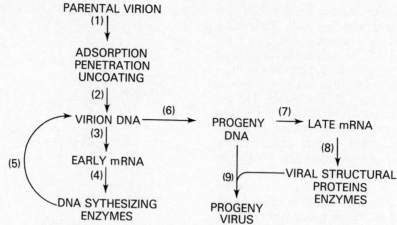

Figure 38–17. Diagram of the replication cycle for viruses containing double-stranded DNA as a genome. These viruses are in Class I. The events are numbered in approximate chronological sequence.

cleave single-stranded or double-stranded DNA at specific sites. This results in specific smaller fragments of DNA which can be sequenced or hybridized with specific mRNA's to locate and map gene products.

Papovaviruses.[10] These viruses contain circular dsDNA of 3 to 3.6 × 10⁶ molecular weight. In the virion and within the nucleus of the infected cell, the viral DNA is condensed with cellular histones into a minichromosome.

If the histones are removed by deproteinization techniques, the majority of the DNA recovered is in a covalently closed, supercoiled state (DNA 1). The supercoiling is a result of a deficiency of turns of one DNA molecule about the other that arises when the daughter DNA molecule is ligated at the termination of synthesis. Thus, the molecule folds back on itself (supercoils) with about 25 negative turns to relieve these topological constraints. Cleav-

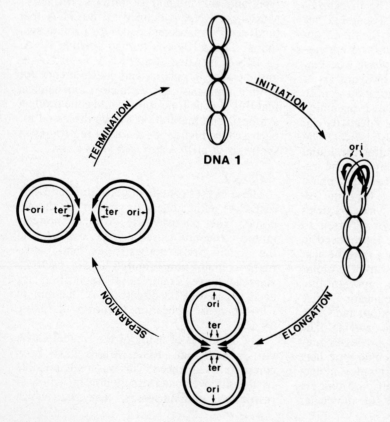

Figure 38–18. Model for papovavirus DNA replication. The replicative intermediate (RI) is the supercoiled monomeric DNA 1 with two growing daughter strands. Replication begins at the origin *(ori)* and proceeds bidirectionally to the termination *(ter)* region. (Adapted from Trapper, D. P., *et al.*, J. Virol., **41**:877, 1982)

age of a single phosphodiester bond in one of the strands relaxes the molecule to a nonsupercoiled circle (DNA 2).

DNA replication occurs on DNA 1 as a template (Fig. 38–18).[8, 11] Replication initiates at a unique site on the circular DNA, the origin of replication (ori) which apparently contains a large palindrome. It requires synthesis of the A gene product, T antigen, and begins with binding of cellular DNA polymerase to the genome. Replication proceeds bidirectionally on both DNA strands in a continuous and discontinuous manner. Discontinuous replication proceeds via synthesis of 80 to 120 nucleotide segments followed by ligation.[30] Each round of replication requires about 15 minutes and ends when the two replicating forks reach a termination point 180° from the origin. At this point the complex consists of one covalently closed parental strand and one newly synthesized daughter strand with a gap of 20 to 75 nucleotides at the termination point. After filling the gap, the strands are ligated to produce the covalently closed, double-stranded genome which rapidly becomes complexed with histones.[9]

Synthesis of papovavirus mRNA is similar to eukaryotic mRNA synthesis in that large-molecular-weight RNA molecules are synthesized and processed by splicing and enzymatic degradation before transport into the cytoplasm.[25] The mRNA's are capped on the 5' end with a methylated guanosine (^{7m}G5'-ppp5' Xm) and contain polyadenylic acid (poly A) on the 3' end. The primary transcripts of early mRNA are at least 50 per cent of the genome size and are transcribed from one strand of the DNA (Fig. 38–19). In processing this molecule, the intervening sequences are excised and the ends are ligated to form the mRNA molecule. The primary transcripts of the late mRNA also are at least 50 per cent of the genome size and are transcribed from the opposite strand of DNA. These, too, are processed by post-transcriptional modification. The papovaviruses code for three structural proteins: VP1, VP2, and VP3. The genetic organization of the SV40 genome is depicted in Figure 38–19. The viral proteins, VP2 and VP3, are synthesized from the same mRNA by using different reading frames and initiation points, whereas VP1 is synthesized from a

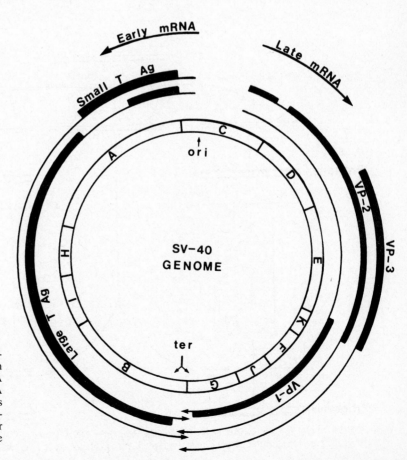

Figure 38–19. Genetic organization of the SV40 genome. Both early and later messenger RNA originates near the origin of DNA replication (ori). The heavy lines represent the protein coding region of the mRNA and the lighter lines show the remainder of the initial transcript.

separate mRNA. Similarly, VP3 also may be synthesized from a separate mRNA.

The viral proteins are translated by the cell machinery. There is no evidence for post-translational modification.

Adenoviruses.[21] The genomes of the adenoviruses are nonpermuted, linear molecules containing 35,000 to 45,000 base pairs with inverted terminal repetitions of 130 to 160 bases.[12] A viral protein is covalently bound to the 5' terminus of each strand, which may facilitate initiation of DNA replication. Figure 38–20 shows that replication can be initiated at either end of the double-stranded genome, following which a daughter strand is synthesized in a 5' to 3' direction with a concomitant displacement of the parental strand.[26] The displaced parental strand then becomes circularized by base pairing of the inverted terminal repetition sequences. Synthesis of a complementary strand of DNA initiates at this double-stranded area and proceeds to produce another daughter molecule. The terminal protein is attached to the nascent DNA strands as a precursor molecule, which subsequently is cleaved as a late step in virion assembly.[38]

It is obvious that initiation can occur at either end of the genomic DNA and utilize the same mechanisms. It also is probable that some molecules will initiate at both ends; in these cases, both parental molecules serve as templates for daughter strand synthesis. Experimental evidence indicates that this is not likely. There is no requirement for a discontinuous mode of DNA synthesis during adenovirus DNA replication.

Adenovirus protein synthesis can be divided into early and late proteins, as can that of all DNA viruses. The adenovirus genome is transcribed by host RNA polymerase II, and both DNA strands encode mRNA's.[41] The early genes involve transcription of at least five transcription units with separate promoters for each. The primary transcripts are synthesized as large-molecular-weight molecules which are then excised and spliced to remove intervening sequences. The mRNA's are capped on the 5' end with a methylated guanosine and contain polyanylate on the 3' end. The late mRNA's all originate at the same promoter located 16.3 map units on the r strand of the genome. The primary transcripts are long molecules that subsequently are spliced to yield the mRNA.[41] The post-transcriptional processing of the

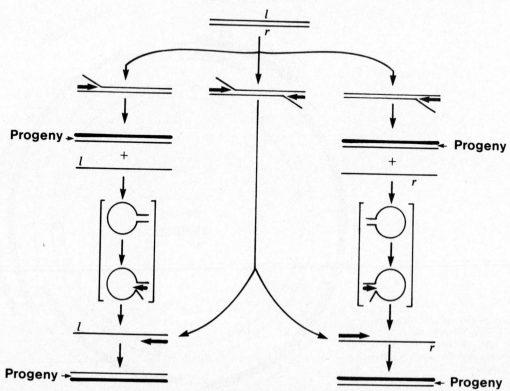

Figure 38–20. Model for adenovirus DNA replication. Daughter DNA molecules are represented by heavy lines and parental strands are represented by light lines. (Adapted from Lechner, R. L., and Kelly, T. J., Jr., Cell **12:**1007, 1977.)

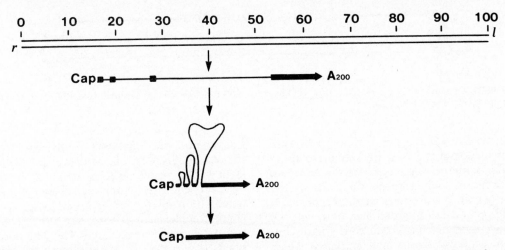

Figure 38–21. Post-transcriptional processing of the adenovirus hexon mRNA. The heavy lines represent the mature mRNA and the lighter lines represent the areas that are excised.

mRNA for the hexon protein, the most abundant capsid protein, is diagrammed in Figure 38–21. All of the late mRNA species contain the same tripartite leader sequences spliced to the body of the RNA.

Herpesviruses.[3] These viruses contain linear, nonpermuted double-stranded DNA with a molecular weight of 80 to 150 × 10⁶ daltons. The physical structure of the genome of the human herpesviruses is diagrammed in Figure 38–22. The genome consists of a long unique sequence (U_L) and a short unique sequence (U_S) bracketed by palindromic sequences. The palindromic sequences bracketing the short unique sequence may be inverted repeat sequences. Herpes simplex viruses and human cytomegalovirus have such inverted repeat sequences bracketing the unique DNA.[36] Because of these inverted repeats, the unique segments can invert relative to each other, thus producing four molecular arrangements that are present in equimolar amounts in any virus suspension. Apparently, all of the isomers are infectious and yield equivalent progeny virus.[35]

Herpesvirus DNA replication involves two phases: (1) during the first round of replication, the newly synthesized DNA is associated with molecules up to twice the genomic size; (2) at later times in infection, the newly synthesized DNA is associated with structures up to 100 times the genomic size.[3] The following replication model has been proposed. After parental DNA enters the nucleus, the ends of molecules are digested by an exonuclease. Since the ends of the molecule are repeats, the DNA forms circles or concatemers. Replication is initiated primarily on the circular molecules, and newly synthesized DNA is associated with concatemers of genome-sized molecules linked covalently. Replication is thought to occur by a rolling circle mechanism. Maturation of the genome from the concatemer requires assembly of the viral capsid and subsequent excision of the genome from the concatemers.

Poxviruses.[28] These are highly complex DNA viruses that are synthesized in the host cell cytoplasm. The genome is double-stranded DNA with a molecular weight of 120 to 150 × 10⁶ daltons. The ends of the genome are covalently closed into a terminal hairpin structure and contain long inverted terminal repeat sequences (Fig. 38–23).[7] The poxviruses have a number of enzymes associated with the virion which are needed for DNA replication. These include: (1) DNA-dependent DNA polymerase, (2) thymidine kinase, (3) single-strand–specific deoxyribonucleases, (4) DNA ligase, and (5) topoisomerase.

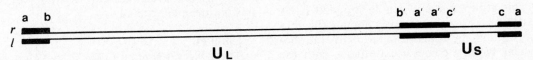

Figure 38–22. Organization of the herpes simplex genome. The genome consists of a long unique region (U_L) and a short unique region (U_S) bracketed by palindromic sequences.

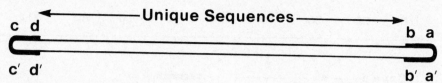

Figure 38-23. Organization of the vaccinia virus genome. The ends of the genome are covalently closed hairpin structures and are of inverted repeat sequences.

The features of the semiconservative replication of poxvirus DNA are similar to those for adenovirus. Initiation apparently occurs at one terminus and synthesis proceeds to the opposite end. It is not clear whether replication is unidirectional or bidirectional; however, the evidence indicates that continuous and discontinuous synthesis occurs concomitantly, which would be compatible with bidirectional replication. The fate and function of the terminal hairpins has not been resolved.[28] Poxvirus mRNA is transcribed and processed by mechanisms analogous to that for eukaryotic cells.

Class II[4]

These viruses contain single-stranded DNA (ssDNA) as the genome and consist of one family, the Parvoviridae. The parvoviruses are the smallest and least complex of the DNA animal viruses. They consist of a nonpermuted, linear, ssDNA genome surrounded by an icosahedral capsid. Both ends of the genome are folded into hairpin structures held together by base-pairing within the first 100 to 120 nucleotides.[4] This group contains two major subgroups: parvoviruses that are autonomous in replication, and those that are defective.

Replication of the parvoviruses occurs in the cell nucleus and utilizes cellular enzymes. DNA synthesis is initiated from the 3' terminal hairpin on the viral strand and proceeds to the other end. There is no evidence for discontinuous synthesis, since DNA synthesis can be initiated at either 3' end.[4] Synthesis of a daughter strand displaces one of the parental strands, so that a unit length, single-stranded molecule is obtained. Since synthesis can initiate at either 3' end, the progeny molecules are complementary, *e.g.*, genomic DNA strands of both polarities are formed. Both strands apparently are infectious.

Class III

This group contains double-stranded RNA (dsRNA) as a genome and contains the reoviruses and the rotaviruses. Most of the molecular biology comes from studies with the reoviruses.[20] The virus consists of 10 dsRNA segments surrounded by a double-layered cap-

sid. There is no envelope. Reoviruses enter the cell by phagocytosis, after which the outer layer of the virion capsid is stripped away by host cell enzymes within the phagocytic vacuole. The resultant subvirus particle, or core, is not completely uncoated, since the genome is not released as naked dsRNA. The core is released into the cytoplasm, where the virion RNA-dependent RNA polymerases transcribe the dsRNA segments into early mRNA, which is extruded from the cores. Electron micrographs have shown mRNA strands being extruded from artificially prepared cores. Apparently all the genomic RNA segments are transcribed, but the amount of each mRNA accumulated is regulated and is proportional to the amount of each protein synthesized. Shortly after infection, all seven structural proteins can be detected in the cytoplasm. Although there is cleavage of proteins to form the mature virion, each mRNA yields a unique viral protein.

Progeny genomic RNA is replicated in a conservative fashion,[20] as diagrammed in Figure 38-24. The (+)RNA segments which are transcribed from the core may be used for mRNA or for progeny genomes. Once the core proteins have been synthesized, the (+)RNA associates with them to form new subvirus particles, after which the enclosed (+)RNA is converted to dsRNA by the polymerase within that core. These cores then can transcribe (+)RNA and thus amplify the replicative process. The core also contains the enzymes necessary to cap and methylate the 5' end of the RNA.

The dsRNA viruses replicate via a (+)RNA intermediate in a conservative fashion. The dsRNA is never fully uncoated, so that cellular enzymes do not gain access to the reovirus genome but only to the (+)RNA templates. The mechanism by which the 10 segments of (+)RNA are assembled into a core particle has not been elucidated.

Class IV

These viruses contain mRNA, (+)RNA, as a genome. The picornaviruses, the togaviruses, and the coronaviruses are well-characterized

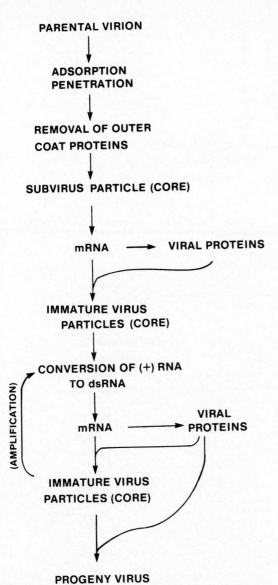

PARENTAL VIRION

↓

**ADSORPTION
PENETRATION**

↓

**REMOVAL OF OUTER
COAT PROTEINS**

↓

SUBVIRUS PARTICLE (CORE)

↓

mRNA → **VIRAL PROTEINS**

↓

**IMMATURE VIRUS
PARTICLES (CORE)**

↓

**CONVERSION OF (+) RNA
TO dsRNA**

(AMPLIFICATION)

↓

mRNA → **VIRAL
PROTEINS**

↓

**IMMATURE VIRUS
PARTICLES (CORE)**

↓

PROGENY VIRUS

Figure 38–24. Schematic representation of the replication cycle for viruses containing double-stranded RNA as a genome. These viruses are in Class III.

members of this class. Unique mechanisms are employed in the replication of the genomic RNA and in the synthesis of viral proteins by the viruses in this class.

Picornaviruses.[34] These are naked icosahedral viruses containing (+)RNA. Since poliovirus has been used as a prototype of the picornaviruses, most of the data presented here will concern poliovirus. Poliovirus contains a single-stranded (+)RNA genome. The 3′ end contains polyadenylic acid and the 5′ end is capped with a covalently linked viral protein (VPg). Figure 38–25 shows a diagram of replication of this group. After adsorption,

penetration, and uncoating, the (+)RNA associates with ribosomes to direct synthesis of viral proteins. A protein that inhibits host cell protein synthesis and an RNA-dependent RNA polymerase are two such proteins. Since the cell does not contain the enzymatic machinery to replicate RNA from an RNA template, synthesis of this polymerase is obligatory to RNA replication. After initial protein synthesis, the genomic RNA directs the replication of (+)RNA. Initially, the genetic information must be transferred to a complementary (−)RNA strand, after which the multiple copies of (+)RNA are synthesized by the polymerase molecules. Figure 38–26 shows that the new strands of (+)RNA are initiated by attachment of the VPg protein, after which the growing strands of (+)RNA are synthesized on the (−)RNA template. This structure is termed the **replicative intermediate (RI).** Each growing strand is attached weakly to the (−)RNA template by the polymerase. The polymerase moves down the template from 3′ to 5′, and the (+)RNA is completed by the addition of a polyadenylate on the 3′ end. Multiple copies of (+)RNA are synthesized simultaneously from a single template. Apparently, the end product of replication is a dsRNA molecule termed the **replicative form (RF).** The exact mechanism for synthesis of the (−)RNA template has not been elucidated; hence, the intermediate is shown in brackets in Figure 38–26. However, the genomic RNA must be copied into complementary RNA to initiate the replicative process.

The genome of poliovirus has been sequenced, and the translation and processing of the viral proteins is becoming clear.[23, 32] As Figure 38–25 shows, the progeny (+)RNA may become genomic RNA for progeny virus or it may serve as mRNA for the synthesis of viral proteins. The progeny RNA that becomes mRNA is identical to that which becomes genomic RNA, except that the VPg on the 5′ end is removed from the mRNA. The ribosomes attach to the 5′ end of the mRNA and traverse almost the entire length of the mRNA to produce a giant polypeptide chain with a molecular weight of about 250,000 daltons. This primary translation product is termed **noncapsid viral protein 00 (NCVP-00),** and it contains all the proteins coded for by the viral genome. NCVP-00 is cleaved *in situ* to produce three large molecules which subsequently are cleaved to produce the **structural** and **nonstructural viral proteins** (Fig. 38–27). The structural proteins are those proteins that are in the virion, while the nonstructural proteins prob-

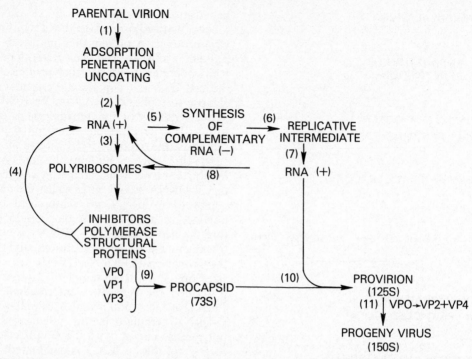

Figure 38–25. Diagram of the replication cycle for viruses that contain (+)RNA as a genome. These viruses are in Class IV. The prototype for this class is poliovirus. The events are numbered in approximate chronological order.

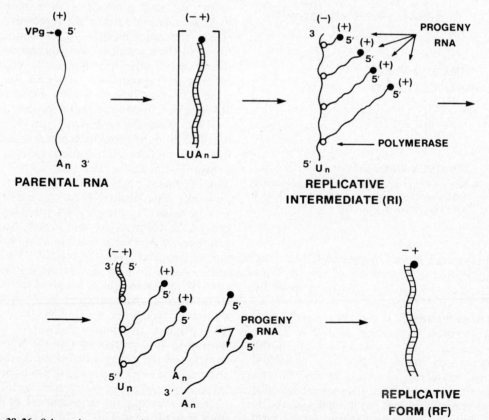

Figure 38–26. Schematic representation of the synthesis of poliovirus RNA from the replicative intermediate (RI). Replication is initiated with the binding of the viral protein g (VPg). The growing (+)RNA strands are attached weakly to the (−)RNA template and are released on completion of synthesis.

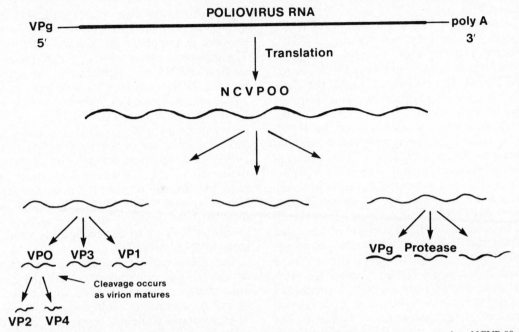

POLIOVIRUS RNA

VPg — poly A
5′ — 3′

Translation

N C V P O O

VPO   VP3   VP1   VPg   Protease

← Cleavage occurs
as virion matures

VP2   VP4

Figure 38–27. Schematic representation of post-translational cleavage of poliovirus precursor proteins. NCVP-00 is a giant precursor protein that is the product of the entire poliovirus genome. It is cleaved to produce viral structural proteins (VP) and other noncapsid viral proteins (NCVP).

ably are enzymes necessary for replication. It initially was assumed that the proteinase responsible for cleavage was host cell–derived. However, proteolytic processing now has been shown to be catalyzed by a virus-coded enzyme. NCVP-00 actually does not exist in the infected cell, since it is cleaved as a nascent polypeptide chain to produce the primary cleavage products. However, it can be demonstrated in cells treated with proteolytic enzyme inhibitors. The final steps in **post-translational cleavage** do not occur until maturation of the virion. Proteins VP-0, VP-1, and VP-3 form a procapsid, after which the RNA is inserted to form the provirion. Protein VP-0 then is cleaved to yield VP-2 and VP-4, at which time the mature virion is completed. The mechanism that directs the (+)RNA to protein synthesis or progeny virus is not clear; however, the (+)RNA associated with the virion has a VPg protein covalently attached to the 5′ terminus. This protein may be needed for virion maturation.

Post-translational cleavage was demonstrated by incubating infected cells for a short period of time with a radioactive amino acid **(pulse labeling),** followed by incubation in the presence of an excess amount of unlabeled amino acid **(chasing).** The radioactive amino acid was incorporated into the proteins being synthesized during the pulse label, after which

the fate of those proteins could be followed. Acrylamide gel electrophoresis revealed that the radioactivity accumulated in large precursor proteins during the pulse label and then subsequently appeared in the viral structural proteins during the chase.

Togaviruses.[39] The togaviruses are enveloped icosahedral viruses that contain single-stranded (+)RNA as a genome. The genomic RNA of most togaviruses contains polyadenylate on the 3′ end and a methylated guanosine cap on the 5′ end. Replication of the togaviruses follows a pathway similar to that of the picornaviruses, and progeny genomic RNA synthesis occurs by a similar replicative intermediate. However, transcription and translation of the mRNA differs. The genomic RNA is a 40 to 42 S molecule that is found in abundance in the infected cell serving both for progeny genomes and for mRNA. Also in the infected cell is a smaller 26 S viral mRNA which is identical to the 3′ third of the 42 S molecule. Both molecules are synthesized from a (−)RNA 42 S template; however, the 26 S molecule is initiated at an internal site. Viral nonstructural proteins are translated from the 5′ two-thirds of the 42 S molecule and the structural proteins are translated from the 26 S molecule. In each case, precursor proteins are translated and subsequently processed by post-translational cleavage.

Class V[22]

These viruses contain genomic RNA that is opposite in polarity to messenger RNA, (−)RNA. Hence, they are termed negative strand viruses. This group includes the orthomyxoviruses, the paramyxoviruses, the rhabdoviruses, the arenaviruses, the bunyaviruses, and the myxoviruses. The replication of the (−)RNA viruses is diagrammed in Figure 38–28. After adsorption, penetration, and uncoating, a virion protein—an RNA transcriptase—remains associated with the (−)RNA. This enzyme is a structural component of the virion and is necessary for infectivity. It transcribes the (−)RNA sequentially from the 3′ end to produce (+)RNA molecules. The same enzyme carries out mRNA synthesis and genomic-length (+)RNA and (−)RNA strand synthesis.[31] It is not certain whether the monocistronic mRNA's are a result of processing of a large precursor molecule or from internal initiation of the polymerase.[1] However, the data indicate that the mRNA molecules are cleaved from the large RNA transcript produced by the transcriptase as it traverses the genome. These molecules then receive polyadenylate at the 3′ end and a methylated guanosine at the 5′ end. The mRNA molecules are translated into proteins that do not require further processing. The transcriptase also must synthesize genomic-length (+)RNA molecules to serve as templates for genome replication. The mechanism that diverts (+)RNA synthesis from mRNA to templates and the reverse has not been elucidated. However, the genomic-length molecules, both (+)RNA and (−)RNA, are in association with the nucleocapsid proteins in the infected cell. It is probable that when the capsid proteins have been produced in excess in the cell, the newly synthesized (+)RNA associates with these proteins and thereby is protected from cleavage.[6] Similarly, if the supply of nucleocapsid proteins has been depleted, the newly synthesized (+)RNA is likely to be processed to produce more mRNA molecules.

The nucleocapsid proteins are synthesized on cytoplasmic polyribosomes, but the envelope proteins are synthesized on ribosomes bound to the rough endoplasmic reticulum. These proteins contain a signal peptide at the amino terminal that promotes binding of the ribosome to the membrane and insertion of the protein into the membrane. The protein subsequently is glycosylated through cellular mechanisms.

Basic similarity in the replication strategy has been demonstrated between the rhabdo-

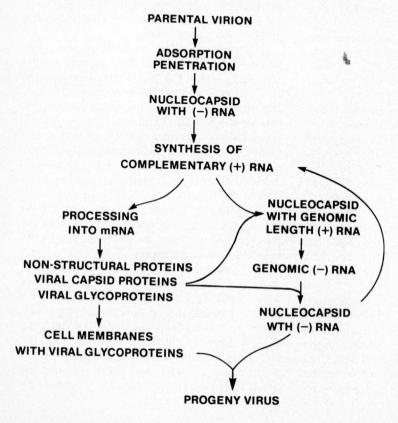

Figure 38–28. Diagram of the replicative cycle for viruses containing (−)RNA as a genome. These are the negative strand viruses and are in Class V.

viruses, and it is anticipated that all negative strand viruses share some common strategies. However, some notable differences do exist. The influenzaviruses replicate eight RNA segments independently and synthesize eight monocistronic mRNA's which are capped at the 5′ end and polyadenylated at the 3′ end.[37]

Class VI[5, 19]

These viruses contain (+)RNA as a genome and replicate through a DNA intermediate. This group is composed of the RNA tumor viruses or retroviruses. Since these viruses contain an enzyme that transcribes DNA from an RNA template (reverse transcriptase), the family name Retroviridae has been chosen. However, the term "RNA tumor virus" is found extensively in the literature. These viruses have been found in most species of animals and birds. The replicative cycle of the RNA tumor viruses is diagrammed in Figure 38–29. After adsorption, penetration, and uncoating, the parental (+)RNA is converted into a base-paired RNA–DNA duplex by the reverse transcriptase. Synthesis of the DNA strand is primed by transfer RNA carried in the virion. A dsDNA molecule then is synthesized from the RNA–DNA complex by the same enzyme. The genetic information contained in the parental (+)RNA is transferred to dsDNA, which subsequently circularizes and becomes integrated into the host cell genome. This viral DNA is called **provirus,** and it is replicated with cell DNA and transferred to each daughter cell.

The viral DNA is transcribed and the (+)RNA is processed like cellular mRNA. Virion RNA is 35 S, whereas the mRNA is 20 S. The mRNA is translated into precursor proteins, which subsequently are cleaved to form the viral proteins. The whole genome is not translated into a giant precursor molecule; however, most of the structural proteins are obtained by post-translational cleavage.[19]

The viral DNA is transcribed into large (+)RNA, which is processed similarly to cellular RNA. Subsequently, the 35 S genomic RNA and the smaller 20 S mRNA are polyadenylated and capped at their 3′ and 5′ termini, and are found in the cytoplasm.

MATURATION AND RELEASE

The maturation processes involve the interaction of the capsid proteins with the genome to form the nucleocapsid, followed by the acquisition of an envelope by some viruses.

Maturation of naked icosahedral viruses is synonymous with assembly of the nucleocap-

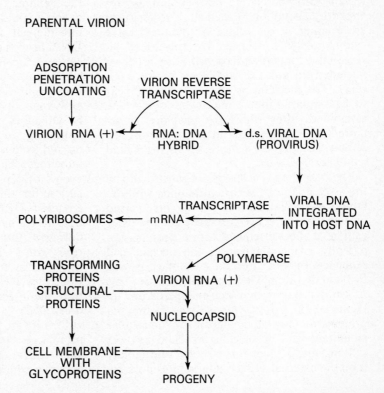

Figure 38–29. Diagram of the replicative cycle of viruses that contain a (+)RNA genome and replicate via a DNA intermediate. These are the RNA tumor viruses and are in Class VI.

sid. The basic mechanisms of assembly appear to be the same, since the icosahedral capsid is specified by the primary amino acid sequences of the capsomers. The capsid polypeptides are synthesized and gain their mature secondary and tertiary configurations as specified by the primary amino acid sequence. These subunits associate to form capsomers and the capsomers aggregate to form empty icosahedral shells, or **procapsids.** This process of assembly is inefficient, since an excess of capsomers remain in the cell. For example, in cells infected with the adenoviruses, 90 per cent or more of the capsid proteins may not be assembled. An infected cell also contains empty and partially assembled capsids. In the case of polioviruses, the genome enters the procapsid to form the virion. The poliovirus procapsid is formed from proteins VP-0, VP-1, and VP-3. The genomic RNA enters the procapsid to form the **provirion**, which does not have the structural integrity of the mature virion, since the genome still is susceptible to RNase. The VP-0 protein is cleaved to form VP-2 and VP-4, at which time virus assembly is completed.

The naked icosahedral viruses generally are released by cellular disruption. Poliovirus is released rapidly by a procedure resembling "reverse phagocytosis," in which vacuoles filled with virus are released at the cell membrane. The adenoviruses and papovaviruses remain localized in the nucleus and are released by disruption of the cell. These viruses are retained in the cells even after extensive cytopathology is evident. The enveloped viruses may contain an icosahedral or a helical nucleocapsid and may be DNA or RNA viruses. The mechanisms of maturation appear to be similar. First, a nucleocapsid must be assembled, after which the envelope is acquired. The icosahedral nucleocapsids are assembled by the same processes as the naked icosahedral viruses.

The helical nucleocapsids are constructed by the association of the structural units with the viral RNA. The binding of the first capsid proteins are sequence-specified, but the association of the subsequent capsid proteins apparently is independent of the nucleic acid sequence. In both cases, the envelope is gained by budding through a cellular membrane. This process is shown by electron microscopy in Figure 38–30. After synthesis, the membrane proteins are inserted into an area of the cellular membrane and become glycosylated by host cell enzymes so that the carbohydrate moiety is on the external surface. During this process, cellular glycoproteins are excluded from this membrane area, and the membrane partially loses its fluidity. Matrix proteins may be associated with the inner layer of the membrane. The nucleocapsid migrates to lie beneath the area of membrane containing the viral glycoproteins, after which the nucleocapsid and the surrounding membrane protrude and the bud close off to form the enveloped virion. The envelope proteins are coded by the virus, but the lipids and carbohydrates are characteristic of the cell.

The site of budding is characteristic of the virus. The herpesviruses bud through the nuclear membrane, the paramyxoviruses bud through the external cell membrane, and the togaviruses bud either through the cell membrane (alphaviruses) or into cytoplasmic vacuoles and the endoplasmic reticulum (flaviviruses). Such viruses are then released to the exterior of the cell.

The process of budding is compatible with the cell's continued existence. Thus, many particles can bud from the infected cell without extensive cell damage.

INFECTIOUS VIRAL NUCLEIC ACID

Since viruses must be able to direct synthesis of their components with the information in the genome, it is feasible that the isolated genome could be infectious if it gained entry into the cell. It was shown that deproteinized DNA from the papovaviruses and RNA from some of the RNA viruses retained infectivity when introduced into the cell. This infectivity was sensitive to nucleases but not to specific antiviral antibody. The ratio of infectious RNA to infectious virus was approximately 10^{-3}, indicating an inefficient process. RNA extracted from some other RNA viruses was not infectious. The elucidation of the molecular events of replication has provided an explanation for this paradox. Those viruses that contain $(+)$RNA as a genome can yield infectious RNA, since the genome serves as mRNA during a normal replicative cycle. Those viruses with $(-)$RNA genomes cannot replicate if the RNA transcriptase has been removed. Infectious DNA has been difficult to obtain from the larger DNA viruses. However, infectious DNA can be obtained from the adenoviruses if care is taken not to remove the viral protein attached to the genome. This protein apparently facilitates the circularization of the genome, which is necessary for replication.

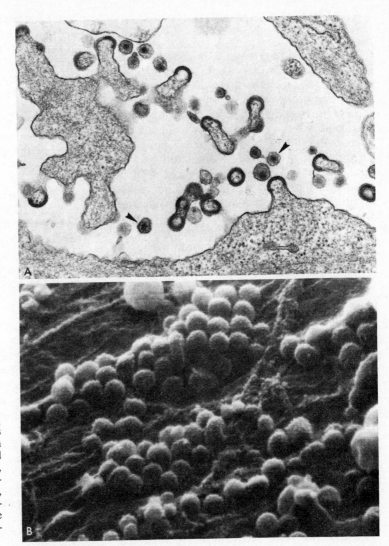

Figure 38–30. Electron micrographs of the budding of visna virus. *A*, Thin section showing the nucleocapsid budding through the membrane, which has thickened due to the incorporation of viral glycoproteins. *B*, Scanning electron micrograph showing the viral buds protruding from the cell membrane. (Courtesy of M. Dubois-Dalcq.)

Cellular Consequences of Viral Infection

Virus replication in the host cell may result in destruction of the cell, in a persistent infection with no apparent damage to the cell, or in transformation of the cell.

CELL DESTRUCTION[27]

The resultant effect of the cytocidal viruses is cell death, which can be observed microscopically as CPE. The histology of the types of CPE has been described previously. The mechanisms responsible for cell death are not known and may vary according to the particular virus. However, there are general mechanisms which may be involved. The virus may code for protein(s) that inhibit cellular RNA and protein synthesis. As a consequence, host DNA synthesis also declines. Such inhibition of host cell macromolecular synthesis eventually results in cell death. Some viral proteins are toxic. As these proteins build up during replication, the toxicity to the host cell is magnified, which may result in death of that cell. For example, the adenovirus penton antigen inhibits cellular DNA, RNA, and protein synthesis. Release of lysosomal enzymes by the cell may lead to cellular destruction. These enzymes may be released due to injury to the lysosomal membrane, or they may be released in an attempt to destroy the virus.

PERSISTENT INFECTIONS[17, 18]

These are differentiated into **steady state** infections, in which all of the cells are infected, and **carrier state** infections, in which a low percentage of the cells is infected. In the steady state cultures, large amounts of virus may be produced, yet the cells continue to divide and appear morphologically normal. These cultures cannot be "cured" of infection by antiviral antibody. Hence, the infection must be passed to daughter cells at the time of cell division. Such infections have been demonstrated with most of the viruses that mature by budding through the cell membrane. In contrast, the carrier state cultures can be "cured" by cloning the cells in the presence of antiviral antibody. These infections usually are maintained by some inhibitor that prevents the virus from infecting most of the cells.

Certainly viruses that cause persistent infections in cell cultures may do the same in the host. These may be manifest as either a latent or a chronic infection. An example of the former is the latency of the herpesviruses. After an acute primary infection, the virus apparently disappears. The acute disease reappears later, due to activation of the latent virus, not exogenous reinfection. During the period of latency, the virus apparently lies dormant in the trigeminal nerve ganglion (for herpes simplex) or the dorsal root ganglion (for herpes zoster), where the virus is not susceptible to the host immune defenses. Upon activation, the virus spreads down the nerves to infect the skin. Activation and recurrent disease occur in the presence of high titers of antiviral antibody.

Chronic infections, in which infectious virus is present and may be shed without producing disease symptoms, also occur. An example of chronic human infections occurs with hepatitis B, where the carrier may shed infectious virus for several years.

TRANSFORMATION

The oncogenic viruses have the property of causing stable heritable changes in their host cells, a process termed transformation. It is thought that viral transformation *in vitro* is analogous to tumor induction in animals, since the transformed cells have gained the properties of neoplastic cells. Some of the key properties of transformed cells are: (1) the loss of contact inhibition; (2) growth to high saturation density; (3) appearance of virus-specific antigens, both tumor (T) antigens and tumor-specific transplantation antigens (TSTA); (4) tumor formation upon injection into a susceptible host; (5) increased agglutinability by plant lectins; and (6) altered cell morphology. In transformed cells, virus-specific nucleic acid sequences have been integrated into the genome. In the case of DNA viruses, the viral DNA can be integrated directly. The RNA tumor viruses must synthesize a DNA copy of their RNA genomes for integration. This is accomplished by the virion reverse transcriptase enzyme. Studies with temperature-sensitive mutants have shown that the maintenance of the transformed state is a viral function and typically can be mapped to a discrete small area of the genome.

LYSOGENY

Although plant viruses have not been discussed here, the property of lysogeny must be discussed, since it results in changes in pathogenic bacteria and may provide a key aspect of the mechanism of pathogenesis. Some bacterial viruses, the temperate bacteriophages, show two responses after infecting a sensitive bacterium: the **lytic** response, which culminates in cell lysis and the release of progeny phage, or a specialized phage-cell interaction termed **lysogeny.** In the lysogenic response the phage nucleic acid becomes **integrated** into the bacterial chromosome, a situation analogous to transformation of eucaryotic cells by the oncogenic viruses. In the integrated form, the phage is termed lysogenic. Lysogenic bacteria appear normal and, under ordinary conditions, cannot be identified as infected. Usually a lysogenic culture will contain free phage in the medium. The lysogenic cells are immune to superinfection by the same phage or closely related phages, but may contain many prophages of different serotypes. Insertion of the phage nucleic acid into the host cell genome is controlled by the integration gene of the phage and occurs after the phage genome circularizes.

The prophage induces new functions in the cell. One of these is the establishment of immunity to superinfection. This immunity is mediated by a repressor protein that exerts control on the phage genome. Also, the phenotype of the cell may be changed by the products of the prophage, a process termed lysogenic conversion. For example, integrated phage genes are responsible for the production of toxin in the toxigenic strains of *Corynebacterium diphtheriae*.

Lysogenic bacteria may undergo spontaneous induction to the lytic state. Thus, a lysogenic culture constantly produces a small amount of virus. Induction can be increased to a high percentage by treating the lysogenic cells with ultraviolet light, x-rays, and other mutagens. These agents apparently interfere with the production or action of the repressor protein, after which the prophage enters the vegetative state.

Viral Genetics

Since viruses are nucleic acid surrounded by a protective coat, they undergo mutations, interact with the host cell nucleic acid, and interact with other viruses in mixedly or multiply infected cells.

When two or more viruses infect the same cell, the result may be (1) independent replication, (2) interference with the replication of either or both viruses, (3) complementation or enhancement of either or both viruses, (4) genetic recombination, or (5) phenotypic mixing.

MUTATIONS

Mutations of animal viruses occur spontaneously, as in any replicating nucleic acid. The frequency of spontaneous mutation varies between one mutation in 10^4 and one in 10^6 gene replications. Mutations also can be induced by treating the virus with mutagens such as nitrous acid, hydroxylamine, nitrosoguanidine, 5-bromodeoxyuridine, or 5-fluorouracil. The last two compounds induce base substitutions in replicating DNA and RNA, respectively.

Many types of viral mutants have been described. These have specific characteristics such as resistance to heat or chemical inactivation or altered growth patterns. **Plaque mutants** exhibit an altered plaque morphology. The reasons for such alterations vary. For instance, the mutant viruses may be more sensitive to the polysaccharide inhibitors in agar; they may exhibit an altered thermolability; or they may differ in the mechanisms of release from the host cell. **Host-dependent** mutants fail to grow in some cells that normally serve as hosts. An example is the PK-negative mutants of rabbitpox virus. These mutants do not grow in pig kidney cells, whereas the wild-type rabbitpox virus does. Hot- or cold-adapted mutants grow better at a higher or lower temperature than wild-type virus. Frequently, selection of cold-adapted mutants results in the attenuation of virulence, as was demonstrated with poliovirus. **Temperature-sensitive (ts)** mutants are conditional lethal mutants that exhibit restricted replication at elevated temperatures (nonpermissive) under which the wild-type virus can replicate; however, they can replicate at lower temperatures (permissive). The ts mutants are mutated such that a protein is produced that is functional at the permissive temperature but not at the nonpermissive temperature. This is caused by a change in the primary amino acid sequence, which results in secondary and tertiary structures that are unstable at the higher temperature. These viruses usually do not replicate as well as the wild-type even at the permissive temperatures, and they rarely are completely restricted at the nonpermissive temperature. Such mutants may be induced and selected in any viral protein, and the function of specific proteins can be isolated for study. As a result, these conditional lethal mutants have been extremely valuable in elucidating the molecular events that occur during replication. The use of ts mutants frequently involves temperature-shift experiments in which viral replication is initiated at either temperature, and the temperature is shifted after a suitable interval to isolate the action or effect of a particular protein. The ts mutants of a particular virus can be localized into groups by complementation so that each group represents a specific function.

INTERACTIONS BETWEEN VIRUSES

Cells that are infected with more than one virus particle of the same type are termed **multiply infected** cells, whereas those infected with more than one type of virus are **mixedly infected** cells. In a multiply or mixedly infected cell, the viruses may interact. This may involve interchange between the nucleic acids to produce a new genome (nucleic acid interactions), or it may involve the "borrowing" of a gene product (gene product interactions). The nucleic acid interactions are known as recombination and reactivation.

Recombination

This involves an exchange of nucleic acid between related infectious viruses so that some progeny contain a unique combination of nucleic acid derived from both parents. These genetically stable progeny are termed recombinants. Intramolecular recombination occurs when the nucleic acid segments are joined covalently into a single molecule, which also may involve segments of viral and host cell nucleic acid. This type of recombination occurs readily with viruses containing DNA and at a low frequency with some (+)RNA viruses. Intramolecular recombination has not been detected with (−)RNA viruses. Recombination has been used extensively to produce genetic maps of the viral genomes by crossing ts mutants. Also, hybrid viruses can be produced experimentally by recombination between two different DNA viruses such as adenoviruses and papovaviruses.

Reassortment is a type of recombination in which the segments of nucleic acid are not joined. This occurs with the viruses that have segmented genomes: influenzaviruses, reoviruses, bunyaviruses, and arenaviruses. In this case, segments of nucleic acid from both parents are encapsidated to form unique, genetically stable progeny. Reassortment may account for the appearance of new influenza strains. A new virus may be produced from a cell infected with influenzaviruses of human and animal origin. Such recombinants have been produced under experimental conditions in the respiratory tract of animals.

Reactivation is recombination involving inactive virus. Multiplicity reactivation is the production of infectious virus by a cell multiply infected with inactivated virus of the same strain and results from recombination of the damaged nucleic acid to produce an infectious genome. In order for multiplicity reactivation to occur, the cell must receive two or more virions that have lethal defects in different genes. **Cross-reactivation** or marker rescue involves recombination between an infectious virus and a related inactivated virus. The two viruses must have distinguishable genetic traits in order to be detected. Infectious progeny is produced that contains genes from the inactivated parent.

GENE PRODUCT INTERACTIONS

These are interactions that involve the sharing of gene products in multiply or mixedly infected cells. Gene product interactions include complementation, interference, and phenotypic mixing.

Complementation

The production of an increased yield from a mixedly infected cell is a result of complementation. Complementation may involve related or unrelated viruses. These may be two defective or conditional lethal viruses, an infectious and an inactivated virus, or an infectious and a defective virus. Since this involves the sharing of viral proteins without alteration of the genome, the progeny of inactive virus will be inactive. There are many specific examples and uses of complementation.

Two Conditional Lethal Mutants. The ts mutants can be divided into groups such that each group consists of mutants in the same gene product. Cells infected with two ts mutants are incubated at the nonpermissive temperature and the production of progeny is monitored. If the ts mutations are in separate genes, complementation can occur and progeny will be produced. However, if the viruses contain mutations in the same gene, complementation cannot occur and progeny cannot be produced.

An Infectious and a Defective Virus. This type of complementation probably occurs frequently in nature, where a defective virus is able to replicate only in the presence of an infectious helper virus. The adeno-associated viruses (AAV) are completely defective and cannot replicate without infectious adenovirus as a helper. In a mixedly infected cell, both adenovirus and AAV will be produced. Similarly, the human adenoviruses cannot replicate in monkey cells unless the monkey cells also are infected with SV40, a papovavirus. When such infections are achieved, the resultant progeny consists of adenovirus and adenovirus:SV40 recombinants. These recombinants also are defective and require SV40 as a helper. This example involves recombination and complementation. Of the RNA tumor viruses, the sarcoma viruses (mammalian and avian) are defective in most cells and cannot replicate unless the cell also is infected with a leukosis virus. The sarcoma viruses cannot direct the synthesis of at least one of the envelope proteins, which can be supplied by the leukosis virus.

Interference

A common result of multiply or mixedly infected cells is the reduction in replication of one of the viruses. Although interferon mediates some interference, there are instances that are not interferon mediated. Interference may occur with homologous or heterologous viruses. An example of heterologous interference is that occurring with Newcastle disease virus (NDV) by rubella virus. Cells infected with rubella virus are subsequently nonpermissive for NDV, although the NDV is capable of adsorbing and entering the cell. A widespread type of homologous interference is that caused by **defective interfering (DI)** particles. During replication of most viruses, DI particles are generated which cannot replicate independently, but can replicate in the presence of infectious homologous virus. Such particles usually contain only a portion of the genetic information of the parent.[24] The DI particles gain the missing functions from the infectious virus, so this also is a form of complementation. Replication of the DI particles interferes with the replication of the infectious virus apparently by favorably competing for the limited amounts of polymerase and nucleocapsid proteins. The DI particles contain the normal capsid proteins, and they interfere specifically with homologous virus replication. In some cases the DI particles can be separated by physical means, whereas in others their presence can only be demonstrated biologically. Interference by DI particles first was demonstrated by von Magnus[40] when he passed influenza virus at high virus-cell ratios. They have been demonstrated subsequently with many viruses. Such particles have been demonstrated *in vivo* and have been postulated as being important in the limitation of acute viral diseases and the establishment of persistent infections; however, their importance in man is not clear.[18]

Phenotypic Mixing

When two closely related viruses infect the same cell, the progeny genomes may be encapsidated with either capsid or a hybrid of both. This altered phenotype is not stable, since there is no genetic change. The mismatching of complete capsids between two viruses is termed **transcapsidation.** The antigenicity and host range will be a function of the capsid; however, the genome will breed true. Another form of phenotypic mixing is the formation of mosaic envelopes. This occurs in cells mixedly infected with viruses that acquire envelopes by budding. The majority of phenotypically mixed particles contain representative antigens from both parents.

Antiviral Agents and Chemotherapy

Although the viruses are totally dependent on the host cell metabolic pathways and structures, there exist biochemical processes essential to the virus but of no consequence to the host cell. It is here that the action of antiviral agents must be focused. There are several compounds that inhibit specific aspects of virus replication. Only those compounds that are selective in action will be discussed. There are many other compounds, such as detergents, sulfonated polysaccharides, heparin, hyaluronic acid, and polyanions, that inhibit a variety of viruses. However, these compounds have little or no chemotherapeutic potential.

Adamantadine

Adamantadine is a stable crystalline amine with an unusual symmetrical structure that inhibits penetration and uncoating of the influenza A virus. Adamantadine also exerts a therapeutic effect if given early during the course of influenza A. This drug has proven highly effective in patients with compromised defenses during epidemics. It also inhibits rubella virus and some of the RNA tumor viruses.

Rifamycins

Rifamycins are products of fermentation by *Streptomyces mediterranei*. These molecules inhibit the reverse transcriptase of the RNA tumor viruses and also block the maturation of the poxviruses by inhibiting the cleavage of viral precursor proteins into coat proteins. The rifamycins also inhibit bacterial DNA polymerase but not mammalian DNA polymerases.

Iododeoxyuridine

Iododeoxyuridine (IUdR or IDU) is a halogenated deoxyribonucleoside that becomes incorporated into DNA, where it inhibits enzymes involved in DNA synthesis and subsequently inhibits DNA synthesis. It is toxic to mammalian cells, since mammalian cell DNA synthesis also is inhibited. IUdR has been useful in areas of limited cell division such as the eye cornea, and it has been used for treatment of herpes keratitis. It also has been effective against herpes simplex encephalitis when the drug is administered systemically, but newer antiviral agents have replaced IUdR for treatment of herpes simplex encephalitis. Other halogenated deoxyribonucleosides that have antiviral activity include bromodeoxyuridine (BUdR) and fluorodeoxyuridine (FUdR).

Cytosine Arabinoside

Cytosine arabinoside (1-β-D-arabinofuranosylcytosine, ara-C) is an analogue of cytosine in which arabinose has been substituted for ribose. Ara-C interferes with all DNA synthesis, but it is more effective against viral DNA than cellular DNA; herpes simplex type 2 is most sensitive to its action. The ara-C is incorporated into DNA and inhibits DNA polymerase. Ara-C is very toxic, partially due to the suppression of the host immune response.

Adenosine Arabinoside

Adenosine arabinoside (9-β-D-arabinofuranosyladenine, ara-A) was synthesized as an anti-cancer drug. The mode of action of ara-A is similar to that of ara-C, and mammalian as well as viral DNA synthesis is inhibited. All DNA viruses except polyomavirus and adenovirus type 3 were found to be inhibited by ara-A, as was Rous sarcoma virus. Ara-A is toxic, but not as toxic as ara-C, and has replaced ara-C in the treatment of severe herpetic infections. It is most effective against the herpes simplex and varicella zoster viruses.

Guanidine and 2-(α-Hydroxybenzyl)-Benzimidazole

These two compounds inhibit the replication of the picornaviruses, but differ in their inhibitory spectrum. They inhibit the synthesis of viral RNA and viral structural proteins, thereby arresting production of progeny virus. Neither drug has been approved for human use.

Thiosemicarbazones

Isatin-β-thiosemicarbazone (IBT) and 1-methylisatin-3-thiosemicarbazone (methisazone) are effective in preventing poxvirus replication by inhibiting the formation of a viral core protein. As a result, the late viral mRNA is degraded, and infectious virus is not produced. These compounds are only effective if used prophylactically. The eradication of smallpox has made this drug obsolete; however, it will be a major line of defense if an outbreak should occur.

Interferon

Interferon is a mammalian cell product that can render a cell refractile to virus infection. After release from infected cells, it is adsorbed to susceptible cells and subsequently induces the synthesis of a cell protein that interferes with viral transcription and translation. Apparently interferon acts on the recipient cell at the cell membrane. This interferon–cell membrane interaction leads to the synthesis of the protein that mediates the antiviral state. It does not have direct antiviral activity. Interferon is species-specific in that interferon prepared in human cells can be adsorbed to and protect other human cells but not cells of other species. Interferon is not virus-specific, so that a cell rendered antiviral by interferon is resistant to a broad spectrum of viruses.

Interferon is synthesized in response to most viral infections. It has several properties that make it worthwhile for possible clinical use. It is highly active so that a small amount can render a large number of cells refractile, weakly antigenic, and nontoxic. Thus, repeated doses can be administered without inducing an immune response or a toxic reaction.

The physical characteristics of interferon and the induction of interferon synthesis are described in detail in Chapter 12.

REFERENCES

1. Ball, L. A., and G. W. Wertz. 1981. VSV RNA synthesis: how can you be positive? Cell **26**:143–144.
2. Baltimore, D. 1971. Expression of animal genomes. Bacteriol. Rev. **35**:235–241.
3. Ben-Porat, T. 1983. Organization and replication of herpesvirus DNA. pp. 147–172. In A. S. Kaplan (Ed.): Organization and Replication of Viral DNA. CRC Press, Boca Raton, Florida.
4. Berns, K. I., and W. W. Hauswirth. 1983. Organization and replication of parvovirus DNA. pp. 3–36. In A. S. Kaplan (Ed.): Organization and Replication of Viral DNA. CRC Press, Boca Raton, Florida.
5. Bishop, J. M. 1978. Retroviruses. Ann. Rev. Biochem. **47**:35–88.
6. Blumberg, B. M., M. Leppert, and D. Kolakofsky. 1981. Interaction of the VSV leader RNA and nucleocapsid protein may control VSV genome replication. Cell **23**:837–845.
7. Dales, S., and B. G. T. Pogo. 1981. The biology of poxviruses. Monogr. Virol. **18**:1–109.
8. Das, G. C., and S. K. Niyogi. 1981. Structure, replication and transcription of the SV40 genome. pp. 187–223. In W. E. Cohn (Ed.): Progress in Nucleic Acid Research and Molecular Biology. Vol. 25. Academic Press, New York.

9. DePamphilis, M. L., *et. al.* 1979. The replication and structure of SV40 chromosomes. Cold Spring Harbor Symp. Quant. Biol. **43**:679–683.

10. DePamphilis, M. L., and P. M. Wassarman. 1983. Organization and replication of papovavirus DNA. pp. 37–114. *In* A. S. Kaplan (Ed.): Organization and Replication of Viral DNA. CRC Press, Boca Raton, Florida.

11. Fareed, G. C., and D. Davoli. 1977. Molecular biology of papovaviruses. Ann. Rev. Biochem. **46**:471–496.

12. Flint, S. J. 1980. Structure and genomic organization of the adenoviruses, pp. 383–442. *In* J. Tooze (Ed.): Molecular Biology of Tumor Viruses. 2nd ed. Cold Spring Harbor Laboratory, Cold Spring Harbor, New York.

13. Gajusek, D. C. 1977. Unconventional viruses and the origin and disappearance of kuru. Science **197**:943–960.

14. Helenius, A., M. Marsh, and J. White. 1980. The entry of viruses into animal cells. Trends in Biochemical Sciences **5**:104–106.

15. Horne, R. W. 1974. Virus Structure. Academic Press, New York.

16. Horne, R. W., and P. Wildy. 1963. Virus structure revealed by negative staining. Adv. Virus Res. **10**:101–170.

17. Hotchin, J. 1971. Persistent and slow virus infections. Monogr. Virol. **3**:1–15.

18. Huang, A. S. 1977. Viral pathogenisis and molecular biology. Bacteriol. Rev. **41**:811–821.

19. Hughes, S. H. 1983. Synthesis, integration and transcription of the retroviral provirus. Curr. Topics Microbiol. Immunol. **103**:23–50.

20. Joklik, W. K. 1981. Structure and function of the reovirus genome. Microbiol. Rev. **45**:483–501.

21. Kelly, T. J., Jr. 1983. Organization and replication of adenovirus DNA. pp. 115–146. *In* A. S. Kaplan (Ed.): Organization and Replication of Viral DNA. CRC Press, Boca Raton, Florida.

22. Kingsbury, D. W., *et. al.* 1978. Paramyxoviridae. Intervirology **10**:137–152.

23. Kitamura, N., *et. al.* 1981. Primary structure, gene organization and polypeptide expression of poliovirus RNA. Nature **291**:547–553.

24. Lazzarine, R. A., J. D. Keene, and M. Schubert. 1981. The origins of defective interfering particles of the negative-strand RNA viruses. Cell **26**:145–154.

25. Leborwitz, P., and S. M. Wissman. 1979. Organization and transcription of the SV40 genome. Curr. Topics Microbiol. Immunol. **87**:43–71.

26. Lechner, R. L., and T. J. Kelly, Jr. 1977. The structure of replicating adenovirus 2 DNA molecules. Cell **12**:1007–1013.

27. Martin, E. M., and I. M. Kerr, 1968. Virus-induced changes in host-cell macromolecular synthesis. Symp. Soc. Gen. Microbiol. **18**:15–26.

28. McFadden, G., and S. Dales. 1983. Organization and replication of poxvirus DNA. pp. 173–190. *In* A. S. Kaplan (Ed.): Organization and Replication of Viral DNA. CRC Press, Boca Raton, Florida.

29. Melnick, J. L. 1982. Taxonomy and nomenclature of viruses, 1982. Prog. Med. Virol. **28**:208–221.

30. Ogawa, T., and T. Okazaki. 1980. Discontinuous DNA replication. Ann. Rev. Biochem. **49**:421–434.

31. Perlman, S. M., and A. S. Huang. 1973. RNA synthesis of vesicular stomatitis virus. V. Interactions between transcription and replication. J. Virol. **12**:1395–1400.

32. Racaniello, V. R., and D. Baltimore. 1981. Molecular cloning of poliovirus cDNA and determination of the complete nucleotide sequence of the viral genome. Proc. Natl Acad. Sci. USA. **78**:5887–5891.

33. Reed, L. J., and H. Meunch. 1938. A simple method of estimating fifty percent endpoints. Amer. J. Hygiene **27**:493–497.

34. Rekosh, D. M. K. 1977. The molecular biology of picornaviruses. pp. 63–110. *In* D. P. Nyak (Ed.): The Molecular Biology of Animal Viruses. Marcel Dekker, New York.

35. Roizman, B., *et. al.* 1979. On the structure, functional equivalence, and replication of the four arrangements of herpes simplex virus DNA. Cold Spring Harbor Symp. Quant. Biol. **43**:809–820.

36. Sheldrik, P., and N. Berthelot. 1974. Inverted repetitions in the chromosomes of HSV. Cold Spring Harbor Symp. Quant. Biol. **39**:667–684.

37. Smith, G. L., and A. J. Hay. 1982. Replication of the influenza virus genome. Virology **118**:96–108.

38. Stillman, B. W. 1981. Adenovirus DNA replication *in vitro*: a protein linked to the 5′ end of nascent DNA strands. J. Virol. **37**:139–148.

39. Strauss, J. H., and E. G. Strauss. 1977. Togaviruses. pp. 111–166. *In* D. P. Nyak (Ed.): The Molecular Biology of Animal Viruses. Marcel Dekker, New York.

40. von Magnus, P. 1951. Propagation of the PR8 strain of influenza in chick embryos. III. Properties of the incomplete virus produced in serial passage of undiluted virus. Acta Pathol. Microbiol. Scand. **29**:156–181.

41. Ziff, E. B. 1980. Transcription and RNA processing by the DNA tumor viruses. Nature (London) **287**:491–496.

CHAPTER 39

The Poxviruses;
The Herpesviruses;
The Papovaviruses;
The Adenoviruses

The viral families whose members contain a DNA genome have been discussed earlier (Chap. 38). Aside from the common feature of their genomic DNA, these viruses exhibit great heterogeneity in morphology and structure and the site of viral maturation. They range in size from among the smallest of viruses (parvoviruses) to the largest and most complex (poxviruses). The nucleocapsid contains DNA—single-stranded in the Parvoviridae, and double-stranded in the remaining families.

The DNA viruses responsible for human disease are found primarily in the families Poxviridae, Herpesviridae, Papovaviridae, and Adenoviridae. Although parvoviruses are known to infect man, as evidenced by shedding in the feces, so far as presently known, they do not cause recognizable disease.[45]

A number of the DNA viruses cause diseases of man and animals that are exanthematous in nature; such viruses are said to be dermatropic because the predominant lesions occur in skin. Certain of these make up the more or less homogeneous poxviruses, having common properties of relatively large size, brick shape, and formation of inclusion bodies within infected cells. Others, the herpesviruses and papovaviruses, are spheroidal, smaller, and less complex, and form both intracytoplasmic and intranuclear inclusion bodies in infected cells.

The adenoviruses are not usually considered to be dermatropic, and are most often found in respiratory and eye infections in man and animals.

While the infection of host cells with virus often results in relatively rapid death, many of the DNA viruses induce a proliferative cellular response, and such viruses are said to be tumorigenic. The proliferative response may be brief and followed by necrotic changes, or it may be prolonged so that hyperplasia is an outstanding feature of the disease. Such response is apparent, though transitory, in smallpox; it is more pronounced in human molluscum contagiosum infections and in rabbit fibroma; in rabbit papilloma and myxoma, the process is quite marked. In most of the natural diseases, the tumors produced are benign, but in a few, as with some herpesviruses, malignancies occur in the natural animal infections and, perhaps, in humans.

The Poxviruses[24, 29]

The viruses that make up the Poxviridae resemble one another morphologically and in the pathogenesis of the diseases they produce, and they are immunologically related to one another. They can be differentiated from one another by host specificity, by specific antigen constitution, and by their growth effects in cell culture or on the chorioallantoic membrane of chick embryos.

The poxviruses are unusual in their morphology, as discussed in Chapter 38. They possess a large DNA genome and exhibit a complex protein structure; many of the proteins have enzymatic function. Unlike other DNA viruses, they replicate in the cytoplasm of infected cells. Most of the poxviruses produce extensive cytopathic effects in the cells they infect; some, on the other hand, stimulate host cell proliferation. In general, poxviruses profoundly affect host cell metabolism by terminating macromolecular synthesis.

The Poxviridae that infect vertebrate animals are classified on the basis of virion morphology and specific antigenic constitution. Six genera are recognized, along with a small number of ungrouped viruses whose taxonomy is uncertain. The classification of vertebrate poxviruses is summarized in Table 39–1.

Morphology

Poxviruses are among the largest of the viruses, and the viral particles are just within the limits of optical resolution. The virion is generally a regular six-sided structure with rounded corners that is often described as brick-shaped, with dimensions of 200 to 250 nm. by 250 to 300 nm. (Fig. 39–1). In some

Table 39–1. **Poxviruses of Vertebrates**

Genus	Virus	Principal Hosts
Orthopoxvirus	Variola	Man
	Vaccinia	—
	Cowpox	Cattle, man
	Monkeypox	Monkeys, man
	Whitepox (?)	Monkeys
	Ectromelia (mousepox)	Mice
Avipoxvirus	Fowlpox	Fowl
Capripoxvirus	Sheeppox	Sheep, goats
Leporipoxvirus	Rabbit myxoma	Rabbits
	Rabbit fibroma	Rabbits
Parapoxvirus	Orf	Sheep, man
	Milkers' node	Cattle, man
Suipoxvirus	Swinepox	Swine
Ungrouped	Molluscum contagiosum	Man
	Yaba and Tanapox	Monkeys, man

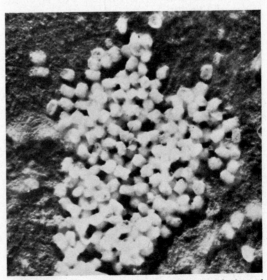

Figure 39–1. Electron micrograph of thin section through the chorioallantoic membrane of a 10-day chicken embryo 24 hours after inoculation with vaccinia virus. The numerous viral particles can be seen to possess a cuboidal or brick shape. × 15,000. (R. W. Wyckoff, Ztsch. Zellforsch., Vol. 38, 1953.)

preparations, the virions appear to be ovoid in shape (Fig. 39–2). The characteristic features of poxviruses are listed in Table 39–2.

Virion morphology is complex, with three major components, as exemplified in *Orthopoxvirus*. The **virion core**, composed of DNA and associated proteins, is biconcave in shape and surrounded by a core membrane. Two **lateral bodies**, located in the concavities of the core, are protein in composition; a **complex envelope** encloses these structures (see Fig. 38–4, p. 721). Superimposed on the external surface of the virion are tubular structures, consisting of a single species of polypeptide. In contrast to other enveloped viruses, the surface membrane of mature virions is synthesized *de novo* in the cytoplasm of the host cell, although an additional surface membrane is acquired if the virion is released by budding through the host cell plasma membrane.

Chemical Composition

As might be expected from their size and complexity, the chemical makeup of poxviruses is more nearly like that of procaryotic cells than other viruses. Proteins are the major constituents, composing about 90 per cent of the particle weight; DNA constitutes about 3 to 4 per cent of the weight, and lipid about 5 per cent.

The genome of poxviruses is dsDNA; the molecular weight varies from $85-90 \times 10^6$ daltons in *Parapoxvirus*, to $160-185 \times 10^6$ in *Avipoxvirus;* that of *Orthopoxvirus* is in the range of $120-130 \times 10^6$ daltons.

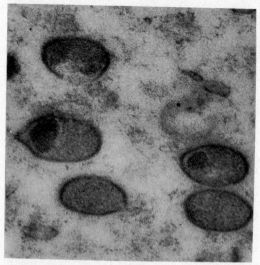

Figure 39–2. Electron micrograph of vaccinia virus in a section of infected chorioallantoic membrane showing the oval shape observed in some preparations. × 53,000. (C. Morgan, *et al.*, J. Exptl. Med. **100**:301, 1954.)

Table 39–2. **Properties of Poxviruses**

Brick-shaped virion, 200–250 × 250–300 nm.
Linear, dsDNA genome
Complex structure
Assembled in cytoplasm
Ether-resistant

Poxvirions possess a great variety of proteins; at least 30 polypeptides have been detected and it is likely that many more are present. Some of the virion proteins have enzymatic activities, *e.g.,* DNA-dependent RNA polymerase, nucleotide phosphohydrolase, deoxyribonuclease, and protein kinase; others represent structural proteins.

Replication

Infection and subsequent replication of poxvirus begins when the virus particle enters the host cell, probably by fusion of the virus envelope with the plasma membrane.[9]

Following uncoating, virion enzymes are released and activated, with subsequent synthesis of early RNA species. Release of core DNA is followed by transcription of early genes, with production of early structural proteins and enzymes associated with DNA synthesis. Progeny DNA is then synthesized, which specifies late RNA species with production of new virion enzymes and the majority of the structural proteins. Virions are assembled in the cell cytoplasm by complex processes that include *de novo* synthesis of viral membranes and the morphogenesis of the mature virion; mature virions are released by cell lysis or by budding through the plasma membrane.

Viruses are frequently seen in the cytoplasm of infected cells as cytoplasmic **inclusion bodies,** known as Guarnieri bodies in variola and vaccinia. These inclusions may be stained with polychrome stains such as Giemsa.

Antigenicity

The great number of proteins contained in poxvirions results in a complex antigenic structure for these viruses. All poxviruses share one or more antigens, while other antigens are specific to the genus or viral subgroup.

Some of the protein antigens are heat-stable, while others are heat-labile. The soluble antigen of variola and vaccinia is found free in infected tissues and appears to be a complex of heat-stable (S) and heat-labile (L) antigens; it is designated LS. These antigens may be demonstrated by complement fixation and probably represent early proteins of the replication cycle. Hemagglutinins are produced that agglutinate fowl erythrocytes, and their activity is specifically inhibited by antibody. Vaccinia virus also produces a protein cytolytic toxin. The protein tubules that appear on the surface membranes are associated with protection, since antibody to the purified material neutralizes viral infectivity.

Pathogenesis of Pox Disease

There is a considerable degree of host specificity among these viruses, but differences in the pathogenesis of the diseases they produce may be considered to be variations on the same theme. The proliferative response alluded to above, for example, is minimal in variola and vaccinia, but in some forms of fowlpox is so marked that the disease has been known as contagious epithelioma.

The viruses may be grouped on the basis of tissue tropisms, *e.g.*, the poxviruses are dermatropic; such tropisms are inferred from the site of the overt or predominant lesion. It is significant, however, that viral replication may occur without obvious damage in cells and tissues, apart from those in which the predominant lesions occur; such replication and dissemination may be an integral part of the pathogenesis of the disease. The occurrence of viremia, for example, exposes the virus to the action of humoral antibody and is fundamental to effective immunity to such a disease.

Many years ago, the sequence of events in the pathogenesis of mousepox was worked out in detail by Fenner, as shown in Figure 39–3.

This animal model of infection serves as a prototype for the exanthematous viral infections of humans, including smallpox. Clearly, during the incubation period of each infection, virus is widely disseminated in the tissues, multiplying in cells of organs and tissues other than the skin before the dermal lesions become apparent. As detailed in the following chapters, analogous phenomena also occur in infections with other kinds of viruses.

Several of the poxviruses infect humans, causing diseases with related clinical features (Table 39–3). Historically the most important of these was smallpox, but with its global eradication, attention has recently focused on the other infections.

SMALLPOX (VARIOLA)[5, 18]

Smallpox is an ancient disease that is known to have occurred in epidemic form in China as early as the twelfth century B.C., and was present in endemic and, from time to time, epidemic form in Asia, Africa, and the Middle East. It was widely disseminated in Europe during the Crusades, and was apparently introduced into the Western Hemisphere in the early sixteenth century, spreading into Central and South America, and the infections continued to be introduced by the slave trade.

Until the early twentieth century, smallpox was a common disease throughout the world. By 1950, immunization and other control

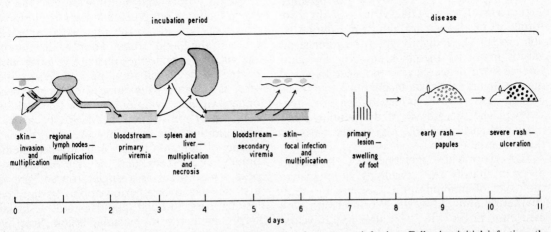

Figure 39–3. Diagrammatic representation of the pathogenesis of mousepox infection. Following initial infection, the virus multiplies in the skin and spreads to the regional lymphatics; it multiplies there within the first two days of the incubation period. The virus is then shed into the blood stream to give a primary viremia in the second and third days, spreading the infection to the spleen and liver, where it multiplies further and produces necrosis. Virus is again shed into the blood stream to give secondary viremia on the fourth and fifth days, spreading the infection to the skin to set up foci of infection on the sixth day. By the seventh day—the end of the incubation period—the primary lesion, a swelling of the footpads, occurs; a papular rash appears by the ninth day, which progresses to severe rash and ulceration by the eleventh day. (Redrawn from Fenner.)

Table 39–3. **Human Poxvirus Infections**

Name	Features
Smallpox (variola)	Exclusively human infection, characterized by contact transmission and generalized infection with pustular skin rash.
Vaccinia	Infection in humans usually purposefully engendered by vaccination. Limited contact transmission; localized infection with solitary pustule. Generalized infection and complications rarely follow vaccination.
Cowpox	Natural disease of cattle (rare), characterized by localized ulcers on teats and udder. Transmission to humans by contact; lesions resemble those of vaccinia.
Monkeypox	Natural disease of monkeys in Africa. Transmitted to man, directly or indirectly. Seen mostly in children. Clinically similar to smallpox, but limited case-to-case spread; mortality about 17%.
Orf	Natural disease of sheep and goats (scabby mouth). Contact transmission to humans, characterized by solitary papular lesions that heal without scars.
Milkers' node	Natural infection of cattle, transmitted to humans by contact. Clinically similar to cowpox, but virus not closely related to cowpox virus.
Molluscum contagiosum	Natural infection of humans, usually affecting children. Contact transmission, characterized by chronic, multiple skin nodules.
Yaba and Tanapox	Natural disease of monkeys, with benign skin tumors. Transmitted to humans, presumably by contact.

measures had largely eliminated smallpox from Europe and North America, but it continued to devastate Asia, Africa, and South America. In the latter areas, epidemics affected millions of persons and caused hundreds of thousands of deaths.

Smallpox occurred in two forms, differing markedly in severity. **Variola major** (malignant smallpox) was characterized by a case-fatality rate ranging from 10 per cent to as much as 40 per cent. The milder form, **variola minor** (alastrim), had a case-fatality rate of perhaps 1 per cent. The causative viruses of the two forms of the disease are almost indistinguishable except for a slightly greater virulence of variola major for the chick embryo. This difference in virulence may be enhanced by varying the temperature of incubation, thus permitting laboratory differentiation of the viruses. The diseases were differentiated on epidemiological grounds, *i.e.,* on the basis of the case-fatality rate.

The worldwide incidence of smallpox dropped sharply as a result of an intensive campaign of immunization, case-finding, and quarantine initiated by the World Health Organization in 1967. In 1977, after just 10 years of this international effort, what proved to be the last known case of smallpox was reported in Somalia.[11] On May 8, 1980, the World Health Assembly declared the global eradication of smallpox.[41] There is, therefore, every hope that smallpox has become a disease of only historical importance. Nevertheless, international surveillance continues, particularly with respect to possible, if unlikely, animal reservoirs of variola or similar viruses.

Smallpox in Man
Variola virus is resistant to drying, and the crusts from pustules are highly infectious. Human infection can be acquired by contact, direct or indirect, with such infectious material. There is reason to believe that in the typical disease primary infection occurs in the respiratory tract with multiplication of the virus in minimal, but possibly infectious, lesions. The virus spreads to the regional lymphatics and into the blood stream; after localization in the viscera, it multiplies during the latter part of the 12-day incubation period. When the virus is released from these sites to give secondary viremia, symptoms appear that include chills, fever, prostration, headache, backache, and vomiting. The secondary viremia gives rise to foci of infection in the skin, mucous membranes, and viscera, and the skin lesions appear. These occur as a single crop and are at first macular; over a period of 5 to 10 days the lesions pass through papular and vesicular stages, ending in the pustular lesion. Scarring typically results from these skin lesions.

Chemotherapy
The most common complication is secondary pyogenic bacterial infection. Antibiotic therapy is effective in minimizing these infections with consequent reduction in residual scarring,

although chemotherapeutic agents are ineffective against the virus infection.

Isatin β-thiosemicarbazone and some closely related compounds have been found to have antiviral activity in experimental poxvirus infections. This compound and its methyl derivative are effective against experimental variola, vaccinia, and cowpox, but inactive against mousepox. N-Methylisatin β-thiosemicarbazone has been tested in man and found to have marked prophylactic value in case contacts. The thiosemicarbazones appear to interfere with production of a core protein. Under experimental conditions, rifamycin is also active against poxviruses, interfering with virus maturation.

Immunity

Smallpox has been the classic example of infectious disease in which recovery is associated with the development of a highly effective and long-lasting immunity, and there is no doubt that the individual remains immune for many years. The immune response is evident in the appearance, during the course of the disease, of complement-fixing and hemagglutinin-inhibiting antibody activity, but these antibodies do not appear to be associated with effective immunity. Protection seems to be correlated with virus-neutralizing antibodies. Unlike complement-fixing and hemagglutinin-inhibiting antibodies that decline to insignificant levels in some 12 months, neutralizing antibodies are demonstrable for years.

There is a high degree of cross-immunity among the various kinds of poxviruses. For example, that between variola and vaccinia is of a high order and allows the use of a mild infection of the latter to produce an effective prophylactic immunity to smallpox in man (see below).

Laboratory Diagnosis[31]

Although smallpox has presumably been eradicated, exanthematous diseases with similar manifestations occur. Smallpox surveillance requires that all suspected cases of smallpox be promptly reported and diagnostic procedures initiated. Diseases that may resemble smallpox include generalized vaccinia, varicella, and, in Africa, human infections with the monkeypox virus.

Because of the possibilities of a laboratory-acquired infection, laboratory diagnosis of suspected smallpox is performed only in laboratories with rigid biocontainment capability, such as those at the Centers for Disease Control in the United States.

Orthopoxviruses can usually be cultivated and identified from clinical specimens such as scrapings, fluids, or crusts of the skin lesions, or from blood during the pre-eruptive phase of disease. Poxviruses can be identified by diagnostic tests that include (1) virus morphology as observed by electron microscopy, (2) antigenic analysis by immunoprecipitation in gels, (3) characteristic pock morphology during growth on the chorioallantoic membrane of chick embryos, and (4) characteristic cytopathogenic effect of tissue-cultured cells.

Poxvirus infection usually engenders antibodies detectable by complement fixation, precipitation, inhibition of viral hemagglutination, and virus neutralization. Diagnosis of smallpox by these serological methods is not satisfactory, however, because of the relatively late appearance of antibodies during the disease.

Experimental Infections

Natural variola infection occurs only in man and monkeys, but the virus is readily cultivable in cell culture or on the chorioallantoic membrane of the embryonated hen's egg, where it produces pock-like lesions (Figs. 39–4, 39–5); it may be maintained in serial passage in the yolk sac. The disease in monkeys is similar to that in man. Only minimal lesions are produced in the rabbit and the calf. It is extremely difficult to pass the infection serially in the rabbit, a characteristic that differentiates variola sharply from vaccinia, and on serial passage in the calf the virus loses its original

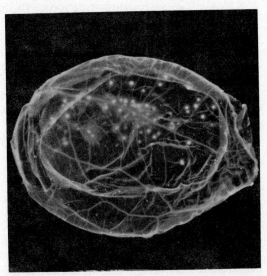

Figure 39–4. The gross appearance of the pock-like lesions produced by variola virus on the chorioallantoic membrane of the embryonated egg after 72 hours' incubation. Hematoxylin and eosin; × 100. (N. Hahon and M. Ratner, J. Bacteriol. **74**:696, 1957.)

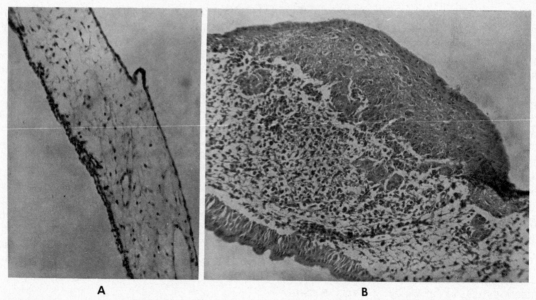

A   B

Figure 39–5. Sections of chorioallantoic membranes of 13-day embryonated eggs. A, Uninoculated; B, section through a variola lesion. Note the thickening of the membrane and discrete area of epithelial hyperplasia. × 100. (U.S. Army photograph, courtesy of Dr. N. Hahon.)

character and becomes vaccinia-like. The adult mouse may be infected by intracerebral inoculation, but massive doses are required to produce regular death patterns; the suckling mouse appears to be more susceptible.

VACCINIA

As noted earlier, recovery from smallpox yields a solid immunity to the disease. The development of such immunity appears to be dependent upon infection with variola or related viruses, of which vaccinia is the most important.

The practice of **variolation,** deliberate inoculation of man by ingestion or by application of the dried crusts of variola pustules to the skin or nasal mucous membranes, was common in the Orient in ancient times. It was introduced into Europe in 1718 by Lady Mary Wortley Montagu, wife of the British ambassador at Constantinople. The infection so produced was usually much less severe than naturally acquired smallpox and the mortality rate considerably less than that of the natural disease.

Meanwhile, it had been observed by a number of persons that those who contracted cowpox from infected cattle did not acquire smallpox upon subsequent exposure. Cowpox is a relatively mild disease in man, rarely fatal, in which the lesion is almost always limited to the site of inoculation. These casual observations were extended by Edward Jenner, who published his classic treatise on the relation of the two diseases in 1796. Prophylaxis of smallpox by inoculation with cowpox, or so-called Jennerian prophylaxis, was favorably received and widely applied.

Vaccinia Virus

It was assumed by Jenner that cowpox virus is variola virus adapted to the bovine host. The cow may be infected with variola, at first with insignificant lesions following intracutaneous inoculation, but on passage in this animal a vesiculopustular eruption is produced, which is similar to, but not identical with, that of naturally occurring cowpox. While variola, vaccinia, cowpox, and mousepox are related immunologically, antigenic differences may be discerned. In this respect vaccinia is found to be more closely related to variola than to cowpox, and in turn cowpox is more closely related to mousepox than to variola. The origin of vaccinia is obscure, but it is not identical with present-day cowpox. Possibly the vaccine strains first used by early vaccinators were poxviruses of other animal species, now extinct.[4] In this connection it is of interest that naturally acquired cowpox in man is somewhat more severe than vaccinia.

Vaccinia in Man

Vaccinia is almost always a purposefully acquired infection to produce immunity to smallpox. From time to time, however, it has occurred in localized epidemic form. It is almost always a mild localized disease in man; generalized vaccinia occurs rarely in the normal individual but may appear when a nonimmune child with previously existing skin lesions, *e.g.,* eczema, acquires vaccinia by contact.

Vaccination

Smallpox vaccine for human use is usually produced by vaccinia infection of calves and is the collected vesicular fluid from the skin lesions of these animals. The virus is inoculated subcutaneously into humans, usually by multiple needle punctures through a drop of vaccine placed on the skin.

After three to four days a papule appears, which becomes vesicular on the sixth or seventh day, progresses to a pustule at 10 to 12 days, and then regresses. Fever may occur from the fourth to eighth day, and there may be some tenderness and enlargement of the regional lymph nodes. The crust that forms on the pustule becomes detached about three weeks after inoculation, leaving a red pitted scar that turns white in time.

The foregoing reaction is that given by a fully susceptible individual and is sometimes called the **primary reaction.** It is modified in the partially or fully immune individual to give a **vaccinoid reaction** in the first instance and an **immune reaction** in the second. The vaccinoid reaction is similar to the primary reaction but accelerated and less severe. While there are gradations in the response, in general the papule appears at two days, and the maximum reaction is reached between three and seven days. The immune reaction consists of the development of a papule or shallow vesicle that reaches its maximum size in 8 to 72 hours, disappears without going through a pustular stage, and leaves no scar.

The protection conferred is of a high order but does not persist as long as that associated with recovery from variola. Susceptible contacts of cases of the disease may also be protected, provided that vaccine is given very early, within 48 hours, in the incubation period.

Although quite rare, complications have followed primary vaccination. Adverse reactions have included generalized vaccinia, postvaccinal encephalitis, and progressive vaccinia; the latter two have been responsible for deaths in vaccinated individuals. The risk of complications now far exceeds that of smallpox infection, and vaccination is not widely practiced;

it is recommended only in laboratory personnel handling the virus.

Experimental Infections

In contrast to variola virus, most laboratory animals may be infected with vaccinia virus, and it is readily cultivable on the chorioallantoic membrane of the embryonated egg, where it produces pocks closely similar to those of variola. The rabbit is the usual experimental animal, and infection is produced by all the customary routes of inoculation. The virus adapts relatively readily to growth on various kinds of tissues, and coincident alterations in virulence have resulted in strains producing encephalitis, orchitis, or pneumonia; strains may differ in other respects, such as pock morphology and heat resistance.

MONKEYPOX[3, 7, 40]

Monkeypox is one of the more recently discovered of the poxvirus diseases occurring in lower animals. The infection results in serious disease in orangutans and other nonhuman primates. The virus resembles variola major in producing pocks on the chorioallantoic membrane of the chick embryo at 38.3°C., but differs from it in producing hemorrhagic necrotic lesions in the rabbit skin and by its serial transmission in rabbits by intradermal inoculation. It is immunologically related to other orthopoxviruses; cynomolgus monkeys are protected against it by immunization with vaccinia or cowpox vaccines.

In 1970, the first human infection with monkeypox virus was recognized in Africa, and by 1982 a total of 62 cases had been reported, most occurring in children; the case-fatality rates have been about 17 per cent. The clinical disease resembles smallpox (Fig. 39–6), but does not usually give rise to secondary cases. Whether the disease is acquired directly from monkeys is not known with certainty, but circulating antibodies have been found in monkeys without overt disease, indicating both clinical and subclinical infections in these animals.

Whitepox Virus[18]

It has long been believed that no animal reservoir exists for the smallpox (variola) virus. Indeed, the eradication program by the World Health Organization was, in part, based on this conclusion. Some doubt was raised when variola-like viruses were isolated from mon-

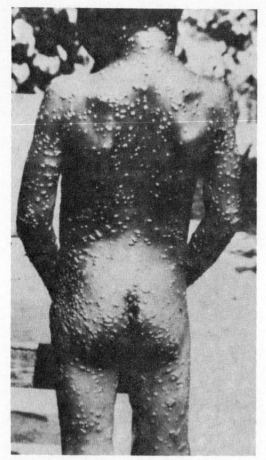

Figure 39–6. Monkeypox in a 7-year-old girl. (J. G. Breman, *et al.,* Bull. Wld Hlth Org. **58**:165, 1980.)

keys, first in Holland and later in Zaire. Because these isolates produced white pocks on chorioallantoic membranes of chick embryos (in common with variola viruses), they were called whitepox viruses. Only six strains have been isolated, two in Holland and four in Africa. The Holland strains almost certainly represent contamination with a true variola virus;[14] the African strains remain enigmatic, but are indistinguishable from variola.

Yaba and Tanapox Viruses[13, 44]
Two other diseases of monkeys caused by poxviruses have been reported. One, designated Tanapox, has been described as occurring in animals and man in the valley of the Tana River in Kenya. The other is a benign tumorous disease of monkeys, caused by the Yaba pox virus. Both may give rise to human infections, acquired from infected nonhuman primates. These viruses seem not to be im-

munologically related to one another or to other poxviruses.

OTHER POXVIRUS DISEASES

Cowpox
Cowpox is a mild, naturally occurring disease of cattle, characterized in the acute form by a vesicular eruption on the udder and teats. It is not a common disease, at least in the acute form. It is transmissible to man, as noted earlier in connection with Jenner's work, and the human disease is somewhat more severe than vaccinia. The virus is distinguished from variola and vaccinia in its hemorrhagic properties, apparent in the pocks formed on the chorioallantoic membrane of the chick embryo, and the vesicle fluid in bovine and human infections may contain blood. There is a cross-immunity between cowpox on the one hand and variola and vaccinia on the other, although minor antigenic differences are demonstrable. Cows may also acquire vaccinia from man.

Molluscum Contagiosum
This is an infectious disease of man caused by poxviruses not yet assigned to a genus. The disease is worldwide in distribution and occurs in both sporadic and epidemic form. The infection is spread by contact, and the disease is characterized by the occurrence of multiple nodules on the face, arms, back, and buttocks that are at first red, then pearly white, and undergo necrosis, with the discharge of caseous material. The disease is chronic, and the lesions persist over several months or years.

The lesion develops in the epidermis as thickened areas of hyperplasia and hypertrophy of the affected cells. These cells are enlarged and practically filled with an acidophilic granular inclusion body, or **molluscum body**, similar to those observed in other pox diseases. The inclusion body contains oval or brick-shaped virions 230 × 330 nm. in size. In ultrathin sections the virions are heterogeneous with respect to contained electron-dense material, and the several morphological types may be interpreted as representing a sequence of developmental stages.

It has not been possible to infect experimental animals with this virus or to grow it on the chorioallantoic membrane of the embryonated egg. Heat-labile soluble antigen, prepared as extracts of macerated infected tissue, fixes complement in the presence of serum from some patients and has been shown to be unrelated to the antigens of *Orthopoxvirus*.

The Herpesviruses[30, 33, 42, 43]

The herpesviruses encompass a large group of viruses affecting a wide variety of animals, including man. The Herpesviridae (Chap. 38) are enveloped icosahedral viruses containing linear, double-stranded DNA. The nucleocapsid is assembled in the nucleus and enveloped by budding through the nuclear membrane. The nucleocapsid is about 100 nm. in diameter, while the enveloped particle is somewhat larger, 120 to 200 nm.; the viruses are ether-sensitive. The characteristics of the human herpesviruses are summarized in Table 39–4.

The herpesviruses normally are lytic for the cells they infect, but an unusual feature of infection is the tendency of the virus to produce persistent or latent infections; in some cases they appear to be oncogenic. The mechanisms of latent infections are of considerable interest in relation to pathogenesis and epidemiology.

The human herpesviruses include the herpes simplex viruses, which cause herpes labialis or herpes genitalis; the varicella-zoster viruses, etiological agents of chickenpox and shingles; the Epstein-Barr virus, which is the agent of infectious mononucleosis and is associated with Burkitt's lymphoma; and cytomegalovirus, which is responsible for cytomegalic inclusion disease (Table 39–5).

Herpesviruses are also responsible for a great variety of animal infections, many of which exhibit a high degree of host-specificity and do not infect man. These viruses include most of the simian herpesviruses, as well as the herpesviruses of domestic and wild animals (cattle, horses, dogs, swine, chickens, and cats) and many lower vertebrates. In many instances, though not always, infections in lower animals are clinically inapparent. One of the simian viruses, designated B virus, was originally isolated from a fatal case of acute ascending myelitis in a laboratory worker who had been bitten by an apparently normal rhesus monkey, and there is reason to believe it is usually a benign disease in these animals, in contrast to the human infection, which has a high mortality rate.

Morphology and Structure

The viruses that make up the Herpesviridae are similar in structure and morphology. The innermost structure of the herpesvirion is the **core**, composed of the DNA genome coiled about a fibrillar protein spool. The surrounding **capsid** is an icosahedron with five capsomeres on each edge; there are 162 capsomeres in the capsid. Surrounding the capsid is the amorphous **tegumen**, variable in thickess and distribution, which is enclosed in the **viral envelope**. The envelope is a trilaminar membrane with glycoprotein spikes projecting from the outer surface (see Fig. 38–2, p. 720).

Replication

The infectious process begins when herpesvirions are adsorbed to receptors on the surface of the host cell. The virions enter the cytoplasm by fusion with the plasma membrane. After the particle is uncoated, the viral DNA–protein complex is translocated to the nucleus. Here the viral DNA is transcribed and mRNA is generated. Viral proteins are formed in the cytoplasm of the host cell, but viral assembly occurs in the nucleus. The capsid is enveloped by budding through the inner lamella of the nuclear membrane. Viral accumulations are then observed between the lamellae of the nuclear membrane and in the cisternae of the endocytoplasmic reticulum (Fig. 39–7).

HERPES SIMPLEX

Herpes simplex is a naturally occurring disease of man characterized by vesicular lesions in the epithelial layers of ectodermal tissue and the presence of intranuclear inclusion bodies in the affected cells. The presence of virus in both the nucleus and the cytoplasm of infected cells can be demonstrated by the fluorescent antibody technique.

Herpes simplex viruses are of two types, designated types 1 and 2 (HSV-1; HSV-2). Although they are immunologically similar, differences can be discerned by a variety of immunological procedures, including viral neutralization, immunofluorescence, and indirect hemagglutination inhibition. In addition, the two types differ in the location of lesions in the disease. Infections by HSV-1 generally

---

Table 39–4. **Properties of Human Herpesviruses**

Spherical virion, 120–200 nm.
Icosahedron, 162 capsomers
Linear, dsDNA genome
Assembled in nucleus of host cell
Enveloped (from nuclear membrane)
Ether-sensitive
Variable host range

Table 39–5. **Human Herpesvirus Infections**

Virus	Disease
Herpes simplex virus type 1	Herpes simplex, usually with oral or facial lesions (herpes labialis; cold sores; fever blisters)
Herpes simplex virus type 2	Herpes simplex, usually with lesions in the genital region (herpes genitalis) Cervical carcinoma (?)
Varicella-zoster virus	Chickenpox (varicella) Shingles (zoster)
Epstein-Barr virus	Infectious mononucleosis Burkitt's lymphoma (?) Nasopharyngeal carcinoma (?)
Cytomegalovirus	Cytomegalic inclusion disease (salivary gland disease) Pneumonitis Mononucleosis

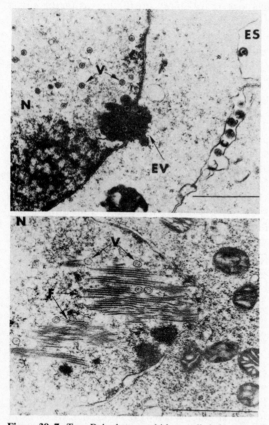

Figure 39–7. *Top,* Baby hamster kidney cells infected with herpes simplex virus type 1. Unenveloped viruses *(V)* are present in the nucleus *(N)*; enveloped virus particles *(EV)* are present at the nuclear membrane and in extracellular spaces *(Es)*. *Bottom,* cells infected with herpes simplex virus type 2. Note the presence of microtubule-like filamentous structures *(F)* in the nucleus. Bar = 1 μm. (S. K. Young, N. H. Rowe, and K. C. Sanderlin, J. Infect. Dis. **135**:486, 1977. Published by the University of Chicago Press. © 1977 by The University of Chicago. All rights reserved.)

occur "above the waist"— in the mouth, on the lips, and at other skin sites. Infections with HSV-2 usually appear "below the waist"— primarily in the genital region. The viruses also differ in other biological properties, such as cytopathic effect in cultured cells, pathogenesis in the chick embryo, and neurotropism in mice.

The Disease in Man[1, 2, 23, 26, 28, 50]

The vesicular lesions of herpes begin as a local burning sensation, followed by the appearance of papules which become vesicular and coalesce to form groups of thin-walled vesicles. The vesicular fluid contains epithelial cells and multinucleated giant cells with inclusions present in nuclei, and the fluid is infectious. The vesicles rupture, scabs are formed, and healing occurs without scarring.

The character of herpetic infections of humans is determined by the type of herpesvirus involved. Infections with HSV-1 tend to be spread by the oral-respiratory route and exhibit the symptoms of classic herpes labialis. On the other hand, HSV-2 infections, often termed herpes genitalis, are usually transmitted by sexual contact and are characterized by lesions in the genital region. These distinctions are not absolute, however; HSV-1 is occasionally found in genital infections and HSV-2 in oral infections. The lesions are similar in both kinds of infection, differing primarily in location.

Herpetic infections in man are manifest in a predictable sequence. Upon first infective contact with herpesvirus, a **primary**, or **initial**, **infection** results, often with severe, sometimes fatal, systemic effects. The primary infection occurs in those individuals without neutralizing serum antibodies and, therefore, without prior infection. A primary infection with one type does not, however, preclude a later primary infection with the other type, since they are not immunologically identical. Following this initial infection, the virus is not eliminated from the host, but rather becomes latent. At a later time, the occult infection may be activated as a **recurrent form**. Recurrent herpes, of either type, is seen in persons with neutralizing serum antibody and is characterized by appearance of local lesions, but with minor or no systemic effects.

Primary Herpes. Acute primary infections with HSV-1 virus occur relatively early in life. Infants have an effective passive immunity, and infection seldom occurs in the first six months of life. By six years of age the proportion of individuals showing the presence of neutralizing antibody is increasing rapidly, and in adults the proportion of immunes is associated with economic status, 50 per cent or more at high economic levels and 90 per cent or more in lower income groups. The incidence of the primary type of infection is not sufficient to account for the high incidence of neutralizing antibody in adults, lending support to the view that most initial infections are subclinical or asymptomatic. Although these inapparent infections may induce antibody formation, not all such infections result in latent carriage of the virus.

In nonimmunes the vesicular eruption commonly occurs in the mouth to give an acute herpetic gingivostomatitis in which the vesicular eruption appears as plaques and shallow ulcers; the tonsillar region may be affected, and the gums are often involved. This condition is to be differentiated from herpangina caused by Coxsackie viruses. The submaxillary lymphatics may become swollen and tender, and there is a constitutional reaction of varying severity, including high fever. Occasionally the virus invades the blood stream to give rise to a generalized vesicular eruption known as eczema herpeticum or Kaposi's varicelliform eruption, which may simulate mild variola, generalized vaccinia, or severe varicella. The eye may be infected, with the production of herpetic keratoconjunctivitis, or the central nervous system involved to give a herpetic meningoencephalitis (Fig. 39–8). There is reason to believe that in the last instance the infection reaches the central nervous system via the peripheral nerves rather than by the

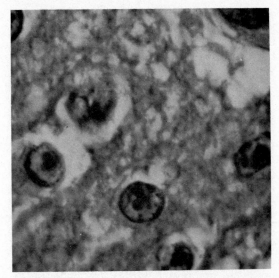

Figure 39–8. Intranuclear herpetic inclusion bodies of the human brain. (Armed Forces Institute of Pathology. No. 102644.)

hematogenous route. While primary herpes may be fatal, it is usually a self-limited infection, persisting for perhaps two weeks.

Herpes genitalis is considered to be a venereally transmitted disease. The disease tends to appear later in life than classic herpes simplex, and coincides with the onset of puberty and active sexual contact. The likelihood of infection is greater with increased sexual activity and number of different sexual partners. Herpes genitalis is now one of the most prevalent venereal diseases in the United States.

In women, the primary disease is usually mild or asymptomatic. The lesions are not unlike those described above and appear in the vulva, vagina, cervix, and perineum. In males the lesions are more obvious and are found on the glans, prepuce, or penile shaft.

Infants born of mothers with genital infections may contract neonatal herpes during passage through the birth canal. Neonatal herpes may be relatively asymptomatic, particularly if maternal antibody is present, or it may constitute a severe systemic disease, often with nervous system involvement, and is sometimes fatal. In surviving infants there may be residual damage to the central nervous system. In the rare cases of infection *in utero,* congenital malformations may result.

Recurrent Herpes.[47] Following primary infection, the disease is usually contained by the combined humoral and cell-mediated immune defenses of the host. Although the immune response results in clinical recovery from the primary infection, it does not result in eradication of the virus. Rather, the virus enters a latent state and can later be activated by a variety of nonspecific stimuli.

The sheltered site for the latent infection appears to be the neurons of the sensory ganglia serving the region of the primary infection. As the primary lesions subside, virus travels along the axons to the ganglia, usually the trigeminal ganglion in the oral primary infection and the sacral ganglion in genital herpes. The nature of the latent virus is not yet settled, but one of two possibilities is thought to obtain. In the first postulated case, a dynamic latent infection is thought to exist in which small numbers of infected cells continue to shed virus over extended periods; however, the host defenses are believed to prevent the appearance of active lesions. An alternative view is that the virus genome exists within the neurons in a nonreplicative or static state, perhaps integrated into the host cell chromosomes. The available evidence tends to support the latter, or static state, hypothesis.

Recurrent herpes then results upon reactivation of the latent infection, brought about in various nonspecific ways. Often the stimulus is a febrile reaction, so that herpes may appear during convalescence from other diseases, or it may follow physical shock, such as chilling; metabolic or hormonal disturbance, such as menstruation; exposure to ultraviolet light; or a wide variety of other stimuli. Individuals vary widely in their susceptibility to recurrent infection, *i.e.*, in the intensity of the nonspecific stimulus required to induce recrudescence.

In recurrent herpes the virus travels along the axons to the peripheral site, where new lesions appear. The disease is usually limited to a local vesicular lesion, presumably because of modification of the disease process by preexisting immunity. The eruption usually appears at mucocutaneous junctures, such as the border of the lips or nares (fever blisters, cold sores). It may also occur on the genitalia (herpes genitalis) of either sex—on the glans penis or corona in the male, and on the labia and lower vaginal mucous membranes in the female. In any case, the lesions tend to recur in the same location in successive recrudescences in a given individual.

Cervical Carcinoma.[20, 35, 39] Particular interest has attached to HSV-2 genital infections in the female in connection with cervical carcinoma. Significant association of genital herpes infection with the development of such carcinomas has been observed, and serological evidence supports an association of the virus with this type of malignancy. In addition, herpes simplex virus DNA can induce changes in animal cells that cause them to be tumorigenic, and virus-specific RNA and viral antigens can be detected in cervical carcinoma cells. In view of these and related observations, there is a presumption favoring a relationship of HSV-2 to at least some cases of cervical carcinoma.

Chemotherapy[19]

The treatment of oral and genital HSV infections with chemotherapeutic agents has not been very successful, despite perennial reports to the contrary. Therapeutic attempts have generally involved the use of nucleoside analogs, interferon, and viral inactivators such as ether or photodynamic inactivation with certain dyes. Topical therapy with chemotherapeutic agents is intended to lessen the severity or reduce the duration of skin lesions, and is without effect on viruses already infecting the neural tissues. In controlled trials with iododeoxyuridine and other nucleoside analogs, little or no beneficial effect is evident.

Systemic treatment has had only limited effect. Results with interferon have been conflicting, while adenine arabinoside may shorten the clinical course in immunosuppressed individuals. Animal trials, using acyclovir (acycloguanosine) and bromovinyldeoxyuridine are promising, but controlled clinical trials are not yet complete. These latter two drugs accumulate specifically in virally infected cells and act by interfering with DNA polymerase, thereby inhibiting viral replication. This specific mode of action against viruses is reminiscent of some of the effective antibacterial drugs.

Greater success has attended the use of local antiviral agents in ocular infections. The drugs most often used have included iododeoxyuridine and vitarabine (Ara-A); acyclovir has been effective topically and holds promise as a systemically administered drug.

Immunity

As indicated above, recovery from primary herpes infection is associated with the appearance of neutralizing antibody in the serum that may be titrated in tissue culture. It modifies subsequent recurrent disease but does not prevent it. Complement-fixing antibody appears concurrently, and both antibodies reach peak titer in two to three weeks. Antibodies to the viral surface glycoproteins are responsible for viral neutralization and are thus believed to be protective. Cellular immunity, indicated in

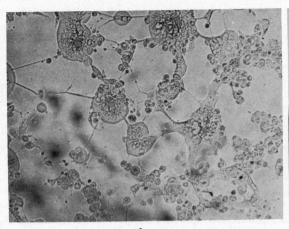 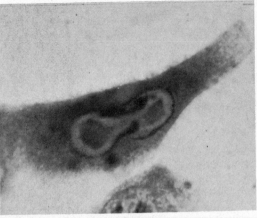

A   B

Figure 39–9. Herpesvirus in HeLa culture. *A*, One kind of cytopathology produced by the virus, characterized by the formation of multinucleated giant cells joined by cytoplasmic bridges. × 100. *B*, An infected cell showing division of the nucleus and an inclusion body in each of the daughter nuclei. × 1000. (A. Gray *et al.*, Arch. ges. Virusforsch. **8**:59, 1958.)

part by the skin reaction and in part by other *in vitro* correlates, appears to be of considerable importance in effective immunity. Cell-mediated immune defects or immunosuppressive therapy lead to increased susceptibility to disseminated herpes infection. There is also evidence to suggest that recurrent herpes may be due to temporary or local diminution of cellular immunity and that this deficiency may be induced by the virus.

Vaccination, with killed or attenuated virus, has yielded immunity in animals, but the possibility of oncogenesis by viral DNA makes these vaccines unsuitable for use in humans. Subunit vaccines, using purified glycoprotein antigens, may offer hope for immunoprophylaxis, but much additional study is required.

Experimental Infections

The virus may be grown on various kinds of tissue cultures, exhibiting cytopathic effects (Fig. 39–9). It may also be cultivated on the chorioallantoic membrane of embryonated hen's egg, forming pock-like plaques on the membrane somewhat different from the larger, deeper necrotic pocks produced by variola and vaccinia viruses. The common laboratory animals, including rabbits, mice, hamsters, and rats, may be infected by various routes of inoculation, with the results depending somewhat upon the relative dermatropic or neurotropic tendencies of the virus strain. Inoculation of the rabbit cornea results in keratoconjunctivitis and corneal opacity. Intracerebral inoculation results in encephalitis, which may also occur in the rabbit following corneal inoculation with a neurotropic strain of the virus.

VARICELLA AND ZOSTER

Varicella (chickenpox) and zoster (shingles) are exanthematous diseases of man characterized by a vesicular eruption and the presence of acidophilic intranuclear inclusion bodies in the affected cells. A single virus is responsible for both disease syndromes, and zoster is considered to be a reactivation form of varicella.

The morphology of the virus particle is closely similar to that of the herpes simplex virus as observed in vesicular fluid, and intranuclear inclusions are produced in cell culture (Fig. 39–10). It is cultured with some difficulty

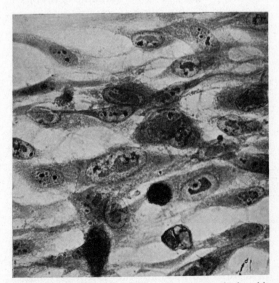

Figure 39–10. Varicella. Fifth culture passage in foreskin tissue of fluid from varicella lesion. Focus of cells with intranuclear inclusions on sixth day after inoculation. × 550. (T. H. Weller, Proc. Soc. Exptl. Biol. Med. **83**:340, 1953.)

in human cell cultures, including human fore-skin, amnion, lung fibroblasts, and primary thyroid cell cultures. Serial passage usually requires transfer of infected cells, but heavily infected thyroid cells have been reported to release infective virus into the medium. It has not been possible to infect experimental animals other than monkeys and guinea pigs.

Varicella

Chickenpox is a common, highly contagious exanthematous disease of childhood which occurs in epidemic form. The infection is usually benign in children, but is more severe in adults and in immunocompromised individuals. After an incubation period of two to three weeks, there is a febrile reaction, and a macular eruption appears that progresses to the vesicular stage and may become pustular. These lesions occur in successive crops and may be observed in all stages of development. The varicella lesion is unilocular even at an early stage and can be distinguished from the early multilocular vesicle of variola-vaccinia infections. In adults, but apparently not in children, a primary varicella pneumonia may be seen in a small portion of those with chickenpox, and is among the more serious complications.

Some neurotropic tendency of the virus is evident in this disease by the rare occurrence of encephalitis as a complication, and there may be neuritis of the cranial nerves. The disease is not affected by antibiotics, but these are useful in minimizing secondary bacterial infection of the lesions. Immune globulin is prophylactic, indicating that immunity to infection is associated with circulating antibody.

Zoster[8]

The vesicular eruption of zoster, or shingles, is substantially identical with that of varicella, but the disease is distinguished from varicella by its sporadic occurrence in adults, inflammation in spinal or extramedullary ganglia accompanied by severe pain localized to some portion of the involved nerve, and the tendency of the vesicular eruption to follow the distribution of one or more cutaneous sensory nerves, usually of the torso.

The disease is initiated by a febrile reaction, general malaise, and extreme tenderness along the dorsal nerve routes. A macular eruption appears within three to four days that becomes vesicular, and pustular when secondary bacterial infection occurs. The dorsal roots of the trunk are most often affected, but involvement of the maxillary or mandibular divisions of the trigeminal nerve may occur, with vesicular lesions in the tonsillar area or buccal mucosa; the ophthalmic division may be affected with scleritis and lesions of the cornea and conjunctiva; or involvement of the geniculate ganglion with corresponding vesicular lesions may occur. Meningoencephalitis is an uncommon complication, and persistent neuralgia tends to occur in older persons. It is clear that the neurotropic tendencies of the virus are much more marked in zoster than in varicella.

Relation of Varicella and Zoster

It has long been apparent that these diseases are intimately related. While varicella occurs largely in children and zoster in adults, the identity of the virus is indicated by the observation that the zoster virus can be transmitted to children, resulting in a primary varicella infection. Zoster occurs predominantly in those individuals, usually older adults, who have had earlier varicella infections, and, in parallel with recurrent herpes, is considered to represent activation of a latent infection.

Following the primary varicella infection, the virus becomes latent in the sensory ganglia; the form of the virus in the ganglion and its mode of transit to this site are not as clear as in herpes simplex infection, but the virus has been isolated from human dorsal root ganglia. Reactivation usually follows a perturbation in cell-mediated immunity, as by immunosuppression or, rarely, by contact with individuals with varicella infection. Thus, zoster is seen in older persons, often in those with malignancy. Cell-mediated immunity, perhaps coupled with circulating antibody, is thought to protect against activation of the latent infection. Chemotherapy with adenine arabinoside or bromovinyldeoxyuridine reduces the duration and severity of illness.

EPSTEIN-BARR VIRUS[25]

The Epstein-Barr (EB) virus was first discovered in the 1960s in continuous culture of cells derived from Burkitt's lymphoma, a tumor appearing mostly in African children. The history and scientific interest in the virus has been linked to its association with this human malignancy. Soon after it was discovered, it became apparent that EB virus was the etiological agent of infectious mononucleosis, a disease long recognized but with an obscure origin.

The possible relationship of EB virus to Burkitt's lymphoma led to extensive studies on the virus that have brought an understanding of its biology and chemistry.

Perhaps the most striking characteristic of EB virus is its ability to enter a latent state in infected cells. A preponderant majority of adult humans have suffered previous EB infections, either as inapparent infections of childhood or as later clinical episodes of infectious mononucleosis. Almost all adults, then, carry EB virus as latent infections in B lymphocytes. Latently infected cells are transformed so that they are capable of sustained growth in tissue culture, in contrast to uninfected B lymphocytes, which rapidly become senescent. In many individuals, EB virus is shed for long periods in the oropharyngeal secretions following primary infection, indicating that some cells are permissive for virus production. The proliferation of virus-infected cells in normal individuals is held in check both by specific immune events and by nonspecific resistance factors, including interferon.

The EB virus is morphologically and structurally similar to other herpesviruses, but it is antigenically unique and thus differentiable. The virion genome is linear, double-stranded DNA. After the virus enters a susceptible cell, the DNA circularizes and persists in the nucleus as an episome, usually in multiple copies. Infected cells also express two viral intranuclear antigens, as well as a new antigen on the cell surface. As will be noted later, these viral characteristics relate to the possible role of EB virus in tumor induction.

INFECTIOUS MONONUCLEOSIS[16]

Infectious mononucleosis is an acute infectious disease occurring in children and young adults, characterized by an increased number of monocytes and large lymphocytes in the blood, angina, lymphadenitis, and the presence of heterophile antibody in the serum.

Etiology
Infectious mononucleosis is a clinical entity of possibly diverse etiology. The vast majority of these infections are, however, characterized by the appearance of heterophile agglutinins (see below) and there is now little doubt that heterophile-positive infectious mononucleosis is due to the EB virus.

An encompassing hypothesis, bolstered by epidemiological, serological, and genetic evidence, has been advanced by Epstein and Achong[15] to explain the interrelationships of the infections caused by EB virus. Epstein-Barr virus infection appears to be worldwide in occurrence and of exceptionally high prevalence, as shown by serological findings.

Very young children are not infected, since they are protected against infection by maternally derived antibodies. As this protection wanes, inapparent infections begin, and in lower socioeconomic groups most children are infected by the age of puberty. The disease is usually without overt signs and affects up to about 80 per cent of the population. In higher socioeconomic groups, many children escape infection during early years and a greater proportion are infected as young adults. In contrast to the usually subclinical childhood infections, about half of those contracting the infection after adolescence develop infectious mononucleosis in clinically observable form. The disease is thought to be transmitted by intimate contact, such as kissing, and has, in fact, been called "kissing disease."

The antibody response to both inapparent and overt infection is marked by the production of virus-specific antibodies. These are protective against subsequent exogenous infection, but the virus is not eliminated. As noted above, the virus is harbored in B lymphocytes as a nonproductive, latent infection, or it may be persistent, as shown by the continued shedding of the virus in oral secretions without other signs of infection.

The Disease in Man
The onset of infectious mononucleosis may be acute or insidious and is characterized by loss of appetite and fatigue. Systemic involvement is indicated by the febrile reaction and symptoms, such as epistaxis, nausea, vomiting, and headache; the cervical lymph nodes become swollen and tender, and there is angina, ranging in severity from mild hyperemia to a pseudomembranous ulcerating form. A cutaneous rash appears in some individuals; there may be conjunctivitis and liver damage, and the central nervous system is occasionally involved. The white blood cell count increases, to as much as 80,000 per cu. mm., with the differential count showing a decrease of polymorphonuclear leucocytes and a marked increase in monocytes, to give a characteristic blood picture.

Serology
Prior to the discovery of the EB virus and the advent of specific serological tests, the serological evidence of infectious mononucleosis was dependent upon the agglutination of sheep erythrocytes by patients' serum—the

Paul-Bunnell test. This nonspecific test is easily performed and still widely used, but is advantageously supplemented with virus-specific procedures. Specific serum antibody response may be detected by indirect immunofluorescence; antibodies may be directed against virion antigens, including the viral capsid antigen (VCA) and the EB nuclear antigen, or against a nonvirion but virus-specified antigen, termed the early antigen (EA). Although virus neutralizing antibody is produced, its detection is technically complex owing to the difficulty in cultivating the virus in vitro.

BURKITT'S LYMPHOMA[10, 51]

Burkitt's lymphoma is a malignant neoplasm of B lymphocytes, found primarily in children in certain areas of Africa and New Guinea. Although its frequency of occurrence is higher in these geographical locations, sporadic cases occur throughout the world. The geographical incidence of the disease prompted the search for a possible viral agent, which culminated in the discovery of the EB virus. Whereas the etiological role of EB virus in Burkitt's lymphoma is not as strongly supported as in infectious mononucleosis, the association is striking. The likelihood is strengthened by similarities in the lymphoproliferative response—malignant in Burkitt's lymphoma but more benign in the case of infectious mononucleosis.

Although EB virus particles cannot be demonstrated within Burkitt's tumor cells in situ, there is immunological evidence for the presence of virus-specified antigens on the cell surface; furthermore, tumor cells produce EB virus when cultured in vitro. This and other evidence is convincing that the EB virus genome is present in tumor cells, existing as a latent infection. It has been noted above that the EB virus is horizontally transmitted and silent EB virus infections occur in a majority of individuals. An important question then arises as to the mechanism of tumor induction in such a small proportion of infected individuals. It is reasonable to assume that in the majority of EB virus infections, the host immune responses, particularly those of cellular immunity, are sufficiently effective to prevent activation as either infectious mononucleosis or tumor induction. Selective impairment of this immunity could lead to tumor formation or to infectious mononucleosis. Malignancy is thought to result from an unusual change in one or a few latently infected cells, possibly a chromosomal translocation, permitting the cell to escape host immune surveillance. It has been suggested that latent infections by EB virus might be an antecedent step in malignant transformation; alternatively, EB virus may be a "passenger" that infects malignant lymphocytes.

In those areas of the world where Burkitt's lymphoma appears in highest incidence, there is an epidemiological association with malaria. It has been proposed that malaria infection may be a precipitating cofactor for tumor production in EB virus–infected individuals. It is of interest that regional eradication of malaria has led to reduced incidence of Burkitt's lymphoma.

The EB virus has also been associated with another malignant disease, nasopharyngeal carcinoma, found in highest incidence in certain Chinese groups. Genetic susceptibility and, possibly, another virus cofactor appear to be the major determinants for tumor induction in these infected individuals.

CYTOMEGALOVIRUS[27, 36]

A disease known as cytomegalic inclusion disease occurs widely in man and a number of animal species. As the name suggests, it is characterized by cellular gigantism and intranuclear inclusions (and sometimes small, compact intracytoplasmic inclusions) present within affected cells. The size and structure of these "owl-eye" inclusions tend to set them apart from inclusions in other viral diseases (Fig. 39–11). The disease is caused by a group of closely related but highly species-specific herpesviruses.

Cytomegaloviruses (CMV) are morphologically and structurally similar to other human herpesviruses, although the genome is larger, about 145×10^6 daltons. In common with other herpesviruses, they produce both persistent and latent infections, in addition to acute infections. They are antigenically distinct from other herpesviruses. All CMV share complement-fixing antigens, but they are otherwise antigenically heterogeneous. Cytomegaloviruses are somewhat unstable, and infectivity is rapidly lost upon storage at $-20°$ or $37°$ C.

The Disease in Man
Although the vast majority of human CMV infections are asymptomatic, individuals at greatest risk of clinically apparent disease are the perinatally infected, the immunosup-

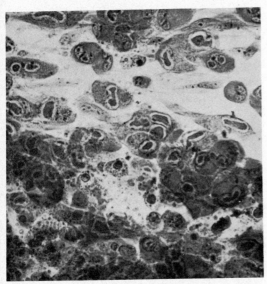

Figure 39–11. Salivary gland virus in human foreskin tissue culture showing the edge of a focal lesion, with central degeneration and infected cells at the periphery. Hematoxylin and eosin; × 360. (T. H. Weller, *et al.* Proc. Soc. Exptl. Biol. Med. **94**:4, 1957.)

pressed, and those receiving blood transfusions or organ transplants. Cytomegalovirus infections are the most frequent perinatally acquired infections and are the infections most often responsible for congenital abnormalities.

Congenital Infections. The fetus may be infected *in utero,* by transmission of CMV through the placenta from the mother; congenital infections occur in about 1 per cent of births. Most infected infants—about 90 per cent—are asymptomatic at birth, although up to 17 per cent may exhibit later neurological symptoms such as decreased mentation and auditory impairment.

Infants that display clinical symptoms at birth are viruric, a condition that may persist for months to years, and viruses are also shed in saliva and nasopharyngeal secretions. Illness in these individuals may range from mild to lethal; prominent findings include hepatosplenomegaly, jaundice, thrombocytopenic purpura, and petechial rash. More serious manifestations arise from chronic intrauterine encephalitis; those severely affected are microcephalic at birth and exhibit optic atrophy, chorioretinitis, and cerebral calcification.

Natal Infections. A substantial number of all infants—up to 20 per cent—are infected at birth by exposure to CMV from the cervical secretions of the mother; others are thought to become infected by ingestion of virus present in mothers' milk. Viruria and shedding of the virus usually begins some weeks post partum and, as in other groups, the vast majority are subclinical. Symptoms of apparent infection in this group include pneumonitis, lymphadenopathy, hepatosplenomegaly, and rash.

It is apparent that CMV infection in pregnant women is an important health problem, primarily because of transmission to their offspring. Cytomegalovirus infections in adults are usually latent and are widespread. Latent infections in women tend to reactivate during pregnancy. While these reactivated infections pose little hazard to the mother, transmission to the offspring is facilitated. In most instances, the mother is immune to effects of CMV, and circulating antibody is usually evident. Maternal immunity, however, does not prevent infection of the fetus, but these infections are usually asymptomatic.

Adult Infections. Serological and cultural surveys indicate that CMV infections of adults are very common. An overwhelming proportion are inapparent, either as latent infection, in which virus is not produced, or as persistent infection with only low levels of virus production and excretion. The proportion of infected individuals rises gradually from childhood and reaches a peak in young adults. In industrialized nations, about 40 per cent of adults are seropositive for CMV, whereas the level often reaches 100 per cent in developing nations with poor socioeconomic conditions. Transmission of the virus is facilitated by close contact between individuals; the incidence rises after puberty, since the virus can be transmitted by sexual contact, either heterosexual or homosexual.

The primary syndrome of CMV infections in otherwise healthy adults is a **mononucleosis** that resembles EB virus mononucleosis, both clinically and epidemiologically. It is characterized by fever and malaise, frequently with mild hepatitis and splenomegaly. As in EB mononucleosis, atypical lymphocytes are increased, but heterophile antibodies are not formed. It is believed that this syndrome usually follows a primary rather than recurrent infection by CMV.

Protection against both perinatal and adult infection is thought to be due to stimulation of cell-mediated immunity. This aspect of immunity is slow to develop in most instances and thought to be attributable to an immunosuppressive effect by the virus. Consonant with these beliefs is the greater incidence of disease observed in persons with malignancies associated with abnormalities of the immune system.

Iatrogenic Infections.[21] Infections with CMV can be transmitted by blood transfusion, particularly when large quantities of blood are transfused. Although most infections of this type are asymptomatic, CMV mononucleosis has been observed in these patients.

There is also a high incidence of CMV infections in recipients of renal transplants, particularly when immunosuppressants are administered; donor kidneys are believed to be the source of virus. Symptoms of overt illness include mononucleosis, hepatitis, or pulmonary disease. Similarly, individuals undergoing immunosuppressive therapy are at higher risk of CMV disease.

Laboratory Diagnosis[46]
Significant aids to the diagnosis of CMV infections include characteristic histopathology of tissue sections, isolation of the virus, and serology.

Virus can usually be isolated from tissues or body fluids, principally urine and throat washings, by inoculating human fibroblast cell cultures; other types of cell cultures routinely used in clinical laboratories will not support growth of CMV. Cytopathic effects by CMV are distinctive, and the virus can be identified by immunofluorescent microscopy.

The most useful serological tests for CMV infection is complement fixation, although a variety of immunofluorescent assays have been advanced that are more accurate and can aid in differentiating primary and recurrent infections.

Immunization[34]
The failure of chemotherapy in CMV infections has prompted interest in immunoprophylaxis. Immunization is seen as particularly advantageous in selected groups, *e.g.*, allograft recipients. Immunization studies have generally employed attenuated strains of CMV that are believed to induce both humoral and cell-mediated immunity. For the most part, these studies have not demonstrated great efficacy and are further inhibited by the antigenic heterogeneity of CMV.

The Papovaviruses[17, 48]

Members of the family Papovaviridae are icosahedral in symmetry, contain circular DNA genomes, and do not possess envelopes. Two genera are recognized: *Papillomavirus,* which causes wart-like growths in man and a variety of animals, and *Miopapovavirus,* which includes several viruses that produce vacuolation in tissue culture cells and a variety of neoplasias in animals; several have been linked to multifocal leukoencephalopathy in man. The important properties of these two genera are shown in Table 39–6.

THE PAPILLOMA VIRUSES[52]

Wart Viruses
For a number of years it was believed that the skin and genital warts of humans were manifestations of a single virus. It is now recognized that there are several types of papilloma viruses that cause these growths. These viruses are, nevertheless, similar and none have been consistently grown in cell cultures; consequently, their biology is not as well understood as that of other papovaviruses. Figure 39–12 shows their typical morphology. The human papilloma viruses have been shown to be infectious in humans, and the disease can be experimentally transmitted from man to man, with production of warts after an

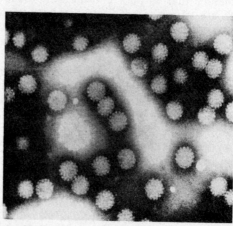

Figure 39–12. Human papillomavirus from a common wart. × 109,000. (H. zur Hausen, Curr. Topics Microbiol. Immunol. **78**:1, 1977.)

Table 39–6. **Properties of Papovaviruses**

	Papillomavirus	Miopapovavirus
Virion size	45 nm.	55 nm.
Capsid	Icosahedron	Icosahedron
Genome	Circular dsDNA, 5×10^6 daltons	Circular dsDNA, 3×10^6 daltons
Replication	Nuclear	Nuclear

incubation period of several months. The tumors are benign and usually occur as solid epithelial proliferations localized in skin and mucosa. The virus is seen in nuclei of infected cells as crystalline aggregates. Three types of tumors are distinguished: flat warts without papillary hyperplasia; common warts with varying degrees of papillary hyperplasia and a verrucous surface; and condyloma acuminata, or genital warts, characterized by marked proliferation and little keratinization.

The infection is transmitted by close contact between individuals, sexual in the case of genital warts; minor skin trauma or irritation are predisposing factors.

Interest has focused on human papilloma viruses as possible initiators of malignant conditions. Indeed, genital warts (but not other skin warts) sometimes exhibit malignant conversion, and many regard condyloma acuminata as premalignant lesions. There is, however, a long latent period, lasting many years before conversion appears. Although malignant cells do arise in these lesions, a role for papilloma viruses in their pathogenesis is only speculative.

HUMAN POLYOMA VIRUSES

A primate polyoma virus, SV40 (simian virus 40), is commonly found in rhesus and cynomolgus monkey kidney tissue, and was originally discovered as a contaminant of monkey kidney cell cultures and of virus vaccines prepared in such cultures. The SV40 virus is readily cultivable in tissue cultures; in cells derived from monkeys, the virus produces a unique cytopathic effect characterized by ballooning and vacuolation of the infected cells. Although these viruses do not cause neoplastic disease in their natural hosts, newborn hamster kidney cells are transformed in tissue culture, and tumors are produced by inoculation of neonatal hamsters. A similar, but not identical, virus has been isolated from human disease, notably from cases of progressive multifocal leukoencephalopathy.

In 1971, two additional human polyoma viruses, designated BK and JC, were isolated from humans; each is antigenically distinct, but they share antigens with one another and with SV40. These primate polyoma viruses thus constitute a cluster of viruses, related in some degree to one another, but immunologically unrelated to the polyoma viruses of lower animals, such as the murine polyoma virus.

Both the BK and JC viruses are widely distributed, and inapparent infections are common in humans, presumably acquired during childhood; the BK virus is apparently not responsible for any known disease process, whereas rare brain infections with JC virus result in progressive multifocal leukoencephalopathy (PML) (Fig. 39–13). The virion of BK and JC viruses hemagglutinates human, guinea

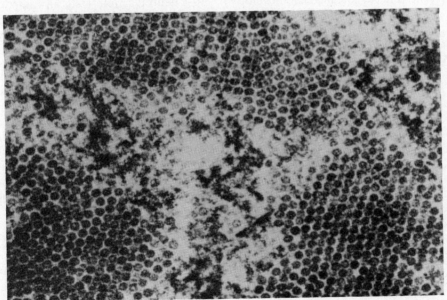

Figure 39–13. Papovavirions in progressive multifocal leukoencephalopathy. Electron micrograph showing a portion of glial nucleus containing crystalline aggregates of viruses. × 71,000. (K. K. Takemoto, Internat. Rev. Exptl Pathol. **18**:281, 1978. Photograph by Dr. Gabrielle Zurhein.)

pig, and chicken erythrocytes; thus, hemagglutination-inhibition by immune serum permits seroepidemiological surveys for their prevalence in human populations. Although not extensive, the available evidence indicates that, by adolescence, antibodies to BK virus appear in 75 per cent or more of the population; the prevalence of JC virus is somewhat less—about 65 to 75 per cent of the adult population possess serum antibodies.

The viruses may be grown in human cells in tissue cultures. The BK virus is rarely shed from infected individuals; most isolations have been from urine of those with defective immunity or undergoing immunosuppressive therapy. The JC virus is more difficult to cultivate, as it grows poorly, and only in primary human fetal glial cell cultures; it has been isolated from brain tissue of PML cases and from the urine of immunosuppressed renal allograft patients.

The JC virus is highly oncogenic in newborn hamsters, particularly by intracerebral inoculation, producing malignant gliomas of diverse histology. This is in contrast to the BK virus, which is only weakly oncogenic in these animals. The BK viruses are, however, capable of transforming hamster cells in culture.

While both JC and BK viruses are capable of infecting man, virus is produced only in those with impaired immune defenses, the infection being latent in normal persons. No significant disease is connected with BK virus infection, but JC virus has been associated with more than a score of PML cases and may stand in causal relation to many of these. This destructive, often fatal, disease of the central nervous system usually is found in individuals with intercurrent diseases that impair immune defense.

The Adenoviruses[32, 37, 38]

The viruses known as the adenoviruses were discovered in 1953, independently and almost simultaneously, by two groups of investigators. When tonsil and adenoid tissue fragments, removed at operation, were cultured as explants in plasma clots a degenerative cytopathology was produced that was transmissible in series in various kinds of tissue cultures. The cytopathic changes included the development of acidophilic swollen nuclei that appeared to contain inclusion bodies. The viruses apparently exist in the form of a latent infection in human adenoid or tonsil tissue.

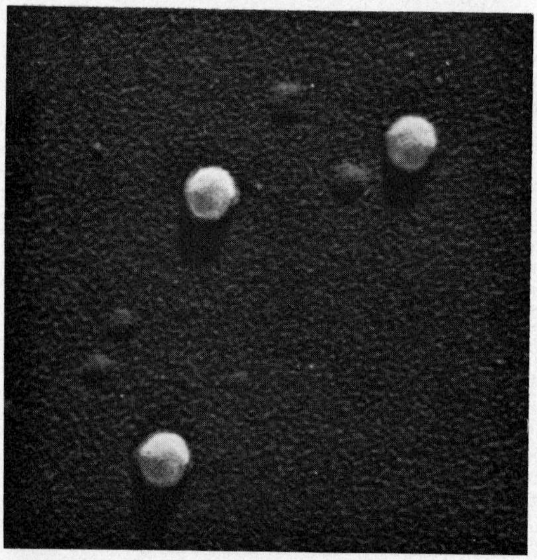

Subsequently, similar viruses have been isolated all over the world. They form a group containing common complement-fixing, soluble antigens, but fall into distinct serotypes by cross-neutralization tests in tissue cultures. They are classified in the family Adenoviridae, with the mammalian types placed in the genus *Mastadenovirus*.

Morphology

The adenoviruses are DNA viruses in which the nucleic acid is linear and double-stranded. Adenovirions are 70 to 90 nm. in diameter (Fig. 39–14) and are not enveloped; the capsid has cubic symmetry and is icosahedral in form. There are 252 capsomers—240 hexons, so designated because they have six identical neighbors, and 12 pentons, each with five neighbors.

Figure 39–14. Electron micrograph of shadow-cast preparation of purified adenovirus. × 17,000. (Tousimis and Hilleman.)

Table 39–7. **Properties of Adenoviruses**

Spherical virion, 70–90 nm.
Icosahedron, 252 capsomers (240 hexons, 12 pentons)
Linear, dsDNA genome
Assembled in nucleus
Nonenveloped
Ether-resistant; acid-stable; heat-sensitive
33 human serotypes

Polypeptide SDS-gel   Structural Unit

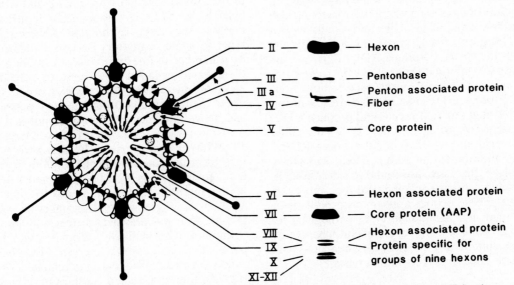

II — Hexon

III — Pentonbase

III a — Penton associated protein

IV — Fiber

V — Core protein

VI — Hexon associated protein

VII — Core protein (AAP)

VIII — Hexon associated protein

IX — Protein specific for

X — groups of nine hexons

XI-XII

Figure 39–15. A model of adenovirus 2. The location of the principal structural proteins (and their SDS gel patterns) are shown. (H. Persson and L. Philipson, Curr. Topics Microbiol. Immunol. **97**:157, 1982.)

The capsomers at the vertices are pentons; projecting from each penton is a "fiber" with a terminal "knob." The properties of adenoviruses are listed in Table 39–7. A model of adenovirus 2 is diagrammed in Figure 39–15.

Adenoviruses may be grown in a variety of cell cultures, of which HeLa cells are among the most susceptible and widely used. Both DNA replication and virion assembly occurs in the nucleus of the host cell, and the virus particles occur in orderly arrays to give a crystalline appearance to the inclusion bodies (Fig. 39–16). The cytopathic effect is characterized by rounding and aggregation of the cells.

Many of the human adenoviruses produce hemagglutinin and some possess receptor-destroying enzyme (RDE). The hemagglutinin is

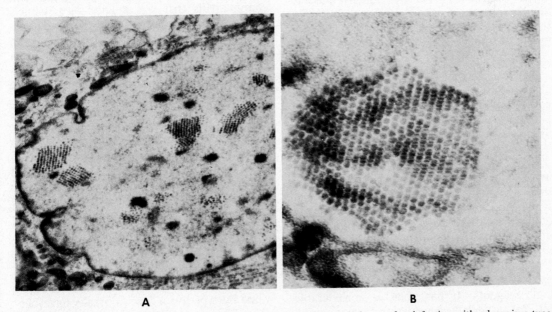

A   B

Figure 39–16. Electron micrographs of ultrathin sections of HeLa cells at 48 hours after infection with adenovirus type 4. *A*, Single particles and packed arrays of particles are distributed throughout the nucleus. *B*, A higher magnification of a similar cell showing the single particles. (A. J. Tousimis, and M. R. Hilleman, Virology **4**:499, 1957.)

associated with the fibers noted above. They may be conveniently divided into four hem-agglutinin (HA) groups, on the basis of agglutination of rhesus and rat erythrocytes, which parallel immunological groupings. The viruses of HA group 1 agglutinate rhesus but not rat cells and do not produce RDE; those of HA group 2 agglutinate rat cells, with some serotypes agglutinating rhesus cells to low titer, and produce RDE; HA group 3 viruses incompletely agglutinate rat cells and produce RDE; those of HA group 4 do not agglutinate either rat or rhesus cells and do not produce RDE.

In addition to the human adenovirus types, similar viruses are also found in lower animals as simian, bovine, canine, murine, and avian types. These do not appear to be pathogenic for man, nor are human types pathogenic for lower animals. The mammalian types often show unilateral serological cross-reactions with one or another of the human types.

Antigenic Structure

At least two kinds of antigens are present in adenoviruses; one is group-specific and the other is type-specific. A soluble, complement-fixing antigen is group-specific and shows cross-reactions between serotypes. Serotypes within the group are differentiated by neutralization tests carried out in tissue culture. The neutralizing activity is associated with the hexons of the viral surface and with the fiber proteins. A total of 33 differentiable serotypes have been described. These types have been given arabic numbers, and appear to be homogeneous even though widely different in temporal and geographical origin.

The Disease in Man

As indicated above, adenoviruses were discovered both as latent infections in normal persons and in association with respiratory disease. The disease produced by these viruses is an acute infection of the mucous membranes of the respiratory tract and of the eye, with involvement of the submucous lymphadenoid tissues of these areas, including the regional lymph nodes. While it is probable that many of them have the capacity to produce similar disease, there is a definite association of certain serotypes with clinical syndromes. Other serotypes, although found in association with disease, have not been shown to be specific etiological agents. It has been of considerable interest, especially considering their ubiquity, that certain of the adenoviruses have been found to be oncogenic in neonatal hamsters.

Acute Respiratory Disease.[6, 49] The adeno-virus strains first isolated from military recruits with acute respiratory disease were type 4, and this serotype, together with types 3 and 7, has been found to be closely associated with the disease. The etiological relation of these serotypes to acute respiratory disease is indicated by a number of lines of evidence. In addition to repeated isolation from cases of such disease, rise in specific antibody titer occurs between paired serums from affected persons, and active immunization of nonimmunes with polyvalent vaccine has been found to protect 50 to 70 per cent or more. Furthermore, serums from patients with acute respiratory disease, taken during World War II and stored in the interim, have been found to contain antibody to these serotypes, suggesting that the infection was prevalent at that time also.

Immunization with live adenovirus vaccine, particularly in military recruits, has been widely practiced. The live, unattenuated virus is given in enteric-coated capsules to induce a mild localized enteric infection; such vaccines yield a high rate of type-specific protection against the respiratory disease.

Types 1, 2, and 5, as well as some others, have been recovered repeatedly from tonsils and adenoids removed surgically from persons not ill with respiratory disease, but these types also have been found in association with febrile respiratory infections occurring, for the most part, in infants.

Pharyngoconjunctival Fever. This is a febrile disease characterized by pharyngitis and conjunctivitis that was defined as a clinical entity in connection with studies on adenoviruses. It occurs in epidemic form, largely in school children, and it is estimated that 50 per cent of exposed nonimmunes develop the disease. Some infections have been traced to contaminated swimming pools. The conjunctivitis is usually unilateral and nonsuppurative, and does not result in corneal damage.

Epidemic Keratoconjunctivitis. This is a highly infectious disease characterized by relatively little ocular exudate, the development of round subepithelial opacities in association with the keratitis, and, often, swelling of the regional lymph nodes. There may also be systemic symptoms, especially headache. The incidence of complications resulting in impairment of vision has been variable.

Most earlier outbreaks of the disease were caused by adenovirus type 8, joined in recent years by type 19; a few outbreaks have been caused by type 4. There is some evidence of an associated genital infection, with the suggestion of a genito-ocular syndrome, as occurs with *Chlamydia trachomatis*.[22]

DNA Viruses and Oncogenesis[10, 12, 20, 35, 39, 51, 52]

As noted earlier, the infection of a host cell with virus often leads to the destruction of the cell and the appearance of new viral particles. Infection with DNA viruses is no exception and the acute infections are usually cytolytic. This is not invariably the case, however. Infections may occur in which the virus is latent or occult, and others in which virus is produced but without destruction of the host cell. These infections, in many cases, are linked to a proliferative cellular response that may extend to the appearance of tumors, either benign or malignant.

The proliferative response ranges from the transient and limited, as seen in smallpox, to a marked but benign hyperplasia, such as that seen in molluscum contagiosum, human warts, and rabbit fibroma. In other instances, malignant tumors may be caused. On the one hand are the rabbit papillomas, beginning as benign tumors with orderly proliferation, but eventually progressing to disorderly growth, invasion of contiguous tissues, metastasis, and development of a malignant process. In other instances, the natural infections exhibit a proliferative response that is malignant substantially from the initiation of infection, as illustrated by the lymphomas induced in certain primates by herpesvirus saimiri.

It has been noted earlier that herpes simplex type 2 and the Epstein-Barr viruses are associated with certain human tumors, and may indeed be the etiological agents of these malignancies. Although the oncogenic potential of DNA viruses in humans is strongly indicated only in these two instances, DNA viruses are known to be etiological agents in several naturally occurring animal diseases. For the most part, the viruses involved are those of the herpes group, and include the virus of monkey lymphoma (herpesvirus saimiri); the Lucké virus, causing adenocarcinoma of frogs; and Marek's virus, an agent inducing an economically important lymphomatosis in fowls.

Although these are the principal naturally occurring malignancies caused by DNA viruses, these and several other DNA viruses are capable of inducing tumorigenesis in animals under artificial conditions. Generally, tumor production is achieved by virus inoculation into immunodeficient animals, usually neonatal hamsters or other newborn rodents.

While animal studies have been informative concerning the role of viruses in oncogenesis, it is the cell-virus interactions that have been of greatest interest and potential in delineating the mechanisms of cellular alterations that lead to tumor formation. When animal cells cultured *in vitro* are infected with oncogenic viruses, a striking series of changes are induced in these cells, and they are said to be transformed. Transformed cells undergo apparently unregulated growth, resulting in disoriented arrays of cells that are piled one upon the other in clusters; this is in contrast to the growth patterns of normal cells, usually characterized by parallel arrangements of elongated cells in sheets of single-cell thickness. Such transformed cells are also capable of prolonged growth, *i.e.*, they may be carried in serial culture and have been said to be "immortal." The plasma membrane of transformed cells is altered, possibly accounting for the peculiar growth patterns, and there is an alteration in the membrane glycolipids and glycoproteins. The cells may also possess new antigens, not detectable in normal cells; these may be located on the cell surface (transplantation antigens) or intracellularly, *e.g.*, the T-antigens. In the great majority of such infections, virus is not detectable, *i.e.*, the infection is not productive, although the virus genome, or a part of it, is present and integrated into the host cell genome. Depending upon the infecting viruses, however, viral antigens may be present in the host cell in a detectable form.

Not all cells are susceptible to transformation by a given virus, however. The adenoviruses, for example, will only transform cells that are nonpermissive for virus production; these include newborn hamster kidney cells and rat embryo fibroblasts. The human papovaviruses are also restricted in host cell range—the JC virus, for instance, will only transform human cells in culture.

Virally transformed cells are considered to be malignant or premalignant, and such cells are often capable of initiating tumors when introduced into suitable, *e.g.*, neonatal, animals.

When cells from virally induced tumors are cultured *in vitro*, they usually have the growth and cell surface characteristics of virally transformed cells. The viral genome can sometimes be shown to be present in integrated form, but virus can only rarely be rescued from such cells. Occasionally, cultured tumor cells yield virus spontaneously, as in SV40-induced tumors, and in other instances, specialized techniques can sometimes induce virus production.

Clearly, then, many of the DNA viruses have oncogenic potential, even though tumors may not be a part of the natural infection. The widespread distribution of herpesvirus infections in man, coupled with their tendency to become latent and their oncogenic potential in cultured cells, has, in particular, prompted intensive studies of their possible role in human cancer.

REFERENCES

1. Allen, W. P., and F. Rapp. 1982. Concept review of genital herpes vaccines. J. Infect. Dis. **145**:413–421.
2. Babiuk, L. A., and B. T. Rouse. 1979. Immune control of herpesvirus latency. Can. J. Microbiol. **25**:267–274.
3. Baxby, D. 1977. Poxvirus hosts and reservoirs. Brief review. Arch. Virol. **55**:169–179.
4. Baxby, D. 1977. The origins of vaccinia virus. J. Infect. Dis. **136**:453–455.
5. Behbehani, A. M. 1983. The smallpox story: life and death of an old disease. Microbiol. Rev. **47**:455–509.
6. Brandt, C. D., et al. 1972. Infections in 18,000 infants and children in a controlled study of respiratory tract disease. II. Variation in adenovirus infections by year and season. Amer. J. Epidemiol. **95**: 218–227.
7. Breman, J. G., et al. 1980. Human monkeypox, 1970–79. Bull. Wld Hlth Org. **58**:165–182.
8. Brown, G. R. 1976. Herpes zoster: correlation of age, sex, distribution, neuralgia, and associated disorders. Southern Med. J. **69**:576–578.
9. Chang, A., and D. H. Metz. 1976. Further investigations on the mode of entry of vaccinia virus into cells. J. Gen. Virol. **32**:275–282.
10. de-Thé, G. 1979. The epidemiology of Burkitt's lymphoma: evidence for a causal association with Epstein-Barr virus. Epidemiol. Rev. **1**:32–54.
11. Deria, A., et al. 1980. The world's last endemic case of smallpox: surveillance and containment measures. Bull. Wld Hlth Org. **58**:279–283.
12. Dougherty, R. M., and M. K. Bradley. 1978. Oncogenicity of human papovaviruses. pp. 424–431. In D. Schlessinger (Ed.): Microbiology—1978. American Society for Microbiology, Washington, D. C.
13. Downie, A. W., et al. 1971. Tanapox: a new disease caused by a pox virus. Brit. Med. J. **1**:363–368.
14. Dumbell, K. R., and J. G. Kapsenberg. 1982. Laboratory investigation of two "whitepox" viruses and comparison with two variola strains from southern India. Bull. Wld Hlth Org. **60**:381–387.
15. Epstein, M. A., and B. G. Achong. 1973. The EB virus. Ann. Rev. Microbiol. **27**:413–436.
16. Epstein, M. A., and B. G. Achong. 1977. Pathogenesis of infectious mononucleosis. Lancet **2**:1270–1273.
17. Fareed, G. C., and D. Davoli. 1977. Molecular biology of papovaviruses. Ann. Rev. Biochem. **46**:471–522.
18. Fenner, F. 1977. The eradication of smallpox. Prog. Med. Virol. **23**:1–21.
19. Field, H. J., and P. Wildy. 1981. Recurrent herpes simplex: the outlook for systemic antiviral agents. Brit. Med. J. **282**:1821–1822.
20. Galloway, D. A., and J. K. McDougall. 1983. The oncogenic potential of herpes simplex viruses: evidence for a "hit-and-run" mechanism. Nature **302**:21–24.
21. Glenn, J. 1981. Cytomegalovirus infections following renal transplantation. Rev. Infect. Dis. **3**:1151–1178.
22. Harnett, G. B., and W. A. Newnham. 1981. Isolation of adenovirus type 19 from the male and female genital tracts. Brit. J. Vener. Dis. **57**:55–57.
23. Haynes, R. E. 1976. The spectrum of herpes simplex virus infections in children. Southern Med. J. **69**:1069–1078.
24. Holowczak, J. A. 1982. Poxvirus DNA. Curr. Topics Microbiol. Immunol. **97**:27–79.
25. Kieff, E., et al. 1982. The biology and chemistry of Epstein-Barr virus. J. Infect. Dis. **146**:506–517.
26. Klein, R. J. 1982. The pathogenesis of acute, latent and recurrent herpes simplex virus infections. Brief review. Arch. Virol. **72**:143–168.
27. Kumar, M. L., and G. A. Nankervis. 1979. Cytomegalovirus infections. Southern Med. J. **72**:854–861.
28. Longson, M. 1978. Persistence in herpes simplex virus infections. Postgrad. Med. J. **54**:603–612.
29. Moss, B. 1974. Reproduction of poxviruses. pp. 405–474. In H. Fraenkel-Conrat and R. R. Wagner (Eds.): Comprehensive Virology. Vol. 3. Plenum Press, New York.
30. Nahmias, A. J., W. R. Dowdle, and R. F. Schinazi (Eds.). 1981. The Human Herpesviruses. An Interdisciplinary Perspective. Elsevier, New York.
31. Nakano, J. H. 1980. Smallpox, monkeypox, vaccinia, and whitepox viruses. pp. 810–822. In E. H. Lennette, et al. (Eds.): Manual of Clinical Microbiology. 3rd ed. American Society for Microbiology, Washington, D. C.
32. Nermut, M. V. 1980. The architecture of adenoviruses: recent views and problems. Brief review. Arch. Virol. **64**:175–196.
33. O'Callaghan, D. J., and C. C. Randall. 1976. Molecular anatomy of herpesviruses: recent studies. Prog. Med. Virol. **22**:152–210.
34. Osborn, J. E. 1981. Cytomegalovirus: pathogenicity, immunology, and vaccine initiatives. J. Infect. Dis. **143**:618–630.
35. Pagano, J. S. 1975. Diseases and mechanisms of persistent DNA virus infection: latency and cellular transformation. J. Infect. Dis. **132**:209–223.
36. Panjvani, Z. F. K., and J. B. Hanshaw. 1981. Cytomegalovirus in the perinatal period. Amer. J. Dis. Children **135**:56–60.
37. Persson, H., and L. Philipson. 1982. Regulation of adenovirus gene expression. Curr. Topics Microbiol. Immunol. **97**:157–203.
38. Philipson, L., U. Petterson, and U. Lindberg. 1975. Molecular biology of adenoviruses. Virol. Monogr. **14**:1–115.
39. Rawls, W. E., S. Baccheti, and F. L. Graham. 1977. Relation of herpes simplex viruses to human malignancy. Curr. Topics Microbiol. Immunol. **77**:71–95.
40. Report. 1972. Monkeypox. Bull. Wld Hlth Org. **46**:569–639.
41. Report. 1980. Global eradication of smallpox. Bull. Wld Hlth Org. **58**:161–163.
42. Roizman, B. (Ed.). 1982. The Herpesviruses. Vol. 1. Plenum Press, New York.
43. Rosenthal, L. J. 1979. Replication of herpesviruses and latency. Can. J. Microbiol. **25**:239–244.
44. Sheek, M. R., A. L. Chapman, and H. A. Wenner. 1975. Human and primate poxviruses. I. Growth characteristics of cytolytic and tumor variants. Arch. Virol. **48**:47–61.

45. Siegl, G. 1976. The parvoviruses. Virol. Monogr. **15**:1–109.

46. Starr, S. E., and H. M. Friedman. 1980. Human cytomegalovirus. pp. 790–797. *In* E. H. Lennette, *et al.* (Eds.): Manual of Clinical Microbiology. 3rd ed. American Society for Microbiology, Washington, D. C.

47. Stevens, J. G. 1975. Latent herpes simplex virus and the nervous system. Curr. Topics Microbiol. Immunol. **70**:31–50.

48. Takemoto, K. K. 1978. Human papovaviruses. Internat. Rev. Exptl Pathol. **18**:281–301.

49. Top, F. H., Jr. 1975. Control of adenovirus acute respiratory disease in U.S. Army trainees. Yale J. Biol. Med. **48**:185–195.

50. Tummon, I. S., D. K. L. Dudley, and J. H. Walters. 1981. Genital herpes simplex. Can. Med. Assn J. **125**:23–29.

51. Ziegler, J. L. 1981. Burkitt's lymphoma. New Engl. J. Med. **305**:735–745.

52. zur Hausen, H. 1977. Human papillomaviruses and their possible role in squamous cell carcinomas. Curr. Topics Microbiol. Immunol. **78**:1–30.

CHAPTER 40

The Orthomyxoviruses; The Paramyxoviruses; The Rhabdoviruses; The Retroviruses

Disease of the respiratory tract in man is of heterogeneous etiology, the causative agents including fungi, rickettsiae, bacteria, and viruses. Acute respiratory disease is thus etiologically complex, though perhaps less so clinically.

Elucidation of the viral etiology of a portion of diseases of this kind was initiated with the isolation and characterization of the influenza virus in 1933; subsequent development of more sophisticated tissue culture techniques made possible wide application of this method and the isolation of a series of hitherto unknown viruses. The extension of readily applicable serological methods of characterization and identification as a corollary to tissue culture methods, and the application of such serological methods to the retrospective diagnosis of infections of this kind, allow estimation of the relative prevalence of such viruses in the host population. In consequence, a general pattern of viral infections of this kind has emerged, although many gaps remain and a considerable portion of undifferentiated acute respiratory disease remains of uncertain etiology.

The viral agents of acute respiratory disease are diverse, including not only the influenza and related viruses of the myxovirus group but also the adenoviruses and certain of the picornaviruses associated with the common cold syndrome. The orthomyxoviruses and paramyxoviruses will be considered in this chapter. Adenoviruses are considered with the DNA viruses in Chapter 39, and the picornaviruses, including those causing respiratory diseases, are discussed in Chapter 41.

The Orthomyxoviruses[27, 55]

The viruses of the Orthomyxoviridae are enveloped RNA viruses in which the nucleic acids are segmented, single-stranded, and of negative polarity. The capsid has helical symmetry with a helix diameter of 9 to 17 nm., and the mature virus particle is enclosed in an envelope derived by budding from the cell membrane.

The Orthomyxoviridae are differentiated from the Paramyxoviridae on the basis of structure, size, and cytopathic effect produced in cell culture. The properties of myxoviruses are listed in Table 40–1 and shown schematically in Figure 40–1. The orthomyxoviruses, which include the influenza viruses, possess a segmented (−)RNA genome; are somewhat more uniform and smaller in size, 80 to 120 nm.; and produce a cytopathic effect that is usually degenerative in type. The paramyxoviruses include the parainfluenza, mumps, measles, and Newcastle disease viruses. They contain a non-segmented (−)RNA genome, are 150 to 300 nm. in size, and produce a cytopathic effect that is syncytial in character; eosinophilic inclusions are found in the cytoplasm of infected cells.

INFLUENZA VIRUSES

Influenza is a widespread disease of man occurring as sporadic interepidemic cases, as periodic epidemics, and in pandemic form. A series of pandemics of influenza have occurred at fairly regular intervals since 1890. In the 1918–1919 pandemic, the disease occurred all over the world, and the estimated number of deaths exceeded 21 million.

The **epidemic periodicity** differs somewhat between the two main types of influenza virus (see below), and epidemics of greater or lesser extent occur at one- to three-year intervals in the case of influenza type A, and at four- to five-year intervals with influenza type B. Epidemic periodicity appears to be due to host population changes, *e.g.*, the accumulation of susceptibles and the subtraction of immunes by death, but pandemic influenza seems to be the result of antigenic changes in the virus of sufficient magnitude that there is little effective cross-immunity between the preexisting and the new antigenic types.

The prevalence of the infection is indicated by the occurrence of serum antibody in practically all adults and in most children over five years of age. It is probable that many infections are subclinical, or mild and regarded as common colds, and that the viruses persist in interepidemic periods in the form of such infections and as sporadic cases. There seems to be no unequivocal evidence of the existence of a chronic carrier state. Persistence of these viruses perhaps contributes to the maintenance of observed antibody titers in the general population.

Morphology and Fine Structure[33, 43, 60]

The influenza viruses are morphologically indistinguishable. Upon primary isolation in the embryonated egg, and often for the first few passages, the virus occurs as both spheres and filaments; both of these forms are infective. The fine structure of the influenza viruses is now reasonably well defined, and is basically that of the enveloped viruses with helical nucleocapsid, as described in Chapter 38 and illustrated diagrammatically in Figures 38–1 and 40–1. The capsid is composed of eight segments of (−)RNA, and is associated with a nucleoprotein (NP). The nucleocapsid is enclosed in a membrane derived from the host plasma membrane during budding. Applied to the inner side of the envelope membrane is a virus-specified, electron-dense layer of protein (M) that represents the outer layer of the virus capsid. Inserted in the outer surface of the

Table 40–1. **Properties of Myxoviruses**

Orthomyxoviruses	Paramyxoviruses
(−)RNA genome; segmented, linear, and single-stranded	(−)RNA genome; nonsegmented, linear, and single-stranded
Helical nucleocapsid	Helical nucleocapsid
Spherical virion, 80–120 nm.	Spherical virion, 150–300 nm.
Transcriptase in virion	Transcriptase in virion
Enveloped (from plasma membrane)	Enveloped (from plasma membrane)
Ether-sensitive	Ether-sensitive

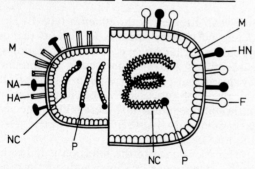

Orthomyxoviruses   Paramyxoviruses

Figure 40–1. Structure of myxoviruses. *P*, RNA polymerase; *NC*, nucleocapsid; *M*, membrane protein. In *Orthomyxovirus*, two glycoproteins are present as spikes on the viral surface, *viz.*, neuraminidase (*NA*) and hemagglutinins (*HA*). In *Paramyxovirus*, the hemagglutinin and neuraminidase activities are located in the glycoprotein *HN*; a glycoprotein (*F*) is responsible for cell fusion, virus penetration, and hemolysis. (R. Rott, Arch. Virol., 59:285, 1979.)

lipid bilayer are two virus-specified glycopeptides, the **hemagglutinin (HA)** and the **neuraminidase (NA)**. Both hemagglutinin and neuraminidase occur as "spikes," or peplomers, projecting from the surface of the virion. Approximately 80 per cent of the spikes are hemagglutinin and 20 per cent are neuraminidase. Three peptides (P1, P2, and P3) are associated with the nucleocapsid and together form the transcriptase required to synthesize mRNA, using the viral RNA genome (vRNA) as a template. These viral components are listed in Table 40–2. In addition to these viral constituents, virus-specified, nonstructural

(NS) proteins have been noted in the nucleolus of infected cells.

The larger gene segments (segments 1 to 6) each encode for a single polypeptide (Table 40–2); the two smaller segments each encode for two polypeptides: segment 7 encodes for a nonstructural protein as well as virion matrix protein, and segment 8 encodes for two nonstructural proteins.

Replication
The replication of influenza virus follows the pattern described in Chapter 38 and outlined in Figure 38–22. Virion components are assembled at the host plasma membrane. The HA and NA proteins migrate to the site of assembly and are inserted into the host cell membrane; during this process they are glycosylated. The M protein accumulates on the inner side of the membrane at the site of future budding and the nucleocapsid components bind to the specifically prepared portion of the host cell membrane. After budding, virions are released from the host cell surface, probably by action of the neuraminidase. The morphology and release of virions are illustrated in Figure 40–2.

Toxicity
Like certain other viruses, the influenza viruses are toxic when administered in high concentrations to experimental animals. The toxicity not only is evident with infective viruses, but persists even after ultraviolet inactivation. Toxicity is overcome by treatment with type-specific antibody, and the evidence

Table 40–2. **Components of the Influenza Virion**

Component	Location	Gene Segment No.	Average Molecular Weight (daltons)	Properties
(–)RNA	Nucleocapsid		$4.8 \times 10^{6*}$	Viral genome; occurs in 8 single-stranded segments
HA	Spike on the virion surface	4	80,000†	Glycoprotein with hemagglutinating properties; activated by host enzymes
NA	Spike on the virion surface	6	60,000	Glycoprotein with neuraminidase (enzymatic) activity; activated by host enzymes
NP	Associated with viral RNA	5	60,000	Protein with affinity for RNA, may link RNA segments
M	Membrane	7	25,000	Membrane (matrix) protein
P1	Nucleocapsid	1	96,000	⎫
P2	Nucleocapsid	2	87,000	⎬ Proteins with transcriptase activity
P3	Nucleocapsid	3	85,000	⎭

*Total molecular weight of the RNA segments.
†Composed of two noncovalently bound subunits, HA_1 (55,000 daltons) and HA_2 (25,000 daltons).

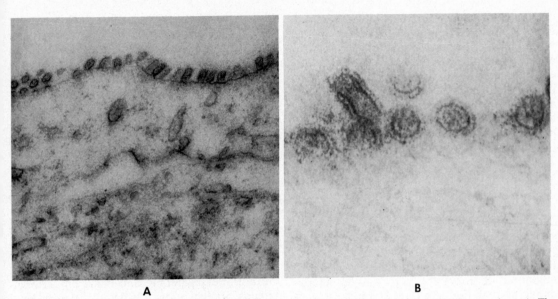

A   B

Figure 40–2. Ultrathin sections of entodermal cells of chorioallantoic membrane infected with influenza virus. *A,* The virus particles in the form of spheres and short rods are on the surface of the cell, and the cell nucleus is below. × 45,000. *B,* A similar preparation at higher magnification showing the spherical bodies to consist of an internal body, a sharply defined dense membrane, and a less dense envelope. The obliquely sectioned rod appears to have an amorphous interior. × 152,000. (C. Morgan, H. M. Rose, and D. H. Moore, J. Exptl. Med. **104:**171, 1956.)

suggests that toxicity is related to the attachment of viral particles to the host cell membrane. Damage resulting from this membrane association may be analogous to that observed in high-multiplicity chlamydial infections noted earlier (Chapter 34).

Hemagglutination

The myxoviruses, when mixed with the red blood cells from many animal species, will effect agglutination of the erythrocytes. Hemagglutination is noted with other viruses, *e.g.,* togaviruses (Chapter 42), but most myxoviruses are distinguished by their content of neuraminidase, an enzyme which degrades the hemagglutinin receptors on the red cell to allow spontaneous elution of the virus. Some other viruses, such as the poxviruses, produce a soluble hemagglutinin, but the virion does not act as the agglutinating agent.

Hemagglutination by influenza virus provides a convenient *in vitro* method for titration of the virus, *viz.,* serial dilutions of virus-containing material in red cell suspensions show an endpoint that is a measure of viral concentration. Agglutination of erythrocytes also occurs about centers of viral replication in infected tissue culture monolayers and is usually apparent before the cytopathic effect. This phenomenon is termed **hemadsorption.**

Viral hemagglutination is specifically inhibited by antiviral serum, and a specific serological test, hemagglutination-inhibition (HI),

has been devised to titrate antiviral antibody (see below). Hemagglutination is due to the presence of hemagglutinin (HA) spikes on the virus that react specifically with neuraminic acid–containing glycoproteins on the erythrocyte surface. These receptors are also present on other host cells, and viral attachment by this mechanism is considered to be the initial step in the infection process, leading to penetration and uncoating. Thus, hemagglutination is intimately related to infectivity, and antibody directed against the specific HA protein is thought to be protective by preventing attachment.

When virus-agglutinated red cells are allowed to stand for a few hours, the virus particles are spontaneously eluted. The elution is referable to the degradation of the specific host receptors by the viral neuraminidase. Red blood cells from which the virus has been eluted are not reagglutinated by the addition of fresh influenza virus. As noted above, the neuraminidase of influenza virus occurs in a set of peplomers on the virus surface that are separate from the HA spikes. Neuraminidase is also produced by a number of bacteria, notably *Vibrio cholerae* and *Clostridium perfringens,* and treatment of erythrocytes by these enzymes also renders the cells inagglutinable by myxoviruses.

Antigenic Structure

Several kinds of antigens are present in influenza viruses, representing the protein components of the virion. A soluble antigen is found both free in infected tissue and in the virus, and is the nucleoprotein (NP) of the nucleocapsid; the NP antigen is the type-specific antigen of the virus and is demonstrable by complement fixation. Antibody to the NP antigen is formed in response to infection, but is not ordinarily encountered in the serum of persons immunized with inactivated or partially purified virus.

A second group of antigens, intimately associated with the virus particle, includes the hemagglutinin and neuraminidase glycoproteins as well as the membrane (M protein) antigen; the M antigen appears to be type-specific, while the others are strain- or subtype-specific. The hemagglutinin can be detected by HI tests, and the neuraminidase by antibody inhibition of enzymatic activity—the neuraminidase-inhibition test. The M antigen reacts in complement fixation and immunodiffusion tests.

Nomenclature.[39] The influenza viruses are separable into at least three main types that are immunologically distinct from one another: type A, which was isolated in 1933; type B, isolated in 1940; and type C, isolated in 1949. Each of these types is distinguished by the specificity of the **nucleoprotein antigen;** within each type, strains or subtypes are set apart by the antigenic specificities contained in the HA and NA antigens. It has become almost axiomatic that a newly isolated strain will not be immunologically identical with strains isolated at other times, because of slight changes in specificity of these latter two antigenic components.

A recently adopted nomenclature for influenza viruses permits the designation of virus strains based in large part on their antigenic differences. The designation includes (1) the type (based on the NP antigen), (2) the animal host of origin (if other than man), (3) geographical origin, (4) strain number, and (5) the year of isolation. In addition, the designation for type A strains contains a notation of the HA and NA subtypes. For example, the human influenza prototype strain responsible for the pandemic of 1957 is designated A/Singapore/1/57 (H2N2), while the prototype strain responsible for the 1968 pandemic is described by A/Hong Kong/1/68 (H3N2).

The antigenic variability of influenza strains, particularly those of type A, has given rise to a terminology peculiar to these viruses. In the two examples given above, it will be noted that there was a significant change in the HA antigen of the strains that appeared in 1968,

i.e., from H2 to H3 specificity. These major antigenic changes probably represent changes due to **genetic recombination**, or **reassortment** (see below and Chapter 38), and are referred to as **antigenic shifts**. Since the human population in 1968 did not possess antibodies against the new antigen (H3), the antigenic shift resulted in a new influenza pandemic. During the interpandemic periods, minor antigenic alterations in the surface antigen also appeared, probably as point mutations in the genome, resulting in minor alterations in the glycoproteins of both the HA and the NA antigens. This **antigenic drift** is observed as small reductions in affinity between the altered antigen and antibody formed against the original strain. For instance, the Hong Kong virus, which appeared in 1968, has undergone drift in both hemagglutinin and neuraminidase antigens, so that viruses isolated in later years, *e.g.,* A/Hong Kong/5/72 (H3N2) and A/England/42/72 (H3N2), react in HI tests with homologous titers several times greater than titers against the original Hong Kong (1968) isolates, even though all are H3N2 subtypes.

Type A influenza virus is the most common cause of influenza in man and shows the greatest strain variability. Beginning with the pandemic of 1918–1919, a succession of shifts in the viral antigens has taken place at about 10-year intervals, as shown in Table 40–3. In 1976, a new strain of influenza virus with new HA and NA antigenic specificities (H1N1) was isolated from military recruits; this represented antigenic shift in both antigens. The strain was similar to influenza viruses known to circulate in swine populations and also resembled the highly virulent strain responsible for the devastating 1918–1919 pandemic. The new strain proved, however, to be less virulent than the Hong Kong strains then prevalent, and did not cause the pandemic that many had expected. Nevertheless, similar viruses with H1N1 antigens appeared in epidemic form in 1977, originating first in China and later in the U.S.S.R., and these "Russian" strains continue to cocirculate with the earlier Hong Kong varieties in the human population.

Type B influenza viruses are also variable, but to a much lesser extent than type A viruses. Thus, no subtypes are distinguished, although it is recognized that antigenic drift occurs, with attendant small alterations in antigenic specificity in strains isolated some years apart. Type C influenza viruses are less common than types A and B, and appear to be more stable; in general, the type C viruses are relatively homogeneous. The type C viruses have not been

Table 40–3. **Antigens of the Major Epidemic Strains of Type A Influenza Viruses**

Epidemic	Subtype Antigens*
1918–1919 (pandemic)	Hsw1N1
1929	H0N1
1947	H1N1
1957 (pandemic)	H2N2
1968 (pandemic)	H3N2
1977	H1N1

*Current terminology combines H0 and Hsw1 into H1. The older terminology is retained here for clarity.

associated with epidemic disease in man, but they may be responsible for a mild type of influenza. Strain designations for types B and C viruses therefore do not include subtype designation, *e.g.*, B/England/5/66 and C/Paris/1/67.

Variation[53]

In addition to antigenic shift and antigenic drift in the HA and NA components, there are several kinds of variations among the influenza viruses, including variations in virion morphology, host range, and pathogenicity.

Upon primary isolation, the virus grows more readily in the amniotic than in the allantoic cavity of embryonated hen's egg, and hemagglutinins are produced that act against guinea pig and human, but not fowl, erythrocytes. After continued adaptive passage in the egg, the virus acquires the capacity to grow in the allantoic cavity and to produce hemagglutinins for fowl erythrocytes. Further passage also often results in the rapid loss of virulence for man.

Antigenic Variation.[9, 41, 62] Variation in the hemagglutinin and neuraminidase glycopeptides of the viral surface is of major importance and occurs with some facility under natural conditions; similar changes may also be experimentally induced. The naturally occurring phenomenon appears to be a continuous variation of antigenic character (antigenic drift), with occasional major changes (antigenic shift) of sufficient magnitude that there is little or no effective cross-immunity as far as man is concerned. Both kinds of antigenic change are apparent in influenza virus type A, but only antigenic drift occurs in types B and C.

Antigenic drift represents minor antigenic changes that occur within a major subtype, such as the Hong Kong strain (H3N2) that appeared in 1968. These changes are noted in both the HA and the NA glycoproteins, are gradual and cumulative, and probably reflect minor mutations in the viral RNA that result

in alterations in some of the amino acids making up the antigen. Thus, the antigens that arise late in the epidemic cycle differ slightly from those that appear early in the cycle. The conventional explanation is that antigenic drift results from interaction between these antigenic mutational events and the pressures of immunological selection, which permits the emergence of viruses with novel antigens in hosts possessing antibodies against the older viruses. Indeed, it may be shown experimentally that variants arise when influenza viruses are propagated in the presence of antibody, both in embryonated eggs and in partially immune animals. The selection of variants by antibody is generally agreed to account for the observation that new antigenic varieties usually supplant the older antigenic forms in human populations.

The second type of antigenic variation in influenza type A is seemingly more complex. It has been noted above that several sharp antigenic changes in the virus occur at intervals, representing substantial alterations in both the hemagglutinating and the neuraminidase antigens, *viz.*, H1N1→H2N2→H3N2 (Table 40–3) and that the appearance of each of these new strains resulted in large pandemics of disease. Those cited represent only the changes observed since isolation of the virus in the early 1930s; similar variations undoubtedly preceded these. The earlier variations can only be inferred from retrospective serological diagnosis in relation to age groups, but there is evidence for recycling of influenza antigens, as in the appearance in 1977 of Russian strains with H1N1 antigens, closely similar to those that circulated in the early 1950s. Fortunately these new strains have not proved to be as virulent as the earlier ones; they have not caused a new pandemic and they have not supplanted the H3N2 strains in the population.

Surveys of serum antibody present in persons of all ages, sorted out with respect to specificity and age group, reflect the temporal presence of the serotypes of influenza A virus. Such data are interpreted in light of the fact that in the past, new virus types rapidly and completely supplanted the previously circulating serotype. In the early 1950's, it was evident that the serum of children contained antibody to the then-prevalent serotype (H1N1); serum of individuals in the 15- to 28-year-old age group contained antibody to the previous serotype as well; and antibody to all serotypes circulating over the past 25 years or so was found in persons at least 30 years of age. Later surveys, subsequent to the appearance of the later Asian strains (H2N2), revealed that antibody to this seemingly new antigenic variety was also present in persons 70 to 90 years of age, suggesting that a similar variety was epidemic in the 1880s.

The validity of these inferences is dependent upon the nature of the immune response in man. Data such as the foregoing, and experimental immunization with monovalent vaccines of representative antigenic varieties, suggest that (1) the initial or childhood experience reflects the dominant antigens of the prevalent strains and is of limited effectiveness, since the disease is most prevalent in this age group; (2) successive subsequent infections with differing antigenic varieties of the virus both reinforce the initial response and broaden it with the acquisition of new antibody specificities; and (3) the wide range of antibody activity in the serum of older persons is a consequence of contact with a broad range of influenza antigens, with continuous reinforcement of prior antibody responses and the development of a progressively more effective immunity.

The mechanism of antigenic shift has been controversial. It has been suggested that these major antigenic changes could arise from the same mechanisms as antigenic drift, *i.e.*, cumulative changes in the antigenic glycopeptides by point mutations or, possibly, by frameshift mutations. The preponderance of evidence is, however, in favor of recombination, or more accurately, reassortment. It will be recalled that the genomic RNA of these viruses is in the form of RNA segments, each coding for different viral proteins. These RNA segments are packaged in the virion just prior to release from the cell. Thus, when virus assembly takes place in a cell mixedly infected with two such viruses, some of the progeny may be hybrids, with RNA segments derived from either parental type. Antigenic hybrids of different influenza A viruses have been produced by mixed infections in the chick embryo and in tissue cultures. Furthermore, animal experiments have shown that hybrid viruses arise under conditions simulating natural transmission, and elegant RNA hybridization studies have established that recombinants arise in natural human infections.[3]

These experiments do not, however, resolve the question of the origin of the new serotypes of influenza A appearing in humans, which is usually associated with the appearance of major epidemics. Perhaps most widely accepted is the hypothesis that these new human strains represent recombinants that arise from mixed infections, in a suitable host, with both human and animal influenza viruses. It is known, for example, that influenza virus of human infections is capable of infecting a number of animal species under natural conditions, and thus recombination with animal viruses in these hosts is probable. The potential of antigenic variation by this mechanism is illustrated by the identification of 12 distinct hemagglutinins and 9 neuraminidases among the influenza viruses of human and animal species.

Parenthetically, it should be noted that antigenic variation of influenza viruses occurs predominantly among the neuraminidase and hemagglutinin antigens. Other viral antigens, such as the nucleoprotein and membrane protein antigens, remain relatively constant.

Infection in Lower Animals[11, 32, 40, 44]

Naturally occurring infections of various domestic animals with type A influenza virus are well known, but a number of related viruses are typically found in lower animals. In addition to fowl plague virus, certain avian influenza viruses are found in chickens, turkeys, and ducks. In domestic mammals, swine influenza has been known since 1918, and horse influenza was described in 1963. Such animal infections may not be reservoirs of human infections in the accepted sense, but could represent sources of new viral antigens as outlined above. The human and lower animal strains are antigenically related; for example, human and avian strains share surface antigens, and recombination occurs between strains. Cross-infection has been produced experimentally, with the production of influenza in human volunteers with horse influenza virus, and ponies have been infected with human strains.

There is therefore the strong possibility that strains of influenza virus with novel HA and NA antigens can arise from infection in animals, principally ducks, chickens, or swine. If these viruses retain pathogenic properties for humans, their introduction into this population could lead to new epidemic or pandemic strains. It is of some theoretical interest that the original influenza outbreaks due to A/H2N2, A/H3N2, and the new A/H1N1 viruses have apparently originated in southern China. This has led to the suggestion that close association of humans with infected swine and ducks in this region may introduce new antigenic types into human populations. It is perhaps significant in this regard that types B and C viruses do not exhibit antigenic shifts, nor do they naturally infect animals.

Experimental Infections. The ferret is highly susceptible to intranasal inoculation with the influenza viruses and may, in fact, be infected by contact. Upon primary isolation from man, effected by the intranasal inoculation of human nasal washings into ferrets, the animals may exhibit few symptoms, but the infection is evident by a rise in antibody titer. On serial passage, virulence increases and there are overt symptoms of disease and lung consolidation.

The embryonated hen's egg may be infected by various routes, but isolation is most often successful by inoculation of the amniotic cavity of 12- to 14-day-old embryos. On passage the virus will grow in the allantoic cavity, in the yolk sac, and on the chorioallantoic membrane. Of these methods of isolation, inoculation of the amniotic cavity of the embryonated egg is regarded as one of the most sensitive.

The Disease in Man[8, 13, 48, 49]

The virus enters the body via the respiratory tract and attaches to host epithelial cells. Viral attachment, which begins the infectious process, is mediated by viral hemagglutins reacting with host cell receptors. The incubation period of influenza is short, one or two days, giving the epidemic and pandemic disease its explosive character. Symptoms referable to the respiratory tract, including nasal, pharyngeal, and laryngeal irritation and associated symptoms, occur but are often subordinate to the constitutional reaction with fever and prostration. The syndrome is variable and not characteristic, and influenza cannot be diagnosed on clinical grounds.

The most common complication, and usually the immediate cause of death in the fatal disease, is pneumonia resulting from secondary bacterial infection, usually due to staphylococci or streptococci. It is also evident that influenza virus alone may produce a fatal pneumonia, as observed in the 1957–1958 epidemic and again in the 1968–1969 epidemic. In such instances there is intense congestion of the trachea, with consolidation and hemorrhage in the lungs but little evidence of cellular reaction.

The pathological effects of influenza viruses are attributable to mechanical damage to the epithelium of the respiratory tract and to the inhibition of phagocytic elements. The defenses of the respiratory tract are thus compromised, leading to secondary bacterial invasion and pneumonia. In addition to these effects, type B influenza frequently is temporally associated with Reye's syndrome, a serious and often fatal disease in children.[30]

Following an epidemic, the disease becomes apparently less prevalent, but this is a consequence of an increasing proportion of clinically mild or inapparent infections. Serological studies have shown that the incidence of infections continues, with persistence during interepidemic periods in smoldering epidemic form. Influenza A epidemics characteristically occur every year or so and type B epidemics at longer intervals. Pandemic influenza arises from antigenic shifts in the virus, with appearance of varieties to which preexisting immunity gives little or no protection, and control of pandemic influenza represents an unsolved problem. Epidemics and pandemics are characterized by an excess in deaths from pneumonia-influenza, a phenomenon illustrated in Figure 40–3.

Chemoprophylaxis[31, 50]

Amantadine and its structural relative, rimantadine, have been found to have antiviral activity for influenza virus in tissue culture and to prevent infection in the mouse. Subsequently, these agents have been shown to be prophylactic against naturally acquired influenza in human volunteers, with relatively mild side effects. The prophylactic effect has been confirmed in a number of field trials, with efficacy as high as 70 per cent. They also have a modest therapeutic effect in influenza infections. Both compounds act by interference with virus uncoating in the infected cells.

Immunity

Recovery from the disease or immunization with inactivated virus results in immunity to influenza. Immunity is expressed as resistance to acquisition of infection or as a modified disease course when infection does occur. Increased resistance is also manifest by a reduction in the amount of virus shed in nasal secretions. There is, then, a profound effect upon the epidemiology of the disease in pop-

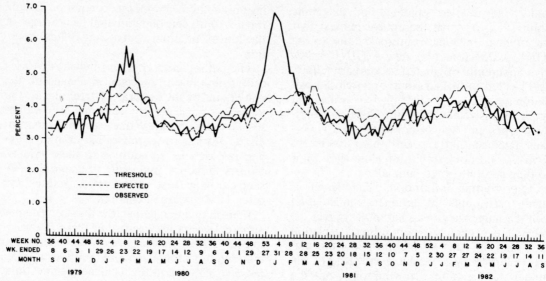

Figure 40–3. Deaths from pneumonia-influenza in 121 cities in the United States, showing excess mortality occurring during epidemic influenza. (Centers for Disease Control, Annual summary 1981: reported morbidity and mortality in the United States. Morbidity and Mortality Weekly Report, Vol. 30, No. 54, 1982.)

ulations with moderate to high levels of herd immunity, since the amount of circulating virus is lowered.

The immune response includes the appearance of antibodies against the NP antigens; these are generally detectable by complement fixation reactions. Effective immunity is, however, associated with antibodies against the hemagglutinating antigen, measured by either HI or virus neutralization. Although some protection, or viral neutralization, is exhibited by antineuraminidase antibodies, their activity in this regard is thought to be due to steric hindrance, since the neuraminidase spikes on the viral surface are in close juxtaposition to the hemagglutinating antigen. Antineuraminidase may play a role, however, in preventing or inhibiting release of virus from infected cells and thus has a modifying action in the disease process.

The presumed role of antibody is to prevent the attachment of virus to epithelial cells through the hemagglutinin. Since this attachment takes place at the surface of respiratory mucous membranes, attention has focused on secretory IgA as an effective antibody in the preliminary stages of infection. There is increasing evidence that **secretory IgA** is a better indicator of influenza immunity than serum antibodies, and this local immunity is considered to be a significant factor in effective immunity to the disease.

Immunity resulting from initial exposure to the virus antigens appears to be of a low order but, as described above, seems to increase in effectiveness with repeated exposure to the virus, so that the total experience of perhaps three decades provides a reasonable measure of effective immunity. This often, but not invariably, modifies subsequent infections so that the disease is subclinical or little more than a mild coryza. Such immunity is not effective, however, against virus strains in which major antigenic changes have occurred.

Prophylactic Immunization[47, 51]

Prophylactic immunization against the disease is accomplished with inactivated vaccine, prepared from virus grown in the allantoic cavity of the embryonated egg and partially purified, commonly by adsorption and elution from chicken red cells. An appreciable degree of effective immunity against homologous or closely related strains of virus is apparent in about a week and persists for some months. The degree of protection conferred is dependent upon the time elapsing between immunization and exposure, and it is estimated that 40 to 70 per cent of persons are protected by immunization. Vaccines employed for human immunization are usually multivalent, containing both type A and type B strains, but the specific virus strains used are periodically changed to reflect the alterations in HA and NA antigens that occur with antigenic shift or drift.

The use of inactivated vaccines has, on occasion, led to adverse effects, as in 1976–1977, when more than 500 cases of Guillain-Barré syndrome appeared among 40 million vaccinees in the United States. The improvement of influenza vaccines has therefore claimed the attention of investigators. More highly purified vaccines have been devised, either by separating the antigenic glycoproteins from the virion (subunit vaccines) or by more effective purification of whole virus vaccines by zonal centrifugation; subunit vaccines appear to be as effective as whole virus vaccines. Attenuated live vaccines hold more promise, since they may be administered intranasally, so as to stimulate secretory immunity as well as serum antibody response. Particular attention has been paid to genetic manipulation of these latter types, especially by recombination, to yield viruses of lowered virulence and with surface antigens tailored to match the prevalent wild viruses.

Laboratory Diagnosis[10]

The differentiation of influenza from a variety of clinically similar conditions is etiological and requires direct or indirect identification of the virus in the laboratory. Direct identification is accomplished most readily by virus isolation. Nasal washings, containing appropriate antibacterial substances, such as a mixture of penicillin and streptomycin, are inoculated into the amniotic cavity of 10- to 11-day-old chick embryos or into primary rhesus monkey kidney tissue culture. Virus, detected by the agglutination of type O human erythrocytes, appears in the amniotic fluid of eggs in two to four days and may be identified by hemagglutination-inhibition using antiserum against known influenza virus. In monkey kidney cell cultures, cytopathic effect is evident within a few days, hemadsorption is demonstrable, and viral hemagglutinins are released into the culture supernatant.

During infection of humans, the presence of the virus is shown indirectly by a rising antibody titer in paired serum specimens, one taken as early as possible in the acute stage of the disease, and the other 10 days to three weeks later. Complement fixation and hemagglutination-inhibition reactions are commonly employed for serological diagnosis. The former is less likely to be affected by minor antigenic differences between the test antigen and the infecting virus; a fourfold or greater rise in titer is regarded as diagnostic.

The Paramyxoviruses[6, 28]

The Paramyxoviridae, like the orthomyxoviruses, are large, enveloped, RNA viruses with a single-stranded RNA genome of negative polarity; a transcriptase is associated with the virion. They differ from orthomyxoviruses, however, in two significant aspects (see Table 40–1 and Fig. 40–1). First, the genomic RNA is not segmented, but is in the form of a single linear strand. Second, the surface glycoprotein spikes differ in form and function. One variety of glycoprotein spikes usually contains both hemagglutinating and neuraminidase (HN) activities. A second group of glycoprotein projections has a cell fusion (F) enzyme that causes fusion of adjacent host cells, leading to **syncytium formation** in cell monolayers. Three genera are recognized: (1) *Paramyxovirus,* which includes the parainfluenza viruses, Newcastle disease virus, and mumps virus; (2) *Pneumovirus,* containing the respiratory syncytial virus; and (3) *Morbillivirus,* containing the measles virus.

PARAINFLUENZA VIRUSES[14]

The viruses of the parainfluenza group are of worldwide occurrence and account for a considerable portion of acute respiratory disease in children, but are by no means unknown in adults. Four antigenic types of parainfluenza viruses are distinguished on the basis of their glycoprotein surface antigens. Although there is some variation in the clinical syndrome produced by each type, the disease often resembles a common cold, with pharyngitis, rhinitis, bronchitis, and fever, and a tendency to be more severe in children. The etiological relation of these viruses to such respiratory disease is indicated by specific antibody response and also by the experimental reproduction of the disease in human volunteers.

Most human infections with parainfluenza viruses are due to types 1, 2, or 3; type 4 is rarely encountered, and illnesses by this type tend to be quite mild. The viruses can be found in respiratory secretions, usually by type-specific immunofluorescence staining, or they may be isolated in monkey kidney tissue cultures. Similar serological tests may be adapted for titration of serum antibodies for serological diagnosis. In either case, however, there is often cross-reactivity between types, as well as with other viruses, so that all serological procedures must be carefully controlled and interpreted. Virus isolation is considered to be the most reliable diagnostic procedure.

Parainfluenza viruses rank second only to respiratory syncytial viruses as the cause of infections of the **lower respiratory tract**. Most lower respiratory infections occur in infants and young children. Reinfections in older children and adults are usually localized in the upper respiratory tract and are not as common as those in younger children. The parainfluenza viruses are often associated with a dramatic disease of children that manifests as **acute laryngotracheobronchitis**, or croup; types 1, 2, and 3 account for about 40 per cent of the cases of croup on a worldwide basis. Although the virus serotypes are closely related, the diseases they cause are often clinically and epidemiologically differentiated.

Parainfluenza Virus Type 1

Infections with the type 1 virus are common in children; there is evidence that about 75 per cent of children have been infected by around 5 years of age. Approximately half of these, however, are inapparent and without outward signs of infection; most of the remainder are mild febrile illnesses. Only about one-fourth of the clinically apparent infections result in more serious illness of the lower respiratory tract, usually bronchitis or pneumonia. A few of the primary infections with this type, up to 3 per cent, develop acute croup. Nevertheless, type 1 parainfluenza virus is the principal cause of this syndrome.

Since the early 1960s, type 1 parainfluenza infections have exhibited an epidemiological pattern characterized by epidemic outbreaks in children that occur in the autumn of alternate, even-numbered years. Expectedly, the incidence of croup follows this same pattern.

The virus is **highly communicable** by direct contact transmission, and a majority of the susceptibles are infected after exposure. Very young children seem to be protected by maternal antibody, and infection rarely is seen in those under 4 months of age. The incidence of infection rises rapidly after this, however, and continues until about 6 years of age. Reinfections may occur in later life, although not as often as with other parainfluenza types; most clinically apparent reinfections involve the upper, rather than the lower, respiratory tract.

Protective immunity is associated with antibody directed against the surface glycoprotein of the hemagglutinin-neuraminidase complex. There is evidence that local antibody, or secretory immunity, is more effective than serum antibody in preventing infection.

A subtype of parainfluenza virus type 1, the Sendai virus, has been an important model for molecular biology of paramyxoviruses. It is the cause of an acute pneumonitis of rodents in many parts of the world, and among swine in Japan. Human infections with Sendai virus have been claimed, and epidemics in Japan and the U.S.S.R. in the 1950s were reportedly due to this virus.

Parainfluenza Virus Type 2

The epidemiology and clinical aspects of type 2 infections are similar to those of type 1 virus, although illness is usually somewhat milder. The acute croup syndrome by this virus is less common than that due to type 1.

The virus commonly affects the same age groups as type 1 virus, and a majority of children are infected by the time they reach school age. Epidemics have usually appeared in alternate years, with a tendency to occur in the autumn of odd-numbered years.

Parainfluenza Virus Type 3

In contrast to types 1 and 2 parainfluenza virus, type 3 is often the cause of severe lower respiratory tract disease in children under 6 months of age. It appears that little protection is afforded by maternal antibody. Most illnesses by this virus type occur in children under 1 year of age, and about 80 per cent of children have experienced infection by 4 years of age. Of these, more than three-fourths develop a febrile illness and a significant portion of these, about one-third, experience bronchitis or pneumonia. Type 3 infections are transmitted more readily than the other types of parainfluenza viruses, and nosocomial outbreaks in hospital nurseries occur with some frequency.

Parainfluenza virus type 3 differs, too, in epidemiological patterns. Epidemic outbreaks are uncommon, and infections occur throughout the year. Many of these sporadic cases occur in older children and adults as reinfections, but they generally are milder than the primary childhood infections.

MUMPS VIRUS

Mumps, or epidemic parotitis, is a highly contagious, widespread, but seldom fatal disease of man that has long been known because of its distinctive clinical character, *i.e.*, swelling and tenderness of the parotid glands and orchitis in a variable but appreciable portion of cases. Some 60 per cent of adults are immune

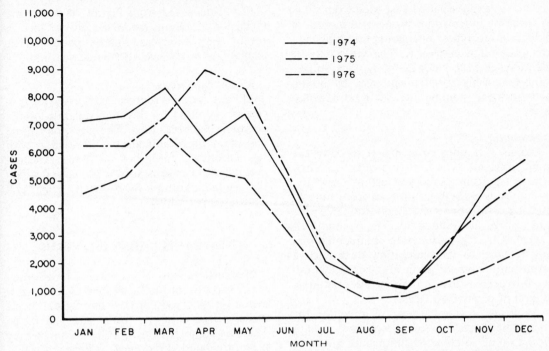

Figure 40–4. The incidence of mumps infection in the United States as shown by the number of cases reported each month, 1974–1976. Note the seasonal variation. (Morbidity and Mortality Weekly Report, Annual Summary, Vol. 25, 1976. Centers for Disease Control, U.S. Public Health Service.)

as compared with 90 per cent immune to measles virus. The disease tends to occur in the winter and early spring (Fig. 40–4).

The mumps virus has the biological and physical properties of other Paramyxoviridae and, with the parainfluenza viruses, is placed in the genus *Paramyxovirus*.

The mumps virus enters the host through the mucous membranes, through attachment mediated by the hemagglutinin-neuraminidase peplomers. Viruses grow in the parotid gland or in the epithelium of the respiratory tract and are then shed into the blood with secondary foci established in other tissues. The virus is found in blood, cerebrospinal fluid, saliva, and urine during the acute phase of the disease, but shedding probably begins several days before clinical symptoms appear. Not all infections are clinically apparent; depending on the age of the host, up to 70 per cent of infections are asymptomatic, yet virus may be shed in urine and respiratory secretions. Thus, the infection may be transmitted from incubating cases and from those with inapparent infections.

The Disease in Man

Mumps occurs only in man, and there is no animal reservoir of infection. The incubation period is about three weeks, in contrast to the short incubation period of other *Paramyxovirus* infections. A febrile reaction usually is seen and is followed within 24 hours by enlargement of the **salivary glands**, usually the parotids, but the sublingual and submaxillary glands may be affected also, and there is an edematous infiltration of the adjacent tissues. The swelling may be bilateral, unilateral, or unilateral followed by involvement of the unaffected side within a few days. It reaches a maximum in 48 hours and persists for one to two weeks, though some evidence of swelling may persist for longer periods. Typical symptoms of mumps, as just described, occur for the most part in children 5 to 10 years of age; infants rarely exhibit this clinical syndrome.

In adults, the complications of mumps are more serious. **Orchitis** occurs in perhaps 20 per cent of cases in young adult males, but the proportion may vary considerably from one outbreak to another, and the involvement is bilateral in only 15 to 20 per cent of those exhibiting orchitis. Sterility is therefore rare.

Symptoms referable to the central nervous system, indicative of meningoencephalitis, occur in a small proportion of cases—perhaps 10 per cent—and usually in older individuals; encephalitis may occur in the absence of parotitis. The pancreas, epididymis, prostate, and ovaries are affected only rarely.

The virus can usually be isolated from saliva or urine by inoculation of one of a variety of tissue culture types, but monkey kidney cells are most often employed. The virus may be identified in such cultures by hemadsorption-inhibition using specific antibody, by immunofluorescent staining, or by neutralization tests.

Immunity

Strains of mumps virus appear to be of the same antigenic type, and recovery from the disease results in a solid and lasting immunity. Immunity is possibly reinforced from time to time by reinfection, and unquestionable second attacks are quite rare. The immunity is indicated by the presence of complement-fixing, hemagglutination-inhibiting, or protective serum antibody. Infection also engenders delayed hypersensitivity to the intradermal inoculation of inactivated virus.

As an aid to the diagnosis of infection, the complement fixation test, employing mumps viral (V) or soluble (S) antigen is the most widely used. Antibody to the S antigen appears earlier, within a few days of onset, and may reach high titer before antibody to V antigen is detectable. Antibody to the S antigen disappears more rapidly, leaving persisting antibody to the V antigen as evidence of past infection.

A fourfold or greater rise in complement-fixing antibody titer between paired serums, taken as early as possible in the disease and two to three weeks after onset, is regarded as diagnostic. Serological diagnosis is not important when the syndrome is typical but is of value in meningoencephalitis appearing in the absence of salivary gland involvement.

Immunization[18]

Two kinds of vaccine are used for active immunization against mumps: one a formalin-inactivated virulent virus, and the other an attenuated live vaccine, prepared from a virus modified by culture in the embryonated egg and chick embryo tissue culture. The immunity produced by the former, as judged by serum-neutralizing antibody, is of limited duration, no antibody being detectable six months after immunization. The attenuated live virus vaccine, in contrast, produces seroconversion in more than 95 per cent of persons inoculated; it is lasting in that neutralizing antibody, as well as effective immunity to disease, persists for at least nine years after immunization, and there is evidence that this immunity is periodically reinforced by subclinical infection in the immunized population.[57]

It will be noted from Figure 40–5 that the incidence of mumps has markedly declined in recent years, a decrease that has paralleled the availability of the live attenuated vaccine.

Model Infections

Mumps may be reproduced in several species of monkeys by direct inoculation of the gland via Stensen's duct. The infection can be passed in these animals by inoculation with suspensions of parotid gland tissue. The experimental disease is similar to natural infections in man, with parotitis, facial edema, and associated pathology.

NEWCASTLE DISEASE VIRUS

Newcastle disease is a disease of birds which is occasionally acquired by man through contact with infected birds. The natural hosts include both domestic fowls and wild birds. There is some reason to believe that it may have originated in Indonesia, where it was first described in 1926. Newcastle disease appeared in England in the same year and was eradicated by slaughter and terminal disinfection. It was first identified in the United States in 1944 but may have been present as early as 1935. The disease has since been reported from all over the world.

Morphology and Cell Culture

The newcastle disease virus is similar to other kinds of *Paramyxovirus*; the virus is 80 to 120 nm. in diameter, but is not necessarily spherical, and may be filamentous or sperm-like in shape. It is usually resistant under both natural and laboratory conditions. In the first instance, poultry quarters may remain infective for many weeks and produce disease in freshly introduced chickens.

The virus is readily cultivable in the embryonated egg and in several kinds of tissue cultures. When it is grown in the allantoic cavity, hemagglutinin is found in the allantoic fluid. Heavily infected allantoic fluid is also toxic, killing mice in one to three days after intravenous inoculation. Intranasal inoculation in this animal produces interstitial pneumonia that is a manifestation of toxicity, for the virus does not multiply in the mouse lung.

The Disease in Man

Human infection is not common and appears to be confined almost exclusively to those who are closely associated with poultry, although laboratory infections have occurred. The incubation period is very short, two days or less;

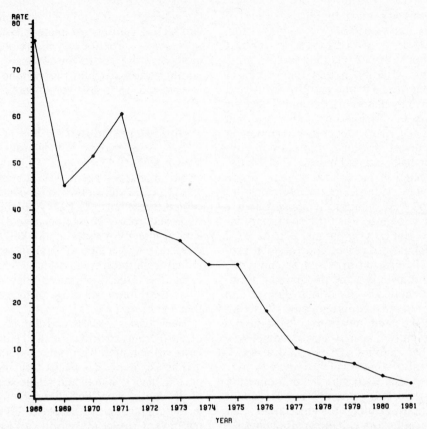

Figure 40–5. Reported cases of mumps in the United States, 1968–1981, per 10^5 population. The incidence has declined 95 per cent since 1968, the year after the live attenuated vaccine was licensed in the United States. (Centers for Disease Control, Annual summary 1981: reported morbidity and mortality in the United States. Morbidity and Mortality Weekly Report, Vol. 30, No. 54, 1982.)

disease is manifest as unilateral conjunctivitis without corneal involvement, and there may be preauricular adenitis, malaise, and chills, but without fever. No fatal cases have been reported, and recovery is complete within two weeks.

Serum antibody may or may not be detectable after recovery, and serodiagnosis is complicated by the presence of nonspecific neutralizing activity in the serum. At least some strains of mumps virus have antigens in common with Newcastle disease virus. In general, serodiagnosis of the human infection is not dependable.

The number of persons exposed to infection is very large. Several million people are intimately associated with the raising and care of chickens in this country, and several hundred thousand others are involved in the processing of poultry. Almost all human cases found thus far have been initial infections acquired from infected birds, and transmission from man to man has not been observed. Neither has there been an instance of human infection acquired from dressed poultry.

RESPIRATORY SYNCYTIAL VIRUS[16, 20, 34]

This virus was first isolated from chimpanzees with respiratory disease and has subsequently been found in children with pneumonia and bronchiolitis, and from adults with mild upper respiratory disease.

Respiratory syncytial virus (RSV), although similar to parainfluenza virus, is sufficiently different that it is classified in the genus *Pneumovirus*. The virus nucleoprotein helix is somewhat smaller than other paramyxoviruses, and neither neuraminidase nor hemagglutinin is apparent in the virion. The F glycoprotein is present and is responsible for the syncytium formation in cell cultures. The virus exhibits some antigenic heterogeneity among strains, but the differences are minimal. Respiratory syncytial virus may be grown in HEp-2 or HeLa cells and is isolated in this way from respiratory secretions; it is tentatively identified by characteristic cytopathic effects, *i.e.,* syncytium formation.

The virus is the most important agent of pneumonitis and bronchiolitis in infants, causing up to 90 per cent of bronchiolitis and as much as 40 per cent of pneumonia in infants. Infections are unusual in that they occur in infants during the first few months of life and are unaffected by maternal antibody. The virus is worldwide in distribution, and serological surveys indicate that infection is common in childhood; about one-half of infants are infected in the first year and most of the remainder are infected in the following year. There is considerable evidence that reinfections are common and that immunity is acquired only by such repeated infections. Most primary infections are clinically apparent, usually as a febrile, respiratory disease. Only a small proportion of these result in life-threatening disease, *viz.*, bronchiolitis and pneumonia. Reinfection seldom leads to serious illness, and most cases resemble common colds. It is concluded that repeated infection yields some degree of immunity that may not be completely protective but modifies subsequent disease.

There is also some evidence that a prior immune response, as occurs in immunization with inactivated RSV, potentiates subsequent RSV infections, leading to suggestions that immunological factors enhance pathogenesis.

MEASLES (RUBEOLA) VIRUS[21, 36, 63]

Measles is one of the commonest diseases of childhood, and prior to the advent of immunization, the number of reported cases often exceeded half a million per year in the United States. Humans appear to be universally highly susceptible to this infection, and the disease confers a solid immunity. These two factors combine to make measles the classic example of periodicity in the prevalence of infectious disease. In the absence of vigorous immunization programs, it has tended to recur in epidemic form at two- to three-year intervals.

Morphology and Cell Culture

The viral etiology of measles has been known since 1911, when the filterable nature of the infectious agent was demonstrated. It was grown in chick embryos and chick embryo cell cultures, but with no cytopathic effect. It remained poorly known because of the necessity for infectivity assay in monkeys until 1954, when it was isolated in human and monkey kidney cell cultures, in which a characteristic cytopathic effect is produced. Figures 40–6 and 40–7 illustrate morphology of measles virus in tissue culture.

The measles virus is classified as a member of the Paramyxoviridae in the genus *Morbillivirus*. In common with other paramyxoviruses it is an enveloped (–)RNA virus in which the nucleic acid is linear and single-stranded, the nucleocapsid is of helical symmetry, and the virion contains a transcriptase. Like the other paramyxoviruses, the virion surface possesses protein spikes with hemagglutinating (H) and cell fusion (F) activities. Unlike the mumps and parainfluenza viruses, however, no neuraminidase has been reported.

In cell culture, the cytopathic effect is syncytial in character, with formation of giant multinucleated cells by cell fusion (Fig. 40–8). Associated with the cell fusion character and the F glycoprotein spike is the capacity of viral particles to bring about hemolysis of certain

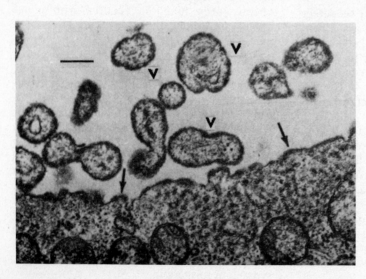

Figure 40–6. Measles virus in tissue culture. Released virions (*V*) exhibit some pleomorphism. Future budding sites (arrows) on the plasma membrane show accumulation of dense material. Bar = 200 nm. Miller, C. A., and C. S. Raine, J. Gen. Virol. **45**:441, 1979.)

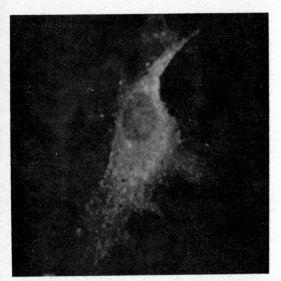

Figure 40–7. Intracellular measles virus in human epithelial cell tissue culture, treated with convalescent serum and with fluorescein-labeled antiglobulin serum. × 480. (Rapp and Gordon.)

kinds of red blood cells, *e.g.*, simian erythrocytes. Complement-fixing antigen is found in culture supernatants, and is most likely the ribonucleoprotein of the capsid. The virus, or its isolated hemagglutinating spikes, agglutinates monkey red blood cells, and hemadsorption occurs in cell culture sheets. Hemagglutination-inhibiting, as well as hemolysin-inhibiting, antibodies occur in antiserums and the cell culture system is used for the titration of

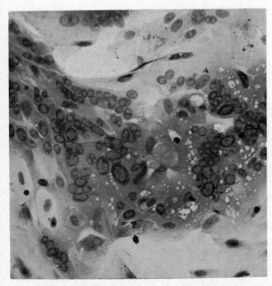

Figure 40–8. Measles virus in human renal cell tissue culture after 20 days' incubation showing multinucleated giant cell formation and nuclear acidophilic masses. (J. F. Enders and T. C. Peebles, Proc. Soc. Exptl. Biol. Med., **86**:277, 1954.)

neutralizing antibody. The virus is antigenically homogeneous, *i.e.*, only one antigenic type is known, and its marked stability in this respect is indicated by the persisting effective immunity.

The measles virus is antigenically related to the viruses of canine distemper and rinderpest, and indistinguishable from them in morphology and cytopathic effect, but the latter two viruses are set apart from the measles virus by failure to show hemagglutination. Distemper is a disease of carnivores, including foxes, wolves, and ferrets, as well as dogs, while rinderpest is a disease of cattle and swine.

The Disease in Man

The infection is probably acquired through the oropharyngeal and ocular pathways. Viral replication occurs in localized areas in the lymphatic system, followed by a transient viremia, during which the virus may be isolated from the blood.

The disease is initiated by prodromal symptoms of a few days' duration which are essentially catarrhal in nature, and include cough and fever. Perhaps the most characteristic lesions—**Koplik spots**—appear on the buccal mucosa during this period. These are focal exudations of serum and epithelial cells, forming vesicles which become necrotic, and their gross appearance is that of a white or bluish-white center on an erythematous area. Koplik spots are diagnostic of measles and occur in 95 per cent or more of cases. Virus is present in the nasopharyngeal and tracheobronchial secretions during the prodromal period and for a day or two after the appearance of the rash.

The characteristic macular or maculopapular rash, which tends to be confluent, appears within one or more days and spreads over the entire body. The capillaries of the corium are affected first; epithelial cells proliferate and a serous exudate spreads into the epidermis, followed by necrosis of the epithelial cells. The rash later becomes vesicular and brownish, followed by desquamation. There is some belief that the rash is not directly mediated by the virus, but may be an allergic phenomenon. Children with depressed T cell function, for example, do not develop rash and their measles attacks are otherwise atypical.

During the course of the disease there is a general lymphoid hyperplasia, and **multinucleate giant cells** are found in the tonsils, adenoids, lymph nodes, spleen, and appendix. Giant cells are also seen in the alveolar and bronchial epithelium in interstitial pneumonitis and in what has been referred to as giant cell pneumonia. There is a reduced resistance to secondary bacterial infection, particularly to bacterial pneumonia, which may be related to the known capacity of these viruses to interfere with certain features of cell-mediated immune response. Encephalomyelitis, with demyelination in the brain and cord, is an uncommon complication, with a case fatality rate of perhaps 20 to 25 per cent; 20 to 50 per cent of the survivors, however, are left with some neurological impairment. It has been established that measles infection is more serious in malnourished children and, curiously, measles appears to precipitate malnutrition, possibly by protein loss from the intestine. Chemotherapy is useful only in minimizing secondary bacterial infection.

Subacute Sclerosing Panencephalitis[7, 15, 17, 24, 56]

This affliction, a fatal central nervous system disease of children and young adults, was long thought to be a viral infection. This view was supported in 1965 when electron microscopy of postmortem specimens revealed the presence, in brain cell nuclei, of tubular structures morphologically resembling paramyxovirus nucleocapsids. Soon thereafter it was found that individuals suffering from subacute sclerosing panencephalitis (SSPE) developed abnormally high serum titers to the complement-fixing and hemagglutinating antigens of the measles virus and, in contrast to acute measles, antibody was present in cerebrospinal fluid as well. Immunofluorescent antibody staining of brain sections established that measles virus antigen was present in nerve cells. Numerous attempts to transfer the virus to animals were largely unsuccessful, but in the late 1960s, specialized techniques in which brain cells were cocultivated with established cell lines resulted in rescue of viruses that are similar to measles virus. The association of measles virus with SSPE now seems reasonably well established.

The mechanism of pathogenesis that leads to SSPE is not yet clear, but it is widely accepted that it represents a **persistent measles virus infection**, without production of mature infectious virus. It has recently been shown that while SSPE patients form antibodies to most measles virion proteins, antibodies directed against the membrane (M), or matrix, protein are significantly lacking; subsequent studies indicate that membrane protein is not produced in the infection. Since M protein plays an essential role in the assembly of virions at the plasma membrane, its absence

can explain the persistent, nonproductive infection with accumulation of other virion components in infected cells. It has been suggested that the failure to produce M protein results from host restriction of M protein synthesis in certain brain cells.

It is possible that measles or similar viruses are involved in other central nervous system disorders. It has been suggested that multiple sclerosis (MS) could be initiated by a persistent virus infection, and high titers of measles antibodies have been found in MS patients.

Immunity

Antibody is not detectable prior to the appearance of the rash, but thereafter the immune response is very rapid, with the appearance of significant titers within 48 hours. Recovery from the disease is associated with a solid immunity, persisting essentially throughout life. This continued immunity may be due to periodic reinforcement by subclinical infection, although some believe that it may be explained by persistent or latent infection. The measles virus is antigenically homogeneous, and complement-fixing, hemagglutination-inhibiting, and neutralizing antibody, though maximal in convalescent serum, is present in almost all adult serums.

Immunization

Passive immunization with pooled gamma globulin following exposure to infection may abort or modify the disease, depending upon how soon it is administered; if the disease is aborted; there is no active immune response. Pooled gamma globulin, *i.e.*, from adult serum, contains relatively high titers of both neutralizing and hemagglutination-inhibiting antibodies.

Active Immunization. Attempts to immunize against measles were initiated as early as 1758, but it was not until the development of methods of virus culture that the preparation of vaccines became practical. Two kinds of vaccines have been developed: one an inactivated unmodified virus, and the other an attenuated living virus.

Inactivated vaccines give relatively little untoward reaction, but have proved to be poor antigens and do not yield high levels of protection. Attenuated live measles vaccines were first licensed in the United States in 1963. They sometimes produce a febrile reaction and, occasionally, rash. Immunity induced by attenuated vaccines appears to be of a high order, with 95 per cent seroconversion, and persists for two years or more. Its efficacy has been

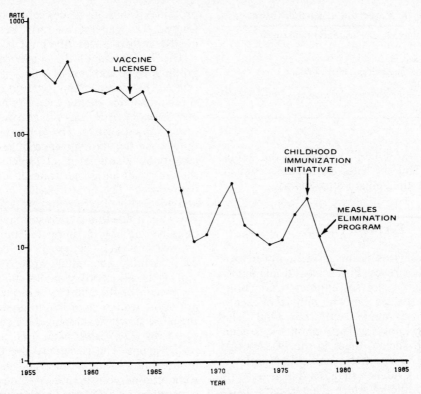

Figure 40–9. The incidence of measles in the United States, 1955–1981, as reported cases per 10^5 population. (Centers for Disease Control, Annual summary 1981: reported morbidity and mortality in the United States. Morbidity and Mortality Weekly Report, Vol. 30, No. 54, 1982.)

apparent in a number of field trials in various countries and through its widespread use in the United States.

Since the introduction of the vaccine the number of reported cases of measles in the United States reached a record low of 1.4 cases per 10^5 population, a 99.5 per cent reduction from the prevaccine period of 1955 to 1962 (Fig. 40–9). Based on the apparent success of immunization campaigns, a federal program was initiated in 1978 aimed at eliminating indigenous measles in the United States. Immunization initiatives have been directed toward preschool children, military personnel, and other young adults, such as those at colleges and universities. Epidemiological evi-

dence supports the view that measles transmission probably could not be maintained in most communities if 50 to 90 per cent of the population were immunized. There is, then, the possibility of the early eradication of indigenous measles.

It is of some interest that immunization programs have markedly changed the epidemiology of measles in the United States. In addition to the significant reduction in both morbidity and mortality, the age of greatest incidence has shifted from the 5- to 9-year-old age group to the 10- to 14-year-old age group, and the two- to three-year periodicity of epidemics has disappeared.

The Rhabdoviruses

The rhabdoviruses are a group of viruses that infect a wide variety of living forms, including plants and insects as well as animals. The viruses are rod-like or bullet-shaped particles, composed of a nucleocapsid of helical symmetry enclosed in a membrane derived by budding from the host cell. Embedded within

the membrane and projecting from the surface are glycoprotein spikes. Like the paramyxoviruses described above, the rhabdovirus nucleocapsid is composed of single-stranded, linear RNA of negative polarity associated with a core protein (Table 40–4).

The family Rhabdoviridae includes the ra-

Table 40–4. **Properties of Rhabdoviruses**

(−)RNA genome; continuous, linear, and single-stranded
Helical nucleocapsid
Rod- or bullet-shaped virion, 80 × 180 nm.
Transcriptase in virion
Enveloped (from plasma or intracytoplasmic membranes)
Ether-sensitive

bies and rabies-related viruses of the genus *Lyssavirus* and the virus of bovine vesicular stomatitis in the genus *Vesiculovirus*.

RABIES VIRUS[1]

The rabies virus is the most highly **neurotropic** of the viruses. Practically all mammals, and some birds, are susceptible to infection, and in most species, but with important exceptions, rabies is almost uniformly fatal. The disease, also known as hydrophobia, has been known from ancient times in the Old World, in Egypt, Greece, Italy, and other parts of Europe; the evidence suggests that it was imported into the Western Hemisphere from Europe. Rabies is essentially a disease of wild animals, principally carnivores and omnivores; the disease is sometimes passed to domestic animals by bite or intimate contact. Humans are usually infected by the bite of infected animals, either wild or domestic, although a few cases have appeared under circumstances suggesting airborne infection, *viz.*, from exposure to bat droppings in caves.

Morphology and Cell Culture[38, 42]
The rabies virus is rod-shaped, 80 by 180 nm., with one end of the particle flat and the other rounded to give a bullet shape characteristic of rhabdoviruses; it sometimes occurs as shorter particles, or as longer filaments. Like other viruses with lipid envelopes, it is ether-sensitive.

The helical nucleocapsid consists of a single-stranded (−)RNA with an associated protein, the N protein, of about 60,000 daltons, together with a smaller minor protein (NS protein). A third protein of the nucleocapsid is longer (L) and is the RNA-dependent RNA polymerase. The nucleocapsid is enclosed within a lipid membrane derived from the host cell that contains two membrane proteins (M1 and M2) of viral origin. A glycoprotein (G protein) occurring within the membrane and projecting as spikes from the surface in hexagonal arrangement is the largest of the virion

proteins. Rabies virus replication is thought to follow the general pattern described for (−)RNA viruses described in Chapter 38.

The N protein of the nucleocapsid is the **group-specific antigen** of rabies virus and is related by complement fixation reaction to similar proteins of the rabies-related viruses, *viz.*, Mokola virus, Lagos bat virus, and certain other animal viruses. The G protein is considered to be the **serotype-specific antigen** and is essentially identical in all rabies viruses, although small antigenic strain differences have been noted. The G protein has **hemagglutinin activity** and is also the antigen responsible for **virus neutralization** by antiserum; it is usually demonstrated by the latter reaction.

The virus may be grown in embryonated eggs. Without adaptation, growth in the chick embryo is sufficiently slow that it is outstripped by growth of the embryo, and yields of virus are poor. It may be grown to greater yields in the more slowly developing duck egg, and duck egg virus (DEV) has been used as an immunizing agent. The virus may also be grown in mouse brain tissue culture and in cultures of some non-nervous tissues, *viz.*, newborn hamster kidney fibroblasts, rabbit endothelium, and the WI-38 strain of human diploid cells, but without cytopathic effect. In such cell cultures the virus is demonstrable by the fluorescent antibody technique.

Pathogenicity[37]
The neurotropism of the rabies virus is evident in the pathogenesis of the disease. At the site of the local injury where it is introduced into the body, the virus multiplies in muscle cells; the virus then invades the peripheral nerves and ascends to the central nervous system. The virus usually enters the central nervous system via the spinal cord and rapidly ascends to the brain. The localization and replication in the brain is responsible for the signs and symptoms of rabies.

Infection results in extensive destruction in the cerebral and cerebellar cortices, midbrain, basal ganglia, pons, and medulla, with neuronal degeneration and demyelination. Similar changes are observed in the spinal cord and are most marked in the posterior horns. There is general hyperemia and mononuclear infiltration, and there may be small perivascular hemorrhages. The extent of these changes is related to the duration of the disease, and when death occurs soon, they may be minimal.

Centrifugal spread follows brain involvement, with the virus descending through neural

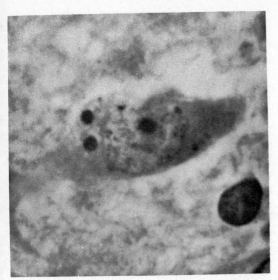

Figure 40–10. Negri bodies in a nerve cell in a section of the brain of a rabid cat. The three dark spherical bodies within the cytoplasm of the cell are Negri bodies. (Schleifstein.)

tissue to involve nerve endings in most peripheral organs and tissues, including skin, muscle, and salivary glands.

Negri Bodies. The acidophilic inclusion body, the Negri body, is pathognomonic of rabies (Fig. 40–10). The matrix of this inclusion appears to be made up of unassembled components of the virus, e.g., ribonucleoprotein. The Negri bodies are found within the cytoplasm of the large ganglion cells; they are round in shape when lying free in the cytoplasm, may be compressed to an oval form by the nucleus, and are elongated when present in the dendrons. There is considerable range in size of Negri bodies, commonly given as 2

to 10 μm., but both smaller and larger bodies may be found. Negri bodies are demonstrable by Giemsa or Seller's stain and by fluorescent antibody staining.

Negri bodies are not invariably present in infections. Many of the viruses infecting wildlife, e.g., skunk and bat strains, do not form Negri bodies. They are also not consistently produced by canine (street) virus or by rabbit-adapted (fixed) strains.

Rabies in Lower Animals[45]

Rabies virus occurs primarily in reservoirs of infection in lower animals, most often carnivorous mammals. The kinds of animals providing the reservoirs differ from one part of the world to another. Two epidemiological forms of animal disease are recognized: the **urban form,** found in domestic animals, and the **wildlife forms** (Fig. 40–11).

In Europe, rabies is present as an enzootic in foxes. The infection in these animals is probably transmitted by biting, since the virus is found in salivary secretions. Fox rabies is almost invariably fatal, and the infection is maintained by continuous transmission.

In North America, the wildlife infection, based on isolation of the virus, appears in a wider variety of animals; in the central and Pacific states, skunks are the predominantly infected variety, with a significant number of infections occurring also in foxes. Raccoons are the principal reservoir in the Southeastern states, and bats carry the infection in most geographical areas. In Canada the disease is enzootic in foxes and skunks.

The infection in wild animals may be regarded as the natural form of the disease. It serves as the source of infection for domestic

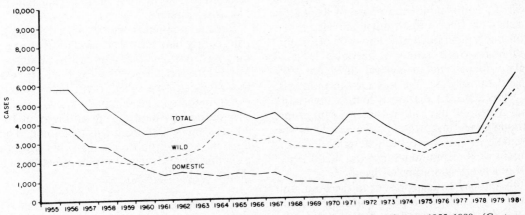

Figure 40–11. Reported cases of rabies in wild and domestic animals in the United States, 1955–1980. (Centers for Disease Control, Annual summary 1980: reported morbidity and mortality in the United States. Morbidity and Mortality Weekly Report, Vol. 29, No. 54, 1981.)

animals, yielding the urban type of disease, the form most important to man. Rabies is usually transmitted to humans by the bite of cats or dogs. Human infections are rare in Europe and the United States, because of animal immunization and other control programs. Only 23 cases of rabies were reported in the United States between 1970 and 1981. In underdeveloped nations where control measures are not widely practiced, human infections are more frequent.

Rabies in Dogs.[26] The infection in dogs is closely similar to that in wild animals and also to the human disease, and may be considered as representative. Dogs are infected by wild animals, or by other dogs, from the bite of an infected animal. Disease is not inevitable; fewer than half of the dogs bitten by a rabid animal later develop the disease. The usual incubation period is 3 to 10 weeks, but may be as short as 10 days, and under experimental conditions is dependent upon the amount of virus inoculated. The virus is present in the saliva prior to the appearance of characteristic clinical signs of the disease, and the animal is infectious during the last three to five days of the incubation period.

The disease takes two forms—one **furious** or **mad rabies**, the other **dumb rabies**—depending upon the prolongation of the excitation period. In furious or mad rabies, the animal at first becomes restless and apprehensive, and may become apathetic or seek out companionship. It then becomes hyperexcitable, responding to minimal stimuli, and runs about snapping and biting without discrimination, apparently oblivious to its surroundings. Beginning paralysis results in drooling of saliva due to inability to swallow, the gait may become abnormal, and the vocal cords are affected to give an eerie quality to the bark or howl. In dumb rabies the phase of excitation is relatively short, the animal appears to be profoundly depressed and unaware of its surroundings, overt paralysis becomes increasingly evident, and in general the more prolonged the disease, the greater the paralysis. In either case the disease is almost invariably fatal within 10 days after onset of symptoms, although rare instances of recovery from the paralytic disease have been described. Occasionally death from rabies may occur suddenly, without overt symptoms of disease.

On autopsy virus is present in the brain and cord, in the salivary and lacrimal glands, and in the kidney and pancreas, but seldom in the blood, and generally is not found in tissues of mesodermal origin. Strains of virus differ somewhat in their tissue affinities, some strains infecting and multiplying in the salivary glands to a greater extent than others.

The clinical features of the disease are characteristic, and the canine infection is diagnosed by the presence of Negri bodies (but not eliminated by their absence) or by isolation of the virus, commonly by intracerebral inoculation of mice. The diagnosis of canine rabies is of practical significance in relation to the institution of prophylactic immunization in humans exposed to infection by the bite of a dog.

Rabies in Bats.[4] The occurrence of bat rabies, or chiropteran rabies, was first recognized in Brazil in 1908. The infection has since been found to be widely distributed in vampire bats. The most important species in this connection is *Desmodus rotundus murinus,* found in South and Central America, and Mexico. Since 1953 the infection has been found in a number of species of nonhemophagous bats in various parts of the United States.

While the furious type of rabies is seen in both naturally and experimentally infected bats and is frequently fatal, an appreciable number survive to become healthy carriers of the virus. Bats are, therefore, an exception to the general rule that the infection is almost always fatal.

During hibernation, the virus persists without multiplication in the brown fat, or hibernation gland. When hibernation is broken and the animal's temperature rises, virus multiplication begins. The virus may then be detectable in other tissues, including nasal mucosa.

The vampire bat bites at night, to transmit the infection to cattle and domestic animals and to man. The fatal paralytic disease in cattle has, in the past, assumed epizootic proportions in the Americas. In most instances, however, infected cattle do not present an infection hazard to humans.

Infected nonhemophagous insectivorous and fruit-eating bats have been found in 15 states, ranging from a number of southern states to Minnesota and east to New England. In Texas, the Mexican free-tailed bat *(Tatarida mexicana)* appears to be relatively heavily infected as indicated by neutralizing antibody in 16 to 70 per cent of the specimens examined. There appears to be little doubt that bats constitute a significant reservoir of rabies infection in the Western Hemisphere.

Attenuation

Alteration of the virulence of rabies virus by serial animal passage is the classic example of attenuation of virulence, and this method was applied by Pasteur in his development of attenuated virus for prophylactic immunization. The canine virus, as encountered in nature, was designated by him **street virus.** On serial passage by intercerebral inoculation into rabbits, this virus becomes progressively less virulent. Virus strains modified in this fashion were termed **fixed virus** by Pasteur.

Fixed virus is characterized by an enhanced neurotropism, an inability to produce Negri bodies in the infected animal, and a reduced ability to invade the salivary glands. Pasteur's original strain of fixed virus, together with many of its substrains, is still available and has gone through more than 2000 passages in the rabbit. These strains vary in virulence, as indicated by differences in incubation period and ability to produce infection by peripheral routes of inoculation in various experimental animals, but in general neurotropism is sufficiently enhanced that strains are avirulent for the rabbit, dog, and man by the subcutaneous route.

The virus may also be adapted to the chick and chick embryo by continuous passage. The best-known adapted strain is the Flury strain. After original isolation it was passed 136 times in chicks without observed changes except for a decrease in incubation period, from 30 to 6 days. Upon repeated further passage in chick embryos its pathogenicity for rabbits and dogs was altered so that it no longer produced disease when given by other than neural routes. Both dogs and rabbits are resistant to intracerebral inoculation with this high egg passage, or HEP, strain. Such attenuated strains are of particular interest as immunizing agents.

The Disease in Man

Human infection with rabies virus is acquired by the bite of an infected animal. The infectiousness of the animal is determined by the presence of virus in the saliva; it may be present for a few days, probably not more than five, prior to the onset of symptoms. This time element is significant, for if the animal does not develop rabies within 10 days, the saliva was probably not infectious at the time of the bite. The incubation period of the human disease ranges from a minimum of two weeks, or possibly slightly less, to as long as five to seven months and is related to the severity and location of the bite and the innervation of the muscle tissue involved. Not all persons bitten by a known rabid animal develop the disease.

Whether or not infection occurs is influenced by factors such as the severity of the wound, the removal of saliva when the bite is through heavy clothing, etc., but among equally severely bitten persons fewer than half may develop the disease. There is evidence that the infection may be acquired by inhalation, as in the laboratory or in caves frequented by bats, and an association between such caves and the occurrence of rabies in foxes has been observed. In this regard, of the 19 cases of human rabies acquired in the United States between 1966 and 1981, bite exposure could not be established in nine cases. Several cases of rabies have apparently been transmitted by corneal transplant from infected donors.

The clinical disease in man is similar to that in the dog. The prodromal symptoms include fever, headache, malaise, nausea, and anorexia; anxiety or depression is common, and there are often sensations of itching, burning, or tingling at the site of the wound. The onset of the excitation phase is gradual and indicated by increasing nervousness and apprehension. The characteristic symptom is the painful spasmodic contraction of the muscles involved in swallowing and the accessory muscles of respiration when fluid comes in contact with the fauces; subsequent suggestion of the act of swallowing may precipitate muscle spasm. It is this feature of the disease that gives it the name hydrophobia. As the disease progresses there may be muscular contractions and tremor, choking, and resulting cyanosis; convulsions occur, and there is often maniacal behavior. Such periods of excitation may be interspersed with lucid intervals. Death usually occurs during convulsions. In some instances the patient survives the period of excitement and becomes apathetic, stupor and coma follow, and an ascending type of paralysis develops. The disease in man has been considered to be invariably fatal but at least two instances of recovery have been described.

Laboratory Diagnosis[23]

The laboratory diagnosis of rabies is usually of primary importance in the animal which has bitten or otherwise exposed humans to the virus. As indicated above, the saliva is infectious prior to the development of symptoms. Premature destruction of the animal is undesirable and if possible the disease should be allowed to develop, if present, to facilitate diagnosis. Such diagnosis, in lower animals or man, is based on the demonstration of Negri bodies by Giemsa or Seller's stain; the fluorescent antibody technique allows the identification of smaller bodies not ordinarily identifiable as Negri bodies. The latter technique may, in fact, be used to identify the virus in the salivary glands of infected animals. The virus may also be isolated by intracerebral inoculation of infant mice and demonstration of Negri bodies in the mouse brain.

Immunity

Complement-fixing and neutralizing antibodies are formed in response to immunization with vaccine and in unimmunized individuals during the course of the disease. The immune response to infection is not an effective one in man, nor does antibody activity have diagnostic value except in animals that recover from the disease, such as bats. Antibody titrations are useful, however, for assaying the response to immunizing preparations, identification of virus by neutralization tests, and other experimental purposes.

Immunoprophylaxis[35, 38]

There seems to be no significant change in the antigenicity of rabies virus on adaptation to give fixed virus, and effective immunization against rabies in man is possible because of the long incubation period, which allows sufficient time to induce an effective immune response. Immunization of dogs and other pets on a mass basis makes possible the control of the urban type of the disease. The immune response to vaccines is not long-lasting, and in the case of dogs must be repeated each year.

The extended incubation period in rabies makes possible the development of an effective immunity even though the immunization is begun after exposure. Pasteur's original method was the daily inoculation of the exposed person with emulsions of fixed virus contained in dried rabbit spinal cord. Later, other vaccines prepared from viruses grown in brains of infected animals and inactivated by various chemical and physical methods were used. Many of these vaccines contained relatively large amounts of nerve tissue, which resulted in complications, usually neuritis or myelitis with occasional permanent damage from immunological cross-reactions.

Vaccines prepared from egg- or cell-cultured virus, and consequently lacking contaminating nerve tissue antigens, are more acceptable immunizing agents. The chick embryo–adapted HEP Flury strain noted above is effective for primary immunization of domestic animals, but not for man or subhuman primates. Vaccine prepared from virus cultured in duck eggs, and inactivated with β-propiolactone, is a more effective immunizing agent and has been widely used for human immunization.

In Europe and the United States these vaccines have now been replaced by the human diploid cell culture vaccines (HDCV), in which virus is grown in human embryo lung cells (WI-38) and inactivated after virus purification. These vaccines have proved to be very effective when given after exposure.

Rabies antiserum contains neutralizing antibody demonstrable experimentally and has been of interest as a prophylactic or an adjunct prophylactic for the human disease. It is evident that if antiserum containing neutralizing antibody is given very soon, within a few days of exposure to infection, it gives an appreciable protective effect, and a combination of antiserum and vaccine often gives better protection than either alone.

In recent years, interest has developed in interferon as a prophylactic agent for rabies. In monkeys, some protection has been noted by administration of human interferon,[58] and combinations of interferon inducers and HDCV provided better protection than vaccine alone.[2] It has been suggested that vaccination not only serves to induce neutralizing antibody but may also induce interferon.

The Retroviruses[5, 29, 61]

The RNA tumor viruses have been known for a number of years, having been first observed in 1908 in association with leukemia of chickens and later, in 1911, as the agent of a sarcoma of chickens. The viruses are widely distributed in nature and are associated with tumor production in a number of animal species, primarily fowl, rodents, and cats.

The viruses of this group are classified in the family Retroviridae, since they contain a **reverse transcriptase,** or RNA-dependent DNA polymerase (Chapter 38); the RNA tumor viruses are contained in the subfamily Oncovirinae. Related viruses in other subfamilies are (1) the Spumovirinae—the foamy viruses, characterized by a syncytial type of cytopathic effect and persistence in their hosts, found in a variety of domestic animals and primates; and (2) the Lentivirinae—the visna virus and related agents that cause respiratory and demyelinating diseases of sheep. The members of these latter two subfamilies are not, strictly speaking, tumor viruses and will not be discussed in this context.

Morphology and Structure

The RNA tumor viruses, also called **oncoviruses,** are spherical in form and about 100 nm. in diameter. The viral genome is composed of two apparently identical subunits of 30 to 40 S, single-stranded RNA. These are linked by hydrogen bonding near their 5′ ends to form a complete 60 to 70 S RNA complex. Associated with this complex are a few smaller RNA molecules that serve as primer for the virion enzyme, reverse transcriptase. It is this latter enzyme that characterizes the retroviruses. Its function is to transcribe viral RNA into a complementary double-stranded DNA molecule. The complementary DNA molecule is integrated into the host cell DNA; in this form it is known as the **provirus.** The provirus serves as the template for transcription of progeny viral RNA, using host cell transcriptase.

The virus is assembled in the cytoplasm and enveloped by budding through the plasma membrane. The host-derived glycolipid membrane contains virus-specified envelope glycoproteins that appear as projections on the virion surface. These glycoproteins are the type-specific antigens of the virus and are responsible for host-range specificity, since they behave as adsorption determinants. Internal structural proteins are not glycosylated, and these constitute the group-specific antigens of the virus. The properties of retroviruses are shown in Table 40–5.

Two principal morphological types of retroviruses are distinguished. Type B particles, exemplified by the mouse mammary tumor virus, contain an eccentric, electron-dense nucleocapsid, while the nucleocapsid of type C viruses is centrally located in the virion. Type

C viruses are the most common and are characteristic of the sarcoma and leukemia viruses of both avian and murine species.

Replication[22]

The replication of RNA tumor viruses is discussed in Chapter 38 (see also Fig. 38–29). After attachment, penetration, and uncoating, complementary viral DNA is transcribed by action of the reverse transcriptase, using virus RNA as a template. Located at both ends of the viral DNA is a region of several hundred base pairs, called the **long terminal repeats (LTR)**, that serve as a promoter to initiate later RNA synthesis. After transport to the nucleus, the viral DNA is integrated into the host DNA in a highly ordered process. The integrated viral DNA, with its LTRs, is termed the provirus and becomes a part of the genetic lineage of the cell, being vertically transmitted to progeny cells.

In productive infections, the viral DNA is transcribed to virus-specified RNA, with subsequent translation of mRNA to form viral proteins. The viral components are assembled in the cytoplasm and the virus is enveloped when it is released by budding through the plasma membrane. Release in this way does not lead to death of the host cell. Released viruses are infective and can be horizontally transmitted among animals.

Retroviruses possess three genes that are required for virus replication and production of the mature virion: *gag, pol,* and *env. Gag* encodes for the nonglycosylated structural proteins, *pol* for the reverse transcriptase, and *env* for the glycosylated proteins of the virion envelope. Many of the oncoviruses are, however, defective in one or more, sometimes all, of these genes required for replication; in such instances, no viral progeny are formed. Some of the defective leukemia and sarcoma viruses can, however, replicate in the presence of an infectious helper virus, which supplies the missing genetic information.

The proviral form of retroviruses is subject to control by regulatory signals contained in the LTRs and to the regulatory events that affect cellular genes. The insertion of provirus into the host genome is also believed to affect the expression of host genes.

Endogenous Viruses[46, 59]

As noted above, infection of a cell with retrovirus is followed by insertion of the provirus into the cell genome and subsequent transmission of the provirus to daughter cells.

Table 40–5. **Properties of Retroviruses**

(+)RNA genome; linear, single-stranded; two identical
  RNA molecules associated by hydrogen bonding
Icosahedral symmetry
Spherical virion, 100 nm.
Reverse transcriptase in virion
Enveloped (from plasma membrane)
Ether-sensitive

When this proviral insertion takes place in germline cells of an animal, the provirus is transmitted to the offspring and to succeeding generations. Such viruses are termed endogenous viruses and may be genetically silent (without the production of new viruses or viral products), or they may be activated, resulting in virus production. In some instances, only defective virus may be produced.

Endogenous viruses are apparently not harmful to the host in which they occur; there is some evidence that they may even be beneficial. Endogenous viruses appear to be ubiquitous in vertebrate species. It is of interest that while endogenous viruses are harmless in their natural host, if the mature and infectious virus is transmitted to a new host species, productive infection and tumorigenesis may ensue.

Endogenous viruses are usually present as only a few copies of provirus per cell. This number may increase by repeated infection of the germline cell. Reinfection can also lead to recombinational events that may give rise to infectious oncogenic viruses, often with increased host range.

Animal Oncoviruses[12, 52]

The viral etiology of avian leukosis was first described in 1908, and the fowl sarcomas, transmissible by cell-free filtrates, were identified by Rous in 1911. Since that time, oncoviruses have been shown to cause neoplastic diseases in a number of animal species. For more than two decades, these animal diseases, particularly those of avian and murine species,

have been extensively studied as models of oncogenesis and as probes for the biochemical and molecular bases of cellular growth and development.

Representative RNA tumor viruses of animals are listed in Table 40–6. These viruses are conveniently separated into two groups, differing in mode of tumorigenesis and the time elapsing between infection and appearance of tumors.

Acute Transforming Viruses. The acute, transforming viruses are those that are capable of transforming cells in culture (Chapter 38) and rapidly induce tumors in animals. They include sarcomagenic viruses of birds, rats, mice, cats, and gibbon apes, as well as the acute leukemogenic viruses of birds.

The acute transforming viruses each possess an **oncogene,** or transforming gene, that is responsible for transformation of cells in culture and for the induction of tumors. The oncogene of the Rous sarcoma virus (RSV), designated *src,* has been intensively studied and may be regarded as a prototype of the transforming genes in RNA tumor viruses. The *src* gene is a part of the RSV genome and is necessary to maintain the oncogenic state of transformed cells; it is not required for replication of the virus. It is of great theoretical significance that there is a normal cell equivalent, or homolog, of the *src* gene, so that the viral gene is now designated *v-src* and its normal cell homolog is *c-src.* The normal cell gene is present in low numbers of copies and is highly conserved. Thus, both avian and mammalian DNA contain *c-src* genes that are

Table 40–6. **Some RNA Tumor Viruses of Animals**

Group	Oncogenicity	Representative Virus
Acute transforming viruses	Avian sarcoma	Rous sarcoma virus Fujinami virus
	Murine sarcoma	Harvey sarcoma virus Kirsten sarcoma virus Moloney sarcoma virus
	Feline sarcoma	Feline sarcoma virus
	Simian sarcoma	Sarcoma virus of wooley monkeys
	Avian leukemia	Myeloblastoma virus Erythroblastosis virus Myelocytomatosis virus
Subacute oncogenic viruses	Avian leukemia	Avian leukosis virus
	Murine leukemia	Murine leukemia virus
	Mouse adenocarcinoma	Mouse mammary tumor virus
	Feline leukemia	Feline leukemia virus
	Bovine leukemia	Bovine leukemia virus
	Ape leukemia	Gibbon ape leukemia virus

largely homologous to the RSV *v-src* gene. The normal cell *c-src* gene also possesses transforming potential.

The gene product of RSV *src* has recently been identified as a phosphoprotein with protein kinase activity, phosphorylating other proteins at their tyrosine residues. The protein kinase activity is localized in the cell membrane and, in ways not yet defined, is either directly or indirectly concerned with transformation of the cell.

It now appears likely that *v-src* genes, or other viral transforming genes, generally known as *onc* genes, represent cellular genes (*c-onc*) appropriated by the provirus from the normal cellular genome by recombination or other means. In this fashion the *c-onc* may be placed under the control of a viral promoter and lead to uncontrolled overproduction of the *c-onc*, now *v-onc*, gene product to result in transformation of the cell. It is presumed that the cellular genes are restricted in normal cells and that their function is to control growth and development of the cell.

Based on recent findings, in which a dozen or more cellular gene sequences have been identified in the genomes of acute transforming viruses, a unified concept is emerging that similarly accounts for transformation by these viruses through the overproduction of transforming proteins.

Subacute Oncogenic Viruses. The second group of RNA tumor viruses, the subacute oncogenic viruses, differ from the acute transforming viruses just described. The subacute viruses, responsible for leukemias of birds, mice, cats, cattle, and gibbon apes, and adenocarcinomas of mice, do not transform cells in culture, nor do they possess transforming genes. Moreover, they are more slowly oncogenic in infected animals.

The mode of tumorigenesis in these viruses is possibly more complex and varied than transforming viruses, and is not as well defined by present knowledge. Several possible mechanisms for oncogenesis have been proposed, each with some supporting evidence. Perhaps the best supported of these hypotheses is the **promoter insertion model.** In this model, it is presumed that the provirus, with potent regulating signals in its LTRs, can influence transcription of adjacent sequences of host DNA. Evidence supporting this hypothesis arises from studies on avian leukosis viruses (ALV). Defective exogenous proviruses have been found in a number of ALV-induced tumors, often without virus gene expression. Thus,

presence of the virus is not required for oncogenesis. Furthermore, the provirus is often integrated into the host genome at a site near or adjacent to a *c-onc* gene. In this instance, the LTR is thought to promote the transcription of adjacent cellular sequences; if these contain a *c-onc* gene, overproduction of the gene products could result, leading to pathogenesis. The presence of defective provirus would appear to potentiate this mode of oncogenesis.

Human Cancer[19, 25, 54]

Many of the malignancies of humans, particularly the leukemias and breast cancer, have similarities to those produced in animals by RNA tumor viruses, a fact that has caused many to search for viral agents in human cancer. Several avenues have been followed to provide evidence for viral etiology, *viz.,* electron microscopic searches for viral particles, identification of viral antigens on tumor cells or antibodies to the virus in serum, the presence in tumor cells of reverse transcriptase activity, and the presence of viral RNA or DNA provirus.

In most instances, the etiological relationships between RNA tumor viruses and human cancer is tenuous at best, but appears to be strongest in human leukemias and lymphomas. Retroviruses have recently been isolated in the United States from human patients with cutaneous T cell leukemia or lymphoma, and a similar virus has been isolated in Japan from patients with adult T cell leukemia. In the latter case, normal human T cells have been transformed by the virus. Thus, there is now a stronger link between retroviruses and one type of human cancer.

REFERENCES

1. Baer, G. M. (Ed.) 1975. The Natural History of Rabies. Vols. I and II. Academic Press, New York.
2. Baer, G. M., *et al.* An effective rabies treatment in exposed monkeys: a single dose of interferon inducer and vaccine. Bull. Wld Hlth Org. **57**:807–813.
3. Bean, W. J., Jr., N. J. Cox, and A. P. Kendal. 1980. Recombination of human influenza A viruses in nature. Nature **284**:638–640.
4. Bigler, W. J., G. L. Hoff, and E. E. Buff. 1975. Chiropteran rabies in Florida: a twenty-year analysis, 1954 to 1973. Amer. J. Trop. Med. Hygiene **24**:347–352.
5. Bishop, J. M. 1980. The molecular basis of oncogenesis by retroviruses. pp. 211–224. *In* H. Smith, J. J. Skehel, and M. J. Turner (Eds.): The Molecular Basis of Microbial Pathogenicity. Verlag Chemie, Weinheim.

6. Choppin, P. W., and A. Scheid. 1980. The role of viral glycoproteins in adsorption, penetration, and pathogenicity of viruses. Rev. Infect. Dis. **2**:40–61.

7. Choppin, P. W., et al. 1981. The functions and inhibition of the membrane glycoproteins of paramyxoviruses and myxoviruses and the role of the measles virus M protein in subacute sclerosing panencephalitis. J. Infect. Dis. **143**:352–363.

8. Couch, R. B. 1981. The effects of influenza on host defenses. J. Infect. Dis. **144**:284–291.

9. Cox, N. J., Z. S. Bai, and A. P. Kendal. 1983. Laboratory-based surveillance of influenza A(H1N1) and A(H3N2) viruses in 1980–81: antigenic and genomic analysis. Bull. Wld Hlth Org. **61**:143–152.

10. Dowdle, W. R., A. P. Kendal, and G. R. Noble. 1980. Influenza virus. pp. 836–844. In E. H. Lennette, et al. (Eds.): Manual of Clinical Microbiology. 3rd ed. American Society for Microbiology, Washington, D.C.

11. Gardner, I. D., and K. F. Shortridge. 1979. Recombination as a mechanism in the evolution of influenza viruses: a two-year study of ducks in Hong Kong. Rev. Infect. Dis. **1**:885–890.

12. Gilden, R. V., and H. Rabin. 1982. Mechanisms of viral tumorigenesis. Adv. Virus Res. **27**:281–334.

13. Glezen, W. P. 1982. Serious morbidity and mortality associated with influenza epidemics. Epidemiol. Rev. **4**:25–44.

14. Glezen, W. P., F. A. Loda, and F. W. Denny. 1976. The parainfluenza viruses. pp. 337–349. In A. S. Evans (Ed.): Viral Infections of Humans, Epidemiology and Control. Plenum Publishing Corp., New York.

15. Haase, A. T., et al. 1981. Measles virus genome in infections of the central nervous system. J. Infect. Dis. **144**:154–160.

16. Hall, C. B. 1980. Prevention of infections with respiratory syncytial virus: the hopes and hurdles ahead. Rev. Infect. Dis. **2**:384–392.

17. Hall, W. W., and P. W. Choppin. 1981. Measles-virus proteins in the brain tissue of patients with subacute sclerosing panencephalitis. Absence of the M protein. New Engl. J. Med. **304**:1152–1155.

18. Hayden, G. F., et al. 1978. Current status of mumps and mumps vaccine in the United States. Pediatrics **62**:965–969.

19. Hehlmann, R. 1976. RNA tumor viruses and human cancer. Curr. Topics Microbiol. Immunol. **73**:141–215.

20. Henderson, F. W., et al. 1979. Respiratory-syncytial-virus infections, reinfections and immunity. A prospective, longitudinal study in young children. New Engl. J. Med. **300**:530–534.

21. Hinman, A. R., et al. 1980. Current features of measles in the United States: feasibility of measles elimination. Epidemiol. Rev. **2**:153–170.

22. Hughes, S. H. 1983. Synthesis, integration, and transcription of the retroviral provirus. Curr. Topics Microbiol. Immunol. **103**:23–49.

23. Johnson, H. N., and R. W. Emmons. 1980. Rabies virus. pp. 875–883. In E. H. Lennette, et al. (Eds.): Manual of Clinical Microbiology. 3rd ed. American Society for Microbiology, Washington, D.C.

24. Johnson, K. P., et al. 1981. Experimental subacute sclerosing panencephalitis: selective disappearance of measles virus matrix protein from the central nervous system. J. Infect. Dis. **144**:161–169.

25. Kalyanaraman, V. S., et al. 1982. A new subtype of human T-cell leukemia virus (HTLV-II) associated with a T-cell variant of hairy cell leukemia. Science **218**:571–573.

26. Kappus, K. D. 1976. Canine rabies in the United States, 1971–1973: study of reported cases with reference to vaccination history. Amer. J. Epidemiol. **103**:242–249.

27. Kilbourne, E. D. (Ed.). 1975. The Influenza Viruses and Influenza. Academic Press, New York.

28. Kingsbury, D. W. 1972. Paramyxovirus replication. Curr. Topics Microbiol. Immunol. **59**:1–33.

29. Klein, P. A., and R. T. Smith. 1977. The role of oncogenic viruses in neoplasia. Ann. Rev. Med. **28**:311–327.

30. LaMontagne, J. R. 1980. Summary of a workshop on influenza B viruses and Reye's syndrome. J. Infect. Dis. **142**:452–465.

31. LaMontagne, J. R., and G. J. Galasso. 1978. Report of a workshop on clinical studies of the efficacy of amantadine and rimantadine against influenza virus. J. Infect. Dis. **138**:928–931.

32. Mau-Liang, W. 1979. Dual recombination as origin of pandemic influenza viruses. Lancet **2**:1077.

33. McCauley, J. W., and B. W. J. Mahy. 1983. Structure and function of the influenza virus genome. Biochem. J. **211**:281–294.

34. McIntosh, K., and J. M. Fishaut. 1980. Immunopathologic mechanisms in lower respiratory tract disease of infants due to respiratory syncytial virus. Prog. Med. Virol. **26**:94–118.

35. Meyer, H. M., Jr. 1980. Rabies vaccine. J. Infect. Dis. **142**:287–289.

36. Morgan, E. M., and F. Rapp. 1977. Measles virus and its associated diseases. Bacteriol. Rev. **41**:636–666.

37. Murphy, F. A. 1977. Rabies pathogenesis. Brief review. Arch. Virol. **54**:279–297.

38. Plotkin, S. A. 1980. Rabies vaccine prepared in human cell cultures: progress and perspectives. Rev. Infect. Dis. **2**:433–448.

39. Report. 1980. A revision of the system of nomenclature for influenza viruses: a WHO memorandum. Bull. Wld Hlth Org. **58**:585–591.

40. Report. 1981. The ecology of influenza viruses: a WHO memorandum. Bull. Wld Hlth Org. **59**:869–873.

41. Report. 1981. The role of genetic and molecular characterization of viruses in relation to influenza surveillance and epidemiology: a WHO memorandum. Bull. Wld Hlth Org. **59**:875–879.

42. Schneider, L. G., and H. Diringer. 1976. Structure and molecular biology of rabies virus. Curr. Topics Microbiol. Immunol. **75**:153–180.

43. Scholtissek, C. 1978. The genome of the influenza virus. Curr. Topics Microbiol. Immunol. **80**:139–169.

44. Shortridge, K. F., and C. H. Stuart-Harris. 1982. An influenza epicentre? Lancet **2**:812–813.

45. Steck, F., and A. Wandeler. 1980. The epidemiology of fox rabies in Europe. Epidemiol. Rev. **2**:71–96.

46. Steffen, D. L., and H. Robinson. 1982. Endogenous retroviruses of mice and chickens. Curr. Topics Microbiol. Immunol. **98**:1–10.

47. Stuart-Harris, C. 1980. The present status of live influenza virus vaccine. J. Infect. Dis. **142**:784–793.

48. Stuart-Harris, C. H. 1979. The influenza viruses and the human respiratory tract. Rev. Infect. Dis. **1**:592–599.

49. Sweet, C., and H. Smith. 1980. Pathogenicity of influenza virus. Microbiol. Rev. **44**:303–330.

50. Symposium. 1980. Amantadine: does it have a role in

the prevention and treatment of influenza? A National Institutes of Health Consensus Development Conference. Ann. Intern. Med. **92**:256–258.

51. Tyrrell, D. A., *et al.* 1981. Development and use of influenza vaccines. Bull. Wld Hlth Org. **59**:165–173.

52. Varmus, H. E. 1982. Form and function of retroviral proviruses. Science **216**:812–820.

53. Ward, C. W. 1981. Structure of the influenza virus hemagglutinin. Curr. Topics Microbiol. Immunol. **94/95**:1–74.

54. Waterson, A. P. 1982. Human cancers and human viruses. Brit. Med J. **284**:446–448.

55. Webster, R. G., and W. J. Bean, Jr. 1978. Genetics of influenza virus. Ann. Rev. Genet. **12**:415–431.

56. Wechsler, S. L., and H. C. Meissner. 1982. Measles and SSPE viruses: similarities and differences. Prog. Med. Virol. **28**:65–95.

57. Weibel, R. E., *et al.* 1975. Long-term follow-up for immunity after monovalent or combined live measles, mumps, and rubella virus vaccines. Pediatrics **56**:380–387.

58. Weinmann, E., M. Majer, and J. Hilfenhaus. 1979. Intramuscular and/or intralumbar postexposure treatment of rabies virus-infected cynomolgus monkeys with human interferon. Infect. Immun. **24**:24–31.

59. Weiss, R. A. 1982. Perspectives on endogenous retroviruses in normal and pathological growth. Curr. Topics Microbiol. Immunol. **98**:127–132.

60. Wrigley, N. G. 1979. Electron microscopy of influenza virus. Brit. Med. Bull. **35**:35–38.

61. Wyke, J. A. 1981. Oncogenic viruses. J. Pathol. **135**:39–85.

62. Young, J. F., U. Desselberger, and P. Palese. 1979. Evolution of human influenza A viruses in nature: sequential mutations in the genomes of new H1N1 isolates. Cell **18**:73–83.

63. Zhdanov, V. M. 1980. The measles virus. Molecular Cellular Biochem. **29**:59–66.

CHAPTER 41

The Picornaviruses;
The Coronaviruses;
The Rotaviruses;
The Hepatitis Viruses

The descriptive term picornaviruses encompasses a group of small *(pico) RNA viruses* which resemble one another closely in morphology and in the cytopathic effect produced in cell cultures. The viruses of this group are classified in several genera of the family Picornaviridae. *Enterovirus* includes the polioviruses, Coxsackie viruses, and echoviruses. *Rhinovirus* contains antigenically diverse viruses etiologically associated with the common cold syndrome; they have also been termed coryzaviruses. Two other genera contain viruses that are primarily animal pathogens: members of *Cardiovirus* cause encephalomyocarditis of lower animals, while members of *Aphthovirus* are responsible for foot and mouth disease of cattle, swine, sheep, and goats. Since human infection with viruses of these latter two groups is rare and generally mild, these viruses will not be described.

The properties of picornaviruses are shown in Table 41–1 and their relationships are summarized in Table 41–2.

Table 41–1. **Properties of Picornaviruses**

(+)RNA genome; single-stranded, nonsegmented; 2.3 to 2.8 $\times$ 10^6 daltons

Spherical virion, 24–30 nm. in diameter

Icosahedral capsid symmetry; 32 capsomers

Assembled in cytoplasm of infected cells

Nonenveloped

Ether-resistant

Table 41–2. **The Principal Picornaviruses**

Genus	Differential Characteristics	Virus Subgroup	Infection
Enterovirus	Resistant to pH 3.0; relatively heat-stable	Polioviruses	Causes poliomyelitis in man. 3 serotypes.
		Coxsackie viruses	Variety of illnesses produced, including herpangina, febrile pharyngitis, epidemic pleurodynia, aseptic meningitis, myocarditis, and epidemic conjunctivitis. Two groups: A (23 serotypes) and B (6 serotypes).
		Echoviruses	Most serious disease produced is meningitis. Enterovirus 70 causes acute hemorrhagic conjunctivitis. 31 serotypes of echoviruses; 4 serotypes of unspecified enteroviruses.
Rhinovirus	Sensitive to pH 3.0; relatively heat-labile	Rhinoviruses	Viruses responsible for most common colds, 90 or more serotypes.

The Polioviruses

Poliomyelitis was differentiated as a clinical entity by Heine in 1840 and described in epidemic form by Medin in 1891. The viral nature of the etiological agent was demonstrated in 1908, when Landsteiner and Popper transmitted the disease to monkeys.

Poliomyelitis is found all over the world, occurring in most endemic areas as a disease of childhood. The age at which primary infection occurs is subject to some variation, however, and is affected by social and economic factors.

The great majority of poliomyelitis infections are symptomless, and clinical disease, paralytic or nonparalytic, appears to be the exception. With the waning of passive immunity of maternal origin, repeated infection, with or without overt disease, results in effective immunity. Even before mass vaccination campaigns were instituted, most adult serums contained neutralizing antibodies. In most areas of the world where vaccination with Salk and Sabin vaccines is practiced, incidence of poliomyelitis has been markedly reduced, and in some areas it has been eliminated. This low incidence can only be maintained, however, by continued effective immunization as new susceptibles appear.

Morphology and Structure[33]

The polioviruses are among the smallest of the viruses, the spherical particles ranging from 22 to 32 nm. in diameter. The ribonucleic acid genome is single-stranded and of negative polarity. In infected host cells, poliovirus parti-

cles often occur in orderly arrays (Fig. 41–1), and the virus has been prepared in the form of bipyramidal crystals.

The primary structure of the poliovirus RNA genome has recently been reported.[20] The viral RNA is composed of 7433 nucleotides. More than 89 per cent of the RNA codes for a large viral polyprotein, which is subsequently cleaved to form the 12 viral polypeptides. These findings may lay the foundation for cloning of virus-specific genome segments in bacteria to produce viral antigens for vaccine production.

Polioviruses, like the other enteroviruses, are acid stable and withstand a relatively wide pH range, from pH 3 to 10. The virus is not destroyed after several days at refrigerator temperature, but is inactivated in 30 minutes at 50° to 55° C. It is resistant to treatment with glycerol, ether, and 1 per cent phenol, but is labile to oxidizing agents, formalin, and ultraviolet irradiation; in water, it is somewhat more resistant to chlorination than vegetative cells of many bacteria.

Tissue Culture. Since 1949, poliovirus has been grown in cultures of a variety of tissues, including human embryonic tissues, human foreskin and testis, monkey kidney and testis, and in HeLa cell culture.

A degenerative type of cytopathology is produced (Fig. 41–2), which is clearly apparent in the fibroblastic outgrowth as a progressive granulation and eventual destruction. The cytopathic effect is more pronounced with some virus strains than others, but pathogenicity in

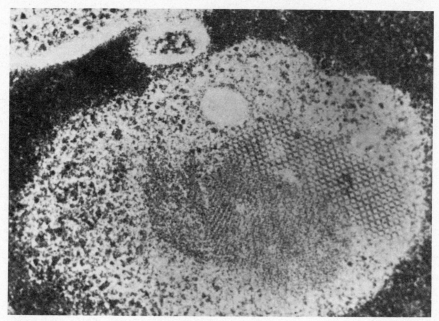

Figure 41–1. Intranuclear crystals in poliovirus-infected cells. × 85,000. (M. Kawanishi, Arch. Virol., **57**:123, 1978.)

tissue culture and virulence for experimental animals are not necessarily parallel.

The cytopathic effect is specifically neutralized by antiserum, providing the basis for tissue culture typing of virus strains and for virus quantitation by the plaque method. There is evidence that the observed cytopathology is in part a toxic effect of some strains of poliovirus in which the toxicity and infectivity are immunologically independent.

Antigenic Types

Polioviruses share common protein antigens that may be detected by complement fixation reactions. They are, however, separated into **three serological types** by the specificity of neutralizing antibody against certain viral proteins. These types are designated by arabic numerals. In those tropical areas where poliomyelitis is not yet controlled, type 1 strains are most often encountered,[28] as they were in

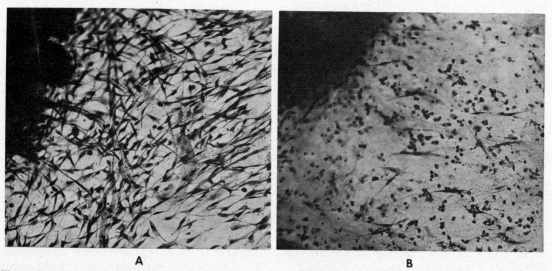

A   B

Figure 41–2. Preparations from roller-tube cultures of human embryonic skin-muscle tissue seven days after cultures were initiated. *A,* Uninoculated culture; *B,* inoculated three days previously with type 1 poliomyelitis virus. Few cells remain in the infected culture, the majority having been destroyed by the cytopathogenic action of the virus. Hematoxylin and eosin. (T. H. Weller, New Engl. J. Med. **249**:186, 1953.)

temperate zones before effective immunization was inaugurated. Serological typing is carried out by antibody neutralization in tissue culture.

Variation

Serial passage in tissue culture may result in changes in virulence for experimental animals. Type 2 strains, carried in human embryonic tissue culture, for example, show a decrease in mouse virulence without a corresponding decrease in virulence for the monkey or alteration in tissue culture infectivity. Variation in virulence for the mammalian host may be accompanied by changes in plaque morphology. Variants of reduced virulence, with abnormal capacity for growth in tissue culture, have been produced by rapid tissue passage with large inoculums. These have been of special interest as immunizing agents (see below).

The Disease in Man[41]

So far as is known, natural infection with poliovirus occurs only in man. The virus is demonstrable in the pharyngeal secretions and stools of clinically apparent cases and in contacts who do not develop the disease. Indeed, the infection is usually inapparent and almost always involves the alimentary tract; paralysis is an uncommon complication of poliovirus infection. Since the virus is shed from the throat and intestinal tract of both asymptomatic and clinical cases, the virus is spread by both **respiratory** and **fecal** routes. This dissemination is facilitated by poor sanitary conditions and crowding. The incubation period is variable, usually one to two weeks, although it may be as long as four or five weeks. The clinical disease is separable into three types: the **abortive,** the **nonparalytic,** and the **paralytic types.**

The initial symptoms of poliomyelitis are those of a mild upper respiratory infection with nonexudative pharyngitis and headache, or gastroenteritis with nausea and vomiting, but with constipation rather than diarrhea; in either case there is a febrile reaction. When the disease does not develop beyond this point, it is known as abortive poliomyelitis, but it cannot be diagnosed as such without isolation of the virus or demonstration of an increase in antibody titer between paired serums.

In some individuals, the disease may progress, with development of symptoms that indicate involvement of the central nervous system; these include pain and stiffness of the muscles of the neck and back and a positive Kernig's sign. This is the nonparalytic type of poliomyelitis. In paralytic poliomyelitis, the most serious form, a flaccid paralysis and muscle spasms occur at the terminal phase of the febrile period. Virus disappears rapidly from the spinal cord but may continue to be eliminated in the feces for some time.

The lesions in paralytic poliomyelitis consist of pathological changes in neurons. The anterior horn of the spinal cord is involved, and the destruction of the large nerve cells giving rise to the motor fibers of the peripheral nerves results in the flaccid paralysis. There is no impairment of mental faculties, and symptoms of encephalitis disappear when the acute stage of the disease subsides. Bulbar poliomyelitis is a consequence of a concentration of neuron destruction in the parts of the medulla containing the motor nuclei of the cranial nerves, with effects ranging from weakness of facial muscles to involvement of the respiratory and vasomotor centers.

Pathogenesis. The pathogenesis of poliomyelitis is best understood in the chimpanzee model. Since this experimental infection appears to be a counterpart of human infection, it has been assumed to represent, in a general way at least, the pathogenesis of the human disease (Fig. 41–3). Within a few days after the ingestion of an infecting dose of poliovirus, high concentrations of virus are demonstrable in the lymphoid tissues in the tonsils and in Peyer's patches in the intestine. Multiplication of the virus and its excretion from these areas account for its appearance in the throat and in the feces. The deeper lymph nodes, cervical and mesenteric, are infected by drainage from these primary sites, and the virus invades the blood stream by way of the lymphatic vessels and the thoracic duct, to produce viremia. The infection is spread via the blood stream to other susceptible tissues. The pathway for invasion of the central nervous system is somewhat uncertain. It may be by way of the blood, but there is also evidence of centripetal spread of the virus along the axons of peripheral nerves.

The virus is present in the feces, and laboratory diagnosis is dependent upon its isolation and serological identification. Monkey kidney, HeLa, WI-38, and human amnion cell cultures appear to be about equally sensitive for isolation. Serological identification consists of virus neutralization in tissue culture by known antiserum.

Predisposing Factors. In the abortive type of disease, the infection progresses no further

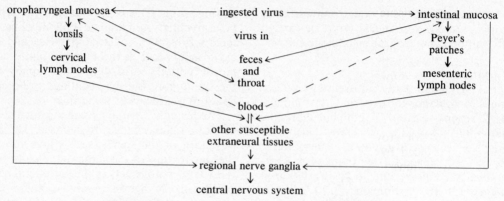

Figure 41–3. The pathogenesis of poliomyelitis (after Sabin).

than the alimentary or viremic phase. There is limited invasion of the central nervous system with reparable damage in nonparalytic poliomyelitis; extensive invasion and destruction within the central nervous system, which may be largely spinal, or bulbar and bulbospinal, occur in the paralytic form. The factors that determine whether the virus is to enter and multiply within the central nervous system are known in only a limited way, and there is a suggestion that adult susceptibility is genetically determined.[56]

There is no doubt that specific immunity plays an important part in limiting the spread of the infection, but certain nonspecific factors are also significant. Evidence from various sources indicates that immunization of children against diphtheria, pertussis, and tetanus may influence to some degree the site of paralysis in cases occurring up to three weeks following inoculation. It is also established that heavy physical exercise during the prodromal stage of the disease results in more severe paralysis; paralysis is also more likely to occur during pregnancy. An increased incidence of the bulbar form of the disease occurs following tonsillectomy or adenoidectomy, possibly by reduction in IgA immune response.

There is also no doubt that age is highly significant in the severity of the disease. Poliomyelitis is generally milder in young children than in adults, as indicated by an increase in both disability and case fatality with increasing age. The incidence of the more severe bulbar type of infection is appreciably greater in the higher age groups, and the case fatality rate is several times greater in adults than in children.

Epidemiology[17, 31]

The influence of social and economic conditions on the epidemiological character of

infectious disease has been discussed elsewhere (Chapter 13) and is nowhere better illustrated than in the changing epidemiological character of poliomyelitis.

The epidemic described by Medin in 1891 in Sweden is regarded as one of the first epidemics of poliomyelitis to occur; the first major epidemic in the United States occurred in 1916. Beginning about the turn of the century the disease began to shift from an endemic form, characterized by sporadic cases, to a form in which cases occurred in epidemics. The endemic form continues to persist in primitive populations, particularly in tropical areas, although epidemics have occurred in parts of Africa and India. Coincident with this change to an epidemic form, the age incidence peak shifted from those under 5 years of age to those in the 5- to 9-year old age group; at the same time, increased numbers of cases appeared in higher age groups and in adults.

This change in epidemiological character appears to be a consequence of social and economic factors which postpone the time of primary exposure to the virus. Under relatively primitive conditions, transfer of infection occurs more readily than under more enlightened hygienic circumstances. Primary infection occurs relatively early in life, so that passive immunity of maternal origin modifies these early immunizing infections. The aggregate result is a population that is immune to epidemic disease without experiencing clinical disease in epidemic form. When first infections are postponed, on the other hand, the threshold density of susceptibles is raised, so that the population becomes susceptible to epidemic disease.

Prophylactic immunization has made it possible, however, to interfere successfully with the development of population susceptibility to epidemic disease. In poliomyelitis, the development of effective immunizing agents and their application on a sufficiently wide scale has resulted in the reversion of this disease to the endemic form. Poliomyelitis is considered to be under control in South Africa, North America, Europe, Russia, and Oceania. Elsewhere, particularly in tropical areas, the disease has not been as well controlled and continues to persist in both endemic and epidemic forms. In the United States, paralytic poliomyelitis has decreased steadily since the 1950s, as shown in Figure 41–4. Since 1973, the number of poliomyelitis cases each year has ranged from 6 to 34.

Experimental Infections

For many years it was believed that only primates could be experimentally infected with poliovirus. Of such animals available for experimental purposes, the chimpanzee is the most susceptible and has, in fact, been infected accidentally in the laboratory; the disease in this animal closely resembles the human disease, as noted above.

In 1939, type 1 poliovirus was adapted from the monkey to the cotton rat and then to mice; later, strains of the other two immunological types were adapted to mice by introduction of the virus directly into the spinal cord. In such rodents the incubation period is 2 to 10 days, there is a varying degree of paralysis, only a few cases recover, and death occurs from respiratory paralysis.

Immunity[42]

The immune response to poliovirus is demonstrable as the presence of complement-fixing and neutralizing antibodies in the serum and a resistance to subsequent infection. Serum antibody fixes complement in the presence of tissue culture antigen, but its specificity may overlap the serotypes of the virus. Complement-fixing antibody declines relatively rapidly, disappearing within a few months to two years. Neutralizing antibody is readily titrated in tissue culture, neutralization of the virus being indicated by the lack of cytopathic effects. In contrast to complement-fixing antibody, it persists in detectable titer for years.

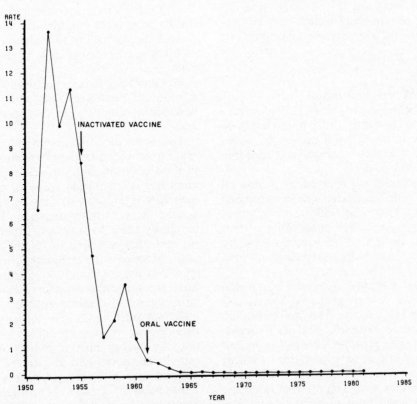

Figure 41–4. Incidence of paralytic poliomyelitis in the United States, 1951–1981 (reported cases per 10^5 population). (Centers for Disease Control, Annual summary 1981: reported morbidity and mortality in the United States. Morbidity and Mortality Weekly Report. Vol. 30, No. 54, 1982.)

Both kinds of antibody appear quite early in the disease, but if acute phase serum is taken early enough, a rise in antibody titer may be shown between this serum and a convalescent serum taken three to four weeks after onset.

The presence of neutralizing serum antibody is associated with effective immunity to the disease. Since infection with poliovirus is initially one of the intestinal and oropharyngeal mucosa, locally formed antibody, or secretory IgA, is considered to play a prominent role in immunity to the disease by preventing the first stage of infection. This antibody response is limited in duration, but a rapid secondary immune response is thought to inhibit initial infection at the mucosal surface; neutralizing antibody, found in the serum, prevents development of the viremic stage.

Although second, and even third, attacks of poliomyelitis have occurred in the same individual, the second attack is probably caused by an immunological type of virus different from that of the prior infection. Monkeys recovered from one attack of the disease are solidly immune to inoculation with the same type of virus, but not to heterologous types. Naturally acquired active immunity in man is probably an immunity to all three types of poliovirus, continuously reinforced by repeated exposure and, usually, asymptomatic infection.

Prophylactic Immunization[17, 26]

Prophylactic immunity may be either passively or actively acquired. Maternal antibody is protective in infants, but protection wanes rapidly and is usually ineffective in children over six months of age.

Active immunity is produced by parenteral inoculation with inactivated vaccine prepared from monkey kidney cell culture or by infections with live attenuated strains of the virus given orally. Both kinds of vaccines must include all three immunological types of the virus to provide broad protection.

Inactivated Vaccine. Vaccines inactivated with formaldehyde were prepared by Salk and are known as Salk vaccine. This kind of vaccine was subjected to extensive field tests, beginning in 1954, and provides an effective immunity. A course of three inoculations reduces the incidence of paralytic disease by 70 to 80 per cent. There is also evidence that when the disease does occur in immunized persons it is less severe. Little secretory IgA is induced by this vaccine, but amounts are sufficient to protect against oropharyngeal colonization; intestinal colonization is probably not prevented. Thus, the vaccine appears to be more effective when used in regions where sanitary conditions prevent fecal-oral spread. For example, extensive studies in Sweden and the Netherlands have shown protection rates as high as 90 to 95 per cent. It is significant that dissemination of wild-type virus has virtually ceased in regions where mass vaccination programs have been inaugurated.

Living Attenuated Vaccine.[6, 37] Virus strains, attenuated in neurovirulence, have been developed as immunizing agents that can be administered by the oral route—the Sabin vaccine.

Such attenuated vaccines have been extensively tested in most areas of the world and have been remarkably effective in reducing the incidence of disease. In the United States, immunization has been largely responsible for the reduction from almost 14,000 cases reported in 1955 to 6 in 1981. The experience has been similar in most other temperate countries with effective programs. In a few instances, the vaccine did not induce high immunity in residents of tropical countries unless multiple doses were administered. The reasons for these vaccine failures are not clear, although the difficulties in maintaining viability of attenuated vaccines may be partly responsible.

Persistent immunity is achieved by oral immunization; neutralizing antibodies have been detected as long as eight years postimmunization.

The antigenic stimulus provided by proliferation of the attenuated vaccine strains *in vivo* differs from that produced by inactivated virus in two significant respects. First, secretory IgA is induced so that immunization is against the alimentary infection. This kind of immunity tends to suppress, if not effectively prevent, dissemination of virulent virus. Second, infection with attenuated virus tends to spread in the community to immunize or reinforce the immunity of others, and attenuated viruses tend to displace virulent virus in the intestinal tract and in the environment. The vaccine also produces an effective immunity in the very young; immune protection of 75 per cent in newborns and 95 per cent in infants three to six months of age has been described. There is, then, considerable evidence that poliomyelitis can be eradicated in effectively immunized populations.

Nevertheless, there are problems, both theoretical and real, with live attenuated vaccines. First, there is the possibility that circulating vaccine strains can mutate to neurovirulence. In rare instances, paralytic poliomyelitis has been found in vaccinees or their contacts. Second, individuals with immune deficiency disease could develop complications from live vaccine strains. In spite of these possibilities, untoward reactions are very rare. In one study· in 13 countries, involving a total population of 509 million persons, the incidence of paralysis was only 0.14 per million per year; even in these instances, not all cases of paralysis were associated with vaccine administration.

The Coxsackie Viruses

The first of what proved to be a new group of viruses was isolated in 1948 from two children ill with disease diagnosed as poliomyelitis. Similar viruses were subsequently isolated in various parts of the world. These viruses make up the somewhat heterogeneous group known as the Coxsackie viruses (the first strains were found in Coxsackie, New York) and are classified in the genus *Enterovirus* of the family Picornaviridae. These viruses have been found most often in feces and in sewage and are isolated from time to time from the throat. They have been found together with poliovirus and during poliomyelitis epidemics in persons not infected with poliovirus. They appear to be most prevalent in the late summer and early fall. Human infections seem to be quite common, as indicated by the presence of antibody to all of the immunological types of these viruses in pooled serums; they are found in man both in association with disease and in healthy persons.

Although similar in size to the polioviruses, Coxsackie viruses are distinct in pathogenicity and immunological character. They are relatively stable over a wide range of temperature and pH, and are relatively resistant to ethyl alcohol, ether, glycerol, and phenolic compounds, but 0.3 per cent formaldehyde is an effective disinfectant.

Infection of cynomolgus monkeys and chimpanzees by the oral route results in a transient febrile reaction. Virus is found in the pharyngeal secretions and stools, there is a specific immune response, and some strains may produce neuron damage on intracerebral inoculation. Of the more common experimental animals, only the newborn mouse and hamster are regularly susceptible to infection. While this limited host range is a definitive characteristic of the Coxsackie viruses, it does not invariably differentiate them from certain other viruses.

Virus Types
Coxsackie viruses are separable into two groups, designated A and B, on the basis of their pathogenicity for the infant mouse and ability to grow in tissue culture. Immunological types are delineated within these groups. The characteristic effect of the viruses of group A in the infant mouse is an inflammatory and degenerative lesion of striated muscle without adverse effect on other tissues. Infected mice show a generalized weakness, flaccid paralysis develops, and death occurs three to four days after inoculation.

In contrast, infection with group B viruses characteristically results in lesions of the central nervous system, with focal leptomeningitis. Characteristic symptoms include muscle tremors, weakness, and spastic paralysis.

There are also differences between the two groups of Coxsackie viruses with respect to growth in tissue culture. Those of group A are, in several instances, not cultivable in tissue cultures; others grow only in human cell lines such as WI-38 (human embryonic lung) or human rhabdomyosarcoma cells.[46] Most group B viruses are cultivable in various kinds of tissue culture, but there is some irregularity in the pattern of susceptibility. Monkey kidney tissue culture, prepared in monolayers, appears to be one of the most generally satisfactory for viruses of group B, and cytopathic effects are produced (Fig. 41–5). Tubular-type aggregations are seen in infected cells, as shown in Figure 41–6.

The viruses in each group are differentiated into serotypes. Group A contains 23 specific serotypes, while 6 serotypes are recognized in group B. These are arbitrarily assigned numbers as type designations, *viz.*, A1, A2, B1, B2, etc. These viruses are then immunologically heterogeneous, although common antigenic components are shared. All type B viruses, for example, show cross-reactivity by

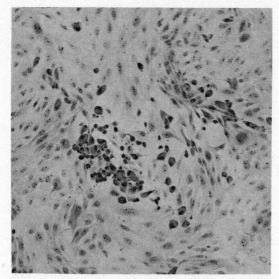

Figure 41–5. Coxsackie virus type B2 in monkey kidney epithelial cell culture. There are focal areas of cytopathology produced 24 hours after inoculation with the virus; the affected cells are rounded and contain crescentia and pyknotic nuclei, and the cytoplasm shows intense eosinophilic staining. (Enders, Ann. Intern. Med. **45**:331, 1956.)

complement fixation and the responsible antigen is also shared with type A9.

Serotypes are separable by complement fixation and by neutralization and protection tests, with substantially the same results. Protective antibody is demonstrable by the neutralization technique, but infant mice cannot be actively immunized and subsequently challenged. An effective passive immunity occurs in infant mice born of and nursed by actively immunized mothers. The protection conferred by active immunity is demonstrable in the chimpanzee as an immunity to challenge inoculation.

The Disease in Man

As indicated above, serological evidence indicates a wide prevalence of human infection with Coxsackie viruses. The infection is seen mostly in children, either as clinical disease or as inapparent infection. The association with poliomyelitis appears to be purely fortuitous, and various attempts to demonstrate a potentiating effect of Coxsackie virus infection on poliomyelitis have given negative results. In fact, an interference between some group B strains and poliovirus occurs in tissue culture, and it has been suggested that Coxsackie virus infection may, on occasion, tend to exclude poliovirus infection.

There are, however, some clinical entities with which Coxsackie viruses have been found to be in close, and probably etiological, relation. These include febrile pharyngitis and herpangina, epidemic pleurodynia, acute hemorrhagic conjunctivitis, polymyositis, some portion of cases of aseptic meningitis, and myocarditis.

Herpangina. This is a febrile disease, usually seen in children, that occurs in both epidemic and sporadic form in many parts of the world. There is often vomiting and abdominal pain, and the characteristic lesion is a small, herpes-like vesicle which breaks down to leave a shallow ulcer. These lesions occur on the edge of the soft palate, on the tonsils, in the pharynx and on the anterior pillars of the fauces. Recovery is usually prompt, within two to three days, and complete. Coxsackie viruses have been isolated from as many as 84 per cent of cases of herpangina examined, and six serotypes, A2, A4, A5, A6, A8, and A10, predominate, although other Coxsackie types, as well as some other enteroviruses, are occasionally found.

There is circumstantial and other evidence, including laboratory infection, indicating that both group A and group B[45] viruses can produce a febrile pharyngitis, particularly in summer, without the identifying herpangina lesion, giving the disease sometimes known as three-day fever or summer grippe. Other, more severe cases of disease have been observed in which herpangina is associated with parotitis.

Epidemic Pleurodynia. This disease was

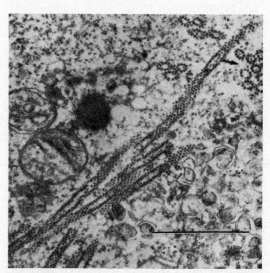

Figure 41–6. Tubules of virus-aggregation in HeLa cells infected with Coxsackie B5. Some tubules are shown in cross-section (arrow). Bar = 1 μm. (M. S. Shahrabadi, and O. Morgante, Virology, **80**:434, 1977.)

first observed in Bornholm, Denmark, in 1930, and is also known as Bornholm disease, epidemic myalgia, and "devil's grip." The disease tends to occur in epidemic form, most commonly in late summer. The incubation period is two to four days, the onset sudden, and the disease characterized by acute pain in the thoracic wall, abdomen, and lower region of the back. It is commonly accompanied by headache, but there are no respiratory or constitutional symptoms. The pain is paroxysmal, lasting a day or more, and the muscles are tender to pressure. There is a tendency to relapse at intervals of a few days or longer, and orchitis and meningeal involvement may occur.

Strains of group B Coxsackie virus have been isolated from the throat or feces in a considerable portion of cases in several epidemics studied. Increase in antibody titer to the virus isolated is observed, and it seems established that these viruses are the etiological agents of this disease.

Aseptic Meningitis.[2,25] Aseptic meningitis is a clinical syndrome rather than an etiological entity and may occur in epidemic form. It is usually mild, with signs and symptoms indicating involvement of the meninges. Fever, headache, nausea, pain in the abdomen, and stiffness of the neck or back usually occur. This disease may be caused by a variety of nonbacterial agents, including Coxsackie viruses. Viruses of group B and at least one of group A (A9) have been isolated from the feces and from the spinal fluid in cases of this disease; neutralizing antibody to the isolated virus occurs in the serum.

Myocarditis.[15, 22] Acute myocarditis of infants has been described from various parts of the world. In many instances, isolation of group B Coxsackie viruses has been reported, and there seems little doubt that neonatal myocarditis can be due to these agents. The association of group B viruses with acute adult myocarditis and pericarditis is not as easily documented, but several recent investigations indicate association between virus infection and myopericarditis as judged by serological evidence of concurrent infection.

Acute Hemorrhagic Conjunctivitis. Acute hemorrhagic conjunctivitis appeared in epidemic form in 1969 in Africa and Southeast Asia. Although the African epidemic and some of the outbreaks in Asia were due to enterovirus 70 (see p. 823), one epidemic in Singapore in 1970 was due to an antigenic variant of Coxsackie A24. Subsequently, this virus has been responsible for epidemics throughout Asia. In some epidemics both Coxsackie A24 and enterovirus 70 have circulated concurrently.

Hand, Foot, and Mouth Disease.[50] This is a disease in which vesicular lesions in the mouth and on the hands and feet are prominent. It appears to be due primarily to Coxsackie A16, but outbreaks in Japan have been due to enterovirus 71.[51] The illness is primarily one of children and is usually mild; it apparently occurs also as a subclinical infection. Although most outbreaks involve only small numbers of cases, several in Japan have been particularly extensive, with many thousands of cases.

The Echoviruses[55]

With the development of practical and generally applicable methods for the isolation of polioviruses from the intestinal tract in tissue culture, a great many isolations of cytopathogenic agents other than poliovirus have been made. These viruses were previously undescribed entities, and while some were found in cases of poliomyelitis, often diagnosed as the nonparalytic type of infection, in many instances there was no specific association with illness, and they were called orphan viruses. Those isolated from man have been named the enteric cytopathogenic human orphan viruses, or more simply as echoviruses. Similar cytopathogenic orphan viruses are found in mon-

keys, cattle, and swine. It is apparent that at least some echoviruses stand in etiological relationship to human disease. As noted earlier, the enteroviruses (other than polioviruses) are quite similar, with respect to both the viruses themselves and the diseases engendered, and it is now the convention to designate new, serologically specific isolates not as echovirus or Coxsackie virus types, but simply as enteroviruses with a numerical designation, *e.g.,* enterovirus 68, 69, etc.

Echoviruses are similar in size to polioviruses and Coxsackie viruses, about 30 nm. in diameter. They are differentiated from one another by their host range and pathogenicity

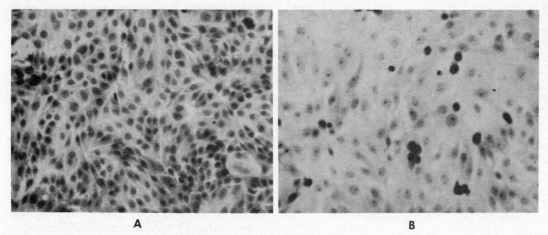

Figure 41–7. The cytopathic effect of echovirus type 1 in culture of monkey kidney epithelial cells. *A,* Uninoculated six-day culture of cells; *B,* 24 hours after the inoculation of virus, a few rounded cells are scattered throughout the field. Carnoy fixation; hematoxylin and eosin. (Melnick: Adv. Virol.)

as expressed in tissue culture, including plaque morphology in monolayer culture, and by separation into antigenic types. Some, though not all, form hemagglutinin and are related to one another in this respect, but not to the influenza virus and other myxoviruses.

Culture

In general, the echoviruses grow more readily on primary isolation in monkey kidney tissue culture than on HeLa cell culture. Growth of echoviruses in monkey kidney cells induces an observable cytopathic effect (Fig. 41–7), and virus is released into the culture fluid. Virus can be detected by complement fixation or serum neutralization tests.

The morphology of plaques formed in monolayer cultures of monkey kidney cells is often a valuable differential characteristic. For example, certain serotypes of echoviruses form slowly developing, irregular plaques of small to medium size that permit their differentiation from polioviruses, as illustrated in Figure 41–8. Several of the echovirus serotypes form large circular plaques, and a few exhibit no plaque formation.

Antigenic Types

The echoviruses and other enteroviruses are separable into serotypes by cross-neutralization tests in tissue culture, and standard antiserums are used for identification. New serotypes continue to be described. A total of 31 echovirus types have been designated, along with four additional enterovirus types, *viz.,* enterovirus 68, 69, 70, and 71.

Strains within a serotype are not necessarily antigenically identical, and those with broader antigenicity than the prototype strain have been called prime strains. Strains within type

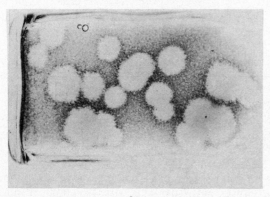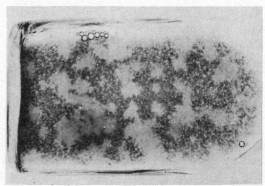

Figure 41–8. The types of plaques produced by poliovirus type 3 *(A)* and echovirus type 6 *(B)* on monolayer cultures of monkey kidney tissue. (Hsiung and Melnick, Virology **1**:533, 1955.)

6 have been studied in this connection, and strains 6' and 6'' have a broader antigenic specificity than that of prototype strain 6. There are cross-reactions among types 1, 8, and 12; echovirus 4 antiserum neutralizes adenovirus 8; and Coxsackie B4 is neutralized by antiserums to several echoviruses.

Pathogenicity

In a general way, the echoviruses are set apart from the Coxsackie viruses by their lack of pathogenicity for the infant mouse, although occasional Coxsackie strains are not pathogenic for the infant mouse on primary isolation. The echoviruses seem to be less virulent than the Coxsackie viruses. The usual infection occurs in children and is subclinical. On occasion, overt disease is produced that includes mild to severe respiratory disease, enteritis, and aseptic meningitis.

Meningitis. Aseptic meningitis is the most serious manifestation of echovirus infection. Cases may occur sporadically, and almost any of the enteroviruses may be involved. Epidemic outbreaks are usually due to types 4, 6, 7, 9, 11, 19, and 30; types 11 and 30 are especially prevalent. Although adults may be affected in many outbreaks, children and neonates seem to suffer higher attack rates. There is a strong suggestion that enterovirus infection of the central nervous system during early life may lead to later neurological impairment.[47] Infections associated with types 4, 9, and 16 have often been characterized by the presence of a rash. The disease syndrome of epidemic pleurodynia, usually associated with Coxsackie virus infection (see above), has also been found to be due to infection with echovirus type 1.

Hemorrhagic Conjunctivitis.[36] In 1969, an acute hemorrhagic conjunctivitis characterized by epidemic spread appeared in West Africa. During the succeeding two years, the disease was found to be broadly distributed in Africa. Another focus appeared in Southeast Asia in 1969, and flared throughout Asia by 1971. In most outbreaks the etiological agent was a new enterovirus of unknown origin, now called enterovirus 70; some of the Asian epidemics have been due to Coxsackie A24, as discussed earlier (p. 821). The disease seems to be primarily tropical, appearing mainly in coastal areas during rainy periods, but has wide geographical distribution. Outside of Africa and Southeast Asia, isolated epidemics have been reported from most parts of the world.

The Common Cold Viruses

The clinical syndrome that characterizes the mild upper respiratory disease called the common cold merges imperceptibly into that of acute respiratory disease, which, as noted elsewhere (Chapter 29), is of diverse etiology. Mild illnesses resulting from infection with the parainfluenza viruses, respiratory syncytial viruses, and adenoviruses may be indistinguishable from the common cold. Nevertheless, the common cold appears to be most often attributable to *Rhinovirus* of the Picornaviridae and to *Coronavirus* of the Coronaviridae.

RHINOVIRUS[4, 23, 40, 49]

The rhinoviruses are ether-stable RNA viruses with a particle size of 18 to 28 nm., characteristic of the picornavirus group. As a subgroup, they are separable from the enteroviruses by their acid lability (pH 3 to 5 for one to three hours) and their relative thermostability at 50°C., which is enhanced by magnesium chloride. Rhinoviruses grow more readily in human embryo tracheal organ culture than in other kinds of tissue culture; some are cultivable in human cell cultures (embryo kidney or diploid cells), while others grow also in monkey kidney and other kinds of cell cultures, with cytopathology manifest as the appearance of ovoid refractile cells (Fig. 41–9). Unlike other picornaviruses, with optimum growth temperatures near 37°C., rhinoviruses grow best at 33° to 34°C. The rhinoviruses are antigenically heterogeneous. At least 115 serotypes have been established and assigned numbers based on the chronology of description. Nevertheless, some antigenic cross-reactions have been noted between serotypes; these serological relationships have recently been clarified, with a suggestion that antigenic groups be established to simplify the typing system.[5]

Pathogenicity[44]

Serological surveys have shown that the distribution of neutralizing antibody in human serums is worldwide, but is not found in serums

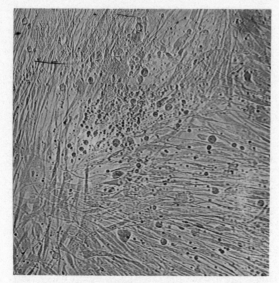

Figure 41–9. The cytopathic effect produced by rhinovirus type 2 in a culture of the W38 strain of human diploid cells. Unstained. (Hamre.)

of lower animals. In addition to the human rhinoviruses, both bovine and equine rhinoviruses have been described. Presumably man is the only host for the human strains. At least two serotypes of the animal rhinovirus have been differentiated, and these can infect humans in populations at risk, such as animal workers.

The significance of human rhinoviruses in the etiology of the common cold has been demonstrated in a number of studies based on isolation and identification of the associated virus. The spectrum of viruses differs between infants and very young children on the one hand, and adults on the other. The parainfluenza viruses, respiratory syncytial viruses, and other myxoviruses assume greater importance in children; rhinoviruses can only be isolated from about 5 per cent of children, but are found in considerably higher numbers in adults with colds.

Rhinoviruses were not reliably isolated from clinically apparent disease using earlier tissue culture methods. The advent of newer techniques, particularly those involving diploid cell lines, has resulted in a higher proportion of positive isolations. The use of human embryo kidney cell cultures at neutral pH and with incubation at lower than usual temperatures (33°C.) has also proved highly successful for isolation.

It is probable that the virulence of the rhinoviruses is not great and that most adults have some degree of partial immunity as indicated by serological surveys. Studies on rhinovirus types 1 and 2 infection in a military population over a 24-week period in winter and spring showed that both viruses were present during 5 of the weeks, and one or the other during 16 weeks, with isolation rates of 12 per cent. The incidence of positive isolations in those with significant antibody titer was only 20 per cent of that in persons showing no antibody. It is likely that the respiratory viruses, including the rhinoviruses, maintain a low level of infection, with the development of clinical disease attributable in part to nonspecific stress.

Transmission

It has long been thought that colds were transmitted primarily by aerosols, generated by coughing or sneezing. Based on recent studies, however, it appears that **hand transmission** is a more efficient mechanism. Nasal secretions contaminate the hands, and viruses are transmitted to other persons or to inanimate objects by hand contact; infection occurs when the recipient transfers the virus to the nasal or conjunctival mucosa.

This mode of transmission suggests that the chain of transmission could be interrupted by the use of antimicrobial hand washes. Dilute iodine solutions effectively inactivate rhinoviruses, and hexachlorophene or benzalkonium chloride in alcohol-water solutions are somewhat less effective.[14]

Immunity

As indicated above, there is an association between pre-existing antibody and resistance to development of disease. Immunization of small numbers of persons with virus vaccine, followed by intranasal challenge, resulted in an approximate tenfold reduction in colds in the vaccinated group as compared to controls. Serum levels of naturally occurring, vaccine-induced, or infection-induced antibodies correlate with occurrence and severity of disease produced by challenge inoculation, although some irregularities are observed. It has also been generally noted that virus is isolated less often from persons possessing serum antibody, and such persons tend to carry and disseminate the virus less frequently. There also is evidence suggesting that immunity is a function of IgA present in nasal secretions.

The possibility of prophylactic immunization against the common cold viruses, perhaps the most common cause of natural infection, has intrigued most workers since the discovery of the rhinoviruses. It seems clear that an appreciable degree of immunity can be developed against individual serotypes, but it has been generally assumed that the large number of these would make immunization impractical. Recent findings suggest, however, that certain serotypes tend to appear with higher frequency and to persist in certain geographical areas.[11] Furthermore, human infection with rhinoviruses may induce cross-reacting, or heterotype, immune responses that would be expected to amplify effective immunity. The possibility of vaccine development may not, therefore, be as bleak as previously supposed.

CORONAVIRUS[24, 48, 54]

A group of human respiratory viruses whose seasonal prevalence differed from that of the rhinoviruses was described in 1966. The human viruses are structurally and morphologically related to a diverse group of animal viruses, affecting a wide range of animal hosts. These viruses are all classified in the family Coronaviridae and are characterized by surface glycoproteins present as spikes projecting from the viral envelope, giving the appearance of a halo (corona) surrounding the particle (Fig. 41–10). The properties of coronaviruses are listed in Table 41–3.

The nucleocapsid of coronaviruses consists of a continuous single-stranded RNA molecule of about 6×10^6 daltons, associated with a phosphorylated capsid protein. The lipid envelope is double-shelled and contains a matrix

Table 41–3. **Properties of Coronaviruses**

(+)RNA genome; single-stranded, nonsegmented; 6×10^6 daltons
Spherical virion, 60–220 nm. in diameter; corona of club-shaped projections, *ca.* 20 nm. in length
Helical capsid symmetry
Capsid assembled in cytoplasm
Envelope consists of two electron-dense shells, derived by budding from intracytoplasmic membranes
Ether-sensitive

glycoprotein of 20,000 to 30,000 molecular weight. One or more high-molecular-weight glycoproteins form the surface projections, or peplomers, and their presence as club-shaped spikes accounts for the halo-like corona that surrounds the particle. These peplomers are likely associated with **hemagglutination, attachment,** and **cell fusion** activities; immunological protection is due to neutralizing antibodies directed against the spike glycoproteins.

Coronaviruses are assembled in the cytoplasm of infected cells and are enveloped when the nucleocapsid migrates to the rough endoplasmic reticulum and buds into the cisterna; they are released from the cell by reverse viropexis. In tissue cultures, persistent infection has been frequently described, but the mechanism of persistence is not clear.

The coronaviruses are best known as animal pathogens, causing natural clinical disease only in the animals from which they have been isolated, and replicating most effectively in tissue culture cell lines from the natural host.

The human coronaviruses are usually responsible for common colds, although some cases of pneumonia and lower respiratory tract infections in children are of coronavirus etiology. They are of worldwide distribution and account for about 15 per cent of common colds. The syndrome is similar to that caused by the rhinoviruses. Coryza is the usual manifestation, but coughs and mucopurulent nasal discharges do not occur. The viruses may be isolated from nasal washings by cultivation in human tracheal organ cultures; some strains, including the prototype strain 229E, will also grow in cell cultures of human origin.

Epidemiological studies indicate that infections by coronaviruses are commonplace. Serum antibodies are highly prevalent in normal human populations and are most frequently found in those between 14 and 24 years of age. The infection appears to be most common in the colder months.[43]

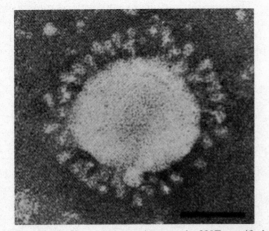

Figure 41–10. Human coronavirus, strain 229E, purified on sucrose gradient. (M. R. Macnaughton, and H. A. Davies, Arch. Virol. **70**:301, 1981.)

At least two serological groups of the respiratory coronaviruses are recognized, based on the surface glycoprotein antigens. In human volunteers, these antigens are protective against homologous, but not heterologous, serogroups.

For the past decade, coronavirus-like particles have been observed in the intestinal contents of individuals suffering from gastroenteritis, with the implication that the viruses are etiologically related to the illness. Similar viruses have also been observed in normal subjects, so that the etiological relationships are somewhat tenuous at present.

Viral Gastroenteritis[3, 9, 30]

Diarrheal diseases of viral etiology are seen frequently in both animals and man, and gastroenteritis is second only to upper respiratory disease as the most common form of human illness. Indeed, various estimates indicate the wide geographical distribution of gastroenteritis; between 500 million and 5 billion diarrheal episodes occur yearly in humans, with 5 to 18 million deaths. Although the affliction is relatively mild and self-limiting in the United States and other industrialized nations, it tends to be more serious in the developing countries.

While a number of agents, including viruses, bacteria, and animal parasites, can cause gastroenteritis, the viruses seem to be of greatest import. A number of viral agents are capable of inducing diarrheal disease. The adenoviruses, picornaviruses, and coronaviruses have been incriminated in outbreaks of enteritis, as noted previously; some others have been due to astroviruses and caliciviruses. The vast majority are, however, caused by members of two virus groups: (1) the Norwalk and Norwalk-like viruses, and (2) the rotaviruses. Figure 41–11 illustrates the comparative morphology of the principal viral agents of gastroenteritis.

The epidemiological patterns of acute gastroenteritis caused by Norwalk-like agents and rotaviruses are somewhat different, and these serve to differentiate the diseases caused by them.

One epidemiological type occurs typically in epidemic form, affecting older children, their family contacts, and adults. The illness, characterized by explosive onset, is self-limiting and generally lasts from 24 to 48 hours. Clinical signs and symptoms include nausea, vomiting, diarrhea, abdominal cramps, headache, and low-grade fever. This form of acute gastroenteritis, frequently known as winter-vomiting disease, is caused by the Norwalk and similar viruses. About one-third of the outbreaks of viral gastroenteritis in the United States are of this type.

A second form of viral gastroenteritis occurs during the colder months of the year as sporadic cases and occasional epidemics, predominantly affecting infants and young children. In this form, diarrhea is generally more severe, and fever and vomiting are more pronounced. Illness is prolonged, lasting from five to eight days, and the accompanying severe dehydration usually requires hospitalization. This form of disease is due to rotaviruses.

NORWALK–LIKE VIRUSES[18]

The current interest in and understanding of viral gastroenteritis can be directly traced to the discovery of the Norwalk agent, responsible for a 1968 epidemic of winter-vomiting

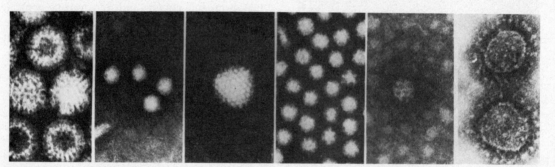

Figure 41–11. Comparative morphology of the principal viruses incriminated in viral gastroenteritis. *From left to right*: rotavirus, Norwalk virus, adenovirus, astrovirus, calicivirus, coronavirus. × 210,000. (A. Murphy, Med. J. Australia, **2**:177, 1981. © The Medical Journal of Australia, reprinted with permission.)

disease in Norwalk, Ohio. Despite repeated trials, the virus has not been cultured in the laboratory. It has been serially transmitted by fecal filtrates to human volunteers, however, and illness develops in about one-half of the volunteers given these filtrates.

The Norwalk virus can be observed, by electron microscopy, in fecal filtrates from infected volunteers and is identified by immunoelectron microscopy. The virus is spherical, about 27 nm. in diameter (see Fig. 41–11), and is resistant to treatment with acid, heat, and ether. The Norwalk virus has not been cultivated in tissue culture nor has disease been produced in laboratory animals; the biology of the Norwalk agent is therefore poorly understood. Similar viruses have been detected in many gastroenteritis outbreaks, all having features in common with the prototype Norwalk virus. Usually named for the location of the outbreak, the Norwalk-like viruses include the Hawaii agent, the Dichling agent, and others; there appears to be considerable antigenic diversity among them, and they are thought to occur as at least three serological types.

The Norwalk and related viruses are spread by the fecal-oral route. Outbreaks have been traced to contaminated drinking water, swimming water, and foods, including shellfish. The infection appears to be globally distributed, and serological studies in the United States suggest that primary infection occurs in adolescence or early adulthood; serum antibody is found in about two-thirds of adults.

Immunity to the Norwalk virus is short-lived. In volunteers recovered from infection, immunity is evident upon challenge after a few weeks, but when challenged after many months, no resistance is observed, even though humoral antibodies can often be demonstrated. As noted above, the attack rate in volunteers is about 50 per cent, and when rechallenged after several months, those who developed illness in the first challenge are again susceptible, while those resistant to the first challenge are unaffected by the second challenge. Paradoxically, the resistant individuals develop no detectable immune response.

ROTAVIRUS[35, 53]

The family Reoviridae comprises three genera, *Rotavirus*, *Reovirus*, and *Orbivirus*, which share the characters of the family as detailed in Chapter 38.

Reovirus are not a significant cause of human illness, although human infections, either subclinical or associated with mild respiratory symptoms, may be relatively common. Most adults, 70 to 80 per cent, possess serum antibodies to these viruses. *Orbivirus* differ morphologically from others in this family, and they multiply in arthropod hosts as well as in vertebrates. For this reason, they are discussed with the arboviruses in Chapter 42; *Reovirus* are not significant human pathogens and will not be discussed.

Rotavirus were discovered in 1973 and soon were established as a significant cause of gastroenteritis in infants. The human rotaviruses appear to be responsible for about half of the cases of gastroenteritis in children between the ages of six months and two years; they are sometimes found in older age groups. The viruses are shed in feces in much larger numbers than the Norwalk agent, and they can be recognized in stool filtrates by immunoelectron microscopy.

Rotaviruses are widely distributed as diarrheal agents in both animals and man, almost invariably affecting the young of the species. The animal and human strains are morphologically similar; the virus is spherical, 70 to 75 nm. in diameter, with a segmented, double-stranded RNA genome. The complete virus particle contains a double-shelled capsid, although both single- and double-shelled particles are seen in diarrheal filtrates. By electron microscopy, the viruses appear in the shape of a wheel, hence the name (Latin *rota*, wheel). The outer shell contains the type-specific antigenic proteins, while group-specific antigens are located in the inner shell. The viruses are not enveloped and are stable to a variety of treatments, *viz.*, mild acids, heat, and ether. The animal and human strains are differentiable by the number of RNA segments in the genome; the human rotavirus genome consists of 11 RNA segments. The properties of human rotaviruses are listed in Table 41–4.

The wild-type human rotaviruses are not efficiently or consistently propagated in tissue

Table 41–4. **Properties of Human Rotaviruses**

RNA genome; double-stranded, occurring in 11 segments
Spherical virion, 70–75 nm.
Capsid contains 32 capsomers
Assembled in cytoplasm
Nonenveloped
Resistant to ether, heat, and mild acids

cultures, although one strain has recently been adapted to cell culture. The animal strains are more consistently grown in this way, and much of our knowledge of rotavirus is based on studies of the animal strains. Human rotaviruses are identified in stool filtrates by immunoelectron microscopy, and this method is commonly used for diagnosis. Radioimmunoassays and enzyme-linked immunosorbent assay (ELISA) techniques have also been adapted for virus detection and identification, often using hyperimmune serum prepared against group-specific antigens from the animal strains.

As noted above, gastroenteritis due to rotavirus is commonly seen as sporadic cases and occasionally as small outbreaks, usually nosocomial in nature. The infection is spread by the fecal-oral route, but can be transmitted from person-to-person by close contact. Adult contacts of infected children sometimes become infected, as indicated by seroconversion, but such illnesses are mild or asymptomatic.

Serological studies have affirmed the widespread occurrence of rotavirus infection. Most adults possess serum antibodies; the prevalence ranges from about 70 per cent in developed countries to perhaps 90 per cent in countries such as India. Infants are apparently protected by maternal antibody during the first few months of life. At least two serotypes of human rotavirus are known, and infection with one type does not provide protection against the other.

Viral Hepatitis[7, 8, 12, 21, 57]

Liver damage with icterus is observed in several infectious diseases, including leptospirosis and yellow fever, but, in addition to these, there is hepatitis of viral etiology. Viral hepatitis is of two kinds, infectious hepatitis and serum hepatitis, each caused by different and unrelated viruses, and differing in epidemiological character. Various kinds of evidence suggest that additional viruses may be responsible for a large portion of transfusion-associated hepatitis cases as well as some that are orally transmitted.

INFECTIOUS HEPATITIS

Infectious hepatitis is a subacute disease of wide distribution, tending to affect children and young adults. Infectious hepatitis may appear in epidemic form within households; in institutions; and in military personnel, as it did in the two World Wars and the war in Korea. Serological studies indicate prevalence as high as 97 per cent in some regions; about 40 per cent of healthy adults in the United States are seropositive. Many of the infections that stimulate this immune response are undoubtedly asymptomatic or mild and unrecognized.

The incubation period of infectious hepatitis varies from one to six weeks, with an average of about four weeks. The disease is one of diffuse involvement of the liver and is separable into two stages, the **pre-icteric** and the **icteric**. The onset is usually abrupt, and symptoms include fever, gastrointestinal distress, headache, anorexia, and lassitude; the postcervical lymph nodes are often involved, and there is leucopenia with relative lymphocytosis. This pre-icteric phase may persist for as long as three weeks but usually lasts for only a few days. Symptoms tend to subside, but there is exacerbation of some, especially those of abdominal discomfort, with the appearance of jaundice, and the liver and spleen are palpable and tender. Examination of biopsy specimens indicates progressive liver damage during the course of the disease, with relatively extensive parenchymal destruction by the time jaundice is apparent, but regeneration occurs subsequently, which is complete in most cases by three months. Consistent with this, there is early evidence of hepatic dysfunction, and bilirubinuria occurs toward the end of the pre-icteric phase of the disease.

The icteric phase may persist for some weeks and is usually followed by uneventful convalescence. It is probable that more than 98 per cent of patients recover completely. Persistent or chronic hepatitis is very rarely observed, and a chronic carrier state is not established. Rare complications of the disease include pneumonia, meningitis, and myelitis.

Hepatitis A Virus

It is customary to designate the virus of infectious hepatitis as hepatitis A virus, or HAV, to distinguish it from the virus of serum hepatitis (hepatitis B, HBV). The virus of hepatitis A has only recently been propagated in cell cultures,[32] so that much of our present knowledge of the virus is derived from morphological and immunological studies in humans and animal models. Chimpanzees and marmosets can be infected experimentally; the marmoset model has been particularly useful, since it opened the way to meaningful immunological studies by providing a ready source of antigen for serology.

Structure and Morphology

Although the viral nature of hepatitis A had been suspected for many years, it was not until 1973 that a morphologically identifiable particle was detected in stools of patients with acute hepatitis A infection. The hepatitis A virus has now been propagated in cell cultures of human and simian origin. The virion is spherical, 27 nm. in diameter; the virus contains nonsegmented, single-stranded RNA and three major proteins. The virus is morphologically and biochemically similar to the enteroviruses, and has recently been classified as an *Enterovirus* (thus becoming enterovirus 72), but continues to be known as hepatitis A virus.[27] Adaptation to cell culture has been an important advance, providing a basis for the biochemical and biophysical characterization of the virus. Passage in cell lines results in reduction in virulence for marmosets; attenuated strains, therefore, hold some promise as immunizing agents.

Immunity

In the marmoset infection model, antibody is produced that neutralizes virus infectivity and reacts with the specific hepatitis A virus antigen (HA–Ag). In the human infection, protective antibodies are produced, a fact that has led to the use of pooled immunoglobulins for passive immunization. The value of pooled immunoglobulin has been repeatedly demonstrated; it probably does not prevent infection, but more likely modifies the disease, thus permitting an active immune response. Effective immunity due to infection has also been demonstrated experimentally in both human volunteers and animal models; the immunity induced provides long-lasting protection against HAV, but offers no protection against hepatitis B virus.

The public health importance of HAV in many parts of the world has prompted vaccine development. The attenuated strains derived by cell culture techniques are being evaluated as vaccines, and it is likely that inactivated virus or purified virus proteins will provide feasible vaccines.

Epidemiology

Hepatitis A infection is prevalent throughout the world, although it appears with greater frequency in lower socioeconomic groups. In the United States, the reported cases of hepatitis A have shown a steady decline since about 1970. Infections tend to be mild or asymptomatic in young children, but severity of the disease increases with age, and young adults are most affected.

Humans can be infected by either parenteral inoculation or ingestion of the virus, and it is probable that the latter route is involved in most naturally occurring infections. Waterborne and foodborne epidemics have been described, and other more direct routes are also indicated. For example, it appears that HAV infection is more common in drug addicts and homosexual males. The virus is fecally excreted, and epidemiological evidence indicates fecal-oral spread.

In human infections, the virus appears in the feces late in the incubation period and continues to be excreted during the acute phase. Viremia is also noted during the late incubation period and during early, pre-icteric stages of the disease.

Laboratory Diagnosis

The laboratory diagnosis of HAV infection is established by demonstration of HAV or HA–Ag in the feces or by serological means.

Since there is no carrier state in HAV infection, the presence of virus or specific viral antigens in excreta is evidence of infection. Their absence does not preclude infection, however, since virus antigens are detected in only 50 per cent or less of those suffering from infection.

The humoral antibody response to infection appears early, and titers rise rapidly and persist for many years, so that simple antibody titrations of paired serums are not usually informative. On the other hand, IgM antibodies arise early in the disease and persist for only a limited time; thus, techniques that measure only HAV-specific IgM are of considerable utility, permitting early and specific serological diagnosis.

SERUM HEPATITIS

Serum hepatitis has been prevalent for many years, and possibly epidemics of jaundice associated with vaccination and the chemotherapy of syphilis were of this nature. There have been many instances of icteric disease following the injection of human blood or blood products, all indicating the presence of an infectious agent in human blood.

The incubation period of serum hepatitis is relatively long, 8 to 22 weeks, usually with insidious onset; the disease is clinically indistinguishable from infectious hepatitis after the onset of symptoms. Both chimpanzees and rhesus monkeys can be experimentally infected; information about the virus has been derived, therefore, from these animal models and from experimental disease in human volunteers.

Hepatitis B Virus[38, 52]

In 1965, Blumberg described an antigenic substance, appearing in the serum of an Australian aborigine, that appeared to be associated with serum hepatitis. This antigen, variously designated Australia (Au) antigen, serum hepatitis (SH) antigen, or hepatitis-associated antigen (HAA), was reported to react with serum from multiply transfused hemophiliacs in microgel precipitation tests. This antigenic reactivity was associated with serum particles found by electron microscopy. The particles were 20 to 25 nm. in diameter and virus-like in morphology, but they did not contain nucleic acids. These early observations stimulated research efforts over the next decade that have led to a clearer understanding of the biochemical and biological events in serum hepatitis and hold promise for control of this widely distributed and serious affliction.

Hepatitis B Virus and Antigens

The virus of hepatitis B has not yet been cultivated *in vitro*, but sophisticated electron microscopy and immunological studies in animal models and in humans have developed a basic knowledge concerning the virus and its components, as well as delineating some of the particulars of the host-parasite relationships.

The hepatitis B virus (HBV) is thought to be represented by **Dane particles**, discovered by Dane and his colleagues. These particles are spherical in form and exhibit a morphological pattern familiar in other viruses. The particle is composed of a core, or nucleocapsid, containing a small, circular, double-stranded DNA genome, with a molecular weight of 1.6 $\times$ 10[6] daltons. Also contained in this structure is a DNA-dependent DNA polymerase. This core is about 27 nm. in diameter and contains

a group-specific antigen, designated the **core antigen**, and abbreviated HBcAg. The nucleocapsid is surrounded by an outer shell, or coat; the complete virion has a diameter of about 42 nm. The hepatitis B virus is, therefore, quite different from the hepatitis A virus, and it is now classified as hepadnavirus type 1; other types of hepadnaviruses are designated to encompass the hepatitis viruses of ducks, ground squirrels, and woodchucks.

The antigens appearing on the outer surface of the HBV particle are designated the **surface antigens**, or HBsAg. As discussed below, HBsAg is antigenically related to the Australia antigen.

Cytological studies have revealed that the core particle containing HBcAg is found in the nucleus of infected cells, *e.g.*, hepatocytes, while the surface antigens, HBsAg, are located in the cytoplasm, where final assembly of virions apparently takes place. These coat antigens are, however, synthesized in great excess in infected cells. When excess HBsAg is released into the serum during the acute phase of the disease, as well as in certain persistent infections, the antigen aggregates to form the serum particles observed by earlier workers. Thus, Australia antigen and HBsAg become more or less synonymous. Electron microscopy of hepatitis serums reveals several kinds of particles with HBsAg-specificity. Perhaps the most numerous are spherical particles, about 22 nm. in diameter; these are seen along with filamentous forms, also about 22 nm. in diameter, but of varying lengths. Dane particles, both "full" and "empty," are also observed; the latter presumably lack the capsid (Fig. 41–12). The serum particles may be detected also by a variety of serological tests for HBsAg (see below). Still another antigen, soluble in nature, is demonstrable by serological, but not microscopic, procedures, and is designated the e antigen (HBeAg); its significance is not yet clear, but it is present in the virion and appears to be a conversion product of HBcAg. The presence of HBeAg is usually indicative of persisting viral replication; such patients are considered to be highly infectious.

Subtypes of the HBsAg have been demonstrated; these have been useful markers for epidemiological studies on the geographical distribution of HBV. A group antigen, designated *a*, is found in all particles. In addition, HBsAg may carry two type-specific subdeterminants, either *d* or *y* and either *w* or *r*. Thus, the antigenic subtypes of HBsAg are four in number: *adw, ayw, adr,* and *ayr*. HBeAg also

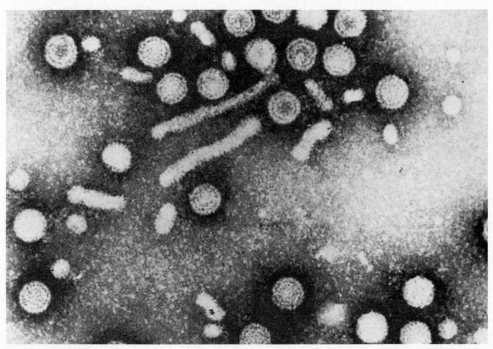

Figure 41–12. Morphological forms of hepatitis B antigen. Note the double-shelled Dane particles; several have been penetrated by the stain to reveal the core. Original magnification × 220,000. (D. J. Almeida, and A. P. Waterson, Amer. J. Med. Sci. **270**:62, 1975. By permission of Slack, Incorporated.)

occurs in three subtypes that are of utility for epidemiological purposes.

The resistance of HBV is of considerable interest as it bears upon the epidemiology of the disease. Since *in vitro* cultivation is not possible, evidence for viral stability and resistance is dependent upon somewhat indirect methods. Numerous studies have confirmed resistance to a wide variety of chemical and physical treatments, including detergents, disinfectants, drying, heat, and both low and high pH.

Epidemiology

Infection with hepatitis B virus is generally manifest in one of several ways, *viz.*, **acute hepatitis, persistent** or **chronic hepatitis**, and **asymptomatic carriage**. In all three categories, HBsAg is present in serum. The distinction between the first two categories is often not clear, *i.e.*, whether chronic persistent hepatitis can lead to chronic active hepatitis. Further, the relationship of these to cirrhosis and to carcinoma of the liver has not been resolved. Extrahepatic manifestations also may be displayed, including polyarteritis nodosa, arthritis, and chronic glomerulonephritis.

Hepatitis B infections exist under natural conditions as both clinical and subclinical cases, presumably circulating by infective routes that involve parenteral introduction. Pertinent modes of transmission include inadequately sterilized needles and surgical instruments; use of contaminated razors; transfusion of infective blood or blood products; tattooing; or abrasions and other wounds, sustained during contact sports and subject to contamination with blood or serum from infected participants. There is also reason to believe that the virus may be transmitted by the gastrointestinal route and by sexual contact, since saliva, menstrual blood, and semen have been established as infective; for example, prevalence is particularly high in homosexual males. Vertical transmission, *i.e.*, from mother to offspring, has been recorded, although it is possible that the infection may be transmitted postpartum by infected maternal blood.[13] Hepatitis B infection becomes occupationally associated in laboratory workers, particularly those employed in blood banks; surgeons; dentists; and those working in hemodialysis units, where quantities of infective blood are handled. Because of the mode of transmission, cases of hepatitis tend to be **sporadic**, unlike the common-source outbreaks so often seen in infectious hepatitis, and are without seasonal variation.

Individuals who are HBsAg-positive are considered to be potentially infectious; it has

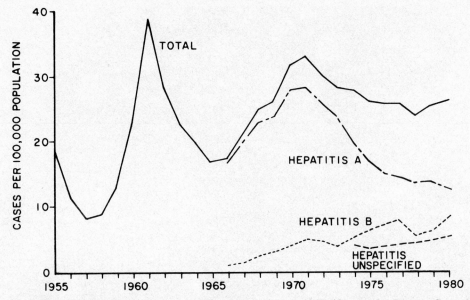

Figure 41–13. Reported cases of hepatitis in the United States, 1955 to 1980. (Centers for Disease Control, Annual summary 1980: reported morbidity and mortality in the United States. Morbidity and Mortality Weekly Report, Vol. 29, No. 54, 1981.)

been found that as little as 0.0001 ml. of infectious plasma can produce clinical disease. Blood bank, laboratory, and surgical practices take cognizance of this by institution of protective measures, such as prohibiting HBsAg-positive individuals from serving as blood donors. As an example of the complexity of this matter, it has been estimated that there are between 400,000 and 800,000 infectious carriers in the United States, and there are perhaps 170 million worldwide. The prevalence of clinically apparent hepatitis in the United States is shown in Figure 41–13.

Serology and Laboratory Diagnosis[16, 58]

The diagnosis of hepatitis type B infections, in the absence of viral isolation, must ultimately depend upon immunological or serological testing. A variety of serological tests have been devised for diagnostic use. These tests are designed to detect HBV antigens, principally HBsAg and HBeAg, or HBV-spe-

cific serum antibodies, such as anti-HBe, anti-HBc, and anti-HBs. Serological tests include gel immunodiffusion; complement fixation; immune adherence, using either antigen- or antibody-coated red blood cells; radioimmunoassay; and counterelectrophoresis. Of these, immunoadherence and radioimmunoassay are both sensitive and rapid.

Table 41–5 displays the principal serological markers of hepatitis B infection and their relationship to infection stages. It should be noted that the presence of antibodies to HBsAg is associated with effective immunity in the recovered host.

Prevention and Control

The prevention of hepatitis type B is primarily dependent upon measures that interrupt the transmission of the virus. Accordingly, incidence of post-transfusion hepatitis may be reduced by effectively screening out donors that carry HBsAg. This is not always effective, leading to the suggestion that additional hep-

Table 41–5. **Serological Markers of Hepatitis B Infection**

HBsAg	HBeAg	Anti-HBe	Anti-HBc	Anti-HBs	Indication
+	+	−	−	−	Incubation period or early acute stage
+	+	−	+	−	Acute stages; carrier state
+	−	+	+	−	Late acute or chronic stages
−	−	+	+	+	Convalescent stage
−	−	−	+	+	Recovered from infection

atitis viruses may be circulating and responsible for a majority of the cases of post-transfusion hepatitis; these are often called non-A, non-B hepatitis viruses (see below).

Other measures that have proved effective for impeding transmission include appropriate sterilization of dental and surgical instruments and the precautions necessary in the transport, handling, and proper disposition of infected serums, saliva, and other biological specimens.

Passive immunization is based upon the protection afforded by anti-HBs antibody. Pooled serum immunoglobulin has been used, with some success, as a prophylactic in populations at risk; better protection is offered by use of pooled serum known to have higher titers of HBs antibody, termed hepatitis immune globulin.

Development of vaccines for active immunization against hepatitis B infection has been slow because of the inability to propagate the virus *in vitro*. Recently, however, subunit vaccines have been prepared by purification of HBsAg found in the serum of chronic human carriers; formalin inactivation of these components destroys infective viruses while preserving immunogenicity.

This vaccine, when given in three doses, engenders protective antibody response in more than 90 per cent of healthy adult recipients. The protective efficacy of the vaccine has been 80 to 95 per cent in field trials in the United States, but the duration of immunity is not yet known. Unfortunately, the vaccine is not effective in eliminating the carrier state.

Pre-exposure vaccination is recommended for high-risk populations, *viz.*, health care workers, hemodialysis patients, homosexually active males, injectable drug users, contacts of carriers, and inmates of correctional institutions. Post-exposure vaccination is warranted in infants born of HBsAg-positive mothers and contacts of active hepatitis B cases. Careful selection of vaccinees is necessary because of the cost and limited availability of the vaccine.

Primary Hepatocellular Carcinoma[59]

In those areas of the world where hepatocellular carcinoma prevalence is high, such as tropical Africa and the Far East, there is a significant association with the markers of hepatitis B infection, *e.g.*, carriage of HBsAg. There is considerable evidence that HBV is an etiological factor in this form of cancer. The frequency of occurrence of HBsAg in hepatoma patients, the higher prevalence of hepatoma in areas where HBV infections are in greater evidence, the integration of HBV–DNA in hepatocellular carcinoma cells, and the release of hepatitis B surface antigens from cell lines derived from hepatocellular carcinomas are suggestive of this association.

Delta Agent[29, 34]

In 1977, a new antigen-antibody system was detected in fulminant hepatitis cases occurring in southern Italy. Designated delta, the antigen now is recognized as belonging to a new and unique virus-like agent that appears to be defective, in that it replicates only in the presence of a helper, the hepatitis B virus.

The delta agent resembles a large particle of HBsAg; it is spherical, 35 to 37 nm. in diameter, and consists of a core containing a very small RNA molecule and the delta antigen. Surrounding the core is a coat composed of HBsAg. The separate viral identity of delta agent is supported by the fact that delta agent RNA does not hybridize with DNA from HBV. Although delta agent does not infect or cause hepatitis in the absence of HBV, simultaneous infection with HBV and delta agent is usually manifest as hepatitis of increased severity.

Delta infection has been described from most parts of the world, but it appears in two epidemiological forms. It is highly endemic in only limited areas, where it is associated with fulminant hepatitis in small outbreaks. In most other regions, only sporadic delta infections appear, usually associated with illicit parenteral drug use. Individuals who are sexually active, particularly homosexual males, also appear to be at greater risk of infection.

NON-A, NON-B HEPATITIS[1, 10, 39]

By employing the serological markers described in foregoing sections, it is now possible to assess with some accuracy the hepatitis infections due to hepatitis A and B viruses. A portion of hepatitis cases, however, cannot be identified as hepatitis A or B, nor can they be assigned to other recognized viruses. Known by the unwieldy name of non-A, non-B hepatitis, these infections often follow blood transfusions or illicit parenteral drug usage and are sometimes termed **post-transfusion hepatitis**. They resemble hepatitis B infections in both clinical appearance and epidemiology, but are not serologically related to either HAV or HBV infections. They are, therefore, diagnosed by exclusion of known viral agents.

Like hepatitis B virus, the hepatitis non-A, non-B (HNANB) viruses have not been propagated *in vitro*, but they have been serially transmitted in chimpanzees and, less reliably, in marmosets. The nature of the virus is enigmatic, but electron microscopy has revealed virus-like particles in liver and serum from both humans and chimpanzees; most of the observed particles have been in the range of 25 to 33 nm. in diameter. Many workers have attempted to devise serological tests for identification of the virus or its products, but these methods are immersed in controversy, and no generally acceptable tests are presently available for identification. Such evidence as is available, including cross-protection tests in chimpanzees, suggests that more than one virus is responsible for this type of hepatitis.

The distribution of HNANB appears to be worldwide. It is estimated that perhaps 20 per cent of clinical cases of hepatitis are due to HNANB viruses, although in some geographical areas its prevalence may be much higher. In Japan, for example, some 50 per cent of hepatitis cases cannot be identified as either hepatitis A or B.

In most instances, HNANB viruses are transmitted by contaminated blood or blood products and by parenteral drug use; sporadic cases also occur in health care workers. In general, the risk factors for HNANB parallel those associated with acquisition of hepatitis B. Although most blood and blood products used in the United States are carefully screened for hepatitis B virus, post-transfusion hepatitis occurs in 5 to 7 per cent of recipients, and 80 to 90 per cent of these infections are attributed to HNANB.

The incubation period for HNANB is similar to that of hepatitis B; clinical findings also resemble those of hepatitis B. The disease is not generally so severe as hepatitis B, although fulminant hepatitis has been observed. The disease may occur in acute or chronic form. There is also some indication of mild or asymptomatic infections, based on elevation of liver enzymes. The widespread distribution of infection is evident, since pooled serum immunoglobulins have a prophylactic effect on development of HNANB, presumably because of protective antibody content.

Epidemic Hepatitis Non-A, Non-B[19]
In parts of Asia and the Middle East, an epidemic form of hepatitis has been recently described that resembles hepatitis A, but without serological evidence of HAV infection.

This epidemic form of hepatitis is thought to be spread by the fecal-oral route, with contaminated water as the most likely vehicle. Although no serological tests are presently available, immune protection in those recovered from the infection is evident. The disease has been experimentally transmitted by ingestion of infective stool filtrates in a human volunteer, with morphological evidence of a virus-like particle in acute phase stools. Whether this form of hepatitis is due to a new kind of hepatitis virus or is a new serotype of hepatitis A is not established.

REFERENCES

1. Aach, R. D., and R. A. Kahn. 1980. Post-transfusion hepatitis: current perspectives. Ann. Intern. Med. **92**:539–546.
2. Andersson, S.-O., B. Björkstén, and L. Å. Burman. 1975. A comparative study of meningoencephalitis epidemics caused by echovirus type 7 and Coxsackievirus type B5. Clinical and virological observations during two epidemics in northern Sweden. Scand. J. Infect. Dis. **7**:233–237.
3. Blacklow, N. R., and G. Cukor. 1981. Viral gastroenteritis. New Engl. J. Med. **304**:397–406.
4. Butterworth, B. E., *et al.* 1976. Replication of rhinoviruses. Brief review. Arch. Virol. **51**:169–189.
5. Cooney, M. K., J. P. Fox, and G. E. Kenny. 1982. Antigenic groupings of 90 rhinovirus serotypes. Infect. Immun. **37**:642–647.
6. Cossart, Y. E. 1977. Evolution of poliovirus since introduction of attenuated vaccine. Brit. Med. J. **1**:1621–1623.
7. Deinhardt, F. 1980. Predictive value of markers of hepatitis virus infection. J. Infect. Dis. **141**:299–305.
8. Deinhardt, F., and I. D. Gust. 1982. Viral hepatitis. Bull. Wld Hlth Org. **60**:661–691.
9. Estes, M. K., and D. Y. Graham. 1979. Epidemic viral gastroenteritis. Amer. J. Med. **66**:1001–1007.
10. Feinman, C. V., *et al.* 1980. Hepatitis non-A, non-B. Can. Med. Assn J. **123**:181–184.
11. Fox, J. P. 1976. Is a rhinovirus vaccine possible? Amer. J. Epidemiol. **103**:345–354.
12. Francis, D. P., and J. E. Maynard. 1979. The transmission and outcome of hepatitis A, B, and non-A, non-B: a review. Epidemiol. Rev. **1**:17–31.
13. Gilbert, G. L. 1981. Vertical transmission of hepatitis B: review of the literature and recommendations for management. Med. J. Australia **1**:280–285.
14. Hendley, J. O., L. A. Mika, and J. M. Gwaltney, Jr. 1978. Evaluation of virucidal compounds for inactivation of rhinovirus on hands. Antimicrob. Agents Chemother. **14**:690–694.
15. Hirschman, S. Z., and G. S. Hammer. 1974. Coxsackie virus myopericarditis. A microbiological and clinical review. Amer. J. Cardiol. **34**:224–232.
16. Hoofnagle, J. H. 1981. Serological markers of hepatitis B virus infection. Ann. Rev. Med. **32**:1–11.
17. Horstmann, D. M. 1982. Control of poliomyelitis: a continuing paradox. J. Infect. Dis. **146**:540–551.
18. Kaplan, J. E., *et al.* 1982. Epidemiology of Norwalk gastroenteritis and the role of Norwalk virus in outbreaks of acute nonbacterial gastroenteritis. Ann. Intern. Med. **96**:756–761.

19. Khuroo, M. S. 1980. Study of an epidemic of non-A, non-B hepatitis. Possibility of another human hepatitis virus distinct from post-transfusion non-A, non-B type. Amer. J. Med. **68**:818–824.

20. Kitamura, N., et al. 1981. Primary structure, gene organization, and polypeptide expression of poliovirus RNA. Nature **291**:547–553.

21. Krugman, S., and D. J. Gocke. 1978. Viral Hepatitis. Major Problems in Internal Medicine, Vol. 15. W. B. Saunders Co., Philadelphia.

22. Lau, R. C. H., and Y. E. Hermon. 1979. The role of Coxsackie B viruses in heart disease in New Zealand. New Zealand Med. J. **90**:375–377.

23. Macnaughton, M. R. 1982. The structure and replication of rhinoviruses. Curr. Topics Microbiol. Immunol. **97**:1–26.

24. Macnaughton, M. R., and H. A. Davies. 1981. Human enteric coronaviruses. Brief review. Arch. Virol. **70**:301–313.

25. Marier, R., et al. 1975. Coxsackievirus B5 infection and aseptic meningitis in neonates and children. Amer. J. Dis. Children **129**:321–325.

26. Melnick, J. L. 1978. Advantages and disadvantages of killed and live poliomyelitis vaccine. Bull. Wld Hlth Org. **56**:21–38.

27. Melnick, J. L. 1982. Classification of hepatitis A virus as enterovirus type 72 and of hepatitis B virus as hepadnavirus type 1. Intervirology **18**:105–106.

28. Metselaar, D. 1976. Possible selection of virulent poliovirus strains in third-world countries. Lancet **1**:174–176.

29. Moestrup, T., et al. 1983. Clinical aspects of delta infection. Brit. Med. J. **286**:87–90.

30. Murphy, A. 1981. Aetiology of viral gastroenteritis. A review. Med. J. Australia **2**:177–182.

31. Nathanson, N., and J. R. Martin. 1979. The epidemiology of poliomyelitis: enigmas surrounding its appearance, epidemicity, and disappearance. Amer. J. Epidemiol. **110**:672–692.

32. Provost, P. J., and M. R. Hilleman. 1979. Propagation of human hepatitis A virus in cell culture in vitro. Proc. Soc. Exptl Biol. Med. **160**:213–221.

33. Putnak, J. R., and B. A. Phillips. 1981. Picornaviral structure and assembly. Microbiol. Rev. **45**:287–315.

34. Raimondo, G., et al. 1982. Multicentre study of prevalence of HBV-associated delta infection and liver disease in drug-addicts. Lancet **1**:249–251.

35. Report. 1980. Rotavirus and other viral diarrhoeas. Bull. Wld Hlth Org. **58**:183–198.

36. Report. 1982. Acute haemorrhagic conjunctivitis. Brit. Med. J. **284**:833–834.

37. Report. 1982. The relation between acute persisting spinal paralysis and poliomyelitis vaccine—results of a ten-year enquiry. Bull. Wld Hlth Org. **60**:231–242.

38. Robinson, W. S. 1977. The genome of hepatitis B virus. Ann. Rev. Microbiol. **31**:357–377.

39. Robinson, W. S. 1982. The enigma of non-A, non-B hepatitis. J. Infect. Dis. **145**:387–395.

40. Roebuck, M. O. 1976. Rhinoviruses in Britain 1963–1973. J. Hygiene **76**:137–146.

41. Sabin, A. B. 1981. Paralytic poliomyelitis: old dogmas and new perspectives. Rev. Infect. Dis. **3**:543–564.

42. Salk, D. 1980. Eradication of poliomyelitis in the United States. I. Live virus vaccine-associated and wild poliovirus disease. II. Experience with killed poliovirus vaccine. III. Poliovaccines—practical considerations. Rev. Infect. Dis. **2**:228–242; 243–257; 258–273.

43. Sarateanu, D. E., and W. Ehrengut. 1980. A two year serological surveillance of coronavirus infections in Hamburg. Infection **8**:70–72.

44. Schieble, J. H. 1980. Rhinoviruses. pp. 829–835. In E. H. Lennette, et al. (Eds.): Manual of Clinical Microbiology. 3rd ed. American Society for Microbiology, Washington, D.C.

45. Schiff, G. M. 1979. Coxsackievirus B epidemic at a boys' camp. Amer. J. Dis. Children **133**:782–785.

46. Schmidt, N. J., H. H. Ho, and E. H. Lennette. 1975. Propagation and isolation of group A Coxsackieviruses in RD cells. J. Clin. Microbiol. **2**:183–185.

47. Sells, C. J., R. L. Carpenter, and C. G. Ray. 1975. Sequelae of central-nervous-system enterovirus infections. New Engl. J. Med. **293**:1–4.

48. Siddell, S., H. Wege, and V. ter Meulen. 1982. The structure and replication of coronaviruses. Curr. Topics Microbiol. Immunol. **99**:131–163.

49. Stott, E. J., and R. A. Killington. 1972. Rhinoviruses. Ann. Rev. Microbiol. **26**:503–524.

50. Tagaya, I., and K. Tachibana. 1975. Epidemic of hand, foot and mouth disease in Japan, 1972–1973: difference in epidemiologic and virologic features from the previous one. Japan. J. Med. Sci. Biol. **28**:231–234.

51. Tagaya, I., R. Takayama, and A. Hagiwara. 1981. A large-scale epidemic of hand, foot and mouth disease associated with enterovirus 71 infection in Japan in 1978. Japan. J. Med. Sci. Biol. **34**:191–196.

52. Tiollais, P., P. Charnay, and G. N. Vyas. 1981. Biology of hepatitis B virus. Science **213**:406–411.

53. Walker-Smith, J. 1978. Rotavirus gastroenteritis. Arch. Dis. Childh. **53**:355–362.

54. Wege, H., S. Siddell, and V. ter Meulen. 1982. The biology and pathogenesis of coronaviruses. Curr. Topics Microbiol. Immunol. **99**:165–200.

55. Wenner, H. A., and A. M. Behbehani. 1968. Echoviruses. Virology Monogr. **1**:1–72.

56. Wyatt, A. V. 1975. Is poliomyelitis a genetically-determined disease? II. A critical examination of the epidemiological data. Med. Hypotheses **1**:23–32.

57. Zuckerman, A. J. 1978. The three types of human viral hepatitis. Bull. Wld Hlth Org. **56**:1–20.

58. Zuckerman, A. J. 1979. Specific serological diagnosis of viral hepatitis. Brit. Med. J. **2**:84–86.

59. Zuckerman, A. J. 1982. Primary hepatocellular carcinoma and hepatitis B virus. Trans. Roy. Soc. Trop. Med. Hygiene **76**:711–718.

CHAPTER 42

The Togaviruses;
The Bunyaviruses;
The Arenaviruses;
The Slow Viruses

An examination of the history of microbiology reveals that as microbial agents of disease were discovered there was a tendency to place these agents into groups that were based, in large measure, upon the natural history of the diseases that they caused. Thus, microorganisms with quite different properties were sometimes assumed to be related to one another because of similarities in pathogenesis and epidemiology. As the agents themselves became better known, classification systems came to be centered upon the common biological and structural features of the microorganisms, bringing order and a clearer understanding of the basic interrelationships. Such an evolution is now taking place in virology as improved observational and biochemical methods permit a better insight into viruses as microorganisms.

In certain instances, however, consideration of the natural history of a group of infectious diseases does permit better recognition of the interrelationships that may exist between different taxonomic groups. So it is with those viruses that have the common feature of infecting both vertebrate and insect hosts as a part of their complex life cycles. Although encompassing several different taxa, these viruses are collectively and informally known as **arboviruses**, or *arthropod-borne viruses*.

Arboviruses occur primarily in infections of lower animals, including mammals and birds, and in arthropods. The last serve as **vectors** to maintain reservoirs of infection in vertebrates and to transmit the infection to man; the human infection is, however, often peripheral to the life history of the virus. These viruses multiply in the arthropod hosts to produce infections that are nonfatal and, so far as is known, asymptomatic. Vertical transmission by **transovarian passage** to offspring is common in ticks, but happens less often in mosquitoes. This kind of transmission is epidemiologically important, since it permits the maintenance of virus in the vector in the absence of vertebrate infection. While the passage of these viruses to vertebrate hosts, including man, is by infected mosquitoes, ticks, or phlebotomus flies, a single virus is transmitted by only one kind of hematophagous vector. The great majority of the arboviruses are mosquito-borne; but a relatively smaller and more homogeneous group is tick-borne.

Since viruses are classified (Chapter 38) largely on the basis of morphology and biochemical makeup, it is to be expected that arboviruses, distinguished by host range and mode of transmission, would include many that

are unrelated in architecture. To a degree, such expectations are met. In many respects, however, there is surprising homogeneity. All appear to be ether-sensitive, heat-labile (56°C.), acid-sensitive RNA viruses. The capsid is surrounded by an envelope, and most are 30 to 50 nm. in diameter, but some are in the range of 70 to 130 nm. Many viruses are cultivable in the chick embryo, in which a fatal infection is produced, and in a variety of cell cultures. The viruses are almost uniformly pathogenic for the suckling mouse; some infect the adult mouse also, producing encephalitis upon intracerebral inoculation. In vertebrate hosts, the consequences of infection range from inapparent disease to systemic infections such as febrile illnesses, severe hemorrhagic fever, and encephalitis that may be highly fatal.

A great many arthropod-borne viruses have been described. Some are found in association with diseases of vertebrates, but others have been encountered only in arthropods. In some of the latter cases, there is serological evidence of vertebrate host infection, but without virus isolation from these hosts; thus, some are still of unknown pathogenicity. Some 488 arboviruses have been described, and probably many more await discovery. As a group they have global distribution, although many are found only in geographical regions that parallel their vector or vertebrate host distribution. Most have been given place names of exotic character.

Viruses that meet the general definition of arboviruses are placed in several of the formal virus families: Togaviridae, Bunyaviridae, and Reoviridae. Almost all of the togaviruses, including the genera *Alphavirus* and *Flavivirus*, are arboviruses, as are the bunyaviruses; only one genus, *Orbivirus*, of the Reoviridae is arthropod-borne. Table 42–1 shows the principal arboviral diseases, their major disease categories, and classification of the viral agents.

Many of the arboviruses, though not all, are **hemagglutinating** for goose or neonatal chick red blood cells. The specificity of the hemagglutination-inhibiting antibody has been particularly useful in the immunological characterization of these viruses, allowing their separation into several groups; *viz., Alphavirus* (formerly group A arboviruses); *Flavivirus* (formerly group B); and *Bunyavirus*; many other viruses either do not form hemagglutinins, or possess hemagglutinins antigenically related to only a few, if any, of the other known viruses. Further subdivision may be

Table 42–1. **The Principal Arboviral Diseases of Man**

Viral Group	Disease Category		
	Encephalitis	*Hemorrhagic Fever*	*Febrile Illness*
Alphavirus (Mosquito-borne)	Western equine encephalitis Eastern equine encephalitis Venezuelan equine encephalitis		Ross River fever Chikungunya O'Nyong-Nyong Semliki Forest Mayaro
Flavivirus (Mosquito-borne)	St. Louis encephalitis Japanese B encephalitis Murray Valley encephalitis Rocio encephalitis	Dengue Yellow fever	Dengue West Nile fever
Orbivirus (Tick-borne)			Colorado tick fever
Bunyavirus (Mosquito-borne)	California encephalitis		
Phlebovirus (Phlebotomus- or mosquito-borne)			Sandfly fever Rift Valley fever
Nairovirus (Tick-borne)		Congo-Crimean hemorrhagic fever	

made on the basis of the specificity of complement-fixing and neutralizing antibodies, but there may be cross-reactions between members of the different hemagglutination-inhibiting groups. Immunological characterization has, however, served to show the close relationship, or even substantial identity, of arboviruses found in widely separated geographical areas.

In this chapter the most important and representative viruses will be considered individually, followed by a summary of their known relationships.

The Togaviruses[13, 16, 21, 41, 52]

As the ultrastructure of viruses became better known, several viruses were found to be similar in architecture to the then recognized antigenic group A and B arboviruses. They differed, however, in that they were not arthropod-borne. In order to accommodate these nonarboviruses in a single taxon based on morphology, the name Togaviridae was proposed as a means of avoiding ecological implications. These are all enveloped viruses with a single-stranded (+)RNA genome. Within the Togaviridae, several genera were established: *Alphavirus*, to contain the older group A arboviruses; *Flavivirus*, to contain the older group B arboviruses; a new genus, *Pestivirus*, for the nonarboviruses causing several animal diseases; and *Rubivirus*, to include the rubella virus, which is not arthropod-borne. The properties of togaviruses are listed in Table 42–2.

Togaviruses are enveloped, and therefore sensitive to ether and detergents; they have a single-stranded (+)RNA genome with a molecular weight of approximately 4 million daltons. The capsid, which has icosahedral symmetry, is from 20 to 40 nm. in diameter and is enclosed in an envelope derived by budding and which may carry glycopeptides as surface projections (Fig. 42–1). By careful treatment, the RNA can be isolated from the virion in infectious form.

Table 42–2. **Properties of the Togaviruses**

Alphavirus *Rubivirus*	*Flavivirus* *Pestivirus*
(−)RNA genome; single- stranded, nonsegmented; 4×10^6 daltons	(+)RNA genome; single- stranded; nonsegmented; 3 to 4×10^6 daltons
Spherical virion, 40–70 nm.	Spherical virion, 40–60 nm.
Icosahedral capsid, 32 or 42 capsomers	Icosahedral capsid
Assembled in cytoplasm	Assembled in cytoplasm
Enveloped, by budding from plasma membrane; glycoprotein peplomers	Enveloped, by budding from intracytoplasmic membrane; glycoprotein peplomers
Ether-sensitive	Ether-sensitive

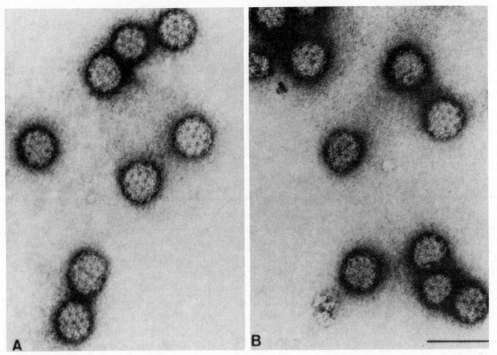

Figure 42–1. The morphology of representative alphaviruses. *A*, Sindbis virus; *B*, Semliki Forest virus, both stained with uranyl acetate. Bar = 100 nm. (P. J. Enzmann and F. Weiland, Virology, **95**:501, 1979.)

The alphaviruses are distinguished by the possession of common hemagglutinins that occur as peplomers on the virion surface; the virion has a diameter of 40 to 70 nm. As noted in Chapter 38, alphaviruses mature by budding through the plasma membrane of their host cells. Mosquitoes are the infected arthropod hosts of these viruses.

The flaviviruses share common hemagglutinins, but these are antigenically distinct from those of alphaviruses. The virion is also somewhat smaller than that of alphaviruses, and the envelope is acquired by budding through the intracytoplasmic membranes into cytoplasmic vacuoles. Although most flaviviruses infect mosquitoes as their arthropod hosts, some are carried by ticks.

The pestiviruses will not be discussed and the rubella virus will be described in a later section, since it is not considered to be an arbovirus.

ALPHAVIRUS

The better known of the viruses of this group are those of the equine encephalitides and certain viruses found largely in Africa and producing dengue-like disease. All are transmitted to vertebrate hosts by **mosquito vectors**.

Only the more important alphaviruses causing human disease are discused here.

While "sleeping sickness," which may be of bacterial or protozoan etiology, has long been known to occur as sporadic cases and in epidemic form, the first encephalitis of probable viral etiology to be described with sufficient accuracy for tentative identification was *encephalitis lethargica* or von Economo's disease. Epidemics first arose in 1915 and continued until 1926, but have not recurred since. Although not bacterial, viral etiology of the disease was never established.

Beginning in the early 1930s, a variety of viruses were isolated that were capable of causing encephalitis. Many of these are related by antigenic character, spread by arthropod vectors, and occur in natural infections of lower animals.

The mosquito-borne *Alphavirus* encephalitides are an important cause of equine and human morbidity in the Americas. The equine encephalitis viruses are responsible for three epidemiological types of disease, each caused by a distinct virus. In Venezuelan equine encephalitis, the epidemic viruses are naturally maintained by a mosquito-equine-mosquito chain. In the other types—western and eastern equine encephalitis—the naturally occurring enzootic chain is maintained by mosquito-bird-mosquito transmission. Equine encephalitis occurs incidentally when the virus is introduced into these populations by infected mosquito vectors; horses play no role in the natural transmission cycle. All of the equine encephalitis viruses infect humans when the viruses are introduced by the bite of mosquitoes that have fed on the infected vertebrate hosts.

WESTERN EQUINE ENCEPHALITIS

The western equine encephalitis (WEE) virion is about 50 nm. in diameter, sensitive to ether and other lipid solvents, and slowly inactivated by formalin. It is readily cultivable in the chick embryo by all routes of inoculation, producing a rapidly fatal infection with generalized hemorrhage, thrombosis, and necrosis. Embryonated egg culture has, however, been largely supplanted by tissue culture techniques. The virus grows readily, and to high titer, in a variety of tissue cultures. Neutralizing antibody may be titrated in such cultures by the plaque reduction test.

The Disease in Man
The incubation period is from less than one to as long as three weeks. The human affection varies from an almost symptomless or abortive form to an acute disease in which the patient becomes comatose within 24 hours; the more severe form usually occurs in infants and young children. The disease is essentially a meningoencephalitis, rarely involving the medulla or spinal cord. In the typical case the prodromal signs and symptoms are usually headache, drowsiness, and fever. Involvement of the central nervous system results in tremor, convulsions, mental confusion, and amnesia, but paralysis is not common, occurring in perhaps 15 per cent of cases; the acute phase lasts from 7 to 10 days. The case-fatality rate is low, generally less than 4 per cent, and recovery is usually uneventful and complete. Serological evidence indicates that many infections with this virus never result in clinical encephalitis, and many others are subclinical.

Experimental Infections
The experimental animal of choice is the mouse, which may be infected by the intranasal, intraperitoneal, or intracerebral route. Following intraperitoneal inoculation, the virus appears in the blood, infects the nasal mucosa, and reaches the central nervous system via the olfactory nerves. Within a few days the animals show such signs of meningoence-

phalitis as spastic muscular contractions and paralysis, followed by prostration and death; the disease in mice is similar to that in man. The inoculation of other animals by the intracutaneous route results in an inapparent infection with viremia to give the kind of infection that probably occurs in animal reservoirs of the virus.

Immunity
Complement-fixing, hemagglutination-inhibiting, and neutralizing antibodies are produced as a result of infection and are associated with a solid immunity. Antibody appears early in the infection, usually within a week of onset, and a rise in titer between paired serums is diagnostic. The complement-fixing antibody usually disappears within a year, but the neutralizing antibody persists for longer periods and is the one titrated in serological surveys.

Epidemiology
In nature, WEE infections occur primarily in wild birds, maintained by mosquito transmission. In the natural history of the disease, infection of horses and man is only incidental. In the United States, infections in humans predominantly occur in areas west of the Mississippi River and are found also in Western Canada. The virus is also present in animal and mosquito reservoirs along the Atlantic and Gulf Coasts. The WEE virus is, however, a minor cause of encephalitis in the United States; only 18 cases were reported in 1981, and none were reported in 1980. Most infections occur in the warmer months, paralleling the presence of mosquitoes.

Hosts. The WEE virus has been recovered from about 20 species of wild birds and at least six species of mammals. There is serological evidence of infection in more than 73 species of wild birds and most common domestic birds and mammals. It has been shown experimentally that the level of viremia is considerably higher in infected wild birds than in domestic birds or mammals, and it may be inferred that mosquitoes are more readily infected by feeding on the former. While this and other evidence leaves little doubt that wild birds are the important natural reservoir of infection, and that infection in mammals and domestic birds does not play a significant part in the transmission cycle, it is not clear which species of wild birds are of primary importance and which are only secondary.

Vectors. Although WEE virus may infect a variety of mosquitoes and bird mites, *Culex tarsalis* is the primary vector in the western part of the country, serving to maintain the natural transmission cycle in birds and transmitting the infection to man and mammals. In the Atlantic and Gulf Coasts, the primary vector is *Culiseta melanura*; this species feeds mostly on birds and is primarily found in swampy areas. Therefore, the virus is not readily transmitted to humans or mammals in these regions. It is also noteworthy that the virus strains found in the eastern states differ antigenically from those isolated in the western states, and there is some evidence that antigenic variation, and possibly virulence, is associated with passage in different vectors.[26]

EASTERN EQUINE ENCEPHALITIS

Eastern equine encephalitis (EEE) is a disease similar to WEE, but differs in its geographical distribution, arthropod vectors, and host range. Human infections occur primarily in Atlantic and Gulf Coast states from New Hampshire to Texas; they have occasionally been found as far west as Wisconsin in this country, in Canada, Mexico, the Caribbean, Central and South America, and in the Philippines.

The EEE virus is closely similar to the WEE virus, producing rapidly fatal infections in the chick embryo as well as cytopathic changes in a variety of tissue cultures. Its pathogenicity for experimental animals parallels that of WEE virus, but it exhibits a somewhat wider host range and is able to infect sheep, cats, and hedgehogs. A comparison of tissue cultures and experimental animals has shown that chick embryo cells are the most sensitive of the tissue cultures and that the suckling mouse is the most susceptible experimental animal host. Chick embryo cell culture of the virus has been used for the preparation of formalin-inactivated vaccine.

Naturally acquired infection occurs in both horses and man. In the former, the disease is substantially identical with that produced by WEE virus, but infections in man are relatively more severe and are characterized by a higher case-fatality rate and a tendency to occur in children. The human disease is rare in the United States; 7 cases were reported in 1980 and none in 1981.

Epidemiology[6]

As in WEE, the natural reservoirs of EEE are wild birds; infection in mammals and domestic birds plays only a minor part in the natural transmission cycle. Transmission to humans and domestic animals is incidental, and occurs only during periods of high prevalence in the natural reservoirs.

Hosts. A wide variety of wild birds have been found with serological evidence of infection by the EEE virus. In a general way, the smaller birds show a higher level of viremia on experimental infection than do larger birds, such as herons and pheasants, and they also tend to be more numerous. Further, the proportion of birds showing serum antibody is greater in migratory birds that winter south of the United States than in birds wintering in the north, suggesting a transmission cycle in Central or South America.

The prevalence of the infection fluctuates somewhat, as indicated by serology and virus isolations in wild birds. During periods of low prevalence, viruses are isolated from less than 1 per cent and antibody is found in 15 to 20 per cent of caught wild birds. During periods of high prevalence, virus has been isolated from as many as 10 per cent of birds examined, and 50 per cent or more show the presence of antibody in the serum. The spill-over of infections to humans is greatest when the prevalence in wild birds is high.

Vectors. The EEE virus has been isolated from many mosquito species, but the predominant vector appears to be *Culiseta melanura*. The proportion of isolations is relatively high from this species, a freshwater-swamp mosquito that bites birds freely. It is believed that *C. melanura* is one of the most important vectors in the maintenance of the natural transmission cycle, but it seldom bites man or domestic animals, and it is probable that other vectors are involved; *Aedes sollicitans*, for example, seems to be an epidemic vector in certain regions.

VENEZUELAN EQUINE ENCEPHALITIS[56]

Venezuelan equine encephalitis (VEE) occurred as an epizootic in horses and mules in Colombia in 1935, and the causative virus was isolated during a similar epizootic in Venezuela in 1938. The disease has also been found elsewhere in South America and has been observed in Mexico, Texas, and Florida.

The infection in man usually results in a relatively mild, influenza-like illness with headache and fever, gastrointestinal disturbance, myalgia, and lethargy, with little or no indication of central nervous system involvement. Such cases occur as a result of naturally acquired infection and have occurred repeatedly as a result of laboratory infection. The disease generally lasts for three to five days, but occasionally longer in more severe cases. Encephalitis is not common, being observed in only about 4 per cent of cases, usually in those under 15 years of age; the fatality rate in encephalitis cases is about 20 per cent. On the other hand, serological evidence indicates that symptomless or subclinical infections in man may be relatively common in endemic areas.

The virus consists of a nucleocapsid with diameter of 35 nm., while the enveloped virus is 55 nm. in diameter. Envelope proteins are responsible for hemagglutination and react in hemagglutination-inhibition, complement-fixation, and neutralization tests. The virus is immunologically distinct from WEE and EEE viruses.

Venezuelan equine encephalitis viruses are properly regarded as a complex of viruses, since several antigenic subtypes may be distinguished, based on neutralization tests. Some of the subtypes differ with respect to host-vector transmission cycles. Subtype varieties IAB and IC are the "epidemic" viruses. Infection by these subtypes is generally of an epidemic nature and is sometimes severe. The viruses infect horses, donkeys, and probably mules, but not cattle. These are considered to be the principal vertebrate reservoirs of the natural infections, although other mammals, both domestic and wild, may become infected. Birds show little evidence of natural infection, and pigeons and doves are refractory to experimental infection. The infection is transmitted to other equines, and to man, by mosquitoes; the virus has been isolated from many mosquito species, but those most often found infected are of the genera *Mansonia, Psorophora*, and *Aedes*. The viruses are naturally maintained by a mosquito-equine-mosquito transmission chain.

The remaining subtypes—ID, IE, II, III, and IV—are often referred to as the enzootic or "nonepidemic" viruses. The natural infection is not one of equines, but is rather one of a variety of rodents in small foci centered in freshwater swamps of coastal areas. Transmission is most often by *Culex* mosquitoes. These viruses are not generally pathogenic for equines; humans may be infected, but the disease is rarely fatal. Peak transmission of both types is seen in the summer months.

The usual laboratory animals are readily infected by peripheral inoculation, producing a high level of viremia and encephalitis, and the most useful experimental animals have been mice and guinea pigs. The virus grows profusely in the chick embryo and is cultivable in a great variety of tissue cultures. Experimental animals may be immunized with formalin-inactivated chick embryo virus, and VEE vaccine has been combined with WEE and EEE vaccines for the immunization of laboratory personnel. An attenuated variant, derived from variety IA, has been shown to infect horses without adverse reaction and to render them resistant to challenge with virulent varieties. Inactivated vaccine has been found to induce neutralizing antibodies in human volunteers.[17]

ROSS RIVER FEVER[1, 16, 58]

Epidemics of polyarthritis have been recognized in Australia since the late 1920s, occurring in the Murray Valley regions of South Australia and Victoria. Sporadic cases of the disease have been noted in the coastal areas of Queensland and New South Wales. Ross River virus (RRV) was isolated from mosquitoes in 1963 in northeast Queensland and linked by serological evidence to epidemic polyarthritis.

Epidemic polyarthritis is a febrile illness characterized in the acute phase by polyarthralgia and rash; mild or asymptomatic infections are more common than the acute form. In eastern Australia, illness is more prevalent in the summer and autumn, and is spread by infected *Aedes vigilax* mosquitoes. The virus is probably maintained in a cycle that involves wild vertebrate animals and a mosquito vector; human infections are incidental to the enzootic cycle in Australia.

Until the late 1970s, Ross River virus infection of humans was largely confined to Australia, New Guinea, and the Solomon Islands, as judged by the presence of neutralizing antibody to RRV in human serum samples. In early 1979, polyarthritis appeared as an explosive epidemic in the Fijian Islands, with more than 30,000 human cases; serological findings indicate that more than half of the population was infected with RRV during the outbreak. A few months later the disease appeared in American Samoa. It is estimated that at least 13,500 persons were infected there, but many infections were clinically mild or inapparent.

These latter epidemics differ somewhat from those that have occurred in Australia. The transmission cycle was thought to involve primarily humans and mosquitoes, since animal reservoirs were not extensively infected. The mosquito vector is uncertain, but *Aedes* species are thought to be responsible for the outbreak in American Samoa.

OTHER ALPHAVIRUSES

Chikungunya Virus

Chikungunya is a dengue-like disease that occurred as an outbreak of infection in the Newala district of Tanganyika (Tanzania) in 1953. The disease in man appears to be a clinical variant of dengue in which the headache is lacking, but retro-orbital and severe joint pains are common. In fact, this virus has been found, together with dengue viruses, in epidemics of dengue fever. The disease has also been noted in other regions, including India and Malaysia, where it is endemic.

The Chikungunya virus has been isolated from the blood of patients with febrile disease and also from *Aedes aegypti*; neutralizing antibody is found in the serum of convalescents. Aedine mosquitoes are the accepted vectors for the natural transmission of the infection. Although it is a member of group A, this virus gives a slight cross-reaction in the neutralization test with dengue type 1, but not with type 2.

Semliki Forest Virus

This virus was isolated in 1942 from *Aedes abnormalis* in the Semliki Forest of western Uganda. It is pathogenic for the mouse by peripheral as well as by intracerebral routes of inoculation and produces fatal infections in guinea pigs, rabbits, and rhesus monkeys on intracerebral inoculation. The brain lesions in infected animals are similar to those produced by the equine encephalomyelitis viruses. The embryonated egg may be infected by various routes of inoculation, and the infection is uniformly fatal to the embryo.

The virus is antigenically distinct and is closely related to the Mayaro virus found in Trinidad. The Kumba virus, isolated from mosquitoes in the Kumba region of Cameroun in West Africa, has been found to be antigenically identical with it. The pathogenicity of the virus for man is shown by the occurrence of human disease in Trinidad and possibly elsewhere in South America, and it is apparent that the infection is widespread in the tropical regions of both continents.

Mayaro Virus

A febrile disease of viral etiology occurred as an outbreak in Mayaro county, Trinidad, and isolation of the causative virus by intra-cerebral inoculation of suckling mice was reported in 1957. The Mayaro virus is closely related to the Semliki Forest virus found earlier in Africa and, if not identical with it, is a closely related variant. An epidemic of febrile disease of apparently the same etiology occurred in the region of the Guama River in Brazil, and surveys have shown that antibody to this virus, and to the Semliki virus, is widely distributed in the Amazon basin.

O'Nyong-Nyong Virus

This virus was isolated from the blood of patients during a major epidemic of febrile dengue-like disease in Uganda and Kenya, and was also found in anopheline mosquitoes. It appears to be endemic in East Africa, and epidemics of illness occur from time to time. Infected suckling mice show a patchy alopecia and retardation of growth, and mouse passage virus may be propagated in chick embryo fibroblast culture, forming plaques in monolayers. In the plaque-inhibition test the virus shows a one-sided relation to Chikungunya and Semliki Forest viruses.

THE MOSQUITO–BORNE FLAVIVIRUSES

Of the mosquito-borne flaviviruses, the classic and longest known is that of yellow fever. The viruses of Japanese B encephalitis, dengue fever, and St. Louis encephalitis are well known and have been studied intensively. Some other flaviviruses, such as West Nile virus, produce mild disease or inapparent infection, as indicated by serological surveys, and are widely distributed in certain areas. *Flavivirus* is made up of at least 26 mosquito-borne viruses, 8 tick-borne viruses, and several more whose vector is not known. Only the more important members are described here.

ST. LOUIS ENCEPHALITIS[35]

The disease known as St. Louis encephalitis (SLE) was first observed in eastern Illinois in 1932 and, in the following year, occurred in epidemic form in and around St. Louis, with an attack rate of 1 per 1000 and a case-fatality rate averaging about 20 per cent. The infection occurs in the central states of the midwest and over the entire western half of this country, coincident with WEE in the latter respect. In the western United States, epidemics have been largely rural, but have also affected urban populations in the midwest and eastern sections. St. Louis encephalitis, together with California encephalitis, WEE, and EEE, make up the most important arthropod-borne viral encephalitides in this country.

The SLE virus was isolated in 1933 by the intracerebral inoculation of monkeys. In many respects it is closely similar to the WEE and EEE viruses described above, and other encephalitis viruses such as Japanese B encephalitis virus, but it is immunologically distinct and differs in its pathogenicity for various experimental animals. The virus is cultivable in chick embryo and mouse embryo tissue culture and in the embryonated hen's egg. The infected chorioallantoic membrane is edematous, with evidence of cell proliferation and focal necrosis. In contrast to the WEE and EEE viruses, SLE virus infection of the embryonated egg does not result in rapid death of the embryo.

Infant mice are the most suspectible of the usual experimental animals and may be infected by all routes of inoculation. Adult mice may be infected by intracerebral or intranasal inoculation. Only an inapparent infection is produced in rabbits, guinea pigs, and various birds.

The Disease in Man

The disease in man is closely similar to WEE, ranging in severity from an abortive type of infection with headache and fever to a severe form with abrupt onset. Symptoms include abdominal and muscular pain, sore throat, conjunctivitis, and signs of neurological disturbance such as ataxia, mental confusion, and occasionally a spastic type of paralysis. The incidence is relatively greater in higher age groups, although there is often a moderately increased incidence in young children. A fulminating type of disease tends to occur in infants, and in a considerable portion of recovered cases, 10 to 40 per cent, there may be evidence of damage to the central nervous system, *e.g.*, mental retardation and hydrocephalus. Recovery in the older age groups is usually complete, with sequelae in 5 per cent or less of survivors, but the case fatality rate rises with age, and recovery is often protracted, up to several months in severe cases. There is evidence that inapparent infection is common; in a 1977 survey in Memphis, Tennessee, the ratio of inapparent to apparent infection was 355:1.

Complement-fixing and neutralizing antibodies appear in the serum by the end of the first week of the disease, and a rise in titer between paired serums is diagnostic. Neutralizing antibody persists for long periods, possibly for life, but complement-fixing antibody declines to insignificant levels within two to three years. There is some epidemiological evidence that previous dengue type 2 infection prevents or modifies infection by SLE virus, but other encephalitis viruses do not have this effect.

Epidemiology

Unlike WEE, which occurs in the summer, SLE tends to occur in late summer and early fall. It is noteworthy that a small number of sporadic cases in one season often presages an epidemic the following year; sporadic cases then follow for several succeeding years. In the western United States, SLE is usually endemic in form, while in the midwest and eastern regions, urban epidemics are more common. Major outbreaks have occurred in this country at about 10-year intervals, beginning in the mid-1950s. In 1974, an epidemic occurred in Memphis, Tennessee, and by 1975, SLE appeared in a number of urban centers in the midwest, from Canada south to Texas, with more than 1800 laboratory-confirmed cases; sporadic cases continued at an increased level for several years.

Hosts. The reservoir of SLE virus infection, like that of WEE and EEE, is in birds, and the disease is transmitted by mosquitoes. The virus has been recovered from several species of birds, and serological evidence of infection has been found in 55 species of wild birds and a number of mammals examined. The level of viremia is relatively low, but mosquitoes seem to be more readily infected with this virus than with others in which a high level of viremia is required for infection of the vector. The more important vertebrate hosts appear to be the small perching birds.

Infected birds become viremic after two to three days and remain infectious for mosquitoes up until about seven days, when antibody production limits the viremic state. After this, the bird may harbor the virus in various organs, but it is probably never again infectious for mosquitoes. After the mosquito feeds on a viremic bird, the virus multiplies in the gut lining and is later transported to the salivary glands; at this point, the virus can be transmitted as the mosquito feeds. The period between virus ingestion and appearance in the salivary gland, the **extrinsic incubation period,** is variable, but it is directly proportional to the environmental temperature. Thus, SLE tends to be more efficiently transmitted in the bird-mosquito-bird chain during the warmer months.

Although a number of birds and other animals may be infected with SLE, man is the only host in which clinical disease appears.

Vectors. Four *Culex* mosquito species are firmly established as vectors for SLE in the United States: *C. tarsalis, C. pipiens, C. quinquefasciatus,* and *C. nigripalpus.* To a significant degree, the epidemiological pattern of the disease is determined by the vector involved in a given area. Two epidemiological forms of SLE are recognized, the urban and the rural types. In the rural disease in the West, the primary vector is *C. tarsalis.* The transmission cycle includes wild birds as reservoirs of infection, maintained by transmission of the virus by *C. tarsalis,* with occasional infections occurring in man. In more densely populated areas of the midwestern and southern states where *C. tarsalis* is seldom present, the urban infection is presumably introduced by wild birds and transmitted to humans primarily by *C. pipiens* and *C. quinquefasciatus,* and outbreaks of the disease in man are associated with the presence of relatively high populations of these mosquitoes. In Florida, the tropical mosquito species, *C. nigripalpus,* has been established as a vector of SLE.

The mechanism of survival of SLE virus during cold periods (overwintering) has long interested epidemiologists. The virus apparently survives in hibernating adult *C. pipiens* mosquitoes,[4] and low rates of transovarial transmission of SLE in *Culex* have also been detected.[19]

JAPANESE B ENCEPHALITIS[23]

Encephalitis has occurred in Japan in the late summer for many years, from time to time assuming serious epidemic form. The disease has been called Japanese B encephalitis (JBE). It also occurs in many parts of the Far East and in the Malaysian peninsula.

The JBE virus, first isolated in 1936 in Japan, is similar to those of the equine encephalitides and SLE in size and properties but has a relatively wider range of pathogenicity for experimental animals. In the rhesus monkey an acute encephalomyelitis, simulating the human disease, is produced following intracerebral or intranasal inoculation and, in contrast with SLE virus, the infection may be carried in monkey passage. The virus is cultivable in the chick embryo and results in death of the embryo within 72 hours; it also grows in a variety of tissue cultures.

The Disease in Man

Infection with JBE virus occurs in man as a symptomless or subclinical infection; an abortive type of disease, in which fever and fleeting signs of central nervous system involvement occur; and as an acute meningoencephalomyelitis. In the last there is extensive cortical damage with focal perivascular infiltration, ganglion cell degeneration, and destruction of the Purkinje cells of the cerebellum; lesions in the cord simulate those of poliomyelitis. The onset may be abrupt or insidious, and symptoms include fever, nausea, and disorientation. In the severe form the neurological symptoms are marked, with spinal rigidity, tremors, convulsions, and spasms. The acute phase may last as long as two weeks, but recovery is usually complete, and neurological or psychotic sequelae occur in fewer than 10 per cent of survivors.

The immune response is evident as the appearance of complement-fixing, hemagglutination-inhibiting, and neutralizing antibodies in the serum and occurs within one to two weeks after onset of the disease. Neutralizing antibody persists for a long time, and the associated immunity to the disease is thought to be relatively permanent. Complement-fixing antibody does not seem to be associated with immunity.

Epidemiology

Natural infections occur in a variety of mammalian hosts, some with disease symptoms, but birds are the principal reservoirs of infection. Mosquitoes serve as the vector for natural transmission. A number of culicine mosquitoes can be infected with the virus and can transmit the infection under experimental conditions. *Culex tritaeniorhynchus* is naturally infected and is one of the principal vectors in South and East Asia. There is now evidence of transovarian passage of JBE virus in this species.[51]

MURRAY VALLEY ENCEPHALITIS[31] (AUSTRALIA ENCEPHALITIS)

Encephalitis of viral etiology has been known in Australia for many years. Beginning in 1917 and continuing until 1926, a series of small epidemics of acute encephalitis, called

Australian X disease, were observed. The early outbreaks occurred largely in children, with high mortality rates, but subsequent epidemics were less severe.

In the summer of 1950–51, an epidemic of encephalitis appeared in the Murray Valley in Victoria, Australia, in which 40 cases were recognized, claiming 17 lives. The infection, considered to be a recrudescence of Australian X disease and now termed Murray Valley encephalitis (MVE), has reappeared at irregular intervals in this region. Occasionally it has expanded beyond the Murray Valley and has been observed in New Guinea as well.

The MVE virus has been isolated by inoculation of chick embryos, growing on the chorioallantoic membrane and killing the embryo in two or three days. It also has been adapted to infant mice, in which it causes a fatal encephalitis after intracerebral challenge. The virus is similar to the JBE virus, but differs immunologically from it.

Immunological response to infection includes the production of complement-fixing, hemagglutination-inhibiting, and neutralizing antibodies; diagnosis is usually by these serological procedures. Surveys in the epidemic areas indicate that about 5 per cent of persons with no history of the disease have significant titers of complement-fixing antibody.

Serological and virological studies following a widespread epidemic in 1974 and 1975 suggest that the virus occurs in horses and birds in the epidemic area. Wild birds, and possibly domestic fowls, are the suspected reservoir hosts and *Culex annulirostris* is considered to be the principal vector.

WEST NILE FEVER

The West Nile virus was first isolated in Uganda in 1940 from a native with mild febrile illness. It has subsequently been found in Egypt and Israel. In contrast to JBE, West Nile fever is rarely fatal and usually takes the form of a febrile disease rather than encephalitis. The incubation period is two to six days, and the illness is characterized by an abrupt onset, fever, drowsiness, abdominal pain, nausea, severe frontal headache, and enlarged lymph nodes. A maculopapular rash may develop, appearing more commonly in children. The acute phase persists for less than a week, but convalescence may be protracted.

The virus is closely similar to the JBE virus, being of the same order of size, and related to it and to SLE virus. Mice may be infected by the intracerebal route, and the virus grows on the chorioallantoic membrane of the chick embryo and in tissue cultures (Fig. 42–2).

The infection is widespread in Africa, probably as inapparent infections, not only in Uganda and Egypt, but also in South Africa and in the Congo and Sudan regions of Central Africa. As many as 70 per cent of persons examined in Egypt show significant antibody titer, and the disease has been studied extensively there. Prevalence is greater during the summer and is sporadic rather than epidemic.

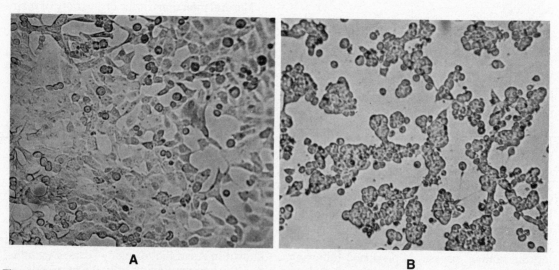

A   **B**

Figure 42–2. The cytopathic effect produced by West Nile virus in HeLa cell culture. *A,* Uninoculated cell culture; *B,* four days after inoculation with virus.

An avian reservoir of infection is suspected, and *Culex univittatus* is regarded as the most probable vector.

ROCIO ENCEPHALITIS[34]

In 1975 and 1976, epidemics of encephalitis resembling SLE and JBE were observed in the coastal areas of Sao Paulo, Brazil. The outbreak was relatively severe, with over 800 clinical cases and 95 deaths, and an overall attack rate of 15 per 1000. The epidemic subsided, and no new cases were found in 1977 and 1978.

A new *Flavivirus* was isolated from human cases; the virus differed antigenically from other members of the genus and was named Rocio virus.

Although not complete, virological, serological, and epidemiological findings suggest an avian reservoir of infection maintained by mosquito transmission, possibly by *Psorophora ferox*.

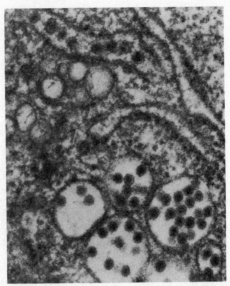

Figure 42–3. Dengue virus, type 2 in infected Raji (lymphoblast) cells. Golgi vesicles contain mostly mature virions, while cisternae of the rough endocytoplasmic reticulum contain immature viruses. × 76,000. (S. Sriurairatna, *et al.*, Infect. Immun., **20**:173, 1978.)

DENGUE[24, 25, 53]

Dengue is an infectious disease transmitted by mosquitoes that is endemic, and often epidemic, in tropical and subtropical climates; it has occasionally occurred also in temperate zones. Epidemics may be very large; it is estimated that there were between one and two million cases in the southern United States during the epidemic of 1922.

Dengue has occurred in epidemics of greater or lesser magnitude in the western Pacific Islands and in Southeast Asia for many years. In the Caribbean, where dengue has long been endemic, a pandemic outbreak of the more serious hemorrhagic form occurred in 1977. The infection entered southeastern Mexico in 1978, and gradually moved northward; in 1980 it was reported in Mexico along the Texas boundary, and 48 cases were confirmed in the Rio Grande Valley of Texas.

Dengue Virus
The virus is similar in morphology to other togaviruses and is approximately 40 to 50 nm. in diameter. The virus is enveloped as it buds from intracytoplasmic membranes and is found in intracellular vesicles as mature virions before being released through the plasma membrane (Figs. 42–3 and 42–4). Four serotypes of dengue virus are distinguished, designated by arabic numerals; even within these types,

however, there is some variation associated with geographical origin. It has been suggested that there is cross-protection between dengue and St. Louis encephalitis, the attack rate in the latter disease being markedly lower in persons showing anti-dengue antibody, and experimental studies have supported this inference.

On primary isolation the dengue virus does not produce cytopathic effect in monkey kidney cell cultures, but grows with cytopathic effect and plaque formation after intracerebral passage in mice. Serotypes are differentiated by neutralizing and complement-fixing antibodies and by hemagglution-inhibition, and seem to be more closely related to one another than to other flaviviruses by the last criterion.

Pathogenicity for Lower Animals
Chimpanzees and several species of monkeys may be asymptomatically infected, but with the production of antibody.

On intracerebral passage in newborn mice, the virus becomes adapted, yielding high titers of virus in the brain and producing motor disturbance and partial flaccid paralysis, often with signs of encephalitis. Adult mice may be infected by intracerebral inoculation of well-adapted strains but are refractory to other routes of inoculation. Intracerebral inoculation with adapted virus may produce fatal paralytic disease in rhesus monkeys, simulating experi-

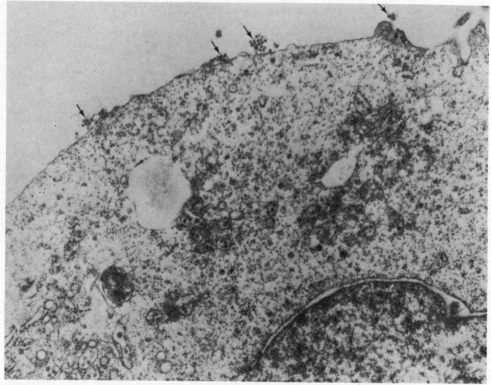

Figure 42–4. Electron micrograph of Raji cell infected with dengue virus, type 2. Dengue virions are clustered on the cell surface (arrows) adjacent to aggregates of the rough endocytoplasmic reticulum, where replication occurs. Extracellular virions are absent from other areas of the cell surface. × 23,500. (S. Sriurairatna, *et al.*, Infect. Immun., **20**:173, 1978.)

mental poliomyelitis. In general, there is no satisfactory experimental animal host for un-modified virus, and infection experiments have been carried out with human volunteers.

Dengue Fever

Illnesses caused by dengue virus may take two forms. Classical dengue fever, the predominant form, is relatively benign and usually is seen in adults and older children. A more severe form, dengue hemorrhagic fever, primarily affects young children and is sometimes accompanied by signs of severe shock. This form has been epidemic for a quarter of a century in the Pacific Islands and Southeast Asia.

In classical dengue fever, the incubation period is usually five to eight days. Prodromal symptoms of headache, backache, and malaise are followed in 6 to 12 hours by abrupt rise in temperature. The acute phase is accompanied by headache, retro-orbital pain, abdominal pain, and severe pain in the muscles and joints that has led to the name "breakbone fever." Maculopapular eruption occurs with variable frequency, appearing about the third day of the disease, spreading from the trunk to the extremities and face, and persisting for three to four days. The febrile period lasts for five or six days and commonly terminates by crisis. Uncomplicated dengue fever is rarely fatal.

Dengue Hemorrhagic Fever

Dengue fever with severe hemorrhage or shock and mortality ranging up to 15 per cent has been known since the turn of the century. The dengue virus etiology of this form of the disease was first recognized in the Philippines in 1956. It has occurred in epidemic form in Southeast Asia, the western Pacific, and, more recently, in the Caribbean. Dengue hemorrhagic fever is most frequent in infants and young children under 12 years of age.

In the initial stages, there is fever, upper respiratory symptoms, headache, and abdominal pain. In this stage the disease is relatively benign, and many recover without further progression. In a proportion of those infected, however, there follows a sudden deterioration, the patient becoming restless, with cold extremities, rapid pulse, and lethargy. The disease is essentially an acute vascular permeability syndrome with plasma leakage and hypovolemic shock, often resulting in death within a short time.

Dengue hemorrhagic fever is almost entirely confined to **indigenous children,** with greatest incidence in those under six to eight years of age and more often affecting females. There is a striking correlation between the severity of disease and preinfection dengue antibody, either passively or actively acquired. Thus, the hemorrhagic fever syndrome is seen in primary dengue infections in very young children with maternal antibody, but in older children the syndrome occurs in those that suffer secondary infections with the virus, particularly with type 2.

Hemorrhagic manifestations are believed to arise from the presence of antibody in the infected host, leading to immunological enhancement of infection. It has been postulated that antibody complexes with, but does not neutralize, the invading virus; virus is then more efficiently phagocytized by mononuclear phagocytes, in which they multiply readily. These cells not only support replication of the virus, but serve to disseminate the virus to many other host tissues, *e.g.,* liver, spleen, and lymphoid tissue. Antibody, therefore, serves to increase the number of cells infected, with an attendant increase in disease severity.

The pathophysiological abnormalities associated with hemorrhagic fever are thought to be due to factors that are released from infected mononuclear phagocytes, resulting in the activation of complement and blood clotting systems and the generation of vascular permeability factors.

Immunity

Recovery from dengue results in a solid, serotype-specific immunity and the appearance of complement-fixing, neutralizing, and hemagglutination-inhibiting antibodies in the serum. Immunity is directed primarily against the homologous serotype and has been shown experimentally to persist for at least 18 months. Convalescents have a considerable degree of initial immunity to all serotypes of virus, but immunity to the heterologous serotypes disappears relatively rapidly. Thus, within two months after recovery, the acquired immunity is probably sufficient to prevent naturally acquired infection with any of the four serotypes. This heterologous immunity wanes within a few months, however, permitting the secondary infections with another serotype

that give rise to hemorrhagic fever. There is as yet no suitable vaccine for human immunization, although attenuated virus vaccines have been tested in monkeys and in a few human volunteers.

Epidemiology

The animal reservoir of dengue virus appears to be man and, possibly, various species of monkeys in which viremic but asymptomatic infection occurs; birds do not seem to be infected. The virus is transmitted by the domestic mosquito, *Aedes aegypti,* and also by *Aedes albopictus,* which exists in the bush or jungle and transmits the infection among primate hosts other than man. Epidemiological observations suggest that *Aedes scutellaris* and *Aedes polynesiensis* may also serve as vectors under natural conditions.

In humans, the viremic period usually begins during the last day of the incubation period and extends for three days or more after onset of the disease. During this time, man is infective for the mosquito. Monkeys are similarly infective, since viremia is demonstrable experimentally for five to eight days after infection. The extrinsic incubation period in the mosquito lasts for 10 days to two weeks, after which the mosquito remains infectious for life; there is, however, no congenital transmission of the virus. Endemic persistence of the infection depends upon climatic conditions that permit mosquitoes to survive throughout the year, together with a sufficient number of newborn mammalian host susceptibles to maintain the transmission cycle.

YELLOW FEVER[60]

Yellow fever is an acute disease, occurring in epidemic and endemic forms, which was first observed in Central America in the seventeenth century. It is uncertain whether the original focus of infection was in Africa or the Western Hemisphere, but in the eighteenth and nineteeth centuries the disease was widely distributed in the Caribbean area, extending to the adjoining coasts of North, Central, and South America. In the nineteenth century, yellow fever spread northward, appearing as epidemics in many northern cities, including Philadelphia, New York, and Baltimore, and resulting in an estimated half-million cases of the disease in the United States.

Yellow fever epidemics in United States military personnel during the Spanish-American War led to the classical studies by the

Yellow Fever Commission of the United States Army under Dr. Walter Reed that demonstrated transmission and the viral nature of the infectious agent.

The virus of yellow fever is one of the smaller viruses. The complete virus is about 40 nm. in diameter with a 35 nm. nucleocapsid. It is relatively labile, being readily inactivated by heating and by the usual disinfectants, but is preserved in 50 per cent glycerol or by lyophilization.

The Disease in Man

The virus of yellow fever is transmitted to man by the bite of infected mosquitoes. After an incubation period of one to three days, the disease begins with sudden onset of headache, backache, rigor, and a rapid rise in temperature. In the first, or congestive, stage there is nausea and vomiting, the face is flushed, and a tendency to hemorrhage becomes apparent. After three or four days the temperature falls, then rises again, and the second stage begins, with venous stasis and a marked tendency to hemorrhage, jaundice, albuminuria, and prostration. In most instances, recovery is rapid and uneventful, but about 5 per cent of the untreated cases end in death, usually by the sixth or seventh day. Many infections, on the other hand, are mild or almost symptomless.

The disease is one of the hematopoietic system; there is little inflammatory reaction, but tissue changes are seen in the liver, kidney, and heart. The characteristic, and pathognomonic, lesion is a hyaline type of necrosis in the midzone of the liver, and the affected cells are known as Councilman bodies (Fig. 42–5). Fatty degeneration occurs in the kidney tubules but is not distinctive, the spleen is hyperemic and shows degenerative changes, and degenerative changes are found in the heart.

Experimental Infections

The human disease is reproduced in the rhesus monkey, and a number of species of monkeys are susceptible to yellow fever; in fact, natural infection is widespread among primates in certain areas (see below). The infant mouse is susceptible to parenteral inoculation; adult mice are infected by intracerebral inoculation but are seldom infected by the intraperitoneal route.

Tissue Culture. Neurotropic virus is cultivable without difficulty in chick embryo tissue cultures that include nerve tissue, but the unadapted pantropic strains may be difficult to grow. The Asibi strain of yellow fever virus was grown first in mouse embryo tissue culture, then in chick embryo tissue culture, and after prolonged passage a variant appeared that had lost both viscerotrophic and neurotropic tendencies. This variant is the 17D strain, now widely used as an immunizing agent. The 17D strain forms plaques in chick embryo cell monolayers and may also be used to titrate neutralizing antibody.

Epidemiology

Yellow fever occurs in animal reservoirs of infection and in infected mosquitoes and is transmitted to the vertebrate host by the insect vector. The epidemiological character of the disease is determined by the species and habitat of both vertebrate and invertebrate hosts and occurs in two epidemiological types: urban yellow fever and jungle yellow fever.

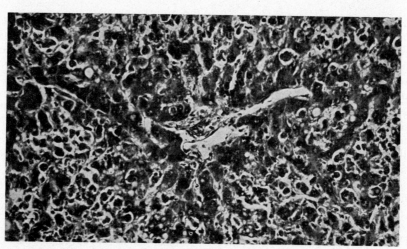

Figure 42–5. Section of liver from a human case of yellow fever. Midzonal necrosis is apparent. Hematoxylin and eosin; reduced from × 235. (Theiler.)

Urban Yellow Fever. In urban yellow fever the virus is transmitted to man by *Aedes aegypti,* and the life history of the virus consists of a man-mosquito-man cycle. The mosquito becomes infected when it bites infected humans; the extrinsic incubation period is 10 to 15 days at tropical temperatures, and the mosquito remains infected for life; there is evidence also of transovarial passage of the virus in the vector. *Aedes* is a domestic mosquito, living largely in and around human habitation, so that the foci of infection are in urban areas and the disease is one of communities. Since direct man-to-man infection does not occur under natural conditions, control of the vector in urban areas allows effective control of the human disease.

Jungle Yellow Fever. In the early 1930s yellow fever occurred in Brazil in the absence of *A. aegypti.* The infection has since been found to persist in nonhuman primate reservoirs and to be transmitted by mosquitoes other than *A. aegypti.* This is sylvan or jungle yellow fever, in which human infection is peripheral to the nature history of the virus. The disease is contracted by humans who enter the forests, such as adult males whose work takes them to such infected areas. This is in contrast with urban yellow fever in which all ages and both sexes are exposed to equal risk. Infection of humans, followed by infection of *A. aegypti,* may, of course, initiate the man-mosquito-man transmission cycle characteristic of urban yellow fever. The endemic foci of jungle yellow fever are in South America, Africa, and Central America, and differ somewhat from one to another of these areas.

South America. The distribution of enzootic infection in South America encompasses the northern coastal countries of South America and the Orinoco and Amazon basins. Within this area forest monkeys appear to be the most important vertebrate host. Other mammalian and avian hosts, although often suspected of involvement, appear not to be significant elements in the natural transmission cycle. Some species of monkeys, especially the howler monkey, *Alouatta,* suffer from epizootics of the disease that are fatal to large numbers of the animals.

Yellow fever virus has been isolated from forest mosquitoes. Species of *Haemagogus* are found in the areas of South America where the infection is endemic and are no doubt the most important vectors in the transmission cycle. These "forest canopy," tree-hole breeding mosquitoes are found in the tops of trees, rarely coming to the ground except at the edge of the forest.

Africa. In Africa, *A. aegypti* is widely distributed, and both the urban and jungle types of yellow fever occur. The endemic area stretches as a band across the continent, generally extending south from about 15° N latitude to the equator. As in South America, the vertebrate hosts in the latter form of the disease are forest primates of many species, including lemurs. *Aedes africanus* is found in many parts of Central Africa and is known to be an important factor in the maintenance of yellow fever virus in the forests of Uganda. Like *Haemagogus* in South America, it is an arboreal mosquito, and it readily bites monkeys, but does not attack man. *Aedes simpsoni,* which bites both monkeys and man, is also present, and is thought to be the mosquito responsible for transmission of the infection from monkeys to man at the edge of the forest.

Immunity

Recovery from yellow fever results in a solid immunity, often said to persist for life, and strains of the virus, even from widely separated areas, are of a single antigenic type. The antibody response is demonstrable as hemagglutination-inhibiting, complement-fixing, and neutralizing antibodies, and the three are not identical. The complement-fixing antibody appears later than neutralizing or hemagglutination-inhibiting antibody and may not occur to significant titer in mild infections; it disappears within a few months. Complement-fixing antibody is usually not formed in response to prophylactic inoculation with the 17D strain of virus and, therefore, has some value in detecting recent natural infections.

The neutralizing and hemagglutination-inhibiting antibodies appear quite early in the disease, often by the fifth day, and persist more or less indefinitely. The titration of these antibodies is used for serological surveys for the prevalence of infection. Neutralizing antibodies are measured by plaque-reduction tests.

Prophylaxis. While vector control suffices to control urban yellow fever, it is ineffective in controlling the jungle type of the disease. In this and certain other circumstances, active prophylactic immunization is required. It was early apparent that inactivated virus does not induce an effective immune response, and living attenuated virus, the 17D strain described above, is generally employed. The immunity produced is effective for a considerable period; persisting antibody titers have been found in immunized persons as long as 19 years after primary inoculation.

THE TICK-BORNE FLAVIVIRUSES[54]

Arboviruses transmitted by various species of ticks are set apart epidemiologically from the mosquito-borne viruses. Some fall into the *Flavivirus* group as a relatively homogeneous subgroup, the Russian spring-summer encephalitis complex, within which the component viruses are more closely related to one another than to the other flaviviruses.

RUSSIAN SPRING-SUMMER ENCEPHALITIS

Russian spring-summer encephalitis (RSSE) was observed in 1937 in the far eastern provinces of the Soviet Union and has subsequently been found in other parts of Russia, in Central Europe, and in Germany.

The virus may be grown on the allantoic membrane of the embryonated egg and in cultures of human embryo muscle tissue, with cytopathic effect. The mouse may be infected by subcutaneous as well as intracerebral inoculation and is extremely susceptible to mouse-adapted virus. The virus is pathogenic for sheep and rhesus monkeys, but not for guinea pigs or rabbits. A number of wild birds and rodents may be infected experimentally to give a symptomless viremia, and many wild rodents are naturally infected.

The Disease in Man

The incubation period is 10 to 14 days, and the febrile disease in man is characterized by signs and symptoms of a meningoencephalitis or polioencephalitis. It varies in severity from an abortive type of perhaps a week's duration, terminating in complete recovery, to a severe fulminating type of meningoencephalitis in which death occurs within a week. In recognized cases, the overall fatality rate is about 30 per cent, but there is a high incidence of antibody in human populations in endemic areas, and it is probable that many infections are symptomless or subclinical.

The disease is characterized by evidence of bulbar involvement and a peripheral type of flaccid paralysis, most often of the brachial and cervical muscles, which may be residual. In fatal cases parenchymatous degenerative changes may be found in the heart, kidney, and liver. The virus is present in the blood and spinal fluid during the course of the disease and has been isolated from the brain at autopsy.

Immunity

An immune response is evident two to three weeks after onset of the disease as complement-fixing and neutralizing antibodies in the serum. The solid immunity to reinfection is long lasting and is associated with the presence of neutralizing serum antibody which reaches peak titer in two to three months. Russian workers have used formalin-inactivated brain and chick embryo vaccines for active immunization.

Epidemiology

The first reported cases of this disease were in persons whose work took them to forested regions, but it is now clear that the distribution of the disease is less restricted, and it has occurred, sometimes in high incidence, in populated areas with greater numbers of infections in children. As noted above, the incidence of serum antibody may be relatively high in endemic areas, and human infection is doubtless more common than the number of clinical cases of the disease would indicate.

Whether or not human infection constitutes a significant reservoir is open to question. Goats are known to be infected and, along with other domestic animals, may be a source of human disease. The virus is infective by the alimentary route, and transmission by the milk of infected animals, especially in urban areas, undoubtedly contributes to human disease and to inapparent but immunizing infections. It is generally believed that wild mammals and birds, in which viremia occurs, constitute a significant reservoir for the arthropod-transmitted infection.

The infection in animal reservoirs is transmitted by ticks, of which *Ixodes persulcatus* is regarded as the principal vector. The infection is congenital in these ticks; infection rates as high as 40 per cent have been found in certain small areas, and there is little doubt that there is an arthropod reservoir of infection.

Human infection is acquired in forests from infected ticks, which act both as reservoirs of infection and as vectors in maintenance of the animal reservoirs of the virus. Infection occurring within populated areas may be transmitted by ingestion of milk, as noted above, and familial outbreaks of the disease have been described.

KYASANUR FOREST DISEASE

Kyasanur Forest disease (KFD) appeared in the Kyasanur Forest in India in 1956. Deaths were widespread in native monkeys, and there was associated illness in man. During early 1957 the epidemic extended over an area of about 500 square miles, and there were 500 human cases of the disease with 70 deaths.

Kyasanur Forest virus is not neurotropic in humans, but affects the hematopoietic system. Following an incubation period of three to seven days after the bite of an infected tick, disease is manifest as fever of sudden onset, headache, nausea, vomiting, myalgia, and prostration. Hemorrhage is the obvious major clinical symptom, with evidence of massive hemorrhage in the chest cavity in fatal cases. The principal source of infection appears to be monkeys, and the virus is transmitted by one of several species of Ixodid ticks.

The viremic period in man is relatively prolonged, and the blood is infectious from 2 days before to as long as 10 days after onset. The KFD virus is cultivable in chick embryo tissue culture, producing cytopathic effects; the mouse may be infected by intracerebral inoculation to produce a disease in three or four days that is characterized by prostration, hind limb paralysis, and tremors. Both complement-fixing and neutralizing antibody, demonstrable in the mouse, are found in convalescents. The virus appears to be antigenically closely related to, but not identical with, the RSSE virus.

POWASSAN ENCEPHALITIS

Powassan virus was found in Ontario in 1958, isolated from a fatal case of encephalitis. It proved to be a flavivirus, closely related to RSSE, and was the first member of the group to be isolated in the Americas. It is found in various forest mammals and their ticks in Canada, and has also been found in the eastern United States.[47] Apparently the same virus was isolated from pools of *Dermacentor andersoni* collected in Colorado some years earlier, but not identified until the Powassan isolate was described.

OMSK HEMORRHAGIC FEVER

This disease was noted soon after World War II in the lake regions of western Siberia. It affected trappers and those in related occupations, and is characterized by fever, headache, vomiting, and diarrhea, with evidence of generalized hemorrhage. Muskrats appear to be the reservoir hosts, and the virus is transmitted to man by contact with infected animals. Some other rodents show serological evidence of infection, and antibodies are sometimes found in domestic animals. Arthropod transmission has not been explicitly demonstrated, but Ixodid ticks are suspected vectors; the virus is also believed to be transmitted by direct contact between animals.

The Orbiviruses[22]

Orbivirus differ from other Reoviridae (*Reovirus* and *Rotavirus*) in that they possess only a single outer capsid; the virion is about 70 nm. in diameter (Chapter 38). These viruses infect both vertebrate and invertebrate hosts (ticks) and are, therefore, appropriately considered with other arboviruses. The most important human disease is Colorado tick fever, but a related virus is responsible for blue tongue disease, an epizootic in asses, zebras, and ungulates in India, Africa, and the United States. The properties of orbiviruses are listed in Table 42–3.

COLORADO TICK FEVER[8, 12, 37]

Colorado tick fever (CTF) occurs in the Rocky Mountain regions of the United States where the tick vector is prevalent. The disease in man was described as a clinical entity in 1930 but probably accounted for some part of febrile disease reported by military personnel in that area in earlier years.

Table 42–3. **Properties of Orbiviruses**

dsDNA genome; nonsegmented, 12×10^6 daltons

Spherical virion, 60–80 nm.

Cubic symmetry, 32 capsomers

Assembled in cytoplasm

Nonenveloped

Ether-sensitive; acid-labile

Colorado tick fever is present in the same geographical regions as Rocky Mountain spotted fever and is clinically similar, except for the absence of rash and a more benign course. The viral nature of the etiological agent was established when it was shown to be filterable and transmissible in series in humans and hamsters. The virus was later adapted to suckling mice by intracerebral passage; these strains grow in chick embryo yolk sac, where they localize in the central nervous system. Mouse-adapted strains are propagated, with cytopathic effect, in several kinds of tissue culture.

Experimental infections produced in rheusus monkeys are essentially asymptomatic, but viremia occurs and persists for four to five weeks.

The Disease in Man

After an incubation period of three to five days following the bite of an infected tick, there is a short febrile phase of two or three days, characterized by chills, fever, headache, and severe, generalized muscular aches. There is then a two- to three-day period of remission, followed by recrudescence of the febrile phase; the disease is, therefore, described as diphasic. Colorado tick fever is sometimes confused with Rocky Mountain spotted fever, particularly in rare cases that develop rash. Convalescence may be relatively prolonged, but is without complications, and recovery is complete; no deaths from CTF have been reported.

The CTF virus persists for several months in the erythrocytes of patients, permitting diagnosis by direct immunofluorescent staining of the virus in blood specimens. The virus may also be isolated from patients, or from infected ticks, by intracerebral inoculation of suckling mice, in which characteristic neurological symptoms are observed. Identification of isolated virus is accomplished by serological procedures, including immunofluorescence microscopy, neutralization of mouse infectivity, plaque-reduction in tissue culture, or complement fixation. The indirect immunofluorescence test is useful for detection of antibody to the virus in patient's serum.

Immunity

Complement-fixing and neutralizing antibodies are produced in response to infection, appearing within two weeks after onset of the disease and persisting for at least three years. Experimental inoculation of human volunteers has shown that there is a solid immunity to reinfection. Chick embryo–adapted virus is attenuated in virulence for humans and has been used as an immunizing agent, producing effective immunity. Formalin-inactivated virus purified from mouse brain also produces immunity of long duration in humans.

Epidemiology

The wood tick, *Dermacentor andersoni*, is naturally infected with CTF virus and is considered to be the primary and, possibly, sole vector of the infection.

A number of possible vertebrate reservoir hosts have been detected, both serologically and by virus isolation. Many rodents are naturally infected; the predominant reservoir host varies with geographical location, but the golden-mantled ground squirrel and the least chipmunk appear to be of greatest significance in most areas.

The natural infection is maintained by a cycle that involves the rodent host and both nymphal and larval stages of the tick vector. The virus overwinters in nymphal stages of *D. andersoni;* in the spring, the nymph infects young rodent hosts, in which an inapparent infection is produced. Larvae of the vector become infected by feeding on these hosts, molt to the nymphal stage, and the cycle is repeated. Human infection by CTF virus is acquired incidentally from the bite of infected ticks. Infections tend to occur in persons exposed to tick bites by occupation, so that adult males are most often affected. In many areas, avocational exposure is common, as among tourists in outdoor recreational areas. The disease is therefore seasonal, with greatest prevalence between March and July in the mountainous regions of the western states, primarily in Colorado. The true incidence is not known, but only 100 to 200 cases are reported each year.

The Bunyaviruses[7, 15]

Included in the informal grouping of arbovirus are the viruses of the family Bunyaviridae, with four recognized genera. The family is a large and complex one, with a number of different viruses and serological groups. The Bunyaviridae are characterized largely on the basis of common properties of the virion, distinguished by the properties listed in Table

Table 42–4. **Properties of Bunyaviruses**

(−)RNA genome; single-stranded; 3 segments;
  6 to 7 × 10⁶ daltons

Spherical virion, 80–110 nm.

Helical capsid, 10–12 nm. diameter

Assembled in cytoplasm

Enveloped by budding from intracytoplasmic membrane

Ether-sensitive

42–4; Figure 42–6 shows the morphology of Rift Valley virus in membrane-bound vacuoles.

The virion contains the single-stranded (−)RNA genome, comprising three segments distinguished by their size—small (S), medium (M), and large (L); the viruses are therefore capable of reassortment. Associated with each RNA species in the nucleocapsid is a protein (N), thought to be the transcriptase. On the outer surface of the virion are two virus-specific glycoproteins, occurring as 5 to 10 nm. spikes.

Four species of Bunyaviridae are now recognized—*Bunyavirus, Phlebovirus, Nairovirus,* and *Uukuvirus*—each distinguished by differences in the molecular details of virion structure and by serological differences. Each genus contains one or more serogroups and these are, in turn, separated into serotypes; each serotype is assigned a name, usually the location of isolation. Although there are more than 200 registered viruses in the Bunyaviridae, only a relative few are of confirmed medical importance as etiological agents of human disease. Only the more important viruses will be described here, including the California serogroup of *Bunyavirus,* the sandfly fever and Rift Valley fever viruses of *Phlebovirus,* and the Congo-Crimean hemorrhagic fever virus of *Nairovirus.*

CALIFORNIA ENCEPHALITIS[27, 41]

Viruses of this subgroup were first isolated from mosquitoes in 1943. They produced encephalitis when inoculated intracerebrally into young mice, cotton rats, and hamsters. The virus grows well in the embryonated hen's egg, but usually without death of the embryo. The California subgroup viruses are immunologically distinct from the other arthropod-borne viruses. The subgroup contains 12 registered viruses, all serologically related to one another, but distinct from other *Bunyavirus;* they

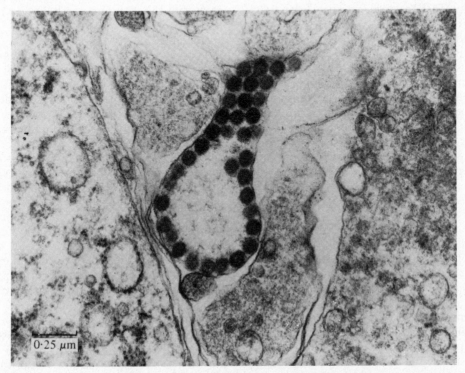

Figure 42–6. Rift Valley fever virus in membrane-bound vacuole in mouse hepatocytes. Bar = 250 nm. (D. S. Ellis, *et al.,* J. Gen. Virol., **42**:329, 1979. Courtesy of Dr. D. S. Ellis, London School of Hygiene and Tropical Medicine.)

are not related to togaviruses. Two members of this serogroup, California encephalitis virus and LaCrosse virus, cause acute infection of the central nervous system; LaCrosse virus is the more important of the two and is responsible for most human infections. Other viruses of this serogroup occur in lower vertebrates and mosquitoes.

Since the middle 1960s, LaCrosse virus has been shown to be responsible for sporadic cases of encephalitis, primarily in children and adolescents. The disease has been most often reported from the north central United States, but serological studies indicate that infection is prevalent as far north as Alaska. Fortunately, the disease is not common in the United States; only 30 to 100 cases are reported annually.

It appears that most human infections are subclinical or mild. Clinically apparent infections range from mild febrile illness with headache, abdominal pains, vomiting, and, later, meningeal irritation, to more severe meningoencephalitis of sudden onset followed by focal or generalized seizures and occasional residual neurological sequelae. The disease is, however, very rarely fatal.

The virus is maintained in small animal reservoirs, including rabbits, ground squirrels, and chipmunks. Transmission between animals and to man is by mosquitoes, principally *Aedes triseriatus*. In this species, transovarial transmission of the virus has been repeatedly demonstrated, and the mosquito is probably the major reservoir host.

Because of the segmented RNA genome, these viruses can undergo genetic reassortment; recombinants between LaCrosse and snowshoe hare viruses have been produced experimentally. Genetic reassortment is believed to explain the diversity of the California subgroup and suggests the possibility that new types may arise in nature.

SANDFLY FEVER[57]

Sandfly fever, or Phlebotomus fever, is an acute nonfatal disease of man. The causal virus is transmitted by a species of sandfly, *Phlebotomus papatasii*. Its geographical distribution is limited by the occurrence of the vector, and it is found in tropical and subtropical regions during the hot dry season. These areas include various portions of the Mediterranean littoral and the Middle and Far East. The Phlebotomus fever serogroup of *Phlebovirus* comprises many serotypes, but two, Naples and Sicilian, are the predominant causes of sandfly fever. Wild-type viruses do not infect the usual laboratory animals, including primates, and are not cultivable in the chick embryo or in tissue culture. Infection has been established by intracerebral inoculation of the newborn mouse, producing encephalitis with lesions occurring predominantly in the hypothalamus and midbrain, after three blind passages in the case of the Sicilian type and one blind passage of the Naples type. Both serotypes have been adapted to weaned mice, by repeated passage in newborn animals. Adapted strains are cultivable in human or mouse kidney cell culture after mouse passage. A cytopathic effect and plaque formation occurs in the human cell cultures after three to four tissue culture passages, but on first passage in mouse cells.

The Disease in Man

The incubation period of sandfly fever is usually three or four days. There may be prodromal malaise and abdominal distress. The symptoms, occurring in various combinations, include nausea, headache, backache, stiffness in the neck and back, pains in the joints, sore throat, and anorexia, but there is no rash. The febrile period lasts from two to four days, and during convalescence there may be diarrhea and weakness. Relapse occurs during convalescence in some small portion of cases, but the disease is rarely if ever fatal.

Immunity

Two or more attacks of the disease may occur during the same season, and this has led to the belief that an effective immunity is not produced by the infection. Controlled experiments in human volunteers, however, have shown that there is a solid immunity to the homologous virus serotype, which persists for a considerable time, but there is substantially no cross-immunity between serotypes. Complement fixation tests, using mouse brain antigen, and mouse protection tests have fully substantiated the antigenic independence of the serotypes. Active immunization of humans with mouse-adapted virus has been demonstrated experimentally, and immunization against the disease may assume some practical importance under certain circumstances.

Epidemiology

There appears to be no verterate host other than man, and *P. papatasii* is the only known vector of the infection. There is some evidence that has been taken to suggest that congenital transmission may occur in the vector, but this has not been established. The seasonal occurrence and short life of the vector, together with the self-limited nature of the infection in man, has been thought to imply some other reservoir of infection, but as yet this remains purely hypothetical.

RIFT VALLEY FEVER[28, 36, 38]

Rift Valley fever (enzootic hepatitis) is a disease of viral etiology that was first observed in 1930 in domestic animals and man in the Rift Valley in Kenya, Central Africa. Serological evidence indicates that the infection is widespread in Africa, occurring in the Sudan, equatorial Africa, and the Republic of South Africa.

The virus is a member of *Phlebovirus* and is cultivable in chick embryo tissue culture and in the chicken embryo. It is pathogenic for most experimental animals except guinea pigs and fowl. Mice are especially susceptible, and the experimental infection is fatal withn four days. Monkeys may be infected with the virus; some infections are febrile, while others are inapparent, but both types are accompanied by viremia.

In East and South Africa, Rift Valley fever has long been endemic, periodically appearing in epizootic episodes primarily affecting sheep and cattle. The mortality in these animals is moderately high, 10 to 20 per cent in mature animals, and up to 90 per cent in the young; abortions are frequent in pregnant animals. Naturally occurring human infections are associated with this animal reservoir; those handling infected animals and carcasses are most often affected. The disease seems to be especially infectious for laboratory workers, and there have been a considerable number of such infections.

In the endemic areas, the disease in humans has long been sporadic, and these cases were usually mild. A major change in the epidemiology of Rift Valley fever occurred in 1977, when infected livestock were inadvertently introduced into Egypt from the Sudan. An epizootic then appeared among sheep, cattle, buffaloes, and camels, with a large number of abortions and deaths. Within a few months of the first animal outbreak, an explosive epidemic occurred among humans in the area and, within a short time, an estimated 18,000 persons suffered from the disease and 598 deaths were reported. The high population densities of humans, domestic animals, and mosquitoes in the affected area are thought to

have contributed to the explosive nature of the epidemic. The disease was again noted among animals during the following summer, and Egypt may now be a new enzootic focus of Rift Valley fever.

In sub-Saharan Africa, the human illness has been relatively mild, occurring in sporadic cases. After an incubation period of five to six days, the disease symptoms range from an influenza-like illness to one with abrupt onset and clinical findings that resemble dengue. The febrile phase lasts only a few days, convalescence is rapid, and recovery complete; Rift Valley fever is rarely fatal. In the Egyptian epidemic, illnesses were much more severe, with complications that included hemorrhagic manifestations, hepatitis, encephalitis, and retinitis; mortality rates were significantly high.

In the South African enzootic areas, the disease is transmitted among animals by hemophagous arthropods. Although a number of mosquito species are capable of transmission, *Culex theileri* is probably the most significant vector among sheep and cattle. Transmission to humans by *Culex theileri* is possible, but most infections appear to be by animal contact. In Egypt, the vector for both animal and human transmission appears to be *Culex pipiens*.

CONGO-CRIMEAN HEMORRHAGIC FEVER[2, 3]

Crimean hemorrhagic fever was first described shortly after World War II in the Crimea. It occurred in early summer among persons in close contact with cattle and other domestic animals. The causative virus was isolated by Russian workers, and serological surveys showed relatively widespread infection in cattle and horses. A similar virus was found in Central Africa in 1956; the two are now known to be identical. The virus was named the Congo-Crimean hemorrhagic fever virus and placed in the genus *Nairovirus* of the family Bunyaviridae.

Virological and serological surveys have confirmed the wide distribution of the virus; it apparently circulates in domestic animals and humans in Africa, Iraq, Russia, and east to Pakistan. It is likely that domestic animals constitute the major reservoir, with transmission effected by a variety of tick vectors, principally *Hyalomma* and *Rhipicephalus* species. The virus is probably maintained in the arthropod vectors by transovarial transmission.

Human disease begins with an influenza-like

illness with fever, headache, and muscle aches. As the disease progresses, a variety of hemorrhagic lesions develop, often followed by hepatorenal failure and involvement of the central nervous system. The mortality rate in recognized cases is substantial, but serological surveys suggest that many infections are mild or inapparent. The human infections may arise from vector transmission, but many cases appear in animal workers under circumstances that suggest infection from handling animal carcasses.

Interrelationships Among Arboviruses[5, 30]

The arthropod-borne viruses (Table 42–5) have in common a reservoir of infection in lower animals, a transmission cycle in which the infection is carried by biting arthropods—mosquitoes, ticks, or sandflies—and a general kind of pathogenesis in which there is viremia in the bird or mammalian host and infection of the viscera or central nervous system, depending upon the relative neurotropism of the virus. As noted earlier, human infection is usually incidental to the natural history of the virus, although under certain circumstances, as in *Aedes*-transmitted yellow fever, man may function as a significant host or even a reservoir of infection.

Immunological relationships among arbovi-

Table 42–5. **Reservoirs, Vectors, and Distribution of Principal Arboviral Diseases**

Disease	Reservoir	Vector	Geographical Distribution
Western equine encephalitis	Wild birds	*Culex tarsalis, Culiseta melanura*	Western United States
Eastern equine encephalitis	Wild birds	*Culiseta melanura, Aedes sollicitans*	Eastern United States, Mexico, Canada, Central and South America, Caribbean
Venezuelan equine encephalitis	Equines	*Psorophora, Mansonia,* and *Aedes* mosquitoes	South America, Mexico, southern United States
Ross River fever	Wild vertebrates, man (?)	*Aedes vigilax*	Australia, Pacific Islands
St. Louis encephalitis	Wild birds	*Culex* mosquitoes	United States
Japanese B encephalitis	Wild birds	*Culex tritaeniorhynchus*	Far East
Murray Valley encephalitis	Wild birds	*Culex annulirostris*	Australia
West Nile fever	Wild birds (?)	*Culex univittatus*	Africa
Rocio encephalitis	Wild birds (?)	*Psorophora ferox* (?)	Brazil
Dengue	Man, monkeys (?)	*Aedes* mosquitoes	Pacific Islands, S.E. Asia, Caribbean, Mexico, southeastern United States
Yellow fever	Man, monkeys	*Aedes, Haemogogus* mosquitoes	South and Central America, Africa
Russian spring-summer encephalitis	Wild rodents, domestic animals	*Ixodes persulcatus*	Asia, Central Europe
Kyasanur Forest disease	Monkeys	Ixodid ticks	India
Powassan encephalitis	Forest mammals	Ticks	North America
Omsk hemorrhagic fever	Muskrats	Ixodid ticks (?)	Siberia
Colorado tick fever	Rodents	*Dermacentor andersoni*	Western United States
California encephalitis	Rodents	*Aedes triseriatus*	Western United States
Sandfly fever	Man	*Phlebotomus papatasii*	Mediterranean, Middle and Far East
Rift Valley fever	Sheep, cattle, camels, buffaloes	*Culex theileri, Culex pipiens*	Africa
Congo-Crimean fever	Domestic animals	*Hyalomma* and *Rhipicephalus* ticks	Asia, Africa

ruses are often of basic significance and are also of practical importance in relation to cross-immunity to infection and to serodiagnosis of disease or serological identification of viruses. These viruses, like many other microorganisms, induce the formation of complement-fixing and neutralizing, or protective, antibodies that may be identical but often are not. In addition, many, but not all, of the arthropod-borne viruses agglutinate goose or neonatal chick red blood cells, and, as in the case of influenza and related viruses, the hemagglutinin is antigenic and stimulates the formation of hemagglutination-inhibiting antibody. The hemagglutinins are present on the virion surface as glycopeptides, while the antigens responsible for complement fixation are probably proteins associated with the viral capsid.

Of the three general kinds of serological reactions that are available for the characterization of these viruses, the hemagglutination-inhibiting antibody is the least specific in that it gives a high proportion of cross-reactions; neutralizing antibody is highly specific; and complement-fixing antibody is intermediate in specificity.

The application of the hemagglutination-inhibiting reaction allows the separation of the arthropod-borne viruses into broad groups as noted earlier. Groups A and B, the latter being considerably the larger, were distinguished first. With the isolation of related strains, the previously ungrouped Bunyamwera virus provided the basis for the *Bunyavirus*. Subgroups within the hemagglutinin groups may be distinguished by cross-reactions in the complement

fixation reaction in which the titer of heterologous reactions is commonly less than that of the homologous reaction. For example, West Nile, St. Louis encephalitis, Japanese B encephalitis, and Murray Valley encephalitis viruses are related with respect to complement-fixing antigens, and yellow fever virus is related to this group and also to dengue. Cross-reactions also occur between the western and eastern varieties of equine encephalitis virus.

When the more highly specific neutralizing antibodies give heterologous reactions, it is generally taken to indicate an extremely close relationship between the viruses. There is, for instance, a partial cross-neutralization between the western and eastern equine encephalitis viruses, and a similar relationshp among the West Nile, Japanese B encephalitis, St. Louis encephalitis, and Murray Valley encephalitis viruses. In the case of Russian spring-summer encephalitis and Kyasanur Forest viruses, the relationship is very close, and the differences among these viruses are considered to be of little more than variant status. Semliki Forest virus and Mayaro virus give essentially complete cross-neutralization reactions and are therefore regarded as practically identical, and Chikungunya virus is either identical with or closely related to them. These relationships, together with those evident in the complement fixation reaction, are indicated as subgroups within the hemagglutinin groups. Such subgroups may not, however, fall entirely within the hemagglutinin groups; for instance, the Chikungunya virus, although closely related to Semliki Forest virus, also cross-reacts to a minor degree with dengue type 1 virus.

The Arenaviruses[14, 42, 45]

The family Arenaviridae contains a small group of viruses of unique morphology and structure placed in a single genus, *Arenavirus*. They are spherical or ovoid and range from 50 to 300 nm. by electron microscopy. The capsid, containing single-stranded, segmented ($-$) RNA, has an electron-dense membrane. Within the capsid are dense granules, about 20 nm. in diameter, that resemble ribosomes. These granules, likened to grains of sand, give the name to the family (Latin *arena,* sand). Surface peplomers of glycopeptides are discernible, but the viruses are not hemagglutinating (Fig. 42–7). The nucleocapsid contains

at least one additional peptide and a glycopeptide. The properties of arenaviruses are listed in Table 42–6.

Among the arenaviruses, some antigenic cross-reactivity is evident in complement fixation reactions, but each is sharply specific by antibody neutralization.

Only a few arenaviruses are responsible for human illnesses. The first described, lymphocytic choriomeningitis virus, is associated with acute benign aseptic meningitis. Two of the viruses, Junin and Machupo, are agents of South American hemorrhagic fevers, and Lassa fever virus produces a severe disease

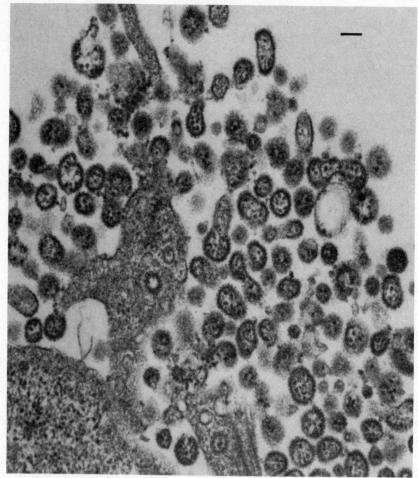

Figure 42–7. Thin section of lymphocytic choriomeningitis virus in infected L cells. The pleomorphic virus particles are in close association with the marginal membrane. Some virions are in the process of budding, while others are lying free. Bar = 100 nm. (G. Muller, *et al.*, Arch. Virol., **75**:229, 1983. Photograph courtesy of Dr. F. Lehmann-Grube.)

first noted in Nigeria in 1969. The remaining members are found in rodents, but are not known to infect man.

LYMPHOCYTIC CHORIOMENINGITIS[10]

This disease was first observed in 1934, and the virus was isolated from a monkey being used in the study of St. Louis encephalitis. The choroid plexuses and meninges were in-

Table 42–6. **Properties of Arenaviruses**

(−)RNA genome; segmented; 3 to 5 × 10⁶ daltons

Spherical or ovoid, 50–300 nm.

Assembled in cytoplasm

Enveloped by budding from plasma membrane

Ether-sensitive, acid-labile

volved and there was lymphocytic infiltration, these characteristics giving the disease its name. The following year it was found to be widespread as an endemic, often symptomless, infection in mice, and in 1936 the virus was isolated from human cases of aseptic meningitis.

Lymphocytic choriomeningitis (LCM) virus may be grown in mouse or chick embryo tissue culture, in Vero cells, and in the embryonated egg. In the egg it does not kill the embryo, and the egg may hatch and the chick survive. Strains of high virulence may grow in chick embryo cell monolayers to give plaques on prolonged incubation, but the virus is generally considered to be noncytopathogenic.

Pathogenicity

The human disease occurs during the cold months of the year, chiefly in adults 20 to 40 years old. It varies in severity from an asymptomatic infection, through a mild influenzalike disease, to aseptic meningitis or meningoencephalitis. The respiratory type may not progress further, and few such cases are recognized as infections with this virus. Alternatively, the respiratory symptoms may be prodromal, and the disease may progress with the appearance of central nervous system involvement within a few days, including sudden severe headache, fever, nausea, and drowsiness, or the meningitis may occur without prodromata. During the febrile stage the virus is present in the blood, nasopahryngeal secretions, and urine, and in the spinal fluid in the meningeal type. Complications are rare, and recovery is usually complete.

Experimental Models

In murine infections, two kinds of disease are observed. In adult mice without previous exposure to the virus, intracerebral inoculation leads to overt disease and fatal choriomeningitis. In these animals, an immune response, both humoral and cell-mediated, is manifest. The syndrome is due not directly to the virus, but to the destructive effects of cell-mediated immunity on infected cells. As would be expected in such animals, immunosuppressive agents protect against pathogenesis in adult animals. When immunologically immature neonatal mice are infected, as occurs in nature, the virus multiples in the host animal without signs of pathogenesis. Infection in this way probably induces a defect in effector T cell function. Under these conditions the virus is harmless for its host, and the asymptomatic animal sheds virus in urine, feces, and nasal secretions, probably for life. A high percentage of wild and laboratory mice, therefore, carry the virus as an endemic infection and represent a natural reservoir of infection.

Immunity

Both complement-fixing and neutralizing antibodies are formed in response to the infection in mature animals. Both appear relatively late, complement-fixing antibody reaching diagnostic levels in three to four weeks and disappearing within a few months, and neutralizing antibody reaching diagnostic titer in seven to eight weeks after onset and persisting for a period of years.

Epidemiology

Mice, dogs, hamsters, and monkeys have been found to be naturally infected with the virus, and it is probable that human infection is most often contracted from mice. The mouse infection is endemic, with the virus transmitted *in utero* or shortly after birth and maintained by healthy carriers. Under some conditions, pet hamsters have been infected, probably from contact with infected mice, and serve as a link to human infections.

The means whereby man contracts the infection from the mouse or other animal is not clearly established, but infected urine is thought to be the usual vehicle, the virus possibly entering the susceptible host through skin abrasions.[55]

It has been noted that passage of LCM virus through hamsters or dogs apparently increases its virulence for humans. A persistent and inapparent infection is produced in these animals and is similarly found in tissue cultures derived from hamsters; such cell cultures exhibit no cytopathology. Laboratory personnel are at significant risk of infection, particularly those working with hamsters or various kinds of hamster tissue cultures. A number of such laboratory-associated infections have been documented.

The infection in man is doubtless much more common than is suggested by the number of clinical cases. Serological surveys in the United States and in Germany have indicated that 3 to 5 per cent of the populations studied possessed neutralizing serum antibodies, and it is probable that many immunizing infections are asymptomatic or are assumed to be influenza or other minor respiratory disease.

SOUTH AMERICAN HEMORRHAGIC FEVERS[54]

Junin Virus

The Junin virus was isolated from cases of Argentinian hemorrhagic fever in 1958 during an epidemic of this disease. The disease is circumscribed in distribution and known to occur only in a limited area of Argentina. It is usually observed in rural areas, and primarily affects male farm workers. Outbreaks occur in late summer and fall, the time when the greatest number of workers are in the fields and when rodent reservoir hosts appear in increasing numbers.

The reservoir hosts apparently are small field rodents that are chronically or persistently infected by the virus. The virus is shed in the urine or other excretions, and man is most likely infected by inhalation or by ingestion of contaminated food or water. The case-fatality rate has been as high as 20 per cent, but in most outbreaks varies from 3 to 15 per cent.

The incubation period of Argentinian hemorrhagic fever varies from 7 to 10 days; the onset is insidious, and symptoms include chills, fever, malaise, headache, myalgia, retroorbital pain, and nausea. Petechiae and lymphoadenopathy are common. After a few days, hemorrhagic manifestations appear and neurological symptoms may follow; death may result from anemic coma or hypovolemic shock.

Machupo Virus

A similar affection, caused by the related Machupo virus, has been endemic in Bolivia since 1958. The transmission cycle is quite similar to Argentinian hemorrhagic fever, except that the rodent reservoir, *Calomys callosus,* lives in close association with man, so that morbidity rates are not weighted by age, sex, or occupation. There is, however, greater prevalence in lower socioeconomic groups, reflecting their greater chance of contact with infected rodents. In addition to the rodent-to-man transmission, there is some evidence of direct man-to-man spread. The mortality rate in Bolivian hemorrhagic fever is somewhat higher than for the Argentinian disease.

LASSA FEVER[11, 18, 32]

In 1969 the first case of Lassa fever was recognized in a nurse who had become infected at a station (Lassa) in Northeast Nigeria. Upon hospitalization in Jos, Nigeria, secondary cases appeared in two nurses at the hospital. Two of the three died, and Lassa virus was isolated from their serum.

In several outbreaks that have followed in Africa since that time, the same general pattern of spread has obtained, *i.e.,* index cases admitted to hospitals have transmitted the infection to other hospital patients, visitors, and personnel. Some other epidemics have been community-associated, following exposure to an index case.

Subsequent studies in Africa have shown, however, that the disease is not spread beyond these secondary cases. Moreover, secondary spread has not been observed from the few cases of Lassa fever exported into the United States, Canada, Great Britain, and Europe. It appears that airborne spread has been exaggerated, and probably occurs principally from cases with pulmonary involvement. Risk of infection is, however, much greater in hospital and laboratory personnel, particularly in those having contact with infected blood, and appropriate isolation and containment precautions are mandatory.

The mode of acquisition of the infection by the primary or index case is unknown, although experience with other arenaviruses has led to the suggestion that rodents may constitute the reservoir of infection. Indeed, the virus has been isolated from the multimammate mouse, *Mastomys natalensis,* in endemic areas of Sierra Leone, but not from a variety of other rodents, bats, or monkeys. Thus a rodent reservoir is likely, and the mode of transmission to man is probably from infected rodent urine, either by direct contact or by contamination of food or dust particles. Man-to-man spread does, however, appear to be established in those epidemics that have been hospital- or community-associated.

In West Africa, the high fatality rates observed in the early outbreaks have continued, at least in the primary cases. The mortality rate in recognized hospitalized cases has varied from 30 to 66 per cent, but is appreciably lower in the secondary cases. As epidemiological and serological data are accumulated, it appears that the spectrum of disease may range from asymptomatic infections through mild disease to severe and fatal illness. It is evident that many mild cases are undiagnosed, so that mortality rates are undoubtedly lower than indicated by published figures. In Sierra Leone, for example, 6 to 13 per cent of surveyed individuals possess complement-fixing antibodies to the virus, while only 0.2 per cent report a history of severe Lassa fever.

Clinical disease has been observed in Nigeria, in Sierra Leone, and in Liberia; it appears to be widespread in West Africa and extends eastward to the Central African Republic.

The incubation period for Lassa fever is from one to two weeks; following insidious onset, the disease is characterized by symptoms of high fever, cough, pharyngitis, tonsillitis (often with white patches), vomiting, abdominal pain and tenderness; and, less often, headache, generalized muscle aches, diarrhea, and conjunctivitis. The acute stage lasts from one to three weeks, and death, if it occurs, is usually in the second week of the disease. Virus is found in the blood, from about the third to fourteenth days. Complement-fixing antibodies are produced, but they do not appear until the second or third week of illness and are, therefore, not useful for diagnosis. Whether convalescent serum is protective is not clear, but it is believed to have had some beneficial effect in a few instances where it has been employed. In experimental Lassa fever in rhesus monkeys, ribovirin has been remarkably effective, suggesting that this drug may prove of value in human infections.[29]

Other Hemorrhagic Fevers[54]

It is already apparent that the clinical syndrome of viral hemorrhagic fever is not restricted in etiology, since it may be due to one of a number of viruses, representing several families, as shown in Table 42–7. A number of epidemiological types are represented among the viral hemorrhagic fevers. Those transmitted by arthropod vectors are caused by togaviruses and bunyaviruses; others are transmitted by contact with infected animal reservoir hosts, *viz.,* South American hemorrhagic fevers and Lassa fever, both caused by arenaviruses.

Two important hemorrhagic fevers are due to viruses that have not yet been classified—hemorrhagic fever with renal syndrome and Marburg-Ebola hemorrhagic fever. Neither appears to be arthropod-borne, but the causative agents are animal viruses transmissible to humans usually by direct contact.

HEMORRHAGIC FEVER WITH RENAL SYNDROME[50, 59]

In the early 1950s, a febrile disease with hemorrhagic manifestations appeared among United Nations troops in Korea, causing serious illness characterized by shock and renal failure and with a mortality rate of 5 to 10 per cent. The disease was named Korean hemorrhagic fever, but has long been known in other parts of Asia and in Europe, under a variety

Table 42–7. **Viral Hemorrhagic Fevers**

Virus Group	Disease
Poxviridae	Smallpox
Togaviridae	Dengue Kyasanur fever Omsk hemorrhagic fever Yellow fever
Bunyaviridae	Congo-Crimean hemorrhagic fever
Arenaviridae	South American hemorrhagic fevers Lassa fever
Unclassified	Hemorrhagic fever with renal syndrome Marburg-Ebola hemorrhagic fever

of names. The epidemiological character of the infection is variable, depending upon the locality where it appears, and the disease is now known as hemorrhagic fever with renal syndrome (HFRS). The earliest recognition of HFRS was in the far eastern parts of the Soviet Union in 1932, where it was extensively studied by Russian workers. Within a few years a similar affliction was reported in Manchuria and in northeast China. Subsequently, epidemics of HFRS have been encountered in Japan, Eastern Europe, and Scandinavia. In all of these areas, sporadic cases also appear, indicating that the infection is endemic in many parts of the world.

Although the viral etiology of HFRS had been suspected for many years, no viral entity had been unequivocally identified prior to the late 1970s. Isolation of the causative agent of Korean hemorrhagic fever (KHF) was reported in 1978. The viral agent was found in the field mouse, *Apodemus agrarius,* and was later propagated in this animal. Subsequently, a mouse-adapted strain was grown in human cell cultures. This virus, named the Hantaan virus, is now accepted as the etiological agent of KHF, based on serological and epidemiological findings. Subsequently, another virus, termed the Puumala agent, has been linked to nephropathia epidemica, the variety of HFRS found in Scandinavia. The latter virus has not been isolated, but the infections are serologically related, and it now appears that at least two serological types of viruses are responsible for HFRS. The Hantaan virus is not yet well characterized, but it is said to resemble orbiviruses.

The Disease in Man

Clinically recognizable HFRS seems to occur in two forms, one severe and more common in eastern Asia, and the second mild, as usually seen in Scandinavia. There is also evidence that many infections are subclinical, since serological surveys in endemic areas show an infection rate of about 4 per cent, many without history of HFRS.

The incubation period of HFRS is usually from two to three weeks, followed by abrupt onset of febrile illness, with fever, headache, muscular pain, and a variety of hemorrhagic manifestations. About one-fifth of the cases will develop more serious disease, characterized by shock, hemorrhage, and renal failure. The acute stage usually lasts from 8 to 10 days and is followed by gradual recovery over a period of several weeks to three months. Mortality is usually less than 5 per cent in treated cases, and complete recovery is the rule except for those with hemorrhages into the central nervous system.

In the mild form, symptoms are similar, but hemorrhage is much less prominent, and illnesses last for only about three weeks. The mortality rate is also much lower, usually less than 0.5 per cent.

Epidemiology

Hemorrhagic fever of this type is essentially a zoonosis, occurring in a number of rodents as an asymptomatic infection. The virus is shed in the feces, and man is infected after contact with rodent excreta, either by aerosol inhalation or by virus penetration of the skin through cuts or abrasions.

As might be expected, HFRS is most often seen in rural areas, particularly among field workers, who are more likely to contact infected rodents. In Korea and China, the reservoir hosts are field mice of the *Apodemus* species, whereas in Scandinavia and some areas of the Soviet Union, bank voles are the predominant reservoir hosts. In rural areas of the Soviet Union, the house rat, *Rattus norvegicus,* seems to be a common reservoir host as well.

An urban type of HFRS has been noted in Korea, China, and Japan. In most urban endemic areas, the principal reservoir host is *Rattus norvegicus.*

The HFRS viruses also have been found in rodents used in medical research, particularly in Korea, Russia, and Finland. These rodent infections have been communicated to laboratory personnel in many instances. As is the case with other hemorrhagic fevers, laboratory manipulations of infected materials also presents a significant risk to hospital laboratory personnel.[33]

MARBURG-EBOLA HEMORRHAGIC FEVER[48, 49]

Human hemorrhagic fever due to Marburg virus was first described in outbreaks in Germany and Yugoslavia in 1967. The primary cases in these outbreaks were linked to African green monkeys imported from Uganda, the infection being traced to contact with infected monkey blood or organs. Of 31 cases identified in these outbreaks, 7 were fatal. In 1975, the disease reappeared in South Africa, with three cases and one death.

From August to November of 1976, severe outbreaks of a similar disease occurred in Zaire and Sudan. The case-fatality rate in Sudan was 53 per cent and 88 per cent in Zaire. The causative agent in these outbreaks is morphologically identical to the Marburg virus, but is antigenically distinct; it has been given the name Ebola virus.

The Marburg and Ebola viruses are morphologically identical, appearing as tubular, sometimes branched, forms in infected tissues (Fig. 42–8). The genome of Ebola virus is single-stranded $(-)$RNA, with molecular weight of 4.0×10^6 daltons;[46] the viruses are not otherwise well characterized.

The clinical features of hemorrhagic fever caused by Marburg and Ebola viruses are also indistinguishable. Following an incubation period of about one week, there is an influenza-like syndrome, followed by sore throat, diarrhea and abdominal pain, maculopapular rash, and bleeding from multiple sites, principally the gastrointestinal tract. Although the case-fatality rate has been high in most outbreaks, serological evidence also indicates mild or subclinical infection in the endemic areas. Recovery, when it occurs, is usually complete, with no long-term sequelae.

The epidemiology of these hemorrhagic fevers resembles that of Lassa fever. There is some suggestion of a rodent reservoir, but most infections are transmitted between individuals by close and frequent contact or, in hospital personnel, by exposure to infected blood or respiratory secretions. So far as can be ascertained, arthropod vectors are not involved in transmission of the viruses.

The Rubella Virus

Rubella, or German measles, is an exanthematous disease of childhood that resembles measles in many respects but is milder, *e.g.,* the catarrhal symptoms of the prodromal stage

are less severe, the subsequent febrile reaction is slight, and the rash is macular, discrete or confluent, resembling that of early measles. Koplik spots are not present, and there is

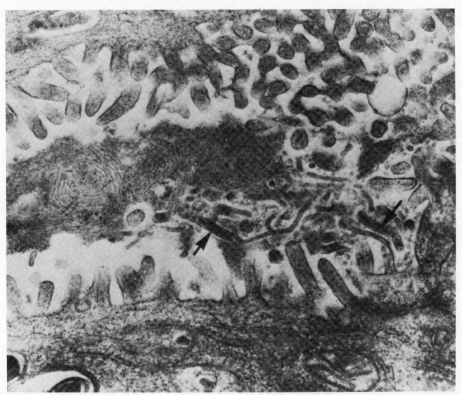

Figure 42–8. Ebola virus in section of liver from infected patient. Tubular forms of the virus are extruded into the bile canaliculus. × 42,000. (D. S. Ellis, *et al.,* J. Clin. Path., **31**:201, 1978. Courtesy of Dr. D. S. Ellis, London School of Hygiene and Tropical Medicine.)

characteristic lymphadenitis affecting the cervical and occipital nodes with swelling persisting for two to three weeks. Because of its mild nature, it is not an important pediatric illness, but it has assumed much greater significance in female adults of the childbearing age group because of its teratogenic effects on the fetus.

Morphology and Cultivation

Rubella virus particles are approximately spherical and are 50 to 75 nm. in diameter. In electron micrographs of negatively stained preparations, the surface of the particle appears rough because of peplomers, and an inner electron-dense core is apparent. In cell cultures, the budding of virus from marginal and intracytoplasmic membranes has been described. Virion morphology is illustrated in Figure 42–9. The contained nucleic acid is single-stranded (+)RNA, and the virus occurs as a single serological type. As noted earlier in this chapter, it is classified as *Rubivirus* in the Togaviridae.

Rubella virus, cultured in many of the commonly used tissue cultures, produces no visible cytopathogenesis. Cytopathic effect, *e.g.,* appearance of ameboid cells and sloughing, is produced only in certain kinds of cell cultures; in rabbit kidney cell cultures, cytopathogenesis is evident within about four days, while several weeks are required for damage to human primary amnion cell cultures. When a cytopathic effect is produced in a reasonable time it allows a practical direct method of titrating neutralizing antibody.

Pathogenicity for Man

As indicated above, rubella is a relatively common childhood affection. Two forms of rubella infection are recognized. **Postnatally acquired rubella** is a relatively benign disease of children and young adults; occasional outbreaks occur in young adults and in hospital environments. **Congenital rubella,** resulting from maternal infection during pregnancy, is associated with fetal abnormalities of varying severity and long-term effect.

The incubation period in postnatally acquired rubella is from two to three weeks, followed by prodromal symptoms of mild respiratory disease with low-grade fever, headache, and malaise. Usually within 24 hours after onset, an erythematous rash appears, spreading to the trunk and extremities, and

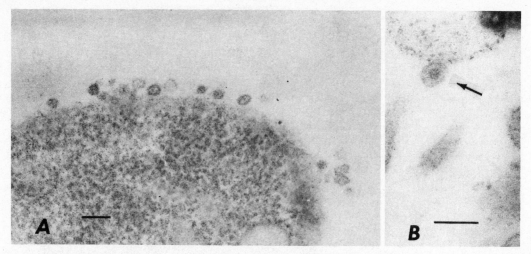

Figure 42–9. Rubella virus growing in African green monkey kidney (Vero) cells. *A,* Virions are adjacent to cell margin following budding. *B,* Higher magnification showing virion morphology (arrow). Bar = 100 nm. (Courtesy of Dr. Gordon Schrank.)

generally lasting for a few days. Virus is found in serum and urine for about a week before the onset of symptoms, but disappears soon after the appearance of rash and coincident with a rise in antibody titer. The virus appears in the nasopharynx during the exanthematous period and is shed for 10 days to two weeks after the appearance of rash.

Congenital Rubella

Intrauterine infection of the fetus apparently occurs readily in consequence of clinical or inapparent maternal infection, as demonstrated by the presence of the virus in aborted fetuses, stillborn infants, and infants with or without abnormalities. In fact, as many as 75 per cent of infected infants were born of mothers with no history of clinical rubella. **Persistent infections** are common, and virus is often found in the nasopharyngeal secretions and in the gastrointestinal tract for some months after birth, in spite of the presence of neutralizing antibody. Persistently infected infants can, thereby, serve to disseminate the virus to others.

The teratogenic mechanisms resulting in associated defects remain speculative. The most obvious teratogenic effects are noted when maternal infection occurs in the first trimester of pregnancy, but more subtle changes are observed when infection takes place during the second trimester. The virus apparently first infects the placenta, and this may be followed by disseminated fetal infection. Embryonic and fetal tissues appear to be generally susceptible to infection, and it has been suggested that viral proliferation interferes with normal cell

growth *in utero,* and possibly also in the postpartum infant. The concurrent presence of antibody and virus has been taken to suggest that antigen-antibody reactions, as well as the direct effects of the virus, may contribute to the observed consequences of fetal infection.

Immunity

The immune response acquired by clinical or inapparent infection is reflected in the appearance of serum antibody, commonly assayed as neutralizing antibody, complement-fixing antibody, and hemagglutination-inhibiting antibody. Antibody appears after the cessation of viremia and is evident about the time the rash appears. Hemagglutination-inhibiting antibody appears first and rises to peak titer in one to three weeks. The appearance of neutralizing antibody and that demonstrable by fluorescence microscopy is somewhat delayed, and complement-fixing antibody is not detectable until 10 days to two weeks after onset of symptoms. The presence of IgM antibody has some diagnostic significance: in primary infections, these antibodies appear a few days before the rash, and are present for only a few weeks; therefore, the presence of hemagglutination-inhibiting IgM antibodies indicates current or recent infection.

Before vaccines were available, immunizing infections occurred through elementary and high school; some 20 per cent of preschool children possessed neutralizing antibody, with the proportion rising to 80 per cent in the 17- to 20-year-old age group. The immune status of women in the childbearing age group, 14 to 44 years, is of special significance because of the teratogenic effects of the infection on the fetus. The age-specific attack rates are consistent with the assumption that neutralizing antibody is associated with effective immunity to the disease.

Vaccines.[43] Immunization against rubella presents a special problem in that the disease is not a serious one, other than its teratogenic effect in pregnant women. Effective vaccines are live, attenuated strains of the rubella virus, and there may be some theoretical risk to the fetus if such vaccines are administered to pregnant women. Immunization in the United States has, therefore, been directed primarily toward younger age groups, on the premise that high levels of herd immunity can prevent the circulation of the virus in all susceptible age groups. The chances for infection in women of childbearing age might thereby be reduced without the necessity of direct immunization. This strategy has been largely successful, as shown by the significant reduction of the incidence of rubella (Fig. 41–10). Although greatly reduced, rubella continues to occur among women of childbearing age, so that current efforts are directed toward vaccination of postpubertal individuals. This approach is now feasible because all available data indicate that the risk of teratogenicity from vaccine use is very small or nonexistent, whereas the frequency of fetal damage from naturally occurring infection contracted during the first trimester is estimated to be in excess of 20 per cent.

A number of strains of the rubella virus, attenuated by prolonged passage in cell cultures, have been developed. Several of these have been used in the United States, but only one is currently licensed, the attenuated RA 27/3 strain, prepared in human diploid cells. When administered subcutaneously to those over one year of age, a single inoculation yields approximately 95 per cent seroconversion as measured by hemagglutination-inhibition. The immunity induced is expected to be long-lived, possibly for life. Vaccinated individuals may shed small amounts of virus from time to time, but there is no evidence of virus transmission to others. Surveillance of women inadvertently immunized during pregnancy has revealed no instance of infants with malformations compatible with congenital rubella syndrome, although a low rate of fetal infection has been documented. It is currently recommended that pregnant women should not be vaccinated, and women should be counseled against becoming pregnant within three months of vaccination.

Even high levels of herd immunity have not always prevented the introduction and spread of rubella virus in certain communities. The protection afforded by herd immunity appears to be less effective than that observed in poliomyelitis.

Experimental Infections

Many attempts have been made to reproduce the disease in experimental animals, but without success. With the availability of virus culture, it has become clear that subhuman primates and nonprimate conventional exper-

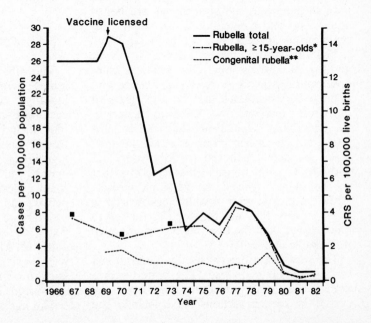

Figure 42–10. Incidence of reported rubella and congenital rubella in the United States, 1966 to 1982. (Morbidity and Mortality Weekly Report, **32**:505, 1983.)

imental animals respond immunologically, often with the production of high-titer neutralizing antibody, but without clinical signs of disease. Of the latter, the ferret appears to be one of the most sensitive experimental animals.

The Slow Viruses[20, 39, 40, 61]

The term "slow infections" was first proposed by Sigurdsson to describe a group of slowly evolving, chronic animal diseases characterized by periods of long latency between infection and the appearance of clinical symptoms, and a protracted clinical course tending to regular and predictable events. The resulting disease was usually severe and often led to death of the host. Among the diseases he described was a central nervous system disease of sheep (rida), probably the disease known as scrapie in other parts of the world. Several years later, the similarities between scrapie and the human disease kuru, found only among the Fore people of New Guinea, were pointed out by Hadlow. In 1966, Gajdusek and associates reported the successful transmission of kuru to chimpanzees and established it as an infectious entity.

Following the stimulus provided by the kuru studies, a number of virus diseases have been found to satisfy the basic definition of slow infections as set forth by Sigurdsson. The term slow virus is now applied to certain of the agents of these affections. "Slow virus" is considered to be a misnomer, since many of the viral agents are capable of rapid replication; nevertheless, the term is now widely used and will undoubtedly continue to be employed until such time as the viral agents are better understood and conventional taxonomic concepts can be applied.

The viral agents of slow infections may be divided into two groups. One group is composed of classic, or conventional viruses, and is quite heterogeneous, not only in terms of the viruses involved, but also with respect to the underlying mechanisms that lead to slow infection. The other group is made up of a series of agents, believed to be viruses, but with strange and unusual characteristics that set them apart from the conventional viruses. Although they are not so well characterized as other viruses, they are regarded as related to one another, and the diseases they cause have remarkable similarity.

The slow infections caused by conventional viruses are quite diverse. The better known human slow virus infections have been discussed in earlier sections, and include the central nervous system diseases of subacute sclerosing panencephalitis following previous infection by the measles virus (Chapter 40) and progressive multifocal leukoencephalopathy associated with papovaviruses (Chapter 39). Others perhaps to be included in this list are congenital rubella infections, brain infections by cytomegaloviruses, and subacute encephalitides due to herpesviruses and adenoviruses. Among the animal diseases of this infection class are the avian leucoses and mouse mammary tumors due to RNA tumor viruses (Chapter 40).

The slow infections due to the unconventional agents (the slow viruses) are noninflammatory subacute degenerative diseases of the central nervous system. Two human diseases, kuru and Creutzfeldt-Jakob disease, and two animal diseases, scrapie and mink encephalopathy, are currently recognized. Their similarities are indicated by the present terminology, which groups them under the rubric of spongiform virus encephalopathies. The discovery that these are infectious diseases of viral etiology has led to questions concerning the possible infectious etiology of other degenerative diseases, such as multiple sclerosis and Parkinson's disease.

SPONGIFORM VIRUS ENCEPHALOPATHIES[9, 44]

The subacute spongiform virus encephalopathies—scrapie, transmissible mink encephalopathy, kuru, and Creutzfeldt-Jakob disease—are categorized by a clinical syndrome that includes progressive cerebellar ataxia, tremors, and postural instability. Histopathological lesions are found primarily in the gray matter and are characterized by severe neuronal vacuolation, astrocytic hypertrophy, gliosis, and status spongiosus. The incubation or latent period is long, from many months to years, depending upon the individual disease and host. Much of the experimental data have been derived from scrapie and experimental kuru in primates, but the similarities between the various agents and diseases are striking.

The agents responsible for these infections

are curious and unusual, and may very well be a new kind of biological form. It has not been possible to identify any recognizable virion by electron microscopy of infected tissues. The only morphological entity that seems to be associated with the infective process is curled membrane fragments that are found in the neuronal vacuoles; presumably these fragments are derived from the vacuolar membrane. Infectivity seems also to be associated with these membrane fragments. Solvents known to disrupt membranes (ether, phenol, urea) destroy infectivity, but other chemical agents that inactivate most viruses, *viz.,* proteolytic enzymes, formaldehyde, deoxyribonuclease, and ribonuclease, are generally without effect on these agents; they are also extremely resistant to ultraviolet irradiation.

The agents have been shown to persist for long periods in tissue explants, but no cytopathic effects are discernible, and no transmission to other cell lines has been found. Identification of the agents is further complicated by the fact that they are not immunogenic, and no antibody is formed. Thus, techniques for morphological and immunological characterization, so valuable with other viruses, are not available.

In the absence of a microscopically identifiable virus particle, no direct measurements of size are possible. A variety of procedures indicate that the scrapie agent exhibits considerable heterogeneity of size, with a minimum diameter of perhaps 4 to 6 nm. and a molecular weight of 50,000 daltons, but the agents of kuru and Creutzfeldt-Jakob disease appear to be larger, failing to pass through membranes of 100 nm. average pore diameter. The scrapie agent has been most extensively studied, and it has recently been shown to possess a protein component that is required for infectivity.

The available evidence, therefore, indicates that these are membrane-associated infectious agents that contain very little, if any, nucleic acids and possess no immunogenic components by conventional measurements. The mode of replication is subject to considerable speculation, and any hypothesis must account for all of these unusual properties.

Scrapie

This slowly progressive disease of sheep, characterized by noninflammatory degeneration of the central nervous system, has been known in Europe for more than 200 years, and has occurred in North America and Australia. Its viral etiology was suggested as early as 1936, and transmission was confirmed within a few years. The susceptibility of sheep to scrapie is, in part, genetically determined, as shown by greater susceptibility of certain breeds; mice are also susceptible to experimental infection, as are hamsters and monkeys. Experimental transmission may be accomplished by parenteral or oral routes, but the natural mode has not been definitely established. The incubation period is long—two to five years in sheep, but four to six months in mice following intracerebral inoculation. The similarities of scrapie to kuru ultimately led to the present state of knowledge concerning the spongiform encephalopathies.

Kuru

Kuru is an invariably fatal disease found only in the Fore people of the eastern highlands of New Guinea. Its distribution and transmission are related to cultural and religious practices of the affected people. Natural transmission was promoted by cannibalistic rituals; women and children are most often affected, probably through inoculation during preparation and because by tradition they consumed brain tissue. These practices have now been virtually abandoned, with resulting disappearance of kuru in the younger population. It seems likely that the disease will now be eradicated. Experimental transmission to chimpanzees and monkeys has been accomplished, with the production of clinical and histopathological events similar to those in man.

The incubation period in intracerebrally inoculated chimpanzees has ranged from 18 to 36 months for primary passage and is about one year for secondary passage. The resulting illness in these animals lasts from about four months to one year, approximately the same duration as human infections.

Creutzfeldt-Jakob Disease

The disease was first recognized by Creutzfeldt in 1920 and by Jakob in 1921. Although the number of recognized cases is not large, it is of wide geographical distribution, in contrast to kuru. The histopathology is, however, similar to that observed in kuru, and it was this similarity that led to the successful attempts to transmit the infection to chimpanzees. Other primates, and guinea pigs, have also been infected. The incubation period in experimentally infected chimpanzees has been recorded as 11 to 14 months; the disease course is shorter than kuru, lasting from four to 12 weeks; secondary passage did not result in shortened incubation times.

REFERENCES

1. Aaskov, J. G., *et al.* 1981. An epidemic of Ross River virus infection in Fiji, 1979. Amer. J. Trop. Med. Hygiene **30**:1053–1059.

2. Al-Tikriti, S. K., *et al.* 1981. Congo/Crimean haemorrhagic fever in Iraq. Bull. Wld Hlth Org. **59**:85–90.

3. Al-Tikriti, S. K., *et al.* 1981. Congo/Crimean haemorrhagic fever in Iraq; a seroepidemiological survey. J. Trop. Med. Hygiene **84**:117–120.

4. Bailey, C. L., *et al.* 1978. Isolation of St. Louis encephalitis virus from overwintering *Culex pipiens* mosquitoes. Science **199**:1346–1349.

5. Berge, T. O. (Ed.). 1975. International Catalogue of Arboviruses Including Certain Other Viruses of Vertebrates. DHEW Publication No. (CDC)75-8301. U.S. Department of Health, Education, and Welfare, Washington, D.C.

6. Bigler, W. J., *et al.* 1976. Endemic eastern equine encephalomyelitis in Florida: a twenty-year analysis, 1955–1974. Amer. J. Trop. Med. Hygiene **25**:884–890.

7. Bishop, D. H. L. 1979. Genetic potential of bunyaviruses. Curr. Topics Microbiol. Immunol. **86**:1–33.

8. Bowen, G. S., *et al.* 1981. The ecology of Colorado tick fever in Rocky Mountain National Park in 1974. II. Infection in small mammals. Amer. J. Trop. Med. Hygiene **30**:490–496.

9. Brown, P. 1980. An epidemiologic critique of Creutzfeldt-Jakob disease. Epidemiol. Rev. **2**:113–135.

10. Buchmeier, M. J., *et al.* 1980. The virology and immunobiology of lymphocytic choriomeningitis virus infection. Adv. Immunol. **30**:275–331.

11. Buckley, S. M., and J. Casals. 1978. Pathobiology of Lassa fever. Internat. Rev. Exptl Pathol. **18**:97–136.

12. Burgdorfer, W. 1977. Tick-borne diseases in the United States: Rocky Mountain spotted fever and Colorado tick fever. Acta Trop. **34**:103–126.

13. Calisher, C. H., *et al.* 1981. Arbovirus subtyping. Applications to epidemiologic studies, availability of reagents, and testing services. Amer. J. Epidemiol. **114**:619–631.

14. Casals, J. 1975. Arenaviruses. Yale J. Biol. Med. **48**:115–140.

15. Clerx, J. P. M., J. Casals, and D. H. L. Bishop. 1981. Structural characteristics of nairoviruses (genus *Nairovirus,* Bunyaviridae). J. Gen. Virol. **55**:165–178.

16. Doherty, R. L. 1977. Arthropod-borne viruses in Australia, 1973–1976. Australian J. Exptl Biol. Med. Sci. **55**:103–130.

17. Edelman, R., *et al.* 1979. Evaluation in humans of a new, inactivated vaccine for Venezuelan equine encephalitis virus (C-84). J. Infect. Dis. **140**:708–715.

18. Emond, R. T. D. 1980. Lassa fever. Roy. Soc. Hlth J. **100**:48–52.

19. Francy, D. B., *et al.* 1981. Transovarial transmission of St. Louis encephalitis virus by *Culex pipiens* complex mosquitoes. Amer. J. Trop. Med. Hygiene **30**:699–705.

20. Fucillo, D. A., J. E. Kurent, and J. L. Sever. 1974. Slow virus diseases. Ann. Rev. Microbiol. **28**:231–264.

21. Garoff, H., C. Kondor-Koch, and H. Riedel. 1982. Structure and assembly of alphaviruses. Curr. Topics Microbiol. Immunol. **99**:1–50.

22. Gorman, B. M. 1979. Variation in orbiviruses. J. Gen. Virol. **44**:1–15.

23. Grossman, R. A., R. Edelman, and D. J. Gould. 1974. Study of Japanese encephalitis virus in Chiangmai Valley, Thailand. VI. Summary and conclusions. Amer. J. Epidemiol. **100**:69–76.

24. Halstead, S. B. 1980. Dengue haemorrhagic fever—a public health problem and a field for research. Bull. Wld Hlth Org. **58**:1–21.

25. Halstead, S. B. 1981. The Alexander D. Langmuir Lecture. The pathogenesis of dengue. Molecular epidemiology in infectious disease. Amer. J. Epidemiol. **114**:632–648.

26. Hayes, C. G. 1978. Variations in biological properties of geographic strains of western equine encephalomyelitis virus before and after passage in *Culex tarsalis* and *Culiseta melanura.* Acta Virol. **22**:401–409.

27. Henderson, B. E., and P. H. Coleman. 1971. The growing importance of California arboviruses in the etiology of human disease. Prog. Med. Virol. **13**:404–461.

28. Hoogstraal, H., *et al.* 1979. Symposium on Rift Valley fever. The Rift Valley fever epizootic in Egypt 1977–78. 2. Ecological and entomological studies. Trans. Roy. Soc. Trop. Med. Hygiene **73**:624–629.

29. Jahrling, P. B., *et al.* 1980. Lassa virus infection of rhesus monkeys: pathogenesis and treatment with ribavirin. J. Infect. Dis. **141**:580–589.

30. Karabatsos, N. (Ed.) 1978. Supplement to international catalogue of arboviruses including certain other viruses of vertebrates. Amer. J. Trop. Med. Hygiene **27**:372–440.

31. Kay, B. H. 1980. Towards prediction and surveillance of Murray Valley encephalitis activity in Australia. Australian J. Exptl Biol. Med. Sci. **58**:67–76.

32. Keane, E., and H. M. Gilles. 1977. Lassa fever in Panguma hospital, Sierra Leone, 1973–6. Brit. Med. J. **1**:1399–1402.

33. Lee, H. W., and K. M. Johnson. 1982. Laboratory-acquired infections with Hantaan virus, the etiologic agent of Korean hemorrhagic fever. J. Infect. Dis. **146**:645–651.

34. Lopes, O. S., *et al.* 1981. Emergence of a new arbovirus disease in Brazil. III. Isolation of Rocio virus from *Psorophoro ferox* (Humboldt, 1819). Amer. J. Epidemiol. **113**:122–125.

35. Luby, J. P. 1979. St. Louis encephalitis. Epidemiol. Rev. **1**:55–73.

36. McIntosh, B. M., *et al.* 1980. Vector studies on Rift Valley fever virus in South Africa. South African Med. J. **58**:127–132.

37. McLean, R. G., *et al.* 1981. The ecology of Colorado tick fever in Rocky Mountain National Park in 1974. I. Objectives, study design, and summary of principal findings. Amer. J. Trop. Med. Hygiene **30**:483–489.

38. Meegan, J. M., *et al.* 1979. Symposium on Rift Valley fever. The Rift Valley fever epizootic in Egypt 1977–78. 1. Description of the epizootic and virological studies. Trans. Roy. Soc. Trop. Med. Hygiene **73**:618–623.

39. ter Meulen, V., and M. Katz (Eds.). 1977. Slow Virus Infections of the Central Nervous System. Springer-Verlag, New York.

40. ter Meulen, V., and W. W. Hall. 1978. Slow virus infections of the nervous system: virological, immunological and pathogenetic considerations. J. Gen. Virol. **41**:1–25.

41. Monath, T. P. 1979. Arthropod-borne encephalitides in the Americas. Bull. Wld Hlth Org. **57**:513–533.

42. Pedersen, I. R. 1979. Structural components and replication of arenaviruses. Adv. Virus Res. **24**:277–330.

43. Preblud, S. R., *et al.* 1980. Rubella vaccination in the

United States: a ten-year review. Epidemiol. Rev. **2**:171–194.

44. Prusiner, S. B. 1982. Novel proteinaceous infectious particles cause scrapie. Science **216**:136–144.
45. Rawls, W. E., M. A. Chan, and S. R. Gee. 1981. Mechanisms of persistence in arenavirus infections: a brief review. Can. J. Microbiol. **27**:568–574.
46. Regnery, R. L., *et al.* 1980. Virion nucleic acid of Ebola virus. J. Virol. **36**:465–469.
47. Report. 1975. Powassan virus isolated from a patient with encephalitis—New York. Morbid. Mortal. Wkly Rep. **24**:379.
48. Report. 1978. Ebola haemorrhagic fever in Sudan, 1976. Bull. Wld Hlth Org. **56**:247–270.
49. Report. 1978. Ebola haemorrhagic fever in Zaire, 1976. Bull. Wld Hlth Org. **56**:271–293.
50. Report. 1983. Haemorrhagic fever with renal syndrome: memorandum from a WHO meeting. Bull. Wld Hlth Org. **61**:269–275.
51. Rosen, L., D. A. Shroyer, and J. C. Lien. 1980. Transovarial transmission of Japanese encephalitis virus by *Culex tritaeniorhynchus* mosquitoes. Amer. J. Trop. Med. Hygiene **29**:711–712.
52. Schlesinger, R. W. (Ed.). 1980. The Togaviruses. Academic Press, London.
53. Schlesinger, R. W. 1977. Dengue viruses. Virol. Monogr. **16**:1–132.
54. Simpson, D. H. I. 1978. Viral haemorrhagic fevers of man. Bull. Wld Hlth Org. **56**:819–832.
55. Skinner, H. H., and E. H. Knight. 1979. Epidermal tissue as a primary site of replication of lymphocytic choriomeningitis virus in small experimental hosts. J. Hygiene (Cambridge) **82**:21–30.
56. Sudia, W. D., and V. F. Newhouse. 1975. Epidemic Venezuelan equine encephalitis in North America: a summary of virus-vector-host relationships. Amer. J. Epidemiol. **101**:1–13.
57. Tesh, R. B., *et al.* 1976. Serological studies on the epidemiology of sandfly fever in the Old World. Bull. Wld Hlth Org. **54**:663–674.
58. Tesh, R. B., *et al.* 1981. Ross River virus (Togaviridae: *Alphavirus*) infection (epidemic polyarthritis) in American Samoa. Trans. Roy. Soc. Trop. Med. Hygiene **75**:426–430.
59. Traub, R., and C. L. Wisseman, Jr. 1978. Korean hemorrhagic fever. J. Infect. Dis. **138**:267–272.
60. Woodall, J. P. 1981. Summary of a symposium on yellow fever. J. Infect. Dis. **144**:87–91.
61. Zeman, W., and E. H. Lennette (Eds.). 1974. Slow Virus Diseases. Williams & Wilkins Co., Baltimore.

Mycology

CHAPTER 43

Medical Mycology: The Pathogenic Fungi and the Pathogenic Actinomycetes

John W. Rippon, Ph.D.

The discovery of the causal relation of certain of the fungi to infectious disease preceded by several years the pioneer work of Pasteur and Koch with the pathogenic bacteria. Schoenlein and Gruby studied the fungus causing favus (*Trichophyton schoenleinii*) in 1839, and in the same year Langenbeck described the yeast-like microorganism of thrush (*Candida albicans*). Gruby isolated the favus fungus on potato slices, rubbed it on the head of a child, and produced the disease. He thus fulfilled Koch's postulates forty years before they were formulated. Prior to this, Bassi had described muscardine of silkworm (caused by *Beauveria bassiana*).

In spite of its earlier beginnings, medical mycology was soon overshadowed by bacteriology and has never received as much attention, though some of the fungal diseases are among the more common infections of man. This is perhaps attributable to the relatively benign nature of the common mycoses, the rarity of the more serious ones, and the morphological basis of the differentiation of these structurally complex forms.

Even a brief consideration of the fungal diseases makes it clear that they fall into four well-defined groups: the superficial, cutaneous, subcutaneous, and systemic mycoses (Table 43–1). The superficial and cutaneous mycoses are by far the more common and are caused for the most part by a relatively homogeneous group of fungi, the dermatophytes. These include the various forms of tinea or ringworm, which are infections of the hair and hair follicles, the superficial infections of the intertriginous or flat areas of the glabrous skin, and the infections of the toe- and fingernails. In general, the lesions are mild, superficial, and restricted. The infections are almost never fatal, although invasion of the brain and heart by *Trichophyton violaceum* has been reported from Russia, Japan, and Rumania. The causative microorganisms have the peculiar ability

Table 43–1. **Clinical Types of Fungal Infections**

Type	Disease	Causative Organism
Superficial infections	Pityriasis versicolor	*Malassezia furfur*
	Piedra	*Trichosporon beigelii* (white)
		Piedraia hortai (black)
Cutaneous infections	Ringworm of scalp, glabrous skin, nails	Dermatophytes (*Macrosporum* sp., *Trichophyton* sp., *Epidermophyton* sp.)
	Candidiasis of skin, mucous membranes, and nails	*Candida albicans* and related species
Subcutaneous infections	Chromoblastomycosis	*Fonsecaea pedrosoi* and related forms
	Mycotic mycetoma	*Pseudallescheria boydii, Madurella mycetomatis*, etc.
	Entomophthoromycosis	*Basidiobolus ranarum*
		Conidiobolus coronatus
	Rhinosporidiosis	*Rhinosporidium seeberi*
	Lobomycosis	*Loboa loboi*
	Sporotrichosis	*Sporothrix schenckii*
Systemic infections	True pathogenic fungal infections	
	Histoplasmosis	*Histoplasma capsulatum*
	Blastomycosis	*Blastomyces dermatitidis*
	Paracoccidioidomycosis	*Paracoccidioides brasiliensis*
	Coccidioidomycosis	*Coccidioides immitis*
	Opportunistic fungal infections	
	Cryptococcosis	*Cryptococcus neoformans*
	Aspergillosis	*Aspergillus fumigatus*, etc.
	Mucormycosis	*Mucor* sp., *Absidia* sp., *Rhizopus* sp.
	Candidiasis, systemic	*Candida albicans*

to digest keratin and are the only group of fungi that have evolved into obligate infectious agents of man or animal. These species have no reservoir other than their infected hosts; however, many other species of dermatophytes have their ultimate reservoir in soil. They are in a sense specialized saprophytes as they do not invade living tissue, deriving their nutrition from the dead cornified material of hair, skin, and nails. Unlike the fungi causing the deep mycoses, however, they are frequently transmitted from one host to another. A yeast, *Candida*, also produces a dermatophyte-like disease.

The deep-seated mycoses are of sporadic distribution, being very common in some parts of the world and unknown in other areas. They include histoplasmosis, blastomycosis, coccidioidomycosis, and paracoccidioidomycosis. The causative fungi appear to be soil-inhabiting saprophytes with peculiar abilities for adaptation to the internal environment of their host and are not transmitted from one individual to another. The species involved exhibit thermal dimorphism; *i.e.*, they exist as conidia-bearing mycelium in soil or culture at 25° C. and transform to parasitic form, usually a budding yeast, at 37° C. Infection follows inhalation of the canidia. Infection by the organism in an endemic area may be very common; however, few infections develop into the severe, deep, spreading, and sometimes fatal disease.

In recent years because of the use of or overuse of antibacterial antibiotics, immunosuppressive agents, cytotoxins, x-irradiation, and steroids, a new category of systemic mycoses has become very prominent. These are the opportunistic fungal infections. There has been a precipitous rise in these diseases. The patient, as a result of underlying disease or medical manipulation, is deprived of his normal defenses. This allows organisms of low inherent virulence to exploit the patient, who is now essentially a "culture medium." Such infections include systemic candidiasis, cryptococcosis, aspergillosis, and mucormycosis. Bacterial infections such as gram-negative septicemia, nocardiosis, *Pseudomonas*, etc.; protozoan infections such as *Pneumocystis carinii*; and viral opportunists such as cytomegalovirus also attack such patients. Multiple infections with various microorganisms are common.

There is a category of diseases that lies between the cutaneous infections and systemic infections. This group is known as the subcutaneous mycoses. It is a very heterogeneous group of fungal and bacterial diseases that are clinically similar. The etiological agents are soil organisms that gain entrance by traumatic implantation and gradually adapt to intratissue existence by various mechanisms, *e.g.,* grains, sclerotic cells, etc. The group includes mycetoma, chromoblastomycosis, sporotrichosis, and similar diseases.

A third group of microorganisms also treated in this chapter are the actinomycetes. These are bacteria which cause fungus-like infections and which were originally considered to be intermediate between fungi and bacteria. Morphologically, physiologically, and biochemically they are bacteria, are susceptible to antibacterial antibiotics, and are in no way related to fungi.

Two of the diseases discussed in this chapter, actinomycosis and candidiasis, are caused by endogenous organisms, that is, species which are part of the normal flora of man. All other fungal and actinomycetous infections are exogenous in origin.

Of the nearly 100,000 species of fungi only a very few are known to be frequent infectious agents of man and higher animals. With the exception of a few anthropophilic (restricted to man) dermatophytes, none of this group is an obligate parasite and most are misplaced soil saprophytes. The dermatophytes are frequently contagious, and man may serve as a disseminator of the species. Infection by the agents of the deep mycoses, however, seems to be a blind alley for the invading organism, for the parasite dies with its host. From a general biological point of view, the pathogenicity of certain fungi is of very minor significance; from that of the parasitized host, man, it is of considerably greater interest. The ability to produce disease in man, then, is an accidental phenomenon not necessary for the dissemination of the fungal species.

The fungi are structurally complex. They produce a variety of reproductive structures associated with sexual and asexual processes (also called teleomorphic and anamorphic stages) in addition to vegetative nonreproductive elements. Their differentiation into genera, species, and varieties is made in large part on a morphological basis, especially the morphology of the reproductive structures. In contrast to the bacteria, the physiological and immunological characteristics of fungi are usually of minor or no importance for purposes of differentiation or identification. The biochemistry of the fungi, and of the molds in particular, has been extensively investigated in connection with the elucidation of decompositions of organic material in nature and their application to industrial fermentation processes. Present knowledge of the respiratory mechanism of the cell and of alcoholic fermentation derives in very large part from studies of yeasts.

The immunological properties of the fungi have been studied also. The allergic phenomena associated with infection by certain of the dermatophytes and yeast-like fungi and frank allergy, *i.e.,* asthma associated with fungal conidia, have been of particular interest. The skin test, complement fixation test, and immunodiffusion test, which are occasionally helpful in diagnosis, have been the subjects of much investigation. Fungi are generally not good antigens, and the role of humoral immune defenses in the resolution of fungal disease is unclear. It appears that the cell-mediated defenses are the chief mechanism of the host for combating fungal invasion.

The tissue response of the host to the offending agent varies widely and depends somewhat on the variety of the invading organism. In dermatophyte infections, erythema is generally produced and is a response to the irritation to the presence of metabolic products of the organism. Occasionally, severe inflammation, followed by scar tissue and keloid formation, will occur. This is the result of an exaggerated inflammatory response and an allergic reaction to the organism and its products.

With organisms that invade living tissue, such as those responsible for subcutaneous and systemic disease, there is generally elicited a rather uniform acute pyogenic response. This usually gives way to a variety of chronic disease responses, listed in Tables 43–2 and 43–3.

Though a great many species of fungi have been described as pathogenic for man and animals, not all are of equal importance. Some, especially among the dermatophytes, are not legitimate species different from those already known. Furthermore, in many cases the fungus described probably had no causal relation to the pathological process from which it was isolated, and in others only one or two cases of infection have even been observed. It is sometimes very difficult to decide whether a fungus isolated from clinical material is of any etiological importance. Table 43–4 outlines laboratory procedures for the diagnosis of fungal infections. The accumulation of large numbers of species of fungi and the minutiae of their morphological differentiation have given medical mycology its complexity. Many skin, sputum, and air contaminants have been written into the literature as disease-producing

Table 43–2. **Tissue Reactions in Fungal Diseases**

Disease Responses and Histological Picture	Fungal Diseases and Agents

Chronic inflammation
  Lymphocytes, plasma cells, neutrophils, and
  fibroblasts; occasionally giant cells
	Rhinosporidium seeberi
	Entomophthoromycosis

Pyogenic reaction
  Acute or chronic, suppurative neutrophilic infiltrate
	Actinomyces israelii: sulfur granules, also lipid-laden
	  peripheral histiocytes
	Nocardia asteroides
	Acute aspergillosis
	Acute candidiasis

Mixed pyogenic and granulomatous reaction
  Neutrophilic infiltration and granulomatous reaction,
  lymphocytes, plasma cells
	Blastomyces dermatitidis
	Paracoccidioides brasiliensis
	Coccidioides immitis: neutrophils, especially at broken
	  spherule
	Sporothrix schenckii: organism rarely seen in tissue
	Chromoblastomycosis: chronic pyogenic and inflammatory
	  reaction, epithelioid cell nodules and giant cells (F.B.)
	Mycetoma: in addition may be large foamy giant cells
	  similar to xanthoma

Pseudoepitheliomatous hyperplasia
  Following chronic inflammation in the skin,
  hyperplasia of epidermal cells, hyperkeratosis,
  extension of rete pegs
	B. dermatitidis
	P. brasiliensis
	Chromoblastomycosis
	C. immitis

Histiocytic granuloma
  Histiocytes frequently with intracellular organisms,
  sometimes becoming multinucleate giant cells
	Histoplasma capsulatum
	Meningeal *C. neoformans*

Granuloma with caseation
  Granulomatous reaction, Langhans' giant cells
  (L.G.C.), central necrosis
	Histoplasma capsulatum
	Coccidioides immitis
	Sometimes pulmonary blastomycosis
	Rarely pulmonary cryptococcosis

Granuloma of "sarcoid" type Non-necrotizing	*Cryptococcus neoformans* Occasionally *Histoplasma capsulatum*

Fibrocaseous pulmonary granuloma, "tuberculoma"	*H. capsulatum:* thick fibrous wall surrounding epithelioid
	  and L.G.C. organisms in soft center, often calcification
	C. immitis: thin fibrous wall, occasionally calcified
	C. neoformans: poorly defined but occasionally
	  encapsulated, fibrosed, and rarely calcified

Thrombotic arteritis
  Thrombosis, purulent coagulative necrosis, invasion of
  vessel
	Aspergillosis
	Mucormycosis
	Acute candidiasis

Fibrosis
  Proliferating fibroblasts, deposition of collagen—
  resembles keloid
	Loboa loboi (lobomycosis)

Sclerosing foreign body granuloma In paranasal sinuses or following viral infection	*Aspergillus* sp.: bizarre hyphae in giant cells

organisms. On the other hand, the potential for invasion is widespread among the "harmless" fungi, much as it is among the "harmless" bacteria. Mushroom fungi have been isolated from heart valves following surgery, just as common soil bacteria (*Serratia marcescens*) have been involved in fatal meningitis after long-term steroid therapy. This emerging spectrum of opportunistic infections by so-called harmless microorganisms has been referred to euphemistically as "diseases of medical progress." Here we shall be concerned only with the more important fungi known to be causally related to human disease. The remainder, including many of the "new" opportunists, are associated with only a small fraction of the fungal diseases of man. These are discussed in specialized texts devoted to the field of medical mycology.[3, 5, 10]

Table 43–3. **Histopathology of Common Systemic Mycoses***

Fungal Form	Disease	Tissue Reaction
Mycelium (nonseptate)	Mucormycosis	Thrombotic arteritis, coagulative necrosis pyogenic reaction (4–7 nm.).
Mycelium (septate)	Aspergillosis Hyphomycosis Phaeohyphomycosis Nocardiosis	Acute pyogenic reaction, coagulative necrosis, suppurative neutrophilic infiltrate. *Aspergillus* and other agents of opportunistic infection have hyaline (clear) hypha, (3–5 nm.) (hyphomycosis); dematiaceous fungi have light brown hyphae in tissue (phaeohyphomycosis). Very thin mycelium (1 nm.) is found in nocardiosis.
Yeast	Histoplasmosis Blastomycosis Paracoccidioidomycosis Cryptococcosis Sporotrichosis	*Histoplasma* is found in histiocytic granuloma (intracellular, 1–3 nm.). Granuloma of tuberculoid type, caseation, calcification. *Blastomyces* is free or intracellular in giant cells (5–8 nm.), mixed pyogenic and granulomatous reaction. *Paracoccidioides* (15–20 nm.) same. *Cryptococcus* (encapsulated, 5–8 nm.) in sarcoid-type granuloma, little infiltrate. *Sporothrix* (2–5 nm.) is found in tuberculoid granuloma with plasma cell infiltrate.
Yeast and mycelium	Candidiasis	Pyogenic reaction, acute suppurative neutrophilic infiltrate (5–7 nm.).
Spherule with endospores	Coccidioidomycosis	Mixed pyogenic and granulomatous reaction similar to that for *Blastomyces* but with calcification (20–80 nm.).

*Hematoxylin-eosin shows fungi not stained or light basophilic; methenamine silver stain shows fungi and bacteria *(Nocardia)* black; periodic acid–Shiff shows fungi red, bacteria not stained.

Table 43–4. **Laboratory Procedures for the Diagnosis of Mycotic Infection**

I. Dermatophyte Infections and Cutaneous Candidiasis

Scraping of skin scales is imperative. One part of the specimen is examined as a KOH mount; the other is cultured on a Sabouraud's slant.
    a. Direct. Dermatophytes appear as branching septate mycelium in skin scales. *Candida* appears as masses of yeasts mixed with hyphal units.
    b. Culture. For dermatophytes, growth occurs in a week to 10 days; identification of species is difficult. *Candida* grows out in 24 to 48 hours and is quickly and easily identified.

II. Systemic Infections

Specimens include sputum, biopsy materials, bronchial brushings, spinal fluid, etc. Four procedures are carried out in the laboratory to assist in the diagnosis of fungal infections: direct examination, histology of biopsy and surgical specimens, culture, and serology. The relative importance of each varies with the disease, but the final criterion for an infection is the isolation and identification of the etiological agent.
  A. True Pathogenic Fungus Infections
    1. Histoplasmosis
      a. Direct. Examination of sputum is usually not rewarding. Sternal puncture is usually positive.
      b. Histology. The yeasts are fairly characteristic and can be identified with a fair degree of accuracy.
      c. Culture. The fungus requires two weeks to two months to grow out.
      d. Serology. Excellent correlation with disease state.
    2. Blastomycosis
      a. Direct. The best way to diagnose disease. KOH mount of sputum or aspiration of skin pustules if present.
      b. Histology. Broad-based budding yeast is quite characteristic.
      c. Culture. Slow—three weeks to three months or more.
      d. Serology. Not meaningful.
    3. Coccidioidomycosis
      a. Direct. Spherules found in sputum, pustules, etc.
      b. Histology. Spherules and endospores are readily identified.
      c. Culture. Rapid—grows out in a short time but is dangerous to handle.
      d. Serology. Excellent correlation to disease state.
  B. Opportunistic Infections

Systemic candidiasis, aspergillosis, mucormycosis, and cryptococcosis are more difficult to diagnose by laboratory procedures than the true pathogenic fungus infections.
    1. Candidiasis. Disseminated disease can be identified by direct examination of biopsy material, lesion material, etc. The organisms appear as yeast and mycelium in tissue, and culture easily. Serology is useful in some disease states. *Candida* is part of the normal flora of sputum, feces, and urine.
    2. Aspergillosis. Invasive pulmonary and disseminated disease is difficult to establish. Cultures of sputum are usually negative, and serology is often negative in immunosuppressed patients. In tissue organisms appear as branching septate mycelium indistinguishable from many other fungi. Culture of organ material is necessary for diagnosis. In aspergilloma, culture is usually negative but serology is positive and can be diagnostic.
    In allergic bronchopulmonary aspergillosis both sputum and serology are positive, as is direct examination of expectorated bronchial mucous plugs.
    3. Mucormycosis. Direct exam and culture of nasal debris in rhinocerebral disease are usually positive. Pulmonary and disseminated disease are usually diagnosed at autopsy. All agents appear as broad nonseptate hyphae in tissue. No serology.
    4. Cryptococcosis. Direct exam of spinal fluid is useful, as is direct exam of cutaneous lesions in disseminated disease. Encapsulated budding yeast is characteristic. Serology for capsular antigen is specific.

The Pathogenic Actinomycetes

The human pathogenic actinomycetes are bacteria and are classified in the order Actinomycetales. This order includes some chronic disease-producing organisms such as the etiological agents of tuberculosis and Hansen's disease (leprosy). By tradition these last two organisms have been studied along with other bacteria. The remaining pathogenic actinomycetes, however, were thought to be transitional forms between bacteria and fungi and were included in the sphere of medical mycology (Table 43–5). The etiological agents of lumpy jaw and actinomycotic mycetoma show some fungus-like characteristics, such as the branching of the organism in tissue, the extensive mycelial network that may occur in tissue or in culture, and the chronicity of the disease produced. However, cell wall analysis shows the presence of the typically bacterial muramic acid, which, along with the lack of a structural nucleus, typical bacterial size, and susceptibility to antibacterial antibiotics, defines these organisms as bacteria and not fungi. As far as their role as a phylogenetic "link" to the fungi is concerned, the presence of typical eucaryotic nuclei and mitochondria in fungous cells makes the derivation of the fungi from procaryotic bacteria independent of other eucaryotic organisms extremely improbable.

Table 43–5. **The Pathogenic Actinomycetes and Their Diseases**

Disease	Organism
Actinomycosis	*Actinomyces israelii* (man)
	Actinomyces bovis (cattle)
	Bifidobacterium adolescentis
	Actinomyces naeslundi
	Actinomyces viscosis
	Arachnica propionicus
Nocardiosis (pulmonary and systemic)	*Nocardia asteroides*
	Nocardia brasiliensis
Mycetoma (actinomycotic)	*Actinomadura madurae*
	Streptomyces somaliensis
	Actinomadura pelletierii
Erythrasma	*Corynebacterium minutissimum*
Cracked heel	*Nocardia keratolytica* (?)
Trichomycosis axillaris	*Corynebacterium tenuis*
Epidemic eczema	*Dermatophilis congolense*

Morphology

The organisms grow in the form of fine straight or wavy nonseptate filaments or hyphae 0.5 to 0.8 μm. in diameter which show both lateral and dichotomous branching and which may grow out from the medium to form an aerial mycelium. On solid mediums the filaments occur in tangled masses, while in liquid mediums there is a tendency to centers or clumps of growth. There are four genera of medical interest: the anaerobic or facultative *Actinomyces* and the aerobic *Nocardia, Streptomyces,* and *Actinomadura*. Classification of species within the genera and even separation of the genera themselves is controversial. The characteristics which follow are generally accepted by workers in the field.

Actinomyces includes organisms which are anaerobic or microaerophilic and non–acid–fast and in which the vegetative mycelium breaks up into bacillary or coccoid elements. The *Nocardia* are aerobic, sometimes partially acid–fast, and they fragment into bacillary or coccoid forms and produce chains of squared spores 1 to 2 μm. long by simple fragmentation of hyphal branches. The tips of other filaments may become swollen and club-shaped. Segmentation of the filaments occurs in some species as early as 24 hours, while in others it is delayed three weeks or more; the segmented filaments fragment to form bacillary bodies 4 to 6 μm. in length which are morphologically indistinguishable from many other bacteria. In most smear preparations of the pathogenic forms, the filaments are broken up and the appearance is that of ordinary bacilli. The cell walls of the nocardioform bacteria contain *meso*-diaminopimelic acid, arabinose, and galactose. The cell itself contains a lipid fraction (LCN) not found in other genera.

In *Streptomyces* there is more aerial mycelium, no fragmenting to bacillary or coccoid forms, and no acid-fastness, and chains of round to oval spores are produced consecutively within a specialized hyphal element. The maturation of the spore-bearing hyphae is often associated with the formation of spirals which range from open, barely perceptible coils to those which are so compressed that adjacent turns are in contact. The spirals may be dextrorse or sinistrorse; and both the direction and the tightness of coiling are constant within species. The spores are more resistant than the filaments and will survive 60° C. for as long as three hours, but are less resistant than bacterial spores. The cell walls of *Streptomyces* species contain LL-diaminopimelic acid and glycine. An additional genus of medical importance is that of *Actinomadura*. These organisms contain *meso*-diaminopimelic acid but no arabinose or LCN, thus separating themselves into a separate genus. All, or practically all, of the actinomycetes are gram-positive, and some of the pathogenic forms of *Nocardia* are partially acid-fast.

Both spores and fragments of mycelium grow in subculture. On solid mediums the growth of the aerobic forms is dry, tough, and leathery, sometimes wrinkled, adherent to and piled above the medium; in many instances it resembles the growth of mycobacteria. In some cases the growth appears powdery or chalky, owing to the formation of aerial mycelium. In liquid mediums growth occurs in the form of a dry, wrinkled surface film or, more often, as flakes or aggregates which adhere to the sides of the flask, especially at the surface, or sink to the bottom.

Pigment formation, with colors ranging over the entire spectrum, is common among the actinomycetes, and differentiation is usually made between pigmentation of the vegetative mycelium and the spore-bearing aerial mycelium, as well as on pigment diffusing into the medium. Soluble purple and brown pigments are often observed on protein-containing mediums. The actinomycetes, especially the saprophytic forms, are physiologically active, utilizing a variety of carbon and nitrogen compounds, and many are actively proteolytic. An earthy to musty odor, like that of freshly turned soil or of a damp basement, is produced by many species. The optimum temperature for growth is usually 20° to 30° C., although some of the pathogenic species grow at 37° C., and thermophilic species, analogous to thermophilic bacteria, are known. The great majority of actinomycetes are aerobic, but some of the pathogenic forms are anaerobic or at least must be cultivated under reduced oxygen tension.

Differentiation of the actinomycetes from one another is determined in part on a morphological and in part on a physiological basis, the latter including pigmentation and proteolytic activity.

Actinomycosis

Lumpy jaw or actinomycosis was once a fairly common disease of cattle and occasionally of man. Today it is an uncommon infection, most often diagnosed in retrospect. This change is largely due to the general betterment of oral hygiene, as the disease is most often associated with carious teeth and to the widespread practice of giving antibiotics for a variety of complaints and infections. The etiological agents *Actinomyces israelii, A. bovis, Bifidobacterium eriksonii (B. adolescentis)*, and others are quite sensitive to most antibacterial antibiotics, including penicillin and the sulfas. Formerly, infection was often associated with tooth extraction or dental surgery, which provided traumatized tissue in which these endogenous organisms could grow. Prophylactic antibiotics following oral procedures have eliminated this hazard, but even today most cases of actinomycosis are associated with dental caries.

Although the disease was undoubtedly observed early in the nineteenth century, actinomycotic tumors being described by Leblanc in 1826 under the name of osteosarcoma, it was first recognized as a specific parasitic disease by Bollinger in 1877. At his instigation the organism was studied by the botanist Harz, who described it and named it *Actinomyces* or ray fungus, because of the ray-like structure of its growth in the tissues, but he did not cultivate it. In 1891 Wolff and Israel isolated a microaerophilic actinomycete from pathological material by anaerobic culture, and in the same year an aerobic actinomycete was isolated by Bostroem from similar sources and named *A. hominis* (sometimes called *A. graminis*). Bostroem's organism has proved to be a contaminant, however, and it is definitely established that the organism isolated by Wolff and Israel was that observed by Bollinger and Harz and the etiological agent of the disease.

Presently, most workers agree that there are two commonly encountered species which cause the disease syndrome "lumpy jaw." *Actinomyces bovis* is the usual cause of actinomycosis in cattle and *A. israelii* the predominant organism in human infection although occasionally found in cattle also. *Bifidobacterium adolescentis, A. naeslundi, A. viscosis,* and *Arachnia propionicus* have also been isolated from actinomycosis, and in recent tabulations from England *A. viscosis* caused more cases of actinomycosis than *A. israelii.*

Morphology and Staining

Actinomycosis is essentially a suppurative process characterized by the presence in pus of yellow granules ("sulfur granules"). These are, in fact, colonies of the bacteria which when examined microscopically are seen to consist of dense rosettes of club-shaped filaments in radial arrangement. The individual rosettes are usually 30 to 40 μm. in diameter but sometimes are as large as 200 μm (Fig. 43–1A). The minute yellow granules, visible to the naked eye, may consist of a single rosette or may be made up of several. The rosette itself is made up of three kinds of structures: a central core of branching filaments, irregularly disposed but with a general radial arrangement; refringent, club-shaped bodies at the periphery, radially arranged; and spherical coccus-like bodies. The granules may be crushed and examined in fresh preparations in which the clubs may be plainly seen (Fig. 43–1B), or a stain such as eosin may be used which colors the sheath of the clubs. The filaments are gram-positive, and the stain is useful for tissue sections; hematoxylin-eosin is quite satisfactory for sections. The organisms are not acid-fast.

The filaments of the central core are branched, are often curved, sometimes spirally, and are thickly interlaced in a network of mycelium. The individual filaments have a granular appearance and, particularly in older granules, segmentation and fragmentation are common, giving the filaments the appearance of chains of cocci. The individual filaments in these granules, as well as the filaments of *Nocardia* species and the various agents found in actinomycotic mycetoma, have an average diameter of 1 μm., or about the diameter of *Escherichia coli*. The filaments in tissue of a fungus and the filaments in granules of mycotic mycetoma are about 4 μm. in diameter. This is a convenient method of assessing the cate-

gory of disease with which one is dealing. Appropriate antibacterial or antimycotic therapy can be instituted before the specific etiological agent has been isolated and identified.

The club-shaped bodies at the margin of the granule are conspicuous by their high light refringency and general structureless, homogeneous appearance (Fig. 43–1B). They are pear-shaped swellings of the terminal ends of the filaments and arise as distinct transformations of these. In young colonies the hyaline substance of which the clubs are composed is soft and may be dissolved in water, but as the age of the colony increases, the clubs become firmer in consistency. The firmness is due to the deposition of $Ca_3(PO_4)_2$. Their formation appears to be associated with the resistance of the tissues; when resistance to invasion is slight, they are absent, filaments alone being found. The clubs have been shown to contain antigen-antibody complexes.

The coccus-like bodies reported by various observers are probably of diverse nature. Such forms may result from the segmentation and fragmentation of filaments; in other cases they may be the ends of clubs appearing in the field of focus of the microscope.

A variety of other microorganisms will be seen in clinical cases of actinomycosis. These include various aerobic and anaerobic micrococci, diphtheroids, gram-negative bacilli, and fusiform bacilli, such as *Actinobacillus actinomycetemcomitans*, which may be a symbiont of some strains of *Actinomyces*. It is probable that the *Actinomyces* species alone could not induce an infectious process, without the other associated flora.

Morphology in Culture. The colonial mor-

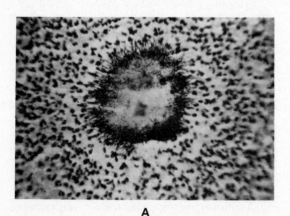

A

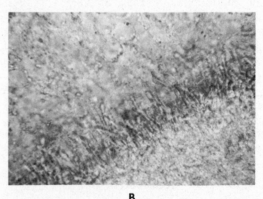

B

Figure 43–1. *A*, Gram stain of granule from actinomycosis. The radiating rays (Actinomyces = ray fungus) are gram positive. × 400. *B*, Wet mount of sulfur granule showing gelatinous club-shaped bodies on periphery of the granule, × 440. (Rippon, J. W.: Medical Mycology, 2nd ed. W. B. Saunders Co., Philadelphia, 1982.)

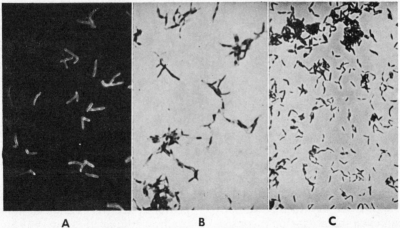

Figure 43–2. *Actinomyces israelii. A,* Darkfield, × 900. *B, C,* Gram stains of rough and smooth cultures, respectively. × 1200. (Rosebury, Epps, and Clark: J. Infect. Dis. **74:**131–149, 1944.)

phology of *A. bovis, A. israelii, A. viscosis,* and *A. naeslundi* grown anaerobically on solid medium is sufficiently distinctive that, with experience and the use of selected physiological characteristics, the organisms can be differentiated from those of contaminating bacteria and from each other.[1, 10] After four to six days' incubation the colonies are often less than 1 mm. in diameter. At this time, all four organisms are usually opaque or dead white, or, rarely, show a slight gray or yellow tinge. *Actinomyces israelii* is generally a rough colony (R form) starting as a mass of branching filaments ("spider" colony or granular colony) with a lace-like border and developing into a lobulated, glistening, "molar tooth" colony. The S variant or serotype II (Figs. 43–2, 43–3) may be transparent, be regular in form, and

resemble *A. bovis*. In broth *A. israelii* grows slowly, forming a hard, granular, fuzzy-edged colony. *Actinomyces bovis* is generally a smooth (S) form in which colonies are at first dewdrop-like and later smooth, convex, and with entire edges. The rare R variant may resemble *A. israelii*. In broth *A. bovis* produces a soft diffuse growth. The common mouth saprophyte, *A. naeslundi,* is generally smooth on agar and rapidly growing, with a diffuse or cloudy appearance in broth. It also grows aerobically after initial isolation; the others are microaerophilic after initial isolation. In physiological tests, *A, israelii* usually ferments xylose and mannitol, reduces nitrate, and does not hydrolyze starch; *A. bovis* hydrolyzes starch, does not reduce nitrates, and does not ferment xylose or mannitol; *A. naeslundi*

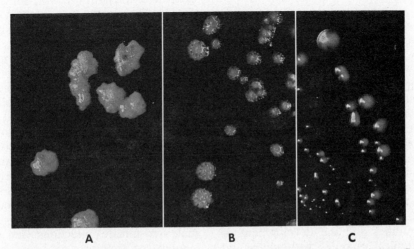

Figure 43–3. Colonies of *Actinomyces israelii* on brain-heart infusion agar after six days' incubation. *A, B,* Rough "molar tooth" types. × 3. *C,* Colonies of the smooth type. × 6. (Rosebury, Epps, and Clark: J. Infect. Dis. **74:**131–149, 1944.)

reduces nitrate, but does not ferment xylose or mannitol *Actinomyces viscosis* is similar to *A. bovis* but ferments raffinose and does not hydrolyze starch. All four organisms are separated from anaerobic diphtheroids by their cell wall composition.[10]

The essential features of the rosette or sulfur granule have been reproduced in cultures. The smaller colonies are rounded masses of branching and interlacing filaments. As the filaments become older they tend to fragment, and the largest colonies are dense opaque masses of short filaments and rod forms. Clubs are not formed in the usual mediums. "Soft" clubs may form in the presence of blood, serum, or ascitic fluid, and even there develop inconsistently. It is generally agreed that club formation in tissue is in large part a host response and is probably an antigen-antibody response akin to the Splendore-Hoepli phenomenon. The latter is observed as eosinophilic radiations seen in tissue infected with *Candida, Sporothrix, Schistosoma* eggs, etc. Stained smears of cultures show largely bacillary forms and a few fragments of branching filaments. The bacillary forms may be diphtheroid in appearance, they stain irregularly, and some have terminal swellings; the last are quite unlike the peripheral clubs of the actinomycetous granules.

Serology

Actinomyces israelii falls into two serotypes. Most infections are caused by the rough colony serotype I. A polyvalent antibody is available for fluorescent staining of *A. israelii* (serotypes I and II) and *A. naeslundi*

Pathogenicity for Experimental Animals

Attempts to infect experimental animals with *A. israelii* have, in general, been disappointing in that only a small proportion of inoculated animals develop the disease, and the lesions are limited and benign. Some success has been found by traumatizing the tissue first and including the associated flora with *A. israelii*. Experimental infection with pure culture has been achieved in mice, using hog gastric mucin to enhance the invasiveness of the organism. Repeated injections of the organism in rabbits and guinea pigs has met with less success. In the experimental disease the essential features of the natural infection are observed, including the formation of tubercle-like nodules and the development of structurally typical granules with clubs and sinus tracts.

Pathogenicity for Man

Infection with *A. israelii* during the first part of the twentieth century was diagnosed much more frequently than it is today. There has been a sharp decrease in the number of cases reported in the United States in contrast to the great increase in true fungal diseases. Probably the most important single cause in the decrease of actinomycosis is the widespread use of antibacterial antibiotics. Nichols and Herrel in 1948 reported on the successful use of penicillin in the disease, and this has been the standard therapy since that time. In patients allergic to penicillin, tetracycline has proved effective. Other antibiotics may be used as adjunct therapy, but alone these are of questionable efficacy. Another important aspect in the decline of infection is the high level of oral hygiene achieved in the developed nations of the world. That this is not the case in emerging nations is attested to by the continued numerous and increasing case reports of actinomycosis and related diseases in these areas.

The disease in man differs in minor respects from that in cattle. Actinomycotic infections of the bone are relatively less frequent, the disease being confined to the softer parts in most cases. There is usually a lesser production of new tissue and a more extensive softening and suppuration. The disease falls into three clinical types. About 60 per cent of the infections are cervicofacial, and this type is often associated with dental defects or accidents and is a chronic, localized form of the disease which is relatively benign and usually susceptible to treatment. Some 14 per cent of the cases are thoracic infections, and 8 to 18 per cent are abdominal infections in which the primary lesion is often in the appendix; in these types prognosis is poor. In recent years the cervicofacial type is often cured before diagnosis is made. For this reason the only forms of the disease that come to the attention of the clinician are the abdominal and thoracic. Draining sinuses are usually found in all types, and abscesses are frequently observed in the liver at autopsy. In recent years many cases of uterine infections have been reportedly associated with the use of the intrauterine device (IUD) for contraception. Generalization by hematogenous spread is occasionally seen and is relatively more common in man than in cattle. Meningitis, endocarditis, genital (both male and female) infections, and a syndrome similar to mycetoma have been reported. The characteristic granules with clubs are usually found in the pus but may be absent occasionally in draining sinuses, especially when the infection has spread rapidly. This is seen particularly in meningitis and empyema. These latter types of disease may terminate fatally in a few weeks through secondary infection or formation of emboli, or may drag along in a chronic form for many years. It is probable that the *Actinomyces* are normal flora of the gastrointestinal and genitourinary tracts as well as the oropharyngeal area. This would account for the observed cases of abdominal (especially in the appendix) and uterine disease in the absence of other symptoms. A few cases of generalized actinomycosis and osseous disease have been attributed to a newly described species, *A. meyeri*.

Immunity

Agglutinins, precipitins, and complement-fixing antibodies have been demonstrated in the serum of patients with actinomycosis. None of the tests are of diagnostic significance. There is little or no evidence that they are involved in combating the disease or protecting the individual against the disease. Active defense against the organism is probably on a cellular level, and it has been suggested that the "clubbing" of the organism seen on the periphery of the granule represents a response to the cellular defense of the host.

Isolation and Diagnosis

As indicated earlier, the demonstration of the typical actinomycetous rosette or sulfur granule in the tissue or pus of a specimen is sufficient to establish a diagnosis of actinomycosis in man. Actinomycosis in cattle may be confused with actinobacillosis. The two are readily differentiated by examination of a gram-stained smear for the presence of gram-positive diphtheroid-like fragments of *Actinomyces* filaments or of gram-negative actinobacilli. As may be inferred from the foregoing discussion, animal inoculation is useless as a diagnostic method. Cultivation of the bacteria is often, though not always, successful. In most laboratories a BHI blood- or Columbia blood-agar plate streaked with lesion material and incubated anaerobically will suffice. By the end of 48 hours spider-like colonies should be transferred for pure culture studies (see Fig. 43–3).

Nocardiosis

Several species of aerobic actinomycetes are capable of causing human disease. All of these organisms are soil organisms and infection is endogenous. It is suggested, however, that *Nocardia asteroides* may be at least a transient member of normal pulmonary flora. Although preexisting lung disease may favor a frank infection by the organism, this is not a necessary prerequisite. *Nocardia asteroides*, *N. brasiliensis*, and *N. caviae* are the accepted etiological agents of the clinical entity nocardiosis. *Nocardia asteroides* is more commonly associated with disease in debilitated patients and thus is an opportunistic organism. The more virulent *N. brasiliensis* can also elicit disease in normal patients, leading to a condition known as pulmonary mycetoma. This type of disease is not infrequently encountered in parts of Mexico. Recently several systemic cases caused by *N. caviae* have been reported.

The genus *Nocardia* was erected by Trevisan in honor of Nocard in 1889. Nocard had earlier described an aerobic, partially acid-fast, branching bacillus from cattle as the causative agent of a disease called farcy. His report concerned an epidemic in cattle on the island of Guadeloupe. The first description of the disease in human patients was made in 1890 by Eppinger, who isolated an aerobic, branching, fungus-like organism from pulmonary and central nervous system lesions. The name *N. asteroides* was first used by Blanchard in 1895 in referring to the *Cladothrix asteroides* described by Eppinger.

The genus *Nocardia* formerly contained various species isolated from the clinical entity mycetoma. Most of these species have been placed in the genus *Streptomyces* or in the genus *Actinomadura* and are discussed under the heading Mycetoma. The remaining species, *N. brasiliensis*, is a common cause of mycetoma and is described with the other agents. This organism can also cause systemic (opportunistic) nocardiosis.

There is a broad spectrum of disease elicited by *N. asteroides* infection. The primary disease, which is pulmonary, is by far the most common manifestation of infection and varies from single lesions and scattered infiltrations to lobar consolidation and cavitation. The disease picture resembles that in tuberculosis, histoplasmosis, or other mycotic infections. *Candida albicans* superinfection may occur in this as in other mycotic diseases, and it is necessary to search thoroughly for an underlying agent.

Hematogenous spread of the infection may result in a secondary infection of the brain. Occasionally, there may be minimal infection in the lung, and the presenting symptoms are extrapulmonary. The kidneys, spleen, liver, and adrenals may be involved; however, in contrast to *A. israelii* infection, bony involvement is rare. The rare reported cases of *N. asteroides* mycetoma are difficult to assess, as there is no clear differentiation from *N. caviae*, an organism frequently reported from mycetoma. Nocardiosis is one of the major hazards as an opportunistic infection in debilitated patients, especially those on steroid or immunosuppressive therapy.

Serology and Immunity

At present there is no standard serological procedure for the diagnosis of this disease, and the question of specific immunity is unclear.

Pathogenicity for Lower Animals

The most frequently involved domestic animal is the dog. Similar types of pathology are seen in both animal and human infections. Cattle are also involved with infection, some in epidemic numbers. The relation of farcy of cattle to *N. asteroides* has been discussed. The organism also infects fish. In all such animals there was a predisposing condition or disease.

Isolation and Diagnosis

In gross examination, lesion material cannot be differentiated from that in other infections caused by pyogenic bacteria. The tissue reaction, like that of *A. israelii,* is of the pyogenic type: acute or chronic suppuration with neutrophilic infiltration. The organism is best seen in tissue sections stained by the Brown and Breen modification of the Gram stain (Fig. 43–4). The Gomori methenamine stain is also useful. Periodic acid-Schiff (PAS) and hematoxylin and eosin (H and E) stains are not helpful. Fine branching filaments, 1 μm. in diameter, are seen coursing through the tissue (Fig. 43–4). There is a lack of agglomeration or granule formation, as is seen in *A. israelii* infection. Otherwise it is not possible to differentiate the two except by culture.

The organism grows well but slowly on all laboratory mediums and is usually not killed by the digestion procedure used on sputa for culture of tubercle bacilli. The classic colony is glabrous, wrinkled, folded, and bright orange. Variations from smooth, glistening yeast-like colonies to dry, powdery colonies with abundant aerial mycelia have been described. The color range recorded includes pink, lavender, salmon, white, buff, and brown.

Prognosis of the disease depends on early

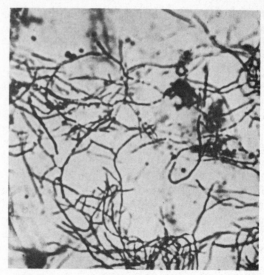

Figure 43–4. *Nocardia asteroides.* Gram stain of sputum. Note the long branched mycelium. × 900.

diagnosis and treatment. There has been a notable lack of success in established infections, especially those with extrapulmonary lesions. Sulfonamides are the favored drugs, particularly sulfadiazine. At present sulfamethoxyzole in combination with trimethoprim is the treatment of choice.

Other Actinomycetous Infections

Erythrasma

This disease was first described by Buchardt in 1859, and the term erythrasma was used by Barensprung in 1862. Skin scales examined by these authors showed delicate filaments which they believed to be of fungal origin. They named the organism *Microsporum minutissimum.* In skin scales and on culture the organisms appear as gram-positive rods and filaments sometimes with granules. The scaling infected area of the patient and the colonies of the organism, when grown on tissue culture medium number 199 agar, show a coral red fluorescence which aids in its diagnosis. The disease itself is characterized by a punctate to palm-sized, well-circumscribed, maculopapular rash on the epidermis. The color varies from light brown to red or reddish brown. The advancing border is serpiginous and erythematous. The lesion is greasy looking and is covered with small furfuraceous scales. The most common form is genitocrural in the male, although other areas and other groups may be affected. It has been found that infection of the toe web may occur in about one-fourth of the population. Systemic erythromycin is the drug of choice. At present the organism is called *Corynebacterium minutissimum.*

Cracked Heel (Pitted Keratolysis)

This disease, also called keratolysis plantare sulcatum, was first described in India, but recently Zaias and co-workers have shown it to be of worldwide distribution. The etiological agent remains obscure but appears to be an actinomycete, either *Nocardia* or *Micromonospora keratolytica.* The bacteria appear to have a lytic action on the horny layer of the epidermis, and the disease is characterized by solution of the thick horny skin of the plantar surface into grooves. The skin cracks along these grooves to form deep fissures on the heel and in the thick sodden skin between the toes. These fissures extend through the corium to the subcutaneous tissues. Secondary infection is common. A similar disease, ulcus interdigitale, may occur on the toes. Treatment consists in good hygiene, the wearing of shoes, and formalin soaks.

Trichomycosis Axillaris

This disease is characterized by yellow *(flava)*, red *(rubra)*, or black *(nigra)* concretions on the shaft of axillary or pubic hair. Perspiration in the affected area may be accordingly discolored and stain the clothing, this being the most common presenting condition. There is no other discomfort to the patient. Recently, an investigation of 100 consecutive patients revealed 28 cases of the flava variety without the patient's being aware of the infection. The disease may be more common than formerly considered. The organism has been named *Corynebacterium tenuis* and the flava variety will fluoresce under the Wood's lamp. It is probable that a number of organisms are involved or are capable of producing the symptoms. Treatment includes depilation, alcoholic formalin solution 1 per cent, and sulfur ointment. McBride has shown that the organism absorbs colored products of the environment and that the different varieties are probably due to the diet of the patient.

Dermatophilosis (Epidemic Eczema, Contagious Dermatitis, Streptotrichosis)

This disease was first described by Van Saceghem in 1915 as a skin disease of cattle. He named the etiologic agent *Dermatophilis congolense.* Other isolates from cattle, sheep, deer, and horses have been given different names, but Gordon concludes they are varia-

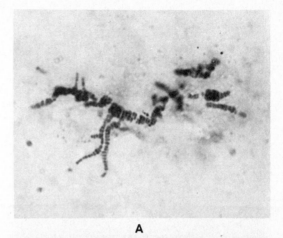

A

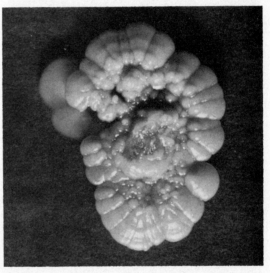

B

Figure 43–5. Dermatophilosis. *A,* Stained smear showing irregular, branched filaments. These are divided both longitudinally and transversely, forming packets of coccoid cells. *B,* Colony of *Dermatophilus congolensis* after five days' growth on brain-heart infusion of glucose blood agar. (Rippon, J. W.: Medical Mycology. 2nd ed. W. B. Saunders Co., Philadelphia, 1982.)

tions of a single species. The organism was first reported in the United States in 1961 and since has been reported from cattle, horse, deer, and man in Texas, Iowa, and New York. It now appears that the organism is of worldwide distribution. Roberts believes the species to be a natural parasite of the epidermis of sheep.

Dermatophilis congolense grows in culture as a moist, lumpy (Fig. 43–5*A*) yellowish colony and microscopically as a branching mycelial mass in which the hyphal elements enlarge and go through a series of longitudinal and transverse divisions (Fig. 43–5*B*) to form a motile coccal form. The motile stage formation

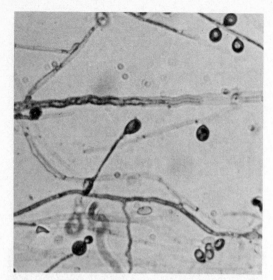

Figure 43–6. *Pseudallescheria boydii.* The colony is mouse-gray and fluffy. Culture mounted in lactophenol–cotton blue solution; single spore on elongate conidiophore. × 400.

is stimulated by low temperature, restricted nutrients, excess aeration, and moisture. The organism is a true epidermal parasite normally not penetrating the dermal-epidermal junction. The disease in sheep is characterized by erythematous, exudative, scaling lesions which develop into pyramidal scabby masses. This condition is sometimes called lumpy wool. The organism is spread by contact and ectoparasites and is favored by cold, damp conditions.

Mycetoma

Mycetoma (fungus tumor, maduromycosis) is a clinical syndrome which may have either a fungal or a bacterial etiology (Tables 43–6 and 43–7). It consists of the clinical triad of tumefaction, sinus tracts, and granular particles. Though the mode of infection, type of tissue reaction, and general course of disease are similar, the choice of treatment depends entirely on knowing whether the infection is bacterial or fungal in origin. The first cases of this infection were reported from southern India (1842 *et seq.*) and became known as Madura foot. It is mainly a disease of tropical climates and appears usually in persons who do not wear shoes. The infection is frequently seen in temperate areas about the Mediterranean and in North Africa, Greece, and Italy. It also regularly occurs in Mexico, Central and South America, and the Caribbean Islands. Cases are sporadically seen in Europe and the United States. Most of the etiological agents are worldwide in distribution, but some are more common in one area than another, such as *Streptomyces somaliensis* in North Africa or *Nocardia brasiliensis* in Mexico.

The disease usually affects the foot, occasionally the hands, and more rarely other parts of the body. There are exceptions, as *Nocardia brasiliensis* is commonly associated with pulmonary infections, from where it may spread systemically. In most cases the organism presumably enters by traumatic implantation into tissue. There is some evidence that it may remain latent for some time, even a period of years, and become active following repeated injury. The part first involved, usually the sole of the foot, shows a small subcutaneous swelling which slowly enlarges and softens to become phlegmonous. It ruptures to the surface, sinus tracts form, and the process burrows into the deeper tissues, producing swelling and distortion of the foot. The bones may or may not be extensively involved. Numerous small eminences are found on the surfaces, each the

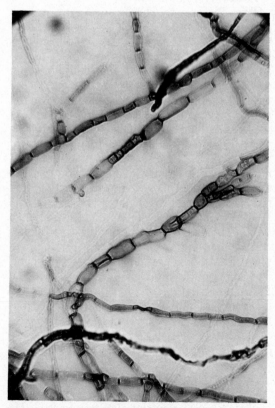

Figure 43–7. *Madurella grisea.* Mycelia of two widths and chains of chlamydospores characteristic of the species. (Rippon, J. W.: Medical Mycology. 2nd ed. W. B. Saunders Co., Philadelphia, 1982.)

Table 43–6. **Actinomycotic Mycetoma**

Species	Grain	Histology [H and E]	Colonial and Microscopic Characteristics	Physiological Profile*							
				C	T	X	St	Gel	U	Ax	L
Nocardia asteroides†	Rare; white soft, irregular, 1 mm.	Homogeneous loose clumps of filaments; rare clubs.	Rapid growth (37° C.); glabrous, folded, heaped; orange-yellow, tan, etc. Short rods and cocci; rare branched filaments; acid-fast.	−	−	−	−‡	−	+	−	+
Nocardia brasiliensis	White to yellow, soft, lobed, 1 mm.	Same as above; clubs common.	Rapid growth (30° C.); colonial and microscopic same as above; acid-fast.	+	+	−	−‡	+	+	−	+
Nocardia caviae	Same as above.	Same as above; clubs occasionally seen	Same as above; acid-fast.	−	−	+	−‡	−	+	−	+
Actinomadura madurae	White, rarely pink, soft, oval to lobed, large, 5 mm.	Center empty, amorphous; dense mantle peripherally; basophilic wide pink border; loose fringe; clubs.	Rapid growth (37° C.); cream white, rarely clot red; wrinkled, glabrous. Delicate nonfragmenting branched filaments; arthrospores; non-acid-fast.	+	+	−	+	+	−	+	−
Actinomadura pelletierii	Red, hard, oval to lobed, small, 1 mm.	Round, homogeneous, dark-staining; light peripheral band; hard—fractures easily; no clubs.	Slow growth (37° C.); small, dry, glabrous; light to garnet red. Delicate nonfragmenting branched filaments; non-acid-fast.	+	+	−	−‡	+	−	−	−
Streptomyces somaliensis	Yellow, hard, round to oval, large, 2 mm.	Variable size; amorphous center; light purple with pink patches; dark filaments at edge, entire; no clubs.	Slow growth (30° C.); cream to brown, wrinkled, glabrous. Delicate nonfragmenting branched filaments; arthrospores; non-acid-fast.	+	+	−	±	+	−	−	−

Actinomyces israelii is also a cause of light-grained mycetoma. Consult text for identification.

*Abbreviations: C = casein; T = tyrosine; X = xanthine; St = starch (amylolytic); Gel = gelatin (proteolytic); U = urea; AX = acid from arabinose and xylose, L = growth in lysozyme; + = positive; − = negative; ± = not determined or variable.
†It is probable that the reports of *N. asteroides* causing mycetoma are cases of infection by *N. caviae.*
‡Some strains are positive.

Table 43–7. Mycotic Mycetoma (Tissue Dimorphic Fungi)

Species	Grain	Histology (H and E)	Colonial and Microscopic Characteristics	Physiological Profile*						
				St	Gel	G	Gal	L	M	S
Pseudallescheria boydii	White, soft, oval to lobed, <2 mm.	Hyaline hyphae, 5 μm; huge swollen cells, <20 μm.; no cement; red border; pink periphery.	Rapid growth (30°–37° C.); fluffy mouse-gray. Large 7 μm. unicellular aleuriospore conidia on simple conidiophore or coremia (see Fig. 31–6); black cleistothecia.	+	+	+	+	0	0	0
Madurella grisea	Black, soft to firm, oval to lobed, <1 mm.	Little dark cement in edge; polygonal cells in periphery; center hyaline mycelium.	Very slow growth (30° C.); leathery tan-gray, later downy. Diffusible pigment. Arthrospore-like heavy septation of mycelium. Mycelium alternates thick to thin (see Fig. 31–7).	+	–	+	+	0	+	+
Madurella mycetomatis	Black, firm to brittle, oval to lobed, <2 mm.	Compact type with brown-staining cement; vesicular type with brown cement only at edge; swollen cells, <15 μm. center hyaline mycelium.	Very slow growth (37° C.); downy, velvety, smooth or ridged; cream apricot to ochre. Diffusible brown pigment; black sclerotia, <2 mm.; rare conidia, phialids.	+	±	+	+	+	+	0
Acremonium kiliense	White, soft, irregular, <1.5 mm.	No cement; hyaline hyphae >4 μm.; swollen cells, >12 μm.	White glabrous colony (30° C.); later downy. Violet pigment diffusible; curved septate; conidia arranged as head on simple conidiophore.	0	±					
Exophiala jeanselmei	Black, soft, irregular to vermiscular.	Helicoid to serpiginous; center often hollow; no cement; vesicular cells, <10 μm.; brown hyphae.	Slow growth (30° C.); leathery black moist, later velvety. Reverse black; toruloid yeast cells, moniliform cells, long tubular phialids.	0	0	+	+	0	+	+
Leptosphoeria senegalensis	Black, soft, irregular, ~1 mm.	Black hyphae; cement in periphery; center hyaline.	Rapid growth; downy gray. Reverse black—rare rose pigment diffusible; black perithecia, <300 μm.; septate ascospores, 25 × 10 μm.							

*Abbreviations: St = starch; Gel = gelatin; G = glucose; Gal = galactose; L = lactose; M = maltose; S = sucrose; + = positive; – = negative; 0 = not determined or variable.

orifice of a sinus. The discharge is a viscid, slightly purulent, often foul-smelling fluid containing granular particles up to 1 mm. in diameter. The presence of these grains separates the mycetomas from pseudomycetomatous conditions observed in yaws, sporotrichosis, etc. In general the actinomycotic mycetoma are characterized by invasion and destruction of bone and a hyperplasia "collar" of tissue around the sinus tract opening. The eumycotic agents less often invade the bony structures.

Examination of the granules will reveal whether the disease is one of the two types of mycetoma or is the mycetoma-like disease, botryomycosis, caused by *Staphylococcus epidermidis* or other bacteria. If the disease is mycetoma, careful examination of the granule (and subsequent confirmation by culture) will reveal which of the two groups is the etiological agent. The most obvious clinical difference in the mycetomas is the color of the grains present in the discharge. These may be white, yellow, red, or black. The grains of microcolonies are composed of mycelial filaments of the organism. One of the agents, *Actinomadura madurae*, has been shown to elaborate a powerful collagenase which is responsible for its ability to infect and cause the disease. If the granule is composed of very thin (1 μm. in diameter) intertwined mycelial elements, often with peripheral club cells, it is bacterial (actinomycotic mycetoma); mycelial elements more than 1 μm. in diameter showing individual cells, septation, and usually chlamydospore production are found in fungal (mycotic mycetoma) infections. Actinomycotic mycetoma is treated with the usual antibacterial antibiotics such as penicillin, tetracyclines, sulfonamides, trimethoprim, and diaminodiphenyl sulfone. Much less success has been observed in the treatment of mycotic mycetoma. Intra-venous amphotericin B has been used, with remission of the disease in some cases. The new imidazole, miconazole, is being given clinical trials, as is ketoconazole. They are effective in some systemic mycoses. There is at present no efficacious treatment for mycotic mycetoma. Amputation as a last resort is often necessary.

The disease is usually local, and secondary abscesses seldom occur, except in cases caused by *N. brasiliensis*. In cases resistant to therapy or with extreme tissue destruction surgical removal of the infected tissues, usually involving amputation, is necessary and curative. Occasionally the organisms associated with mycetoma may be involved in quite different infectious processes, such as *P. boydii* in prostate, eye, pulmonary, and systemic infections.

Laboratory Diagnosis

As indicated above, the mycetomas are characterized by the presence of granules in the discharge (see Tables 43–6 and 43–7). The grains may be hard and are usually treated with strong (20 per cent) sodium hydroxide to dissolve the pigment and debris and to permit examination in a wet mount (unstained) for the presence of tangled mycelial filaments. Clubs may be observed in actinomycetous infections, and thalloconidia (sclerocysts), heavy-walled homogeneous structures, are found in *Madurella* and other fungus infections. For differentiation and identification, culture is necessary on enriched meat mediums (BHI agar) for actinomycetes, and Sabouraud's agar in the case of fungal etiology. Serology has been little used in mycetomas. Usually no antibody titers can be detected except in the more extensive infections, as occurs in *N. brasiliensis* pulmonary and systemic involvement.

The Pathogenic Fungi

The fungi proper, or Eumycetes, are quite distinct from the true bacteria in size, cell structure, nuclear structure, and chemical composition. Differences in cell wall composition and nuclear structure were previously discussed under the section on actinomycetes. Though fungi are essentially single-celled organisms, in some fungal species the cells may show various degrees of specialization. The simplest morphological form is the single-celled building yeast. Elongation of the cell without separation of newly formed cells results in a thread-like hypha. An intertwined mass of **hyphae** is called a **mycelium**. The mycelial mat is known as a **thallus** and, in most of the fungi discussed here, consists of a loose network of hyphae. In some higher forms, hyphae are cemented together to form large, structurally complex fruiting bodies, such as the mushrooms and puffballs. Some of the giant puffballs *(Calvatia)* may weigh more than 60 pounds. Even though attaining such great size, all fungi are still primitive organisms: any separated single cell from a 60-pound puffball can regrow the entire structure. This is called reversible specialization. This ability separates the fungi, protozoa, and algae from higher forms, such as trees and mammals, in which specialization of cells into tissues is not reversible.

Two main structural types of mycelium may be distinguished. In one of these the cells making up the hyphae are not separated by cross-walls or septa, making possible the characteristic flowing of protoplasm and nuclei through the structure. Such a structure is said to be **nonseptate** or **coenocytic** and is characteristic of the phylum Zygomycota. This group contains the agents of mucormycosis. In the majority of fungi, however, the hyphae are **septate**, each cell separated from the other by cross-walls. The septations have "holes" in them so that there may be free flow of cytoplasmic material. Nuclear migration is possible in the Ascomycota, which have a large pore in the intercellular septa. In this phylum are the dermatophytes, *Histoplasma, Blastomyces, Aspergillus,* and many other medically important fungi. A special structure, comprising the dolipore and parenthesome, prohibits nuclear migration in the Basidiomycota. Each basidiomycete cell contains two dissimilar nuclei (dikaryon), one derived from one parent or mating type and the other from the other parent. The mycelium of this latter group may also show a special bridge structure connecting one cell to the cell next in line. This is called a clamp connection and is involved in nuclear transfer to a newly formed cell. The phylum Basidiomycota contain smuts, rusts, mushrooms, and *Cryptococcus neoformans.* Thus these three main classes of fungi may be distinguished in part on the basis of the structure of the mature nonconidiating hyphae, though this is not one of the main characteristics upon which their mycological differentiation is made.

The mycelium is further differentiated into two general types which differ in function. One of these, the **vegetative mycelium**, consists of masses of hyphae within the colony, adjacent to and growing into the substrate, and is concerned with the assimilation of food materials. Fragments of such mycelia will reproduce if transferred. The other type, the **reproductive mycelium**, usually extends into the air to form an aerial mycelium and gives rise to reproductive bodies—**conidia** or spores. The mode of conidia or spore formation and the structure of the conidia or spore-bearing elements are the characteristics by which the fungi are differentiated, classified, and identified. Many fungi have two methods of reproduction: the most common being asexual, now called the **anamorph state**; the other being sexual or the **teleomorph state**. In general, the asexual conidia are seen in the laboratory and are the forms used for identification.

In addition to conidiation and the vegetative growth of hyphae, many species of fungi reproduce by the separation of cells, known as **oidia**, from any part of the mycelium. These vegetative reproductive forms may give rise to new mycelium or reproduce themselves by budding like the yeasts, according to the environment in which they are placed. *Candida, Mucor,* and *Histoplasma* are capable of sustained yeast-like growth, depending on the environment.

Spore and Conidia Formation

Two kinds of spores are to be distinguished. The sexual spores (teleomorph) are produced by the fusion of two cells, which may or may not come from different thalli. The asexual (anamorph) conidia arise by differentiation of the cells of the hyphae without fusion. If a sexual spore is produced only with a nucleus from another mating type, the fungus is said to be **heterothallic**. If any nucleus from within the same thallus will serve in forming sex spores, the fungus is **homothallic**. Fungi for which both sexual and asexual types of spore formation are known are "perfect fungi" and may be further differentiated on the basis of differences in the fruiting body that results from sexual fusion. Differences in type, size, and color of sexual cells along with other morphological characteristics are used in classifying the organism into phylum, class, order, family, genus, and species. The three phyla of fungi which have species involved in human infections are distinguished by their method of sex spore formation. These are Zygomycota, Ascomycota, and Basidiomycota. A fourth group is the form-phylum Deuteromycota, or Fungi Imperfecti. In this group no "perfect" or sexual (teleomorph) state has yet been found.

Sexual Spore Formation. The most common members of the Zygomycota that are of medical importance are species of the genera *Mucor* and *Rhizopus.* These molds produce a sexual spore known as a zygospore by the fusion of neighboring filaments of the same or different thalli. It is usually hard and black. When mature it cracks open to give rise to a sporangium and sporangiospores. These are similar to the asexual method of reproduction in these species. The Ascomycota, which include a number of genera of plant pathogens and animal pathogens, certain strains of *Penicillium* and *Aspergillus,* and many of the yeasts, form sexual spores known as ascospores because they are contained in an ascus or sac. Their formation is simplest in the yeasts. Two contiguous cells fuse by means of minute tube-like processes, the nuclei unite, and the resulting single diploid nucleus divides several times to give four or eight haploid nuclei. Reserve material accumulates about each nucleus, a spore wall is formed, and the cell containing this is the ascus. In most of the Ascomycota the process is somewhat more complex, and the cells which fuse may be distinguishable and are termed the archegonium and antheridium. The cell resulting from this fusion gives rise to new hyphae. It then goes through a complex structural development called crozier formation, with the next to last cell being binucleate. These nuclei fuse and then divide to form the ascospores.

The basidiospores, the reproductive unit of the Basidiomycota, are also formed by a complex process including clamp connection formation, by which one nucleus of a mated pair travels from one cell to a newly formed cell. The other nucleus goes by the "center road" through the middle of the cell to the newly formed cell. Each cell contains two dissimilar haploid nuclei (dikaryon condition). The nuclei finally fuse in a club-like structure called a basidium and give rise to four externally attached basidiospores. They, like most all other fungal spores, are haploid. Basidia line the gills of the mushrooms, are found in crypts inside puffballs, and line the spores in Boletes. So far, only a few of the Basidiomycetes have been involved in human infection, *e.g., Cryptococcus neoformans.* The Ascomycetes include *Piedraia hortai* (black piedra), *Pseudallescheria boydii* (mycetoma), and the dermatophytes (usually known by their anamorph name) *Histoplasma* and *Blastomyces.* The Zygomycota are represented by *Mucor, Rhizopus,* and *Basidiobolus.* Many pathogenic fungi have no known sexual phase and are classed as Fungi Imperfecti.

Fungi Imperfecti. The "imperfect fungi" or Fungi Imperfecti (Deuteromycota) have only an anamorph state. They reproduce asexually, usually by conidia. The group is necessarily provisional, and various species of fungi are removed from it from time to time as their teleomorph or sexual phases are discovered. The classification of the organisms in the Deu-

teromycota is based on asexual conidia-type formation, color, shape, size, etc. Often an organism will be given a name based on its anamorph characteristics before its sexual stage is known. Later, when a teleomorph stage is discovered, a name descriptive and taxonomically meaningful will also be given to it. This sometimes leads to two names for the same organism. It may be confusing at first, but it is taxonomically legal, for example, for the dermatophyte anamorph state to be *Microsporum gypseum* and its teleomorph (sexual or "perfect") state to be *Nannizzia gypsea.* To add to the confusion, the organism we call *M. gypseum* is the anamorph stage of two species of perfect fungi, *N. gypsea* and *N. incurvata.* This emphasizes the concept of Fungi Imperfecti as being simply a convenient descriptive filing cabinet for species waiting to be assigned to meaningful categories when their sexual mechanisms are discovered.

The Deuteromycota contains two classes of medically important fungi: the Blastomycetes, which include *Candida* sp. and other anamorph yeasts, and the Hyphomycetes, which include mycelial fungi. This latter class contains two important families: the Moniliaceae, which have colorless (hyaline) cell walls, and the Dematiaceae, which have pigmented brown cell walls or conidia. In tissue, mycelium of organisms of the latter family are thus brown and the infection called phaeohyphomycosis.

Microscopic Examination. The methods used in the microscopic examination of the fungi vary somewhat according to the nature of the material and the purpose of the examination. In general, the staining methods so used in the study of the bacteria are not applicable; the fungi are almost all gram-positive and may be found in gram-stained smears, but their morphology is obscured. Wet mounts, unstained or lightly stained, are most informative.

Specimens. Open or draining lesions are almost always so heavily contaminated by secondary bacterial invasion that fungi are very difficult to find. In material from surgically opened lesions they are usually demonstrable though not so numerous as bacteria in corresponding bacterial infections. A simple method to show the yeast cells, mycetoma granules, or mycelial units in pus, exudate, or sputum is to treat the specimen with potassium hydroxide (KOH mount) in the manner described below. In the dermatomycoses, secondary bacterial infection ordinarily does not interfere with the microscopic demonstration of the fungus elements. The dermatophytes live in keratin material exclusively, and specimens should be taken from scrapings of horny layers, tops of vesicles, scrapings from nail plates, and infected hair.

The material to be examined should be mounted in strong (10 to 20 per cent) potassium hydroxide. This dissolves or makes translucent the tissue elements, and the fungi are readily observed when examined as a wet unstained preparation. Antiformin or lactophenol may be used instead of potassium hydroxide. Care must be taken to distinguish between conidia and fat globules and between mycelium and fibrin strands; a mycelium-like structure ("mosaic fungus") may be formed in some skin scale preparations, and presumably is cholesterol crystals. Only with experience do these and other artifacts become recognizable and distinguishable from fungi. Fungi may be demonstrated in tissue sections, in the walls of abscesses, and in granulomatous tissue by the Hotchkiss-MacManis (periodic acid–Schiff), the Gridley (a modified PAS), or the Gomori (methenamine silver) stain. Gomori's stain is recommended for finding the few organisms in a large specimen, and Gridley's for distinguishing the detail of fungus structure. The Gomori also stains the actinomycetes, but the others do not. The Gram stain of Brown and Breen's modification is also recommended for the actinomycetes.

Cultures. A bit of growth is removed from the colony, teased apart in a drop of water, and examined as a wet preparation. While the various structures may be seen, the arrangement of the elements is seriously disturbed. Slide cultures show the structure and arrangement of the growth and may be made into permanent mounts. These cultures are prepared by adding a bit of growth to a small portion of agar on a slide. A coverslip is placed on top, and the slide is incubated in a moist petri dish. After a week or more when spores are mature, the cover slip and mediums are gently removed. A drop of lactophenol–cotton blue is added and the coverslip replaced. Some of the mycelium will have adhered to the slide, and the spore heads, conidiophores, etc., will be intact and in their characteristic arrangement. The slide cultures are especially recommended for identification of dermatophytes. They are not recommended for *Coccidioides, Histoplasma,* etc.

Cultivation

Most of the fungi grow rapidly, but the pathogenic forms usually grow relatively slowly. Four to six weeks' incubation or more

may be necessary.[1, 2] The morphology is markedly affected by the type of medium on which the organisms are grown. In general, they show no unusual nutritive requirements and grow readily on all the usual bacteriological mediums, especially if a sugar is added. Sabouraud's medium, a peptone-glucose agar, is perhaps the most widely used medium in medical mycology for the isolation and maintenance of cultures, especially the dermatophytes. Since all the morphological descriptions of dermatophytes and systemic invading fungi have been made on colonies growing on Sabouraud's media, this agar, though not the best medium for the growth of fungi, is nonetheless the "standard" agar for the diagnostic laboratory. Similarly, Czapek-Dox medium is the standard for the description of *Aspergillus* and *Penicillium* species.

In present laboratory practice, antibiotics are added to make the medium selective for a particular group of organisms. For dermatophytes and the mycelial stage of the thermal dimorphic fungi, Sabouraud's medium with chloramphenicol and cycloheximide (Actidione) is used. The former suppresses the growth of bacteria and the latter the growth of contaminant fungi. Some pathogenic fungi will not grow on Actidione medium, *e.g., Candida tropicalis,* the yeast stage of *Histoplasma* and *Blastomyces,* and *Cryptococcus neoformans.* Furthermore, in culturing for opportunistic fungal infections, mycotic keratitis, etc., the etiological agents would also be suppressed. Therefore the following guide can be used for the diagnostic mycology laboratory. For dermatophytes, Sabouraud's agar with antibiotics is sufficient. For other types of infection the same medium is used in addition to a blood agar plate without antibiotics. All mediums are incubated at 25° C. When growth appears, a portion is transferred to a plain Sabouraud's plate or slant and another portion is planted as a slide culture. This will allow for the three main elements of fungal identification: the color, morphology, and consistency of the colony obverse, the color of the reverse, and the microscopic appearance of the hyphae with conidia *in situ.* All of the actinomycetes are inhibited by chloramphenicol. If these organisms are suspected, other culture methods must be used.

Classification

The fungi to be discussed in this section will be arranged as to the clinical location of their site of infection. The categories are as follows:

Superficial Mycoses: Only the outermost layers of skin (stratum corneum) or hair are involved, and there is practically no host reaction to the parasite. Examples are piedra and pityriasis versicolor.

Cutaneous Mycoses: The infection is limited to the superficial layers of the skin (stratum corneum) with little or no invasion of living cells. There may be significant, and occasionally severe, host inflammatory reaction to the presence of the organism. The dermatophyte and dermal *Candida* infections are included in this category.

A purely arbitrary category is that of "yeast infections." It is considered separately because of the diverse clinical conditions that may be involved. The etiological agents are *Candida* species. Other yeasts are strictly opportunists.

Subcutaneous Mycoses: In this category are diseases in which the organism has been implanted into subcutaneous tissue. Usually the infection is limited to the site of entry and a long clinical course may ensue. Chromoblastomycosis, mycetoma, entomophthoromycosis, and sporotrichosis are examples.

Systemic Mycoses: The most dangerous and often fatal disease-producing organisms are in this category. Entrance of the organism is usually through the lung, and the disease may spread to other parts of the body. The diseases of the thermal dimorphic organisms (histoplasmosis, blastomycosis, coccidioidomycosis) are included. Also in this group are the opportunistic infections. These organisms are not dimorphic as are the etiological agents of the above-mentioned diseases. If they exist as mycelium when growing saprophytically, they will also exist as a mycelium when invading the debilitated host. Such diseases include aspergillosis, mucormycosis, and cryptococcosis. The latter is a yeast found in pigeon dung and is also a yeast in cases of human infection. *Candida*, a yeast, shows a transformation to an elongate mycelium when it colonizes tissue. This is a nutrition-induced transformation and both yeast and mycelial units will be found in infected tissue. *Trichosporon beigelii* also demonstrates this nutrition-induced dimorphism.

Rare Mycoses: The mycoses that are not often encountered and the organisms not usually considered pathogenic are included. These may be soil organisms responding to an unusual environment after accidental implantation or invasion of a debilitated host. Such diseases as penicillosis, cercosporamycosis, and cladosporiosis are considered. They are grouped in two general categories: hyphomycosis, in which the cell wall of the hypha is colorless, and phaeohyphomycosis, in which the cell wall is brown.[10]

THE SUPERFICIAL MYCOSES

Pityriasis Versicolor (Tinea Versicolor)

The is a common, worldwide fungal infection. It is most common, however, in tropical areas. The disease is characterized by yellow to brown patches or continuous scaling over the trunk and occasionally the legs, face, and neck. The affected area fluoresces a golden yellow when irradiated with a filtered ultraviolet lamp, "Wood's light" (peak at 365 nm.). Susceptibility to the disease is probably genetic and may be related to the rate of epidermal growth and desquamation. High endogenous or administered cortisone levels may also predispose to the disease. The etiological agent is the lipophilic yeast *Malassezia furfur*, a part of the normal skin flora. A related species, *M. ovalis*, is also often involved. It will not grow on ordinary mediums, as it usually requires some lipid additives. Diagnosis is easily made by examining the scales in a KOH mount (Fig. 43–8). Short, thick hyphal elements and associated round forms are seen. Successful treatment includes sodium hyposulfite solution (20 per cent) or keratolytic agents, such as Whitfield's ointment. The infection usually recurs.

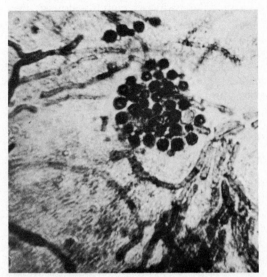

Figure 43–8. Skin scale from pityriasis versicolor. Short branched mycelium and small yeast-like cell are diagnostic of this disease. Methenamine silver; × 400.

Tinea Nigra

The disease tinea nigra manifests itself as dark blotches on the palms of the hands and rarely elsewhere on the body. In a KOH mount the organism appears as brown, branched hyphae, 2 to 3 μm. in diameter. Though most common in the tropics, occasional cases occur in the United States. The etiological agents are members of the family Dematiaceae (brown-walled hyphomycetes). *Exophiala werneckii* is commonly found in Central and South America, while the variant *mansonii* is encountered in India, tropical Asia, and Africa. These are probably variants of the same species. The colonies grow slowly on cycloheximide agar, and are dark, greenish black, and moist. Microscopically numerous, dark, one- and two-celled budding conidia are seen on dark mycelium. Keratolytic fungicides, such as Whitfield's ointment, may be used in treatment. The main importance of tinea nigra is that it has been misdiagnosed as malignant melanoma. This has led to needless mutilative surgery.

Piedra

This disease is a fungal infection of the hair, characterized by nodules on the distal shaft. Two types are encountered. White piedra, in which soft light-colored nodules form, is principally found in temperate regions. The etiological agent, *Trichosporon beigelii* is sensitive to cycloheximide but will grow on most other mediums. It produces a soft, creamy, rapidly growing colony which becomes yellowish gray. Microscopically, it is composed of hyaline septate mycelium that fragments into oval arthrospores. *Trichosporon beigelii* is separated from other members of the genus by its lack of fermentation of sugars, its lack of growth on potassium nitrate, and its carbon assimilation pattern. This species has been involved in opportunistic systemic infections as well. It is part of the normal yeast flora of the skin, mouth, and intestinal tract.

Black piedra is a hard, black or brown nodule caused by the ascomycete *Piedraia hortai* (Fig. 43–9). This disease is mainly tropical, being found in Latin America, Asia, and Africa. It also infects primates other than man. The organism grows slowly on cycloheximide agar, producing a greenish to rusty black, hard, raised colony. The colony is composed of dark mycelium and chlamydospores. Asci are seen in culture and in the mass growing on the hair shaft. Treatment consists in shaving off the hair.

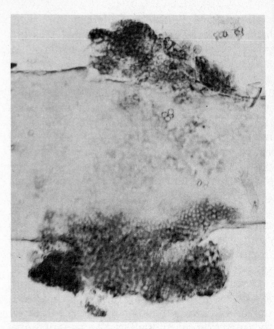

Figure 43–9. Black piedra knob on hair shaft. *Piedraia hortai.* × 100.

THE CUTANEOUS INFECTIONS (DERMATOPHYTOSES)

By far the most common type of fungal disease of man is dermatophytosis. It is a superficial infection of the keratinized epidermis and keratinized epidermal appendages, i.e., the hair, hairsheaths, and nails. The severity of the infection depends for the most part on the location of the lesion and the species of fungus involved. Though certain other fungi, notably *Candida*, produce clinically similar diseases, a more or less homogeneous group of fungi, the dermatophytes, is responsible for the great majority of cases. The ability of these microorganisms to invade and parasitize the cornified tissues is closely associated with, and dependent upon, their common physiological characteristic: the utilization of the highly insoluble scleroprotein keratin. The utilization of keratin is biologically rare and is shared by the dermatophytes (family Gymnoascaceae) with only a few species of saprophytic fungi (notably the family Onygenaceae) and certain insects, including the clothes moth (Tinea), the carpet beetles (Dermestes), and the biting lice (Mallophaga).

Though on the one hand, the various species of dermatophytes produce infections that are clinically characteristic, on the other hand, a single species may produce a variety of diseases, each with its characteristic pathology depending on the site of infection. For example, *Trichophyton rubrum* may cause tinea corporis, tinea cruris, tinea manuum, tinea unguium, or tinea pedis, each a distinct disease. However, another species may cause the identical diseases, but its response to therapy or tendency to recur may be different. Furthermore, other conditions such as chemical dermatitis, neurodermatitis, and certain types of allergy may closely simulate dermatophytosis, but do not, of course, respond to treatment with antifungal drugs. Demonstration of the causative fungus by direct microscopic examination of pathological material and by isolation and culture is, therefore, essential to establish a correct diagnosis and institute proper therapy.

The antibiotic griseofulvin has proved to be a highly effective chemotherapeutic agent for the treatment of the dermatomycoses, but cure commonly requires prolonged (3 to 10 weeks') administration by mouth. There may be severe side effects from the use of this drug. These are very rare, however. The antifungal effect of the antibiotic is reflected in morphological changes in the infecting fungus, both *in vivo* and *in vitro*, and appears to be the result of interference with nucleic acid synthesis. Tolnaftate (Tinactin), haloprogin, and miconazole are topical agents useful in most infections other than nail and hair. The latter two are also effective in dermal *Candida* infections. Thiabendazole has also been used in resistant cases. Recently, the imidazoles, clotrimazole and miconazole, have been successfully utilized as topical agents. Ketoconazole, given orally, can be used in recalcitrant infections.

The dermatophytes were classed until recently as Fungi Imperfecti. Through the work of Stockdale, Gentles, and others, it has been demonstrated that many have a teleomorph or sexual state (and hence a perfect state name). This observation was first made by Nanizzi in 1927 but was ignored. As a result of these observations, many of the organisms are known by two names. In clinical dermatology the older, imperfect (anamorph) state name is still in common usage and probably will remain so. Most of the organisms shown to have a perfect stage are heterothallic and will not show ascus formation except when grown with the opposite mating type. Even then, gymnothecia (the fruiting body containing the asci) formation usually occurs only on mediums containing a mixture of keratin and soil. A list of the known dermatophytes and their perfect stages is given in Table 43–8. Many related organisms have been isolated from the soil, but as yet have not or have only rarely been isolated from lesion material.

The dermatophytes differ from most other pathogenic fungi in that the cells are multinucleate, usually containing four to six nuclei, and division is amitotic. Arthroconidia, chlamydoconidia, and the individual cells of the macroconidia are also multinucleate, but the microconidia contain but a single nucleus. The

Table 43–8. **The Ascigerous Genera and Species of Dermatophytes**

Teleomorph State	Anamorph State
Arthroderma	*Trichophyton*
A. benhamiae Ajello and Cheng 1967	*T. mentagrophytes*
A. ciferrii Varsavsky and Ajello 1964	*T. georgiae*
A. flavescens Padhye et Carmichael 1971	*T. flavescens*
A. gertleri Bohme 1967	*T. vanbreuseghemii*
A. gloriae Ajello 1967	*T. gloriae*
A. insingulare Padhye and Carmichael 1972	*T. terrestre*
A. lenticularum Pore, Tsao and Plunkett 1965	*T. terrestre*
A. quadrifidum Dawson and Gentles 1961	*T. terrestre*
A. simii Stockdale, Mackenzie, and Austwick 1965	*T. simii*
A. uncinatum Dawson and Gentles 1959	*T. ajelloi*
A. vanbreuseghemii Takashio 1973	*T. mentagrophytes*
Nannizzia	*Microsporum*
N. borellii Moraes, Padhye, et Ajello 1975	*M. amazonicum*
N. cajetana Ajello 1961	*M. cookei*
N. fulva Stockdale 1963	*M. fulvum*
N. grubia Georg, Ajello, Friedman, and Brinkman 1967	*M. vanbreuseghemii*
N. gypsea Stockdale 1963	*M. gypseum*
N. incurvata Stockdale 1961	*M. gypseum*
N. obtusa Dawson and Gentles 1961	*M. nanum*
N. otae Hasegawa and Usui 1974	*M. canis*
N. perisicolor Stockdale 1967	*M. persicolor*
N. racemosa Rush-Munro, Smith, and Borelli 1970	*M. racemosum*

(Rippon, J. W.: Medical Mycology. 2nd ed. W. B. Saunders Co., Philadelphia, 1982.)

group is a homogeneous one, immunologically as well as morphologically and physiologically. Only recently have some physiological differences been found which are an aid in identification. These will be discussed later.

Differentiation of Genera and Species[9]

David Gruby in 1841 described the fungal etiology of favus. Culturing the fungus from an infected lesion, he reproduced the disease by inoculation into normal skin. After this time, many fungi were isolated from similar lesions. Some were the responsible agents, many were contaminants, and practically all were given different names without regard to proper taxonomic procedures. Some order was brought about by the work of the French dermatologist Sabouraud. The classification of Sabouraud, presented in 1910 and somewhat modified by him later, is the most generally used. The system was extensively revised by Emmons and Conant, who reduced to synonomy many varieties of the same species. Presently, work on the ascigerous state and physiological differences will help in establishing species lines. As of now, we are still dependent on differences in colonial and microscopic morphology, pigment, conidia types, etc.

Differential Characteristics. Very many different kinds of dermatophytes have been described, some estimate as many as 200 or more, but many "new" species have been inadequately studied and often represent minor variants of established species. A number of physiological studies have been carried out, and it has been found that certain species or strains are distinguished by requirements for vitamins or amino acids. These might provide a basis for identification, but so far at least, physiological characteristics have not been as useful for the differentiation of these forms as they often are for the characterization of bacteria.

Those characteristics established by the work of Georg and Camp and found to be useful are listed in Table 43–9. The test is carried out by planting the organism on deficient mediums.

While growing on the skin and its appendages, the thallus is differentiated only into hyphae and arthroconidia, the latter arising by fragmentation of the mycelium. Arthroconidia production is particularly well developed in the etiological agents of tinea capitis. This in a sense is its parasitic stage, as dermatophytes do not produce arthroconidia when growing

Table 43–9. Nutritional Differentiation of Dermatophytes

Species	Requirement
T. verrucosum	Inositol and usually thiamine
T. tonsurans	Thiamine
T. megninii	L-Histidine
T. equinum	Nicotinic acid
T. violaceum	Thiamine

saprophytically in soil or in culture. The variety of differentiated structures, including microconidia or macroconidia and vegetative structures, such as spirals, pectinate bodies, nodular organs, and racquet mycelium, appear in cultivation on artificial mediums. The differences are no doubt a consequence of the nutritional state of the substrate.

Primary differentiation into the three imperfect genera, *Trichophyton, Microsporum,* and *Epidermophyton,* is morphological, being based on the character of the macroconidia. The first two genera listed above (the third does not invade hair) differ with respect to size and arrangement of the arthroconidia formed in the hairs. The genus *Microsporum* includes the small conidia type (3 to 4 μm. in diameter) and the genus *Trichophyton,* the large type (7 to 8 μm. in diameter). This distinction is not absolute, for the very common species *Trichophyton mentagrophytes* forms small conidia on hair. Furthermore, the conidia differ in arrangement. While the mycelium of *Microsporum* grows within the hairs, conidia are formed only outside the hair and occur in irregular clusters in a kind of mosaic arrangement. The conidia of *Trichophyton,* on the other hand, occur in chains inside (endothrix) or outside (ectothrix) the hair (see Table 43–10).

Further differentiation of the organisms is made on the basis of location of the arthroconidia with respect to the hair. The endothrix type (sometimes called black-dot ringworm) grows within the hair, and mycelium and chains of arthroconidia are found there (Fig. 43–10). The hair often breaks off at the scalp line and produces an area of alopecia (usually cuboidal and accompanied by a kerion) and black dots of hair stubble. The ectothrix type forms the arthroconidia only on the surface of the hair, though the mycelium grows inside (Fig. 43–11). A third type is found in favus (T. *schoenleinii*) in which the organism grows in the hair but produces no conidia, only "air bubbles" in the hair shaft. The hair does not break off, but instead loses its color and luster

Table 43–10. **The Common Dermatophytes and Their Diseases**

			Species	Disease in Man	Geographical Distribution
Invading the Hair and Hair Follicles	Small Conidia Varieties	Ectothrix Type	*Microsporum audounii** (Fig. 43–11)	Prepubertal ringworm of the scalp; suppuration rare; child to child	Commonest in Europe, producing about 90 per cent of infections; in U.S. 50 per cent, becoming rare
			Microsporum canis* (Fig. 43–12)	Prepubertal ringworm of scalp and glabrous skin; suppuration not infrequent; kerion occasional; from pets	Uncommon in Europe, except England and Scandinavia; responsible for about half the infections in U.S
			Microsporum gypseum (Fig. 43–13)	Ringworm of the scalp and glabrous skin; suppuration and kerion common; from soil	Relatively rare in U.S.; common in South America
			Microsporum fulvum	Ringworm similar to that of M. *gypseum*	Same as above
			Microsporum ferrugineum*	Similar to M. *audouinii*	Africa, India, China, Japan
	Large Conidia Varieties	Endothrix Type	*Trichophyton tonsurans*	Black-dot ringworm of the scalp; smooth skin; sycosis; tinea unguium; suppuration common; the hair follicles are atrophied	Common in Europe, Russia, Near East, Mexico, Puerto Rico, and South America, but uncommon in U.S. until recently
			Trichophyton violaceum (Fig. 43–10)	Black-dot endothrix in both scalp and smooth skin; onychomycosis; suppuration is the rule and kerion frequent	Common in southern Europe, the Balkans, and the Far East, rare in the U.S.
			Trichophyton soudanense *Trichophyton gourvilii* *Trichophyton yaoundei* }	Inflammatory, scarring ringworm of scalp	Central and West Africa
		Ectothrix Type	*Trichophyton mentagrophytes* var *interdigitale* (Fig. 43–14)	Commonest cause of intertriginous dermatophytosis of the foot ("athlete's foot"); ringworm of the smooth skin; suppurative folliculitis in scalp and beard	Ubiquitous
			Trichophyton verrucosum	Ringworm of the scalp and smooth skin; suppurative folliculitis in scalp and beard; from cattle	Ubiquitous
			Trichophyton megninii	Sycosis is the most common lesion; infection of smooth skin and nails	Sporadic distribution; Portugal, Sardinia
	No. Conidia in Hair		*Trichophyton schoenleinii** (Fig. 43–15)	Favus in both scalp and smooth skin; scutulum and kerion	Europe, Near East, Mediterranean region; rare in U.S.
Rare in Hair			*Trichophyton rubrum* (Fig. 43–17)	Psoriasis-like lesions of smooth skin; tinea unguium; mild suppurative folliculitis in beard; rare invasion of scalp hair endo- and ectothrix described; endoectothrix in villous hair	Ubiquitous
Not Invading the Hair and Hair Follicles			*Epidermophyton floccosum* (Fig. 43–16)	Cause of classic eczema marginatum of crural region; causes minority of cases of intertriginous dermatophytosis of foot; not known to infect hair and hair follicles	Ubiquitous, but more common in tropics
			Trichophyton concentricum	Cause of tinea imbricata; infection of hair and nails uncertain	Common in South Pacific islands, Far East, India, Ceylon; reported in west coast of Central America and northwest coast of South America

*Infected hairs show fluorescence by Wood's lamp. (Rippon, J. W.: Medical Mycology. 2nd ed. W. B. Saunders Co., Philadelphia, 1982.)

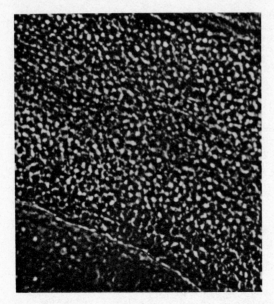

Figure 43–10. Endothrix tinea capitis *(T. violaceum)*. Chains of arthrospores within the hair shaft. × 100.

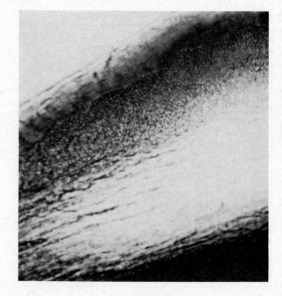

Figure 43–11. Ectothrix tinea capitis *(Microsporum audouini)*. The mycelium is in the hair shaft with mosaic arrangement of arthrospores around hair shaft. × 400.

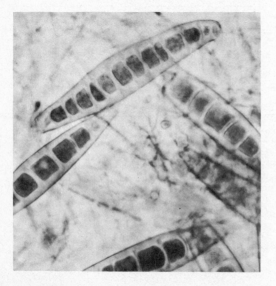

Figure 43–12. *Microsporum canis* macroaleuriospores. The colony is fluffy white with a chrome yellow reverse. Both micro- and macroaleuriospores are found. Lactophenol–cotton blue; × 400.

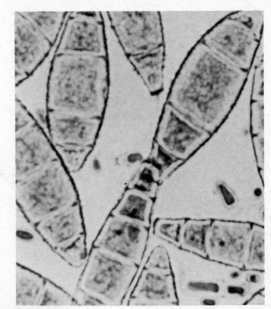

Figure 43–13. *Microsporum gypseum (Nannizzia incurvata)* macroaleuriospores from the cinnamon-colored powdered colony. Lactophenol-cotton blue; × 400.

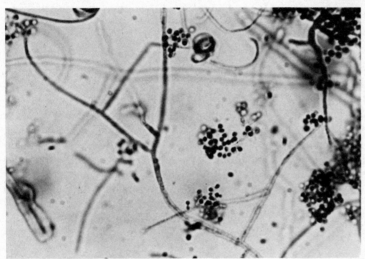

Figure 43–14. *Trichophyton mentagrophytes*. Globose microaleuriospores "en grappe" (in clusters) and spiral mycelium identify this fungus. The pencil-shaped macroaleuriospores are identical to those of *T. rubrum*. (Rippon, J. W.: Medical Mycology. 2nd ed. W. B. Saunders Co., Philadelphia, 1982.)

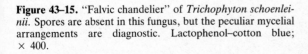

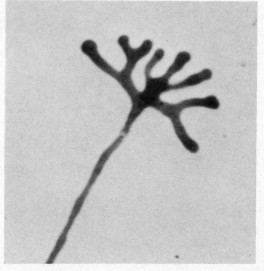

Figure 43–15. "Falvic chandelier" of *Trichophyton schoenleinii*. Spores are absent in this fungus, but the peculiar mycelial arrangements are diagnostic. Lactophenol–cotton blue; × 400.

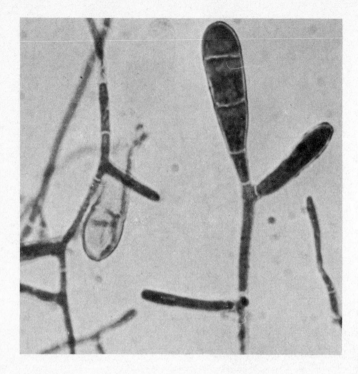

Figure 43–16. *Epidermophyton floccusum,* with its pyriform macroaleuriospores. Micro-aleuriospores are absent. The colony is restricted, grainy, and chartreuse in color.

and appears as a patch of gray hair. *T. rubrum* rarely invades hair, but in such infections it produces endo- and ectothrix arthroconidia.

It will be clear that differentiation of these genera may be approximated by, first, the clinical character of the disease and, second, the direct microscopic examination of epilated infected hairs, but identification is possible only by culture. In general, *Trichophyton* infections show a characteristic tendency to produce an inflammatory reaction with deep infiltration of the skin that is not usually produced by *Microsporum* infections. This difference is of some value in distinguishing between *Microsporum* infections and infections of the scalp with small-conidia ectothrix *Trichophyton.* The animal strains of *Microsporum* such as *Microsporum canis,* however, also elicit inflammatory reactions. A severe inflammatory reaction with a raised mass of tissue, usually suppurating at many points, is called a kerion. Excessive fibrous scar tissue following an infection is called keloid formation.

Epidermophyton invades the superficial lay-

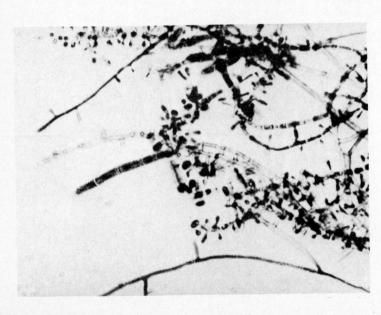

Figure 43–17. *Trichophyton rubrum* in rare granular form showing macroaleuriospores and "tear drop" microaleuriospores. × 440. (Rippon, J. W.: Medical Mycology. 2nd ed. W. B. Saunders Co., Philadelphia, 1982.)

ers of the skin in tinea corporis, and in scales of the epidermis taken from the periphery of the lesion, the fungi are found as articulated filaments of mycelium breaking up into chains of round to oval arthroconidia. It does not invade hair.

Pathogenicity

The majority of dermatophytes grow readily on laboratory mediums and also grow on such substrates as cereal grains, shed hair, horn debris, and sterilized fragments of straw in moist tubes and will remain viable in litter containing such materials for two to three years. If protected from dryness they may live on the wooden floors of shower rooms, dressing rooms, and dressing cabins, and on mats, etc., for a considerable time. If by chance they come in contact with a suitable host (source of keratin) they may again take up residence on that individual and set up an infection. Whereas many species have a soil reservoir, a few, particularly some agents of tinea capitis, have evolved an almost totally parasitic life cycle and probably do not have a soil reservoir.

The dermatophytoses show, in many instances, a pronounced age and sex distribution, and there is some difference in the geographical distribution of the various species. Common ringworm or "gray patch" (*Microsporum audouini*) of the scalp is confined to the young, occurring more often in boys than in girls, and it is rare after puberty. Others, such as the *Epidermophyton* infection, occur for the most part in adult males. The distribution of intertriginous dermatophytosis of the feet, commonly known as "athlete's foot," in the young adult male is probably in large part an expression of risk of exposure. M. *canis* is more common in this country than in Europe, except England, and the reverse is true of *T. schoenleinii*, while *T. concentricum* is well known in the tropics and certain parts of the Far East and Panama but is rare in temperate climates. *Microsporum ferrugeneum* is found almost exclusively in China and Japan.

Some dermatophyte species appear to be so closely adapted to man that they are unable to infect lower animals; human infection is transmitted by contact. These organisms are termed anthropophilic dermatophytes. (Table 43–11). These include *M. audouini, T. rubrum,* and *T. schoenleinii*. Others not only produce infections in experimental animals, but also animals such as the cat and dog are natural hosts, and humans may acquire infection from them. An example is *M. canis*. The reservoir of animal-type dermatophytes is of considerable epidemiological importance. One survey showed, for example, that 37 per cent of cats and 22 per cent of dogs examined at random in the United States were infected. Organisms such as *Microsporum namum* are commonly found infecting pigs but not man. All these are referred to as zoophilic dermatophytes (see Table 43–9). Some are regularly contracted from the soil, such as *Microsporum gypseum*, and are termed geophilic.

There is also a high degree of specificity as to the tissues attacked. While, as indicated earlier, these fungi are well adapted to parasitize the horny layer of the epidermis, they

Table 43–11. **Ecology of Human Dermatophyte Species**

Anthropophilic	Zoophilic	Geophilic
Cosmopolitan Species		
E. floccosum	M. canis	M. gypseum
M. audouinii	M. gallinae	M. fulvum
T. mentagrophytes	T. mentagrophytes	T. ajelloi
var. interdigitale	var. mentagrophytes	T. terestre
T. rubrum	T. verrucosum	
T. schoenleinii	T. equinum	
T. tonsurans	M. nanum	
T. violaceum		
Rare and Geographically Limited Species		
M. ferrugineum	M. distortum	Microsporum
T. concentricum	T. erinacei	racemosum
T. gourvillii	T. simii	
T. megninii	M. persicolor	
T. soudanense		
T. yaoundei		

(Rippon, J. W.: Medical Mycology. 2nd Ed. W. B. Saunders Co., Philadelphia, 1982.)

appear to be unable to invade and infect other organs of the body. The intravenous injection of *Microsporum* conidia or emulsions of virulent *T. mentagrophytes* does not produce an infection of the internal organs of susceptible animals; rather, the microorganisms introduced tend to become localized in the skin and to develop where it is damaged as by scarification. However, it has been shown that dermatophytes, as well as several saprophytes, can be "trained" to assume a yeast-like phase similar to the deep-infecting fungi. In this transient condition the organisms can invade deep tissues of experimental animals.

Growth of the fungus in the skin and hair is more or less equal in all directions, and the lesions produced tend to have a circular (ring) form. For this reason the Greeks named the disease herpes, a term which still persists though modified as herpes tonsurans, herpes circinatus, or herpes desquamans to distinguish the dermatophytoses from herpetic infection of virus etiology. The Romans associated the lesions with lice and named the condition tinea, meaning any small insect larva (worm). This name is likewise in common use. The English ringworm is, of course, a combination of the Greek and Roman terms.

The clinical conditions produced are termed: tinea pedis (athlete's foot); tinea corporis (ringworm of body); tinea capitis (ringworm of the scalp); tinea cruris (ringworm of the groin or "jock itch," also commonly caused by *Candida*); and tinea unguium (ringworm of the nail). Onychomycosis, a similar condition, can be caused by *Candida, Scopulariopsis*, or other fungi. Tinea imbricata, a special concentric ring form on the skin of the body, is caused only by *Trichophyton concentricum,* and tinea favosa, a particular chronic destructive disease of the scalp (favus) is caused only by *T. schoenleinii.*

With any species of dermatophyte, infection begins in the horny layer of the epidermis. Those that infect the hair follicles, hair, and nails soon invade these structures, often producing little more than a scaling of the surrounding epidermis. Those that remain in the epidermis affect the drier parts of the skin, including the palmar and plantar surfaces, or the moister regions in the inguinocrural fold and the interdigital spaces. Thus a wide variety of clinical types may be observed, but the differences are more apparent than real, for the pathological changes are fundamentally the same in all types.

It was observed by Margarot and Devoze in 1925 that infected hairs and fungal cultures show fluorescence in ultraviolet light.* This empirical observation has proved to be of very considerable practical value, especially in *Microsporum* ringworm of the scalp, although hairs infected with *M. gypseum* and *M. fulvum* often do not have this property. It is generally agreed that all hairs infected with *Microsporum* show a brilliant greenish fluorescence. It has been found that the fluorescence is due to the presence of a substance (a pteridine) in the hair which can be extracted either with warm water after preliminary ether extraction or with dilute alkali.

Immunity

Though an acquired immunity to infection has been demonstrated in experimental animals by a number of workers, the status of an effective immunity in man is uncertain. There have been some enthusiastic reports of the efficacy of vaccine therapy which are, perhaps, open to question. Demonstration of IgG antibodies in some infected patients has been possible but the relation to disease and immunity is unclear. Normal serum appears to have some inhibitory effect on the growth of dermatophytes.

Hypersensitivity, however, is a common, though not invariable, manifestation of the immune response to dermatophyte infection. Hypersensitivity is manifested in two ways. One of these is the appearance of secondary, sterile lesions on parts of the body remote from the infection. These are termed "ids," in a general sense mycid or dermatophytid, and more specifically microsporid, trichophytid, and epidermophytid. A similar condition, candidid, may result from a *Candida* infection. The mycid takes the form of a symmetrical eruption over relatively large areas, usually of the trunk, as a rash. The eruption may be vesicular with sterile content, papular, or lichenoid and is sometimes localized at the follicular pores. A rather frequent occurrence is a sterile vesicular eruption on the hands secondary to infection of the feet. It has been postulated that bits of mycelial debris from the lesion enter the blood stream and are eventually deposited in the skin, where they induce the local allergic response with destruction of the fungal elements. This view is based in part

---

*"Black light," commonly known as Wood's light because the radiation is filtered through Wood's nickel oxide glass, which holds back almost all the visible rays but passes the longer ultraviolet rays (peak at 365 nm.).

on a number of successful isolations of these fungi from the blood stream during the development of infection in experimental animals. It is not known what part, if any, soluble substances liberated by the dissolution of the fungi play in the phenomenon. These play an important part in the local inflammation seen, however.

Hypersensitivity may also be demonstrated by the injection or application of preparations of dermatophyte cultures analogous to tuberculin and called trichophytin. The local and constitutional reactions that are produced with trichophytin are much the same as those to tuberculin. The test does not differentiate between *Microsporum* and *Trichophyton* or their species, for all appear to contain a common or very closely related antigen. It is also unreliable as a test for present infection. The reaction is so common in the adult population that the trichophytin test is part of the battery of tests used to evaluate the immune responsiveness of a patient. In some instances the differentiation of immediate and delayed response of the test in persons infected by dermatophytes is of some interest. Whereas almost all patients with established dermatophyte infection will have a delayed trichophytin reaction, persons with chronic *T. rubrum* infections frequently show an immediate wheal in response to trichophytin injection and essentially no delayed response. The relation of this to the chronicity of their disease is unknown but is interesting to speculate upon. It may indicate a specific anergy to the antigens of the infecting organism. This anergy is sometimes found in chronic mucocutaneous candidosis as well.

Laboratory Diagnosis

As indicated earlier, classification of the dermatophytes is based largely on colonial morphology on Sabouraud's agar, color of the reverse, and difference in conidia type seen in microscopic slide cultures. Requirements for vitamins and amino acids and sexual mating are the only new tools to help in distinguishing species. These are of value in only a few cases. Laboratory diagnosis, then, is still a matter of looking at gross and microscopic morphology, an exercise in contemplative observation.

The specimen material must be chosen with some care and taken in abundance for both microscopic examination and culture. In ringworm of the scalp, epilated stumps of hairs may be taken and, in addition, scutula in favus and the contents of abscesses should be taken when the infection is suppurative. In infections of the smooth skin, scrapings from the scaly types should be taken from the margins, rolling toward the normal skin. The tops of vesicles may be clipped with small scissors in the vesicular type of infection, especially of the feet. Macerated epithelium may be taken from intertriginous infections, and nail scrapings and subungual hyperkeratotic masses from tinea unguium. The fungous elements are often difficult to demonstrate microscopically in the latter case.

For direct microscopic examination the material is placed on a slide, a few drops of strong (10 to 20 per cent) potassium hydroxide solution added, the specimen covered with a coverglass, and the preparation heated slightly. Mycelial elements and spores may be found in such specimens (Fig. 43–18). Permanent stained preparations may be made by mounting in Amann's medium, a lactic acid–glycerol–phenol solution containing cotton blue.

General Methods of Cultivation

Cultivation and methods of identification have been noted in the introduction to fungi. As noted there, a specimen is planted on Sabouraud's agar with antibiotics and left to incubate for two weeks or more. At the first signs of growth, transfers to Sabouraud's slants and slide cultures are made (Fig. 43–19). Thereafter, gross and microscopic observations can be made and the species identified.

THE PATHOGENIC YEASTS

The term "yeast" or "yeast-like" is the vernacular for a unicellular, nucleated organism which reproduces by budding. Such a defini-

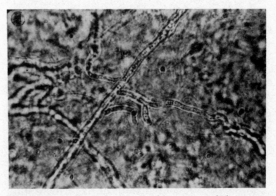

Figure 43–18. Potassium hydroxide mount of tinea corporis. Note refractile, branching, septate hyphae. × 440. (Rippon, J. W.: Medical Mycology. 2nd ed. W. B. Saunders Co., Philadelphia, 1982.)

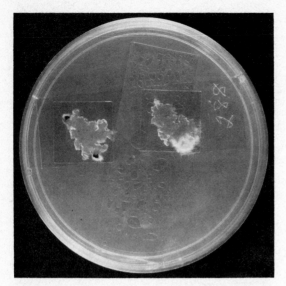

Figure 43–19. Slide culture. The right-hand side is Sabouraud's glucose agar and the left is cornmeal with 1 per cent dextrose. The latter stimulates pigment production in *Trichophyton rubrum.* (Rippon, J. W.: Medical Mycology. 2nd ed. W. B. Saunders Co., Philadelphia, 1982.)

tion is generally recognized as inadequate. Some yeasts reproduce by fission, many produce mycelium or pseudomycelium under appropriate conditions, and hyphomycetes (mycelial fungi) may exist in a unicellular yeast-like form which reproduces by budding, *viz.,* the oidia described in the previous section. On the basis of sexual spore formation, some yeasts are Ascomycota, others are Basidiomycota, (the ballistosporangenous yeasts), and still others have not been shown to have a sexual stage and are grouped with the Fungi Imperfecti. Clearly, then the term "yeast" is of somewhat uncertain significance. As commonly used, the term "yeast" refers to those organisms which exist usually or predominantly in a yeast-like form.

The yeasts belong in three fungal phyla: the basidiospore-forming yeasts or Sporobolomycetaceae in the class Basidiomycota, the ascospore-forming yeasts Endomycetaceae in the class Ascomycota, and the asporogenous yeasts Cryptococcaceae in the Deuteromycota (Table 43–12). This last group contains the human pathogens. The industrial yeasts are perhaps the most familiar organisms. *Saccharomyces cerevisiae*, a member of the Ascomycota, is the common brewing yeast. It produces carbon dioxide and alcohol in its fermentation and occurs as two types: the top yeasts, which are found in the froth on the surface of the fermenting mixture, and the bottom yeasts, which sink to the bottom. Bread yeasts are

usually top strains of *S. cerevisiae.* Another species of this genus, *S. ellipsoideus,* is the common wine yeast, occurring naturally on grapes and in the soil of vineyards, and its varieties are names for the various types of wine which they produce. These organisms are "perfect" yeasts, the cell body becoming an ascus during sexual union. Still other yeasts are lactose-fermenters and are associated with the preparation of fermented milk beverages, such as kefir and koumiss. These are used in southeastern Europe and Asia for the production of beverages. Perhaps the commonest yeasts encountered as contamination in bacterial cultures, found growing on foods, and seen as normal flora of the skin are the asporogenous Rhodotorulae; the pink or coral pigmented forms most often observed are *Rhodotorula flava* or *R. glutinis.* These have sometimes been found as opportunistic infecting organisms isolated from blood or cerebrospinal fluid.

In view of the ubiquitous distribution of yeasts, not only in air, dust, and soil, but on the surface of the body and in the mouth, intestinal tract, and vagina, it is not surprising that these forms have been found in a variety of pathological processes. A great number of species have been described, most of them inadequately, in this connection. In many instances the yeast probably had no etiological relation to the disease, and in others the same yeast has been repeatedly described as a new species, thus giving rise to several synonymous names, and a very long list of "pathogenic" yeasts has accumulated.

Critical examination and consideration has now made it clear that only a very few species of yeasts are actually pathogenic for man and animals and in almost all cases these may be considered opportunistic infections. The yeasts of medical importance produce a wide variety of diseases. These are listed in the accompanying outline with basic differentiation and the classification generally accepted.

Candidiasis will be discussed in this section, the other pathogenic yeasts elsewhere.

Candidiasis

"Monilia" is a *nomen absurdum* perpetrated in the nineteenth century. Unfortunately, the term is still used by clinicians and the public. Mycologically, the word *Monilia* refers to a fungus growing on rotting wood, first described by Persoon. It is also the imperfect stage of *Neurospora* and *Sclerotinia* ("peach mummies"). The correct term for the human disease is candidiasis.

Table 43–12. **Classification of Medically Important Yeasts of the Form-Phylum Deuteromycota**

Form-Class: Blastomycetes

Form-Family: Cryptococcaceae

Genus 1: *Cryptococcus.* Unicellular budding cells only; reproduce by blastoconidia pinched off the mother cell. Most are urease-positive. Cell surrounded by a heteropolysaccharide capsule and produces starchlike compounds; carotenoid pigments are usually lacking. Inositol is assimilated; sugars are not fermented.
    Example: *Cryptococcus neoformans* (cryptococcal meningitis).
Genus 2: *Malassezia.* Mostly unicellular budding cells which reproduce by blastoconidia that develop from a reduced phialide. Cells may adhere, forming short hyphal strands. Growth stimulated by lipids. There is no fermentative ability.
    Example: *Malassezia furfur* (pityriasis versicolor)
Genus 3: *Rhodotorula.* Unicellular budding forms that rarely produce pseudomycelium, are generally encapsulated, but do not produce starchlike substance. They do not assimilate inositol or ferment sugars. Carotenoid pigments are produced.
    Example: *Rhodotorula rubra* (rare pulmonary and systemic infections)
Genus 4: *Candida.* Reproduction is by pinched blastoconidia. They may form pseudomycelium or true mycelium; urease is generally negative; capsules are not formed; starch or carotenoid pigments are not produced; inositol is not assimilated.
    Example: *Candida albicans* (candidiasis)
Genus 5: *Trichosporon.* Reproduction is by blastoconidia and arthroconidia. Mycelium and pseudomycelium are formed.
    Example: *Trichosporon beigelii* (white piedra and systemic infections)
Genus 6: *Geotrichum.* Reproduction is by arthroconidia only. A true mycelium is formed.
    Example: *Geotrichum candidum* (rare pulmonary geotrichosis)

(Rippon, J. W.: Medical Mycology. 2nd ed. W. B. Saunders Co., Philadelphia, 1982.)

Candidiasis is one of the most frequently encountered of the fungal diseases. This is particularly true in the category of opportunistic infections. The species *Candida albicans,* which is responsible for most infectious processes, is endogenous in man. It is part of the normal flora of the buccal cavity, large intestine, and vagina. Under ordinary circumstances it is held in check by normal body defenses and other members of the normal flora. If this balance is changed, as in debilitation of defenses, overdose of antibiotics, or local physiological change, the organism begins to proliferate at a rapid rate and establishes an infection. Not only is it ubiquitous, it is the most variable of organisms in the clinical manifestations it may assume. Most commonly, it is associated with intertriginous dermatophyte-like infection, as well as onychomycosis, foot infection, vaginitis, and thrush. It may also be involved in bronchitis, pneumonitis, and rarely meningitis, endocarditis, and systemic involvement. This latter category is particularly prevalent in opportunistic infections. Such infections are increasingly common in patients following heart surgery, organ transplant, long-term steroid therapy, immunosuppressive therapy, and hyperalimentation.

The organism displays a nutritionally governed type of dimorphism. Under favorable conditions of growth in the presence of fermentable carbohydrate, the organism grows as a budding yeast. In mediums without fermentable carbohydrate and with semi-anaerobic conditions and/or a high nitrogen content, the yeast elongates, forming pseudomycelium and mycelium accompanied by blastoconidia and chlamydoconidia production (Fig. 43–20). Pseudomycelium and mycelium formation is also an index of colonization of tissue. The appearance of yeast forms alone usually means a saprophytic existence. The presence of both yeasts and mycelium in sputum, blood, urine,

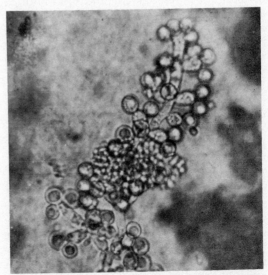

Figure 43–20. Live colony of *Candida albicans* which has produced a thick-walled chlamydospore and small blastospores on cornmeal agar. (S. Macmillan.)

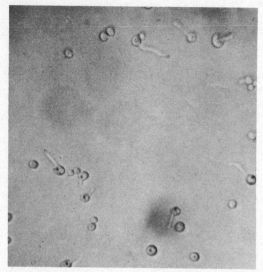

Figure 43–21. Sprout mycelium (R–B phenomenon) of *Candida albicans* after two hours in egg white or serum at 37 °C. × 400.

or stool specimens indicates colonization. When *C. albicans* is mixed with egg albumin or serum and incubated at 37° C., the yeast cells show "sprout" mycelium (Fig. 43–21). This Reynolds-Braude phenomenon affords a rapid diagnostic procedure. In tissue, elongation to form mycelium is commonly encountered. In experimental candidiasis, mycelium conversion occurred within two hours in the kidney after injection of *C. albicans* yeast.

The first description of a fungus of this type occurring in disease was that of Langenbeck, who in 1839 found it in patches on the mucous membranes of the mouth and elsewhere at autopsy. Gruby (1842) confirmed this finding, and the organism was named *Oidium albicans* by Robin four years later. The generic name *Candida* was proposed by Burkhout in 1923 and has come to be commonly used.

The Causative Organism

In addition to the original *Candida albicans*, a considerable number of species of *Candida* have been described, including *C. krusei*, *C. parapsilosis*, *C. tropicalis*, and *C. stellatoidea*. The second most commonly encountered pathogen is *C. tropicalis*. It may be missed if the specimen is planted on a cycloheximide medium, as it is sensitive to this chemical. Together with *C. albicans* it is considered virulent and can cause disease when injected into experimental animals. The other *Candida* are rarely isolated from disease processes. Some normal skin contaminants such as *C. parapsi-*

losis account for most *Candida* heart valve involvement, however. In fact, a large proportion of the current literature on these organisms is devoted to their differentiation, identification, and classification.[1, 2, 7, 10] Differentiation is made on the basis of various cultural characters, such as pellicle formation in liquid mediums, gelatin liquefaction, and differential fermentations and assimilations. The last is the most practical laboratory method. Fermentation and assimilation patterns as used in classification are found in the yeasts by Lodder.[7] The R–B egg test described above is the most rapid method of identifying *C. albicans*.

These various strains are immunologically related and show marked cross-reactions, but the group is not homogeneous. A detailed antigenic analysis has shown the essential identity of *C. albicans* and *C. tropicalis* and common antigens with *C. stellatoidea*. Similar studies by Hasenclever and his associates with *C. albicans*, for which chlamydoconidia production is the usual criterion for identification, showed that it is separable into two antigenic types, designated groups A and B. *Candida tropicalis* falls into group A and *C. stellatoidea* into group B. Strains of *C. tropicalis* and *C. stellatoidea*, as well as *C. albicans* strains of both groups, are virulent for the mouse, but the virulence of *C. albicans* for the rabbit appears to be significantly greater than that of the other species.

Serology

With the increased incidence of opportunistic infections, a serological test for systemic infection has become extremely important. The immunodiffusion test has therefore been developed. In this test, which uses the cell sap (S antigen), precipitin bands form in gel only in cases of systemic candidiasis and long-term chronic mucocutaneous disease. It is rarely positive in absence of infection but may be negative in cases of anergy or long-term immunosuppressive therapy.

Pathogenicity

Candida organisms are commonly present in the skin, mouth, vagina, and the intestinal tract in normal persons and are probably not highly virulent with respect to initiation of an infectious process. In fact, as in many of the mycoses, there is frequently a history of a debilitated condition or other predisposing factors, as noted previously. *Candida* infections have occasionally heralded prediabetic diathesis and hypoparathyroidism before the disease was clinically apparent. In some instances in which they are associated with the development of a pathological process, there is some doubt as to their etiological role; in many others it is clearly evident that they are primary invaders and responsible etiological agents. Several workers have demonstrated humoral anti-*Candida* factors. Unlike induced antibody, these remain at a particular level in normal individuals and are low or absent in diabetes, lymphoblastomas, and other diseases. Transferrin, clumping factor, etc., are among the factors described.

Infections of the Mucous Membranes. Candidiasis of the mucous membranes is known as **thrush** and is one of the common infections of newborn infants. After the establishment of the normal bacterial flora, thrush is of very rare occurrence. Thrush occurs more frequently in bottle-fed than in breast-fed babies, and the lesions not infrequently spread to the pharynx and even the esophagus. In older children or adults the appearance of thrush is associated with polyendocrine disorders, defects of immune mechanisms, or other serious malfunctions. Sometimes the disease progresses to chronic mucocutaneous candidiasis, a manifestation of a variety of underlying diseases. In adults, thrush may occur terminal to wasting diseases such as tuberculosis and cancer; dryness of the mouth associated with prolonged coma or near-coma appears to favor infection. It also occurs with some frequency as a mild vaginal infection in pregnant women which may or may not be associated with infection of the anus. Pruritis ani, a severe itching irritation of the anus due to colonization and the metabolic products of *Candida,* is a frequent complication of broad-spectrum antibiotics.

In the majority of cases the infection in the newborn is mild and remains localized. Occasionally it may spread to other mucous membranes and to the skin, with the development of a generalized cutaneous eruption, intertriginous lesions, and *Candida* granuloma; such cases are sometimes fatal. In the cutaneous form in infants this is to be distinguished from infantile eczema and allergic hypersensitivities. The most common predisposing malady for cutaneous candidosis is diabetes. Hematogenous spread with metastasis and abscess formation in the viscera has been observed.

The lesions of thrush appear as soft whitish patches on the tongue and pharynx, composed largely of fungal growth. They are readily removed and leave an eroded surface. There is some resemblance to a diphtheritic membrane, and lesions in the throat and on the tonsils have no doubt been mistaken for diphtheria. However, it is much easier to peel off the membrane in candidiasis. On microscopic examination of the membranous material in wet preparation, the observation of a tangled mass of segmented mycelium admixed with budding yeast-like cells, desquamated epithelium, and leucocytes establishes the diagnosis. The fungus may be cultivated on Sabouraud's agar, but isolation in pure culture is more readily accomplished with cycloheximide agar. The isolated fungus must be differentiated from other yeasts.

Dermatocandidiasis. *Candida albicans* is also causally associated with eczema-like lesions of the moist skin similar to those produced by *E. floccosum.* Infection of the folds between the fingers, erosio interdigitalis blastomycetica, is more common than dermatophytosis of this region, and is found most often in those whose hands are frequently wet. Perlèche, an infection of the angles of the mouth, is another form of intertrigo produced by these fungi. Ill-fitting dentures may lead to local lesions under the plates. Candidids, sterile vesicular or exudative lesions which appear on the hands secondary to a focus of infection elsewhere, are analogous to trichophytids and are a result of hypersensitivity.

The nails, chiefly of the fingers, are also attacked by *C. albicans* with the production of chronic onychia. The condition is differentiated clinically from tinea unguium by retention of the luster of the infected nail and the absence of yellowish discoloration, crumbling, and thickening of the soft tissues, as is seen in dermatophyte infection of the nail. The nail shows transverse ridges and eventually becomes thickened, distorted, and brownish in color, with frequent involvement of the surrounding nail bed (paronychia). Like interdigital infections, the infection is found most often in those whose hands are often wet.

On microscopic examination of nail and skin scrapings cleared in 10 per cent potassium hydroxide, hyphae may be present together with the budding yeast-like cells.

Candida granuloma is a chronic infection producing large granulomas on the skin. The patients usually have some immune defect. Chronic mucocutaneous candidiasis is also associated with a variety of immune defects, leucocyte dysfunction, etc. In some of these patients a specific IgG has been demonstrated which inhibits the *Candida* clumping effect of normal serum. Clumping appears to be intimately involved with phagocytosis of the organism.

Pulmonary Candidiasis. There appears to be a distinct type of candidiasis of the respiratory tract. This is an opportunistic infection and is associated with some underlying disease or treatment regimen. At present it is most frequently encountered in leukemia and lymphoma patients on cytotoxic therapy or in persons with diseases that require immunosuppression. Pulmonary disease in such patients is rare and represents miliary hematogeneous spread from some other focus of infection, usually the intestine. Sputum cultures are usually negative.

The fungus may be demonstrated by direct microscopic examination and culture, but such findings must be interpreted with caution. The organism is frequently found in sputum in other diseases, especially tuberculosis or chronic obstructive lung disease. It is recommended that the throat be cleansed by gargling before the sputum is collected and that other contamination be avoided. The presence of mycelial elements as well as yeast forms in fresh sputum samples is an indication of colonization by the organism (Fig. 43–22). This finding is difficult to assess, since colonization as thrush-like patches on the trachea in several pulmonary conditions occurs without discern-

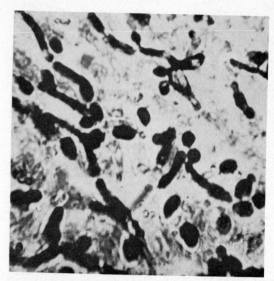

Figure 43–23. Candidiasis of kidney showing elongation of cells to form pseudomycelium and mycelium. In histologic sections from candidiasis, a mixture of yeast forms and hyphae is always present. Gram stain; × 600.

able harm to the patient. However, such patches on the esophagus are to be taken more seriously, as they may herald a rapidly fatal disease process.

Systemic Candidiasis. Systemic disease was of rare occurrence before the advent of antibiotics, macrodisruptive drugs, and surgical procedures. In the immunosuppressed patient or those on cytotoxin therapy, systemic candidiasis may result from invasion from the normal flora of the intestinal tract or rarely from generalization of an esophageal, genitourinary, or pulmonary infection. It is not infrequently the terminal event in leukemia and lymphoma patients. In tissue sections the organism is seen as a mixture of yeasts and hyphae (Fig. 43–23).

The presence of endocarditis following heart surgery is not uncommon, and in drug addicts it may develop on healthy valves. Septicemia and systemic colonization are not uncommon sequelae to long-term use of indwelling catheters. Candidiasis is such a common complication of hyperalimentation therapy as to contraindicate its use in many instances. These latter types of infections in a patient with normal cellular defenses can be cleared by removal of the portal of entry (intravenous needles, catheters, etc.) and the use of very low doses of amphotericin B. Systemic disease in the compromised patient usually requires full-dose amphotericin B. Cutaneous, mucocutaneous, and vaginal diseases respond to

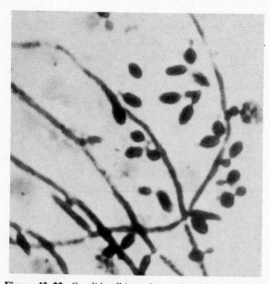

Figure 43–22. *Candida albicans* in a stained sputum specimen. The presence of hyphal elements in addition to the yeast forms indicates colonization of tissue by the organism. The patient had thrush-like lesions of the trachea. Neutrophils were also present. Gram stain; × 600.

topical nystatin and sometimes gentian violet. This latter group of patients benefit from use of ketoconazole. This oral drug is of limited value in the compromised patient and may suppress adrenal function.

The other "pathogenic yeasts" are more obviously opportunistic agents and are discussed under that heading.

THE SUBCUTANEOUS MYCOSES

Subcutaneous mycosis refers to a group of fungal diseases in which both the skin and subcutaneous tissue are involved but dissemination to the internal organs does not usually occur. The etiological agents are classified among several unrelated genera. They have the following characteristics in common: (1) they are primarily soil saprophytes of very low–grade virulence and invasive ability, and (2) in most human and animal infections they gain access as a result of traumatic implantation into the tissue. The list of organisms isolated from or designated as the cause of such conditions is long and varied. Blue-green algae in monkeys and dogs, *Prototheca zopfii* (an algae) and celery blight *(Mycocentrospora acerina)* in man, and *Beauveria* (a beetle fungus) in man and turtles are just a few of the interesting ones listed. This indicates that many, if not all, organisms have a potential to establish local infections under certain circumstances, depending on their adaptability and the response of the host.

Tissue response to these agents varies as to the etiological agent in question. In most cases the lesion tends to be localized, and the reactions that develop are similar to those elicited by a foreign body. Details of tissue response are discussed below.

The major disease types are chromoblastomycosis, sporotrichosis, mycetoma, lobomycosis, rhinosporidiosis, and the recently described and relatively rare entomophthoromycosis. Infection by agents of some of these groups is accompanied by a type of dimorphism. The organisms undergo a morphogenesis from their saprophytic form into a tissue stage. In chromoblastomycosis and mycetoma the response seems to be to complex tissue factors and is called tissue dimorphism. In the former, "sclerotic" cells are formed, in the latter granules (microcolonies) similar to those found in actinomycosis are found. The formation of yeast cells by *Sporothrix schenckii* can be termed an example of thermal dimorph-

ism. Mycetoma was discussed with the actinomycetes. The other organisms will be treated here.

Chromoblastomycosis

Chromoblastomycosis was discovered by Pedroso in 1911, but his observations were not reported until 1920. The first case in the literature was reported from Boston by Medlar in 1915. The geographical distribution is wide, however, with the greatest number of cases being found in the tropics.

Etiology

The causative fungi are closely related to the *Cladosporium* group of the Dematiaceae (Fungi Imperfecti). There are four common agents of the disease: *Fonsecaea pedrosoi, F. compacta, Cladosporium carrionii,* and *Phialophora verrucosa. Fonsecaea pedrosoi* accounts for the majority of infections. Three types of conidiation are observed, the predominant type differing from one strain to another. This has led to the splitting of strains into several genera with considerable confusion resulting. The new genus *Fonsecaea* was created by Negroni in 1936 and has gained general acceptance. Since the teleomorph (sexual) stage is unknown, true species lines cannot be definitely established. The more common etiological agents and their type of conidiation are listed in the table below.

The *(a)* cladosporium type of conidiation is characterized by chains of acropetelously budding conidia resembling *Penicillium;* the *(b)* rhinocladiella conidia type has single conidia around the septa and terminus of the fertile mycelium; and the *(c)* phialophora type has a group of conidia emerging from a vase-shaped phialid (Fig. 43–24*A, B*).

The organisms all have in common very slow growth of a gray to black-brown colony, lack of gelatin liquefaction, and identical tissue phase morphology. The fungus is a brown

Conidia Type	Species
a. Cladosporium	1. *Phialophora verrucosa (c* only) 2. *Cladosporium carrionii (a* and rarely *c)*
b. Rhinocladiella	3. *Fonsecaea pedrosoi (a, b, c).* Conidium is more elongate than in *F. compacta; c* sporulation is rare.
c. Phialophora	4. *Fonsecaea compacta (a, b, c).* Conidia in chains are round and closely packed.

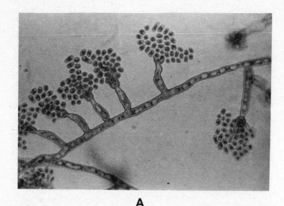
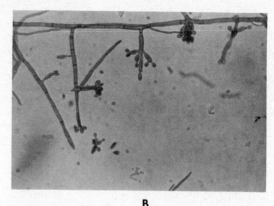

A   B

Figure 43–24. Chromoblastomycosis. Sporulation types. *A, Phialophora verrucosa.* Accumulation of conidia around flaring lips of phialid. × 400. *B, Fonsecaea pedrosoi.* Cladosporium (middle branching) and Rhinocladiella (left side not branching) conidiation. (Rippon, J. W.: Medical Mycology. 2nd ed. W. B. Saunders Co., Philadelphia, 1982.)

sclerotic cell (Medlar bodies, copper pennies) which divides by central planate septation of the yeast-like cell (Fig. 43–25). There is no budding. The granule, which is always brown, is easily seen in unstained material or in H and E–stained tissue sections. In some types of the disease other morphological forms of the fungus may be found. Mixed mycelium and yeast are seen in cystic disease, and mycelium alone are found in cladosporiosis of the brain (see Miscellaneous Mycoses) and opportunistic infections. The latter diseases are more correctly called phaeohyphomycoses and may occur in immunosuppressed patients.

Pathogenicity for Man

The disease is an infectious granuloma of the skin and subcutaneous tissues. It occurs usually, though not always, on the feet and legs. It ordinarily begins with a small warty growth on the foot and extends upward through the development of satellite lesions. This type of chromoblastomycosis is referred to as verrucous dermatitis. It usually remains localized; however, metastases to the brain and other organs are known. The disease develops very slowly; usually the case is of 10 to 15 years' duration at the time of examination, and some are known to have persisted for as long as 40 years. In advanced cases there is some elephantiasis of the affected limb, and great numbers of lesions. These vary somewhat and are of four general types: hard, elevated, pigmented nodules; large, cauliflower-like, prominent tumors; moderately elevated, dull red, scaly patches; and discrete or verrucous hyperkeratotic growths. The lesions are readily traumatized, and the disease may be complicated by secondary bacterial infection and ul-

ceration. The sclerotic cells appear as spherical brown bodies, perhaps 12 μm. in diameter, with a thick cell wall and granular protoplasm, and often show internal septation. They may be observed in biopsy specimens either within giant cells or free in the tissues, and are demonstrable in the epithelial debris obtained by scraping the lesions. The fungus may be cultured from such scrapings or from infected tissue. Chemotherapy with 5-fluorocytosine appears to be efficacious. The response to iodides, amphotericin B, and thiabendazole has been unsatisfactory. Early lesions can be removed surgically.

There appears to be no evidence of spread of the infection from one person to another.

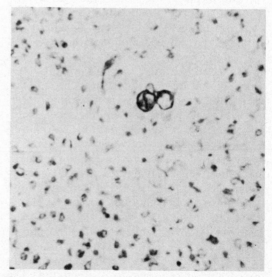

Figure 43–25. Chromomycosis. Brown granule with rounded cells showing planate division. *Phialophora verrucosa.* Hematoxylin and eosin; × 400.

Since the disease tends to occur on the legs and feet of barefoot outdoor laborers in the tropics, it seems probable that the fungi are saprophytes normally present in soil or decomposing organic matter (they have been isolated from lumber, where they cause "blueing"). When introduced into the skin by a splinter or thorn or through some minor abrasion, they may at times cause disease. For this reason, the disease occurs with some frequency among people in temperate climates who handle or come in contact with lumber, *e.g.,* gluteal disease from Finnish saunas. There appears to be good evidence at present for lymphatic and hematogenous spread of the disease in some cases. Involvement of the conjunctiva and central nervous system has been recorded, although there is some confusion in reported cases with cladosporiosis. *Fonsecaea pedrosoi* has been isolated from the lungs in rare cases, and the possibility of a pulmonary portal of entry must be considered. Chromoblastomycosis with sclerotic cells has been observed in rats, toads, and frogs. The same fungal species have been isolated from terminally ill, debilitated patients. In these cases the patient's resistance is low and the fungi grow as mycelium (phaeohyphomycosis).

Sporotrichosis

Sporotrichosis was first recognized by Schenck in the United States in 1898 and a few years later in France by Beurmann and Ramond. It has since been found all over the world, though the majority of reported cases are from the United States, especially from the Mississippi and Missouri Valleys, and from Mexico and South America. It occurs as an occupational disease in pottery workers, basket weavers, etc. The source of infection is the packing material, reeds, and sedges. The organism is favored by moderate temperature and high relative humidity. Epidemics have resulted from the growth of the organism on timbers in mine shafts.

Fungi of the genus *Sporothrix* are characterized by the production of pear-shaped conidia directly from the mycelium on small stems called denticles. These arise both laterally and at the tips of delicate sterigmata on a conidiophore and are described as "palm tree–like." After conidiation, the conidiophore may expand sympodially to form another apex and conidiate again (Fig. 43–26). The characteristic arrangement is not apparent in smears or tease mounts from cultures as the conidia are usually

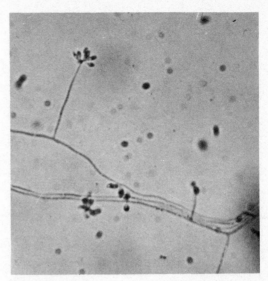

Figure 43–26. *Sporothrix schenckii* mycelium with delicate conidiophore and conidia (note "roping"). Lactophenol–cotton blue; × 400.

found free. However, the arrangement is readily demonstrable in slide cultures. The hyphae are considerably more slender, 2 μm. in diameter, than those of most molds and often form rope-like strands. The character of the growth on agar is different from that of other molds; the colony is first soft and creamy in consistency, becoming more firm as the culture grows older, and there is no cottony mass of aerial mycelium. The growth also becomes darker with age, being at first a light tan which deepens to a dark brown or even almost black. When cultured on blood cystine agar at 37° C., it grows as a budding yeast and is quite as "yeast-like" as *Histoplasma.* (see Table 43–14, p. 918). Mycelium is not formed in the tissues, and the parasitic phase of the fungus is a cigar-shaped body resembling an elongated yeast cell, 1 to 3 μm. in breadth and 10 to 20 μm. in length (Fig. 43–27). These bodies are found within leucocytes or free within tissue. They reproduce by budding and are rarely observed in human infections. Occasionally, so-called asteroid bodies, consisting of a central fungal cell with eosinophilic material radiating from it, are seen in human tissue sections and material from experimentally infected rat testes. This probably represents an immune complex. Because the organism is seldom seen in tissue, diagnosis is dependent on growing the organism.

The organism described by Schenck was named *Sporotrichum schenckii.* That isolated in France was supposed to be a different spe-

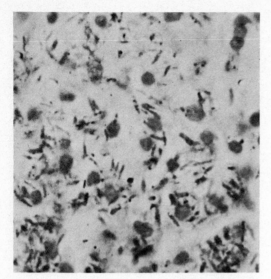

Figure 43–27. Sporotrichosis. Gram stain of heavily infected tissue showing elongate yeast-like cells.

cies and came to be known as *S. beurmanni.* The differences between the two are in pigmentation *(S. schenckii* being the lighter), the formation of fewer lateral spores by *S. schenckii,* and the fermentation of sucrose but not lactose by *S. beurmanni* and the reverse by *S. schenckii.* There also appear to be some differences in the clinical type of disease produced. These differences are not constant, however, being subject to environmental modification, and it is apparent that the two are but a single species, *S. schenckii.* The name *S. beurmanni* continues to persist in the literature, however, giving the impression of two recognized species. The fungus infecting horses, *S. equi,* is also identical with *S. schenckii.* In re-evaluating the genus *Sporotrichum,* Carmichael concluded that the etiological agent of sporotrichosis was more closely allied to another genus, *Sporothrix.* It is now considered that the correct epithet of the organism is *Sporothrix schenckii.* Mariat has noted the similarity of the organism to the imperfect stage of certain species of *Ceratocystis.* Further work may reveal the perfect stage of *S. schenckii* to be an ascomycete in the genus *Ceratocystis.*

Pathogenicity for Man
The most common form of sporotrichosis in this country is lymphocutaneous. The primary lesion, appearing at the site of some minor injury, fails to heal, ulcerates, and is followed by the appearance of a series of subcutaneous abscesses along the course of the regional lymphatics. The subcutaneous lymph vessels can often be traced as reddened lines. In the series of cases reported by Gonzales Bonavides, the disease occurred on the hand in 37.5 per cent, on the forearm in 25 per cent, on the arm in 6 per cent, and on the leg in 9 per cent, with lymphangitic extension in 37.5 per cent. Infection seldom extends beyond the regional lymph nodes, and cases of generalized hematogenous infection are uncommon. A second form, the fixed cutaneous form, occurs frequently in Mexico and South America. This form of the disease may represent previous sensitization to the organism as it occurs in highly endemic areas.

Metastatic lesions of sporotrichosis may appear in the joints most commonly, or in the liver or the lungs. The firm nodules in the skin are suggestive of syphilitic gummata, and probably some cases of sporotrichosis have been so diagnosed. Ocular sporotrichosis also occurs but is uncommon, and primary pulmonary disease is being seen more regularly, particularly in urban alcoholics. The most devastating form of the disease is known as gummatous sporotrichosis. In this form large areas of skin, subcutaneous tissue, and muscle "melt away," similar to the gumma occurring in tertiary syphilis.

Epidemiology
In the great majority of cases, the fungus is introduced into the tissues from plants through some abrasion. The disease has been observed in florists and the fungus isolated from sphagnum moss. There are reports in the older literature of man to man and animal to man transmission but these often lack validation. The organism has been observed growing free on grains, sedges, rose thorns, and meat in cold storage lockers. The fungus lives a saprophytic existence in nature, occasionally setting up an infection in man when mechanically introduced into the tissues. Isolation of the organism from soil has been made many times. Very few of these isolants, however, are able to grow at 37° C. or are pathogenic for experimental animals. As with other fungal infections, therefore, man acts as a selective agent for the "pathogenic" strains.

Diagnosis
The diagnosis of sporotrichosis is established by demonstration of the fungus. The cigar-shaped parasitic cell is gram-positive, but may be found only rarely in gram-stained pus smears. These forms are relatively infrequent

in human material, and sporotrichosis is not excluded by failure to find them. The fungus is readily cultivated on Sabouraud's medium with cycloheximide from pus aspirated from unopened lesions. Rats are highly susceptible to infection, and inoculation of rat testes is of considerable diagnostic value. Injection of male rats intraperitoneally and intratesticularly with lesion material or culture results in a pronounced orchitis and generalized peritonitis with minute nodules on all peritoneal surfaces. The cigar-shaped cells are present in abundance in the rat lesion material and may be found readily in gram-stained smears.

Treatment of choice is still potassium iodide. When this fails and particularly in systemic infections, amphotericin B, dihydroxy-stilbamidine, or thiabendazole may be utilized.

Immunity

There is an immune response to infection manifested by the appearance of agglutinins (for conidia), complement-fixing antibodies, and gel-diffusion precipitins. They are of some diagnostic value, though the first two are somewhat nonspecific in that serums from persons with thrush or actinomycosis may give positive reactions; the gel-diffusion is the most specific, but it is usually negative in early lymphocutaneous disease. A fluorescent antibody test has been used and is helpful in the diagnosis on tissue sections.

Entomophthoromycosis

Lie-Kian-Joe and Emmons first described the entity subcutaneous phycomycosis in 1946. Since then several hundred more cases have been diagnosed, and it may become a significant disease in tropical medicine. The accepted name for the disease is now entomophthoromycosis basidiobolae. Although it was first described in Indonesia, it is now known in many African countries, southeast Asia, and India. In Africa it coincides with the geographical range of Burkitt's sarcoma; an insect vector has been postulated for both. The etiological agent was the first designated *Basidiobolus ranarum,* a fungus associated with frogs and beetles, but the taxonomy is still in doubt. The disease is a long chronic process, often showing swelling of the arms, neck, chest, and trunk. The lesion involves the subcutaneous tissues and remains localized. Tissue section shows broad hyphae (20 μm.) surrounded by an envelope of eosinophilic material. This is probably an immune complex similar to the Splen-

dore-Hoepli phenomenon. The lesion is a granuloma composed of chronic inflammatory infiltrate, foreign-body giant cells, fibroblasts, and thick-walled capillaries. Many of the cases seem to have healed spontaneously or were lost to follow-up. Some have responded to potassium iodide therapy. Nothing is yet established as far as serology is concerned.

The etiological agents of this disease and of entomophthoromycosis conidiobolae (discussed below) are both members of order Entomophthorales. This and the order Mucorales are found in the phylum Zygomycota. The mucorales are often associated with opportunistic infection whereas the subcutaneous diseases discussed are not considered opportunistic. Therefore two categories have been designated: (1) mucormycosis, an opportunistic infection caused by members of the Mucorales, and (2) entomophthoromycosis, caused by members of the Entomophthorales. The correct term for the disease caused by *B. ranarum* is entomophthoromycosis basidiobolae. The second disease of this group is very rare and has always involved the nose, and was called rhinoentomophthoromycosis. The correct epithet would be entomophthoromycosis conidiobolae.

The latter infection is a chronic granulomatous disease so far found only in the nasal submucosa. It is caused by another member of the Entomophthorales, the spider parasite *Conidiobolus coronatus* and has been isolated from nasal polyps in horses also. In tissue section the pathology of the tissue and morphology of the organism is identical to entomophthoromycosis basidiobolae. Both *Conidiobolus* and *Basidiobolus* are easily cultured on the usual laboratory mediums.

Lobomycosis

This disease was first described in 1931 by Jorge Lobo in Brazil, and at first was thought to be a form of paracoccidioidomycosis. It is now known to be a different disease. The terms keloid blastomycosis or Lobo's disease are sometimes used. In lesions characteristic chains of yeast cells of uniform size (10 μm.) are found (Fig. 43–28). The tissue reaction is that of exaggerated fibrous hyperplasia resulting in keloid formation. In tissue section the organisms are very numerous. The disease is restricted to the subepidermal tissue and does not become systemic. So far, human cases have been found only in northern South America, especially Brazil and Surinam, and in Central

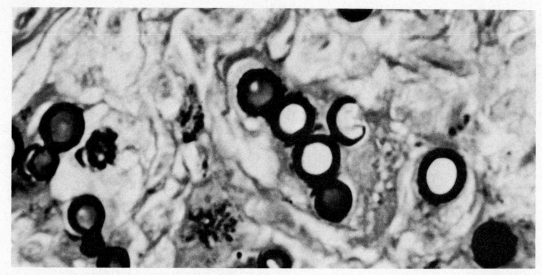

Figure 43–28. Lobomycosis, showing chains of round cells in skin biopsy. Note the distorted arrangement of collagen in this keloid induced by the infection. × 400.

America (a few). It has also been commonly observed in dolphins off the coast of Florida and South America. The organism has not as yet been cultured. For lack of specific identity, it is called *Loboa loboi.*

Rhinosporidiosis

Rhinosporidium seeberi is the name given to the agent of a chronic granulomatous disease characterized by production of polyps or other manifestations of hyperplasia on mucous membrane surfaces. The disease is characterized by friable, highly vascular, sessile or pedunculated polyps which may appear on almost any mucosal surface. The nose, nasopharynx, or soft palate is most often involved. The conjunctiva and lacrimal sac are also commonly involved. Lesions have been found on larynx, penis, vagina, rectum, and skin. The disease was first discovered in Argentina by Posadas in 1892 and reported by Seeber in 1900. About 2000 cases were recorded to 1964, when Karunaratne[6] reviewed the world literature. Of these, 88 per cent were from India and Ceylon. Rhinosporidiosis is also found with some frequency in the Choco Valley of Argentina and in Brazil, Colombia, and Venezuela. Data on about 40 cases have been published from the United States. Scattered cases occur throughout the world.

Histologically, a typical tumor is composed of squamous or columnar epithelium showing a stroma of connective tissue, capillaries, and fungal spherules. The spherules are 10 to 200 μm. in diameter and may contain 16,000 to 20,000 endospores (Fig. 43–29). The cycle of development is similar to that in coccidioidomycosis. The organism has never been cultured. Some claims of successful *in vitro* multiplication have been made, but these await confirmation. Some authors describe a protozoan-like karyosome along with a nucleus. The organism seems to be associated with stagnant water and may be a natural parasite of fish or other aquatic life.

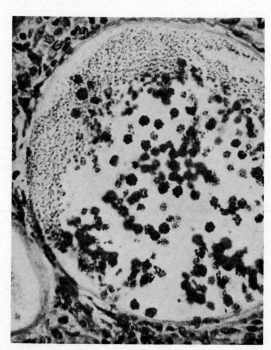

Figure 43–29. Giant spherule of rhinosporidiosis in nasal polyp. Hematoxylin and eosin; × 400.

THE SYSTEMIC MYCOSES

The systemic mycoses involve any or all of the internal organs of the body as well as cutaneous, subcutaneous, and skeletal systems. The usual portal of entry for the etiological agents involved is the lung, in contrast to the other mycoses. Infections are extremely common, especially in the United States, but the vast majority of cases are inapparent. In asymptomatic disease the diagnosis is most often made through a number of tests. Sensitization, which reflects present or previous experience with the organisms, is detected by means of skin test or other serological procedures. Its occurrence may be revealed by the presence of healed lesions observed in roentgenographic examination or at autopsy after death due to other causes. If the infection is symptomatic, the clinical signs may be those of a mild, self-limited disease, or the infection may become progressive with severe symptoms, tissue damage, and frequently death.

The organisms involved often show a predilection for a particular organ or type of tissue. *Histoplasma capsulatum* is an intracellular parasite of the reticuloendothelial system; *Cryptococcus neoformans* prefers the central nervous system; and *Blastomyces dermatitidis* usually involves cutaneous and mucocutaneous tissue and bones. On the other hand, any one of the organisms can elicit the same type of symptomatology and tissue response and can mimic many other systemic or cutaneous diseases.

The systemic mycoses are of two general categories (Table 43–13). The first involves organisms which, with sufficient infecting dose, will infect normal, healthy individuals and are called the true pathogenic fungus infections. All of these have the common attribute of changing their morphology in the infecting process. These are the thermal or tissue dimorphic fungi and include histoplasmosis, paracoccidioidomycosis, blastomycosis, and coccidioidomycosis (see Table 43–14). In the second category of disease are the opportunistic infections. The mycelial fungi involved in these processes, aspergillosis and mucormycosis, do not change morphology in the infection. These species are thermal and tissue tolerant but still unable to infect unless the patient's defenses are lowered or the patient is debilitated. For this reason they are called opportunistic infections. These include systemic candidiasis, aspergillosis, mucormycosis, and cryptococcosis. In addition to lack of dimorphism and inability to invade a normal host, there is a third difference between opportunists and true pathogenic fungi. The etiological agents of the dimorphic systemic mycoses have geographically restricted ranges, whereas the opportunists are ubiquitous and omnipresent.

In a certain sense all fungal diseases are "opportunistic." The normal, well-nourished

Table 43–13. **The Systemic Mycoses**

	True Pathogenic Fungus Infections	Opportunistic Fungus Infections
Diseases	Histoplasmosis Blastomycosis* Paracoccidioidomycosis Coccidioidomycosis	Aspergillosis Candidiasis Mucormycosis Cryptococcosis*
Host	Normal	Abrogated
Portal of entry	Primary infection pulmonary	Various
Prognosis	99% of cases resolve spontaneously	Recovery depends on severity of impairment of host defenses
Immunity	Resolution imparts strong specific immunity	No specific resistance to reinfection
Host response	Tuberculoid granuloma; also mixed pyogenic	Depends on degree of impairment—necrosis to pyogenic to granulomatous
Morphology in tissue	All agents show dimorphism to a tissue form	No change in morphology†
Distribution	Geographically restricted	Ubiquitous

(Rippon, J. W.: Medical Mycology. 2nd ed. W. B. Saunders Co., Philadelphia, 1982.)

*These diseases have significant exceptions to the usual patterns.

†*Candida* spp. are found as mixed yeast and mycelial elements in tissue, except *C. glabrata* and *C. famata*, which are yeasts only.

adult encountering pathogenic fungi is able to cope with them (except in overwhelming exposure), often asymptomatically. Mild or transient debilitation may allow an organism to become established. This debilitation ranges from slight malnutrition to genetic, physiological, or iatrogenic immune deficiency. The most frequent "opportunist" is *Candida,* previously discussed. Cryptococcosis is somewhat intermediate. Infections are most often associated with underlying disease, but sometimes apparently normal people acquire the infection. *Aspergillus* and *Mucor* species have a very specific set of predisposing conditions that precede infection.

THE TRUE PATHOGENIC FUNGUS INFECTIONS

One of the most remarkable and interesting phenomena exhibited by the fungi that infect man is **dimorphism** (Table 43–14). The organisms involved exist in a saprophytic or mycelial phase in nature but undergo a morphogenesis to a parasitic stage during the process of infection. The change is apparently an adaptation to an unfavorable environment and to a degree is inherent in almost all fungi. Several harmless saprophytes and dermatophytes have been induced into a transient yeast-like stage in which they can invade deep organs of experimental animals. The ability of the four species to change morphology and

cause infection seems to be an accidental phenomenon. Infection as far as the organisms is concerned is a blind alley as it does not appear to be necessary for the maintenance or dissemination of the species. The soil form produces the infectious conidia, man to man transmission is essentially unknown, and the organism usually dies with its host.

The factors that have been cited as important in bringing about the transformation of the saprophytic to the parasitic stage are several. The first and most important is temperature tolerance. If it cannot grow at 37°C., it cannot invade. The second is tissue tolerance; it must have the ability to grow in the reduced oxidation-reduction potentials of living tissue. The third is to be able to survive and overcome the cellular defense mechanisms of the host. The true pathogenic fungi are both temperature tolerant and tissue tolerant. The latter is doubtless involved in morphogenesis to a parasitic stage. To a certain extent these fungi overcome the defenses of the normal host and may cause a serious, sometimes fatal infection. The opportunists are thermotolerant but limited in ability for tissue tolerance and for overcoming cellular defenses. Therefore, only debilitated patients are invaded.

Among the true pathogenic fungi there may be ancillary factors necessary but parasitic stage growth *in vitro* and *in vivo* is governed by temperature. This has been shown by injecting poikilothermic animals with the organisms (either growth phase). In animals incu-

Table 43–14. **The Dimorphic Pathogenic Fungi**

Disease and Etiological Agent	Saprophytic Phase (25°C.)	Parasitic Phase (37°C.)
	Systemic Thermal Dimorphic Fungi	
Blastomycosis *Blastomyces dermatitidis*	Septate mycelium; conidia are pyriform, globose, or double. Colonies are white or beige, fluffy or glabrous.	Budding yeast with broad based bud, 8 to 20 μ.
Histoplasmosis *Histoplasma capsulatum*	Septate mycelium, microconidia, tuberculate macroconidia. Colonies are white or buff, fluffy.	Small, single budded yeast, 1 to 5 μ; 5 to 12 μ in var. *duboisii.*
Coccidioidomycosis *Coccidioides immitis*	Septate mycelium, fragment to arthroconidia. Colonies are buff or white, fluffy or "moth-eaten."	Spherules 10 to 80 μ. Endospores produced.
Paracoccidioidomycosis *Paracoccidioides brasiliensis*	Smiliar to *Blastomyces dermatitidis.*	Large, multiple budding yeasts 20 to 60 μ.
	Subcutaneous Thermal Dimorphic Fungus	
Sporotrichosis *Sporothrix schenckii*	Septate, delicate mycelium; conidia on denticles from delicate conidiophores. Colonies are verrucous, black, white, or grey; glabrous or fluffy.	Fusiform, oval budding yeasts, 5 to 8 μ.

(Rippon, J. W.: Medical Mycology. 2nd ed. W. B. Saunders Co., Philadelphia, 1982.)

bated at 25°C., infection occurred with mycelium in the tissues; if they were incubated at 37°C., infection was accompanied by transformation to yeast stage growth. It has been speculated that a temperature-sensitive enzymatic pathway is involved. Perhaps this is in the terminal respiratory chain and possibly involves ubiquinone. Its production in fungi responds both to temperature and to oxidation-reduction of the environment. The thermal dimorphic fungi are a well-delineated group and are described in Table 43–14. Most of these diseases are treated with amphotericin B.

Blastomycosis

The fungal disease known as blastomycosis was first observed in Baltimore in 1894 by Gilchrist and is also called Gilchrist's disease. The great majority of cases have been found in the United States, concentrated in the north central and eastern states, hence the former name North American blastomycosis. The disease has often been observed in the area on the western shores of Lake Michigan and is also called Chicago disease. At least a dozen cases have been reported and substantiated from Africa, Israel, Saudi Arabia, and Poland, which considerably extends its endemic range. Analysis of presumptive and inadequately described cases is difficult because of the usual failure to distinguish this disease from European blastomycosis (cryptococcosis), or African histoplasmosis (large yeast *H. capsulatum* var. *duboisii*). *Blastomyces dermatitidis* may also exist in a small yeast form, which is difficult to differentiate in tissue from the histoplasmosis organism.

The Causative Organism

This fungus was isolated in 1896 by Gilchrist and Stokes from a second case of the disease and named *Blastomyces dermatitidis*. It is dimorphic, occurring only as a unicellular, budding, yeast-like form in the tissues or *in vitro* at 37°C., but as a mycelial form in culture at 25°C. The unicellular form may be observed in potassium hydroxide preparations of pus or sputum. The cells are large, 8 to 10 μm. in diameter (Fig. 43–30), are round or oval, have double contoured walls, and are multinucleate. They show a single broad-based bud. The granular content of the cells distinguishes them from air bubbles or fat droplets, and identification is practically certain if budding cells are found. The teleomorph state has been de-

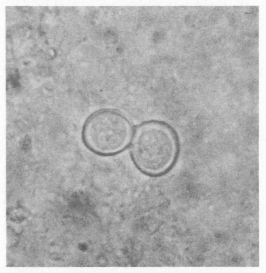

Figure 43–30. Potassium hydroxide preparation of pus showing yeast phase of *Blastomyces dermatitidis*. Note the broad-based bud and thick wall. × 400.

scribed as *Ajellomyces dermatitidis* and is placed in the family Gymnoascaceae of the phylum Ascomycota. The organism is, therefore, closely related to the dermatophytes.

Colonial Morphology. This unicellular morphology also occurs in cultures on nutrient or Sabouraud's agar, microscopic examination showing budding cells with a few rudimentary hyphae. The colony developing at 37°C. is wrinkled and waxy and somewhat similar in appearance to those of the tubercle bacillus. In culture on Sabouraud's agar at 25°C. the mycelial form appears. The colonial morphology is somewhat variable, and three types are distinguished. The "mealy" type is most often observed in primary isolation cultures and is similar to the growth on blood agar; microscopically the fungus is transitional between the unicellular and mycelial forms, with many of the cells tending to form articulated chains. After one or two transfers, the growth may assume a prickly surface, the prickles or spicules consisting of closely packed mycelial filaments which tend to become loose and cottony with continued incubation. The coloring is quite variable, from browns to tans to whites. The third type, sometimes observed on primary isolation and commonly found on laboratory cultures that are frequently transferred, is characterized by a white colony growth with abundant aerial mycelium; in these colonies the unicellular form has completely disappeared and growth consists of septate hyphae. Conidia of the chrysosporium type, 2 to 8 μm.

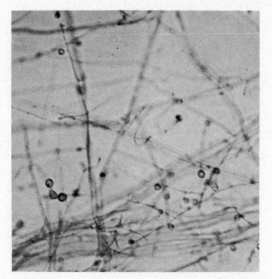

Figure 43–31. Mycelial phase of *Blastomyces dermatitidis*. Chrysosporum type of conidia. Lactophenol–cotton blue; × 400.

in diameter, are borne on lateral conidiophores (Fig. 43–31). They are not diagnostic, as they look similar to other fungal species. The mycelial form reverts to the unicellular yeast-like type in experimental infections or when cultivated on practically any medium at 37°C., and demonstration of dimorphism is necessary for diagnosis. The organisms has been recovered only a few times in nature; the yeast cells lyse in soil. An odd metabolic product of its metabolism is ethylene.

Pathogenicity for Man

There are three types of disease processes: (1) primary pulmonary, (2) secondary cutaneous, and (3) systemic. All infections are acquired through the pulmonary route, but the first symptoms are frequently cutaneous. Primary cutaneous disease may occur but is extremely rare; some five authenticated cases appear in the literature. The secondary skin lesion begins as a small, firm papule about which satellite nodules develop, enlarging with coalescence. The process breaks down in the center and becomes suppurative, with discharge of pus through small fistulas. The inflammatory reaction is granulomatous, with connective tissue formation, proliferation of the epithelium (pseudoepitheliomatous hyperplasia), and mononuclear infiltration; sometimes there is also giant cell formation. The fungus is found in the pus of minute miliary abscesses, which are a characteristic pathological feature. As the disease progresses, there-

fore, a large elevated mass of tissue, with an irregular ulcerated surface, is formed and oozes pus from multiple small openings upon pressure. The resemblance to epithelioma or tuberculous ulcer is sometimes striking. Lesions with pronounced epithelial proliferation simulate tuberculosis verrucosa. The process spreads slowly through the subcutaneous tissues. There is healing in the center of the lesions with scar formation. Biopsy for histological or cultural examination should be taken from the active edge of the lesion. The organisms are very few in tissue sections. The very rare primary inoculation blastomycosis of the skin is a chancriform lesion with numerous organisms present and local lymphadenopathy.

Primary infection of the lungs often closely resembles tuberculosis or histoplasmosis clinically. There is cough, pain in the chest, weakness, sometimes hemoptysis, and productive sputum late in the disease. The radiologic picture is variable in that there may be focal or diffuse consolidation, and the abscesses may be miliary or there may be larger nodules. Often a "crab claw" shadow of the hilum will suggest carcinoma. Cavitation occurs but is limited to small areas. The microscopic picture also resembles tuberculosis, and sometimes it is difficult to differentiate unless the budding cells are found. Primary infection is often asymptomatic—the first manifestations are those of secondary skin involvement. This is similar to the clinical course seen in paracoccidioidomycosis.

With generalization from primary foci of infection, multiple small abscesses of hematogenous origin occur throughout the body. They are most common in the subcutaneous tissues and differ from the skin lesions in that they develop without pain or marked erythema, are soft, and evacuate considerable quantities of pus when opened. In contrast to the skin lesions, which most commonly occur on exposed parts of the body, the secondary subcutaneous abscesses are usually found in covered areas. Secondary abscesses also commonly develop in the bones and viscera, in muscles, under the periosteum, and especially in the prostate. The eye may rarely be affected. The disease may be chronic and persist for years, but in the generalized infection there is a septic febrile reaction and the case-fatality rate is high. The diamidines stilbamidine and dihydroxystilbamidine have therapeutic activity, but relapses are not uncommon. Currently amphotericin B is the drug of choice, except in uncomplicated pulmonary infection where the less toxic drug dihydroxystilbamidine is useful. Males are much more prone to progressive and disseminated disease than are females, and most are in the 20- to 50-year-old group.

Unlike other systemic mycoses (histoplasmosis, coccidioidomycosis), infection with *B. dermatitidis* is a progressive disease; since spontaneous remission is uncommon, it most often requires treatment.

Pathogenicity for Lower Animals

The inoculation of experimental animals is not uniformly successful and has no diagnostic utility. Mice are more susceptible than are guinea pigs, and rabbits are almost completely resistant. Small caseous nodules develop on the peritoneal surfaces of intraperitoneally inoculated animals, and the type of tissue reaction varies with the resistance of the animal and the virulence of the strain of fungus from frank abscess formation to tubercle-like lesions. Natural infection occurs in a variety of animals. In endemic areas the disease is very common in dogs. It also occurs with some frequency in horses.

Immunity

There appears to be a strong resistance to the initial infection by the host. However, once the organism is established there is a long chronic relentless course eventually leading to dissemination. Spontaneous resolution of infections, commonly seen in histoplasmosis and coccidioidomycosis, is rarely encountered in blastomycosis. At present there is no meaningful complement fixation test or skin sensitivity test. Thus diagnostic, prognostic, and epidemiological evaluation is unavailable for this disease, in contrast to histoplasmosis or coccidioidomycosis. A fluorescent antibody test is available for histological examination.

Diagnosis

As indicated above, the yeast-like unicellular form of the fungus can be demonstrated by direct microscopic examination of pus or sputum mounted in potassium hydroxide. Positive complement fixation and skin tests are of no value in pulmonary and systemic infections as presently done. An unequivocal diagnosis can be established, however, only by isolation and identification of *B. dermatitidis*. This is usually not difficult, as the fungus grows readily on cycloheximide agar at room temperature. After growth has been established, it is necessary to confirm the diagnosis by demonstrating dimorphism to the yeast stage. This is done by taking mycelium from the cycloheximide blood-agar plate and planting on plain agar and incubating for several weeks at 37°C. The yeast stage of both *Blastomyces* and *Histoplasma* is sensitive to cycloheximide.

Coccidioidomycosis

Coccidioidomycosis was first observed in Argentina in 1892 by Posados and by Wernicke; two years later it was described independently in California by Rixford. The causative organism was thought to be a protozoan and named *Coccidioides immitis*. In the tissue phase it resembled the coccidia group of protozoan parasites, a group that includes *Eimeria coccidiosis* of chickens and such other bird pathogens as *Isospora*. Ophuls and Moffitt demonstrated by culture that it is a fungus, but this does not invalidate the name. Its relationship to other fungi is uncertain. Though originally reported from South America, the disease appears to be uncommon there. It is most prevalent in the San Joaquin Valley in California and in the dry regions of the southwestern United States and north central Mexico. There are scattered areas of endemicity in Guatemala, Honduras, Colombia, Venezuela, Bolivia, and Argentina. The organism is associated with a particular ecological niche known as the Lower Sonoran life zone. This zone includes desert rodents, the creosote plant, and a highly alkaline salt soil having high boron content. Reports of rare cases in other parts of the world are probably the result of transmission by fomites. A coccidioides-like disease is recognized in Russia, the etiology of which is not yet well described.

The Causative Organism: Parasitic Stage

This fungus differs markedly from the yeast-like fungi in that it never reproduces by budding, and it differs from most other pathogenic fungi in that it reproduces within the tissues exclusively by a process of endogenous spore formation. The newly liberated spores are small mononucleate spheres 1 to 3 μm. in diameter and appear as a central, deeply stained mass of protoplasm surrounded by a double-contoured cell wall. The cell enlarges, soon becoming multinucleate, and eventually reaches a diameter of 50 to 60 μm. A central vacuole appears early and in later stages occupies a large portion of the cell, the protoplasm appearing as a thin peripheral layer.

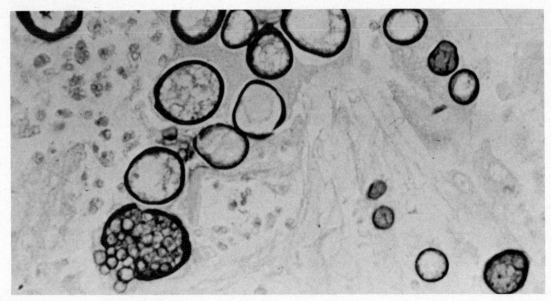

Figure 43–32. Lung tissue showing various stages of development of *Coccidioides immitis* spherules. Some are young and newly released, while others are organizing cytoplasm into cleavage planes for endospore production. One spherule is breaking and releasing mature endospores. Gridley stain; × 440.

The peripheral protoplasm becomes vacuolated by cleavage planes, and an indefinite number of multinucleate protospores becomes delimited. The protospores in turn subdivide to form spores and the entire cell assumes a function similar to that of a sporangium. With rupture of the cell wall the mature spores are liberated, and the developmental cycle begins again (Fig. 43–32). It is at the time of rupture that neutrophils invade the area and may phagocytize and kill the newly released endospores. A similar type of spherule-endospore cycle occurs in rhinosporidiosis. Spherules are also found in adiospiromycosis but these contain no endospores. All of these forms may be observed in the tissues and in pus, though recently disseminated spores are difficult to demonstrate. Hyphal forms have been observed in old necrotic tissue but are very rare. The morphological phase found in the tissues can be produced *in vitro* by culturing at 37°C. or 40°C.

The Causative Organism: Saprophytic Stage

The fungus will grow on a variety of sugar-containing mediums, but Sabouraud's agar is the medium of choice. It grows best at 25°C., under aerobic conditions. On artificial culture mediums the growth is that of a mold. The colony may be smooth and waxy when young, aerial mycelium is soon formed, and it becomes gray or brownish in color. Fragmentation with the formation of arthroconidia begins on side branches (Fig. 43–33). The arthroconidia are barrel- or cask-shaped, are thick-walled, and have an empty space between successive conidia. On any medium, but particularly Converse broth with increased CO_2 tension at 37 to 40°C., *C. immitis* will convert from the mycelial to the spherule stage of growth.

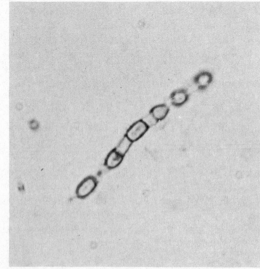

Figure 43–33. Mycelial phase of *Coccidioides immitis* at 25° C. Barrel-shaped arthrospores with empty cells in between. Lactophenol–cotton blue; × 400.

Pathogenicity for Man

For many. years infection with *C. immitis* was known only as coccidioidal granuloma, a severe disease in which the case-fatality rate was thought to be 90 per cent or more. Infection with this fungus is, however, much more prevalent and less severe than had been supposed. It is estimated that 20 to 40 million people in the southwestern United States have or have had coccidioidomycosis. Healed lesions of coccidioidal granuloma are found at autopsy of persons who have died of other causes, and similar arrested lesions have been produced in white rats. Furthermore, it was shown by Dickson in 1937 that the disease may take a second form (known as "valley fever" or "desert rheumatism"), a benign, acute, self-limited respiratory infection, in addition to the chronic, progressive granulomatous disease. He suggested that these be designated primary and secondary or progressive coccidioidomycosis, respectively, and these terms are now in general use. It is now felt that the experience of the benign self-limited disease confers a rather effective immunity. Coccidioidomycosis is the most virulent and most dangerous of all the fungal diseases. Many laboratory accidents have occurred, some fatal. Though the dissemination rate is less than or near 1 per cent, it may be 10 times that in dark-skinned individuals. Any extension beyond the benign self-limited disease must be considered very dangerous for the patient and treated as such. In South America the infection is known as Posada's disease.

Primary Coccidioidomycosis.

The infection is acquired by inhalation of the conidia. The disease varies in severity in recognized cases from that of a common cold to that of cases resembling influenza with pneumonia, cavitation, and high fever. In a small proportion of the cases, possibly 5 per cent, an exanthem-like erythema nodosum or erythema multiforme occurs. This form of disease is known as "the bumps," desert rheumatism, valley fever, San Joaquin fever, etc. Persons showing this allergic response very rarely develop serious progressive disease. Many infections are symptomless, however. In a group of 1351 cases studied by Smith *et al.*, 60 per cent were symptomless, and dissemination with development of the progressive disease occurred in about 1 per cent of the clinically apparent infections. They also noted that dissemination occurred 10 times as frequently in blacks, Mexicans, Portuguese, or Indians as in whites. Minor "epidemics" may occur when people come into contact with areas heavily contaminated. Goldstein and Louie reported that, of several thousand soldiers exposed during military training in an endemic desert area, 75 contracted clinically significant disease. All but one made rapid progress to complete recovery, but the remaining individual developed a generalized infection and coccidioidal granuloma. Almost all personnel, however, became skin test-positive. A similar incident occurred in a prisoner-of-war camp near Florence, Arizona, and in a housing development called Paradise Valley near Phoenix, Arizona. The disease is also a major problem in northern Mexico. Spontaneous recovery is the rule, and only rarely does the disease progress to the secondary type. Residual pulmonary lesions, closely resembling healed tuberculosis or histoplasmosis lesions, are common. In all three diseases, healing granuloma tend to calcify.

Secondary or Progressive Coccidioidomycosis.

The progressive type of infection results in cutaneous, subcutaneous, visceral, osseous, and central nervous system lesions, as well as extension of lesions into the lungs. If the disease is well established in the lung, it seldom remains exclusively pulmonary. The cutaneous type closely resembles blastomycosis but is a much more severe disease, with fever and a greater tendency to hematogenous spread. Elsewhere the lesions closely resemble those of tuberculosis, and, in fact, differentiation from that disease may often be possible only by demonstration of the fungus. Meningeal involvement is often fatal. Amphotericin B is reported to be an effective chemotherapeutic agent in the disseminated infection, but a more effective drug is greatly needed. As in the treatment of all systemic fungal diseases, the toxicity, especially the nephrotoxicity, is a serious side effect. Other side effects are fever, anemia, phlebitis, and various allergic responses. When used intrathecally, arachnoiditis may result, which may have paraplegia as a sequel.

Pathogenicity for Lower Animals

The disease occurs naturally in domestic animals, including cattle, sheep, and dogs, and also in certain wild rodents in endemic areas. The latter include three species of pocket mice, *Perognathus baileyi,* *P. penicillatus,* and *P. intermedius;* the kangaroo rat, *Dipodomys merriani;* and the grasshopper mouse, *Onychomys torridus.* The disease can be disseminated to a new area from the carcass of an animal that has died from it. Experimental animals are readily infected; both rabbits and guinea pigs are susceptible to intraperitoneal inoculation and mice to intracerebral inoculation. Mice, inoculated intracerebrally or intraperitoneally, are used for virulence assay. Sometimes the spherules attain a size of 100 μm. or more in mice.

Immunity

It is now apparent that infection with *C. immitis* can take a mild form from which spontaneous recovery is the rule. Arrested lesions occur with frequency. This indicates that there is an appreciable natural resistance to infection; it also indicates that an effective immunity results from the cleared initial infection, as progressive disease is relatively rare and reinfection essentially unknown.

The immune response is manifested in part as the development of a hypersensitivity to the parasite. Coccidioidin is, like tuberculin (OT), prepared from liquid cultures of the parasite. There is some difficulty in reproducing potencies. An immunologically active polysaccharide appears to make up at least a part of the active principle, producing both skin reactions and precipitin reaction. Coccidioidin is inoculated intradermally, a positive reaction appearing in 24 to 48 hours. The hypersensitivity appears in a few days to a few weeks after infection, recent infections and severe infections resulting in stronger reactions than old infections and mild infections, respectively. The test appears to be highly specific, though there is as yet some disagreement as to its interpretation.

Humoral antibodies are formed also. Complement fixation and precipitin tests, using an autolysate of culture as the antigen, have been developed and are specific. In general, serum antibody is not detectable prior to the development of skin sensitivity. Precipitin appears first and is demonstrable in 50 per cent of cases by the end of the first week of the disease and in 90 per cent or more by the third week, and then gradually falls until no titer is demonstrable after seven months. The complement fixation reaction becomes positive more slowly, with about 8 per cent positive reactions by the end of the first week, and 90 per cent by the third month. Fall in titer may become apparent by the second month and most antibody has disappeared by the sixth to eighth month. In secondary and disseminated disease the CF titer stays the same or rises. Thus the titer of complement-fixing antibody has considerable prognostic significance; rising titer is indicative of the development of the progressive granulomatous form of the disease, often before this is evident clinically. Gel-diffusion tests, fluorescent antibody techniques, and latex particle agglutination tests have been developed.

Diagnosis

The laboratory diagnosis of coccidioidomycosis is dependent upon the demonstration of the parasite. The diagnostic value of a positive coccidioidin reaction is limited because it persists long after resolution of the disease. As indicated earlier, the fungus may be found on direct microscopic examination of pus, spinal fluid, and tissues but may be difficult to demonstrate in the sputum. A KOH preparation is particularly useful. Lactophenol–cotton blue or Mallory's eosin and methylene blue may be used for staining. Though *C. immitis* grows without difficulty on sugar-containing mediums, it has been cultured in a surprisingly small proportion of cases. It grows on cycloheximide medium. There is a very considerable hazard in culturing the fungus owing to the infectivity of the spores, and special precautions are required.

Epidemiology

In the endemic areas of the southwestern United States, the proportion of reactors to the coccidioidin test is high, ranging from 46 to 90 per cent. The prevalence of infection in these regions appears, therefore, to be much higher than suspected earlier. A very large proportion of these reactors have no history of coccidioidomycosis. It has been estimated that only 40 per cent of infected persons have clinical symptoms and only 5 per cent have sufficiently severe disease to be diagnosed.

Though, as indicated earlier, the disease occurs in domestic animals and certain wild rodents, there is no evidence of direct transmission of the infection from animals to man, although dead animals may contaminate the soil in which they are buried. It seems likely that both man and animals are infected by the inhalation of spores contained in dust; there is frequently a history of exposure to dust storms in human cases, and the fungus has been isolated directly from dust. *Coccidioides immitis* is a saprophyte which infects animals and man by chance; the reservoir of infection appears to be the soil. A mild disease is produced in some desert rodents. These may carry the organism from place to place and act as a vector of transmission. During the summer the sun sterilizes the desert soil of *C. immitis*, but it survives and proliferates in rodent burrows.

Paracoccidioidomycosis

The disease known as paracoccidioidal granuloma, Lutz's disease, or South American blastomycosis occurs in Brazil and elsewhere in South America and in Mexico. The endemic regions are warm, wet tropical or subtropical rain forests. The causative organism is *Paracoccidioides brasiliensis*. It has been recovered from soil. This is a yeast-like fungus, proliferating by multiple budding in the tissues (Fig. 43–34), grows in a compact cerebriform colony on Sabouraud's agar, eventually producing a white aerial mycelium and single or double conidia shaped similarly to those of *B. dermatitidis* (see Table 43–14).

The disease is clinically similar to coccidioidomycosis and blastomycosis. The primary infection, often inapparent, is pulmonary, and as in blastomycosis, healed lesions do not calcify. The fungus is then probably transported by macrophages to the oral and gingival mucosa. At these points ulcerative granulomatous lesions are produced. Often these spread to the tongue, lips, and nose. Lymphatic involvement is a characteristic of the disease. The infection spreads via the lymphatics to produce lesions of the viscera and, often, pulmonary involvement. It is often fatal if untreated. Guinea pigs are usually infected by intratesticular inoculation and may also be infected by intratracheal inoculation. Natural infections in animals are unknown. The fungus will grow readily on agar mediums. A fluorescent antibody diagnostic technique has been described, and an immunodiffusion test and skin test antigen have been produced. These are specific for the disease. It appears that, similar to histoplasmosis, inapparent infection is more common than previously suspected, and only the rare severe forms have previously been recognized. Skin test sensitivity shows about a 50:50 sex distribution of reactors within endemic areas. However, 90 per cent of all clinical cases are in males. In almost all fungal diseases males are more frequently involved than females. Some female hormones are thought to be inhibitory to the growth of fungi.

Diagnosis is established by microscopic demonstration of the multiple budding cells (in contrast to the single budding cells of *B. dermatitidis*) in material from the lesions or by culture. Treatment formerly consisted of 4 gm of sulfadiazine a day for life, but amphotericin B and ketoconazole offer hope of clinical cures.

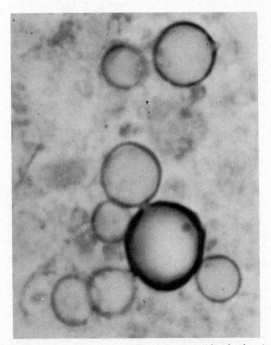

Figure 43–34. Giant yeast cells of *Paracoccidioides brasiliensis* showing multiple budding "Mickey Mouse form." Sometimes the buds are small and of uniform size. This is termed the "pilot wheel" form. Gridley stain; × 400. (P. Graff.)

Histoplasmosis

This organism was discovered in 1906 in Panama by Darling. He observed it in sections of tissues taken postmortem from three cases of what appeared to be visceral leishmaniasis. He named it *Histoplasma capsulatum* (plasmodium within histiocytes and having an unstained area—"capsule"). The first case in the United States was reported in 1926. By 1946 only about 70 cases had been recorded. All of these were of the severe forms of the disease. In 1945 Christie published an important paper on calcifications in lungs of tuberculin-negative patients in Tennessee. In the next year Palmer published a larger study. By skin testing it was shown that these cases represented the benign form of histoplasmosis and that the disease is extremely common in endemic areas.

Healed lesions of pulmonary infections are frequently found at autopsy in areas where the disease is prevalent. The prevalence of the infection is shown by skin testing for hypersensitivity to the microorganism. It is now believed that in the United States 40 million people have or have had histoplasmosis, most residing in the Ohio and Mississippi River valley areas. The disease has been studied most intensively in the United States, but apparently its distribution is worldwide.

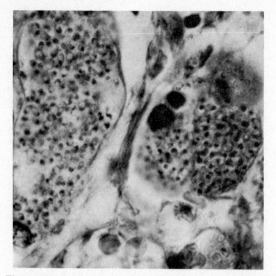

Figure 43–35. *Histoplasma capsulatum.* Yeast-like cells in macrophages of the bone marrow in systemic histoplasmosis. Hematoxylin and eosin; × 1000. (Humphreys.)

The Causative Organism

The organism appears in the tissues as a small, oval, yeast-like cell 2 to 4 μm. in diameter with the appearance of a capsule, although there is none. The unstained area represents cell wall (Fig. 43–35). In tissue stained with Giemsa stain it is difficult to distinguish the organism from that of leishmaniasis except for the karyosome bar in the latter. Larger strains, up to 15 μm. in diameter, are found in duboisii histoplasmosis (*H. capsulatum* var. *duboisii*) (Fig. 43–36). In stained preparations the central stained mass is surrounded by a clear zone. The organism is usually intracellular, in the mononuclear leucocytes in the peripheral blood and in the macrophages else-

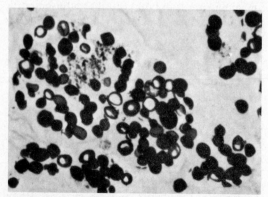

Figure 43–36. Giant yeast cells of *Histoplasma capsulatum* var. *duboisii.* Duboisii histoplasmosis. From a gluteal biopsy of the baboon housed in a Lansing, Michigan, zoo. Methenamine silver; × 440.

where, especially those of the bone marrow and spleen. Because of this characteristic intracellular position of the parasite, the disease is sometimes called reticuloendothelial cytomycosis, or simply cytomycosis. The common worldwide histoplasmosis is caused by *H. capsulatum.* The duboisii form differs by its larger yeast form (var. *duboisii*). This form has also been found in Japan and will probably be isolated in other parts of the world. A second species, *H. farciminosum,* causes farcy in horses and is found around the Mediterranean area and East Africa. It differs from the other two in having smooth-walled macroconidia in its saprophytic stage. The anamorph (formerly called "perfect" or "sexual") state of *H. capsulatum* has been described. It is one of the heterothallic Gymnoascaceae called *Ajellomyces capsulatus.* It is closely related to the dermatophytes and the anamorph state of *Blastomyces dermatitidis.*

The microorganism is cultivable from the blood or biopsy specimens, or it may be isolated from the sputum in pulmonary infections. Soil or pathological material from patients can be inoculated into animals. It grows in the yeast-like form seen in the tissues in blood-agar cultures at 37° C. (Fig. 43–37) and in tissue culture, but on Sabouraud's cycloheximide agar a mycelial form is assumed and the colonies are mold-like, white or tan, and cottony with aerial mycelium when incubated at 25° C. Macroconidia are formed in abundance. At first they are smooth and pyriform, but as they mature they become larger, 7 to 15 μm. in length, thick-walled, and tuberculate with finger-like protuberances, sometimes as much as 6μm. long. Microconidia are also present (Fig. 43–38).

Pathogenicity for Man

Three types of disease are generally recognized. The acute pulmonary type is characterized by sudden onset of malaise, fever, cough, chest pains, chills, sweats, and dyspnea, ranging in severity from severe flu syndrome to subclinical involvement. In this most common form the attack is followed by quick recovery, and a fairly strong immunity develops. It is essentially similar to the primary benign form of coccidioidomycosis. Progressive disease occurs in only 0.1 to 0.2 per cent of cases. The focal granuloma is associated with lymphadenitis of the hilar lymph nodes which then heals, often with calcification, and leaves a lesion roentgenographically identical to those of tuberculosis. Calcifications are also found in the spleen. In all its forms, histoplasmosis

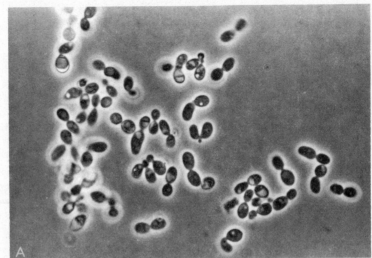

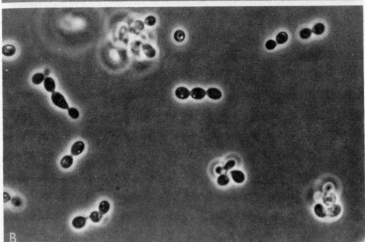

Figure 43–37. Histoplasmosis. Microscopic morphology of yeast form cells from culture. Phase microscopy, × 800. (Courtesy of M. Berliner.) (Rippon, J. W.: Medical Mycology. 2nd ed. W. B. Saunders Co., Philadelphia, 1982.)

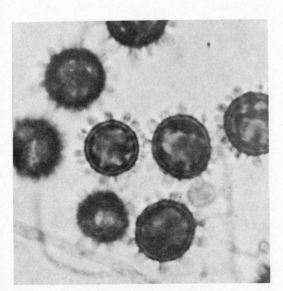

Figure 43–38. *Histoplasma capsulatum.* Mycelial stage showing tuberculate macroaleuriospores and microaleuriospores. Lactophenol–cotton blue; × 400.

mimics tuberculosis. The disease is highly endemic in the midwestern United States, where it is common in children and is called summer flu or summer illness. Almost all cases resolve uneventfully.

The second type of disease, chronic progressive pulmonary histoplasmosis, may present as an exaggeration of the symptoms given above. It is usually found in middle-aged males and is heralded by persistently positive results for the complement fixation test. The disease progresses, like tuberculosis, to necrosis, caseation, and cavitation. The process is usually very slow. The lesion in the lung is called a histoplasmoma and similar in morphology to a tuberculoma.

The third form of the disease is disseminated histoplasmosis, which may develop at any age, but is commonly seen in infants, severely debilitated older patients, or middle-aged adult males. It has a rapid, fulminating, fatal course or may wax and wane over a period of years. This occurs most commonly in adults. Affected children are usually physiologically defective and their disease has a rapid downhill course. This form of the disease is also seen in older people, particularly poor-risk patients, who may have lymphoma, Hodgkin's disease, diabetes, etc. Some of these represent reactivation of old histoplasma granulomas formed many years previously. The third patient-type seen is the middle-aged male patient with an old pulmonary infection which disseminates by extension. Such patients usually have chronic obstructive lung disease or "smoker's" emphysema. Dissemination may involve any organ, but especially the spleen and liver. The first clinical signs may be lesions on mucocutaneous areas.

It is apparent that histoplasmosis is always a generalized infection of the reticuloendothelial system, the parasites being especially numerous in tissues rich in these cells, such as the spleen and bone marrow. Systemic symptoms are not perceptible, however. Although there may be wide dissemination within phagocytes following initial infection, most of these heal immediately without establishment of a disease process. In most cases there are nodules or extensive areas of necrosis in one or more organs, but in some instances only a single organ, such as the adrenals, has been infected. These necrotic lesions usually consist of a central area of necrosis surrounded by granulation tissue containing large numbers of macrophages and ingested parasites. In some instances the parasite has been found to be limited to such areas, while in others it is

widely distributed in the macrophage system as well. Infection of the central nervous system is relatively rare but has been observed. That such dissemination is common even in resolved cases is evident from studies on routine autopsies, in which calcified lesions of the spleen have commonly been found. These represent resolved lesions of several decades earlier.

Experimentally infected animals give a positive reaction to the intradermal inoculation of a preparation of liquid culture of *H. capsulatum* analogous to old tuberculin and coccidioidin and designated histoplasmin. In areas in which the disease is endemic, positive reactions are correlated with the incidence of pulmonary calcification in tuberculin-negative individuals. The association of positive histoplasmin reactions with calcified nodules in the lungs suggests that, as in the case of coccidioidomycosis, histoplasmosis is not a rare, highly fatal disease, but one which is widespread in certain geographical areas in a mild pulmonary form. That such reactors are or have been actually infected is difficult to demonstrate on any large scale, but infection has been shown in a sufficient number of cases to strongly support such an inference. Precipitins are produced early in the disease and disappear fairly rapidly. The complement-fixing antibody titer rises somewhat later and disappears later, usually by five to seven months. If the complement-fixing titer persists or rises, the prognosis is poor. Precipitating antibodies demonstrable by the gel-diffusion technique are also present. Two lines may be formed: the so-called m line near the antigen-containing well indicates experience with the disease, and the thin h line nearer to the serum-containing well correlates with active disease (Fig. 43–39). The fluorescent antibody technique is useful in the diagnosis of histoplasmosis.

The treatment of choice is amphotericin B in the usual course given for systemic fungal disease, 0.6 mg./kg. body weight to a total of 1 to 3 gm. There are some severe side effects from amphotericin B therapy.

Pathogenicity for Lower Animals

A variety of animals have been found to be naturally infected, including dogs and cats, wild rodents, and other wild animals. An association with bats and bat caves has been well established. The microorganism has been isolated from bat tissue, but the role of these animals as a reservoir and in the dissemination of the infection remains to be determined. The bats may act as vectors carrying the organism from one cave to another. Mice have been

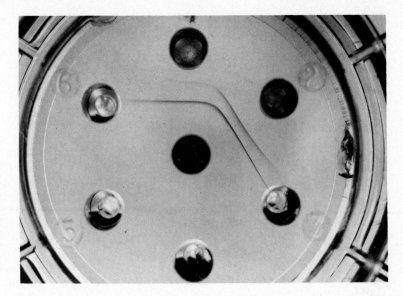

Figure 43–39. Histoplasmosis. Immunodiffusion plate with a known positive serum in one outer well and an unknown one in an adjacent well. The antigen is in the center well. Note the lines of identity in the two tests. The h line is the finer line near the serum-containing well. The m line is near the antigen-containing well. (Rippon, J. W.: Medical Mycology. 2nd ed. W. B. Saunders Co., Philadelphia, 1982.)

infected experimentally by exposure to soil contaminated with the microorganism and when housed in bat caves. Experimental animals are infected with some facility, a localized lesion being produced at the site of subcutaneous inoculation in guinea pigs and rabbits and generalized infection in dogs and rats. Both yeast-like and mycelial forms are infectious experimentally.

Epidemiology

The infection is airborne and is contracted by inhalation. Infection is associated with point sources such as chicken coops, pigeon roosts, starling roosts, bat-infested caves, and old decaying wooden structures where excreta and other decomposing organic matter under conditions of high humidity provide a nidus of infection. The infection tends to occur in rural areas and in low-lying river country. There is a large endemic area of infection in the United States that includes Missouri, Tennessee, Kentucky, Arkansas, and adjacent areas in adjoining states in which the proportion of positive reactors to the histoplasmin test ranges from 50 to over 90 per cent. This is in sharp contrast with the area from the Great Lakes to the Pacific coast and from Colorado to the Canadian border, in which the proportion of reactors is less than 2 per cent. Within the endemic area the proportion of reactors increases with age, from 5 per cent at 2 years, through 60 per cent at 18 years, to 75 to 90 per cent at age 55 and over. It has been postulated that the high endemic areas of the Ohio-Mississippi river valleys are related to the great concentration of starlings (*Sturnus vulgaris*) in those regions.

Only sporadic cases have been reported from Europe. Consistent with this, the reactor rates are less than 2 per cent. However, in occasional isolated areas, such as Burma, the Philippines, and northern Italy, rates as high as 20 per cent have been observed. The disease is worldwide and has been found in all continents, countries, islands, etc., where looked for and if the ecological life zone exists.

Histoplasmosis duboisii, while primarily found in Africa has also been described in Japan. It is known as cave disease because it has often been contracted in caves infested with bats. It differs markedly from American histoplasmosis. The manifestations are primarily cutaneous and osseous, though inhalation of spores is the mode of primary infection. The yeasts are quite large (12 to 18 μm.) compared to small yeasts of *H. capsulatum*. The large yeast form is called *H. capsulatum* var. *duboisii*.

Diagnosis

Microscopic demonstration of the fungus is highly suggestive of the disease, but culture and identification are required to establish the diagnosis. *Histoplasma capsulatum* has been isolated by blood culture in generalized infections and from biopsy specimens; sternal puncture may prove useful. It may be isolated fairly easily from sputum in cases of pulmonary infection by inoculation of yeast peptone phosphate agar (YPP) or blood agar. The recommended procedure is to put the specimen on both YPP and blood agar and incubate at 25° C. Examination for characteristic tuberculate macroconidia and demonstration of dimorphism at 37° C. establish the identity of the organism. Other fungal species have identical tuberculate macroconidia.

OPPORTUNISTIC SYSTEMIC MYCOSES

Cryptococcosis

Although cryptococcosis may occur in the apparently healthy individual, the disease is also commonly an opportunistic infection and associated with steroid, cytotoxin, and x-ray therapy. Even the apparently normal patients probably have some as yet undefined, immunological defect. In Europe it is known as "malade signal" (signal disease), as it signals an underlying debilitation. The etiological agent is *Cryptococcus neoformans*. It has a worldwide distribution and is associated with the filth of pigeons.

Primary Pulmonary and Cutaneous Cryptococcosis (European Blastomycosis)

What was probably the first yeast infection of proved etiology was a fatal generalized disease observed by Busse and by Buschke in 1893. They published reports of the case separately and called it systemic blastomycosis; subsequently, this form of disease and cutaneous cryptococcosis has been generally known as European blastomycosis in the literature. From ulcers on the face and neck, the infection spread to the cervical lymph nodes, and the causative organism was isolated first from a secondary tibial abscess, then from the primary ulcers, and shortly before death from the blood stream. The primary infection is now known always to be in the lungs. The infection may be inapparent and become manifest only when transported to another locus, as the skin. Here a focus of infection is established which may then spread to other areas. Sometimes granulomata are found involving the spleen, kidneys, liver, and mesenteric lymphatics.

The microorganisms are found in exudates and in mucoid masses of gelatinous material as round to oval cells, 5 to 6 μm in diameter, surrounded by a mucilaginous sheath. The gelatinous material in which they may be embedded is a product of the fungus and called a capsule. The capsular material stains specifically by the mucicarmine method. It is reported that the cells may be stained specifically in tissue sections and smears by the fluorescent antibody technique. They are readily cultivated on most ordinary mediums as a smooth white or very light tan colony without distinguishing features. The organism will not grow on mediums containing cycloheximide. More recently, especially in the United States, the more common presenting form of cryptococcosis has been meningeal.

Cryptococcus Meningitis

The primary pulmonary infection may be inapparent and meningitis the first sign of disease. The symptoms are those of brain involvement, especially intracranial pressure. Brain tumor may be closely simulated in some cases, and the disease develops slowly, usually without febrile reaction or other signs of infection; a case of 16 years' duration has been reported. The pathological picture is that of chronic leptomeningitis with thickened meninges adherent to the cerebral cortex and showing diffuse or focal granulomatous lesions. The cerebral cortex is invaded in about half the cases; the lesions are sometimes granulomatous but more often cystic, and there is little if any inflammatory reaction (Fig. 43–40). The granulomatous lesions of both meninges and brain contain large accumulations of macrophages which phagocytose the fungus. The cystic lesions consist of enormous numbers of yeast cells embedded in a gelatinous matrix. The yeast is usually present in the spinal fluid in pure culture and may be observed in wet unstained preparations of the centrifuged sediment in a drop of India ink (Fig. 43–41). There is a strong association of cryptococcal

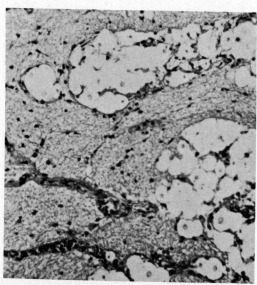

Figure 43–40. *Cryptococcus neoformans* in optic nerve. Spaces represent areas occupied by capsular material. Note lack of cellular reaction. Periodic acid–Schiff hematoxylin; × 400.

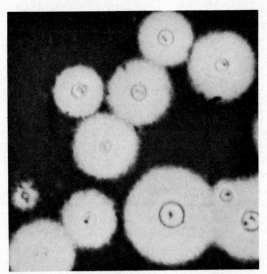

Figure 43–41. India ink preparation of *Cryptococcus neoformans.* Yeast cell in center surrounded by capsule. It is the only medically important fungus that is encapsulated. × 800.

infection with such debilitating diseases as lymphomas and leukemias, and such patients run a particular danger of having a rapidly fatal infection. There is reason to believe that infection is more common than has been supposed, perhaps 2000 for every proven case. Current estimates indicate 15,000 subclinical or clinical cases per year in New York City alone. The portal of entry is the lung. In dried pigeon debris the yeast is small, about 1 μm. in size, and thus can be inhaled into the alveolar spaces. Unlike histoplasmosis, blastomycosis, or coccidioidomycosis, there is so little tissue reaction that a skin test has not as yet been developed and healed cryptococcal lesions rarely calcify. Subclinical infections resolve spontaneously, but clinical disease is almost always fatal if untreated; however, combined 5-fluorocytosine and amphotericin B therapy has been reported to be effective. Old resolved cryptococcal granulomata are not infrequently observed as incidental findings in routine autopsies.

Pathogenicity for Lower Animals. Infection occurs in lower animals, notably in the lungs and nasal granulomata of horses, and cryptococcus has been described as the etiological agent in a severe outbreak of bovine mastitis. There is no reason to believe, however, that lower animals constitute a reservoir of human infection. The organism has been isolated from soil and is the source of both human and animal infection. There is a close association of the organism with pigeon droppings. In areas crusted with bird dung, such as sills, ledges, attics (but infrequently in enriched soil), the organisms can easily be found if looked for, and in large numbers. Point source infections have been documented in New York and Chicago as well as many other places. The organism does not appear to grow in the pigeon body itself, just in the filth left by the bird. The microorganism is virulent for mice with an LD_{50} of about 1000 cells on intracerebral inoculation. Following intraperitoneal inoculation it produces a generalized infection that spreads to the central nervous system. Experimental infection has also been produced in marmosets *(Leontocebus geoffroyi)* by feeding them large numbers of the microorganisms. Some immunity has been achieved in experimental animals, but effective antibodies in human infections are highly debatable. Serological procedures are now reliable. These include both a latex agglutination test for the presence of antigen in spinal fluid and serum and a fluorescent antibody technique. Clearing of antigen and appearance of antibody (complement-fixing) indicates a good prognosis. If the spinal fluid clears of antigen and the serum does not, it may indicate a persistent extracranial focus of infection. A nonantibody anticryptococcal factor in human serum has been reported.

The Causative Organism. For some time the relationship of these clinically diverse infections was not realized, and the yeast of the disease in Europe (European blastomycosis) was known as *Cryptococcus hominis* and that in America (torula meningitis) as *Torula histolytica.* In 1934, however, Benham showed that strains of the two yeasts were essentially identical, the difference in pathogenicity being one of degree only. Similar observations have been reported by others. It seems established, therefore, that these diseases are caused by the same etiological agent and, furthermore, that only a single species of yeast is involved.

Cryptococcus neoformans characteristically assimilates (but does not ferment) glucose and sucrose, but not lactose or melibiose. It is the only member of the genus pathogenic for mice. The genus members characteristically produce urease and assimilate inositol, and this, together with their lack of mycelium production, separates them from the genus *Candida.* Nonpathogenic species, including *C. laurentii, C. albicus,* and *C. luteolus,* are valid species that are found as common saprophytes but which differ from *C. neoformans* in the above physiological tests. The heavily encapsulated forms are poor immunizing antigens, but satisfactory antiserums may be prepared in the rabbit with poorly encapsulated forms. The organism gives a Quellung reaction in homologous antiserum. There are at least four immunological types, designated A, B, C, and D, depending upon the polysaccharide capsular antigen. The polysaccharides are closely related chemically, all containing xylose, mannose, galactose, and a uronic acid. Recently the anamorph state of the organism has been found and called *Filobasidiella neoformans*. The teleomorph state is related to the smuts in the class Basidiomycota.

Other Yeasts. *Candida glabrata* was isolated from animal infection in 1939. It is a small (3 to 4 μm.) intracellular parasite, and infection in tissue somewhat resembles histoplasmosis. The organism is fairly commonly isolated from urine and sputum and may be involved in infections as an opportunist. Quantitatively it is the most numerous yeast encountered as normal flora of the skin and buccal cavity. It has been isolated from uncomplicated meningitis as the cause of death. The organism, like *Cryptococcus*, is always a yeast form. It produces a pasty white to gray colony and ferments only glucose and trehalose. A similar species, *C. pintolopesii*, is found in the mouse alimentary tract and may lead to confusion in experimental infection by human pathogenic fungi.

Geotrichosis

Geotrichosis is a rare infection of the oral, intestinal, bronchial, or pulmonary system by a semiyeast organism, *Geotrichum candidum*. The nomenclatural synonymy and relationships, number of species, etc., are much debated. Geotrichosis seems to have been differentiated from candidiasis in 1842. Bronchial geotrichosis is a rare but fairly well-delineated entity. Chronic bronchitis with persistent expectoration of mucoid sputum and with little or no rise in temperature is the general symptomatology. Oral geotrichosis resembles oral candidiasis, as do the rarely reported beer yeast *(Saccharomyces cerevisiae)* oral and bronchial infections. Other sites of infection have been reported, but the status is provisional as the organism is a common contaminant. It is easily isolated from feces, cottage cheese, and tomatoes. The colony is white and mealy. The barrel-shaped arthroconidia similar to *Coccidioides* (but lacking the empty space between cells) can be seen under the microscope.

Aspergillosis

The common blue-green mold seen on damp bread, bacon, or most any organic material is usually a member of the genus *Aspergillus*. The other common blue-green fungus is *Penicillium* species. Together these organisms constitute the most omnipresent and ubiquitously distributed molds in the world. With every breath, we inhale some conidia of one or more species. Most of the time these conidia are disposed of without injury to the host. In some individuals and under certain conditions, these organisms may provoke injury to man in one of two ways: allergic response to the presence of the conidia or, much more rarely, invasion of pulmonary or other tissue.

Of the two groups, *Aspergillus* is more commonly associated with infection than *Penicillium*, and one species, *A. fumigatus*, is highly pathogenic for birds and also occasionally for man. There are over 600 species of the genus *Aspergillus*, of which a dozen or more have been described as responsible for infection. Of the more than 700 species of *Penicillium*, only a few have been isolated from the very rare disease penicilliosis. Though the genus names are in the family Moniliaceae, order Moniliales, class Hyphomycetes, of the Deuteromycota, a few of each genus produce a sexual (teleomorph) stage. The sexual spore is an ascus and the group, therefore, is in the phylum Ascomycota, order Eurotiales.

Pathogenicity for Lower Animals

Aspergillosis of domesticated birds, pigeons, ducks, penguins, and chickens is not uncommon and at times assumes economic importance. Three types of infection commonly occur: infection of the air sacs and both nodular and pneumonic forms of lung infection. A fourth type, aspergillar meningitis, is found with some frequency in certain bird groups under certain conditions, *e.g.*, penguins in zoos. Infection of the air sacs takes the form of a superficial infection of the epithelial lining, which becomes thickened and covered with a mat of green conidiating mycelium. In the nodular form of the disease, tubercle-like masses of infiltrated tissue, necrotic in the center, are formed. A diffuse infiltrate is formed in the pneumonic form, and the lung tissue is consolidated and grayish white in color. The pneumonic disease sometimes assumes epidemic form in chicks and is known as "brooder pneumonia." The source of infection is usually moldy grain or straw. The fungus may also invade the egg during incubation, with infection of the embryo. Cattle, sheep, and especially horses develop aspergillosis, though less commonly than birds. The lesions are pulmonary and may be either nodular or pneumonic. *Aspergillus* also causes mycotic abortion in these animals.

Strains of infectious aspergilli vary widely in their pathogenicity when tested by inoculation of experimental animals. In general, those isolated from infections are quite virulent, while those found in air and elsewhere are of low virulence. With virulent strains a fulminating, rapidly fatal pneumonia may be produced in pigeons by inhalation of spores, while the feeding of grain overgrown with the mold often produces an infection of the air sacs. Intravenous inoculation of pigeons results in an acute infection with multiple miliary abscesses, especially in the lungs, if the dose is not too large. Otherwise, rapid toxic death occurs. Rabbits inoculated intravenously with conidia suspensions of virulent strains usually die in three to five days, with multiple abscess formation, notably in the kidney, whereas subcutaneous or intraperitoneal inoculation produces localized lesions which may or may not be fatal. The subject of *Aspergillus* pathogenicity is one of the most enigmatic in the study of the fungi. Some isolates of a species can be injected in large numbers and produce no disease; other isolates of the same species are as virulent or more so than *Coccidioides immitis*. Many *Aspergillus* and *Penicillium* species can be induced into a yeast-like growth similar to that of *Blastomyces dermatitidis* in which they are very invasive for the deep organs of experimental animals.

Pathogenicity for Man

Human cases of aspergillosis are most frequently infections of the external ear (otomycosis). The disease varies from a plugging of the external meatus with a mass of mycelium to ulceration of the walls and even penetration of the middle ear; the mild cases are the most numerous. It is fascinating to look through an otoscope and see the external auditory canal lined with the delicate, beautifully architectured fruiting heads of an *Aspergillus*. While *A. fumigatus* is the most common invader, *A. terreus*, *A. flavus*, and *A. niger* are sometimes found. All these species are thermotolerant and to a degree tissue tolerant and able to circumvent host defenses—the three attributes necessary for an infectious agent.

Aspergillosis broadly defined is a group of diseases in which members of the genus *Aspergillus* are involved. This is no better illustrated than in the variety of human pulmonary and systemic conditions involving aspergilli. The two broad categories of disease are allergic and infectious—and there may be symptoms

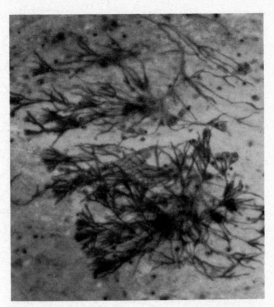

Figure 43–42. *Aspergillus fumigatus* growing in gelatinous bronchial plug from a case of bronchopulmonary aspergillosis. Tissue is not directly invaded, the disease being an allergic response to the presence of the growing organism. Direct mount, methylene blue; × 400.

of both. Roughly divided there are four clinical forms.

Aspergillus Asthma. This occurs as a sensitization of atopic patients to the inhalation of conidia of the organisms. Precipitating antibodies are rarely present, although IgE antibodies can be demonstrated.

Bronchopulmonary Aspergillosis. In this disease the fungi grow as mycelium within the lumen of the bronchiole (Fig. 43–42). Often there is plugging and a characteristic x-ray picture. The disease is an allergy, and an Arthus reaction occurs on the surface of the bronchus. Precipitating antibodies are present, as well as IgE antibodies. Both of the above-mentioned are allergic diseases and are treated with steroids.

Colonizing Aspergillosis: Aspergilloma. This occurs more commonly as a "fungus ball" in pulmonary cavities or in nasal sinuses. The organism colonizes a preformed cavity such as those of old tuberculous, sarcoid, or other origin. There is essentially no invasion of living tissue. Surgical removal is indicated, as exsanguinating hemoptysis is a constant danger. IgG antibodies are present, as demonstrated by immunodiffusion.

Invasive Aspergillosis. This is a rare and often fatal infection. Mycelial elements invade the tissue and may rapidly spread to become systemic (Fig. 43–43). This is an opportunistic disease of debilitated patients, frequently oc-

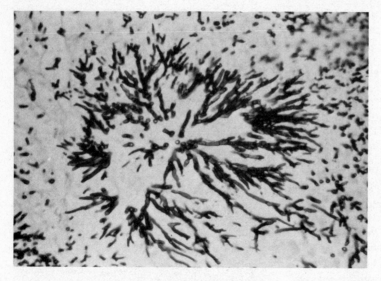

Figure 43–43. Invasive aspergillosis of the lung. The dichotomously branched mycelium is radiating from the central area where the initial infection began in an alveolar space. It subsequently invaded lung parenchyma, occluded vessels and metastasized to heart, kidney, liver, and brain. Methenamine silver, × 440.

curring in lymphoma and leukemia patients, organ transplant patients, and others on immunosuppressive therapy. The mycelium rarely is found in the sputum, which makes diagnosis particularly difficult in this form of disease. Most patients are too debilitated to mount an antibody response so serological procedures are not helpful. Often even repeated cultures are negative so that diagnosis is sometimes not made until necropsy.

Other Aspergilloses. Very rarely aspergillosis may take other forms in man. The occurrence of *Aspergillus* in mycetoma has been noted, and a case of chronic suppuration with discharge of grains has been reported. Rarely it may assume an acute disseminated form, including involvement of the central nervous system. It is not infrequently isolated as the cause of keratitis of the lens following a puncture wound of the eye, and primary cutaneous disease has been reported.

A final word must be said about the constant danger of aspergilli and other common soil fungi to debilitated patients. *Aspergillus fumigatus* is a thermophilic fungus, growing well at 37°C., and it also produces a potent endotoxin. It and many other saprophytes readily invade patients on cytopathic drugs, nitrogen mustard, antimetabolites, or anti-immune drugs (Imuran), or patients with debilitating diseases, particularly neoplasms, less so those with diabetes. Many organ-transplant failures have resulted from infection by "saprophytes." Treatment of choice is amphotericin B, but the fatality rate is high.

Mucormycosis

Mucormycosis has been a very rare infection. It occurs largely as a mycotic complication of chronic debilitating disease, most often uncontrolled diabetes but also amebic colitis and kwashiorkor. With the introduction into general use of therapeutic agents such as antibiotics, corticosteroids, and antileukemic drugs the infection has been found more often, so much so that it is considered to be a "new disease."

There are four types of disease, each of which has a particular predisposing condition. These are (1) acidotic diabetic (or acidosis of some other cause) associated with rhinocerebral disease, (2) leukemia or lymphoma with pulmonary disease, (3) malnutrition in children with gastric and intestinal disease, and (4) cutaneous infection as a complication in burn patients.

In the acidotic patient, primary infection begins in the nose, or rarely the ear, where spores germinate and the mycelial growth invades the mucous membrane and may extend into the adjacent sinuses, orbital cavity, or cerebral tissue. Most acidotic patients have ketone bodies in their serums. The pathogenic Mucorales are among the rare organisms that have the enzyme ketoreductase. This type of infection is almost always caused by *Rhizopus oryzae* or *Absidia corymbifera*.

In pulmonary disease of leukemia and lymphoma patients, primary infection occurs in the lung, where growth on the bronchial mucosa penetrates the wall to the hilar tissue or lobar pneumonia may result. The fungus appears to have a special affinity for arteries, with penetration into the lumen to produce thrombosis and infarction. Often the lungs show large areas of necrosis and cavitation. It may reach the central nervous system via ophthalmic and internal carotid arteries to produce a meningoencephalitis.

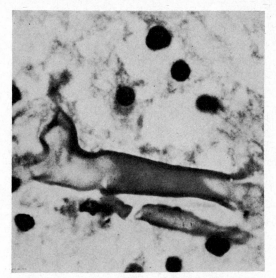

Figure 43–44. Mucormycosis showing broad nonseptate mycelium in brain tissue. Periodic acid–Schiff hematoxylin; × 800.

In gastric disease of malnourished children the gastric or intestinal mucosa is invaded. The organism may be ingested with moldy food.

In tissue the organism appears as broad, distorted, nonseptate hyphae (Fig. 43–44). Most cases are diagnosed at autopsy, the tissue having been thoroughly soaked in formaldehyde and no cultures obtainable. Most species grow readily on mediums without cycloheximide. Members of the genera *Mucor*, *Absidia*, and *Rhizopus* have most often been isolated. They are members of the order Mucorales of the class Zygomycota. As with the pathogenic aspergilli, the Mucorales involved in human disease are thermotolerant and to a degree tissue tolerant and resistant to cellular host defenses.

Mycotic abortion of sheep and cattle caused by the Mucorales is frequently described. Experimental infections are easy to produce.

MISCELLANEOUS MYCOSES

Various other fungi have occasionally been described as producing human disease. Though hundreds of fungal species have been recorded as isolated from lesions, it is quite difficult to assess their significance in the disease process. If the organism is isolated more than once and in quantity from exposed lesions or sputa and all other etiologies have been ruled out, it may be considered as responsible. However, if the organism is isolated from a closed body cavity, lesion, or blood culture, it must be considered as a strong suspect in the disease process.

Below are listed some rarely encountered fungal diseases in which fungi have been isolated with sufficient frequency to establish their potential invasive ability.

A variety of organisms have been isolated from such infections. These include protothecosis, a chronic granulomatous skin infection caused by the colorless algae *Prototheca zopfii*, or infection with blue-green algae, mushroom fungi, etc. An increasingly common opportunist of the lungs is the organism *Pneumocystis carinii*. It now appears to be a fungus and has chitin in its cell wall. It may well be a "link" between the fungi and protozoa.

Adiaspiromycosis

This is a pulmonary disease found in many species of rodents throughout the world. It has rarely been described in man. The conidia (2 to 4 μm.) of the soil fungus are inhaled into the lungs, where they enlarge to a huge spherule. Development stops at this point and no endospores or buds are produced. The name adiaconidia refers to the enlargement then arrest of a fungal conidium growth. There is little host reaction. Adiaconidia can be produced *in vitro* by incubation at 40°C. The fungi involved were described as two species by Emmons and named *Haplosporangium parvum* and *H. crescens*. The names *Chrysosporium parvum* and *C. parvum* var. *crescens* are now accepted. The former has adiaconidia up to 40 μm. and the latter up to 500 μm. (Fig. 43–45). Otherwise there is no difference between them. The organisms are soil saprophytes and grow on medium as a fluffy white colony producing single small (3 to 7 μm.) conidia on a conidiophore. These are correctly called chrysoconidia, as are the mycelial conidia of *Blastomyces dermatitidis*. *Chrysosporium parvum* is found in the southwestern United States; the variety *crescens* is worldwide in distribution.

Penicilliosis and Hyphomycosis

The ubiquity of species of *Penicillium* and their constant contamination of instruments, wounds, urine, sputum, etc., makes the establishment of this diagnosis very difficult. *Penicillium marneffei* is found as a yeast-like invasive pathogen of Asian rodents and rarely man. Substantiated infection of the cornea and the external ear, a few mycetomas, and very rare pulmonary and systemic infections are recorded for a variety of *Penicillium* species. The pathological picture is similar to that of aspergillosis. The related genus *Scopulariopsis*, especially the species *S. brevicaulis*, is a not

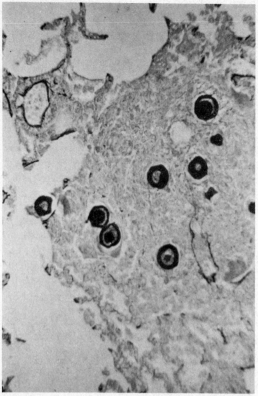

Figure 43–45. Adiospiromycosis spherules in the rat lung. Note the absence of endospores. (Rippon, J. W.: Medical Mycology. 2nd ed. W. B. Saunders Co., Philadelphia, 1982.)

uncommon agent of onychomycosis and paronychia, characterized by much inflammation and pus. This species also has been involved in cutaneous infections and systemic disease of the opportunistic type. *Fusarium* species have also been recovered from mycotic keratitis and a few cases of disseminated opportunistic infection. In the latter form they are identical to *Aspergillus* species in pathological specimens. For this reason, if septate mycelium alone is seen in tissue, the disease should be called hyphomycosis (clear-walled fungi) until the exact etiology is identified by culture on serology. If the walls are pigmented (brown), the disease is called phaeohyphomycosis.

Phaeohyphomycosis

Species of the genus Cladosporium, especially *C. bantianum*, have been isolated several times from cerebral and pulmonary lesions. Many cases have been fatal. The disease is called black degeneration of the brain for its most apparent pathological picture. The lesions usually are localized and encapsulated. In tissue sections, multiseptate, brown, distorted hyphae are seen. The organism (a De-

matiaceae, Deuteromycota) grows well as a black velvety colony on mediums without cycloheximide. It is pathogenic for experimental animals and is neurotropic. *Alternaria* species, another dematiacious fungus, has been recorded from at least three cases of subcutaneous infection involving the nose. Infection followed trauma or surgery. Cutaneous disease has also been reported. This only emphasizes that many potentially pathogenic fungi exist in nature awaiting only the proper circumstances in order to evoke disease.

Mycotic Infections of the Eye

Introduction of fungal conidia into the cornea by abrasion or secondary to herpetic lesions is not an uncommon occurrence. Establishment of the infection is enhanced by the overuse of steroids. The organisms involved are most often soil saprophytes, such as *Aspergillus*, *Fusarium*, and *Curvularia*. The infection is usually localized but may destroy the cornea or spread to the rest of the eye. Hematogenous spread of pathogenic fungi from other loci to the eye is known but is very rare. A condition, histoplasma uveitis, is recognized by ophthalmologists, but a causal relationship to *Histoplasma capsulatum* has yet to be demonstrated conclusively. Treatment of corneal infection was usually by irrigation with nystatin or amphotericin B solutions. A 15 per cent suspension of pimaricin (Natamycin) is now considered the treatment of choice.

FUNGAL ALLERGENS

A number of nonpathogenic fungi can cause considerable distress to particular patients. This is expressed as allergic reactions to their presence rather than as frank infection. There is a gamut of symptoms for the atopic patient, from those such as hay fever, vasomotor rhinitis, and asthma, to severe and debilitating farmer's lung. The organisms involved in the former conditions are common airborne contaminants, such as *Alternaria, Cladosporium, Aspergillus, Helminthosporium, Penicillium* etc. In more severe allergic phenomena, such as byssinosis (cotton-dust disease) and bagassosis (exposure to sugar cane bagasse), a mixed fungal flora has been incriminated in addition to the pneumoconiosis due to fibers. Maple bark stripper's disease is due to inhalation of spores of *Coniosporum corticale*.

A very important allergic disease is farmer's lung. Repeated exposure to moldy hay causes a diffuse granulomatous reaction and interstitial fibrosis. Progressive pulmonary fibrosis may result in a crippling, sometimes fatal pathological condition in the lung. The disease is most often associated with inhalation of spores of the thermophilic actinomycetes *Micromonospora faeni* and *Thermoactinomyces vulgaris*. Some patients may be exposed for years and are not atopic. There is a sudden onset of symptoms and rapid progression to death. The exact mechanism of the disease is unknown. In urban areas it has been associated with moldy air conditioners.

REFERENCES

1. Beneke, E. S., and A. L. Rogers. 1980. Medical Mycology Manual. 4th ed. Burgess, Minneapolis.

2. Campbell, M. C., and J. L. Stewart. 1980. The Medical Mycology Handbook. John Wiley & Sons, New York.

3. Conant, N. F., *et al.* 1971. Manual of Clinical Mycology. 3rd ed. W. B. Saunders Co., Philadelphia.

4. Diamond, R. 1977. Immunology of Invasive Fungal Diseases. *In* R. A. Good (Ed.), Comprehensive Immunology. Plenum Press, New York.

5. Emmons, C. W., *et al.* 1977. Medical Mycology. 3rd ed. Lea & Febiger, Philadelphia.

6. Karunaratne, W. A. E. 1964. Rhinosporidiosis in Man. The Athlone Press, London.

7. Lodder, J. (Ed.). 1970. The Yeasts. North Holland Publications, Amsterdam.

8. McGinnis, M. R. 1980. Laboratory Handbook of Medical Mycology. Academic Press, New York.

9. Rebell, G., and D. Taplin. 1970. Dermatophytes. University of Miami Press, Miami, Florida.

10. Rippon, J. W. 1982. Medical Mycology: The Pathogenic Fungi and the Pathogenic Actinomycetes. 2nd ed. W. B. Saunders Co., Philadelphia.

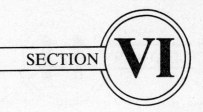

Parasitology

CHAPTER 44

Medical Parasitology

Donald G. Dusanic, Ph.D.

Medical parasitology is a subdiscipline of microbiology concerned with parasites, which are animal agents of human disease. It is probably one of the oldest medical subjects studied, since parasites were recognized by the ancient Egyptians, Greeks, and Romans. Subsequent descriptions of life cycles and control measures were recorded long before any detailed information was available for other microbial pathogens. Although infections by these animal agents have generally been regarded as the specialty of researchers and practioners in tropical medicine, some are relatively common in temperate and arctic regions. Indeed, they also occur in countries with comparatively high standards of living and medical care. Immigration and travel by resi-

dents of these countries to endemic areas increase the frequency with which the parasites are encountered by physicians. Annually, four and a half to five million Americans and equally large numbers of individuals from other developed nations travel to conduct business or vacation in these areas.

Many parasitic infections are difficult to treat, prevent, and control. They represent some of the world's most important public health problems. Table 44–1 contains data compiled by the Rockefeller Foundation and provides conservative estimates of 12 of the more common parasitic diseases of humans.[16] Recognizing the importance of these diseases, the World Health Organization created the Special Programme for Research and Training

Table 44–1. **Prevalence and Mortality of Human Infections by Animal Parasites**

Disease	Infections (thousands of persons/year)	Disease (thousands of cases/year)	Deaths (thousands/year)
African trypanosomiasis	1,000	10	5
American trypanosomiasis	12,000	1,200	60
Amebiasis	400,000	1,500	30
Giardiasis	200,000	500	Very low
Leishmaniasis	12,000	12,000	5
Malaria	800,00	150,000	1,200
Ascariasis	1,000,000	1,000	20
Filariasis	250,000	2,000–3,000	Low
Hookworm	900,000	1,500	50–60
Onchocerciasis	30,000	200–500	20–50
Trichuriasis	500,000	100	Low
Schistosomiasis	200,000	20,000	500–1,000

in Tropical Diseases, especially malaria, trypanosomiasis, leishmaniasis, schistosomiasis, and filariasis. The intent of this program is to support international research and training in medical parasitology and ultimately to control these diseases.

Parasitism by protozoa and helminths, like that of other microbial agents, involves intimate and dynamic interactions between the parasites and their hosts. While some parasites have lost certain sensory or digestive functions, adaptations evolved that exquisitely fitted them for this mode of existence. Complex life cycles, efficient methods of reproduction, specialized organelles, and stages that exist inside or outside of the hosts illustrate some characteristics that enhance the probabilities of survival of these parasitic species. In some respects, the parasites are similar to their human hosts. Like their hosts, they are composed of eucaryotic cells that employ similar metabolic pathways for energy production and biosynthesis. Such similarities may be responsible for the toxicity of some chemotherapeutics for humans.

Less apparent biochemical differences between the parasites and their hosts have been found to be responsible for the selective toxicities of effective drugs. Carbohydrate metabolism of trematodes is regulated by phosphofructokinase. Trivalent antimonials, which have been used in the treatment of schistosomiasis, inhibit the enzyme and glycolysis by the worms. Phosphofructokinase of the schistosome has been shown to be more sensitive to these arsenicals than the same enzyme from the host.[17] Humans utilize preformed folate, while malarial parasites synthesize tetrahydrofolate. The enzyme dihydropteroate synthetase mediates the reaction and is sensitive to antimalarial sulfones and sulfonamides.[42] The ac-

tion of some compounds may also be related to a difference between their uptake by the parasites and the hosts. Tryparsamide, an arsenical used in the treatment of African sleeping sickness, inhibits sulfhydryl-containing enzymes of the trypanosomes by virtue of a stimulated pinocytosis of the drug by the parasites.[72] Consideration of such differences may provide a more rational and less empirical methodology for the design and development of new antiparasitic compounds in the future.

Although many viral and bacterial diseases have been controlled by vaccination, such is not the case with animal parasites of man. Protozoa and helminths represent mosaics of antigens and provoke immunological responses, but they persist in their hosts for long periods of time. Frequently, such infected hosts display resistance to reinfection, while the resident parasite populations employ a variety of strategies to elude the immunological responses. There are numerous examples of protozoan and helminth parasites that occupy intracellular sites in the host. This niche provides shelter from the cellular and humoral immune responses. Malarial parasites reside in liver cells or erythrocytes. *Leishmania* species invade and reproduce in macrophages. *Trypanosoma cruzi* strains exhibit tissue tropisms and may be found in macrophages, muscle, and other cells of the host. *Toxoplasma gondii* does not show a marked tissue specificity, but may be found in virtually every type of cell. Among the helminths, *Trichinella spiralis* larvae penetrate host muscle cells, causing damage to myofibers, increases in the numbers of nuclei and mitochondria, and elevated activities of lysosomal enzymes. This is followed by the development of a double-layered membrane around each larva and the transformation to a nurse cell. Other intracellular parasites do not appear to induce such profound changes, but appear to resist enzymatic destruction after fusion of the phagosomes and lysosomes, exit the phagolysosome and multiply in the cytoplasmic matrix, prevent fusion of the phagosomes and lysosomes, or after active penetration, simply proliferate in the host cell cytoplasm.[21, 88]

Patients with African sleeping sickness present infections with periodic increases and subsequent decreases in the numbers of parasites in their blood. These characteristic waves of parasitemia represent populations of trypanosomes with new variant antigens present as compact glycoprotein surface coats covering the parasites. The host synthesizes antibody against the variant antigen and eliminates the trypanosomes of the specific type, while a population with a new-variant glycoprotein coat emerges to generate the next wave of parasites. This antigenic diversity has a genetic basis and seems to be a nonrandom process, since the sequence of trypanosome variant antigenic types appears predetermined.[25] Antigenic variation seems to be a major mechanism for the continued survival of these parasites in the immune hosts. It has also been characterized in other protozoa and a similar process described in the helminths.[24]

The persistence of adult schistosomes in humans appears to be due at least in part to the adsorption of host proteins to the surfaces of the worms.[8] These adsorbed coats with host antigenic determinants may block the reactions of antibodies with the worms. Studies have shown that eosinophils, neutrophils, or mononuclear phagocytes in the presence of antibody and/or complement kill the invading schistosomes (schistosomules).[23] These schistosomules lack adsorbed host protein and may be killed by such reactions, and the infected host appears resistant to reinfection.

Other properties of the parasites may also permit avoidance of the immune responses. They release exoantigens that may block immunological reactions. Antigen-antibody complexes formed on their surfaces may migrate and be shed or internalized by the parasites without any detrimental effects, while new antigenic determinants may be exposed by this process.

Concurrent with this avoidance, parasites are able to induce immunological unresponsiveness in their hosts. Such immunosuppression may involve B or T lymphocytes, accessory cells, and suppressor T cells. Parasite-mediated suppression is a feature of diffuse cutaneous leishmaniasis and is expressed in the symptoms and pathology. During the course of this disease, the host is not able to control the parasite and lesions spread and fail to heal. Studies in experimental animals indicate that populations of suppressor T cells develop that alter skin-test responses and depress both T and B cell responses. Immunosuppression has been demonstrated in many protozoan and helminth infections. The inabilities of the host to resolve these infections may be due in part to such suppression.

Frequently, individuals are infected by more than one species of parasite, and the clinical findings may be complex. Malnutrition, a common condition of persons from underdeveloped countries, may intensify the effects of the infections. The pathology and symptoms characteristic of each parasitic disease are the result of the location and behavior of the parasites in the hosts, their relatively large sizes, motility, elaborated toxic products, competition with the hosts for nutrients, and hypersensitivity responses to their antigens.

Immunoglobulins and cell-mediated immunity may be directed against more than one stage of a parasite during an infection. These responses may be elicited against internal or surface antigens or released or secreted exoantigens. The reactions between these parasite antigens and the host form the basis for serological and skin tests (immediate and delayed hypersensitivities) employed in the diagnoses of the diseases. Such procedures may occasionally be misleading, since antigens of a particular parasite may give cross-reactions with antibody against antigens of closely related or totally unrelated organisms. It is also possible that antibody titers may reflect a past experience with a parasite in an individual completely cured of the infection. False-negative reactions in immunodiagnostic tests may also occur in subjects who are immunologically compromised or unresponsive.

A presumptive diagnosis utilizes a thorough case history, which includes past travel, activities, and dietary habits. It examines the physical status and symptoms presented and the results of selected clinical tests. Definitive diagnosis is made by the demonstration of the parasite or its products in specimens (biopsy, aspirate, blood, stool, or urine) obtained from the patient. Serological tests on small (1 to 2 ml.) serum samples may be requested from state health laboratories. These requests and samples are forwarded to the Centers for Disease Control in Atlanta, Georgia. During the chronic stages of many infections, the parasites, ova, cysts, or larvae may be difficult to detect. In such cases, the clinical and serological findings dictate the treatment.

Drugs are currently available for the prevention and treatment of many parasitic diseases. Surgical procedures may be required to resolve other parasitic infections. Chemotherapy may be advisable for patients who do not return to endemic areas, but sound medical judgment may dictate alternative approaches for the management of resident patients who are continually exposed to the parasites.

Control of a parasite in an endemic area usually requires a combination of measures. These are determined by its life cycle, available technologies, and resources. A coordinated management and field program may approach the control by educating the resident population, treating infected individuals, eradicating vectors and reservoir hosts, and instituting effective sanitary practices and facilities.

Larval and adult stages of arthropods are also agents of human diseases. Some species invade tissues, sensitize the hosts with secretions while biting, or release or inject poisons in defense. Others serve as vectors for the transmission of animal parasites. Only these vectors will be considered in this chapter, while reference is made to other sources for a more complete coverage of both groups. Over 150 protozoa and helminths have been reported from man and approximately one third of these are commonly found parasites. The organisms included in this chapter were selected as representative examples of specific groups of parasites and as the causal agents of important human diseases.

The Protozoa

The protozoa are a diverse group of single-celled animals. Like the higher animals, they display eucaryotic morphology and functional adaptations to a free-living or parasitic existence. Many thousand species of protozoa have been described, though less than 35 well defined species are known to parasitize man. They constitute an exceedingly heterogenous group of organisms, varying in size from that of the larger bacteria to several millimeters in diameter, in complexity of structure from a simple, formless cell like *Entamoeba histolytica* to organisms of far greater intricacy than many metazoa, and in life cycle from the binary fission of *Trichomonas vaginalis* to the alternation of hosts and of asexual and sexual reproduction exhibited by the malarial parasites.

The systematics of the protozoa is complex and no single scheme of classification is uniformly acceptable. Division of the phylum Protozoa into four subphyla and a single parasite with uncertain taxonomic affinities constitutes the organization for the following protozoan parasites of humans.

1. Subphylum Sarcodina (amebae), characterized by the ability to produce from the cell transient fingerlike protoplasmic processes (pseudopodia) for the engulfment of food and for locomotion. Many free-living species as well as parasitic forms exist. The parasites characteristically are simple in appearance without morphologically complex organelles and multiply without any known sexual stages. All have a motile trophozoite stage during which multiplication is by binary fission. Many species also form a cyst in which stage two or more nuclear divisions may take place preceding the multiplication effected when the cyst infects the host. Amebae of man are primarily found in the digestive tract.

2. Subphylum Ciliophora (ciliates), having numerous, short, bristlelike, cytoplasmic locomotor organelles termed cilia. Most have two types of nuclei (macronucleus and micronucleus) with multiplication by binary fission and with conjugation in some forms. There are many free-living, commensal and symbiotic species with but a single form, *Balantidium coli*, occurring as a bona fide parasite of man.

3. Subphylum Mastigophora (the flagellates), characteristically having throughout or at some point in their life cycle relatively long, filamentous protoplasmic processes used in locomotion. These flagella may be multiple or single. Those intracellular parasitic stages lacking flagella may be recognized by a parabasal body, a rod-like structure associated with the flagellar origin. Division is by binary fission. Evidence for a sexual cycle in the hemoflagellates has been presented but is not wholly acceptable. Numerous free-living, parasitic, and commensal species exist. Flagellates parasitizing man are found in the intestinal and genital tracts, free in the circulation, and as intracellular parasites primarily of the lymphoid-microphage system.

4. Subphylum Sporozoa, an artificial polyphyletic grouping of parasites characterized by the lack of well-defined organelles of locomo-

tion and with an alternation of sexual and asexual reproduction. All members of this group are parasitic and many produce structures of varied morphology that have been designated as spores and that contain one to many infective individuals termed sporozoites. The malaria parasites *(Plasmodia)* and the intestinal coccidia of man belong to this group.

Pneumocystis carinii is superficially similar to the Sporozoa and usually considered in parasitology texts. It is presented separately in this section, until it is adequately classified.

THE INTESTINAL AMEBAE

SARCODINA

Entamoeba histolytica

Lewis in 19870 and Cunningham in 1871 first reported amebae, probably the nonpathogenic *Entamoeba coli*, in human feces. Lösch in 1875 described what were apparently *E. histolytica* in the stools and intestinal ulcers in a fatal case of dysentery. He found similar ulcers containing the amebae in an artificially infected dog.

Characteristics and Life Cycle. The active ameba as seen in the intestinal ulcers of dysentery cases is a granular colorless or pale greenish mass of cytoplasm, 15 to 50 (usually 20 to 30) μm. in diameter. It has no definite shape. Locomotion is accomplished by the sudden extrusion of clear projections of cytoplasm, the pseudopodia, the remainder of the cell body following these pseudopodia in a flowing motion. The granular cytoplasm often contains red blood cells or debris of tissue cells in various stages of digestion. These are the food engulfed by the ameba. The nucleus may be visible as a delicate ring of granules. Reproduction in this stage is by binary fission, the nucleus undergoing a type of mitosis and the cytoplasm then dividing to produce two daughter amebae like the original. In organisms fixed and stained with hematoxylin the nuclear structure is characteristic, consisting of a thin peripheral layer of fine black granules and a central small black dot, the karyosome (see Fig. 44–1). The entire nucleus is generally 4 to 5 μm. in diameter.

Infected persons with diarrhea or dysentery pass active ameboid parasites in their stools.

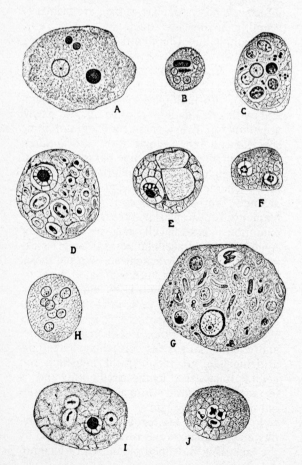

Figure 44–1. The amebae living in man. *A,* Active ameboid form of *Entamoeba histolytica* containing three red blood cells. *B,* Mature quadrinucleate cyst of same containing two chromatoids. *Entamoeba hartmanni* is similar but has smaller nuclei. *C,* Active ameboid form of *Entamoeba gingivalis. D,* Active ameboid form of *Iodamoeba williamsi* containing many intestinal bacteria. *E,* Cyst of same showing large double vacuole which in life was filled with glycogen. *F,* Ameboid form of *Dientamoeba fragilis* containing two nuclei. *G,* Large active ameboid form of *Entamoeba coli* containing intestinal bacteria and debris. *H,* Mature octonucleate cyst of same. *I,* Ameboid form of *Endolimax nana. J,* Mature quadrinucleate cyst of same. *A, B, C, G,* and *H,* about × 1300. (Dobell.) *D, E, F,* and *J,* × 3000. (Taliaferro and Becker.) *I,* × 3000. (Taliaferro in Hegner and Taliaferro's *Human Protozoology,* 1924, courtesy of The Macmillan Company.)

In the intestinal lumen of a carrier, however, the ameba loses its ingested food particles, shrinks to a diameter of 10 to 20 μm. (rarely less), rounds up and becomes essentially non-motile, sending out only an occasional pseudopodium. This is the precystic stage, which soon secretes about itself a clear wall, becoming the partially resistant cyst. In its passage down the intestine the cyst continues to develop, acquiring a vacuole of glycogen and one or more ovoid rods of black-staining material, the chromatoid bodies. The nucleus divides into two and then four, all resembling the nucleus of the active ameboid stage though considerably smaller. In the mature cyst the glycogen vacuole soon disappears, and the chromatoid bodies persist at most for a few days.

The cyst is the infective stage, since most or all of the active ameboid stages are destroyed by gastric juice. As studied in culture, excystment consists of the emergence of a quadrinucleate organism that by a complicated division process produces eight small amebae. These are the stages that initiate a new infection.

Boeck and Drbohlav in 1925 cultivated *E. histolytica* in Locke's solution and inactivated serum tubed over egg slants. Various modifications have been introduced, the most important being the addition of powdered rich starch, which the amebae ingest avidly. Cleveland and Collier used liver infusion agar slants overlaid with serum-saline. Balamuth devised a valuable monophasic medium consisting of buffered aqueous egg yolk infusion, with or without liver extract.

These mediums do not permit pure culture, for the amebae are dependent on living bacteria for growth. The protozoan *Trypanosoma cruzi* has also been utilized as an associate for culture of the amebae. Shaffer and Frye obtained amebic growth in the presence of antibiotic-inhibited bacteria. Cell-free mediums and techniques have been developed for the cultivation of *E. histolytica*.[29] These amebae grow under anaerobic conditions at a pH of approximately 7.0. Niacin or nicotinamide is essential for their axenic cultivation. Strains of axenically cultivated amebae have been immunologically analyzed for common and unique antigenic components.[22]

Amebiasis and Amebic Dysentery. The amebae normally inhabit the large intestine. While some workers believe that they proliferate only in the tissues, the evidence indicates that they may also multiply in the intestinal lumen, living, as in culture, on a diet of microorganisms.

In the wall of the colon the parasites are found in necrotic, usually noninflammatory lesions varying from minute erosive patches to more or less extensive, undermined ulcers of the submucosa. The abundance and severity of the lesions determine the clinical picture. The great majority of infected individuals are carriers exhibiting no symptoms. Clinical cases range from moderate diarrhea to acute dysentery with passage of blood and mucus, extreme weakness, and, not infrequently, death. A varying proportion of individuals with amebic dysentery show necrotic abscesses of the liver, or may show a generalized hepatitis of amebic etiology. Initially the liver abscesses are bacteria-free but may become contaminated secondarily. These also occur occasionally in individuals who give no history of intestinal symptoms of infection. Lung abscesses, usually produced by extension from the liver through the diaphragm, occur in a small number of individuals, and abscesses have been reported in practically every organ of the body. The distribution of lesions in 320 cases of amebiasis detected in 17,598 necropsies in Guatemala is shown in Table 44–2. It was considered the main disease in 285 of these cases.[20]

The host-parasite relationships in amebiasis are complex and not completely understood.[35] Strains of *E. histolytica* vary in pathogenicity.[69] Some human strains are attenuated by cultivation and they may or may not be pathogenic in laboratory animals. Bacterial associates appear to interact synergistically with amebae, since extensive lesions are not produced by pathogenic parasites in bacteria-free guinea pigs.[79] Other factors such as enzymes may also be important in tissue invasion, but it has been shown that both pathogenic and nonpathogenic *E. histolytica* may possess proteases and mucopolysaccharidases.[54, 70]

Immunity. There is no direct evidence of acquired immunity to infection with *E. histo-*

Table 44–2. **Distribution of Lesions in** *Entamoeba histolytica* **Infections**

Site of Lesion	No. Cases
Colon	274
Liver	16
Colon and liver	19
Liver and lung	4
Colon and brain	2
Colon and lung	1
Colon and inguinoscrotal skin	1
Liver and brain	1
Colon, liver, and lung	1
Colon, cervix, and vagina	1

lytica. Natives of hyperendemic regions show acute dysentery less frequently than aliens, possibly as a result of acquired immunity. Serum antibody response to the infection is evidenced by the complement fixation test, which is positive in over 80 per cent of infected individuals. Coproantibodies of the IgG, IgM, and IgA classes have also been found in the stools of individuals with amebic dysentery.[62] Sera from infected individuals will inhibit to varying degrees the ability of amebae in culture to ingest erythrocytes or can be shown to immobilize their locomotor activities. Antibodies from infected individuals when labeled by fluorescein have considerable specificity for the infecting species and a degree of strain specificity. Immune precipitates in a gel-diffusion system on a micro scale also show species specificity. Cell mediated immune responses based on the macrophage migration inhibition test are altered in amebic patients. There does not appear to be a correlation between the degree of migration inhibition and the serum antibody titers in those with amebic colitis, but both are greater in patients with amebic abscesses.[92]

Diagnosis. Diagnosis of infection with *E. histolytica* depends upon the finding of characteristic organisms in the stools and their morphological differentiation from the nonpathogenic amebae occurring in human feces. Cultivation has been utilized, but in culture *E. histolytica* resembles the nonpathogenic *E. coli* so closely that differential diagnosis is often very difficult. Direct smears of fresh loose stools in warm saline may reveal the active ameboid stages. They may also be found in material taken directly from lesions in the lower bowel with the aid of the proctoscope. The M.I.F. stain of Sapero, Lawless, and Strome is valuable for temporary preparations, although permanent smears stained with iron hematoxylin give the best differentiation. In well-formed stools cysts may be expected, and these are most easily identified in iodine solutions, such as D'Antoni's iodine. The formalin-ether concentration method of Ritchie (for cysts) and the M.I.F. concentration method of Blagg and co-workers (for both cysts and trophozoites) are excellent for diagnosis of the light infections that may be missed by direct examination. The P.V.A. preservation technique of Brooke and associates permits shipment of material to a laboratory for examination. *Entamoeba histolytica* appears irregularly in the stools and, whatever the technique, repeated examinations are often necessary to establish a diagnosis. It should be re-empha-

sized that recovery of the organisms is only the first step in diagnosis of *E. histolytica* infection. The final step is the identification of the parasites, a task requiring abundant experience. Some concept of the variation between individuals can be gained by examining photomicrographs. However, considerable experience is needed to exclude the commensals and smaller related forms such as *E. hartmanni*. When parasites cannot be found in the stools, but liver abscesses are suspected, diagnosis may be based on the presence of amebae in aspirates of abscesses or on positive serological tests and symptoms.

Serological tests are now available that are of considerable aid in diagnosis amebiasis. These include commercially available latex agglutination, indirect hemagglutination, complement fixation, double diffusion, immunoelectrophoresis, indirect fluorescence antibody tests, and the enzyme-linked immunosorbent assay. The methods are highly specific but vary in sensitivity. Since the antibodies persist for varying periods of time after termination of infection, these serological techniques are not in themselves adequate for diagnosis of active infection. However, symptoms of liver abscess, physical findings, and a positive serological test may dictate that treatment should be initiated.

Chemotherapy. Treatment may not be advisable for an individual with an asymptomatic *E. histolytica* infection who resides in an endemic area, since reinfection is likely to occur. However, even asymptomatic infections should be treated when they are diagnosed in individuals who are not likely to be reinfected. Metronidazole (Flagyl) and tinidazole (Fasigyn) are employed in the treatment of amebiasis. Although metronidazole may elicit side effects, tinidazole appears to be relatively well tolerated when administered in doses of 50 to 60 mg/kg body weight for three days for intestinal infections or for five days for extraintestinal amebiasis. Some cases of amebic abscesses do not respond to these drugs, and other chemotherapeutics such as emetine and chloroquine may be required.

Epidemiology and Control. The active ameboid stages of *E. histolytica* die quickly after exit from the body, for they are very susceptible to drying and to changes in temperature and salt concentration. Since they are destroyed by gastric juice, they are not usually infective when swallowed. The amebic dysentery patient is therefore practically harmless as a source of infection, since only the ameboid stages occur in his stools. The cysts passed by carriers, while not at all comparable to bacterial spores in resistance, show considerably less susceptibility to conditions outside the body than do the ameboid stages. Studies utilizing cysts from culture tested for viability by cultivation show survival of several months in water at 0° C., three days at 30° C., 30 minutes at 40° C., and five minutes at 50° C. Cysts of *E. histolytica* are somewhat more resistant to chlorine than are enteric bacteria. It is believed that ordinary residual chlorine concentrations are unable to destroy amebic cysts, but that hyperchlorination is effective.

In general, the spread of *E. histolytica* resembles that of intestinal bacterial infections, utilizing any means by which fecal contamination reaches the human mouth. Most important are drinking water, food handlers, and houseflies. Swimming pools, though not definitely incriminated, are a potential source of infection. Viable cysts have been found in the droppings of houseflies one to two days after exposure, and flies have been held responsible for at least one important outbreak. It is still a common infection in the United States, and it is a fallacy to consider it predominantly an exotic infection.[6]

The distribution of *E. histolytica* is worldwide, but temperate regions have usually a low incidence of infection. Surveys indicate a general infection rate in the United States of 4 to 10 per cent, though in some southern localities the incidence has approached 40 per cent. These figures include *E. hartmanni* (see below) and are probably about twice the incidence of *E. histolytica* alone. In the tropics the carrier rate is generally very high, often exceeding 50 per cent. Humans carriers are the only important source of infection, although *E. histolytica* occurs naturally in lower animals, particularly rats, dogs, and monkeys.

Control of the spread of *E. histolytica* is not basically different from that of other human enteric infections. The high incidence of carriers not known to have had clinical dysentery complicates the problem, but it is ultimately a matter of prevention of contamination of food or water by feces.

PRIMARY AMEBIC MENINGOENCEPHALITIS

Since 1965, isolated cases and small epidemics of fatal meningoencephalitis of man have been recognized as being caused by free-living amebae. These are generally considered to be of the Hartmanella (Acanthamoeba)—Naegleria group, abundant and ubiquitous in natural bodies of fresh water. Those affected have usually been healthy children or young adults, with a history of swimming in fresh water during the week before onset of symptoms. Death occurs in 3 to 14 days despite therapy. The portal of entry is probably the nasal mucosa with invasions of the central nervous system producing meningitis or hemorrhagic encephalitis with spinal-fluid findings of acute purulent meningitis. At autopsy numerous amebae may be found in the exudate and may be identified on culture.[32, 71]

Other Species of Amebae Parasitic in Man

Six other species of amebae live in the human intestine. With the exception of *Dientamoeba fragilis*, these are nonpathogenic and are of medical interest only because they must be differentiated from *E. histolytica*.

Entamoeba hartmanni, long considered a small race of *E. histolytica*, has been shown to be a distinct species. It differs from *E. histolytica* in size, the cysts being always less than 10 μm. in diameter, and in size of the nuclei, which are slightly more than half the diameter of those in *E. histolytica*. Usually it is not distinguished from *E. histolytica* in diagnostic work, but in a few surveys it has been found to make up about half the infections of the histolytica type. It is nonpathogenic and can be cultured only with difficulty.

Entamoeba coli, a common species, differs from *E. histolytica* in several characteristics. The stained nucleus shows thicker peripheral chromatin blocks and a larger and usually noncentral karyosome. The ameboid stage is sluggishly and usually nonprogressively motile with blunt, slowly extruded pseudopodia. It ingests bacteria and other particles but rarely red blood cells. The spherical cysts average somewhat larger, 10 to 33 μm. in diameter, contain eight nuclei in the mature stage, and may show chromatoid bodies with pointed or "splintered" ends.

Entamoeba polecki, a parasite of hogs and monkeys similar to *E. coli* but producing uninucleate cysts, has been found very rarely in man.

Endolimax nana is smaller, 6 to 15 μm. in diameter in the ameboid stage. The stained nucleus shows no peripheral chromatin but a very large, nearly central karyosome. Movement is sluggishly progressive, and bacteria are ingested. The spherical or ovoid cyst is 5 to 14 μm. in diameter, containing one to four minute nuclei and sometimes small spherical or rodlike chromatoid bodies.

Iodamoeba bütschlii measures 8 to 20 μm. in diameter in the ameboid stage. The stained nucleus shows a large central karyosome surrounded by a layer of granules. Movement and inclusions are like those of *E. coli.* The cyst is irregular in shape, 5 to 20 μm. in diameter, and contains one or rarely two nuclei. Minute granules may be seen, but the most striking feature of the cyst is a large glycogen mass, staining dark brown with iodine.

Dientamoeba fragilis, seldom reported in the general population though sometimes common in institutions, is a very small form, 5 to 12 μm. in diameter. It usually shows two nuclei, each containing a large multiple karyosome. It moves actively, ingesting bacteria. It has been associated with acute dysentery, and it has been suggested that it may produce low-grade constant irritation with fibrotic changes producing an appendicitis. It is considered by some protozoologists to be an aberrant flagellate rather than a true ameba. No cyst stage is known and the binucleate trophozoite is readily destroyed. One investigation suggests that *D. fragilis* is transmitted via the egg of the pinworm of man, *Enterobius vermicularis.*[18] Precedent for this is found in the cycle of *Histomonas meleagridis,* an ameba-like, pathogenic flagellate of the turkey that is transmitted through an Ascarid egg.

Entamoeba gingivalis, probably the first parasitic ameba seen, was reported by Gros in 1849 from the tartar between the teeth. It has no known cyst stage and apparently is transmitted in the ameboid stage by contact. Formerly suspected of an etiological role in pyorrhea, it is now considered harmless.

CILIOPHORA

Balantidium coli is the largest protozoan parasite found in the intestine of man, reaching a size of 150 by 120 μm. The organisms may cause an acute bloody dysentery similar to amebiasis, commonly penetrating the muscularis mucosae and occasionally perforating the intestine.[5] Carrier infections without symptoms occur in man, and the world incidence is estimated at less than 0.7 per cent. Swine are almost universally infected and human infection usually derives from food or water contaminated with the resistant cysts from this source. Moderate to severe pathology is produced in other primates, and infections naturally occur in the rhesus monkey, chimpanzee, dog, and Norway rat. *Balantidium* may be cultivated on a variety of mediums. Tetracy-

clines and diiodohydroxyquin have been used in the successful treatment of infections.

INTESTINAL FLAGELLATES

MASTIGOPHORA

The mastigophora of the digestive tract and genital organs, illustrated in Figure 44–2, are typically lumen parasites. The common cosmopolitan species of enteric flagellates, *Chilomastix mesnili, Trichromonas hominis,* and *Giardia lamblia,* are host-specific, although a number of less common and less specific coprophagic forms are found in man. None are generally considered as important pathogens. However, *Giardia* is commonly associated with erosion of the epithelium of the duodenum and also with an irritation of the gallbladder. There is evidence that in certain instances *Giardia* is capable of deep invasion of the mucosa. Although the significance of this is not clear, it suggests that it is potentially a more important human pathogen than has previously been suspected.[12, 66] Intense infections in children are considered by some to cause dysentery, celiac syndrome, or a sprue-like condition. The parasites and the associated intestinal symptoms disappear following treatment with tinidazole. Epidemics of giardiasis occur in the United States, with outbreaks recorded in Colorado in 1965 and 1974, and an extensive outbreak occurred in Rome, New York, in 1975. In the latter, over 4800 of the population of 46,000 became ill, with the probability that a much larger number harbored

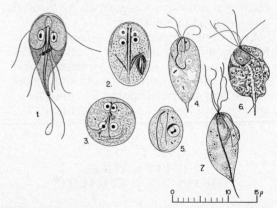

Figure 44–2. Flagellates of the human intestine and genital tract, hematoxylin stain. *1, Giardia lamblia,* trophozoite. *2* and *3, G. lamblia,* cysts. *4, Chilomastix mesnili,* trophozoite. *5, C. mesnili,* cyst. *6, Trichromonas hominis. 7, T. vaginalis.* (Hunter, Swartzwelder, and Clyde, *Tropical Medicine.* 5th ed. W. B. Saunders Co., Philadelphia, 1976.)

asymptomatic infections. Severe giardiasis in groups of American visitors to the Soviet Union has been recorded on a number of occasions.[14] In almost all of the outbreaks recorded, tap water is the likely source of infection.

Trichomonas vaginalis is a cosmopolitan common parasite of the vagina and male genital tract. Infection is commonly symptomless but may produce in the female a severe vaginitis and in the male may occasionally be associated with a urethritis. Transmission occurs primarily through sexual intercourse, as the parasite has no resistant stage. Variation in virulence is related to the strain of the parasite. It is interesting that infected individuals also are usually infected with the nonpathogenic buccal flagellate, *Trichomonas tenax*. Metronidazole (Flagyl) is the drug of choice in treatment.

Chilomastix and *Giardia* are spread by ingestion of material contaminated with human feces containing their cysts. Trichomonas has no resistant cyst, but the trophozoite may remain viable for more than an hour on dry fomites.

HEMOFLAGELLATES

MASTIGOPHORA

The flagellate protozoa occurring in the blood stream or as intracellular parasites of man are termed hemoflagellates. All are members of the family Trypanosomidae. The proper classification of these organisms has been the subect of controversy for many years. The currently accepted classification of the parasites causing African sleeping sickness demands a quadrinominal nomenclature. The flagellates belong to the genus *Trypanosoma* and the subgenus *Trypanozoon*. Their species designation derives from the fact that cyclical development of the *brucei* species occurs in the midgut and salivary glands of the vector. The subspecies identifies the two trypanosomes that cause the disease in man and are considered separate nosodemes. Hence, the accepted names for these parasites are *Trypanosoma trypanozoon brucei gambiense* and *Trypanosoma trypanozoon brucei rhodesiense*. For the sake of brevity, these trypanosomes will be referred to as *Trypanosoma gambiense* and *Trypanosoma rhodesiense* in the text. Similarly, the subgenera of *Trypanosoma (Schizotrypanum) cruzi* and *Trypanosoma (Herpetosoma) rangeli* will also be omitted. The

intracellular *Leishmania* are under study to clarify the taxonomy of this genus. *Leishmania donovani*, *Leishmania tropica*, *Leishmania mexicana*, and *Leishmania braziliensis* are reviewed to illustrate the various forms of the disease, but this coverage is not a complete description of all of the parasites of the *Leishmania* complexes infecting man. The hemoflagellates probably evolved from parasites of the intestinal tract of insects and those parasitizing man still require blood-sucking insect vectors or intermediate hosts for normal transmission.[38] During their life cycles hemoflagellates display a variety of morphological types in regular stages. On microscopic examination of fixed and Giemsa-stained preparations of these stages, organelles are observed which are common to each. There is a falgellum, an associated kinetoplast that is part of the mitochondrium of the parasite, a nucleus, and cytoplasmic granules of varying sizes. The position of the flagellum and the kinetoplast defines each of the stages (Fig. 44–3). The trypomastigote has a flagellum that is inserted into the posterior end of the cell and is attached along its entire length. It usually extends anteriorly beyond the cell and the parasite moves in the direction of this free flagellum. The kinetoplast is located in the posterior end of the cell. It is always found in the region of flagellar insertion. The epimastigote exhibits a free flagellum inserted into the cell near the nucleus and an adjacent kinetoplast, while the flagellum of the promastigote originates near the anterior end of the cell and the associated kinetoplast is near it, distant from the nucleus. A shortened flagellum may be seen in the smaller ovoid amastigote along with the kinetoplast and nucleus. The identification of these forms in blood, aspirates, or tissue preparations is important in diagnosis.

The medically important hemoflagellates can be divided into three groups in two genera. The African trypanosomes, *T. gambiense* and *T. rhodesiense* and related forms, are present in the vertebrate hosts in the trypomastigote form. In the invertebrate vector, the parasites multiply as trypomastigotes and epimastigotes, later differentiating into metatrypanosomes or metacyclic trypomastigotes. The metacyclic trypomastigote is the infective form of the trypanosomes which initiates the infection in the vertebrate host. *Trypanosoma cruzi*, the causal agent of American trypanosomiasis, proceeds through all four of these stages in the vertebrate host, while epimastigote and metacyclic trypomastigotes occur in the inverte-

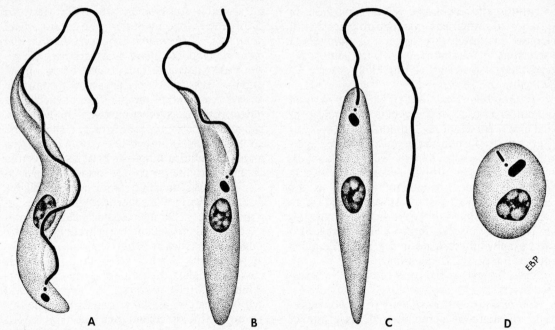

Figure 44–3. Morphological types of hemoflagellates. *A,* Trypomastigote stage. *B,* Epimastigote stage. *C,* Promastigote stage. *D,* Amastigote stage.

brate. Only amastigotes are present in vertebrates infected by *Leishmania* and infective promastigotes in the invertebrate. Amastigote stages are intracellular and the flagellated stages reside in the body fluids of the vertebrate hosts, while only flagellated forms occur in the insect vectors.

Reproduction of all forms is by binary fission. The nucleus, blepharoplast, and parabasal body divide, a new flagellum arises from one blepharoplast, and the cytoplasm divides longitudinally to produce two daughter cells. In the species with which we are concerned, the leishmaniform stages are intracellular in the vertebrate host. The flagellated stages inhabit body fluids of vertebrates or the alimentary tract of insects.

THE TRYPANOSOMES

Trypanosoma gambiense and *Trypanosoma rhodesiense*

In 1910, Stephens and Fantham studied a new disease in humans from East Africa that was more severe than Gambian sleeping sickness, more virulent in laboratory animals, and transmitted by different species of tsetse flies. Because they believed it also differed morphologically from *T. gambiense,* they named it *T. rhodesiense.* Ford observed, in the blood of a Gambian native, a flagellate that was de-

scribed by Dutton in 1902 as *T. gambiense.* In 1903, Castellani observed similar flagellates in the cerebrospinal fluid of a sleeping sickness patient in Uganda. Bruce and Nabarro, in 1903, transmitted *T. gambiense* to monkeys with a tsetse fly, and Kleine, in 1909, showed that the parasites underwent a cyclic development in the fly.

Characteristics and Life Cyles. The life cycles of both *T. gambiense* and *T. rhodesiense* are similar. Species of *Glossina* (tsetse flies) acquire the infection by ingesting a blood meal containing trypanosomes. The parasites multiply in the gut of the fly by binary fission of the trypomastigote stage. These forms are called procyclic stages. Subsequently, they migrate to the salivary glands, where division continues by parasites that have transformed into epimastigotes. After three to five weeks, depending on the temperature, the flagellates change to metacyclic forms. When the tsetse bites a suitable host, the metacyclic stages are injected. They multiply locally as trypomastigotes, and a chancre develops in the area. The trypanosomes invade the lymphatics and then the blood stream, finally entering the tissue spaces and central nervous system.

Epimastigotes have been cultivated on blood agar media at 27° C., and differentiation to the metacyclic stage has been achieved in tsetse fly tissue culture. Blood stream–form trypomastigotes of this group have been grown in tissue culture.[47] In culture and in the hosts, epimastigote forms possess functional mitochondria and cytochrone systems. Blood stream forms lack functional mitochondria and cytochrome systems. They utilize relatively large quantities of glucose and produce pyruvate via the Embden-Meyerhof pathway and a glycerolphosphate oxidase pathway. Protein is endocytosed and the trypomastigotes are capable of deaminating tryrosine and tryptophan, which may yield pharmacologically active compounds such as indole ethanol (tryptophol). This compound induces sleep, convulsions, and respiratory depression in experimental animals. These types of nutrient depletions and released toxic metabolites may be important in the pathogenesis of the African trypanosome infections and those of other parasites.[73]

African trypanosomiasis is endemic in the equatorial zone. *T. gambiense* occurs in central and western Africa and *T. rhodesiense* in the eastern portion of the continent. The disease produced by *T. gambiense* and *T. rhodesiense* is similar, but it progresses more rapidly in the *T. rhodesiense* infection. The disease begins when the infected tsetse bites. The injected trypanosomes localize and multiply at the site of the bite and a chancre develops. The incubation period varies from two to three weeks to several months in Gambian sleeping sickness and from two to three weeks in *T. rhodesiense* infections. A systemic parasitemia develops and the trypanosomes can also be detected in the lymph. Irregular fever is generally the first symptom. The fever later fluctuates during *T. gambiense* infections and is more persistent during *T. rhodesiense* infections. As the trypanosomes multiply, lymphadenopathy is detected. Enlarged posterior cervical lymph nodes (Winterbottom's sign) are characteristic of the disease. Splenomegaly, anemia, and wasting are observed. Cardiac injury and edema may occur. The sleeping sickness stage ensues and trypanosomes are found in the cerebrospinal fluid. Lesions develop in the central nervous system and result in somnolence, apathy, tremors, weakness, and, occasionally, mania and other violent behavior. Coma and death are the final outcome of infection by either parasite. Typically, the Gambian infection runs its course during a period of several months to years, while in *T. rhodesiense*–infected individuals, the disease develops more quickly, and death occurs within three to four weeks after the onset of symptoms.

Immunity. Spontaneous recovery is said to occur in African sleeping sickness, although such cases have not been documented. Typically, infected individuals exhibit a relapsing type of infection. After a period of unchecked multiplication, the trypanosomes are destroyed by antibiodies directed against antigenic determinants on their surfaces. These antigens are glycoproteins that form a compact layer atop the cell membrane of the parasite, called a surface coat. Elevated levels of immunoglobulins are detected during the course of the infection. These in part display specificity against the surface coat antigens and the trypanosomes with the homologous determinants are eliminated by lysis and agglutination. The parasites are able to alter the glycoprotein determinants. This antigenic variation permits the trypanosomes to escape the host immune responses and allows a second population with a new variant antigen to appear in the blood.[25, 30, 36] The antibody eliminates parasites of the variant antigenic type against which it was synthesized, but it does not induce the process of antigenic variation, since this has been shown to occur in the absence of antibody. Successive host immune responses to new variant antigens are responsible for the waves of parasitemia observed during the infection and until the host dies.

Diagnosis. In formulating a progressive diagnosis of African trypanosomiasis, it is important to be aware of the travel history of the patient. The physician should query regarding the countries of residence or visited and whether the subject was limited to urban areas or traveled in rural areas where contact with infected tsetse flies would be more likely. Differential diagnosis may be difficult, since physical findings and symptoms may suggest the disease, but may be caused by other infectious agents. An indirect hemagglutination test is currently commercially available, but usually is not readily accessible. Serum samples may be sent to the state health laboratory for serological testing. Definitive diagnosis is made on finding the trypanosomes in the blood, lymph node fluid, or cerebrospinal fluid. Motile organisms may be seen during microscopic examinations of the blood or fluids. Centrifugation provides a more sensitive microscopic method for detecting the parasites that sediment in the buffy coats atop the red cells or the sediments of the fluid speciments. Thick or thin dry films stained with Wright's or Giemsa stain permit the identification of the organisms, but *T. gambiense* can not be differentiated from *T. rhodesiense* morphologically (Fig. 44–4). The trypanosomes frequently are

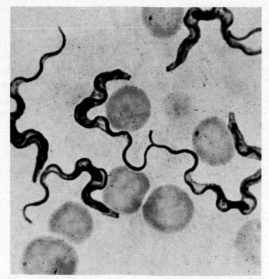

Figure 44–4. *Trypanosoma gambiense* in stained blood film. About × 2000.

scarce and repeated sampling may be necessary. Negative findings are of little diagnostic significance.

Epidemiology and Control. Rare instances of probable venereal infection have been reported. However, the normal transfer of infection occurs by the bite of tsetse flies as described above. Two species of flies are of most importance, *Glossina palpalis* in West Africa and *G. morsitans* in East Africa, where the more virulent Rhodesian form of the disease occurs. Other species of importance are *G. tachinoides, G. swynnertoni, G. pallidipes,* and *G. austeni.* These insects are relatives of the commonly housefly. They are limited to tropical Africa and a small area in South Arabia, and the human disease is confined to their range. They resemble the housefly in appearance except for the long narrow proboscis, which is held straight forward from the head, and the manner of folding the wings at rest, flat on the back with one directly above the other. Both males and females bite and can transmit the disease. They bite exclusively by day. The larvae develop completely in the body of the female, are deposited singly on loose soil or sand in well-shaded places, and quickly burrow into the soil to pupate. After four to eight weeks the adults emerge. *Glossina palpalis* breeds almost entirely near water and is thus more limited in local distribution than *G. morsitans,* which is less dependent on shade and moisture.

The variety of control methods in use testifies to their relative ineffectivenss. Antigenic variation by the African trypanosomes have prevented the development of vaccines against sleeping sickness. Several drugs are available for the treatment of infected individuals in areas where they serve as reservoirs for *T. gambiense.* Three drugs are currently in use and all exhibit toxic side effects. They should be administered with close attention to the patient. Suramin and pentamidine are useful during the first stage of the infections, before there is central nervous system involvement. The latter drug has been administered to hundreds of thousands of Africans in mass treatment campaigns, which reduced the prevalence of the disease. Melarsoprol, an arsenical that passes the blood-brain barrier, is used to treat patients with central nervous system disease. Treatment with this compound should be initiated one week after the start of suramin therapy.

Wild animals act as reservoirs for *T. rhodesiense.* In some areas mass destruction of the reservoir game animals has been attempted, but the success of this measure is doubtful. Where the human and animal infection rates are particularly high, wholesale removal of human populations has been carried out. Control of migrants, a perpetual problem in much of Africa, is utilized in some districts in an effort to minimize spread of the disease.

The life cycle and complex behavior of the tsetse flies make their control exceedingly difficult. Traps and hand-catching have greatly reduced the fly population in some regions. Inspection and fumigation of vehicles have been used to limit the spread of tsetse. The best single method is clearing of forest and brush, particularly along streams and around villages, which destroys the breeding and resting places of the flies.

Trypanosoma cruzi

Chagas, in 1909, discovered intermediate stage flagellates in the hindgut of the bug *Triatoma megista* in Brazil. He showed the infectivity of these flagellates for mammals and later found trypaniform stages in children with a characteristic disease, now known as Chagas' disease. He named the organism *Schizotrypanum cruzi* after his former teacher.

Characteristics and Life Cycle. Slender trypomastigotes are observed in the blood within one week after infection by *T. cruzi.* Within two weeks, shorter and broader forms can be seen that are believed to be stages responsible for infections in the vector. These trypomastigotes are smaller than those of *T. gambiense,* having pointed ends and very large kinetoplasts. In methanol-fixed Giemsa-stained blood films *T. cruzi* frequently assume a C shape. They are not known to divide in the blood, but invade cells, differentiate into amastigotes, and undergo intracellular mutliplication. These amastigotes are 3 to 5 μm in diameter and as their numbers increase, the cell dies. The amastigotes transform to promastigotes, then to epimastigotes, and finally to trypomastigotes, which circulate in the blood and invade other cells. *T. cruzi* is infective for a wide range of mammalian hosts, and strains have been described that are predominantly myotrophic or reticulotrophic parasites. The Tulahuén strain (Fig. 44–5) from Chile exhibits a reticulotropism and may cause enlargement of the liver and spleen, as well as engorgement of the bone marrow. Its pathology resembles that of visceral leishmaniasis.

When the infected vertebrate host is fed upon by a triatomid bug of the family Reduviidae, trypomastigotes are ingested with the blood meal. These transform into epimastigotes and multiply in the midgut. Within two weeks, the epimastigotes differentiate into metacyclic trypomastigotes, which are released with the feces while the bug feeds. The vectors generally cohabit with man and feed at night. They usually bite the victim on the face and are commonly known as assassin or kissing bugs in the United States and barbieros or vinchucas in South America. The metacyclic trypomastigotes enter the wound caused by the bite or penetrate the mucosae, particularly about the eye, nose or mouth. A chagoma, or inflammatory reaction, develops at the site of the initial infection and the parasites multiply locally in cells. They are released into the blood stream and disseminated throughout the host. Transmission of *T. cruzi* may also occur during sexual intercourse, transplacentally to infants from infected mothers during parturition or when nursing, and via blood transfusions.

T. cruzi epimastigotes are easily cultivated in diphasic blood agar and liquid nutrient mediums at 27° C. Metacyclic trypomastigotes can be grown in liquid mediums with and without extracts of triatomid bugs or in triatomid bug tissue cultures. Amastigote stages will grow in special liquid culture mediums, and the complete vertebrate cycle occurs in tissue cultures incubated at 37° C.

Culture form epimastigotes and blood stream–form trypomastigotes utilize glucose aerobically and significant quantities in the pentose pathway. An active cytochrome system has also been demonstrated in both stages. Differences in the activities of the pathways in various strains of *T. cruzi* may be related to the relative pathogenicity of each.

Chagas' Disease. Chagas described the infection from a region having serious endemic goiter, and most of his cases had marked thyroid pathology. It has since been shown in other regions that the goitrous manifestations he described are not part of Chagas' disease. The incubation period is one to two weeks. Irregular fever and edema, particularly of the eyelids (Romaña's sign), characterize the acute phase, and there is considerable enlargement of lymph nodes, spleen, and liver toward the end of this period. A period of latent disease may persist for years or throughout life following the acute phase of the infection with few trypomastigotes present in the blood, or the host may exhibit the chronic form of the disease, most often characterized by myocarditis. The destruction of muscle and ganglionic cells may also cause megacolon, megaesophagus, and the enlargement of other organs. Individuals with chronic Chagas' disease have shortened life expectancies, with death usually occurring as a result of heart failure.

Immunity. The occurrence of latent and chronic *T. cruzi* infections and the concurrent immunological responses indicate that infected humans exert a level of control over the parasites. Immunologically compromised experimental animals have higher parasitemias and greater numbers of amastigotes in the tissues than infected immunocompetent controls.

Infected Kupffer cell

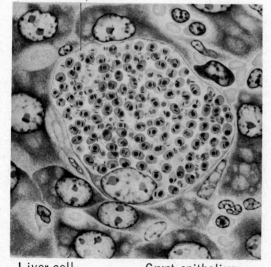

Liver cell   Crypt epithelium →

Figure 44–5. Amastigotes of the Tulahuén strain of *Trypanosoma cruzi* in a Kupffer cell of liver. (Taliaferro and Pizzi.)

Studies with attenuated vaccines (*i.e.,* irradiated parasites unable to reproduce in recipient animals) or relatively nonpathogenic strains of *T. cruzi* (*i.e.,* a strain isolated from mammals in Maryland) show that these preparations confer a demonstrable immunity to challenge infections with the homologous and heterologous virulent parasites. Immunization of laboratory animals with killed trypanosomes, cell fractions, and purified components of the parasites elicit varying levels of resistance, but none provide complete protection against infection. Humoral antibodies synthesized by the human host fix complement and lyse trypanosomes. Agglutinins and precipitins are also detected during the acute and chronic stages of the infections. The passive transfer of serum from animals that survive acute infections to recipient animals results in lower parasitemias and increased survival when compared with similarly challenged untreated controls. Spleen cells, polymorphonuclear leucocytes, eosinophils, and macrophages in the presence of specific antibody damage parasites.[82] In addition, spleen cells from infected mice exhibit decreased responsiveness to T and B cell specific mitogens during the acute phase of the infection in mice, which returns to normal levels during the chronic phase.[56, 81] This suppression appears to be due to soluble suppressive factors and may involve adherent cells (macrophages). The return of normal T and B cell functions during the chronic phase suggest that the disease is regulated immunologically by the host.

Diagnosis. Parasites may be detected in stained blood films during the acute phase of Chagas' disease. However, they may be difficult to demonstrate during the latent and chronic stages of the infection. Hemoculture, the inoculation of a patient's blood into rabbit blood–nutrient agar slants, may permit the growth of epimastigotes, which can be found after two to three weeks of incubation at 27°C. Xenodiagnosis provides a more sensitive test. Laboratory-reared triatomid bugs are permitted to feed on the patient and the contents of their intestines are examined microscopically for flagellates after 10 to 14 days.

Complement fixation, indirect hemagglutination, latex agglutination, and indirect immunofluorescence tests are commercially available as kits, and the enzyme-linked immunosorbent assay is established as a sensitive serodiagnostic technique.[2] When parasites can not be found, diagnosis may depend on indications of possible exposure, the symptoms presented by the patient, and a positive serological test.

Epidemiology and Control. Infection is normally acquired from infected bugs as described above, although occasionally the disease is acquired by direct contamination of mucosae, as in the congenital infection of infants. The major vectors for *T. cruzi* are species belonging to the genera *Triatoma, Panstrongylus* and *Rhodnius* of the family Reduviidae. These insects are members of the order Hemiptera, or True Bugs, to which belong also bedbugs and many others. They are large insects with an elongated, cone-shaped head. Most species are predatory on other insects, but some live on vertebrate blood. They inhabit the nests of various animals and may occur in human houses of poor construction, usually mud and stick or stone with thatched roofs, which provide refuge. The total life cycle, involving egg, larval, nymphal and adult stages, occupies 6 to 10 months.

The human disease is widespread in South and Central America but of low incidence in most areas. It has been reported from every country in the Western Hemisphere, with the exception of Canada, Honduras, and the Guianas, as a sylvatic infection. *Trypanosoma cruzi* has been reported in Arizona, California, Georgia, Louisiana, Maryland, New Mexico, and Texas.[95] In addition, two indigenous cases have been recorded in human beings in Texas.[96] The possibility that more extensive infections occur than are reported in suggested by the fact that patients in the eastern United States suffering from a diffuse myocarditis have been found to react positively to serological tests for *T. cruzi*.[34]

Successful control of Chagas' disease has not been attained. The most effective strategy is the improvement of houses to exclude the triatomid bugs. Currently, Nifurtimox, a nitrofuran derivative, is the only drug available for the treatment of Chagas' disease. It is relatively ineffective in chronic infections, and some strains of *T. cruzi* resist treatment.

Trypanosoma rangeli

Tejera, in 1920, described from a vector of *T. cruzi* in Venezuela a flagellate that he named *T. rangeli*. In 1942, this was obtained from humans by xenodiagnosis, and since that time has been reported widely from Central and South America in the areas in which *Rhodnius prolixus*, its vector, occurs. Trypanosome division takes place in the peripheral circulation of man, dog, and monkeys with no leishmaniform stages demonstrated. No clinical manifestations are known and two experimental infections in man were without symptoms. In contrast to *T. cruzi, T. rangeli* is transmitted to man through the bite of the insect. Morphologically, the trypomastigotes of *T. rangeli* can be distinguished from *T. cruzi* on the basis of their larger size and their smaller terminal kinetoplast. Dual infections by *T. rangeli* and *T. cruzi* are possible in many areas, and cross-reactions may give false-positive reactions in some serological tests for Chagas' disease. Monoclonal antibodies have been used to distinguish between the two species.[2, 3]

Other Species of Trypanosoma

A number of important diseases of domestic animals are caused by species of *Trypanosoma* similar to *T. gambiense* and *T. rhodesiense*. Nagana, a fatal disease of livestock, is caused by *T. brucei* and prevents the raising of cattle in vast areas of Africa. A number of other species transmitted by tsetse flies are important disease agents of animals in Africa. *Trypanosoma evansi* causes a disease of horses, camels, and mules known as "surra," which is widespread in Asia, extending to Russia, Arabia, and Madagascar.

THE LEISHMANIAS

Leishmania donovani

Leishman and Donovan, in 1903, described oval parasites of the macrophages in cases of kala-azar in India. These were recognized as mastigophora when Rogers showed that they developed into motile flagellates in culture.

Characteristics and Life Cycle. In the human disease, kala-azar, the parasites occur as amastigotes 3 to 5 μm. long, in macrophages, where they are indistinguishable from the same stage of *T. cruzi*, as shown in Figure 44–6. They multiply by binary fission until the cytoplasm of the host cell is crowded, when they escape to infect new cells. While the parasites predominate in internal organs, they occur in the skin macrophages as well, and it is probably from this site that the intermediate hosts, sandflies of the genus Phlebotomus, become infected. The parasites transform into the promastigote stage, 14 to 20 μm. long, and multiply in the midgut and foregut of the insect, which becomes infective after a week or more. The flagellates, injected by the bite of the fly into a new host, re-establish the vertebrate phase of the cycle.

Leishmania donovani promastigotes and those of other species can be cultivated at 21 to 27°C in liquid of diphasic media supplemented with rabbit blood or serum. Attenuation occurs after continued subcultivation, and cyclical passage through a vertebrate host is required to maintain the virulence of the parasites. Amastigotes can be grown at 37°C in macrophage cultures. *Leishmania* promasti-

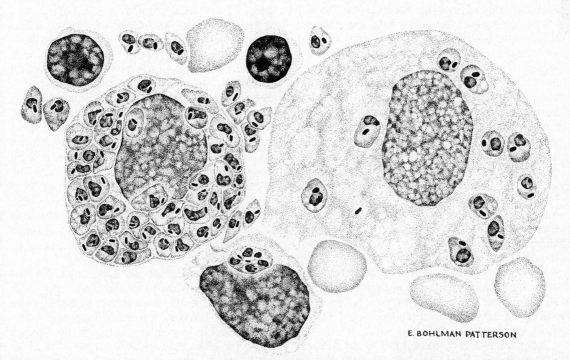

E. BOHLMAN PATTERSON

Figure 44–6. *Leishmania donovani,* free and in phagocytes, in Giemsa-stained smear of spleen. Camera lucida; about × 2000.

gotes catabolize glucose at a higher rate than amastigotes and respiratory rates are as much as tenfold greater in these forms. Oxygen consumption is inhibited by cyanide and iodoacetate, while carbon dioxide, pyruvate, and succinate are major end products. Both amastigotes and promastigotes appear to secrete large quantities of proteins, which may have a role in the disease produced by each species.[43]

Kala-azar. Visceral leishmaniasis, or kala-azar, is usually a chronic disease. Typically it begins, after an incubation period of one to four months (sometimes much longer), with a high temperature, followed by an irregular fever. The spleen and liver enlarge greatly with hyperplasia of the parasitized macrophage system. Wasting, emaciation, and edema are common. Dysentery often occurs as a result of heavy infection in the intestinal wall. The skin is typically dusky in hue, whence the name kala-azar, meaning "black fever." The skin is infected with the parasite but usually does not show lesions until months after systemic recovery when depigmented areas appear, later often becoming slightly raised papules. Anemia and leucopenia are characteristic. Adrenal insufficiency has been reported. Death is the rule in untreated cases, usually as a result of secondary infection.

Immunity. Treated or spontaneously cured kala-azar is apparently followed by a lasting, solid immunity, for second infections are exceedingly rare. However, vaccines have failed to protect against or ameliorate the disease. While antibody is synthesized during visceral leishmaniasis, resistance is not passively transferred. The humoral antibody responses are useful in the serodiagnosis of cases in which amastigotes are difficult to detect. Resistance is believed to be cell-mediated. Since the amastigotes reside and multiply within macrophages, the effector mechanisms of parasite killing are assumed to operate in these cells. Support for this is provided by experiments with *L. tropica* in which lymphokines from sensitized T lymphocytes were used to activate macrophages in suspension cultures. Fewer of these cells were infected than controls after challenge with the parasites. Multiplication of the amastigotes in the lymphokine-treated cells was inhibited. In cells exposed to lymphokines after they were infected, multiplication was also inhibited and parasites were eliminated within 72 hours by 75 to 80 per cent of the macrophages.[67]

Diagnosis and Treatment. Crucial laboratory diagnosis of kala-azar may be obtained by the finding of parasites in biopsies of skin, spleen, liver, or bone marrow. Sternal bone marrow puncture is a reliable and safe procedure. Blood cultures may be positive. In addition, a group of nonspecific serological reactions has shown great value. These reactions depend on the fact that the serum euglobulin is greatly increased in amount in cases of kala-azar. In the formol gel test (Napier's aldehyde reaction), positive serums form an opaque gel when formalin is added. In the antimony test, a pentavalent antimonial drug causes a heavy flocculent precipitate in serums of patients. These tests are positive in over 80 per cent of cases and give false positives only occasionally with other diseases, especially schistosomiasis and malaria. The enzyme-linked immunosorbent assay, countercurrent immunoelectrophoresis, and indirect immunofluorescence are the most sensitive serological tests.

Pentavalent antimonials are the drugs of choice in the treatment of visceral leishmaniasis. Meglumine antimoniate (Glucantime) and sodium stibogluconate (Pentostam) exhibit similar efficacies and toxicities. Treatment regimens vary from small daily doses administered over a period of 30 days to larger doses given on alternative days for shorter periods. Pentamidine, allopurinol, and amphotericin B can be used to treat infections that do not respond to antimonials. Successful treatment is often followed by dermal leishmaniasis, which may persist for several months.

Epidemiology and Control. Kala-azar has been reported in China, India, southern Russia, Mesopotamia, the Mediterranean littoral, southern Arabia, Equatorial Africa, and parts of South and Central America. In Asia it is apparently a disease of man, though various lower animals, particularly dogs, hamsters, and mice, are susceptible. Infection may occur at any age but is most common in older children and young adults. In the Mediterranean area, however, it is primarily a disease of small children. Here dogs are commonly infected and apparently serve as the reservoir, since, unlike children, they show abundant parasites in the skin. The parasite in the Mediterranean area is *L. infantum* and in South America *L. chagasi*.

Factors of seasonal and geographical distribution early pointed to sandflies as probable vectors, and it was soon shown that they were susceptible, developing heavy intestinal infections when fed on individuals with the disease. In these flies the pharynx often becomes blocked with the simple flagellate stages, and in their vigorous efforts to feed, the "blocked" flies apparently are more likely to inject parasites.

The sandfly vectors belong to the genus *Phlebotomus* of the family of small flies, Psychodidae. The most important species are *Phlebotomus argentipes* in India, *P. chinensis* in China, and *P. major* and *P. perniciosus* in the Mediterranean region. The vectors in other areas are as yet unknown. The adult flies are minute, night-biting insects. They fly weakly and travel very short distances but penetrate ordinary window screening with ease. The larvae develop in loose damp soil or debris, mostly in cracks in walls, cliffs, caves, etc., the entire life cycle requiring one to two months.

The transmitting insects can be controlled by removing potential breeding places or by spraying with residual insecticides. Treatment of human cases is also widely used for control of the spread of kala-azar.

Leishmania tropica

Leishmania tropica was discovered by Wright, in 1903, in an Armenian patient in Boston. Morphologically and culturally identical with *L. donovani*, it differs in infecting primarily the skin, where it proliferates in the macrophages of the subcutaneous tissue. In man, dogs, and wild rodents it produces large single or multiple ulcers, usually of exposed parts of the skin, known as oriental sore. These lesions appear after an incubation period of 10 days to several months. They increase to a diameter of 1 to 3 cm. and heal spontaneously after several months to leave a disfiguring scar. Permanent immunity follows infection, and deliberate induction of sores on unexposed parts of the body has long been practiced in the Middle East to avoid the disfigurement of exposed scars. Transmission can be effected by direct contact, fomites, and houseflies, but the principal spread is undoubtedly by sandflies in a manner similar to that in kala-azar. Oriental sore occurs in southern Asia, southern Russia, the Near East, equatorial Africa, and the Mediterranean region, the principal vectors being *P. sergenti*, *P. papatasii*, and, probably, *P. caucasicus*. Laboratory diagnosis is made by identification of the parasites in stained smears of scrapings from the lesions. Reliable diagnosis of oriental sore has been reported with an intradermal test. Since it is often very difficult to detect parasites in the lesions, such a procedure would be valuable. Local or systemic administration of antimony compounds are usually effective in treatment.

Leishmania mexicana. Cutaneous leishmaniasis in the New World is caused by *L. mexicana*. Geographically, the disease is found throughout Central and South America. It is commonly referred to as chiclero's ulcer in some localities, since *L. mexicana* infection is common among forest workers who harvest chicle. Promastigotes develop in blood agar and liquid media at 27°C. and amastigotes in explanted macrophages. Amastigotes of *L. mexicana* are larger than those of other *Leishmania*. They also have a vacuolated cytoplasm and differ in the position of the kinetoplast and the nucleus. Individuals infected with the parasite present with a single or limited number of skin lesions. Disfiguring ulceration frequently occurs on the ear, and rarely cases of diffuse cutaneous leishmaniasis are encountered. Metastatic lesions occur in wild hosts, but are not seen in humans.

Leishmania braziliensis

Morphologically this species is indistinguishable from *L. tropica* and *L. donovani*, and its primary lesion closely resembles that of *L. tropica*. Superficial granular or moist ulcers may occur at any skin site. In some endemic areas the parasite characteristically migrates to secondary foci, particularly mucocutaneous junctions, causing extensive destructive erosion of the nasopharynx, larynx, and associated structures, with facial disfigurement. Metastatic lesions occur with probable spread through the lymphatics, and leishmanias have been recovered from the peripheral blood. Diagnosis and treatment are the same as used for the other leishmanias. Recovery from infection confers a long-lasting immunity to reinfection. Cross-immunity is not found to occur between species of Leishmania, and infection with *L. mexicana* does not protect against *L. braziliensis*. An intradermal test, the Montenegro reaction, utilizing an antigen derived from cultured leishmanias, is also of value. The disease is known by a variety of names throughout its range, including uta, espundia, and mucocutaneous leishmaniasis, and has a distribution ranging from Argentina north into the Yucatan Peninsula of Mexico.

SPOROZOA

Malarial Parasites

With the exception of an uncommon coccidial parasite, and the related *Toxoplasma* that until recently was unclassified, the only sporozoa infecting man are the malarial parasites. They were first recognized by Laveran in 1880, and the life cycle in human erythrocytes was described by Golgi. Manson's suggestions led Ross to the demonstration in 1898 of mosquito transmission of avian malaria, and Grassi, Bignami, and Bastianelli later in the same year showed the mechanism of spread of human malaria. Man harbors four species of malarial parasites, of which *Plasmodium vivax* will serve as an example.

Characteristics and Life Cycle. In fresh preparations of infected blood the parasites of *P. vivax* appear as clear areas in the erythrocytes. They contain yellow or brown granules of pigment, a digestion product of hemoglobin that has been identified as hematin. In Giemsa-stained blood films the parasites show blue cytoplasm and violet-red nuclei. The earliest stage in the erythrocyte, the ring stage, consists of a thin ring of cytoplasm with a nucleus at one side (Fig. 44–7). The parasite grows, becoming an irregular uninucleate body containing several brown pigment granules. This stage is known as the trophozoite. The parasitized cell has now enlarged somewhat and may show scattered throughout its cytoplasm minute red granules or Schüffner's dots, which are believed to be the result of injury to the cell. The parasite continues to grow, phagocytizing the erythrocyte hemoglobin, which it digests, thereby accumulating more pigment. Eventually it nearly fills the erythrocyte, which is now about one and one-half times its normal diameter. The nucleus divides repeatedly until 12 to 24, usually about 16, nuclei are present. This is the schizont stage. Finally, in the segmenter stage, the cytoplasm divides, a portion surrounding each nucleus. The pigment is left in a dense clump, and the cell disintegrates to release the daughter cells, or merozoites, into the plasma. Here they invade fresh erythrocytes and repeat the cycle. The above process of growth and multiple fission is known as schizogony. It occupies, in *P. vivax*, about 48 hours, and the growth is regulated by the daily cycle of activity of the host, so that segmentation usually occurs at about the same time every other day.

After several schizogonic cycles a difference may be noted in the infection. Some ameboid stages, instead of becoming schizonts and undergoing asexual reproduction, develop into large uninucleate parasites with scattered pigment granules. These are the sexual stages. The female, or macrogametocyte, shows a compact, dark red nucleus and intense blue cytoplasm. The male, or microgametocyte, has a more diffuse, less deeply stained nucleus, and the cytoplasm is paler, often pinkish rather than blue. The gametocytes undergo no further development in man, eventually degenerating or being destroyed unless they are taken up by a susceptible mosquito.

Gametes are produced in the stomach of the mosquito. The macrogametocyte escapes from the erythrocyte and becomes a single macrogamete, corresponding to a metazoan ovum. The microgametocyte produces at its surface, by a process generally called "exflagellation," four to eight long, whip-like microgametes, counterparts of the spermatozoa of higher animals. One of these actively wriggling microgametes fertilizes a macrogamete. The resulting spherical zygote transforms into a fusiform ookinete that actively passes the epithelial cells of the mosquito stomach. An oocyst begins to develop on the outside of the stomach one to two days after ingestion of the blood meal. Growth results in an oocyst that comes to rest on the outside of the stomach. Other authors believe that a fusiform ookinete is formed that actively penetrates the epithelial cells. The above process in the mosquito occupies one to two days. Nuclear multiplication occurs and the oocyst grows until a diameter of about 50 μm. is attained. The oocyst now contains many hundreds of nuclei. Each acquires a bit of cytoplasm and becomes a spindle-shaped body, about 8 μm. long, the sporozoite. With the rupture of the oocyst, these sporozoites scatter throughout the body of the mosquito. Many accumulate in the salivary glands, where they are injected into man by the biting mosquito. The complete development in the mosquito requires from one to two weeks; 25° C. is said to be the optimal temperature, no development occurring below 15° C. nor above 30° C.

For many years it was believed that the sporozoites entered erythrocytes to initiate the schizogonic cycle described above. Indirect evidence suggested that the parasites underwent a different type of development before invading the blood. This development was first discovered in a malarial infection of birds.[50] The sporozoites were found to enter fixed tissue cells where, as cryptozoites, they undergo a type of schizogony fundamentally like that in erythrocytes except that no pigment is produced. Segmentation produces merozoites, which invade new macrophages and repeat the cycle. Some of the second generation merozoites enter erythrocytes to establish the blood schizogony. Others continue to reproduce in tissue cells as exoerythrocytic stages, probably throughout the whole course

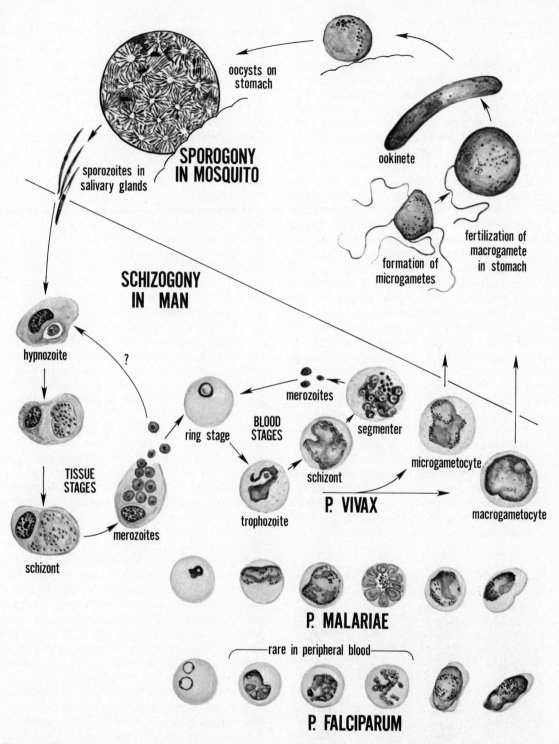

oocysts on
stomach

**SPOROGONY
IN MOSQUITO**

sporozoites in
salivary glands

ookinete

fertilization of
macrogamete
in stomach

formation of
microgametes

**SCHIZOGONY
IN MAN**

hypnozoite

?

merozoites

**BLOOD
STAGES**

ring stage

segmenter

microgametocyte

**TISSUE
STAGES**

schizont

trophozoite

P. VIVAX

macrogametocyte

merozoites

schizont

P. MALARIAE

rare in peripheral blood

P. FALCIPARUM

Figure 44–7. Life cycle and comparative morphology of malarial parasites of man. (Schizogonic blood stages × 2000 are redrawn from C. G. Huff: Manual of Medical Parasitology; original drawing by E. Hanford.)

of infection, and may repeatedly give rise to new schizonts in erythrocytes. The cryptozoites and later exoerythrocytic stages are resistant to drugs effective against the blood parasites.

Until 1948, neither cryptozoites nor later exoerythrocytic stages had been observed in mammalian malarias. They were observed first in monkey malaria and later in a human volunteer infected with enormous numbers of sporozoites of *P. vivax*. Large schizonts were found in the liver 5 to 10 days after sporozoite inoculation. Unlike those in avian malarias, which occur in macrophages, the cryptozoites in *P. vivax* were said to be in hepatic cells. The parasites observed appeared to constitute a second generation of reproduction, but no organisms had been observed before the fifth day of infection.

In experimental infections with simian malaria, schizonts have been observed in the liver three and one-half months after infection, indicating persistence of the tissue parasites during and after the acute blood infection.

Sporozoites initiate schizogony similar to that observed in avian malarias, but in liver cells (Fig. 44–8). After about nine days, released merozoites infect erythrocytes and begin the erythrocytic cycle in *P. vivax* infections. Shortt and Garnham proposed that other merozoites infect liver cells and continue the exoerythrocytic or tissue cycle.[87] More recently, Krotoski and co-workers, using histological and immunofluorescence techniques, detected 2.5 μm. pre-erythrocytic stages of a simian malaria as early as 36 hours after the inoculation of large numbers of sporozoites.[57, 58] Uni-

nuclear stages approximately 4 to 5 μm. in diameter named "hypnozoites" were observed 3 to 105 days after infection. The persistent and dormant hypnozoites were also demonstrated in chimpanzees infected with *P. vivax*. They were not found in malarias caused by nonrelapsing species. A question mark is displayed on the tissue phase of the infection in Figure 44–7 because these studies have opened the question of whether merozoites from exoerythrocytic schizonts can reinfect liver cells as described in the cycle proposed by Shortt and Garnham.

Human malarial parasites can be continuously cultivated in thin layers of erythrocytes overlaid with tissue culture medium under conditions of reduced oxygen. Modifications of this technique provide increased yields of erythrocytic stages. Methods for the synchronization of the parasites allow analyses of specific developmental forms. As suggested by the conditions of the culture system, glycolysis is a major pathway in the metabolism of glucose, with the production of lactic acid. Amino acids are provided by the digestion of hemoglobin and evidenced by the appearance of the pigment, hemozoin, in the infected red cells.

The life cycles and morphology of the other human malarial parasites in erythrocytes are fundamentally similar to those of *P. vivax*. *Plasmodium malariae* requires 72 hours for the completion of schizogony. The erythrocytic parasites show several differences of diagnostic value. No granules of the type of Schüffner's dots are seen in the infected cells. The cells are not enlarged during growth of the parasites. The older trophozoite is not ameboid like that of *P. vivax* but commonly exhibits a "band" form across the parasitized cell. The segmenter produces 6 to 14, usually 8, merozoites, arranged in a "rosette" form. The gametocytes are small, and the pigment typically occurs in abundant, large dark granules; the optimal temperature for sporogony in the mosquito is said to be about 22° C., and sporogony is slow, requiring three weeks or more.

Plasmodium falciparum, like *P. malariae*, causes no enlargement of the infected cells, but some parasitized cells show granules, Maurer's dots, which correspond to the Schüffner's dots of *P. vivax*. Schizogony results in 6 to 24 merozoites. The schizonts and segmenters typically accumulate in capillaries of internal organs, appearing in the peripheral blood only in very heavy infections. Normally, therefore, only ring stages and gametocytes are seen in blood films. Infection of erythrocytes by two or more rings is common and the rings often

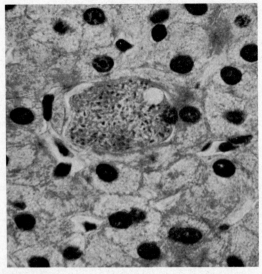

Figure 44–8. Schizont of *Plasmodium vivax* in liver section. (Courtesy of Col. H. E. Shortt.)

contain two nuclei. The gametocytes are distinctive, exhibiting a characteristic sausage shape that distorts or obliterates the infected cell. Because of their shape, they are commonly called "crescents." The pigment is finely granular or amorphous in appearance and in the gametocytes it is typically concentrated about the nucleus. The optimal temperature for sporogony is said to be 29° C.

Plasmodium ovale is a rare species showing similarities to both *P. vivax* and *P. malariae* but characterized chiefly by the fact that the infected cell is often distorted into an oval. Its significance is not known, although many investigators consider it an aberrant type of *P. vivax*.

Malaria. Vivax malaria, or benign tertian malaria, is featured by typical chills and fever occurring at the time of segmentation of the peripheral blood parasites. These paroxysms begin with an acute, shaking chill while the temperature is rising. A "hot stage" occurs at the fever peak, the patient feeling unbearably hot and the oral temperature usually reaching 104° or 105° F. This gives way to a "sweating stage" during which the fever falls rapidly to normal or slightly below. Parasite products or red blood cell contents released at disruption of the infected cells are presumably responsible for the paroxysm. Paroxysms coincide, as stated above, with the time of parasite segmentation. Hence they occur every 48 hours if all the parasites reproduce on the same day. Often, however, distinct broods of parasites segment on alternate days. Vivax malaria commonly shows quotidian (daily) chills for several days followed by the suppression of one brood of parasites with resultant tertian chills (every other day). Between paroxysms the patient feels and appears normal.

Significant anemia occurs commonly in vivax malaria but is rarely serious unless other factors are involved. A week or more after the beginning of an attack, particularly in children, the spleen usually enlarges and remains enlarged for two to six months after termination of the attack. The untreated attack typically lasts three to six weeks, often with temporary cessations of clinical activity. It is followed by a period of latency during which parasites cannot be found microscopically in the peripheral blood. During part of this time large transfusions of blood from the infected person fail to induce infection in recipients. This suggests that exoerythrocytic stages are responsible for maintenance of infection during latency. In many cases renewal of clinical activity, or relapse, occurs after 2 to 10 months

of latency, the clinical picture resembling that in the primary attack. The infection usually dies out after two to three years, and no further relapses occur.

Because of the 72-hour cycle of reproduction, malaria due to *P. malariae* is known as quartan malaria, the chills occurring every third day. It is basically similar to vivax malaria, though the paroxysms are often more severe. The incubation period is usually long, three weeks or more, and the period of clinical activity typically lasts for several months. Relapses are uncommon, but latent infection may persist for many years, as shown by the occasional development of quartan malaria in recipients of blood transfusions from persons who have not shown evidence of infection for 30 years or more. A nephrotic syndrome in children and young adults infected with *P. malariae* has been recognized as a relatively common result of infection. The pathology is that of an immune complex, glomerular nephritis, involving specific malarial antigen, antibody, and complement.[48] Although this may progress to chronic glomerulonephritis with renal failure, prompt antimalarial chemotherapy in children is followed by recovery.

Falciparum malaria is widely known as malignant tertian or estivo-autumnal malaria. As noted above, *P. falciparum* is characterized by accumulation of erythrocytic stages in internal organs. As a result, in addition to or instead of the typical paroxysms, which are quotidian or tertian, various local manifestations of the disease may be prominent. This is especially true in the tropics, where such "pernicious" malaria may follow a series of typical chills. The most common types are algid (cold) malaria, gastrointestinal manifestations, and cerebral malaria with coma and often death. These peculiarities of falciparum malaria make it the cause of most of the deaths attributable to human malarial infection and an important factor in many deaths traced to other diseases. Blackwater fever is a dangerous hemoglobinuria associated with falciparum malaria. This syndrome involves a rapid lysis of erythrocytes with large quantities of hemoglobin and its breakdown products in the blood and urine. Death usually occurs as a result of renal failure. The condition is usually seen in individuals subject to repeated infection and is believed to be the result of an autoimmune response. *Plasmodium falciparum* infections rarely relapse and rarely persist more than a year or two. It is believed that the exoerythrocytic stages do not persist after the cycle in erythrocytes has begun.

Immunity. Examples of innate immunity are provided by differences between the susceptibilities of the normal population and individuals with hereditary anemias. Persons with sickle cell anemia possess hemoglobin that has a valine substituted for a glutamic acid in the molecule. This substitution alters the capacity of the abnormal hemoglobin to carry oxygen. Life expectancy of homozygous individuals is greatly reduced, while heterozygous persons survive, since only a portion of their hemoglobin has the valine substitution. The abnormal hemoglobin precipitates at low pH and low oxygen tension. These conditions are present in the vacuoles of the parasites. The sickle cell hemoglobin assumes an insoluble form, unaffected by the hydrolytic enzymes; thus, its component amino acids are not provided to the parasites. Damage also occurs to membranes of the parasites because of the form of the hemoglobin. Individuals with sickle cell hemoglobin are less susceptible to infections by *P. falciparum*, and in Africa, the parasite appears to have selected for the gene in the populations.

Infections by malarial parasites are also dependent upon the presence of appropriate receptors on the erythrocyte surfaces. Individuals with Duffy blood group determinants are susceptible to *P. vivax* infections, while those who are Duffy-negative are refractory. Almost all Europeans and Asians have the determinants, but Africans lack them and are resistant to vivax malaria.

Acquired immunity to malaria is evident in recovered individuals who are resistant to reinfection. This immunity persists for a few months after the parasites have been eliminated. Antibodies against sporozoites are found in the serum of persons living in endemic areas.[74] Infants are protected by maternal antibodies. Humans immunized with attenuated sporozoites are resistant to infections by the same stage.[76] Antigens inducing these responses are located on the surface membranes of the sporozoites. In rodents, monoclonal antibody has been shown to react on the surfaces, neutralize infectivity, and, when passively transferred, protect against infection.[27, 75, 101]

Immune responses are also directed against tissue and blood stages of the parasites. The hypnozoites and liver schizonts are, by virtue of their intracellular locations, sheltered from antibodies and cellular responses. If all merozoites produced during the erythrocytic cycle were successful at invading red blood cells, the host would soon succumb to an overwhelming parasitemia. This does not occur, but rather many merozoites and parasitized erythrocytes are phagocytosed and digested by macrophages of the spleen, liver, bone marrow, and other organs. Passively transferred serum from recovered animals protects normal recipients. Such serum contains agglutinating and opsonizing antibodies. Specific antibody-dependent cell-mediated cytotoxicity is observed in malaria.[15] Peripheral blood lymphocytes and homologous antisera from infected Gambian children and adults markedly limit *P. falciparum* multiplication in cultures, when compared with Gambian lymphocytes and serum from Europeans, lymphocytes, or the serum alone in control cultures. Interestingly, studies in rodents and primates indicate that recrudescent populations of malarial parasites are able to undergo antigen variation, which suggests a possible mechanism to evade these immunological responses.[24, 63]

Diagnosis. Laboratory diagnosis of acute malaria rests on the finding of parasites in peripheral blood films. They are most easily identified in thin films stained with Giemsa, but, since parasites are often scanty in the peripheral blood, dehemoglobinized thick films, similarly stained, are widely used. The rapid staining method of Field is of especial value for such preparations. The fact that parasite morphology is abnormal in thick films is offset by the much greater volume of blood that can be examined in a comparable time. In surveys the characteristic spleen enlargement is a nonspecific, but highly suggestive indication of current or recent malarial infection. Because it usually persists for several months, it affords a more stable index of the infection rate in an area than do clinical or parasitological surveys. The indirect fluorescent antibody test for malaria has become an important diagnostic and epidemiological tool, and is available as a commercial kit. In the United States it has in recent years been of importance in tracing sources of transfusion-induced malaria.

Chemotherapy. Treatment of malaria for centuries depended on the bark or extracts of the bark of cinchona trees. The main active principle in cinchona bark is the alkaloid quinine. Quinine neither prevents nor cures the natural infection, but rapidly suppresses the number of blood parasites below the density necessary to produce symptoms. The synthetic drug quinacrine (Atabrine) has similar action, and in addition it can cure falciparum malaria. Chloroquine and camoquin, developed in large-scale World War II research, have properties like of those of quinacrine but are more effective. Paludrine, a product of British wartime research, is a very effective suppressive for vivax malaria and is both prophylactic and curative for *P. falciparum* infection. The distantly related Daraprim (pyrimethamine) has similar but stronger action. These two drugs suffer from the disadvantages that they act slowly and that the parasites may become resistant to them.

The above drugs taken continuously during exposure to vivax malaria act as suppressives, holding the infection down to subclinical levels. They do not prevent or cure the infection. Primaquine, however, destroys the exoerythrocytic stages and if given prior to invasion of the erythrocytes will prevent clinical malaria from occurring. It is also used in conjunction with drugs effective against the erythrocytic stages to cure established vivax infection, since elimination of the persistent exoerythrocytic stages is mandatory to prevent relapse.

As with other microorganisms, inheritable drug resistance can be induced in the plasmodia. Development of pyrimethamine resistance in both *P. vivax* and *P. falciparum* has been observed on a number of occasions, and particularly virulent strains of chloroquine-resistant *P. falciparum* have been recovered in Colombia and Thailand and are apparently widespread in Southeast Asia.[80, 100] The former retained sensitivity to pyrimethamine and the latter is resistant to pyrimethamine, but Atabrine-sensitive. Because of the acute onset and fatal consequence of cerebral involvement, drug sensitivity tests are mandatory in management of this infection. A relatively simple culture technique to determine chloroquine resistance or susceptibility is a practical method for the diagnostic laboratory.

As a result of United States participation in the war in Vietnam, malaria in servicemen increased extensively (Fig. 44–9). Returning asymptomatic servicemen had malaria relapses after discharge, some with fatal results, if chloroquine-resistant *Plasmodium falciparum* was the cause and the nature of their infection was not recognized. Others with latent infections contributed to blood banks with the result that acute malaria developed in nonimmune

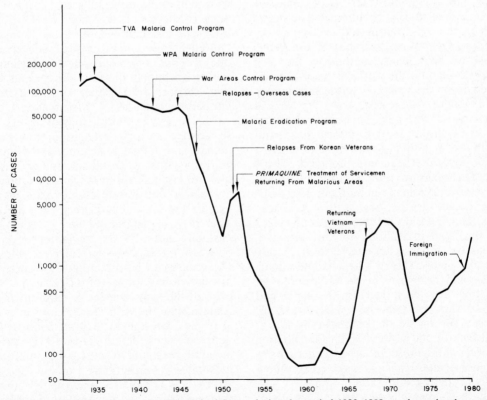

Figure 44–9. The prevalence of malaria in the United States during the period 1933–1980, as shown by the number of reported cases. The influence of control programs, chemotherapy, and the importation of cases can be interpreted from the graph. (Centers for Disease Control, Morbidity and Mortality Weekly Report, Annual Summary 1980, Vol. 29, 1981.)

civilian recipients of whole blood transfusions. There was a rise in needle-induced malaria among those narcotic addicts sharing contaminated syringes.

Epidemiology and Control. Malaria is the most common infectious disease of man, occurring throughout the warmer regions of the world and extending well into the temperate zones to occupy a large part of the land area between 60° N. and 40° S. latitude. The principal factor in distribution of the infection is climate, which affects both the distribution and abundance of the mosquito hosts and the development of the parasite in the mosquito. Although *P. malariae* occurs in chimpanzees, the human malarial parasites are not generally found in lower animals. Man is therefore the primary reservoir of infections. While it has not been possible to detect any resistance to infection based on age, racial immunity with a biochemical basis exists. In endemic areas, adults who have been repeatedly infected do not exhibit clinical malaria. Such resistance may be directed against specific stages (*i.e.,* sporozoites, merozoites, etc.), as described above.

Barring rare congenital cases, blood transfusions, and accidental transfers of blood, as by drug addicts sharing contaminated syringes, human malaria is transmitted exclusively by the bites of certain mosquitoes of the genus *Anopheles.* This genus, comprising over 300 species throughout the world, is readily distinguished from the common house mosquitoes of the genera *Culex* and *Aedes* by several characteristics. The adult generally rests at an angle to the surface, with proboscis, head, and body in a straight line, whereas the others rest parallel, with the head and proboscis turned down. The wings are usually spotted, those of other mosquitoes being unmarked. The palps of the female are as long as the proboscis, giving the impression of three long appendages from the head in addition to the antennae, whereas the other genera have short, barely noticeable palps. The eggs bear inflated floats and are laid singly on the water, whereas in *Culex* they are laid in rafts on the water and in *Aedes* they are deposited singly on damp surfaces. The larvae of *Anopheles* lie flat at the surface of the water, feeding on floating particles, while those of other genera hang down in the water from an elongated breathing tube and usually feed on the bottom.

Only the female mosquitoes feed on blood, most *Anopheles* biting at dusk or in the night. The breeding places vary greatly in character, almost any type of water collection serving to support the larvae of one or more species of *Anopheles.* Most species, however, are quite specific in the types of water collections they choose. The principal malarial vector in the southeastern United States, *Anopheles quadrimaculatus,* breeds chiefly around the debris- and weed-covered edges of swamps, ponds, and sluggish streams. Important malarial vectors, however, are found in hill streams (*A. minimus* in Southern Asia), brackish marshes (*A. atroparvus* in Europe), small temporary pools (*A. gambiae* in Africa), water held in plants growing in the tops of trees (*A. bellator* in Trinidad), etc.

Not all species of *Anopheles* serve equally efficiently as vectors of malaria, about 75 being considered dangerous carriers in one or more regions. The chief determining factors are abundance, contact with man, and susceptibility. The last varies greatly among species and among populations within species. Little is known of the factors in human malaria, but simple genetic differences have been shown to determine susceptibility of some *Culex* mosquitoes to avian malaria. In most situations that have been adequately studied, contact with man is the principal factor in the importance of species of *Anopheles.* Several susceptible species are abundant in the southeastern United States, but in most of this area only one, *A. quadrimaculatus,* shows sufficient preference for human blood to serve as an important carrier. In Europe, species (formerly lumped together as *A. maculipennis)* distinguishable only by morphology of the egg differ so greatly in their relative preferences for human and animal blood that some are dangerous vectors, while others, equally susceptible, are insignificant in the spread of malaria.

Malaria control rests largely on the interruption of the mosquito phase of the life cycle. This may be accomplished by reduction in mosquito numbers or prevention of contact between mosquitoes and man. If mosquito reduction is to be attempted, the differences in relative importance of different species, or even of the same species in different regions, require that the principal vectors in a given area be determined before control is attempted. Such determination is of value in avoiding waste of resources on unimportant mosquitoes. Furthermore, unplanned control efforts may completely miss the principal vectors and have even, on occasion, made matters worse by favoring the breeding of dangerous species. The "natural index" of infection, determined by examining stomachs and salivary glands of wild-caught female mosquitoes for oocysts and sporozoites of malarial parasites, is the best guide to relative importance of a species. Unfortunately, the figure is often so low that dissection of large numbers of mosquitoes is required. In such cases expediency may justify indirect measures. Susceptibility may be determined by exposure of laboratory-reared mosquitoes to carriers and dissection of the fed females for stages of the parasite ("experimental index"). Contact with man may be measured by the location of resting mosquitoes (*e.g.*, in houses as against stables) or by precipitin tests on fed mosquitoes to determine the type of blood they contain.

If control is to be applied to the breeding of mosquitoes, the habits of the important vectors in an area must be determined. Elimination of breeding places is the method of choice in many regions. Water collections may be destroyed by drainage or filling. Salinity may be controlled by tidegates. Breeding around the margins of reservoirs may be eliminated by water-level fluctuations. Shade may be increased or decreased by control of vegetation. Streams may be cleared or periodically sluiced. Specific methods, it will be obvious, depend on local conditions and the habits of the mosquitoes involved. Several effective poisons (larvicides) are available for attack on the aquatic stages. Oils sprayed on the water surface are toxic to the eggs, larvae, and pupae. A minor method of local value is the stocking of ponds and pools with top-feeding minnows, *Gambusia* or *Lebistes*, which eat mosquito larvae.

Elimination of the adult mosquitoes is also an important technique for malaria control. The insecticides lindane and dieldrin have given malariologists a weapon of tremendous value. Sprayed on walls, screens, etc., they kill adult mosquitoes that rest on these surfaces, even several months after application. For those species of *Anopheles* that enter houses to bite man, these insecticides have already demonstrated their value as an inexpensive and highly effective tool in malaria control. Malaria is no longer endemic in the United States and only sporadic cases of exotic origin are found today. The problem of malaria eradication is complicated by the development of drug resistance among the plasmodia. *Plasmodium falciparum* from various areas of Southeast Asia are resistant to chloroquine, other synthetic antimalarials, and quinine. Another complication has been the development of insecticide resistance in anophelene mosquitoes. At the end of 1958 only three resistant species were known and in the following year an additional 14 species of anophelene mosquitoes resistant to dieldrin and/or DDT were described. Another difficulty is that simian malarians (*P. cynomolgi* and *P. knowlesi*) may be transmitted to man and produce clinical disease.

Malarial Parasites of Lower Animals. Malarial parasites fundamentally like those of man occur in apes, monkeys, bats, rodents, birds, and lizards. Since lower animal hosts are not readily infected with the human malarial parasites, the natural parasites of monkeys, birds, and rodents have been widely used experimentally. The species most widely studied are *P. brasilianum*, *P. knowlesi*, and *P. cynomolgi* of monkeys, *P. cathemerium*, *P. relictum*, *P. gallinaceum*, and *P. lophurae* of birds, and *P. berghei* of rats and mice.

INTESTINAL SPOROZOANS

Babesia

The *Babesia* are Sporozoa with life cycles similar to the *Plasmodium*. The parasites are pyriform to round in shape, approximately 1 to 2 μm in width by 2 to 4 μm in length. They are observed singly or in pairs within erythrocytes and multiply by binary fission or budding. *Babesia* resemble ring stages of malarial parasites in blood films after Wright's or Giemsa staining. When the parasites are ingested with the blood meal of a hard tick (*e.g.*, species of *Ixodes, Boophilus*), schizogony occurs in the gut and merozoites are produced that reinfect epithelial cells or enter the hemolymph. They are carried to other tissues of the tick and multiply. In the process, ova are invaded and a similar intestinal cycle occurs in the developing larval ticks (transovarian transmission). Infected stages of vermicules enter the salivary glands and are transmitted when the tick bites.

Texas cattle fever caused by *B. bigemina* represents an economically important disease characterized by the massive destruction of erythrocytes and high mortality rates. Human babesiosis caused by *B. microti*, typically a parasite of rodents, has been diagnosed in residents of the northeastern coastal areas of the United States. Indirect immunofluorescence tests provide evidence of current or past infections by *B. microti*. Effective chemotherapeutics are not available, although chloroquine and pentamidine are used to treat infections. These drugs appear to provide symptomatic relief without elimination of the parasites.

Toxoplasma gondii

Toxoplasma gondii was discovered in 1908 in rodents by Nicolle and Manceaux in Africa and Splendore in Brazil. The first clearly recognized human case of disease due to this parasite was reported by Wolf and Cowen in 1937.

The elucidation of the life cycle by several investigators identifies *Toxoplasma* as a coccidian whose sexual reproduction occurs in the intestinal epithelium of the domestic cat. Asexual stages reproducing in the tissues of man may cause extreme pathology.

Characteristics and Life Cycle. *Toxoplasma gondii* is an intracellular parasite with a crescent or oval-shaped body, 5 to 7 μm. in length by 2 to 4 μm. in width. In Giemsa-stained preparations, the cytoplasm appears blue and the nucleus is reddish (Fig. 44–10). Both intestinal and extraintestinal infections by *T. gondii* occur in felines, while only extraintestinal sites are infected in birds, reptiles, and mammals.[36, 37] Domestic cats are important in the life cycle and serve as one of the sources of human infections. After the cat ingests *T. gondii*, the intestinal epithelial cells are invaded and schizogony and gametogony proceed. Trophozoites develop into schizonts that produce merozoites. Other intestinal cells are invaded and gametocytes develop in some of these. Gametes are formed and fertilization results in zygotes, which proceed to develop into sporoblasts. These sporoblasts differentiate into oocysts containing two sporocysts with four sporozoites each. Oocysts are released into the lumen of the cat intestine and are passed with the feces. Some parasites leave the intestine and infect cells of other tissues. Forms called tachyzoites, which multiply rapidly, are detected early after invasion and cause lesions in the tissues. Following this acute phase of the infection and the initiation of the immune response, the parasites encyst in muscle and brain cells, multiply at a slower rate, and are termed bradyzoites. These two forms of *Toxoplasma* differ also in their infectivity.

The resistant oocysts are infective for a wide range of hosts. When ingested by cats, the process is repeated, but if consumed by humans or other mammals, only the extraintestinal infection occurs. Tachyzoites and, later, bradyzoites are present in the tissues. Man and other mammals may also be infected by tachyzoites and bradyzoites ingested in raw or undercooked contaminated meats. Transplacental transmission occurs in all hosts. Rodents are important sources of infection for cats and acquire the infection as oocysts from raw meat scraps or by cannibalism. Cattle appear to become infected by ingesting oocysts from moist soil, forage, or silage contaminated with oocysts from feline feces.

Toxoplasma gondii can be maintained in laboratory rodents and in tissue cultures. They infect cells by being phagocytosed, even by cells normally not phagocytic. Membranes of the parasite-containing phagosomes become associated with the endoplasmic reticulum and mitochondria, but do not fuse with lysosomes.[46] A variety of cells are susceptible but macrophages, connective tissue cells, muscle cells, neurons, and microglia are usually infected. Although the tachyzoites and bradyzoites reproduce intracellularly, they are frequently found free in body fluids. During chronic infections, the bradyzoites occur primarily within intracellular cysts.

In the cat the cycle is that of a typical coccidian parasite with the production of resistant oocysts containing infective sporozoites. This stage passes to the external environment in the cat feces and remains infective for weeks in moist soil. If ingested by man or many other animals, tissue invasion and asexual reproduction of the parasite occur.[36, 37, 51, 52]

Toxoplasmosis. Although toxoplasmosis is one of the most common infections of man, it only rarely gives rise to acute disease. Antibodies are found in 17 to 50 per cent of

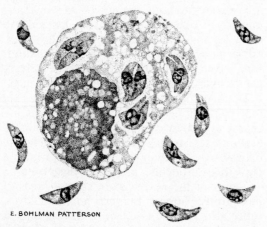

E. BOHLMAN PATTERSON

Figure 44–10. *Toxoplasma gondii,* free and in cell, from mouse brain smear. Giemsa, camera lucida; about × 2000.

population groups tested in the United States.[11] Most of the clinical cases occur in newborn infants infected congenitally during late fetal development. The active lesions predominate in the central nervous system and eyes, causing blindness, gross defects of the brain, and, not infrequently, death. Infection of adults is usually subclinical, but pneumonitis, enlargement of lymph nodes and spleen, fever, and a maculopapular rash may be exhibited. A severe chorioretinitis may result from infection of the eyes. With widespread use of immunosuppressive agents, increasing numbers of cases of adults with acute toxoplasmosis have been found with all tissues infected by the opportunistic organism.

Recovery is accompanied by immunity to reinfection, while bradyzoites remain within cysts in the tissues. This type of premunition or nonsterile immunity is also seen in experimental animals, and a degree of resistance can also be demonstrated after immunization with killed parasite materials. Cell-mediated immune responses are important in protecting animals, but passively transferred convalescent serum prolongs the survival of recipients. If infection is acquired before pregnancy, maternal immunity protects the fetus. When the infection occurs during pregnancy, the fetus may be infected congenitally by tachyzoites. Testing of pregnant females would be useful as a part of prenatal care to minimize the possibilities of infections in those who are serologically negative and to initiate treatment in those who acquire the infection. In humans, both early IgM and later IgG antibodies are synthesized, which is useful in serodiagnostic tests.

Laboratory diagnosis requires isolation of the organisms or immunological tests. In neonatal cases it is usually possible to demonstrate the organisms by inoculation of immunosuppressed laboratory mice. While all mammals and birds tested have been found susceptible, mice are preferred for isolation of the parasites because they are free from natural infection. Complement fixation may be used, and is available from commercial sources, as are indirect hemagglutination, latex agglutination, direct agglutination, and indirect immunofluorescence tests and enzyme-linked immunosorbent assays. One of the most reliable tests is the dye inhibition reaction of Sabin and Feldman. This depends on the fact that *Toxoplasma* in the peritoneal exudate of mice stain well with alkaline methylene blue in normal serum but not in immune serum. An accessory factor, present in fresh normal serum, but destroyed by heat or by storage, is essential to the reaction. The test becomes positive two weeks or more after onset, reaching a titer of 1:256 or higher, and remains positive for many years. A rise in IgG antibody titers during an infection or the presence of IgM antibody to *T. gondii* is diagnostic.

Both acute and subacute toxoplasmoses have been treated with combinations of sulfadiazine and pyrimethamine. Treatment destroys the parasites in experimental animals and, though beneficial in some human infections, toxic side effects may occur with irreparable damage to the brain and eye.

Epidemiology. Perhaps the most vexing question occupying investigators of toxoplasmosis has been the method or methods of natural transmission. It was clear that congenital infection of human embryos occurred, but it was equally clear that other routes of infection existed. The parasite is extremely abundant in nature. Surveys with the dye test show that up to 60 per cent or more of human populations have been infected. Investigations in various parts of the United States have revealed past infection rates of 17 to 35 per cent, with rates of over 65 per cent in the age group above 40. A wide variety of wild and domestic birds and mammals show evidence of infection, often with high incidence. Human congenital infections have been associated with home environs in which mice and other vertebrates had abnormally high incidences of infection. The cysts in muscle are infective by mouth, and epidemiological evidence suggesting that infection might be acquired from undercooked pork has been reinforced by the finding of viable *Toxoplasma* in samples of meat from 22 per cent of hogs from one slaughterhouse. However, orthodox Jews sometimes show evidence of a high incidence of infection, and some species of herbivorous animals are commonly infected, so it is obvious that pork or other meats are not the only important source of infection.

The discovery of the oocyst in cat feces and the determination that this stage is infective by ingestion has resolved this enigma. It is probable that the relatively resistant cyst is infective by direct fecal contamination or may also be transmitted by house and filth flies. Mice and other small mammals with tissue stages are ingested by cats and develop through the sexual cycle. They, like the cats, are extremely important in the epidemiology of the disease. Toxoplasmosis should be considered one of the zoonoses in which man is only one of a large number of species in which organisms of the asexual stage may invade and reproduce without completing the parasitic life cycle.

Sarcocystis

Species of *Sarcocystis* were found as cysts in herbivores. It was not realized until relatively recently that these cysts actually contained bradyzoites. Species of parasites found in the intestinal epithelium which produced oocysts in humans were incorrectly identified as members of a genus *Isospora*. When such cysts are ingested, bradyzoites develop into gametocytes, then gametes, and subsequently into sporoblasts and oocysts, illustrating the intestinal cycle in the definitive host. In humans, these species include *S. suihominis* and *S. hominis,* which may cause diarrheas of limited durations.[31] These infections are treated symptomatically. Cysts identified as *S. lindemani* and of other species have been reported in a number of instances from man, but they do not appear to cause identifiable symptoms. They may be present as fusiform tubes, round in cross section, and several centimeters in length in the striated muscles. They are referred to as "Meischer's tubes" or sarcocysts. Sickle-shaped bradyzoites, 12 to 16 μm. in length, occupy compartments within the cysts.

PNEUMOCYSTIS CARINII

Infection with *Pneumocystis*, a parasite of uncertain taxonomic status, is associated with highly contagious, epidemic, infantile, interstitial, plasma-cell pneumonia. Immunosuppressed or immunodeficient individuals are extremely susceptible to the infection. The organisms are ovoid or crescent-shaped, 1 to 3 μm. in diameter, and are commonly seen in rosettes of eight individuals within a membrane, free or within phagocytes. The organism is the etiological agent of the disease, which in younger infants frequently terminates in death. It has also been described from a wide variety of wild and domestic mammals. Although widely distributed, infection is rarely diagnosed. Pentamidine and supportive measures may be used to treat infections, but a combination of trimethoprim and sulfamethoxazole is effective and less toxic in the treatment of children and adults.

The Metazoa

All phyla of animals other than protozoa are commonly designated by the term Metazoa, and it will be convenient to mention certain general characteristics of the parasites of man, mostly known as "worms," which belong to this aggregate. They are usually macroscopic in size, ranging from about a millimeter to several meters in length. Their structure is generally complex, and their life cycles vary from the simple production of infective egg or larvae to complex alternation of generations involving as many as three different hosts. An important general characteristic is that multiplication usually does not occur in the human body, so that infection does not increase in intensity in the absence of re-exposure. Some of the worms parasitic in vertebrates have been cultivated. A substantial body of information has been accumulated on the metabolism and the immunological interactions with their hosts from studies conducted both *in vitro* and in experimental animals. The quantity of information and the great variety of metazoan parasites of man makes it impossible to discuss them extensively in a small space. Therefore, representative examples will be used wherever possible. For fuller discussions the reader is referred to general texts.

PLATYHELMINTHES

The phylum Platyhelminthes, or "flatworms," is distinguished from other phyla of animals by several characteristics. They are bilaterally symmetrical and composed of the three primitive germ layers of tissues—ectoderm, endoderm, and mesoderm. The body cavity is not lined with mesoderm, as in higher forms, but filled with a spongy mass of cells, the parenchyma. The digestive tract is absent or, if present, lacks an anus, solid wastes being regurgitated through the mouth. There are three major classes of Platyhelminths. The Turbellaria are free-living or external parasites of aquatic animals. The remaining classes, the Trematoda (flukes) and the Cestoda (tapeworms), which will be reviewed in part in this section, are all parasites.

TREMATODA

The trematodes infect a variety of sites in the human host. Examples are covered of flukes whose adult stages localize in the lungs, intestine, liver, and blood stream. The lung fluke, *Paragonimus westermani,* and the blood fluke, *Schistosoma mansoni,* are reviewed in somewhat more detail to illustrate various facets of the host-trematode relationship. Some similarities will be obvious between species, but major and subtle differences exist that define the character of each parasite and the disease caused by it.

Paragonimus westermani

The adult worm, found by Westerman in 1877 in the lungs of a tiger, was described by Kerbert in 1878. Nakagawa, Yokogawa, and others elucidated the life cycle. Several species have been described which show minor morphological differences.

Characteristics and Life Cycle. The adult lung fluke is an ovoid reddish worm, 7 to 12 mm. long by 3 to 6 mm. in diameter, covered with a tegument that is studded with spines. The anatomy of a flattened specimen is shown in Figure 44–11. Two muscular suckers are present, the acetabulum on the ventral surface, and the anterior sucker, perforated by the mouth, at the anterior end. The mouth opens into a muscular pharynx, followed by a thin esophagus. This divides into two blind intestinal ceca extending down the sides of the body. The nervous system is simple, and no special sense organs are present. The excretory system consists of a bladder opening at the posterior end and receiving collecting tubules which extend throughout the body, terminating in characteristic "flame cells." The circulatory system is rudimentary, consisting of indefinite channels through the parenchyma.

The adult fluke is hermaphroditic, both male and female reproductive systems occurring in the same individual. These systems are typically elaborate and, as in most flukes, are the most prominent structures of the body. In the female system a single ovary connects via an oviduct with the ootype, where the eggs are formed and receive their shells. In its course the oviduct receives the common vitelline duct, into which shell material comes from the branched vitellaria, glands occupying the sides of the dorsal surface of the body. The oviduct also has a diverticulum, the seminal receptacle, in which sperms are stored. An inconspicuous duct of unknown function, Laurer's canal, runs from the oviduct to an opening on the dorsal surface of the body. The ootype, surrounded by gland cells, Mehlis' gland, opens into the uterus, a long coiled tube which carries the completed eggs to the common genital pore near the acetabulum.

The male reproductive system consists of paired testes in the posterior part of the body, connecting by vasa efferentia with the vas deferens, which empties into the common genital pore along with the uterus. Part of the vas deferens is widened into a sperm reservoir, the seminal vesicle, and a more distal portion is the glandular prostatic region. The terminal portion forms a muscular copulatory organ, the cirrus.

The eggs produced by adult worms in the lung are coughed up and either escape in the sputum or are swallowed and passed in the feces. They are ovoid, averaging 60 by 90 μm. in size, and show a removable cap, the operculum, at one end. The embryos are undeveloped at the time of escape from the host. They develop in from two to six weeks in water, where the eggs hatch by the opening of the operculum to release a free-swimming ciliated larva, the miracidium. This larva survives only a few hours unless it succeeds in penetrating the tissues of a suitable intermediate host. Various snails of the genera *Melania* and *Pomatiopsis* can serve as hosts. In the lymph spaces of the snail the miracidium becomes an irregular, thin-walled sac, the sporocyst, growing to a final length of about 0.4 mm. Cell masses within the sporocyst enlarge, developing in about one month into 12 or more rediae. These escape by rupture of the sporocyst and grow to a length of about 0.3 mm. They differ from the sporocyst principally in having a rudimentary digestive tract and a birth pore. By a reproductive process similar to that in the sporocyst the first generation redia produces 12 or more second generation rediae. These escape by way of the birth pore and grow to a length of about 0.5 mm. Within each second-generation redia arise 20 or more tailed larvae, or cercariae. The cercaria is essentially a rudimentary adult worm. It differs principally in having a small tail and two types of penetration organs, a stylet in the mouth region and several gland cells, opening at the anterior end, which secrete histolytic enzymes. About three months after invasion of the snail by miracidia the cercariae escape and move about in the water, dying in one or two days unless they find a suitable second intermediate host, a crayfish or crab of any of various genera, such as *Astacus* and *Potamon* in the Far East. The cercaria penetrates the softer part of

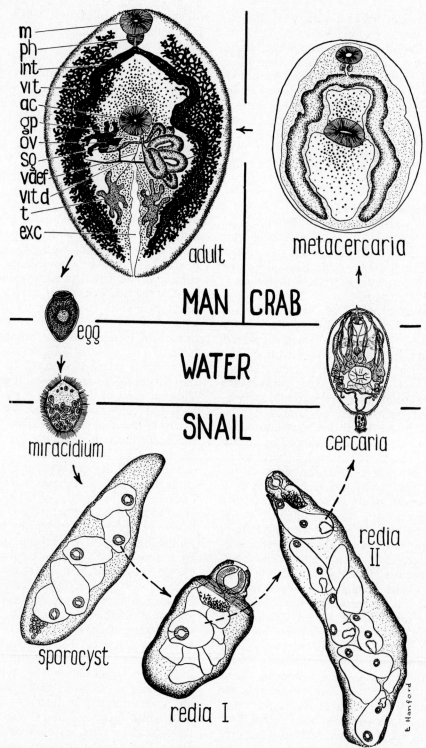

Figure 44–11. Life cycle and morphology of *Paragonimus. m,* Mouth; *ph,* pharynx; *int,* intestinal cecum; *vit,* vitellaria; *ac,* acetabulum; *gp,* genital pore; *ov,* ovary; *sg,* ootype; *vdef,* vas deferens; *vitd,* vitelline duct; *t,* testis; *exc,* excretory bladder. Larval stages, × 120; adult worm, × 7. (Larval stages redrawn from Ameel, 1934.)

the integument of a crab, loses its tail, and grows in the tissues into the metacercaria, a near-spherical body about 0.4 mm. in diameter enclosed in a cyst wall. The full development requires about one month, after which the metacercaria is infective when eaten by man. In the small intestine the cyst wall softens, releasing the metacercaria, which penetrates the wall of the small intestine and reaches the abdominal cavity within a few hours. It wanders rather aimlessly but usually passes through the diaphragm within a few days and invades the lung, where it becomes encapsulated by the tissues and grows to the adult stage. Considering this apparently random migration it is interesting to note that the pleural cysts commonly contain two or three adults. After about six weeks eggs may be found in the sputum.

Paragonimiasis. The adult worms in the lung, and particularly the secretions and eggs they produce, cause tissue destruction, inflammation, and hemorrhage. Local pneumonic processes with cough and bloody sputum are characteristic. As in most worm infections, the damage is roughly proportional to the number of organisms present. In severe cases, weakness and even death may result from the extensive lung injury. Aberrant worms in other tissues, such as the brain, may produce local injury.

There is no evidence concerning acquired immunity to *Paragonimus*. Human infections have been shown to persist at least six years in the absence of re-exposure, but it is said that they often clear up after several years.

Diagnosis of lung fluke infection depends on the finding and identification of characteristic eggs in the sputum or feces. As in other trematode infections, the size and structure of the eggs are characteristic. Other trematode eggs may occur in the feces, but only those of *Paragonimus* normally occur in the sputum. Immediate hypersensitivity reactions are detected in infected individuals injected intradermally with extracts of adult worms. Cross-reactions occur in persons infected by *Clonorchis*. Complement-fixing antibodies are synthesized before eggs are produced and disappear shortly after the worms are eliminated. Specific immunodiagnosis is possible, using micro-Ouchterlony methods or immunoelectrophoretic patterns of human sera reacted with *Paragonimus* antigens.[98]

Epidemiology and Control. Various mammals are susceptible to *Paragonimus* infection. Cats, dogs, mink, muskrats, and man are the usual natural hosts. Infection in lower animals is known in Asia, Africa, and North and South America, including the United States. Pulmonary infections by *P. mexicanus* are found in the Americas and the Caribbean. Abdominal lesions are detected and occasionally cerebral hemorrhages are fatal. Other species cause infections in Africa. Human infection is limited by food habits, occurring commonly only in the Far East. The metacercariae in infected crustacea are destroyed only by thorough cooking or considerable exposure to pickling sauces, and in the endemic areas freshwater crabs, raw or slightly pickled, are considered a delicacy. It should be emphasized that the asexual reproduction in snails is obligate and that only the metacercariae and possibly the cercariae are infective for mammals. Thus, direct transfer from mammal to mammal does not occur, and numerical increase of an individual infection is unknown in the absence of re-exposure.

Chloroquine, in addition to its antimalarial activity, has been utilized with some success in a number of helminth infections including paragonimiasis. It is beneficial in early pulmonary infection but of dubious value in long-established infection or in ectopic cerebral parasitism. Good clinical results have also been reported with bithionol.

Chemotherapy of human infections is useless for control, both because of its unreliability and because lower animals are an important reservoir. Destruction of snails has generally failed. The only effective control measure known is education to the dangers of eating improperly cooked freshwater crustacea. It should be noted here that while such modification of food habits is the best control method for all human trematode infections except the blood flukes, established habits and prejudices often interpose difficulties in its execution.

Fasciolopsis buski

The large adults of this species attain a length of 7 cm. (Fig. 44–12). They are found attached to the mucosa of the small intestine of man and the pig. The infection is most common in China but occurs in other parts of Asia. The large eggs (average 140 by 80 μm.) escape in the feces (Fig. 44–13) and develop in water, where the miracidia invade snails of the genera *Segmentina* and *Planorbis*. The development in the snail, like that of *Paragonimus*, comprises a sporocyst generation and two generations of rediae. The long-tailed cercariae encyst as metacercariae on aquatic plants, particularly the water chestnuts. These plants, eaten raw or peeled with the teeth,

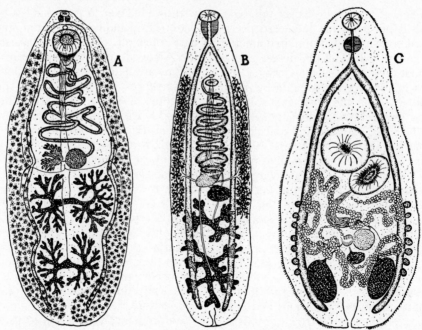

Figure 44–12. Trematode parasites of man. Note difference in magnification. *A, Fasciolopsis buski,* × 3. *B, Clonorchis sinensis,* × 5. *C, Heterophyes heterophyes,* × 60.

convey the infection to man or the pig. Symptoms are generally related to the intensity of infection. They consist of intestinal disturbances and generalized edema. The latter has been attributed to toxemia but may be merely nutritional, resulting from the food-robbing of the host by the worms. Severe infections may cause death. As in many other intestinal worm infections, hexylresorcinol is therapeutically efficient. Control is achieved by treatment of human infections, proper sewage disposal, and

education to the dangers of eating raw plants from contaminated water. The problem is complicated by the practice, common in endemic areas, of using human feces as fertilizer.

Fasciola hepatica infects the livers of sheep and cattle, causing "liver rot," and is of great economic importance. It is important also because it was the first trematode whose life cycle was described. Occasional human cases are known, usually contracted by eating fresh watercress to which metacercarial cysts are at-

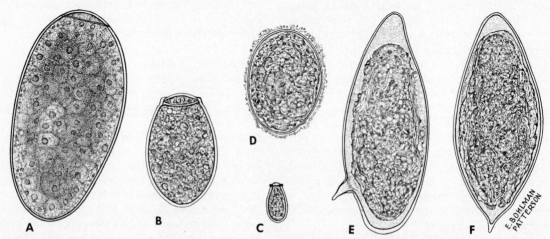

Figure 44–13. Trematode eggs in optical section. *A, Fasciolopsis buski. B, Paragonimus westermani. C, Clonorchis sinensis. D, Schistosoma japonicum* (note that the shell has the halo of debris usually seen when this egg is found). *E. Schistosoma mansoni. F, Schistosoma haematobium.* Camera lucida; about × 310.

tached. Human infection is relatively frequent and clinically important in Cuba, Chile, southern France, and other scattered areas where sheep or cattle husbandry accompanies the raising of leafy vegetable crops commonly eaten uncooked. *Fasciola gigantica* and *Fascioloides magna* of herbivores also occasionally infect man. Another economically important parasite of the liver of herbivores, *Dicrocoelium dendriticum,* has been found rarely in man.

Heterophyes heterophyes

Heterophyes heterophyes is a small trematode, about 1.5 mm. long, of the intestine of man, cats, dogs, and other fish-eating mammals in Egypt, Asia Minor, and Asia. The eggs are small, averaging 25 by 16 μm. Metacercariae are ingested by man in insufficiently cooked or salted fish. The adult trematodes produce only minor gastrointestinal disturbances, but it is reported that the eggs are often deposited deep in the mucosa, whence they reach the general circulation and are localized in various distant tissues. The inflammation in these tissues, particularly the myocardium and brain, is said occasionally to cause serious symptoms or death. Several related species attack man. The most important of these is *Metagonimus yokogawai,* which occurs in man and other fish-eating animals in the Balkans, the Middle East, and Asia. A number of heterophyid flukes whose eggs cause extensive ectopic lesions have also been reported from man in the Philippines.

Other Intestinal Trematodes

Several species of *Echinostoma, Echinochasmus,* and *Euparyphium* occasionally parasitize man. They are elongate trematodes with a ring of large spines on the head region. The human infection is acquired by ingestion of raw snails or mussels containing the metacercariae. Various mammals and birds are the normal hosts of the adult worms. Occasional human infections are also reported with *Gastrodiscus hominis* and *Watsonius watsoni.* Their life cycles are unknown, but since they chiefly parasitize herbivorous mammals it is presumed that the metacercariae are found on plants.

Clonorchis sinensis

The Chinese liver fluke, *Clonorchis sinensis,* is a thin, elongate trematode, 1 to 2 cm. in length. The adult worm inhabits the smaller bile ducts of man, cats, dogs, and other fish-eating mammals in China and Japan. The operculate eggs, averaging 29 by 17 μm., pass out with the bile and escape in the feces. They are fully developed but do not hatch in the water. Upon ingestion by suitable snails, usually of the genera *Parafossarulus* and *Bithynia,* they hatch, and the miracidia become sporocysts in the lymph spaces. Rediae produced in the sporocyst give rise to long-tailed cercariae. These encyst as metacercariae in the tissues and on the skin and scales of various freshwater fish. Metacercariae ingested by man hatch in the small intestine, and the young worms migrate up the bile ducts to develop into adults three to four weeks later. In rabbits experimentally infected, the young worms complete migration to the liver in hosts whose bile ducts have been ligated. Consequently, passage through the circulatory system to the liver or direct migration through the intestinal wall to the peritoneal cavity and into the liver surface may also occur. Thorough cooking (100° C. for 15 minutes) is necessary to destroy the metacercariae. Infection of man occurs by ingestion of the metacercariae, possibly in drinking water or by contamination of the fingers in handling infected fish, but usually by consumption of insufficiently pickled or cooked fish, a favorite article of diet in the endemic regions. Hazards are increased in these areas by the practice of propagating fish for market in ponds fertilized with human feces.

Human infection is characterized by proliferation of the bile-duct epithelium and of the surrounding connective tissue. This results in liver cirrhosis, destroying liver parenchyma and obstructing portal blood flow. Intestinal disturbances, liver enlargement, and ascites are the common symptoms, while severe infections may cause death.

Although a variety of chemotherapeutic agents have been used for liver fluke infections of man, no reliable agent for the treatment of clonorchiasis is available. Surgery may be required to remove worms involved in the blockage of bile ducts in acute cholangitis. Diagnosis depends on the identification of eggs obtained from feces or by duodenal intubation. There have been a number of efforts to develop practical immunodiagnostic methods for clonorchiasis. However, most of these crossreact with other trematode infections, such as paragonimiasis and schistosomiasis. A purified antigen prepared from adult clonorchis and consisting primarily of a polyglucose has been shown to have high specificity when used in a complement fixation test in this infection.[85] Control, as in the trematode infections discussed above, depends principally on education concerning avoidance of undercooked infected food, in this case freshwater fish.

A closely related species, *Opisthorchis viverrini*, is of considerable importance in northern Thailand, where it infects 25 per cent of the population. *Opisthorchis felineus* and *O. tenuicollis* infect fish-eating mammals and, less commonly, man in parts of Central Europe and Asia.

Human Blood Flukes: The Schistosomes

The prevalence of infection of man with the several species of schistosomes, as well as the chronic debilitating disease produced, places these organisms among the world's most important infectious agents. Control measures and treatment of the individual are still inadequate. Bilharz, in 1852, first described trematodes in the veins of an Egyptian, and subsequently infection with the schistosomes was termed "bilharziasis" in much of the medical literature. The worms are usually found in pairs in the portal venous system or in veins of the vesical plexus with the female held in the ventrally grooved male gynecophoral canal (Fig. 44–14). The split body of the male suggests the generic name for the group and, unlike the other trematodes mentioned, all blood flukes are dioecious. The adults attach to the walls of the blood vessels with their suckers and migrate to the smaller venules in copula for egg deposition. Occasionally they may develop in ectopic sites, probably being carried there by the circulation prior to attaining maturity. The blood flukes rely on a supply of carbohydrate and utilize glucose from the blood. Glucose is consumed at a rate of approximately 20 per cent of the dry weight of the worms per hour via the glycolytic pathway. Lactate is the principal product of glycolysis, and the metabolism is not affected by oxygen. In addition they ingest erythrocytes and possess enzymes for the hydrolysis of globin. *Schistosoma mansoni* is used here as an example of the group.

Morphology and Life Cycle. The paired adults of *S. mansoni* are normally found in the smaller mesenteric veins. The cylindrical female is 1 to 1.5 cm. in length by about 0.25 mm. in diameter. An anterior sucker surrounds the mouth and shortly behind it is a stalked acetabulum. The intestinal ceca unite before the middle of the body to form a single tube continuing to the posterior end. An oval ovary lies immediately anterior to the union of the intestinal ceca, and the uterus, containing eggs, extends forward to open behind the acetabulum. The posterior half of the body is occupied by vitellaria. The male is shorter than the female, about 1 cm. long by about 1 mm.

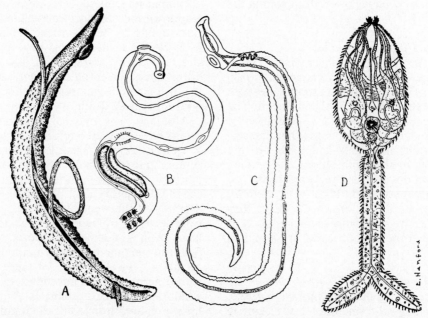

Figure 44–14. *Schistosoma mansoni.* Note differences in magnification. *A,* Adult worms, × 8. *B,* Anterior end of female worm, × 20. *C,* Adult male, × 10. *D,* cercaria, × 180. (*A* and *C* redrawn from Mason-Bahr. *D* redrawn from Cort.)

in diameter, its integument covered with coarse tubercles. The suckers and alimentary tract are similar to those of the female. The reproductive system consists of a cluster of eight or nine testes in the anterior region emptying into a seminal vesicle, which opens to the outside just behind the ventral sucker.

Schistosoma mansoni has large eggs, averaging 150 by 65 μm. with no operculum but with a prominent spine at the side. They are deposited in the fine venules of the mesenteric veins in the wall of the intestine, where they lodge after the retreat of the ovipositing worms and the collapse of the vessels which had been distended by the worm body. The lateral spine aids in fixing the egg in the vessel and by a combination of events, probably including secretion of lytic substances by the developing embryo, the egg passes through the vessel wall. From the tissues the eggs continue migration through the mucosa and into the lumen of the intestine. They are mature at the time they leave the body in the feces. On dilution of the feces with water the shell ruptures, releasing the miracidium. In suitable snails, Biomphalaria in Africa and *Biomphalaria glabrata* in the Western Hemisphere, the miracidium penetrates and two generations of sporocysts are produced resulting, after about six weeks, in the production of cercariae with long, forked tails. Escaping into the water the cercariae swim actively or rest at the surface, dying in about three days if they do not reach a susceptible final host. Coming in contact with human skin they attach and actively penetrate the skin. The epidermis is passed quickly and cercariae shed their tails and may reach lymph vessels in the dermis within 15 minutes or less. This rapid invasion of the unbroken host skin is accomplished through the use of cercarial enzymes as well as by muscular activity. A major feature of cercarial morphology is the possession of sets of large unicellular "penetration glands" which are the source of mucoid secretions, collagenase-like proteases, and mucopolysaccharidases, all presumed to be of importance in invasiveness of these parasites. The parasite is carried via lymph and blood to the portal veins in the liver, where maturation occurs and the adult forms mate and migrate distally in the portal system to the mesenteric veins. Four to eight weeks after infection the sexually mature worms begin egg production. The infection may persist for over 25 years without re-exposure.

The other species of human blood flukes differ from *S. mansoni* in size, details of morphology, egg structure, location in the definitive hosts, types of snail hosts, and geographical distribution. *Schistosoma haematobium* adults occur predominantly in the venules of the urinary bladder wall, the eggs escaping in the urine. The eggs are large, 150 by 60 μm., with a terminal spine. The male, 1 to 1.5 cm. long, is covered with fine tuberculations and has four large testes. The female is about 2 cm. long. Snails of the genera *Physopsis* and *Bulinus* serve as intermediate hosts.

Schistosoma japonicum occurs in the venules of the intestine. The eggs average 80 by 65 μm., with a small lateral knob rather than a spine. They escape in the feces, the miracidium invading snails of the genus *Onocomelania*. The male is 1 to 2 cm. long, with a smooth integument, and has seven or eight testes. The female is 1 to 2.5 cm. long.

Schistosomiasis. The disease produced by the schistosomes varies with the infecting species, the number of adult worms present, and the duration of infection. The pathology may conveniently be divided into the incubation period, from skin penetration to egg deposition, the acute stage, and the chronic stage. At the inception of the incubation period, skin penetration may cause a mild transient dermatitis. In the forms normally parasitizing man this is less severe than that produced in man by the penetration of cercariae normally parasitizing other vertebrates (see below). The larvae in passing through the lung may cause an eosinophilic infiltration and while developing in the portal system, parasite metabolic products cause a toxic hepatitis often accompanied by irregularly fluctuating fever and allergic manifestations such as urticaria. This is followed by the acute stage in which eggs are actively deposited in the tissues and are extruded into the lumen of the intestine or bladder. During this period trauma may produce intestinal hemorrhage and pseudodysentery in *S. mansoni* and *S. japonicum* infections. Hematuria is characteristic of this stage of *S. haematobium* infections.

Even in these early stages numerous eggs may escape into the circulation rather than migrate through tissues to organ lumina. These embolic eggs lodge in numbers in the liver, where they become enclosed in small granulomata (pseudotubercles) and in *S. haematobium* and *S. japonicum*, numbers commonly pass to the lung. In many instances in *S. japonicum*, relatively large numbers reach the brain, producing the symptomatology of cerebral damage. The chronic stage is due to the host's reaction to continuous egg-produced tissue damage. In *S. mansoni* the wall of the large intestine becomes thickened with scar tissue and rectal polyps of connective tissue with eggs may be extensive. Similarly, impairment of the small intestine and thickening occur with *S. japonicum,* and in both, fibrosis of the liver is a most important sequel. With *S. haematobium* the wall of the urinary bladder is greatly thickened with fibrous connective tissue and the urethral lumen is commonly reduced. The external genitalia are also commonly involved. Carcinomas of the rectum, liver, and urinary bladder are often observed and in some areas a high correlation between these malignant conditions and schistosomiasis is claimed. Concomitant with the liver damage found in *S. mansoni* and *S. japonicum* infections, circulatory impairment produces portal hypertension, splenic enlargement, esophageal varices, and ascites.

To a considerable degree the pathology of schistosomiasis is immunological in nature. The granulomatous response of the host to eggs in tissue is a manifestation of delayed hypersensitivity.[94] Epidemiological and experimental evidence indicates that populations may develop tolerance to some of the antigens concerned.[60] There have also been demonstrated anti-DNA antibodies in infections of man with *S. mansoni* or *S. japonicum* and in laboratory-induced infection in small mammals.[45] The production of such antibodies is characteristic of a number of diseases, including systemic lupus erythematosus, and is often accompanied by glomerulonephritis of immune complex origin. Renal disease with glomerulonephritis is associated with hepatosplenic schistosomiasis.[13] As briefly summarized above, the pathology produced varies with time and also with the different site of egg deposition by the different species of adult worm. Another important species difference in the disease is the fact that the female *S. japonicum* produces 10 times the number of eggs per day as the *S. masoni* female. Egg production of the female *S. haematobium* is believed to be intermediate between these.

Immunity. Direct evidence of functional immunity to schistosomes in man is lacking. Children and young adults commonly have severe infections which may terminate fatally. Some infected adults are found without symptoms of progressive disease under conditions where it may be assumed that they have periodic exposure to reinfection with *S. japonicum* or *S. mansoni.* Animals cured of initial infection show some resistance to reinfection and, in monkeys, some individuals surviving initial infection are strongly immune to massive reinfection[93] Monkeys inoculated with a nonhuman Taiwan strain of *S. japonicum* exhibit resistance to infection with a human strain from Japan. Mice immunized with cercariae of *S. mansoni* that were attenuated by exposure to cobalt radiation display immunity to reinfection with untreated cercariae.[49, 91]

The infected human is exposed to a variety of stages of the schistosomes: cercariae, schistosomules (developing immature schistosomes), adults, and ova.[59] Antibodies in the serum of infected individuals react with antigens of each. Precipitins and agglutinins are detected with cercariae, precipitins with schistosomules and adults, and circumoval precipitins with ova.[55] Complement fixation is demonstrable, and antigens and immune complexes are found in the serum of infected mice.[84] Complement, IgG1, IgG2a, IgM, and IgA are detected in the circulating complexes. Immune complexes formed with IgE are detected in the blood of infected rats and interact with macrophages in cytotoxic reactions with schistosomules.[19] The mouse and rat models clearly differ. *S. mansoni* persist in the mouse, but are eliminated by the rat during the first month of the infection. B cell–deficient infected mice display the same level of immunity as intact controls, while B cell–deficient rats are less resistant to reinfections.[7, 61] Antibody-dependent cell-mediated cytotoxicity of schistosomules occurs with granulocytes.[5] Eosinophils appear to be the most active effector cells and complement enhances killing of the schistosomules.[4] Resistance to the killing increases with increasing age of the worms; 2-hour schistosomules are more efficiently killed than worms cultivated for 24 hours.[68] Eosinophilia is observed during schistosome infections. The resistance shown by humans with established infections may be mediated by such humoral and cellular interactions directed in part against the developing schistosomules.

Diagnosis. Laboratory diagnosis is based on the finding of characteristic eggs in the feces, urine, rectal biopsy, or rarely, liver biopsy. In very early or in late chronic stages the eggs may not readily be found, and multiple examinations plus concentration techniques must be routine for diagnosis of individual infections. Immunological techniques are also valuable both for the individual diagnosis and for epidemiological surveys. These include the production of precipitate about viable or lyophilized eggs (circumoval precipitin reaction), high-titer hemagglutination of erythrocytes sensitized with adult antigens, intradermal reaction to adult antigens, binding of fluorescent antibody by preserved cercariae, and a variety of other methods including complement fixation and gel-precipitation techniques. Some of the reactions are group-specific, persist after cure, or are negative in a high percentage of the lower age group. The circumoval, fluorescent antibody, and intradermal tests are of practical value if their limitations are understood.

Therapy. Trivalent antimonials have been used to treat all three species of schistosomes. Sodium antimony tartrate (tartar emetic) is injected intravenously on alternate days during a one-month treatment regime. Stibophen (Fuadin), an intramuscularly injected antimonial, sterilizes the female worms and reduces symptoms referable to damage by the deposited ova. However, the cure rate is lower than obtained with tartar emetic and when not properly administered, the worms are believed to recover. These compounds are extremely toxic, and other drugs are currently in use to treat each of the species: oxamniquine for the treatment of *S. mansoni* infections, metrifonate for *S. haematobium*, and niridazole for *S. japonicum*. Praziquantel (Biltricide) is effective against all species of schistosomes, when administered in one oral dose of 40 mg./kg. for *S. mansoni* and *S. haematobium* or two doses of 30 mg./kg. for *S. japonicum*.[39] Few severe toxic reactions are reported in trials; it has not yet been approved for use in the United States.

Epidemiology and Control. Humans are infected with schistosomes by contact of the skin with water containing the cercariae. This occurs especially in the working of rice fields fertilized with human feces, but also in bathing and chance contact. Infection may be acquired from drinking water and rarely as an intra-uterine infection. Man is the only important reservoir of *S. mansoni* and *S. haematobium* infection, although both occur naturally in monkeys, and rodent infections of *S. mansoni* have been described. The disease is for these two species perpetuated by the promiscuous discharge of urine and feces by man or their deliberate use as fertilizer in the cultivation of rice, sugar cane, and similar crops. Infection of streams and irrigation canals used for ablution and the washing of clothes is important in maintenance of the infection. In contrast to these forms, *S. japonicum* has numerous reservoir hosts among domestic and wild mammals which pass eggs in feces and may maintain the infection in man's absence. *Schistosoma mansoni* is widely distributed throughout Africa wherever suitable snail intermediate hosts are found. The delta of the Nile is an endemic area of primary importance; it is common throughout tropical Africa to South Africa and in much of its range coexists with *S. haematobium*. Importation of *S. mansoni* with slaves established the disease in Brazil, Venezuela, Surinam, and the West Indies, including Puerto Rico. The present distribution of *S. haematobium* includes not only all of Africa suitable for its development but also much of the Middle East, as well as small endemic areas in Portugal, and India. *Schistosoma japonicum* is limited to the Far East with important endemic areas in the Philippines, China, the Celebes, and Japan. A number of small foci have been found in Thailand and Laos, and a strain primarily parasitizing dogs and rats is found in Taiwan.

Control of schistosomiasis depends on destruction of the snail intermediate hosts, prevention of access of eggs to water containing snails, or avoiding contact with cercaria-containing waters. Some limited success has been obtained in snail control using copper sulfate or sodium pentachlorophenate as molluscidides. Periodic drying of irrigation ditches is of some value for the control of snails transmitting *S. mansoni* and *S. haematobium* but of little value in *S. japonicum* control as the snail host is operculate and resists desiccation. As it does not survive well in ponds or in well-drained areas, ponding and drainage are utilized in control. Safe sewage disposal and increased sanitation have not met with outstanding success as control measures, since the customs of the people as well as the economics of the endemic areas operate against these methods. Avoidance of contact with infected water is difficult in some areas, since it is also associated with religious habits of ablution; in other areas only infected waters are available for drinking and general cleansing, and it has not been economically possible to provide safe water supplies.

Other Schistosome Species. A number of species commonly parasitizing ungulates of Africa and India, including *S. bovis* and *S. spindale*, have been reported as occurring in man. Several hundred cases of *S. intercalatum* in man have been reported from tropical Africa. This form has a terminal-spined egg slightly larger than that of *S. haematobium*. The eggs are passed in the feces rather than in the urine.

Schistosome Dermatitis. Several species of schistosomes, especially in the genus *Trichobilharzia*, may invade the skin of man to cause severe allergic dermatitis. These worms, which normally parasitize birds or lower mammals, apparently cannot mature in man. While dermatitis-producing schistosomes have been recorded from scattered areas throughout the world, excepting Africa, they are prominent only in parts of Europe and North America. Certain lakes in the north central states, particularly in Michigan and Wisconsin, were formerly notorious for the "swimmer's itch" contracted by bathers. Although snail destruction with copper salts has successfully controlled the infection in some of these areas, this type of cercarial dermatitis continues to be a serious problem over much of this area. The dermatitis can be treated with anti-allergic ointments. One of the parasites producing schistosome dermatitis, *Schistosomatium douthitti* is of especial interest because it is easily studied in laboratory mice. Avian schistosomes causing dermatitis are also contacted on saltwater beaches of Hawaii, California, and the eastern United States.

CESTODA

The Cestoda or tapeworms are all parasitic. The adults usually reside in the alimentary tract of the definitive host and the larval stages infest the tissues of an intermediate host. The ribbon-like adult tapeworm generally consists of a scolex at its anterior end which anchors the parasite to the host, a neck or growing region, and a strobila consisting of segments or proglottids. These develop sexually and are pushed back from the growing region. The proglottids nearest the neck are immature, while those intermediate on the strobila are mature and contain a complete reproductive system. Gravid proglottids are located at the posterior end of the strobila. The nervous and excretory systems are shared by the whole organism. There is no alimentary tract, but the entire body surface is highly specialized for the absorption of soluble nutrients. Two orders of tapeworms, the Pseudophyllidea and Cyclophyllidea contain human parasites. The Pseudophyllidea are discussed later (see *Diphyllobothrium latum*). Most of the tapeworms of man belong to the Cyclophyllidea, of which *Taenia solium* will serve as an example.

Taenia solium

The pork tapeworm, *Taenia solium,* was known in ancient times. Küchenmeister, in 1855, first suspected its relationship to "bladderworms" in pork and demonstrated their transformation into the adult worms in the intestine of a condemned criminal.

Characteristics and Life Cycle. In the intestine of man the adult *T. solium* attains a length of 2 to 3 meters. The scolex is a rounded cubical organ approximately 1 mm. in diameter bearing four large cup-like suckers and a rostellum with 20 to 35 hooks (Fig. 44–15). Mature proglottids average 0.5 cm. square. The genital pore occurs on either side of the proglottid, alternating irregularly from segment to segment. The male reproductive system consists of small follicular testes scattered throughout the dorsal part of the segment. They empty through masa efferentia into a coiled vas deferens which ends in the muscular copulatory organ or cirrus at the genital pore. The vagina extends from the genital pore to the ootype in the posterior central part of the segment. Ovaries are on either side of the ootype and vitellaria are located behind it.

As the proglottids move toward the posterior end of the worm, the uterus fills with eggs. There are about 10 branches on each side of the uterus, and the gravid proglottids measure 0.5 cm. in width by 1 cm. in length. These gravid segments detach and are void with the feces. They may break before or after being void and release large numbers of eggs. The eggs average 35 μm. in diameter and possess a thick shell. The embryo or onchosphere within each egg bears six hooks.

When the eggs are ingested by the intermediate host, the pig, they hatch in the intestine. The onchospheres penetrate the intestinal wall and enter the lymph or blood. They are carried to various tissues in the body and develop into infective cysticerci or bladderworms. Each cysticercus consists of a scolex like that of the adult, a short neck, and a fluid-filled sac or bladder about 1 cm. in diameter. The scolex is invaginated into the bladder when the cysticercus is in the host tissue.

When man ingests the cysticercus in undercooked pork, the bladder is digested, the scolex evaginates, and the worm attaches to the intestinal wall. The adult tapeworm develops by growth from the neck region. Within two months after infection, gravid proglottids and eggs are present in the feces. The *T. solium* infection may last for many years.

The Human Disease. Adult pork tapeworms usually occur singly in the intestine of man. They often cause no noticeable symptoms, though general intestinal discomfort may occur, and in children nervous disturbances are sometimes seen. The ravenous appetite popularly associated with tapeworm infections

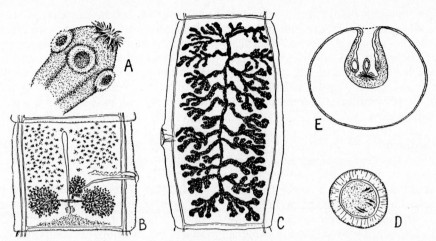

Figure 44–15. *Taenia solium. A,* Scolex, × 20. *B,* Mature proglottid, × 5. *C,* Gravid proglottid, × 5. *D,* Egg, × 500. *E,* Cysticercus, × 5. (Adapted from various sources.)

is actually uncommon, loss of appetite being more frequently observed. In contrast with infection by the adult worm, tissue infection with the cysticerci (cysticercosis) is dangerous. The larvae act like benign tumors; growth is slow and terminates naturally with full development. The injury results from pressure, and its seriousness, therefore, depends on the location of the larvae. In most muscles and connective tissues they are of no consequence, but larvae in the eye may affect vision. In the brain they may give rise to epilepsy or other manifestations of local pressure.

Cattle exhibit resistance to reinfection by *T. saginata.* There are relatively few instances of multiple infections with adult *T. solium* in humans. It appears from studies with other cestodes that rejection of the parasites is immunologically mediated and that the responsible antigens are located in the scolex and neck region.[33] Antibodies are detected in individuals with cysticercosis by a variety of serological tests. An indirect hemagglutination test is available commercially, and both complement fixing and precipitating antibodies can be demonstrated in laboratory assays. Differences have been reported in the immune responses of humans with cysticerosis with respect to antibody titers, responsiveness to specific antigens, the presence of particular classes of immunoglobulins, and the severity of their symptoms. Immunodiffusion and immunoelectrophoretic analyses indicate that all cysticerci are not identical, but share approximately one third of their antigens.[97] The variability in the responsiveness of humans and the disease may be due to antigenic variability in the cysticerci.

Laboratory diagnosis of intestinal infection with *T. solium* is based on recovery of eggs or gravid proglottids from the feces. The eggs are not distinguishable from those of the beef tapeworm (see below), but the gravid segments can be identified by the smaller number of uterine branches, about 10 on each side as against more than 15 in the beef tapeworm. Diagnosis of the cysticercus infection is rarely made before operation or necropsy, but the immunological reactions mentioned above have been used. Niclosamide, an oral drug, is used to eliminate the adult worms, but there is no treatment available for cysticercosis except surgical removal of the bladderworms.

Epidemiology and Control. The larvae of *T. solium* occur most commonly in pigs but are found also in man, monkeys, sheep, camels, and dogs. In Berlin before 1850, 2 per cent of human autopsies showed the cysticerci, but the incidence is now much lower. Pigs acquire the infection by contamination of their food or water with human feces. In some areas of the tropics and the Far East, pigs, because of their coprophagic habits, are responsible for the relative cleanliness around small rural villages. Larval infections in man are incurred chiefly by contamination of food, water, or fingers with eggs from human feces, but it is also possible that in the intestine of an individual harboring the adult worm the eggs may hatch without reaching the outside. Whether or not eggs must leave the body before they are infective, a person with the adult worm in his intestine is a constant hazard to himself as well as others. Man, the only known host for the adult tapeworm, acquires the infection by ingestion of undercooked pork, which often contains large numbers of larvae. Freezing and thorough cooking kill the larvae, but ordinary pickling and smoking are ineffective. Government meat inspection reveals most infected carcasses and has been the most effective single control measure. Other control methods are directed at the prevention of contact between pigs and human feces.

Taenia saginata

The beef tapeworm, *Taenia saginata*, resembles *T. solium* in morphology and life cycle, but several differences are noteworthy. The scolex is "unarmed," lacking the hooked rostellum of *T. solium*. The adult worm is usually about 5 meters long, but occasionally is much longer. The gravid proglottids are distinguished from those of *T. solium* by a larger number of uterine branches, usually 15 to 20 on each side. Man is the only known host of the adult. The cysticerci develop in cattle and other ruminants, human infection resulting chiefly from consumption of undercooked beef. Rare cases of human infection with the larvae have been claimed, but it is probable that they were abnormal cysticerci of *T. solium*.

Echinococcus granulosus

The adult of *Echinococcus granulosus* inhabits the intestines of dogs and related species. It is a minute worm 0.25 to 0.5 cm. in length, consisting of an "armed" scolex and three proglottids, one immature, one mature, and one gravid. Large numbers of the adults may occur in the intestine of an infected dog.

The natural intermediate hosts are sheep, cattle, and other ruminants, but a wide variety of animals are susceptible, including man, in whom the larva causes a serious disease. This larva is markedly different from those of the beef and pork tapeworms discussed above. In the viscera of an infected animal it attains a diameter of about 1 cm. after five to six months. It is infective after eight months or more but continues to grow, often, after several years, reaching a diameter of more than 20 cm. The larva, known as a "hydatid cyst," is a spherical, fluid-filled sac composed of a thick cuticular wall with a thin germinative epithelium on its inside surface. From this germinative epithelium are formed two types of structures. Buds may appear and grow into stalked vesicles, brood capsules, on the inner surface of which stalked cysticercus-like "scolices" are produced. These brood capsules may become detached as daughter cysts, enlarge, and produce brood capsules and scolices within themselves. In the large cysts there may thus be produced many thousand infective scolices, each of which can develop into an adult worm if the cyst is eaten by a dog feeding on the viscera of an infected animal. Thus *E. granulosus* differs from *T. solium* chiefly in the fact that multiplication occurs in the larval as well as the adult stage. The predominant site of larval infection is in the liver. The lung is next in importance, and cysts may occur also in practically every other organ.

Hydatid Disease in Man. Echinococcosis, or hydatid disease, is characterized by two general types of manifestations. First, hypersensitivity develops to components of the hydatid fluid, and accidental rupture of a cyst may cause serious, even fatal reactions. Second, and most important, the growing cyst acts like a tumor, the injury resulting from pressure effects and depending on the localization of the cyst. Rupture of a cyst may give rise to new cysts produced from scolices, daughter cysts, or fragments of germinative epithelium. Osseous cysts, occurring in bone, may weaken the bone by erosion of its structure.

Direct evidence of acquired immunity to larval infections is not available, but in immunized sheep, the cysts develop abnormally. When *E. granulosus* is cultured in the presence of serum from infected sheep, some die as onchospheres within 24 hours, some die during differentiation into cysts, and some develop normally but have precipitates in the outer cyst layers.[44] Host immunoglobulins are found in the hydatid cyst fluid. Dogs immunized with larval antigens resist infections with adult *E. granulosus*.

Diagnosis of hydatid disease is generally based on information provided by the patient indicating residence in an endemic area and possible exposure, the presence of a space-occupying lesion, and positive immunological reactions. The Casoni intradermal test is useful, but remains positive after removal of the cysts and gives cross-reactions in individuals with cysticercosis. Specificity has been improved in antigen kits from commercial sources. Indirect hemagglutination, latex agglutination, and complement fixation tests are also available for serodiagnosis.

Hydatid cysts are removed surgically with extreme care to avoid their rupture, since the contents are capable of metastatic growth. The fluid may also induce systemic anaphylaxis. Mebendazole administered over long periods is also considered an effective treatment.

Epidemiology and Control. The normal life cycle of *E. granulosus* involves dogs and sheep or cattle, man being an accidental host of the larva. For this reason, the infection is most common in the great grazing regions of the world, particularly Australia and New Zealand, North and South Africa, Iceland, and southern South America. The incidence in cattle and sheep occasionally exceeds 50 per cent. Various wild mammals may also be involved among them moose, reindeer, and wolves in northern North America. Transmission of *Echinococcus* eggs to food by sarcophagic flies from dog feces has been experimentally demonstrated and may be presumed to occur naturally.

In the United States infection has been found in man in a recently recognized, large endemic focus in the Central Valley of California. Lesser areas in Utah involving human cases have also been described. The infection has been maintained by the sheepherders of Basque origin who commonly allow the sheepherding dogs to consume sheep carcasses. High levels of infection in coyotes also occur in these areas.[65]

Control of the infection in domestic animals depends chiefly on preventing dogs from eating offal. Possibly infected waste material should be buried or burned. Prophylaxis of human infection requires measures to reduce the chance of contamination of human food and water by feces of dogs.

Echinococcus multilocularis

The adult of *E. multilocularis* differs from *E. granulosus* only in fine morphological detail. The larva, however, develops differently from the discrete, spherical cyst produced by the latter, forming an alveolar cyst which spreads malignantly as a foaming mass of minute, budding globules, each containing, in the normal hosts, a few scolices. The liver is usually infected, and it is extensively destroyed by the exuberant growth of the larval tissue.

Echinococcus multilocularis has been found in central Europe and the Aleutian Islands but probably also occurs in northern Asia. The adult hosts are foxes, and the larvae normally parasitize wild rodents. Sporadic larval infections occur in man, causing usually fatal destruction of liver tissue.

Alveolar hydatid was known in man for nearly a century before, in 1951, Rausch and Schiller recognized it as a distinct species. It had previously been considered an abnormal form of *E. granulosus*. The name *E. alveolaris* has also been applied to it.

Hymenolepis nana

The human dwarf tapeworm, *Hymenolepis nana*, is a small worm, 1 to 4 cm. in length, with mature proglottids 0.5 to 1 mm. in breadth. The scolex is similar to that of *T. solium* but smaller, about 0.25 mm. in diameter. The mature proglottids are markedly different in appearance from those of *T. solium*, the width being more than four times the length. Three large testes occur in each segment. The uterus in the gravid segment is a large, irregular sac. The gravid segments are usually destroyed in the intestine, releasing the eggs, which are found in the feces.

Hymenolepis nana is unique among human tapeworms in not requiring an intermediate host. Ingested eggs hatch in the intestine of man to release an embryo which invades the tissues of an intestinal villus. Here, in about four days, it develops into a cysticercoid, a larva with a small bladder and a solid tail. This larva breaks out of the intestinal wall, attaches to the mucosa, and develops into the adult worm. Eggs are found in the feces about two weeks after infection. It is reported that several types of insects can serve as intermediate hosts, but they are probably unimportant in human spread of the parasite. Large numbers of worms are commonly found in an infected individual, and they may give rise to intestinal and nervous disturbances in children. Epileptiform convulsions may occur. Niclosamide is used for elmination of the worms.

Hymenolepis nana occurs naturally in man, monkeys, and rodents. The parasite is cosmopolitan. It is by far the most common tapeworm of man in the United States, especially prevalent in children, but occurring in all age groups. Age resistance has not been shown in man but is experimentally demonstrable in rats and mice.

The lack of an intermediate host permits direct spread from man to man. It is not known whether the eggs can hatch without having reached the outside. However, an infected individual is particularly liable to reinfection from fingers contaminated with his own feces.

The closely related *Hymenolepis diminuta* of rats and mice is transmitted by several species of insect intermediate hosts. Occasional human infections have been reported mostly in children.

Tapeworms of Lower Animals

Species of the genus *Multiceps* exhibit the adult stage in dogs and larval stages in sheep. The larva, known as a coenurus, resembles a cysticercus but has a number of scolices attached to a single bladder. In the brains of sheep the larvae produce a fatal disease. Occasional cases have been reported in man.

Taenia pisiformis is a common tapeworm of dogs and cats, the larvae developing in the abdominal cavity of rabbits. *Taenia taeniaeformis* occurs commonly in the intestine of cats. The larvae, strobilocerci, normally develop in the liver of rats or mice.

Dipylidium caninum, a common parasite of the intestines of dogs and cats, measures 10 to 50 cm. in length. Each elongate, rounded mature proglottid contains two sets of reproductive systems, one opening on each side of the segment. The uterus breaks up into pouches, each containing several eggs. Dog lice and various species of fleas serve as intermediate hosts, the cysticercoids in the insects being infective when ingested. Young children occasionally harbor the adult tapeworm.

Diphyllobothrium latum

The fish tapeworm *Diphyllobothrium latum* (or *Dibothriocephalus latus*) is the most important human parasite in the order Pseudophyllidea. It differs markedly in structure and life cycle from the species discussed above. It is a more primitive type, in many respects showing strong resemblances to the trematodes.

Morphology and Life Cycle. The adult worm in the intestine of man is very large, often exceeding 10 meters in length. The scolex is an elongate ovoid structure, about 1 by 2.5 mm. in dimensions, bearing, instead of the circular suckers of the cyclophyllidea, two elongated grooves which serve as attachment organs (Fig. 44–16). The mature proglottid is broader than long, about 4 by 10 mm. in size. The small testes are scattered throughout the lateral dorsal regions, emptying the fine ducts into the vas deferens. This coiled tube runs from the posterior center of the segment forward to the muscular cirrus, which opens into the ventral genital pore in the middle of the anterior region. The vagina extends from the genital pore back to the large ootype in the center of the posterior region. The ovaries lie on either side of the ootype, and the vitellaria are small follicles scattered throughout the lateral ventral regions. Arising from the ootype, the egg-filled uterus coils throughout the center of the proglottid, ending at the uterine pore just behind the genital pore. This permits escape of the eggs without rupture of the proglottid, so that, contrary to the usual situation as seen in *T. solium,* the eggs are released into the intestinal contents and escape in the feces. The spent proglottids at the end of the worm break off and are passed in the feces.

The egg is underdeveloped when it escapes in the feces, embryonation requiring a week or more in water. Like the eggs of most trematodes it is ovoid, with an operculum. Average measurements are 65 by 45 μm. Hatching occurs by opening of the operculum to release a free-swimming, spherical, onchosphere covered with long cilia. This embryo, the coracidium, dies within a few days unless it is ingested by a suitable small crustacean, one of several species of copepods of the genera *Cyclops* and *Diaptomus.* Losing its cilia, the embryo reaches the body cavity of the copepod and becomes, in two to three weeks, an elongated solid body with a round

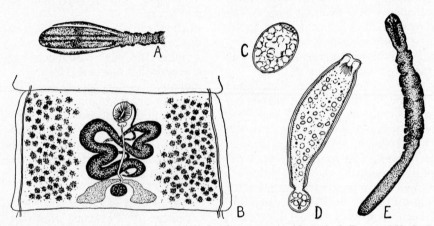

Figure 44–16. *Diphyllobothrium latum. A,* Scolex, × 10. *B,* Mature proglottid, × 6. *C,* Egg, × 250. *D,* Procercoid × 100. *E,* Sparganum, × 8.

tail bearing the six hooks seen in the embryo. This stage, the procercoid, is about 0.5 mm. long.

If the infected copepod is eaten by a fish, the procercoid penetrates the wall of the intestine and reaches the viscera or muscles. Here, in a week or more, it transforms into the sparganum, a worm-like stage 0.5 to 2 cm. long with a rudimentary scolex at the anterior end. This stage, ingested by man in undercooked fish, develops to the adult worm in the intestine, and eggs may be found in the feces after three weeks or more. If the infected fish is eaten by another fish, the spargana become established in the tissues of the second fish and remain infective for man. Human infections have been known to persist for years.

The Human Disease. *Diphyllobothrium latum* commonly produces multiple infections, a number of worms occurring in the same intestine. The adult worms usually cause no symptoms, though in heavy infections intestinal disturbances may occur, sometimes with generalized edema. A small proportion of infected individuals show severe anemia, indistinguishable from pernicious anemia. It has been shown that the tapeworm concentrates vitamin B_{12} in its tissues, and it is clear that the consequent deprivation of a susceptible individual precipitates the anemia. Satisfactory data on acquired immunity are not available. Laboratory diagnosis depends on identification of the eggs in fecal smears. As with the other tapeworms, niclosamide is the drug of choice.

Epidemiology and Control. The adult worm parasitizes man, cats, dogs, bears, and other fish-eating mammals, but man is probably the principal source of infection in endemic areas. Susceptible copepods are widespread, and a variety of fishes can serve as second intermediate hosts. Endemic centers are known in northern and central Europe, northern Asia, Japan, parts of Africa, and the Great Lakes region of North America. Infection is especially widespread in Finland, where the incidence has been estimated at 20 to 25 per cent and where most of the cases of tapeworm anemia have been reported. Personal protection depends on thorough cooking or freezing of fish from endemic areas and care in handling of such fish. Other control methods are aimed at reducing the pollution of bodies of water with untreated human feces and at the supervision of transportation of possibly infected fish.

Related Species. Several related species of tapeworms, normally parasites of lower animals, are reported occasionally in man. Man also occasionally harbors the spargana of several species of *Diphyllobothrium,* normally parasites of the dog and other carnivores. *Diphyllobothrium mansoni* is a common example. Infection with these larvae in the subcutaneous tissues, muscles, or eye is known as sparganosis. Among the larvae infecting man is the very rare parasite, *Sparganum proliferum,* which multiplies enormously in the subcutaneous tissues and may cause death. The adult of this species is unknown. Larval infections with *Diphyllobothrium* usually result from ingestion of copepods in drinking water. In parts of the Orient split frogs are sometimes used as poultices, and human sparganosis has resulted from the migration of spargana from the frog tissues into the exposed tissues of man.

NEMATODA

All the important human parasites in the phylum Nemathelminthes (Aschelminthes of some authors) belong to the class Nematoda. They are cylindrical, elongate worms, unsegmented and with a body cavity which is not lined with a peritoneum of mesodermal origin as in higher animals. Symmetry is primitively bilateral. Male and female reproductive systems usually occur in separate individuals noticeably different in general appearance. In some parasitic forms, parthenogenesis and protandry occur. Free-living nematodes are among the most numerous of animals and are found in a tremendous variety of habitats. Parasitic species in plants and animals are also abundant, and wild vertebrates are usually parasitized, as are many invertebrates. Nematodes are important as disease agents of most domestic animals, and the majority of mankind is infected with one or more species.

The structure of the nematodes parasitizing man varies greatly, and in size alone species occur which are too small to be readily seen with the unaided eye, as well as forms over 1 meter in length. The life cycles are also varied from simple direct forms of development to those requiring several hosts. Among the simple forms, the pinworm of man, *Enterobius vermicularis,* will serve to illustrate the morphology and life history.

A word of caution is necessary here. The order of presentation of species in this section, based primarily on life cycles, cuts sharply across the lines of zoological classification, separating closely related types and bringing together types of very different structure.

Enterobius vermicularis

The human pinworm, *Enterobius vermicularis,* normally inhabits the upper large intestine of man, occasionally invading the female genitourinary system. The female worm, about 1 cm. long by 0.5 mm. in diameter, is a spindle-shaped organism with a long, pointed tail (see Fig. 44–17). The outer covering is a smooth, impervious, flexible cuticle, characteristic of nematodes in general. This cuticle, together with the fact that the body musculature is exclusively longitudinal, gives the worms a characteristic bending, wriggling type of movement. Among nematodes the cuticle shows great variety of external structures—knobs, fins, papillae, etc.—which are of value in technical identification of species. The alimentary tract consists of a mouth at the anterior end, a musculature esophagus with a posterior bulbous enlargement, and a thin-walled intestine emptying through the anus near the posterior end. The female reproductive system empties through a short vagina a little in front of the middle of the body. Extending forward and back from the vagina are two separate egg-producing systems (one to several in other nematodes). Each consists of a broad uterus filled with eggs, followed by a short narrow oviduct, which terminates in a long, thin ovary coiled about in the body cavity.

The male worm is smaller than the female, 2 to 5 mm. in length and 0.1 to 0.2 mm. in diameter, the posterior end coiled into a tight spiral and lacking the pin-like tail of the female. The male reproductive system is a single tube consisting of a testis, a vas deferens, a seminal vesicle, and a muscular ejaculatory duct, provided with glands, which empties with the intestine into a cloaca. A sharp copulatory spicule can be extruded through the anus. The posterior end has minute expansions (more prominent in many other nematodes) which form a clasping bursa used in copulation.

Some of the eggs escape in the intestine, passing out in the feces, but usually the gravid females migrate out of the anus to release their eggs on the surrounding skin. The eggs average 55 by 25 μm. in size, usually show mature embryos when passed, and are infective within a few hours. Ingested by man they hatch in the small intestine, where the worms mature and mate before passing down to the large intestine. Eggs appear in the feces about two weeks after infection. The adults in the intestine are short-lived, but infection is maintained or increased in the individual by self-infection. Hatching of eggs on the perianal surfaces with subsequent migration of larvae into the anus (described as "retroinfection") occurs in related species, and it has been suggested this may also occur in man.

Pinworm Infection in Man. The adult worms in the intestine have little or no effect on the host. However, they occur in the vermiform appendix, and since they are said to be more common in diseased than in normal appendices, they have been suspected of an etiological role in appendicitis. During the nocturnal emergence of the female and with egg deposition in the perianal region, itching occurs which may be intense, leading to scratching, scarification, weeping eczema, and bacterial infection. Worms may enter the female genitalia and cause similar irritation and occasionally migrate into the peritoneal cavity via the fallopian tubes. In children pruritus ani, sleeplessness, and resulting irritability are common. A slight eosinophilia may accompany infections, but information is not available on resistance to the parasites in humans. Adults are less susceptible to pinworm infections than children, and the mechanism of this age-related difference is not known.

Diagnosis is based on identification of eggs in the feces or from the perianal skin. The

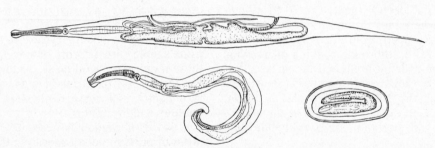

Figure 44–17. *Enterobius vermicularis. Top,* female, × 15. *Left,* adult male, × 15. *Right,* egg, × 300. (Redrawn from Faust after Leuckart.)

best method utilizes a strip of cellophane tape. The gummed side is pressed repeatedly on the perianal skin and then applied to a microscopic slide for examination.

Epidemiology and Control. Man is the only host of *E. vermicularis*. The eggs are resistant to drying and may contaminate clothing, bedding, and house dust, thus maintaining a constant source of infection in homes and institutions. The parasite is cosmopolitan. It is especially common in children, probably largely because their unsanitary habits allow greater chances of spread. A single oral dose of mebendazole is recommended for treatment, but reinfection is a common occurrence. Treatment may be repeated if the infection and symptoms reappear. Effective control measures are not currently available.

Related Species. Similar nematodes occur in many lower animals and are sometimes economically important as minor disease agents. *Syphacia obvelata,* a species found in rats and mice, is an occasional parasite of man and may readily be obtained for study from rodents. The eggs resemble those of *E. vermicularis* but are twice as large.

Trichuris trichiura

Trichuris trichiura is a frequent inhabitant of the cecum, appendix, and upper colon of man. The anterior three-fifths of the adult worm, containing the nonmuscular esophagus, is attenuated, and the general appearance of the body has given rise to the common name "whipworm." Male and female worms are similar in size, 3 to 5 cm. long. The adult worms, embedded in the intestinal mucosa, have been accused of a role in the pathogenesis of appendicitis, but the evidence is inconclusive. Light infections are common throughout the population of the world's tropics and subtropics, are relatively without symptoms, and are unimportant to the infected individual. However, heavy infections, particularly in children, cause a hyperemic mucosa of the colon and rectum, chronic diarrhea, extensive inflammation, and rectal prolapse. In the past, trichuriasis was difficult to treat. Mebendazole has little toxicity for the patient, and twice-daily doses over a three-day period are effective in eliminating the worms. The eggs passed in the feces are thick-walled, with a plug at either end, 53 by 22 μm. in size (Fig. 44–18). They are very resistant, surviving for months in contaminated soil. The embryos, undeveloped at the time of passage, require two weeks to several months, depending on temperature and humidity, to reach the infective stage. Ingested with contaminated food or water, they produce adult worms in the intestine. *Trichuris trichiura* infection is worldwide but especially abundant in the tropics and subtropics because of poor sanitation and the effect of climate on development of the eggs.

Capillaria philippinensis

An acute, usually fatal disease caused by invasion of the intestinal mucosa by large numbers of this small (4 to 5 mm.) nematode occurred in the Philippines in the period 1967

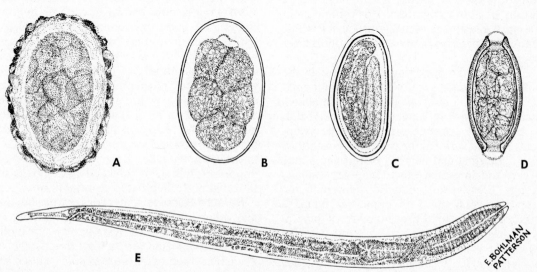

Figure 44–18. Nematode eggs and larvae. *A, Ascaris lumbricoides. B, Necator americanus. C, Enterobius vermicularis. D, Trichuris trichiura. E, Strongyloides stercoralis* (rhabditiform larva). × 400.

to 1969. The disease is characterized by protracted, profuse diarrhea and the resulting electrolyte imbalance and hypoproteinemia. Intestinal capillariasis has since been reported from other areas of Asia. Its overwhelming aspects are due to internal autoinfection.[26] Diagnosis is readily made by finding characteristic eggs and often larvae in the stool. Treatment with mebendazole is effective and results in few relapses. Infection is acquired by eating freshwater or brackish water raw fish containing infective larvae. Birds are believed to be the natural definitive hosts, and fish-eating and water birds have been infected in the laboratory.

Ascaris lumbricoides

Widely known simply as the "roundworm" of man, *Ascaris lumbricoides* is a large parasite of the small intestine. The white or flesh-colored females measure 20 cm. or more in length by 5 mm. in diameter; in males, 16 cm. by 3 mm. The characteristic eggs, 45 to 75 μm. by 35 to 50 μm., have a smooth inner and a roughly tuberculated outer shell. They are undeveloped when passed in the feces. In soil or water they become infective in nine days or more, depending on environmental conditions. They may survive for several years despite drying, bacterial contamination, or adverse chemical conditions. Ingested in food or water they hatch in the intestine. The embryos, however, do not develop directly into adults in this site. Gaining access to the circulation they are carried to the lungs and escape into the air spaces. Via the trachea they reach the pharynx and are swallowed. Partial development occurs during the above migration. It is completed in the small intestine, where egg-producing adults are found about two and one-half months after infection.

Passage of the migrating larvae through the lung may produce severe bronchopneumonia. Larvae filtered out of the circulation in abnormal sites induce inflammatory lesions. Adult worms in the intestine often cause no symptoms. Particularly in heavy infections, however, intestinal and nervous disturbances may occur, and intestinal obstruction occasionally results. Massive infection of children in the tropics is common, with numerous fatalities occurring prior to the availability of piperazine. The drug acts as a myoneural blocking agent for *Ascaris,* and the paralyzed worms are eliminated by normal peristalsis as they are no longer able to maintain their position in the intestine. Consequently, chemotherapeutic methods now are effective in infections which previously necessitated surgical intervention to eliminate intestinal obstruction by worms. Various other injuries result from migration of the adult worms out of the normal habitat into the appendix, the bile ducts, the upper alimentary or respiratory tracts, or the genitourinary system, or through the intestinal wall into the abdominal cavity. Hypersensitivity develops in infected persons and in laboratory workers who have handled the worms, and severe anaphylactic reactions may occur in such individuals. It has been suggested that in the northern hemisphere a high percentage of individuals with bronchial asthma have nematode parasites, which accounts for their allergic condition. *Ascaris* may be the most common cause, with *Strongyloides stercoralis* and *Necator americanus* also being implicated.[90]

Acquired immunity has not been observed in man, but experimental animals exhibit partial resistance to reinfection with related parasites. Antibodies are detectable by various tests after either infection or vaccination with worm extracts, and considerable investigation has been devoted to antigenic analysis. An allergic skin test has been used in diagnosis but is often positive in uninfected individuals who have acquired hypersensitivity from contact with the parasite. Laboratory diagnosis is preferably based on the finding of eggs in stools. However, a small proportion of cases harbor only male worms, and in such cases the immunological tests can be used.

Piperazine and mebendazole are effective in removing the adult worms from the intestine.

Man is the only known host of *A. lumbricoides.* Infection predominates in children; that this results in part from age resistance is suggested by the marked age resistance of lower animals to related parasites. Infection is worldwide but most prevalent in the tropics and subtropics, where sanitary and climatic conditions favor its dissemination. Control depends on the reduction of soil contamination by proper sewage disposal and treatment of infected individuals. Raw vegetables are an important source of infection and should be thoroughly washed before consumption.

Related Species. Cats, dogs, cattle, horses, and other lower animals harbor a number of closely related species. Rare human infections have been reported with at least three of these. A distinct race of *A. lumbricoides* causes severe pneumonitis in young pigs, known as "thumps." In man the eggs hatch and the larvae reach the lung, but adult worms do not become established in the intestine. Similarly, the human *A. lumbricoides* develops only to the lung stage in pigs. The adults of the pig *Ascaris* are easily obtained from slaughterhouses for laboratory study.

Visceral Larva Migrans. Visceral larva migrans has been recognized only recently as a clinical entity and the nematodes responsible are close relatives of *Ascaris*. The species most often involved are *Toxocara canis* and *T. cati*, the extremely common ascarids of the dog and cat. The larvae do not mature in man but wander extensively through the tissues producing lesions and granulomata in the brain, eye, liver, lung, or other sites. The symptoms produced may be minor except for eosinophilia or may involve hepatomegaly, pulmonary infiltration, cough, hyperglobulinemia, and allergic manifestations. Diagnosis is difficult but may be made on recovery of larvae in sectioned biopsy material with recognition of the larvae, as shown in Figure 44–19. Serological reactions are of value in diagnosis but give cross-reactions with *Ascaris*. There is no specific therapy. Children with a history of dirt eating and an association with household pets run a risk of serious infection, emphasizing the need for anthelminthic treatment of dogs and cats.

Large nematode larvae causing eosinophilic granulomas and acute abdominal syndromes in man have been identified as *Anisakis*. *Anisakis* and several other genera are parasites of marine animals. These relatives of the ascarid worms utilize crustaceans and marine fish in their life cycles; humans become infected when they eat raw or undercooked fish.[99] The disease is most common in the Far East, but is also found in Europe and the United States.[53]

The larvae of *Angiostrongylus cantonensis*, a lungworm of rats, cause eosinophilic meningoencephalitis in man. Epidemic outbreaks as well as isolated occurrences are found throughout the Pacific islands and in Southeast Asia.[1] Other species, *A. malaysiense* and *A. costaricensis*, the latter from Costa Rica and other Central American countries, also cause angiostrongyloidiasis. The infection is acquired by the ingestion of raw freshwater or terrestrial snails, slugs, or prawns containing infective larvae.[1, 83]

Hookworms

The two important hookworms of man, *Ancylostoma duodenale* and *Necator americanus*, will be discussed together. Known since antiquity, human hookworms were first accurately described by Dubini in 1843. Their relationship to disease was definitely shown by Perroncito in 1880, and the life cycle was elaborated by Looss.

Characteristics and Life Cycle. The adults of *A. duodenale* from the human small intestine are shown in Figure 44–20. The female measures 1 to 1.5 cm. in length by about 0.5 mm. in diameter. The double reproductive system coils abundantly throughout the body cavity. Two pairs of prominent unicellular glands are seen in the anterior half of the body, one excretory in function, the other secreting histolytic enzymes. The dorsally directed mouth is characterized by two pairs of ventral teeth (replaced in *N. americanus* by curved cutting plates). The male measures a little less than 1 cm. in length by about 0.4 mm. in diameter. The reproductive system shows a long, muscular ejaculatory duct, a prominent seminal vesicle, and a coiled testis. At the posterior end of the male worm is a broad, flat clasping apparatus, the copulatory bursa, composed of cuticle supported by finger-like rays of tissue. *Ancylostoma duodenale* and *N. americanus* can be identified by details of structure of this bursa as well as by the differences in buccal teeth noted above.

The thin-walled eggs measure about 38 by 58 μm. Those of the two species of human hookworms cannot be distinguished microscopically from one another. They are usually in early stages of development upon escape from the body, maturing and hatching within

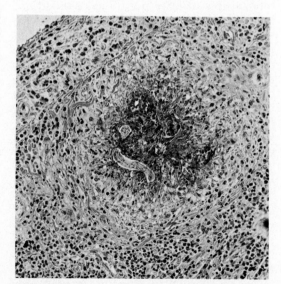

Figure 44–19. Human visceral larva migrans. Liver section showing granulomatous area containing *Toxocara canis* larva. × 105. (Beaver)

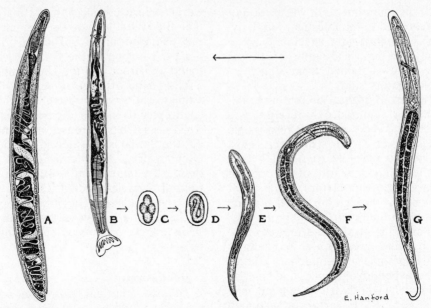

Figure 44–20. Life cycle of a hookworm, *Ancylostoma duodenale*. Note difference in magnification. *A*, Female worm. *B*, Male worm. *C* and *D*, Eggs. *E*, First stage larva. *F*, Second stage larva. *G*, Infective larva. *A* and *B*, × 10. *C* to *G*, × 250. (Adapted from Looss.)

24 hours if conditions are favorable in the soil. The larva, about 0.25 mm. in length, feeds on fecal material and grows in three days or more to a length of about 0.4 mm. After molting, it continues to grow until, by the fifth day or later, it measures about 0.6 mm. These two stages, characterized by a bulbous esophagus, are known as rhabditiform larvae. The third stage, resulting from a second molt, is a thinner form with a closed mouth and a less bulbous esophagus. It is usually still surrounded by a "sheath," the molted skin of the preceding stage. This is the filariform larva, the infective stage for man. It does not feed but may survive long periods in the soil under favorable conditions. If the infective larva comes in contact with human skin, it actively penetrates through the epidermis, reaches the circulation, and is carried to the lungs. Here, like the migrating larva of *Ascaris,* it breaks out in the air spaces and reaches the intestine via the trachea and esophagus. After two further molts, the worms are mature. Egg production begins about one month after infection.

Hookworm Disease. Penetration of the skin by hookworm larvae produces a dermatitis known as ground itch or miner's itch. This is severe enough in some previously exposed individuals to be incapacitating. The adult hookworms live attached to the mucosa of the small intestine, feeding on blood and bits of tissue. They move about frequently, leaving bleeding wounds in the intestinal mucosa. The chronic loss of blood causes a microcytic hypochromic anemia and edema, resulting, in severe cases, in retardation of growth and mental development and in weakness and general debilitation. In many areas where hookworm disease is of importance, this anemia is intensified by virtue of the fact that nutritionally the population receives a relatively inadequate supply of available food iron. The additional loss of large quantities of blood and iron through hookworm infection produces the severe anemias often seen. Intestinal disturbances are seen in heavy infections. Death, except in infants and young children, is rarely a direct result of hookworm disease, but the condition often contributes to death from other causes. In infected persons, the symptoms are directly related to the intensity of infection, which, because of the necessary development outside the body, is stable unless re-exposure occurs. Individuals with fewer than 25 *N. americanus* virtually never show symptoms. Those with between 25 and 100 worms show borderline effects. With more than 100 worms some clinical injury is almost always detectable. *Ancylostoma duodenale* is more harmful, about half as many worms being required to produce a given effect. Normally, infection is maintained by constant re-exposure. In previously infected persons living under conditions which prevent additional infection, however, it has been shown that about one-half of the worms are lost in six months and about three-quarters in two years. A smaller number persist for as long as 12 years.

Immunity. Dogs acquire resistance against hookworms by repeated reinfections with small numbers of filariform larvae. Immunization with irradiated larvae which are unable to develop to adults induces a high level of immunity against *A. caninum.* It is not known if humans can develop a similar protective response, but partial protection has been reported. In endemic areas, hookworm incidence may be high, but there may also be a low intensity of infection, in part due to frequent periodic exposures to small numbers of filariaform larvae.

Passively transferred immune serum confers some protection in puppies against dog hookworm infections. In humans, there is an eosinophilia and a variety of immunoglobulins are elicited during the infections. Antigen-antibody reactions produce precipitates at the exterior openings of the larvae and react with the cuticle. Complement-fixing antibodies are utilized in serological tests. IgE levels are elevated and reactions are directed against the larvae. Both immediate and delayed hypersensitivity are also detected against these larval antigens.

Diagnosis. Diagnosis of hookworm infection is based on recovery of characteristic eggs from the feces. Direct fecal smears were formerly used, but many infections with fewer than 25 worms are not detected with this method. Because the number of hookworms present in an infected individual is so important, several quantitative diagnostic methods have been devised. In the Stoll method a measured quantity (4 ml.) of feces is mixed with dilute NaOH solution (56 ml.), and all the eggs in a known sample volume (0.075 ml.) of this suspension are counted. The Lane method, or D.C.F. (direct centrifugal flotation), can be applied to lighter infections. One milliliter of feces washed by centrifugation is mixed with brine and recentrifuged with a coverslip on top of the tube. The eggs rise and can be counted on the coverslip. A relatively simple and accurate densitometric technique has also been devised. Figures obtained by either of these methods are expressed as the number of eggs per milliliter of feces. A single female *N. americanus* produces about 45 eggs per ml. of feces (about 6000 eggs per day) so that 25 worms (male and female) produce about 600 eggs per ml. and 100 worms produce

about 2500 eggs per ml. *Ancylostoma duodenale* produces about twice as many eggs per worm, but because of the greater pathogenicity of this species the egg output gives a roughly equivalent index of the severity of infection in both species.

Mebendazole is effective in eliminating hookworms from the intestine. Supportive treatment with ferrous sulfate supplements dietary iron and helps to increase hemoglobin levels.

Epidemiology and Control. Man is the reservoir of infection with both *A. duodenale* and *N. americanus.* Many studies have been conducted on the habits and requirements of hookworm larvae in the soil. The optimal temperatures are about 75°F. for *A. duodenale* and about 80°F. for *N. americanus.* Consistent high temperatures, about 100°F., are unfavorable. At 60°F. development is prolonged to two weeks or more, and below 50°F. there is little or no development. Continued temperatures below 40°F. kill the larvae. Moisture is essential to survival of the soil stages, but they die under water and are scattered by heavy rain. The type of soil is significant, probably largely in relation to its waterholding properties. Coarse sand and heavy clay are unfavorable, optimal development occurring in light sand or sandy loam. A large proportion of the infective larvae die within the first two weeks, but a few survive for several months under favorable conditions. Although lateral migration from the site of development is insignificant, the filariform larvae can move considerable distances vertically in the soil. Unless excessive drying occurs, they remain at the surface, where the chance of contact with human skin is greatest.

In addition to the environmental requirements of the larvae, various human factors affect the distribution of hookworm infection. Fecal disposal practices and the use of shoes are among the most important. All these factors combine to make hookworm infection a problem of the rural parts of warm countries. Exceptions occur in mines and tunnel-building operations, where local conditions may be favorable despite a generally unsuitable environment. *Necator americanus* is the hookworm of central and southern Africa, the Western Hemisphere, and southern India. Throughout the rest of southern Asia it is mixed with *A. duodenale,* and a few foci of *A. duodenale* occur in South America. In most of Asia, southern Europe, European mines, and North Africa only *A. duodenale* is found.

In the southern United States hookworm infection is most common in children, largely because adults are protected from infection by wearing shoes. That age resistance, if it exists at all, is a minor factor is shown by the fact that in countries where the whole population goes without shoes, infection may predominate in adults.

Control depends on the reduction of soil contamination by treatment of cases and proper fecal disposal and on the prevention of contact between human skin and the soil. Chemical destruction of larvae in the soil has been of use only in particular cases, such as mines. Education is the major weapon in hookworm control, for the chief problems are sociological, and biological knowledge of the parasite is adequate to insure successful hookworm eradication if the habits of infected populations can be sufficiently influenced. Treatment of cases has an important place in hookworm control programs. Formerly it was customary to treat all infected members of a community, or even the whole community (mass treatment), if sample diagnoses showed abundant and heavy infections. Current opinion favors treatment of only the clinically significant cases. In most regions the treatment of a small proportion of the population can eliminate most of the egg production.

Related Nematodes of Lower Animals. Various animals harbor hookworms. Two species, *Ancylostoma braziliense* and *A. caninum* of dogs and cats, occasionally invade the skin of man. They are unable to develop further, and their wandering in the subcutaneous tissues produces a serpiginous dermatitis known as creeping eruption or cutaneous larva migrans. Closely related species, *A. malayanum* and *A. ceylonicum,* have been reported from man in the Far East. Other, more distantly related parasites such as the numerous species of *Trichostrongylus* are disease agents of ruminants and are incidental parasites of man. One species, *T. orientalis,* is more common in man than in other animals. Heavy infections in man may produce diarrhea and high eosinophilia. The eggs resemble those of the hookworms but may be distinguished from them by their larger size and slightly different shape.

Studies have been made of the mechanisms involved in the exsheathment or cuticle shedding necessary between developmental stages of nematodes. The fluids responsible for this are believed important in stimulating the antibodies producing functional immunity to several of these infections. Extensive studies on the development of living nematode vaccines for use in veterinary medication are in progress, as in some forms it is believed that only antigenic stimulation by such metabolic products can produce significant immunity.

Strongyloides stercoralis

Strongyloides stercoralis is a common intestinal parasite of man in warm countries. It exhibits a life cycle of extreme complexity, involving reproduction by adults in the soil as well as in the human intestine. Investigators working with different species of *Strongyloides* disagree on fundamental points and it is not clear whether or not these disagreements result from specific differences in the worms studied.

Only female worms are found in the intestine of man. They are thin, transparent worms 2 to 2.5 mm. long by about 0.05 mm. in diameter. They lie buried in the mucosa of the small intestine, and the thin-shelled eggs are deposited in the tissues, where they hatch to release rhabditiform larvae very similar to those of hookworms. Escaping in the feces the larvae undergo one of two types of development. They may molt to filariform larvae, which penetrate the skin to establish infection. Alternatively, they may develop into the free-living males and females. The free-living female is stouter than the parasitic female and about 1 mm. long. The male is somewhat smaller, about 0.7 mm. in length. It is believed that male gonads develop first, then produce sperm, which are stored, and subsequently the female reproductive system develops. Eggs produced by the free-living female hatch to release rhabditiform larvae which may continue the free-living cycle or may develop into infective larvae. The infective larvae, whether produced by free-living adults or developed directly from the rhabditiform larvae in the feces, penetrate the skin of man and reach the intestine via the circulation and lungs as in the hookworms. Male worms have not been found in the intestine, but "parasitic" males like those in the soil have been reported in the lung in abnormal hosts. Since investigation of a related species in rats has shown that a single infective larva can give rise to a female in the intestine producing fertile eggs, it is clear that the parasitic males are not essential in all species of *Strongyloides*. Oviposition in the lung has also been reported. A final complication is introduced by the reports that rhabditiform larvae might transform into infective larvae in the colon and penetrate its wall or the perianal skin (autoinfection cycle) to produce hyperinfections (Fig. 44–21).

Penetration of the skin by the larvae causes

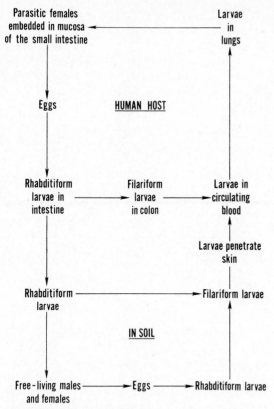

Figure 44–21. Diagrammatic representation of the life cycle of *Strongyloides stercoralis*.

dermatitis, and passage through the lung may give rise to bronchopneumonia. The parasitic females cause intestinal disturbances characterized chiefly by diarrhea. However, larvae may be delayed in their migration through the lungs and there develop into adults. Reproduction occurs as in the intestinal phase and the prognosis in such infections is poor. Damage to the intestinal mucosa by adults and larvae may in some cases result in ulceration leading to a fatal septicemias. Intestinal infections may persist for many years. Laboratory diagnosis is based on identification of the rhabditiform larvae in the feces. These can be distinguished from hookworm larvae occasionally encountered in stool specimens by the shorter buccal cavities and a notch in the tails of *Strongyloides*. Thiabendazole is the most effective drug for therapy of *S. stercoralis*, although it is not completely efficient in eliminating infection.

The epidemiology of *S. stercoralis* infection is similar to that of hookworm, and the same sanitary control measures apply. Dogs are infected with a strain indistinguishable from the form found in man and may be of some consequence in its maintenance. *Strongyloides ratti*

of rats is a similar form which can produce local allergic manifestations in man and cutaneous eruptions similar to those of the hookworms.

Trichinella spiralis

The "trichina" worm, *Trichinella spiralis*, was first seen in human muscles at necropsy by Tiedemann in 1821. Leuckart and others worked out the life cycle.[40] The adult forms are intestinal parasites of man and many other mammals, but their sojourn in the intestine is so brief that the more persistent larval infection in the muscles receives the main emphasis. The infective stage for man is a larva in the muscles of the hog. This stage is a minute coiled worm, about 1 mm. in length, enclosed in a lemon-shaped fibrous cyst, 0.25 by 0.5 mm. in dimensions, localized within muscle cells where it remains viable and infective for years. When ingested by a susceptible host, the larvae are digested free of the muscle. They penetrate the intestinal epithelium and molt to become adult males and females within two days. The male is a thin, transparent worm about 1.5 by 0.04 mm. (Fig. 44–22). The anterior half of the body is occupied by a nonmuscular esophagus like that of the closely related *Trichuris trichiura*. At the posterior end are two pear-shaped clasping lobes. The female is about 4 by 0.06 mm. in size. After fertilization, the females burrow into the mucosa, where, after about one week, they begin to deposit minute larvae, about 0.1 mm. in length, in the tissues. These larvae reach the general circulation and are filtered out in the skeletal muscles, cardiac muscle, the central nervous system, and other sites. In most tissues they die, but in skeletal muscle they grow in about two weeks to the infective stage. One month after infection, they are within a modified muscle (nurse) cell, which supports the nutritional requirements of each larvae. Later, the larvae may die and be calcified, but most remain infective for periods of months to years. Any skeletal muscle may be infected, but the larvae are most abundant in the diaphragm, intercostals, tongue, larynx, and eye muscles.

Meanwhile the adults have disappeared from the intestine. Most of the males die and are passed out within a week after infection. The females have largely disappeared within a month. It will be seen that the complete life cycle occurs in a single individual, for infective larvae are produced in the tissues of the same host which harbors the adults in its intestine.

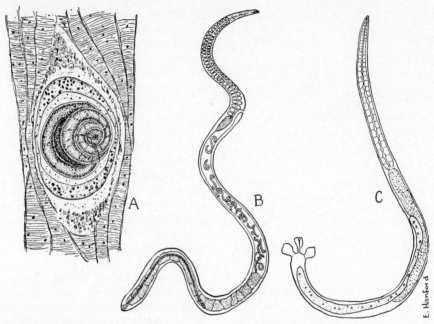

Figure 44–22. *Trichinella spiralis. A,* Larva in muscle, × 100. *B,* Adult female, × 50. *C,* Adult male, × 50.

Trichinosis. Although the incidence of infection in a population may be high, the usual infection with *Trichinella* is without detectable symptoms and the damage to the host is probably insignificant. However, severe cases resulting from relatively massive infection occur and are characterized by two phases. Intense infection with the adult worms produces gastrointestinal disturbances, usually with diarrhea. Occasionally the injury to the intestine is so severe as to result in death within a few days after infection. Muscle invasion by the larvae leads to varied signs of toxemia, hypersensitivity, and muscle injury. Heavy infections cause death or chronic illness. The severity of the disease is proportional to the number of larvae ingested, and many mild cases undoubtedly escape detection.

Laboratory rodents infected with *T. spiralis* are resistant to reinfection by the parasite. A variety of humoral antibodies are synthesized and some appear to act in concert with lymphocytes to mediate the resistance. Antigens of each developmental stage of the worms provoke responses which eliminate the parasites or interfere with their functions. Bell and colleagues defined four protective responses which operate in the intestine of the immune host: (1) rapid expulsion of the larvae, (2) antipreadult immunity, (3) anti-adult immunity, and (4) antifecundity effects.[8, 9] Animals immunized with larvae rapidly expel 95 per cent of an oral challenge within 24 hours.

Preadults and adults elicit similar responses which cause an expulsion of the adults from the intestine and reduce worm fecundity. The combined effects of immunization with larvae, preadults, and adults provides a sterile immunity against infections with large numbers of infective larvae. High, intermediate, and low responder strains of inbred mice exhibit fast, moderate, or slow elimination of primary *Trichinella* infections with variable effects on the preadults, adults, and fecundity.[10] Appropriate F_1 crosses of the mouse strains and assessments of the infections in immunized progeny indicate that multiple genes regulate the intestinal immune responses. While the genes regulating immunity are not linked to the major histocompatibility complex, they may be associated. Protective antigens isolated from soluble proteins of *T. spiralis* muscle larvae by immunoabsorbent affinity techniques have molecular weights ranging from 11,000 to 105,000 daltons.[28]

Modulation of the immune responses is an important facet of the host-*Trichinella* interactions. Cell-mediated immunity and antibody responses to T cell–dependent antigens are epressed, while those which are T cell–independent are unaffected in infected mice. Homologous antibody titers increase and hypersensitivity reactions to worm antigens develop during the infections in experimental animals and humans. Precipitins and skin test reactions are detectable two to three weeks after infection and persist for several years. The complement fixation test, bentonite, latex, and cholesterol flocculation tests are negative two to three months after infection and are indicative of current or recent trichinosis. Countercurrent immunoelectrophoresis and double diffusion kits are currently available from commercial sources for diagnosis. Eosinophilia is often greater than 20 per cent during infections, but definitive diagnoses are made by identifying larvae in biopsy specimens from skeletal muscles. Treatment is symptomatic at this time, since the larvae are unaffected by drugs. However, thiabendazole is effective against the adult worms if diagnosis is made soon after infection.[89]

Trichinella spiralis occurs principally in man, hogs, rats, and bears, although experimental infection has been produced in many species of mammals and birds. Human infection follows the consumption of undercooked pork (more rarely the meat of other animals, such as bears), while pigs acquire the parasite from garbage containing pork scraps or, less commonly, by eating carcasses of infected rats. Infection through the ingestion of larvae that pass out in feces has also been demonstrated and may be of some importance in the infec-

tion of coprophagous swine. In the United States as well as in the arctic regions a significant sylvatic infection in carnivores exists. *Trichinella spiralis* is worldwide in distribution, though infection in the tropics is rare. Various surveys in the United States, using routine necropsy examination of human diaphragms, have revealed a reduction in incidence to 4.1 per cent by 1970 from earlier surveys that indicated infection rates of at least three times as great. Clinical disease has become relatively rare in the United States, with slightly more than 100 cases reported annually and with few deaths as a result of infection (Fig. 44–23). Pork sausages and pork adulteration of beef products are the main sources of infection, and most infections can be traced to commercial sources.

Personal protection can be assured by thorough cooking of pork products, including hamburger of unknown composition. Government meat inspection does not attempt to detect *Trichinella*, for examination guaranteeing safety is considered impractical, but refrigeration for 24 hours at −18°C. destroys most of the larvae. Laws which forbid the feeding of raw garbage to hogs have been successful in reducing the incidence of infection.

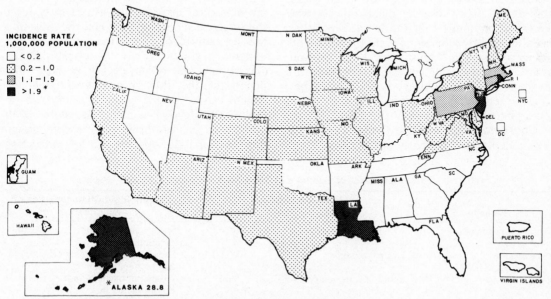

The highest incidence rates for trichinosis were observed for Alaska, New Jersey, Rhode Island, and Louisiana. A moderately high mean incidence was observed for Connecticut, Massachusetts, and Pennsylvania. In 16 states, no cases were reported for the past 5 years.

In 1980, 18 common-source outbreaks involving at least 2 cases each, accounted for 58.4% of all cases. The majority of infections were acquired from pork products purchased from commercial sources; however, 12 cases were acquired from the meat of wild animals.

Figure 4–23. The reported average cases of trichinosis per 1,000,000 population in the United States for the period 1976–1980. (Centers for Disease Control, Morbidity and Mortality Report, Annual Summary 1980, Vol. 29, 1981.)

THE FILARIA

Seven species of nematodes belonging to this group are important parasites of man. All produce motile embryos termed microfilariae which are produced in large numbers by the female in the host tissues and are released within a sheath (believed to be an elongate eggshell) or unsheathed. Microfilariae migrate or are carried by the circulation to the skin or to peripheral vascular beds, where they may be ingested by bloodsucking arthropods. Within this insect intermediate host the microfilariae transform without multiplication into infective larvae, become associated with the insect mouthparts, and may then be transmitted by the insect to the definitive host. After an incubation period and growth, which is little understood and may take as much as a year, the filaria may be found in their final sites of parasitism and are producing larvae. The locations of the adult worms and the microfilariae in the human host, along with some morphological features of the larvae important in the microscopic identification of the parasites, are presented in Table 44–3.

Wuchereria bancrofti

Of the several species of filaria mentioned above, *Wuchereria bancrofti* is by far the more important. The disease elephantiasis was known in antiquity, but the larvae were first seen in 1863 by Demarquay and the adults by Bancroft in 1876. Manson, in 1878, showed that development of the larvae took place in mosquitoes. This discovery is noteworthy because it represents the first incrimination of an insect in the transmission of disease.

Characteristics and Life Cycle. The adults live coiled in the lymph nodes of man. They are thread-like translucent worms, the female 7 to 10 cm. long by 0.25 mm. in diameter, the male 4 cm. by 0.1 mm. The egg, covered by a thin membrane, hatches in the uterus or in the host tissues to release an active embryo about 0.2 mm. long. This embryo, known as a microfilaria, escapes into the lymph and enters the circulating blood by way of the thoracic duct (Fig. 44–24). In most regions the embryos of *W. bancrofti* show marked nocturnal periodicity, occurring in the peripheral blood almost exclusively at night. In many of the South Pacific islands, however, they appear in the blood at all hours. Extensive study has failed to provide a satisfactory explanation of this periodicity, although there is suggestive evidence that daytime activity induces accumulation of the microfilariae in capillaries of the lung.

The microfilaria develops no further in the circulating blood. If ingested by a susceptible mosquito, however, it undergoes a series of transformations in the tissues of the insect. Within a day, the larva leaves the stomach of the mosquito and invades the thoracic muscles. Here it develops into a stout "sausage larva," which, after a second molt, elongates to form the infective stage, a thin worm 1.5 to 2 mm. in length. This infective larva leaves the muscles and migrates to the proboscis sheath of the mosquito, arriving six days or more after the infective blood meal. When the mosquito takes a new blood meal, the infective larva, apparently stimulated by the warmth of the skin, breaks out of the proboscis sheath and penetrates the skin, probably through the wound caused by the biting mosquito, to establish an infection in man. The early development of the worms in man is not known, but microfilariae appear in the circulating

Table 44–3. **Characteristics of Adults and Microfilariae Causing Human Diseases**

Parasite	Location in Body		Morphologic Characteristics of Microfilariae
	Adults	Microfilariae	
Wuchereria bancrofti	Lymphatic vessels	Blood	Sheath, nuclei do not extend to tip of pointed tail
Brugia malayi	Lymphatic vessels	Blood	Sheath, tail blunt with swellings at two terminal nuclei
Onchocerca vulvulus	Subcutaneous nodules	Skin	Unsheath, nuclei do not extend to tip of pointed tail
Acanthocheilonema streptocerca	Subcutaneous nodules	Skin	Unsheath, nuclei extend to tip of blunt tail
Mansonella ozzardi	Pleural or peritoneal cavities	Blood	Unsheath, nuclei do not extend to tip of pointed tail
Acanthocheilonema perstans	Pleural or peritoneal cavities	Blood	Unsheath, nuclei extend to tip of pointed tail
Loa loa	Connective tissues	Blood	Sheath, nuclei extend to tip of pointed tail

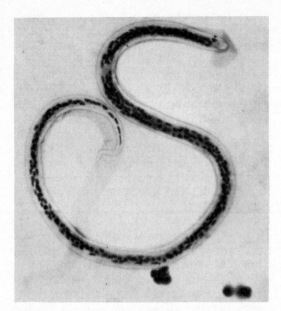

Figure 44–24. Microfilaria of *Wuchereria bancrofti* in thick blood film. × 300.

blood several months after infection. In the related species, *Brugia malayi* (see below), development to the adult stage requires about 80 days in experimental animals. Although the longevity of the adult worms in the lymphatics has not been determined, they probably live for several years.

Filariasis. The adult worms are most prevalent in the lymph nodes of the inguinal region, but they are also found in lymphatics elsewhere in the body. They induce inflammation and fibrosis in the infected nodes. The consequent restriction of lymph flow causes edema, lymphangitis, lymphadenitis, and elephantiasis. Secondary infection of the lymphatics with streptococci and staphylococci is often significant. Long-standing cases sometimes show enormous enlargement of the scrotum, vulva, legs, or breasts.

While some patients with chronic bancroftian filariasis display an eosinophilia, most infected individuals do not show altered accounts of eosinophils, neutrophils, or mononuclear cells, and total peripheral blood leucocytes remain comparable to those of uninfected individuals in endemic areas. *Wuchereria bancrofti* cannot be maintained in the laboratory. Birds can be infected with *B. malayi,* and this parasite is frequently utilized in studies because, like other filarial species, it contains group-specific antigens which cross-react with antibodies to *W. bancrofti.* Using such antigen preparations, it has been found that IgM, IgG,

and IgE antibodies specific for the parasite are elevated in infected individuals, but IgM and the C3 component of complement appear to be lower than in uninfected subjects.[77] Persons with concurrent fevers and chronic lymphatic pathology have lower IgG titers to adult filarial antigens, and the lowest levels are found in patients with microfilaremias. Antibody-dependent cell-mediated adhesion and cytotoxicity are observed during infections. Neutrophils and eosinophils adhere to parasites in the presence of IgG from microfilaremic patients. However, eosinophils alone have no effect on the microfilariae *in vitro,* while neutrophils kill the larvae.[64]

Laboratory diagnosis is based on the identification of microfilariae in fresh blood specimens or in thick blood films. Low-density microfilaremias are detected using more sensitive filtration procedures that concentrate the microfilariae from a larger volumes of blood specimens on filters. Microfilariae are often not detected in early infection or in long-standing cases which present extensive tissue damage. There are a variety of serological tests (complement fixation, indirect immunofluorescence, microfilarial agglutination tests, and enzyme-linked immunosorbent assays) and skin tests that employ *B. malayi* or filaria of lower animals. False-positive reactions may occur because of these and other nematode infections. In serological studies on bancroftian and malayan filariasis patients using indirect immunofluorescence and microfilarial agglutination tests with *B. malayi* antigens, titers of antibodies against adult worms appear to be useful indicators of infection, while antibody levels against microfilariae correlate with the severity of the disease.[41]

Treatment for bancroftian and malayan filariasis involves the administration of diethylcarbamazine three times daily for two weeks. Toxic side effects include fever, nausea, and skin rashes. In the event of relapses, the treatment may be repeated.

Epidemiology and Control. Man is the only known host of the adult worm. A large number of mosquitoes of the genera *Culex, Aedes, Mansonia,* and *Anopheles* support development of the larvae, but the most important are *Aedes polynesiensis* in the South Pacific islands, *Anopheles gambiae* in West Africa, and *Culex quinquefasciatus (C. fatigans)* elsewhere. There is an interesting correlation between the habits of the mosquito hosts and the periodicity of the microfilariae discussed above. *Aedes polynesiensis* bites by day, and it is in the regions where this mosquito transmits *W. bancrofti* that the microfilariae are found in the peripheral blood at all hours. In other regions, where the principal vectors attack man in the evening or at night, the microfilariae show a marked nocturnal periodicity.

Wuchereria bancrofti is a parasite of warm countries, occurring widely throughout the tropics and subtropics. Climate favors the production of mosquitoes and the development of larvae of *W. bancrofti* in the insect, and the poorer housing of the tropics permits greater contact between mosquitoes and man. The slow development of human infections, the lack of multiplication of *W. bancrofti* in the mosquito hosts, and other hazards combine to limit dissemination of the parasite. As a consequence the infection seems to die out in an area unless there are many human cases and abundant mosquitoes. The former endemic center in the United States, around Charleston, South Carolina, where the incidence was 20 to 30 per cent before 1920, now shows no cases. Control is a matter of mosquito reduction, protection from mosquito bites, attention being directed to the habits of the particular vectors in any area, and chemotherapy of cases.

Other Species of Filarial Worms

Brugia malayi is very similar to *W. bancrofti* and is widely distributed in southeast Asia, the China Sea area, and Eastern India, often occurring with *W. bancrofti*. In some areas it is transmitted by mosquitoes of the genus *Mansonia,* whose larvae obtain oxygen from subaquatic vegetation, posing additional problems of control. A similar parasite, *B. pahangi,* of Malaya is common in wild and domestic mammals and, in man, may produce the symptoms of tropical eosinophilia and eosinophil lung.

Onchocerciasis is a major health problem in Central Africa, where over 30 million individuals are afflicted with the disease. In the Western Hemisphere, approximately one million inhabitants of Mexico, Guatemala, Venezuela, and Colombia are infected with *Onchocerca vulvulus.* The filaria was first described by Leuckart in Ghana in 1893 and by Robles in Guatemala in 1915.

The adults are found in subcutaneous nodules. The tightly coiled females are 33 to 50 mm. by 270 to 400 μm., and the associated males, 19 to 42 mm. by 130 to 210 μm. Microfilariae are produced that migrate in the subcutaneous tissues. They are not found in the circulating blood, but concentrate in the skin. When bitten by a female blackfly of the genus *Simulium,* the ingested larvae invade the intersyncytial elements of the thoracic muscle fibers and undergo two molts during a period of about six days. The resulting infective larvae travel to the labium and are transmitted when the blackfly takes another blood meal. They infect the wound, develop into adults, and mate. They may live for years in the subcutaneous tissue. Generally, in less than a year, fibrous connective tissue nodules are formed about the worms in response to secreted products.

Immediate hypersensitivity reactions are observed when individuals infected with *Onchocerca* are skin tested with extracts of adult worms or with excretion and secretion products of the microfilariae.[86] Various levels of cross-reactions occur with each type of preparation because of antigens shared by other species of Filaria. Such cross-reactions are also common in serodiagnostic tests conducted by immunofluorescence, complement fixation, indirect hemagglutination, and enzyme-linked immunosorbent assay with frozen sections of adult worms, microfilariae, or soluble antigens of these stages from human or animal filaria. *Onchocerca* antigens are detected in the circulating blood of patients using antiserum against the homologous adult worms.[78] Blood from patients with other nematode infections cross-react with these antiserums. This research emphasizes the difficulties associated with the reliable immunodiagnosis of filarial infections.

Onchocerciasis is caused in part by the microfilariae, which induce inflammation and hypersensitivity reactions. Subcutaneous tissue nodules, rashes, and lesions of the eye represent major signs and symptoms of the disease. In Central and South America nodules of various sizes occur on the upper body and head, and in Africa nodules appear on the lower body. In African patients, lymphatic involvement may lead to enlargement of the scrotum. Itching and rashes may develop on the skin, which subsequently undergoes sclerotic changes. Microfilariae invade the eyes. Corneal lesions and opacity reflect the effects of motile and dying microfilariae. Vascularization of the cornea may obscure vision. Degeneration of the iris, glaucoma, acute inflammation, and degeneration of the optic nerve may result in blindness.

Diagnosis is made by superficial biopsy of

the skin in the areas of the nodules. The biopsied material is teased in saline and examined microscopically for microfilariae. Giemsa-stained imprints of the biopsied skin may also be examined to identify the microfilariae. Treatment may involve surgical removal of the nodules to reduce the numbers of microfilariae and hence the possibility of eye involvement. Suramin kills adults and microfilariae, but because of toxic effects, diethylcarbamazine—which is effective against microfilariae—should be used in cases without eye involvement. Suramin may be administered in cases which relapse. Hypersensitivity reactions may accompany treatment with either drug and may be controlled with corticosteroids.

The larvae of blackflies require fast-flowing mountain streams for development. The distribution of these intermediate hosts determines the endemic areas. Man is the only known definitive host and attempts have been made to control the disease by surgical removal of nodules, chemotherapy, and insecticide applications to eliminate the vectors.

Loa loa is found in the subcutaneous tissues of a variety of primates, including man, and is limited to West and Central Africa, where it is transmitted by the biting deerfly *Chrysops*. It has been called the "eye worm" because of the frequency with which it may be found passing under the conjunctiva of the eye surface, and it is also associated with a fugitive "calabar" swelling presumed to be due to reaction of the host to the metabolic products of the migrating adult worm. The circulating microfilariae have a diurnal periodicity.

Acanthocheilonema streptocerca is found in the dermal and subcutaneous connective tissue and its unsheathed microfilariae are in the superficial layers of the dermis. It is limited in distribution to parts of Central Africa. *Acanthocheilonema perstans* has a wide distribution in tropical Africa and is also present in coastal areas of South America and the West Indies. Its microfilariae are nonperiodic and unsheathed, and are found in the peripheral blood. The adults are found associated with the peritoneal cavity, in mesentery, in retroperitoneal tissues, in the pericardium, or occasionally in subcutaneous cysts. Infections are often without symptoms but may be associated with sensitization phenomena and rarely with more serious or fatal complications. *Mansonella ozzardi* is also found in the tropical areas of the Western Hemisphere, occupies body cavities, and has circulating, unsheathed, non-periodic microfilariae. No symptoms are associated with infection. Both species of *Acanthocheilonema* and *Mansonella* are transmitted by gnats of the genus *Culicoides*.

Numerous species of filarial worms of mammals and birds are distributed over the world. One of these, *Dirofilaria immitis*, is an important pathogen of dogs, the adult worms living in and occluding the vessels of the heart. Antigen prepared from *Dirofilaria* has been used in intradermal and serological tests for the diagnosis of filariasis in man. As indicated above the specificity of the reactions is low.

Dracunculus medinensis, the Guinea worm, is a common parasite of man in the Middle East, Africa, India, and Indonesia. It was also endemic in the tropics of the Western Hemisphere. Estimates indicate nearly 50 million cases in these areas. Although a tissue parasite resembling the filaria, it does not have a true microfilarial stage. The small male worms are rarely seen. The females, after several months' development in internal connective tissues, appear in the subcutaneous tissues, usually of the leg. They are large worms, averaging about 1 m. in length, often visible through the skin as they lie in the tissues. The skin of the host ulcerates at the anterior end of the worm, and larvae escape, usually when the leg is submerged in water. These larvae develop in copepods, *e.g.*, cyclops, and human infection follows ingestion of the parasitized copepods in drinking water. The human infection, possibly the "fiery serpent" of the Bible, is associated with severe sensitivity reactions immediately preceding initial blister formation and larval release by the female. In some regions the female worm is gradually removed from the tissues by rolling it up on a stick. Thiabendazole and niridazole have been used in treatment of dracunculiasis, and antihistamines may be used to relieve the sensitivity phenomena.

Drugs for Parasitic Infections. The drugs suggested in the text for treatment may not be the current drugs of choice. It is imperative to recognize that new drugs frequently become available and to determine the drug presently recommended for treatment, the dosages, routes of administration, possible side effects, and contraindications. A relatively large number of the drugs recommended for specific infections are not officially approved by the U.S. Food and Drug Administration. Unapproved drugs that are considered the treatments of choice can in many instances be obtained (with recommendations for their administration) as investigational drugs from the Parasitic Diseases Branch of the United States Public Health Service, Center for Disease Control, in Atlanta, Georgia.

References

1. Alicata, J. E. 1962. *Angiostrongylus cantonensis* (Nematoda: Metastrongylidae) as a causative agent of eosinophilic meningoencephalitis of man in Hawaii and Tahiti. Can. J. Zool. **40**:5–8.
2. Anthony, R. L., *et al.* 1979. Use of the micro-ELISA for quantitating antibody to *Trypanosoma cruzi* and *Trypanosoma rangeli*. Amer. J. Trop. Med. Hygiene **28**:969–973.
3. Anthony, R. L., *et al.* 1981. Antigenic differentiation of *Trypanosoma cruzi* and *Trypanosoma rangeli* by means of monoclonal-hybridoma antibodies. Amer. J. Trop. Med. Hygiene **30**:1192–1197.
4. Anwar, A. R. E., *et al.* 1979. Killing of schistosomula of *Schistosoma mansoni* coated with antibody and/or complement by human leucocytes *in vitro*: requirements for complement in preferential killing by eosinophils. J. Immunol. **122**:628–637.
5. Arean, V. M., and E. Koppisch. 1956. Balantidiasis: a review and report of cases. Amer. J. Pathol **32**: 1089–1115.
6. Barrett-Connor, E. 1971. Amebiasis, today, in the United States. Calif. Med. **114**:1–6.
7. Bazin, H., *et al.* 1980. Effects of neonatal injection of anti-μ antibodies on immunity to schistosomes (*S. mansoni*) in the rat. J. Immunol. **124**:2373–2376.
8. Bell, R. G., *et al.* 1979. *Trichinella spiralis:* multiple phase specific anti-parasite responses mediate the intestinal components of protective immunity in the rat. Exptl Parasitol. **47**:140–157.
9. Bell, R. G., *et al.* 1979. *Trichinella spiralis:* role of different life cycle phases in the induction, maintenance, and expression of rapid expulsion in rats. Exptl Parasitol. **48**:51–60.
10. Bell, R. G., et al. 1982. *Trichinella spiralis:* genetic basis for differential expression of phase-specific intestinal immunity in inbred mice. Exptl Parasitol. **53**:315–325.
11. Boughton, C. R. 1970. Toxoplasmosis. Med. J. Australia **2**:418–421.
12. Brandborg, L. L., *et al.* 1967. Histological demonstration of mucosal invasion by *Giardia lamblia* in man. Gastroenterology **52**:143–150.
13. Brito, T. J., *et al.* 1970. Advanced kidney disease in patients with hepatosplenic Manson's schistosomiasis. Revta. Inst. Med. Trop. Sao Paulo **12**:225–235.
14. Brodsky, R. E., H. C. Spencer, and M. G. Schultz. 1974. Giardiasis in American travelers to the Soviet Union. J. Infect. Dis. **130**:319–323.
15. Brown, J., and M. E. Smalley, 1980. Specific antibody-dependent cellular cytotoxicity in human malaria. Clin. Exptl Immunol. **41**:423–429.
16. Bruer, J. The Great Neglected Diseases. A Progress Report. June 1982, pp. 26–28. RF Illustrated. Rockefeller Foundation, New York.
17. Bueding, E. 1968. Responses of trematodes to pharmacological agents. pp. 551–55. *In* M. Florkin and B. T. Scheer (Eds.): Chemical Zoology. Academic Press, New York.
18. Burrows, R. B., and M. A. Swerdlow. 1956. *Enterobius vermicularis* as a probable vector of *Dientamoeba fragilis*. Amer. J. Trop. Med. Hygiene **5**:258–265.
19. Capron, A., *et al.* 1977. IgE and cells in schistosomiasis. Amer. J. Trop. Med. Hygiene **26** (Suppl.): 39–46.
20. Castro Malsonado, H. F. 1974. Anatomic and pathological findings in amebiasis, report of 320 cases. pp. 44–68. *In* C. A. Padilla y Padilla and G. M. Padilla (Eds.): Amebiasis in Man. Epidemiology, Therapeutics, Clinical Correlations and Prophylaxis. Charles C Thomas, Springfield, Ill.
21. Change, K. P., and D. M. Dwyer. 1976. Multiplication of a human parasite (*Leishmania donovani*) in phagolysosomes of hamster macrophages *in vitro.* Science **193**:678–680.
22. Chang, S. M., *et al.* 1980. Antigenic analyses of two axenized strains of *Entamoeba histolytica* by two-dimensional immunoelectrophoresis. Amer. J. Trop. Med. Hygiene **28**:845–853.
23. Clegg, J. A. 1974. Host antigens and the immune response in schistosomiasis. pp. 161–176. *In* Parasites in the Immunized Host: Mechanisms of Survival. Associated Scientific Publishers, Amsterdam.
24. Cox, H. W. 1962. The behavior of *Plasmodium berghei* strains isolated from relapse infections of white mice. J. Protozool. **9**:114–118.
25. Cross, G. A. M. *et al.* 1980. An introduction to antigenic variation in trypanosomes. Amer. J. Trop. Med. Hygiene **29**:1027–1032.
26. Cross, J. H., *et al.* 1970. A new epidemic diarrheal disease caused by the nematode *Capillaria philippinensis.* Industry and Tropical Health. Vol. 7. Industrial Council for Tropical Health, Harvard School of Public Health, Boston.
27. Danforth, H. D., *et al.* 1982. Production of monoclonal antibodies by hybridomas sensitized to *Plasmodium berghei.* J. Parasitol. **68**:1029–1033.
28. Despommier, D. D., and Leccetti, A. 1981. *Trichinella spiralis:* partial characterization of antigens isolated by immuno-affinity chromatography from large particle fractions of the muscle larvae. J. Parasitol. **67**:332–339.
29. Diamond, L. D. 1968. Techniques of axenic cultivation of *Entamoeba histolytica* Schaudin, 1903 and *E. histolytica*-like amebae. J. Parasitol. **54**:1047–2056.
30. Doyle, J. J. 1977. Antigenic variation in salivarian trypanosomes. pp. 27–63. *In* L. H. Miller, J. A. Pindo, and J. J. McKelvey, Jr. (Eds.): Blood Parasites of Animals and Man. Adv. Exptl. Med. Biol., Vol. 93. Plenum Press, New York.
31. Dubey, J. P. 1977. *Toxoplasma, Hammondia, Besnoitia, Sarcocystis,* and other tissue cyst-forming coccidia of man and animals. pp. 101–237. *In* J. P. Kreier (Ed.): Parasitic Protozoa. Vol. III. Academic Press, New York.
32. Duma, R. J., *et al.* 1969. Primary amebic meningoencephalitis. New Engl. J. Med. **281**:1315–1323.
33. Elowni, E. E. 1982. *Hymenolypis diminuta:* the origin of protective antigen. Exptl Parasitol. **53**: 157–163.
34. Farrar, W. E., *et al.* 1963. Serologic evidence of human infections with *Trypanosoma cruzi* in Georgia. Amer. J. Hygiene **78**:166–172.
35. Faust, E. C. 1961. The multiple facets of *Entamobea histolytica* infection. Internat. Rev. Trop. Med. **1**: 43–76.

36. Frenkel, J. K. 1973. Toxoplasmosis: parasite life cycle, pathology, and immunology. pp. 343–410. *In* D. M. Hammond with P. L. Long (Eds.): The Coccidia. Eimeria, Isospora, Toxoplasma and Related Genera. University Park Press, Baltimore.

37. Frenkel, J. K., J. P. Dubey, and N. L. Miller, 1970. *Toxoplasma gondii* in cats: fecal stages identified as coccidian oöcysts. Science **167**:893–896.

38. Fulton, J. D. 1960. Some aspects of research on trypanosomes. pp. 11–23. *In* L. E. Stauber (Ed.): Host Influence on Parasite Physiology. Rutgers University Press, New Brunswick, N.J.

39. Gonnert, R., and P. Andrews. 1977. Praziquantel, a new broad-spectrum antischistosomal agent. Ztschr. Parasitkde **52**:129–150.

40. Gould, S. E. 1970. Trichinosis in Man and Animals. Charles C Thomas, Springfield, Ill.

41. Grove, D. I., and R. S. Davis. 1978. Serological diagnosis of bancroftian and malayan filariasis. Amer. J. Trop. Med. Hygiene **27**:508–513.

42. Gutteridge, W. E., and G. H. Coombs. 1977. Biochemistry of Parasitic Protozoa. University Park Press, Baltimore.

43. Hart, D. T., and G. H. Coombs. 1982. *Leishmania mexicana:* energy metabolism of amastigotes and promastigotes. Exptl Parasitol. **54**:397–409.

44. Heath, D. D., and S. B. Lawrence, 1981. *Echinococcus granulosus* cysts: early development in the presence of serum from infected sheep. Internat. J. Parasitol. **11**:261–266.

45. Hillyer, G. V. 1971. Deoxyribonucleic acid (DNA) and antibodies to DNA in the serum of hamsters and man infected with schistosomes. Proc. Soc. Exptl Biol. Med. **136**:880–883.

46. Hirsch, J. G., et al. 1974. Interactions in vitro between *Toxoplasma gondii* and mouse cells. pp. 205–223. *In* R. Porter and J. Knight (Eds.): Parasites in the Immunized Host: Mechanisms of Survival. Ciba Foundation Symposium No. 25 (new series). Associated Scientific Publishers, Amsterdam.

47. Hirumi, H., et al. 1977. African trypanosomes: cultivation of animal-infective *Trypanosoma brucei in vitro*. Science **196**:992–994.

48. Houba, V., et al. 1971. Immunoglobulin classes and complement in biopsies of Nigerian children with the nephrotic syndrome. Clin. Exptl. Immunol. **8**:761–774.

49. Hsü, H. F., and S. Y. Li Hsü. 1960. New approach to immunization against *Schistosoma japonicum*. Science **133**:766.

50. Huff, C. G., and W. Bloom, 1935. A malarial parasite infecting all blood and blood-forming cells of birds. J. Infect. Dis. **57**:315–336.

51. Hutchison, W. M. 1967. The nematode transmission of *Toxoplasma gondii*. Trans. Roy. Soc. Trop. Med. Hygiene **61**:80–89.

52. Hutchison, W. M., and J. F. Dunachie. 1971. The life cycle of the coccidian parasite, *Toxoplasma gondii*, in the domestic cat. Trans. Roy. Soc. Trop. Med. Hygiene **65**:380–399.

53. Jackson, G. J. 1975. The "new disease" status of human anisakiasis and North American cases: a review. J. Milk Food Techn. **38**:769–773.

54. Jaramalinta, R., and B. G. Maegraith. 1960. Hyaluronidase activity in stock cultures of *Entamoeba histolytica*. Ann. Trop. Med. Parasitol. **54**:118–128.

55. Kagan, I. G. 1958. Contributions to the immunology and serology of schistosomiasis. *In* Symposium: Resistance and immunity in parasitic infections. Rice Inst. Pam. **45**:151–183.

56. Kierszenbaum, F. 1982. Immunologic deficiency during experimental Chagas' disease (*Trypanosoma cruzi* infection): role of adherent nonspecific esterase-positive splenic cells. J. Immunol. **129**:2202–2205.

57. Krotoski, W. A., et al. 1982. Observations on early and late postsporozoite tissue stages in primate malaria. II. The hypnozoite of *Plasmodium cynomolgi bastianellii* from 3 to 105 days after infection, and detection of 36- to 40-hour pre-erythrocyte forms. Amer. J. Trop. Med. Hygiene **31**:211–225.

58. Krotoski, W. A., et al. 1982. Demonstration of hypnozoites in sporozoite-transmitted *Plasmodium vivax* infections. Amer. J. Trop. Med. Hygiene **31**:1291–1293.

59. Lewert, R. M. 1958. Invasiveness of helminth larvae. *In* Symposium: Resistance and immunity in parasitic infections. Rice Inst. Pam. **45**:97–133.

60. Lewert, R. M., and S. Mandlowitz. 1969. Schistosomiasis: prenatal induction of tolerance to antigens. Nature **224**:1029–1030.

61. Maddison, S. E., et al. 1981. Acquired immunity in B cell deficient mice to challenge exposure following primary infection with *Schistosoma mansoni*. Amer. J. Trop. Med. Hygiene **30**:609–615.

62. Martinez-Cairo, C. S., et al. 1979. Coproantibodies in intestinal amoebiasis. Arch. Invest. Méd. **10**:121–126.

63. McLean, S. A., et al. 1982. *Plasmodium chabaudi:* antigenic variation during recrudescent parasitemias in mice. Exptl Parasitol. **54**:296–302.

64. Mehta, K., et al. 1981. Antibody-dependent cell-mediated effects in bancroftian filariasis. Immunology **43**:117–123.

65. Miller, C. W., R. Ruppaner, and C. W. Schwabe. 1971. Hydatid disease in California: study of hospital records, 1960 through 1969. Amer. J. Trop. Med. Hygiene **20**:904–913.

66. Morecki, R., and J. G. Parker. 1967. Ultrastructural studies of the human *Giardia lamblia* and subjacent jejunal mucosa in a subject with steatorrhea. Gastroenterology **52**:151–164.

67. Nacy, C. A., et al. 1981. Intracellular replication and lymphokine-induced destruction of *Leishmania tropica* in C3H/HeN mouse macrophages. J: Immunol. **127**:2381–2386.

68. Navato-Silva, E., et al. 1980. *Schistosoma mansoni:* comparison of the killing effect of granulocytes and complement with or without antibody on fresh or cultured schistosomula in vitro. Amer. J. Trop. Med. Hygiene **29**:1263–1267.

69. Neal, R. A. 1956. Strain variation in *Entamoeba histolytica*. Parasitology. **46**:173–191.

70. Neal, R. A. 1960. Enzymic proteolysis by *Entamoeba histolytica;* biochemical characteristics and relationship with invasiveness. Parasitology **50**:531–550.

71. Nelson, E. C., and M. M. Jones. 1970. Culture isolation of agents of primary amebic meningoencephalitis. J. Parasitol. **56** Sec. II:248.

72. Newton, B. A. 1974. The chemotherapy of trypanosomiasis: towards a more rational approach. pp. 285–307. *In* Trypanosomiasis and Leishmaniasis with Special Reference to Chagas' Disease. Ciba Foundation Symposium 20 (new series). Associated Scientific Publishers, Amsterdam.

73. Newton, B. A. 1979. The metabolism of African

trypanosomes in relation to pathogenic mechanisms. pp. 17–22. *In* Losos, G., and A. Chouinard (Eds.): Pathogenicity of Trypanosomes. International Development Research Center, Ottawa.

74. Nordin, E. H., *et al.* 1979. Antibodies to sporozoites: their frequency and occurrence in individuals living in areas of hyperendemic malaria. Science **206**: 597–599.

75. Nordin, E. H., and R. S. Neussenzweig. 1978. Stage specific antigens on the surface membrane of sporozoites of malarial parasites. Nature (London) **274**:55–57.

76. Nussenzweig, R., J. Vanderberg, and H. Most. 1969. Protective immunity produced by the injections of x-irradiated sporozoites of *Plasmodium berghei.* Milit. Med. **134**:1176–1182.

77. Ottesen, E. A., *et al.* 1982. Endemic filariasis on a Pacific island. II. Immunoglobulin, complement, and specific antifilarial IgG, IgM, and IgE antibodies. Amer. J. Trop. Med. Hygiene **31**:953–961.

78. Ouaissi, A., *et al.* 1981. Detection of circulating antigens in onchocerciasis. Amer. J. Trop. Med. Hygiene **30**:1211–1218.

79. Phillips, B. P., *et al.* 1955, 1958. Studies on the ameba-bacteria relationship in amebiasis. I. Comparative results of the intracecal inoculation of germ-free, monocontaminated, and conventional guinea pigs with *Entamoeba histolytica.* II. Some concepts on the etiology of the disease. Amer. J. Trop. Med. Hygiene **4**:675–692; **7**: 392–399.

80. Powell, R. D., *et al.* 1964. Studies on a strain of chloroquin-resistant *Plasmodium falciparum* from Thailand. Bull. Wld Hlth Org. **30**:29–44.

81. Ramos, C., *et al.* 1979. Suppressor cells present in the spleens of Trypanosoma cruzi infected mice. J. Immunol. **122**:1243–1247.

82. Rimoldi, M. T., *et al.* 1981. *Trypanosoma cruzi:* sequence of phagocytosis and cytotoxicity by human polymorphonuclear leucocytes. Immunology. **42**:521–527.

83. Rosen, L., *et al.* 1967. Studies on eosinophilic meningitis. 3. Epidemiologic and clinical observations on Pacific islands and the possible role of *Angiostrongylus cantonensis.* Amer. J. Epidemiol. **85**:17–44.

84. Santoro, F., *et al.* 1979. *Schistosoma mansoni:* circulating antigens and immune complexes in infected mice. Exptl Parasitol. **47**:392–402.

85. Sawada, T., *et al.* 1965. The isolation and purification of antigen from adult *Clonorchis sinensis* for complement fixation and precipitant tests. Exptl Parasitol. **17**:340–349.

86. Schiller, E. L., *et al.* 1980. Intradermal reactivity of excretory and secretory products of onchocercal microfilariae. Amer. J. Trop. Med. Hygiene **29**: 1215–1219.

87. Shortt, H. E., and P. C. C. Garnham. 1948. Demonstration of a persisting erythrocyte cycle in *Plasmodium cynomolgi* and its bearing on the production of relapses. Brit. Med. J. **1**:1225–1232.

88. Stewart, G. L., and S. Holmes Giannini. 1982. *Sarcocystis, Trypanosoma, Toxoplasma, Ancylostoma,* and *Trichinella* spp.: a review of intracellular parasites of striated muscle. Exptl Parasitol. **53**: 406–447.

89. Stone, O. J., *et al.* 1964. Thiabendazole—probable cure for trichinosis: report of first case. J. Amer. Med. Assn **187**:536–537.

90. Tullis, D. C. 1970. Bronchial asthma associated with intestinal parasites. New Engl. J. Med. **282**: 370–372.

91. Villella, J. B., H. J. Gomberg, and S. E. Gould. 1961. Immunization to *Schistosoma mansoni* in mice inoculated with radiated cercariae. Science **134**:1073–1075.

92. Vinayak, V. K., *et al.* 1980. Cellular and humoral responses in amoebic patients. Trop. Geographic Med. **24**:298–302.

93. Vogel, H. 1958. Acquired immunity to Schistosoma infection in experimental animals. Bull. Wld Hlth Org. **18**:1097–1103.

94. Warren, K. S., E. O. Domingo, and B. T. Cowan, 1967. Granuloma formation around schistosome eggs as a manifestation of delayed hypersensitivity. Amer. J. Pathol. **51**:735–748.

95. Wood, S. F., and F. D. Wood. 1961. Observations on vectors of Chagas' disease in the United States. Amer. J. Trop. Med. Hygiene **10**:155–165.

96. Woody, N. C., and H. B. Woody. 1961. American trypanosomiasis. I. Clinical and epidemiologic background of Chagas' disease in the United States. J. Pediat. **58**:568–580.

97. Yakoleff-Greenhouse, V., *et al.* 1982. Analysis of antigenic variation in cysticerci of *Taenia solium.* J. Parasitol. **68**:39–47.

98. Yogore, M. G., R. M. Lewert, and E. D. Madraso. 1965. Immunodiffusion studies on paragonimiasis. Amer. J. Trop. Med. Hygiene **14**:586–591.

99. Yokogawa, M., and H. Yoshimura. 1965. Anisakis-like larvae causing eosinophilic granulomata in the stomach of man. Amer. J. Trop. Med. Hygiene **14**:770–773.

100. Young, M. D., and D. V. Moore. 1961. Chloroquin resistance in *Plasmodium falciparum.* Amer. J. Trop. Med. Hygiene **10**:317–320.

101. Yoshida, N., *et al.* 1980. Hybridoma produces protective antibodies directed against the sporozoite stage of malaria parasite. Science **207**:71–73.

Index

Page numbers in *italics* refer to illustrations; page numbers followed by t refer to tables.